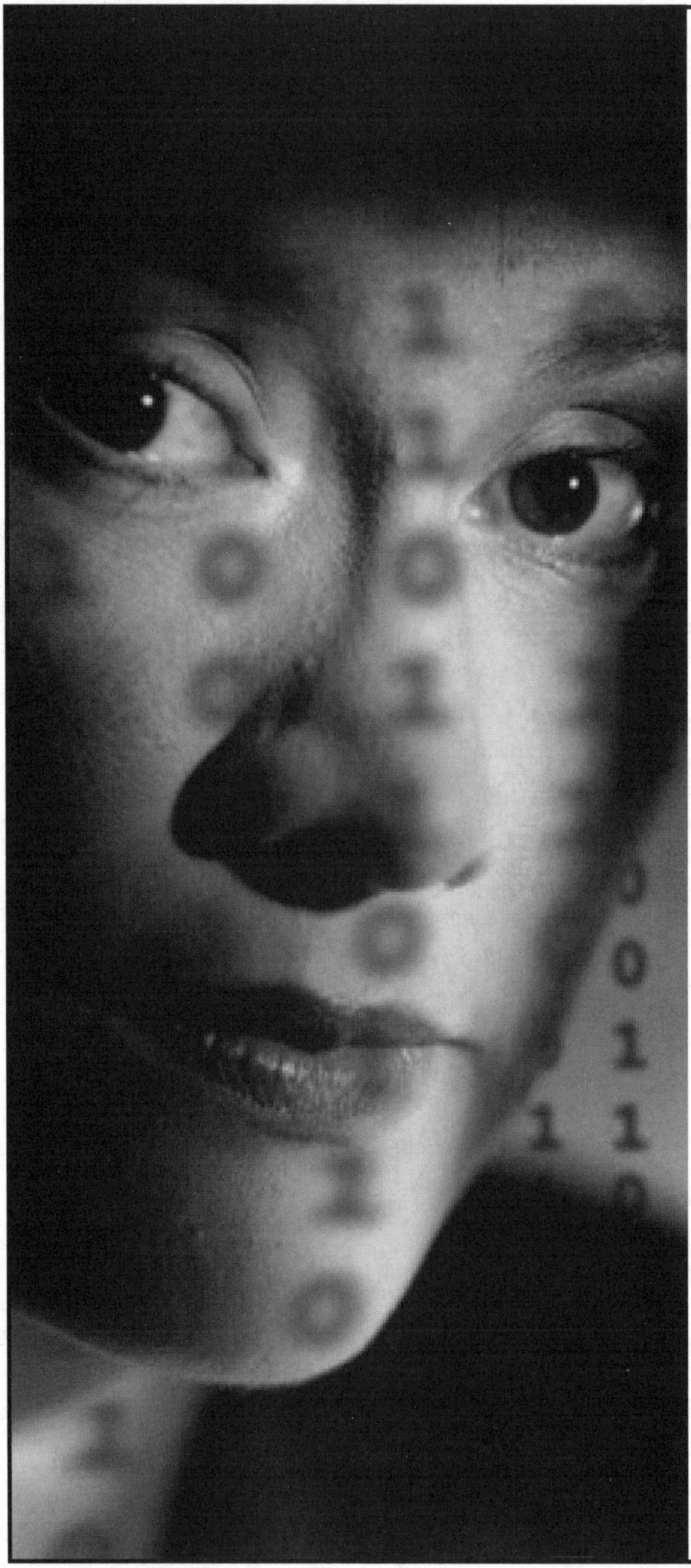

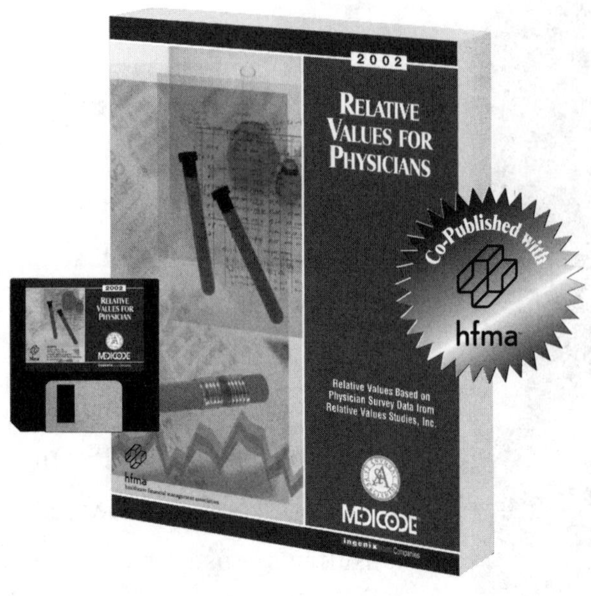

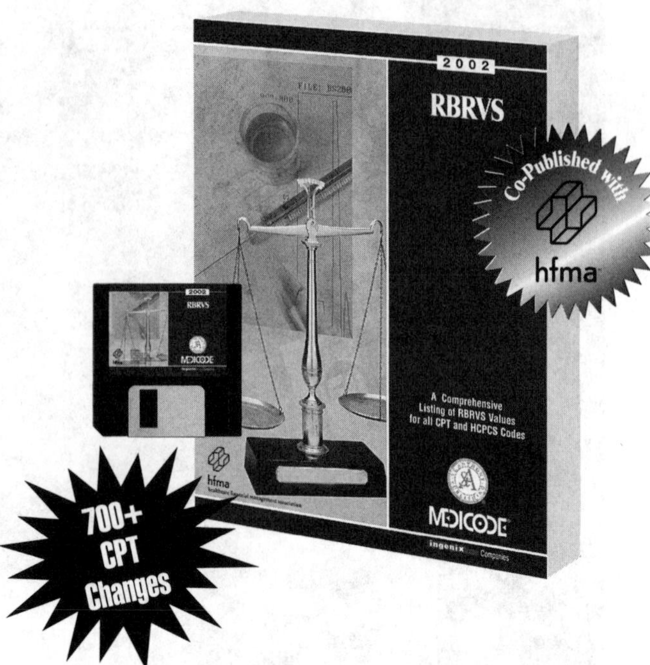

A Complete Relative Value Scale Developed with Direct Physician Input

Relative Values for Physicians

Establish, defend, and negotiate fees using a resource that physician offices like yours have relied on for over 15 years.

- Reference relative values for CPT and HCPCS Level II codes.
- Incorporate relative value units developed through physician surveys.
- Establish relative values based on the clinical skill and knowledge needed to perform a procedure. Subjective charge data is eliminated.
- Value codes relative to one another. Surgery codes are valued relative to surgery codes, E/M codes are valued relative to E/M codes, etc.

ISBN: 1-56337-401-3 — Item No. 4322 **$269.95**

ASCII Data File (Includes Book): Item No. 4320 **$599.95**

Available: December 2001 — 5 CEUs from AAPC

The Most Comprehensive RBRVS Available

RBRVS

RBRVS is now the most widely used relative value scale in existence and is the system CMS (formerly HCFA) uses to calculate Medicare fees. This is the data you need to reference when negotiating contracts with your payers, conducting fee schedule reviews, or auditing current reimbursements.

RBRVS contains relative value units for all procedures valued by CMS in the *Medicare Physician Fee Schedule*, as well as the relative values for those codes not valued by CMS ("gap" codes). These "gap" codes have been developed using the same methodology used to develop the values for Medicare covered services.

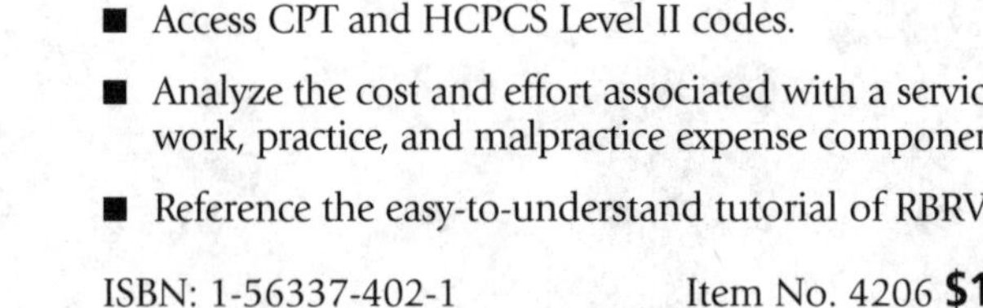

- Reference the same relative value units used by over 60% of the major U.S. HMOs.
- Access CPT and HCPCS Level II codes.
- Analyze the cost and effort associated with a service with work, practice, and malpractice expense components.
- Reference the easy-to-understand tutorial of RBRVS.

ISBN: 1-56337-402-1 — Item No. 4206 **$199.95**

ASCII Data File (Includes Book): Item No. 4323 **$599.95**

Available: December 2001 — 5 CEUs from AAPC

Order Toll-Free 1-800-765-6588

Also Available from your Medical Bookstore or Distributor

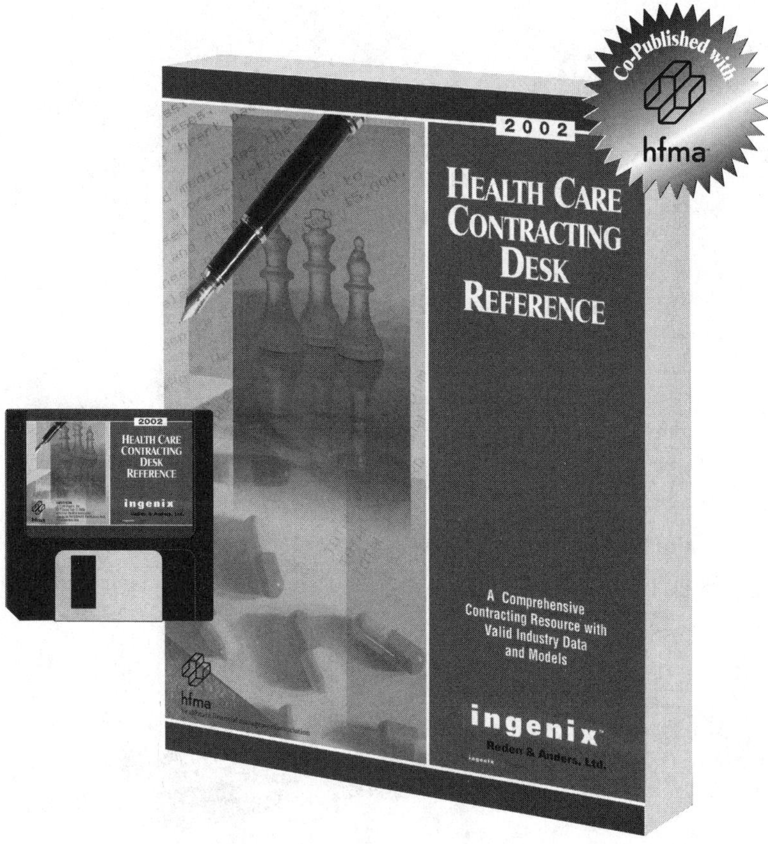

Negotiate Better Health Care Contracts Now

Health Care Contracting Desk Reference

To be successful in today's quickly evolving and competitive marketplace, health care professionals need to negotiate favorable contracts. *Health Care Contracting Desk Reference* has made it easy to understand each component and nuance of capitation, fee-for-service, facility, and ancillary services contracts so you can make educated decisions that will benefit your bottom line.

- Reference proprietary inpatient, outpatient, and physician utilization data in print or ASCII formats.
- Analyze utilization data for separate Medicare and commercial patient populations.
- Access Utilization per Thousand for…
  - Top 50 DRGs
  - Top 50 outpatient surgeries.
  - Top 200+ CPT codes performed by physicians.
- Know what to expect during the negotiation process.
- Understand individual contract elements.
- Reference sample contract language for each type of contract.

ISBN: 1-56337-420-X Item No. 5481 **$399.95**

Available: October 2001

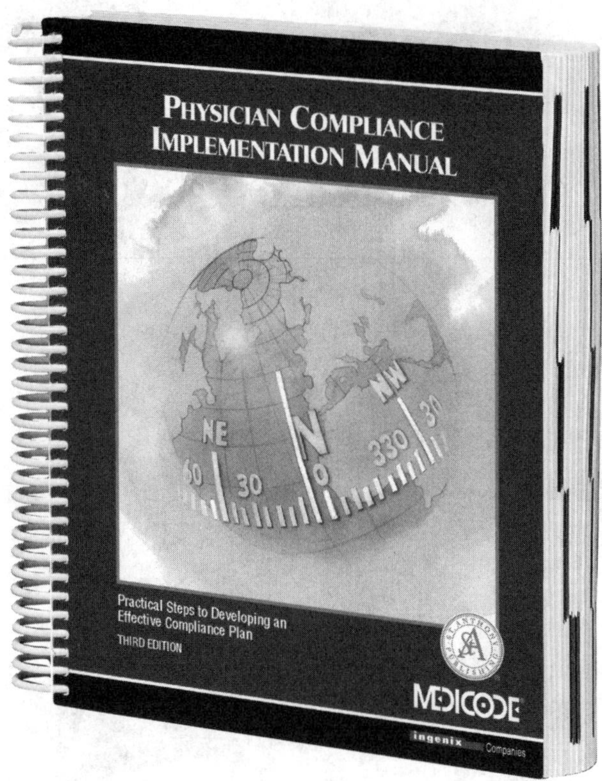

Step-By-Step Instructions

Physician Compliance Implemantation Manual, 3rd Edition

This best-selling manual walks you through each of the seven Office of Inspector General's (OIG) compliance program elements and shows you how to implement a compliance plan based on you unique needs.

- **CMS (Formerly HCFA) Final Compliance Guidelines for Physicians.** Follow CMS' (Formerly HCFA) recommendations for effective compliance programs.
- **Customizable Forms and Worksheets on Diskette.** Provides sample forms and writing policies found in the book in an electronic format that can easily be customized. It will also include a corrective action log and materials to be used during training sessions.
- **OIG Outline and Recommendations.** Shows you how to reduce errors, implement effective compliance policies and procedures, monitor and document your compliance "track record", and avoid penalties if an auditor targets your practice.
- **Glossary of Compliance Terms.** Enables you to learn the definitions and implications of compliance's quickly developing language.
- **Resource Section.** Provides help when you are stumped and don't know where to go for answers.

ISBN: 1-563329-790-6 Item No. 4288 **$159.95**

Available: October 2001 5 CEUs from AAPC 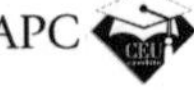

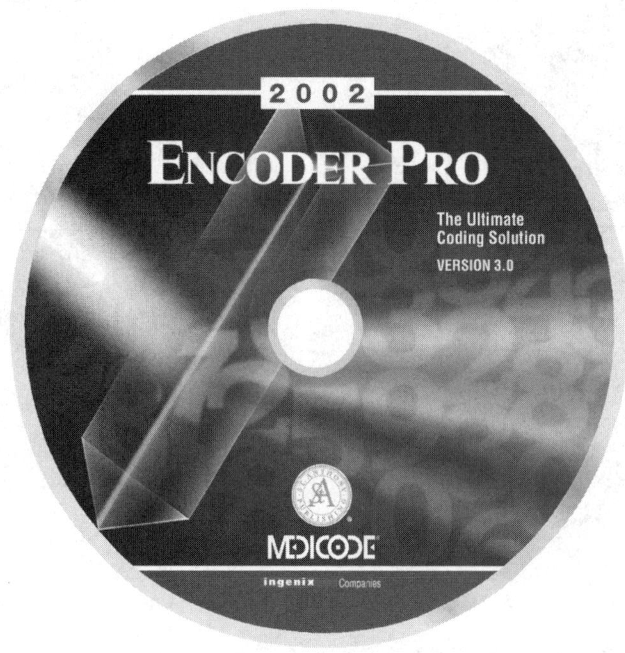

An Entire Coding Library at your Fingertips!

Encoder Pro

Encoder Pro is the ultimate coding solution. In either the local (CD) or ASP deployment (online), *Encoder Pro* gives you an entire coding library at your fingertips. Now powered with Ingenix's CodeLogic™ search technology for even faster more complete code lookup.

This powerful tool gives you:

- **NEW — Ingenix's CodeLogic™ Technology**. New search capabilities allow you to code simultaneously across all three code sets with built-in spell-check, abbreviation, and narrow functions for finding the right codes even faster.
- **HCFA-1500 Form.** New format makes it much easier to create, edit and print.
- **Bookmarks and Sticky Notes.** Easily track your code searches and customize the information you'll need to code correctly every time.
- **HCPCS and CPT Cross Codes.** Justify code selection with all corresponding codes for CPT and HCPCS procedures.
- **Surgical and Procedural Cross Codes.** Find all the CPT add-on codes for primary procedures and verify the right match between code sets.
- **Medicare CCI Unbundling Edits.** Stop billing errors by seeing which CPT codes should no be billed together.
- **CPT and HCPCS Modifiers.**

$499.95 (Single User Pricing)

◆ *Call for multi-user pricing*

Available: October 2001 — 8 CEUs from AAPC

Local Deployment (CD) — Item No. 2717

ASP Deployment (Online) — Item No. 7575

LOCAL DEPLOYMENT Recommended Hardware	ASP DEPLOYMENT Recommended Hardware
• 256 MB of RAM	• 128 MB of RAM
• 800X600 SVGA	• PII 233 MHZ
• PIII 800 MHZ	• 800X600SVGA
• 125 MB Disk Space	• 60 MB Disk Space

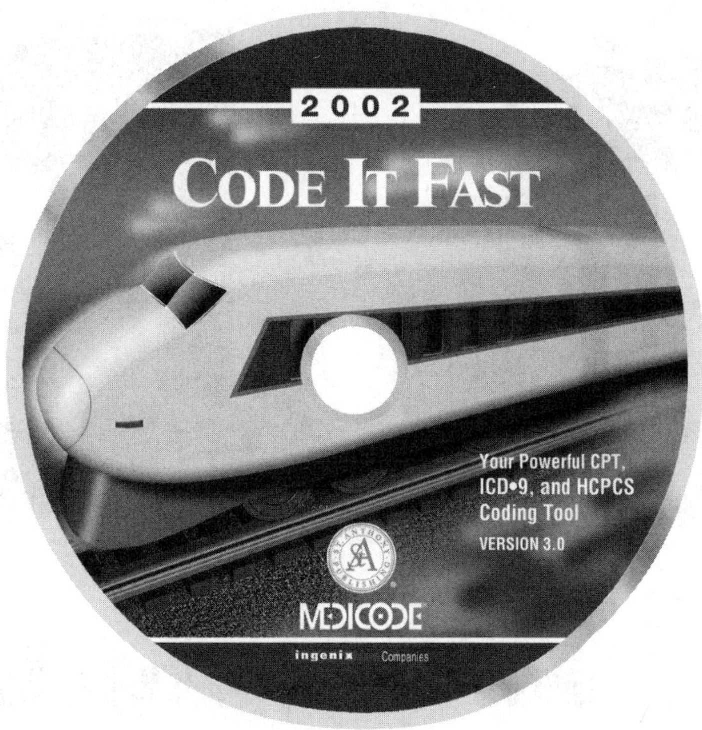

Get All Your Codes Books on CD!

Code It Fast

Code It Fast speeds code lookup for ICD-9, CPT, and HCPCS codes in one easy-to-use program.

- **Web-enabled Version.** Launch Code It Fast ASP directly from your desktop and enjoy Live data updates and fast search capablilities. Requires dial-up ISP connection.
- **Smart Search Engine.** Code across all three code sets. Employs a built in spell-check and narrow function for finding the right codes fast.
- **CPT and HCPCS Modifiers.**
- **ICD-9 Code Annotations and Icons.**
- **Notepad Functionality.**
- **Bookmarks and Sticky Notes.**
- **Definitions, Key Points, Tips and Glossaries.**

$249.95 (Single User Pricing)

Local Deployment (CD) Item No. 3310

ASP Deployment (Online) Item No. 7566

Available: Now

◆ *Call for multi-user pricing*

St. Anthony Publishing/Medicode 2002 Publications

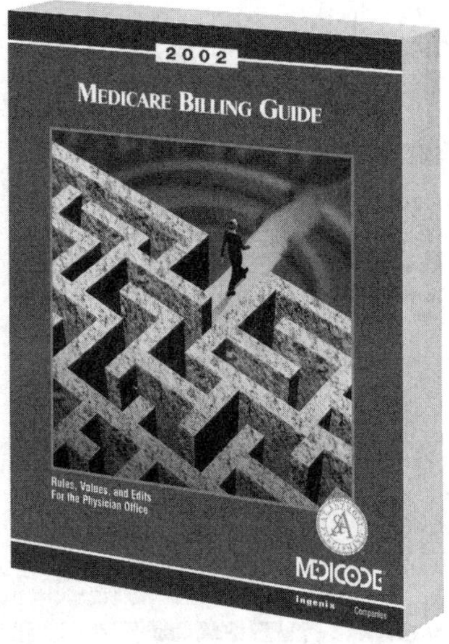

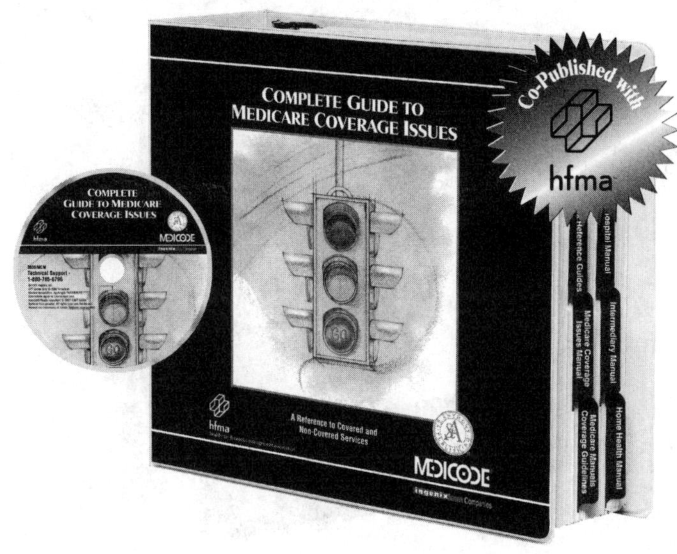

Learn how to Comply with Medicare Regulations

Medicare Billing Guide

Ideal for the physician office or small groups, this guide takes complex Medicare payment information and puts it into easy-to-understand charts and icons.

- **NEW — Overview of Balanced Budget Act.** Understand how it will affect you.
- **NEW — MCM and CIM.** Learn what the rules are for your codes.
- **EXCLUSIVE — Medicare edits at a glance with easy-to-read icons.** Instant reference to identify modifier rules and coverage issues.
- **Organized like CPT.** Its organization makes it very easy to cross-reference information in CPT.
- **Breakout RVUs for Work, Practice Expense, and Malpractice.** Newly revised GPCI (Geographic Practice Cost Indices) to convert the RVUs for your area, calculate payment, and predict cash flow.

ISBN: 1-56337-394-7 Item No. 2994 **$99.95**

Available: February 2002 5 CEUs from AAPC

Know What Medicare Will and Will Not Cover Before Submitting the Claim

Complete Guide to Medicare Coverage Issues

This color-coded, updateable guide will help you determine whether or not to issue an advance beneficiary notice to the Medicare beneficiary. It provides detailed, national coverage policies for medical services, items and procedures based on HCFA's official source documents.

- **Color Coded Coverage Prompts.** See at a glance whether an item or procedure has restricted coverage.
- **Quick Reference Guides.** Quickly identify noncovered procedures and services, including OCE edits.
- ***Coverage Alert* Newsletter.** Get advance notice of national decisions, *Federal Register* notices, rule summaries, OIG issues related to coverage and medical necessity and implementation dates for recently finalized coverage decisions.
- **Searchable CD-ROM with Full Text of the Guide.**
- **Updates for One Full Year.**

Item No. 3036 **$279.95**

Available: Now 5 CEUs from AAPC 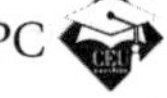

Order Toll-Free 1-800-765-6588

Also Available from your Medical Bookstore or Distributor

090101

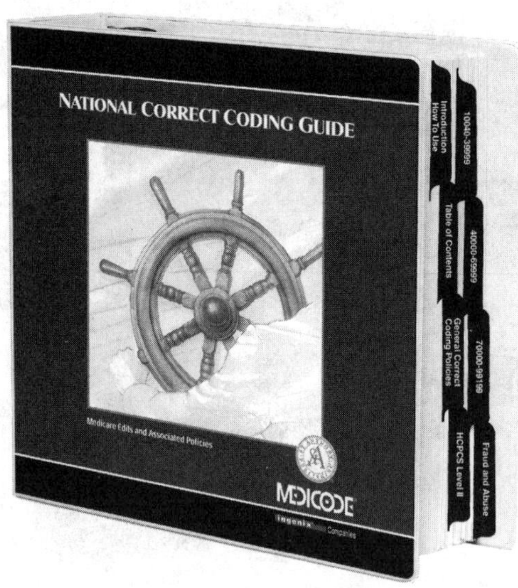

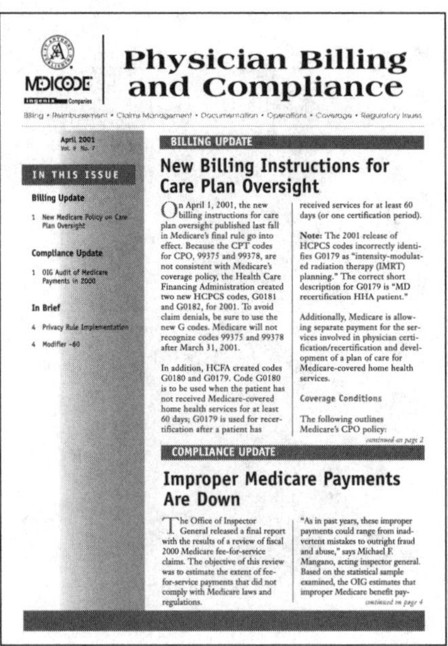

MEDICODE

Physician Billing and Compliance

Billing • Reimbursement • Claims Management • Documentation • Operations • Coverage • Regulatory Issues

April 2001
Vol. 9 No. 7

IN THIS ISSUE

Billing Update

1 New Medicare Policy on Care Plan Oversight

Compliance Update

1 OIG Audit of Medicare Payments in 2000

In Brief

4 Privacy Rule Implementation

4 Modifier -60

BILLING UPDATE

New Billing Instructions for Care Plan Oversight

On April 1, 2001, the new billing instructions for care plan oversight published last fall in Medicare's final rule go into effect. Because the CPT codes for CPO, 99375 and 99378, are not consistent with Medicare's coverage policy, the Health Care Financing Administration created two new HCPCS codes, G0181 and G0182, for 2001. To avoid claim denials, be sure to use the new G codes. Medicare will not recognize codes 99375 and 99378 after March 31, 2001.

In addition, HCFA created codes G0180 and G0179. Code G0180 is to be used when the patient has not received Medicare-covered home health services for at least 60 days; G0179 is used for recertification after a patient has received services for at least 60 days (or one certification period).

Note: The 2001 release of HCPCS codes incorrectly identifies G0179 as "intensity-modulated radiation therapy (IMRT) planning." The correct short description for G0179 is "MD recertification HHA patient."

Additionally, Medicare is allowing separate payment for the services involved in physician certification/recertification and development of a plan of care for Medicare-covered home health services.

Coverage Conditions

The following outlines Medicare's CPO policy:

continued on page 2

COMPLIANCE UPDATE

Improper Medicare Payments Are Down

The Office of Inspector General released a final report with the results of a review of fiscal 2000 Medicare fee-for-service claims. The objective of this review was to estimate the extent of fee-for-service payments that did not comply with Medicare laws and regulations.

"As in past years, these improper payments could range from inadvertent mistakes to outright fraud and abuse," says Michael F. Mangano, acting inspector general. Based on the statistical sample examined, the OIG estimates that improper Medicare benefit pay-

continued on page 4

A Guide to HCFA's National Correct Coding Edits

National Correct Coding Guide

This easy-to-understand manual condenses CMS's (formerly HCFA) National Correct Coding Initiative (NCCI) edit policy manual into an easy-to-manage, user-friendly guide. Learn and understand the impact of NCCI on physician billing and coding practices. Know that you have correctly coded each service for reimbursement in compliance with CMS's policy. This guide is useful in coding and expediting all claims, not just Medicare Part B.

- **Complete listing.** Medicare Correct Coding Edits including surgery, medicine, laboratory, radiology and HCPCS.
- **Policy Symbols by Each Edit.** Correctly code your service for reimbursement in compliance with CMS's policies to prevent claim rejection, delays and audits.
- **Explains Medicare's NCCI.** Understand exactly how these policies affect coding. Take the mystery out of NCCI.
- **Fraud & Abuse Overview.** Learn and understand the magnitude and implications of the NCCI and the impact on physician billing and coding practices.
- **State-by-State Directory.** Know whom to call with questions.
- **Quarterly updates for one full year.** Keep you current with CMS's revisions to the CCI.

Item No. 3038 **$229.95**

Available: Now 5 CEUs from AAPC

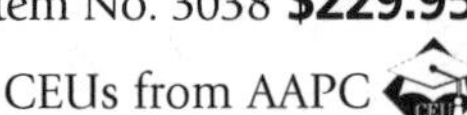

Get Practical Billing Operations and Compliance Tips — Every Month

Physician Billing and Compliance

Physician Billing and Compliance providesexpert advice and "how-to" instruction on submittingclean claims, running an efficient billing operation, and minimizing your risk for fraud and abuse. We help youget the reimbursement you deserve for the services you provide.

Inside each monthly issue you'll find:

- **In-depth Analysis of Physician Billing Issues.** Submit claim forms right the first time and immediately reduce billing errors, claim denials, and underpayments.
- **Operational Strategies for Your Billing Department and Accounts Receivable.** Learn to efficiently and economically manage your billing department and billing staff.
- **Compliance Issues of Importance.** Learn easy self-auditing methods to help reduce your audit liability.
- **Billing Tips from Our Billing Experts.** Learn the latest rules on billing modifiers, DME, nonphysician provider services, office-based tests, and more.

Item No. 4017 **$159.95**

Available: Now Up to 10 CEUs from AAPC

Unparalleled Clinical Coding Expertise

Our in-house technical staff includes nurses, medical records experts, billing service managers, consultants, and auditors who are credentialed, field-tested experts. (CPC, CPC-H, CCS, CCS-P, RHIT, RHIA, RN, LPN)

Order Toll-Free 1-800-765-6588

Also Available from your Medical Bookstore or Distributor

090101

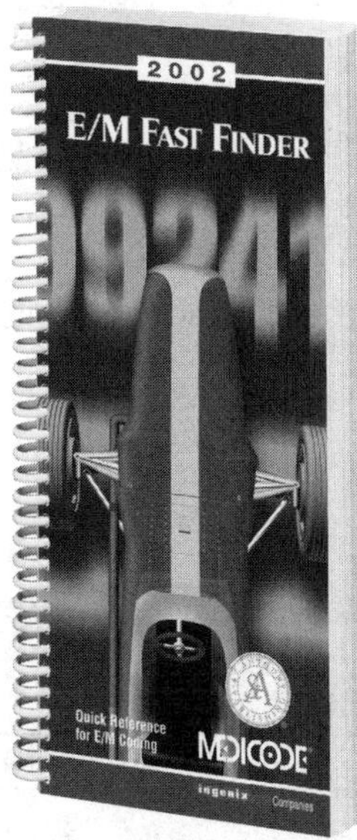

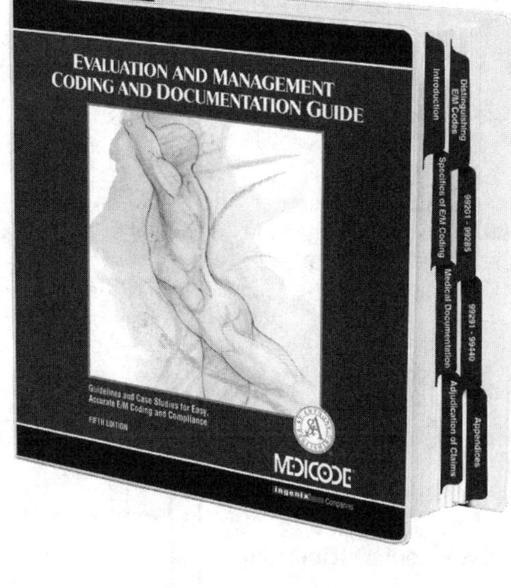

Quick Reference For E/M Coding

E/M Fast Finder

This pocket-sized resource is an invaluable tool when assigning E/M codes.

- **Updated with 2002 E/M Codes.** Make coding decisions with confidence.
- **Organized by Site of Service for Quick Code Access.**
- **Quick Reference Graphs.** Simplify the process of selecting appropriate codes via the level of history, exam, and medical decision-making criteria.
- **Two Color Key.** Issues are highlighted for ease of use.
- **Step-by-Step Instructions.** Easy to follow instructions and a sample worksheet walks you through the steps needed to properly use the fast finder.
- **Abbreviation Key.** List of commonly used and accepted medical abbreviations makes this a perfect tool for a beginner or an experienced physician.

ISBN: 1-56337-422-6 Item No. 2885 **$29.95**

Available: December 2001 1 CEU from AAPC

E/M Coding Made Easy!

Evaluation and Management Coding and Documentation Guide

This comprehensive, updateable guide to CMS (formerly HCFA) E/M guidelines provides instructions for correctly documenting each level of E/M service and helps users stay current with timely revisions.

- **Real-Life Clinical Case Studies Updated for 2002.** Illustrates how to apply the guidelines in everyday situations. Use them to train your staff.
- **Crosswalk between the 1995 and 1997 E/M Guidelines.** Helps you prepare for the transition to stricter documentation requirements ahead.
- **Self-Audit Forms.** Create a checklist of important documentation needed to support the appropriate level of E/M service.
- **Handy E/M Fast Finder.** A portable reference, organized by place of service, and illustrated with tables. Practitioners can take E/M Fast Finder with them into the exam room.
- **Updates for One Full Year.** When new guidelines are released you will be updated automatically…enabling you to stay in compliance.
- **Real-Life Audit Scenarios.** Helps you uncover areas of risk in your own organization so you can fix problems now — not after fines or penalties.

ISBN: 1-56329-714-0 Item No. 3022 **$129.95**

Available: Now 5 CEUs from AAPC 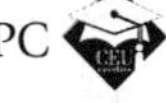

4 Easy Ways to Order

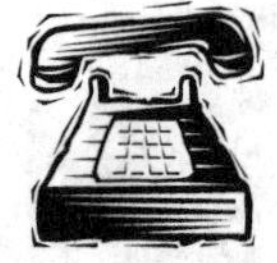

CALL toll-free
800.765.6588 and mention the source code from your mailing label

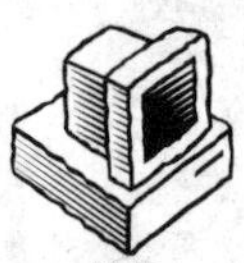

SHOP on line at
www.IngenixOnLine.com

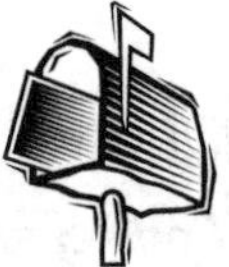

MAIL this form with payment and/or purchase order to:
PO Box 27116
Salt Lake City, UT 84127-0116

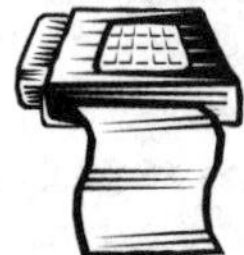

FAX this order form with credit card information and/or purchase order to 801.982.4033

Shipping and Handling	
No. of Items	**Fee**
1	9.95
2-4	11.95
5-7	14.95
8-10	19.95
11+	Call

Publication Order and Fax Form

FOBA3

Customer No.__________ Purchase Order No.__________
(Attach copy of Purchase Order)

Contact Name __________

Company__________ Title__________

Address __________
(no P.O. Boxes, please)

City__________ State____ Zip__________

Phone (____)__________ Fax (____)__________
(in case we have questions about your order)

IMPORTANT: Email required for order confirmation and select product delivery.

Email __________

❑ Yes, I want to receive Product Updates and Information

❑ Yes, I want to receive Ingenix New Product Announcements and Special Offers

Item #	Qty	Item Description	Price	Total
4025	1	(SAMPLE) DRG Guidebook	$89.95	$89.95

Sub Total

OH and VA residents please add applicable sales tax

Shipping & handling (see chart)
(11 plus units, foreign and Canadian orders, please call for shipping costs)

Total enclosed

Payment Options:

❍ Bill Me. (St. Anthony, Medicode, CHIPS & St. Anthony Consulting are doing business as Ingenix).

❍ Check enclosed. (Make payable to Ingenix, Inc.) Check #__________

❍ Charge my: ❍ MasterCard ❍ VISA ❍ AMEX ❍ Discover

Card # | | | | | | | | | | | | | | | | | Exp. Date: | | | (MM YR)

Signature __________

100% Money Back Guarantee

If our merchandise ever fails to meet your expectations, please contact our Customer Service Department at (800) 765-6588 for an immediate response. We will resolve any concern without hesitation.

All prices subject to change without notice.

2002

RBRVS

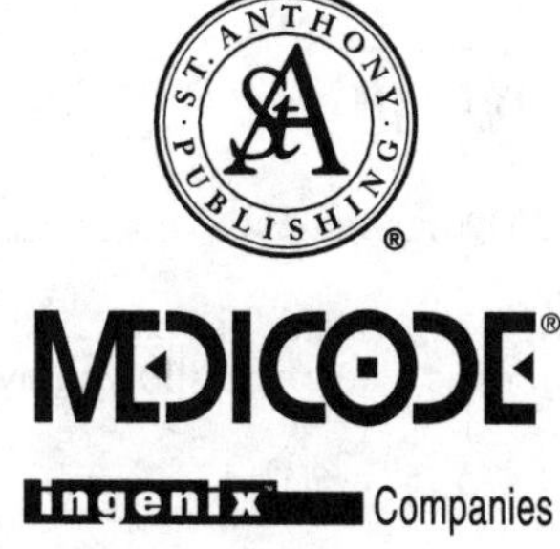

Publisher's Notice

The Ingenix 2002 *RBRVS* is designed to provide accurate and authoritative information in regard to the subject covered. Every reasonable effort has been made to ensure the accuracy of the information within these pages. However, the ultimate responsibility for accuracy lies with the user.

Ingenix,Inc., its employees, agents and staff make no representation, guarantee or warranty, expressed or implied, that this compilation is error-free or that the use of this publication will prevent differences of opinion or disputes with Medicare or third-party payers, and will bear no responsibility for the results or consequences of its use.

Ingenix Publishing Group combines the expertise and industry experience of Medicode, St. Anthony Publishing, Cambridge Health Economics (CHEG), and the Center for Healthcare Industry Performance Studies (CHIPS), bringing you the most powerful and useful sources of data obtainable in healthcare. Ingenix Publishing Group's line of products provides leading healthcare information and analysis for the clinical and financial decision support market.

Ingenix maintains the largest database of charge data, clinical measurements, and audited healthcare financial records in the healthcare industry. With Ingenix's expert analyses and robust data sets you are assured the most relevant and current decision support information available.

American Medical Association Notice

Acknowledgements

Susan P. Seare	*Publisher*
Ralph S. Wankier, MBA	*Product Director, Benchmark Product Line*
Melissa Fonnesbeck	*Product Manager*
Lynn Speirs	*Senior Director of Publishing*
Lauri Gray, RHIT, CPC	*Technical Editor*
Chris B. Frazier, MA, CPC	*Project Editor*
Carla Gee	*Data Analysis*
Kerrie Hornsby	*Desktop Publishing Manager*
Gregory Kemp	*Desktop Publishing Specialist*

If you have questions or comments regarding this publication write to:

Product Manager, RBRVS
Ingenix, Inc.
2525 Lake Park Blvd.
Salt Lake City, UT 84120
Ph: 800-999-4600

Or e-mail: melissa.fonnesbeck@ingenix.com

We appreciate and acknowledge the Healthcare Financial Management Association (HFMA) and its team of reviewers for this publication:

Wendy Trout, *Director of Corporate Compliance, Wellspan Health*
Clinnie Biggs, Jr., *Certified Management Consultant, Deloitte & Touche, LLP*

Copyright

ISBN 1-56337-402-1

Contents

Preface

The Ingenix *RBRVS* contains data developed by Ingenix, Inc., using methodology developed by the Cambridge Health Economics Group (CHEG). CHEG is the expert in Resource-Based Relative Value Scale (RBRVS) methodology. The company was founded in 1988 by members of the original Harvard University RBRVS studies team. CHEG specialists have vast knowledge and experience in the development and application of value scales. These value scales may be used to evaluate pricing of professional healthcare services, develop fees and rates for services, measure provider productivity, assess profitability, and profile costs.

In order to develop the values for the physician services found in RBRVS, the Harvard University studies team first identified and defined three distinct components affecting the value of each service or procedure. These three components include physician work, practice expense, and malpractice insurance. Relative Value Units (RVUs) were then assigned to each component for each distinct Medicare-covered service. A distinct service is defined as each unique CPT or HCPCS code. Federal law requires Medicare to breakout the individual RVUs assigned to each component for each unique CPT or HCPCS code. The sum of the RVUs for each of the three components found in RBRVS comprises the total value of each physician service.

These three components are also used by the Centers for Medicare and Medicaid Services (CMS) (formerly HCFA) to assign dollar values to each CPT or HCPCS code. However, geographic practice cost indices (GPCIs) must also be applied to each component prior to converting the fee to a dollar amount. Once the GPCIs are factored into the equation, the geographic specific dollar amount can be calculated by multiplying the GPCI adjusted total value by the dollar conversion factor. These dollar amounts then become the reimbursement rates found in the geographic or locality specific Medicare Fee Schedule (MFS).

Even though RBRVS was developed specifically for assigning reimbursement rates to Medicare covered services, over 60 percent of non-Medicare payers use Medicare RBRVS to establish fees or maximum allowables for physician services. This works well for those services covered by Medicare; however, because Medicare does not cover all services and relative values were originally developed only for Medicare covered services, the MFS has holes or gaps. In order to create a complete RBRVS fee schedule, these Medicare non-covered services needed to have relative values assigned. Over the past decade, CHEG has filled these gaps using the same methodology used to develop the values for Medicare covered services.

The Ingenix *RBRVS* includes values for more than 3,000 Level I and II gap codes not included in the MFS in addition to all MFS Level I and II codes. Whenever possible, the same methodology for valuing these gap codes has been used. However, modifications to this methodology have been made for some services, such as laboratory, durable medical equipment, medical supplies, prosthetics, orthotics, and drugs and biologicals. For specific information on the methodology used to value these types of services, see the introductions to the Laboratory and HCPCS Level II sections. *RBRVS* is the most comprehensive resource-based relative value scale available. Here are the *RBRVS* features:

- All physician services, including those not part of the MFS
- Clinical laboratory services
- Level II codes, such as durable medical equipment (DME), medical and surgical supplies, and transportation
- J codes (injectable drugs)

Introduction

Development

The Ingenix *RBRVS* incorporates the relative values produced by the Centers for Medicare and Medicaid Services (CMS) (formerly HCFA) Medicare Fee Schedule (MFS) into a comprehensive reference of RBRVS relative values. However, as users of the MFS are acutely aware, not all services are valued under Medicare's RBRVS system. In order to produce a complete fee schedule based on RBRVS, the codes not valued by Medicare, sometimes referred to as "gap" codes, need to be valued.

Realizing the importance and power of the Resource-Based Relative Value Scale (RBRVS), Ingenix Publishing Group has teamed with the most respected developers of the RBRVS scale, Cambridge Health Economics Group (CHEG).

CHEG's core expertise is in the use of RBRVS to assess the resource costs required to deliver physician services. Ingenix uses this expertise to provide a wide range of RBRVS applications, including pricing of healthcare services, measurement of provider productivity, profitability assessment, and cost and utilization profiling.

With the founders of CHEG, a robust and compatible relative value scale was developed for those services not covered by Medicare. Using the same proprietary methodology used to develop the original RBRVS, Ingenix's proprietary database of values enables a more complete and comprehensive application of the RBRVS system.

Please note that the Medicare values included in this book are those available at the time of printing. CMS may issue corrections throughout the year. Check the CMS website at www.cms.gov for any changes throughout the year.

How to Use This Book

The Ingenix *RBRVS*, while primarily intended as a reference book for reimbursement, also can be used for other applications that will be described later in the introduction. Because it contains relative value information for all Level I and II codes, it can be used as a reference for Medicare, Medicaid, and private sector payers. However, because of the variability among private sector payers, the information used may need adjusting in its application. The Ingenix *RBRVS* provides a number of scenarios as examples of the varying payer methodologies. However, in applying RBRVS information to specific payers, it is important to first understand how RBRVS was intended to be applied and how it is currently being applied by CMS in administering the MFS. Only after the Medicare methodology is fully understood can one apply RBRVS to other payers and understand and adjust for their differing reimbursement methodologies.

This introduction will address the following:

Medicare and RBRVS — This section provides a short history of the development of RBRVS and describes the process by which RVUs are transformed into the geographic specific dollar amounts reimbursed by Medicare.

Private Sector Payers and RBRVS — Private sector payers may or may not apply RBRVS using the same rules and assumptions applied to the MFS. This section will present some of the more common variables. However, because of the number of variables, it is not possible to describe them all. It is therefore critical before contracting with any payer to obtain a complete written description of their rules and assumptions.

Capitation and RBRVS — Although capitation is an alternative to fee-for-service (FFS) reimbursement, reimbursement rates under a capitated system must still be analyzed to determine if payment levels are adequate to cover the value of the services provided. RBRVS is an excellent tool for this type of analysis. A discussion of capitated contracts in relation to RBRVS is included in this section.

Determining Your Gross Conversion Factor — Many RBRVS guides provide instruction only on developing a gross conversion factor. While this is still helpful as a rough analysis of your fees and payer proposals, it is not the most accurate method for evaluating your fee schedule or payer proposals. However, in the absence of good information on the frequency of services, this may be the only method available for calculating a conversion factor. Therefore, a description is included in this section.

Determining Your Frequency-Adjusted Conversion Factor — If good information is available on the frequency of services provided, a frequency-adjusted conversion factor should be developed. This section provides detailed information on why and how this type of conversion factor is used.

Developing an RBRVS Fee Schedule — This section describes how to develop an RBRVS fee schedule using either a gross conversion factor or a frequency-adjusted conversion factor.

Productivity Measurement — RBRVS is useful in analyzing productivity, particularly in a multi-provider and/or multi-specialty practice or clinic. Practices with capitation contracts may wish to use RBRVS-based productivity measures to distribute the capitation payment. This section will provide some examples of how to develop productivity measures and how to apply them.

Cost/Benefit Analysis — The four-year transition to resource-based relative value units for the practice expense component that began in 1999 is now complete. This change may have a significant effect on reimbursement not only from Medicare but from private sector payers as well. The effect on individual providers will depend on each provider's mix of services and the sites where the services are performed. In general, providers who furnish more office-based services will experience higher reimbursement rates for those services, while those who furnish more facility-based services will experience lower reimbursement rates. Continued evaluation of the relative costs and benefits of moving some services currently provided outside the physician office to the physician office is recommended. This section provides examples of how to use RBRVS for cost/benefit analysis.

Five-Year Review Process — Medicare has just completed the second five-year review of physician work RVUs. Significant changes have been made to the work value of hundreds of codes. Reviewing the effect of these changes on Medicare reimbursements and commercial payer contracts based on RBRVS is more critical than ever. This section explains the Five-Year Review Process.

Medicare Sustainable Growth Rate (SGR) — For the first time in several years there has been a reduction of the Medicare Conversion Factor. This is a result of legislation aimed at controlling the actual growth in aggregate Medicare expenditures for physicians' services. Legislation requires yearly review and adjustment of expenditures to meet SGR targets. Expenditures are manipulated by adjusting the conversion factor. This section explains factors affecting SGR and the effect on the conversion factor.

RBRVS Terminology — RBRVS has its own vocabulary. Without an understanding of these terms and acronyms, it is difficult, even impossible, to understand Medicare's methodology much less the differing applications of private sector payers. Although each term will be defined when it is presented, this section lists each term alphabetically so that all relevant terms and acronyms can be easily accessed for quick reference.

Medicare and RBRVS

For most of Medicare's history, physicians were paid using a methodology referred to as the "customary, prevailing, and reasonable" (CPR) charge system. The CPR methodology was similar to that used by private sector payers, who refer to their methodology as the "usual, customary, and reasonable" (UCR) charge system. Essentially, under both systems physician services were reimbursed based on the physician's actual fees. Neither system made any attempt to reimburse physician services based on the work required for each service.

However, as healthcare costs skyrocketed in the 1970s and 1980s, both government and private sector payers began evaluating alternative reimbursement methodologies. A number of alternatives to Medicare's CPR system were proposed and evaluated, including revamping the CPR system; using a diagnosis related group (DRG) approach similar to that used for inpatient hospital services; using a capitated payment system similar to those being experimented with in the private sector; or developing a new payment schedule based on the relative values of services provided. Eventually, after years of heated debate and study, a resource-based relative value scale (RBRVS) was adopted by Medicare in 1992 and phased in over a five-year period.

The current RBRVS system ranks services according to the relative costs required to provide them. These costs are defined in terms of units, with more complex, more time-consuming services having higher unit values than less complex, less time-consuming services. Furthermore, each service is compared to all other physician services so that each service is given a value that reflects its cost or value when compared to all other physician services.

For example, a single layer laceration repair of the finger might have a value of five, while an open reduction and internal fixation of a wrist fracture might have a value of 15. These values are directly related to the differing levels of complexity and the amount of time required to perform the procedures.

Medicare's RBRVS has divided cost into three distinct components affecting the value of each service. These three components include physician work, practice expense, and malpractice insurance. Each of these components has been assigned separate relative value units (RVUs).

Physician work, referred to in the table as "work value," reflects the cost of the physician's time and skill. For example, the time and skill required to perform a new patient comprehensive eye exam (92004) might have a work value of two, whereas an extracapsular cataract extraction (66984) might have a work value of 10.

Practice expense (PE) reflects the cost of the physician's rent, staff, supplies, equipment, and other overhead associated with the service. Until 1999, PE costs were determined by historical physician charges. A 50 percent site-of-service reduction was applied to only 675 codes. These site-of-service reductions were applied to those services that were determined by Medicare as being performed in the physician office at least 50 percent of the time. However, in 1999, Medicare began a four-year phase-in of resource-based practice expense units. This phase-in is now complete and PE as of 2002 is 100 percent resource-based. Because PE is dependent upon site of service, implementation of the resource-based PE required that the PE component be subdivided into non-facility PE and facility PE. Non-facility PE, identified in the table as "non-fac PE," reflects the cost of providing this service in the physician's office, patient's home, or residential care setting. Facility PE, identified in the table as "fac PE," reflects the cost of providing the service in a hospital, ambulatory surgery center (ASC), or skilled nursing facility (SNF). Some services are routinely performed in the physician office, but may on occasion be performed in another facility. For these services two different PE values are listed with the non-facility having a higher value than the facility PE. For example, closed treatment of a non-displaced wrist fracture (25600) might have a PE value of four when performed in the physician's office; however, the same service provided in a hospital emergency room might have a PE value of two. When the service is routinely provided outside the physician office, the values listed in these two columns will be the same. For example, a cholecystectomy (47600) will have the same value listed in both columns because it cannot be performed in the physician's office.

Malpractice insurance, identified as "malpractice" in the table, reflects the relative risk or professional liability associated with the service. Services involving lower risk or professional liability have lower values than those with higher risk or professional liability. For example, a lumbar puncture (62270) has a lower relative risk than a laminectomy for excision of an intraspinal neoplasm (63275), which is reflected in the values assigned to the malpractice component for each procedure.

The sum of these three components—physician work, practice expense (non-facility or facility), and malpractice insurance—reflect the total value of the service or the total relative value units (RVUs). Because practice expense has been subdivided into two categories, two total values are available for each service. The non-facility total value, identified in the table as "non-fac total," reflects the total value of the service when provided in the physician's office, patient's home, or other non-hospital setting; while the facility total value, identified in the table as "fac total," represents the total value of services provided in a hospital, ASC, or SNF. These totals are the units used by Medicare to determine the actual dollar payment for the service.

However, prior to determining the dollar payment, additional adjustments must be made to each of the three components. Because cost varies according to geographic location, each component of the total value must be adjusted to reflect these geographic differences. Therefore, prior to calculating the Medicare reimbursement rate, each of the three components must be adjusted by locality using the Geographic Practice Cost Indices (GPCI). GPCIs were developed according to statute and are revised every three years. The revisions are implemented in a step fashion over a three-year period in order to reduce the overall impact of any changes. GPCIs are listed in the table on page 26 and are used as follows:

Step 1 (multiply)

GPCI for work value	x	work value	=	geographically adjusted work value (A)
GPCI for practice expense	x	practice expense	=	geographically adjusted practice expense value (facility value or non-facility) (B)
GPCI for malpractice	x	malpractice value	=	geographically adjusted malpractice value (C)

Step 2 (add)

A + B + C = geographically adjusted (GPCI) total value

Using the GPCI total value, the actual Medicare dollar amount for a given locality is calculated after applying the Medicare conversion factor. Medicare currently has a single conversion factor for all types of services except anesthesia. The conversion factor represents the dollar value of each relative value unit. For example, if the Medicare conversion factor is $30, then a GPCI total value of 10 represents a dollar value of $300 for the service. This $300 is the Medicare fee or Medicare allowable for a given locality. This is calculated as follows:

Step 3 (multiply)

Geographically adjusted total value x Medicare conversion factor = Locality specific Medicare fee

Private Sector Payers and RBRVS

While over 60 percent of all private sector payers use RBRVS for pricing, the methodology used to establish reimbursement rates may differ considerably from Medicare's methodology. Key differences involve the application of GPCIs, the application of facility and non-facility practice expense RVUs, and the conversion factor.

GPCIs may or may not be applied by private sector payers. One key to determining whether GPCIs are factored into the reimbursement rate is how the payer describes the reimbursement methodology. If the payer describes the reimbursement rate as a percent of Medicare, GPCIs have usually been factored into the reimbursement rate. Therefore, if the payer describes the reimbursement as 120 percent of Medicare, the reimbursement rate is probably GPCI adjusted. However, this should be verified by requesting the reimbursement rates for five to 10 CPT codes. Use the methodology described in the first section of the introduction, Medicare and RBRVS, to determine the GPCI adjusted Medicare fee, then multiply the Medicare fee by 120 percent. If the fees are GPCI adjusted, your calculated rates and the payer's rates will be equal. If they are not GPCI adjusted, your calculated rates will be higher or lower than the payer's rates.

If the payer describes his reimbursement methodology using a conversion factor, GPCIs may or may not be factored into the reimbursement rate. Once again, it will be necessary to request reimbursement rates for five to 10 CPT codes and perform the same calculations described above. Use the methodology described in the Medicare and RBRVS section; however, this time instead of using the Medicare conversion factor, the private payer conversion factor would be used. If the fees are GPCI adjusted your calculated rates and the payer's rates will be equal. If they are not GPCI adjusted, your calculated rates will be higher or lower than the payer's rates.

In addition to performing these calculations to verify whether GPCIs are factored into the reimbursement rates, a written description of the payment methodology should be requested from the payer and included in any contract. This description should specifically state whether the rates are GPCI adjusted.

However, because of the additional calculations required to adjust for geographic cost differences using GPCIs, many payers elect to adjust for geographic differences using different conversion factors for different geographic areas. For example, a payer has beneficiaries in two localities. Locality One has costs twice that of Locality Two. If Locality Two represents the base rate and has a conversion factor of $40, then Locality One will have a conversion factor of $80 (2 X $40). If the payer expands to a third locality where costs are 1.25 times that of the base reimbursement rate, then Locality Three will have a conversion factor of $50 (1.25 X $40).

Even though Medicare uses one conversion factor for all services except anesthesia, private sector payers may have multiple conversion factors within a single locality. There are two common scenarios. First, private sector payers may apply a higher conversion factor for care provided by primary care physicians than they do for specialists. Second, private sector payers may apply a higher conversion factor based on type of service. The most common adjustment is to use a higher conversion factor for evaluation and management services and a lower conversion factor for all other services.

Another area where private payer methodology may differ from Medicare is in the definition of non-facility PE and facility PE. With the elimination of the 50 percent site of service differential for practice expense (PE) in 1999 and the adoption of two resource-based PE RVUs for each service, private sector payers may choose to use only one of the two RVUs in calculating all reimbursement. In other words, some private sector payers may select either the non-facility or the facility PE and use that single PE to calculate total RVUs regardless of whether the service was performed in the physician's office or in a hospital setting. Other payers may opt to implement PE RVUs exactly as Medicare has, tying reimbursement to the site-of-service. All payers using RBRVS-based fee schedules should be contacted to determine how they are handling the physician expense component if this is not specifically addressed in the contract.

Whenever changes are made to the RBRVS fee schedule, it is important to contact payers and request a written description of how these changes will be applied to your contracts. It is also important to monitor payments to verify that payments are being made as intended.

Capitated Contracts and RBRVS

Over the last few years, payment for services using capitation has become more common. Recent studies indicate more than 30 percent of HMOs use capitation for physician payment. In order to determine whether the capitated rate is adequate to cover the value of the physician services provided, some type of uniform measure must be applied to analyze the proposed capitation rate.

RBRVS provides a uniform measurement scale for analyzing proposed capitation rates. It also can be used to assess physician work and distribute capitation payments among providers. In addition, since capitation shifts risk from the payer to the provider, RBRVS can be used as a tool for analyzing the long-term cost-effectiveness of various treatment options when multiple treatment options are available.

In order to use RBRVS to analyze capitation proposals, it is first necessary to understand this type of payment system. Capitation is a system in which a fixed rate is paid, usually on a monthly basis, for each plan enrollee covered under the capitation agreement. All of the payer's membership may be capitated or only a portion of the membership (e.g., all those who live in a specific geographic area, all those who participate in a specific plan, or all Medicare enrollees). Instead of receiving payment on a fee-for-service basis, the provider is paid a fixed amount based on the number of members covered under the capitation agreement. While the reimbursement rate should be based on historical utilization and should approximate reimbursement levels based on a discounted fee schedule, there is no guarantee that payment will equal what was previously reimbursed on a service-by-service basis.

There are two basic methods used by payers to calculate the capitation payment. The more common method is to establish a fixed rate per member per month (PMPM). For example, the payer may contract with a group of orthopedic surgeons at a rate of $1.25/PMPM for all necessary orthopedic services. This PMPM is paid regardless of the actual services provided to the covered membership. Another method involves paying a fixed rate based on a percent of premium for each plan enrollee. For example, the same group of orthopedic surgeons may agree to accept 1.25 percent of the average monthly premiums for a defined membership. If the average monthly premium per member is $100, then the group is paid the same $1.25. However, the PMPM will fluctuate depending on increases or decreases in the average monthly premium. For example, an increase in the average monthly premium to $105 would result in an increase in the PMPM to $1.3125, while a decrease in the average monthly premium to $95 would result in a decrease in the PMPM to $1.1825.

Using RBRVS to Establish a Capitation Rate

1. Obtain at least one year of historical information regarding the capitated membership from the payer, including monthly membership and a monthly frequency of services by CPT code.

2. Using a spreadsheet, enter each CPT code identified in the historical information and the frequency of each CPT code (use at least a one year total).

3. Determine the total RVUs for each procedure. Because there are two total RVU amounts, one for facility-based procedures and one for non-facility-based procedures, several different approaches might be used. One approach would be to use the total RVU that is most appropriate for each service. For example, if closed treatment of a wrist fracture (25600) is usually performed in the office, use the total non-facility RVU. However, if it is usually performed in the hospital, use the total facility RVU. Another approach might be to use actual experience to determine which total RVU amount to use. This could be obtained from internal data or requested from the payer. For example, if it is determined from internal data that procedure 25600 is performed in a hospital setting 40 percent of the time and in an office setting 60 percent of the time, and the total number of times that service was performed during the year is 10, then use the total facility RVU for a frequency of four and total non-facility RVU for a frequency of six. A third approach would be to select either the total facility RVU or the total non-facility RVU and use the same RVU for all services regardless of where they are performed. Examples of each approach are provided in the following tables.

Table 1. Determining Total RVUs Based on Most Frequent Site of Service

CPT code	Frequency	RVU	Total RVU
99213	50	1.39	69.50
25600	10	7.505	75.00
27788	8	9.68	77.44
27236	5	30.77	153.85
73070	10	0.73	7.30
29345	10	3.10	31.00
Total	93		414.09

Table 2. Determine Total RVUs Based on Actual Site of Service Experience

CPT code	Frequency	Total Non-fac RVU	% Non-fac	Total Fac RVU	% Fac	Total RVU
99213	50	1.39	100%	0.94	0%	69.50
25600	10	7.50	60%	6.07	40%	69.28
27788	8	11.71	30%	9.68	70%	77.44
27236	5	30.77	0%	30.77	100%	153.85
73070	10	0.73	100%	0.73	0%	7.30
29345	10	3.10	80%	2.61	20%	30.02
Total	93					407.39

Table 3. Determining Total RVUs Using Facility Site of Service

CPT code	Frequency	RVU	Total RVU
99213	50	0.94	47.00
25600	10	6.07	60.70
27788	8	9.68	77.44
27236	5	30.77	153.85
73070	10	0.73	7.30
29345	10	2.61	26.10
Total	93		372.39

4. Determine the total yearly reimbursement by multiplying covered membership by the proposed PMPM times the number of months being reviewed. For example, if the total covered monthly membership is 1,000 patients and the PMPM is $1.25, then total yearly (12 month) reimbursement is 1,000 x $1.25 x 12 = $15,000.

5. Calculate the conversion factor by dividing the total yearly reimbursement by the total RVUs for all services performed. For example, if RVUs were calculated using the facility RVU for all services regardless of actual site of service (see Table 3 in Step 3), then the total reimbursement of $15,000 would be divided by 372.39 and the conversion factor for this

capitation contract would be $40.28. If the RVUs were calculated using actual site of service experience (see Table 2 in Step 3), then the total reimbursement of $15,000 would be divided by 407.39 and the conversion factor would be $36.82.

6. If you already have a fee schedule based on RBRVS, the capitated conversion factor can be compared to your fee-for-service conversion factor. If the payer uses RBRVS, the capitated conversion factor should also be compared to the payer's fee-for-service conversion factor. If you do not have an RBRVS-based fee schedule or have not previously determined how your fee schedule converts to RBRVS, this will need to be done so that you have a basis for comparison (see "Developing an RBRVS Fee Schedule").

Determining a Gross Conversion Factor

Because so many private sector payers use RBRVS to determine reimbursement rates, all providers should evaluate their fee schedule by determining their gross conversion factor. Whether or not you continue to use your current fee schedule or convert to a RBRVS-based fee schedule, determining your gross conversion factor will allow you to quickly analyze payer proposals based on RBRVS. For example, if you know that your undiscounted fees reflect a gross conversion factor of $50, you can quickly determine that a payer proposal of $40 will represent approximately a 20 percent discount. If you determine that a 20 percent discount is not acceptable, then no further analysis would be required. If you determine that a 20 percent discount is acceptable, a more detailed analysis should always be performed to determine whether the payer's rates are GPCI adjusted and whether the payer uses the total non-facility RVU, the total facility RVU, or bases payment on the actual site of service.

See Table 4 for an example of a gross conversion factor worksheet.

Table 4: Determining a Gross Conversion Factor

CPT Code	Current Fee	Total Non-Fac RVU	Total Fac RVU	Non-Fac Conversion Factor	Fac Conversion Factor
11640	$ 300	4.14	2.92	72.4638	102.7397
12002	$ 160	4.22	2.96	37.9147	54.0541
17000	$ 70	1.73	0.919	40.4624	76.9231
25600	$ 445	7.50	6.07	59.3333	73.3114
27236	$ 2,990	30.77	30.77	97.1726	97.1726
27788	$ 590	11.71	9.68	50.3843	60.9504
29345	$ 185	3.10	2.61	59.6774	70.8812
31622	$ 625	6.61	4.12	94.5537	151.6990
33513	$ 6,525	52.76	52.76	123.6732	123.6732
45385	$ 1,080	15.78	7.95	68.4411	135.8491
49505	$ 1,215	12.83	12.38	94.6999	98.1422
52601	$ 2,145	21.27	21.27	100.8463	100.8463
58150	$ 2,445	24.67	24.67	99.1082	99.1082
58670	$ 1,210	9.88	9.88	122.4696	122.4696
59400	$ 2,369	42.61	42.61	55.5973	55.5973
62270	$ 170	5.27	1.67	32.2581	101.7964
63030	$ 3,950	24.13	24.13	163.6966	163.6966
66984	$ 2,445	18.49	18.49	132.2336	132.2336
69436	$ 500	4.15	4.15	120.4819	120.4819
73070	$ 78	0.73	0.73	106.8493	106.8493
93526	$ 1,195	8.80	8.80	135.7955	135.7955
97010	$ 8	0.11	0.11	72.7273	72.7273
99213	$ 53	1.39	0.94	38.1295	56.3830
99223	$ 196	4.17	4.17	47.0024	47.0024
99244	$ 192	4.54	3.69	42.2907	52.0325
Total	$ 31,154	327.36	310.48		
Gross Conversion Factors				96.9038	104.3459

Determining A Frequency-Adjusted Conversion Factor

A gross conversion factor will only give a rough approximation of the conversion factor required to maintain income at the level currently generated using a non-RBRVS-based fee schedule. A more accurate conversion factor is one that is frequency-adjusted. Look at the "Non-facility Conversion Factors" in the preceding worksheet. As you can see, the procedure specific conversion factor required to establish a reimbursement rate at current non-RBRVS levels varies significantly from a low of 32.2581 for procedure 62270 to a high of 163.6966 for procedure 63030. The gross conversion factor of 96.9038 when applied to each of these procedures will significantly alter the fee schedule rates for both of these procedures. Using the gross conversion factor from the table above results in a much lower fee for 63030, $2338.29 as compared to the previous fee of $3950.00, and a much higher fee for 62270, $510.68 as compared to the previous fee of $170. However, the total income generated by these two services is tied not only to the fee for each, but also to the number of times each service is performed.

This can be illustrated using a simple example with codes 99213 and 27788. Assume that the provider performs only these two procedures at the frequency listed in the examples. The following is what will occur to total income using a gross conversion factor and using a frequency-adjusted conversion factor:

1. Determine the gross conversion factor:

CPT Code	Current Fee	Total Non-Fac RVU	Non-Fac Conversion Factor
27788	$ 590	11.71	50.3843
99213	$ 53	1.39	38.1295
Total	$ 643	13.10	
Gross Conversion Factor			49.0840

The gross conversion factor (53.2285) is derived by dividing the total of current fees ($643) by the total non-facility RVUs (12.08).

Total Current Fees/Total Non-facility RVUs = Gross Conversion Factor

2. Calculate the total income generated by all services by including frequencies for each service performed.

CPT Code	Frequency	Current Fee	Total Non-Fac RVU	Total Income
27788	8	$ 590	11.71	$ 4,720
99213	100	$ 53	1.39	$ 5,300
Total Income All Services				$ 10,020

Frequency x Current Fee = Total Income

3. Calculate the total income generated by all services using RBRVS and the gross conversion factor:

CPT Code	Frequency	Total Non-Fac RVU	NF Gross CF	RBRVS-Based Fee Using Gross CF	Total RBRVS Income Using Gross CF
27788	8	11.71	49.0840	574.77	4,598.19
99213	100	1.39	49.0840	68.23	6,822.67
Total Income Using RBRVS-Based Fee And Gross CF					$11,420.86

Frequency x RBRVS-Based Fee Using Gross Conversion Factor (CF) = Total RBRVS Income

As can be seen in this simple example, using a gross CF will not produce the same amount of income as the current non-RBRVS-based fee schedule. In this example the income using a gross CF factor is higher, but, depending on the actual frequencies of the services in your practice, using a gross CF to develop a new fee schedule could also result in lower income.

4. Determine the frequency-adjusted conversion factor:

CPT Code	Frequency	Current Fee	Total Non-Fac RVU	Total Non-RBRVS-Based Fees	Total Non-Fac RVU
27788	8	$ 590	11.71	$ 4,720.00	93.68
99213	100	$ 53	1.39	$ 5,300.00	139.00
Totals				$ 10,020.00	232.68
Frequency-Adjusted CF = $10,020/232.68				43.0634	

Total Non-RBRVS-Based Fees / Total Non-facility RVUs = Frequency-Adjusted CF

5. Calculate total income using frequency-adjusted conversion factor:

CPT Code	Frequency	Current Fee	Total Non-Fac RVU	Total Non-RBRVS-Based Fees	Total Non-Fac RVU	NF Adj RVU	RBRVS-Based Fee Using Adj CF	Total RBRVS-Based Fee Using Adj CF
27788	8	$ 590	11.71	$ 4,720.00	93.68	43.0634	$504.27	$ 4,034.18
99213	100	$ 53	1.39	$ 5,300.00	139.00	43.0634	$ 59.86	$ 5,985.81
Total Income				10,020.00				10,019.99

As is evident from this simple example, using a frequency-adjusted conversion factor generates the same total income for the provider as was previously generated using a non-RBRVS-based fee schedule. It does so by redistributing the income between the two procedures. Previously code 27788 had generated $4,720.00 in income, but using an RBRVS-based fee it now generates on $4,034.18. However, code 99213, which had previously generated only $5,300 in income, now generates $5,985.81.

Because one goal of developing an RBRVS-based fee schedule is to develop fees that will generate the same total income as was previously generated by the non-RBRVS-based fee schedule, a frequency-adjusted conversion factor should be used whenever possible. Below is a table listing a more extensive example of how to determine your frequency-adjusted conversion factor.

CPT Code	Frequency	Current Fee	Total Non-Fac RVU	Total Fac RVU	Current Fee x Frequency	Total Non-Fac RVU x Frequency	Total Fac RVU x Frequency
11640	10	$ 300	4.14	2.92	$ 3,000	41.40	29.20
12002	15	$ 160	4.22	2.96	$ 2,400	63.30	44.40
17000	25	$ 70	1.73	0.91	$ 1,750	43.25	22.75
25600	10	$ 445	7.5	6.07	$ 4,450	75.00	60.70
27236	5	$ 2,990	30.77	30.77	$ 14,950	153.85	153.85
27788	8	$ 590	11.71	9.68	$ 4,720	93.68	77.44
29345	10	$ 185	3.1	2.61	$ 1,850	31.00	26.10
31622	5	$ 625	6.61	4.12	$ 3,125	33.05	20.6
33513	3	$ 6,525	52.76	52.76	$ 19,575	158.28	158.28
45385	10	$ 1,080	15.78	7.95	$ 10,800	157.80	79.50
49505	7	$ 1,215	12.83	12.38	$ 8,505	89.81	86.66
52601	7	$ 2,145	21.27	21.27	$ 15,015	148.89	148.89
58150	10	$ 2,445	24.67	24.67	$ 24,450	246.70	246.70
58670	10	$ 1,210	9.88	9.88	$ 12,100	98.80	98.80
59400	20	$ 2,369	42.61	42.61	$ 47,380	852.20	852.20
62270	5	$ 170	5.27	1.67	$ 850	26.35	8.35
63030	3	$ 3,950	24.13	24.13	$ 11,850	72.39	72.39
66984	10	$ 2,445	18.49	18.49	$ 24,450	184.9	184.90
69436	20	$ 500	4.15	4.15	$ 10,000	83.00	83.00
73070	10	$ 78	0.73	0.73	$ 780	7.30	7.30
93526-26	10	$ 1,195	8.8	8.8	$ 11,950	88.00	88.00
97010	5	$ 8	0.11	0.11	$ 40	0.55	0.55
99213	100	$ 53	1.39	0.94	$ 5,300	139.00	94.00
99223	15	$ 196	4.17	4.17	$ 2,940	62.55	62.55
99244	25	$ 192	4.54	3.69	$ 4,800	113.50	92.25
Total					$ 247,030	3,064.55	2,799.36
Frequency-Adjusted Conversion Factors						$80.6089	$88.2452

Developing an RBRVS-Based Fee Schedule

The following steps are necessary to develop an RBRVS-Based Fee Schedule, to determine a gross conversion factor, or to determine a frequency-adjusted conversion factor.

1. Identify by CPT procedure code all services performed by the provider during the past year
2. List the frequency of each service
3. List your current fee for each service
4. List the total non-facility RVU and/or total facility RVU for each service. (Note: the example provided lists both; however, use the total RVU amount, which reflects the usual practices of your providers, since only one conversion factor should be developed. Both are listed in our examples to show differences in the two RVU amounts and how they affect the resulting conversion factor.)

To determine a gross conversion factor (use only if frequencies are not available):

1. Determine the sum of all fees
2. Add the total non-facility RVUs
3. Add the total facility RVUs
4. Divide the sum of all fees by the sum of total non-facility RVUs, this is the conversion factor for non-facility services
5. Divide the sum of all fees by the sum of total facility RVUs, this is the conversion factor for facility services

To determine a frequency-adjusted conversion factor:

1. Multiply the fee for each service by the frequency
2. Multiply the total non-facility RVU by the frequency
3. Multiply the total facility RVU by the frequency
4. Add the results in each of these columns to obtain frequency-adjusted totals
5. Divide the sum of the frequency-adjusted fees by the sum of the frequency-adjusted non-facility RVUs and by the sum of the frequency-adjusted facility RVUs. These two results are the frequency-adjusted conversion factors

To convert to an RBRVS fee schedule:

1. Determine either the gross conversion factor or frequency-adjusted conversion factor as described in the preceding information
2. Multiply each service by the conversion factor. In this example, the non-facility frequency-adjusted conversion factor has been used after rounding to the nearest hundredth
3. The result is the RBRVS fee for each service
4. It is recommended that the current fee and the income generated by those fees (total income using current fee schedule) be included when developing an RBRVS-based fee schedule. These can be used as a validity check

CPT Code	Frequency	Total Non-Fac RVU	Non-Fac Freq Adj Conversion Factor	Current Fee	RBRVS Fee	Total Income Using Current Fee Schedule	Total Income Using RBRVS-Based Fee Schedule
11640	10	4.14	$80.6089	$300	$333.72	$3,000	$3,337
12002	15	4.22	$80.6089	$160	$340.17	$2,400	$5,103
17000	25	1.73	$80.6089	$70	$139.45	$1,750	$3,486
25600	10	7.5	$80.6089	$445	$604.57	$4,450	$6,046
27236	5	30.77	$80.6089	$2,990	$2,480.34	$14,950	$12,402
27788	8	11.71	$80.6089	$590	$943.93	$4,720	$7,551
29345	10	3.1	$80.6089	$185	$249.89	$1,850	$2,499
31622	5	6.61	$80.6089	$625	$532.82	$3,125	$2,664
33513	3	52.76	$80.6089	$6,525	$4,252.93	$19,575	$12,759
45385	10	15.78	$80.6089	$1,080	$1,272.01	$10,800	$12,720
49505	7	12.83	$80.6089	$1,215	$1,034.21	$8,505	$7,239
52601	7	21.27	$80.6089	$2,145	$1,714.55	$15,015	$12,002
58150	10	24.67	$80.6089	$2,445	$1,988.62	$24,450	$19,886
58670	10	9.88	$80.6089	$1,210	$796.42	$12,100	$7,964
59400	20	42.61	$80.6089	$2,369	$3,434.75	$47,380	$68,695
62270	5	5.27	$80.6089	$170	$424.81	$850	$2,124
63030	3	24.13	$80.6089	$3,950	$1,945.09	$11,850	$5,835
66984	10	18.49	$80.6089	$2,445	$1,490.46	$24,450	$14,905
69436	20	4.15	$80.6089	$500	$334.53	$10,000	$6,691
73070	10	0.73	$80.6089	$78	$58.84	$780	$588
93526	10	8.8	$80.6089	$1,195	$709.36	$11,950	$7,094
97010	5	0.11	$80.6089	$8	$8.87	$40	$44
99213	100	1.39	$80.6089	$53	$112.05	$5,300	$11,205
99223	15	4.17	$80.6089	$196	$336.14	$2,940	$5,042
99244	25	4.54	$80.6089	$192	$365.96	$4,800	$9,149
Total						$247,030	$247,030

Introduction

Productivity Analysis Using RBRVS

RBRVS is also a useful tool for analyzing productivity. For this analysis, physician work RVUs are the best indicator of physician productivity. Productivity should be measured for each physician on a monthly basis. This data can be used to analyze monthly trends for each physician and compare physician workloads in a multi-physician practice. The workload comparison is especially helpful for capitated services where physicians are not paid on a fee-for-service basis. The productivity information can be used to distribute capitation payments.

Steps required to analyze monthly productivity:

1. Identify each service provided by each physician by CPT code
2. Determine the work RVU for each service
3. Determine the frequency of each service for each physician
4. Multiply the frequency of each service times the work RVU
5. Total the monthly work RVU for each physician

CPT Code	Work RVU	Frequency Physician 1	Frequency Physician 2	Total RVU Physician 1	Total RVU Physician 2
12002	1.86	10	2	18.60	3.72
12041	2.37	5	0	11.85	0.00
17000	0.60	25	10	15.00	6.00
17003	0.15	15	8	2.25	1.20
17110	0.65	8	10	5.20	6.50
36533	5.32	0	2	0.00	10.64
38500	3.75	0	2	0.00	7.50
46935	2.43	3	0	7.29	0.00
47605	14.69	3	4	37.08	58.76
49505	7.60	5	8	32.45	60.80
47563	11.94	10	8	119.40	95.52
64721	4.29	2	5	8.58	21.45
99203	1.34	25	30	33.50	40.20
99204	2.00	10	6	20.00	12.00
99212	0.45	25	30	11.25	13.50
99213	0.67	60	65	40.20	43.55
99214	1.10	25	20	27.50	22.00
99243	1.72	5	6	8.60	10.32
99244	2.58	7	10	18.06	25.80
99253	1.82	3	5	5.46	9.10
99254	2.64	2	7	5.28	18.48
Total Work RVU				440.04	467.04

To distribute a capitation payment based on the preceding productivity analysis:

1. Add the total work RVUs for each physician to determine the total work RVUs for the practice. For example:
   Physician 1 + Physician 2 = Total Work RVUs (440.04 + 467.04 = 907.08)

2. Divide the total work RVUs for each physician by the total work RVUs for the practice to determine the percentage of the capitation payment each physician should receive:
   Physician 1 440.04 / 907.08 = 48.5 percent
   Physician 2 467.04 / 907.08 = 51.5 percent

3. Multiply the percentage determined in Step 2 by the capitation payment. If the capitation payment is $15,000 for the month, the distribution would be as follows:
   Physician 1 $15,000 x 48.5 percent = $7,277
   Physician 2 $15,000 x 51.5 percent = $7,723

Productivity analysis has other uses as well. It can be used to identify trends. For example, most practices experience periods of higher utilization and periods of lower utilization. Monthly productivity analysis identifies these trends and allows the practice to plan for these variations. The practice can use the monthly productivity information to allocate funds to cover fixed costs during the periods of lower utilization. This information might also be helpful in addressing non-financial aspects of the practice, such as staffing requirements.

Cost/Benefit Analysis

The transition to resource-based relative value units for practice expense is now complete. It began in 1999 and was fully phased in as of January 1, 2002. This change may effect reimbursement rates for individual providers. Generally, the effect will be dependent on the mix of services provided and the sites where those services are performed. Providers who furnish more office-based services are expected to experience increases in Medicare payments, while those who provide primarily facility-based services are expected to see decreases. Because many private sector payers also use RBRVS-based fee schedules, these changes are expected to carry over into the private sector as well.

If your practice has not yet evaluated the effects of this change, it should do so now to determine if it would be beneficial to shift some services from the facility setting to the office setting. However, this should not be done without evaluating all costs and benefits associated with moving selected services. The process for analyzing costs and benefits is outlined below.

Steps required to analyze potential additional revenue include:

1. List all services currently performed by the provider by CPT code. Include a short written description of the service

2. Have the provider identify any services currently being performed in a facility setting that could be performed in an office setting

3. List the frequency of each service provided in a facility setting. For those services that are currently provided in both settings, be careful to list only the facility frequencies

4. For services that can be provided in the office only part of the time, list the percent of the time the service could be provided in the office

5. List the non-facility and facility practice expense RVUs for each service in separate columns

6. Subtract the non-facility PE RVU from the facility PE RVU. This difference is the additional value of performing the service in an office setting. (Note: Some services may need to be analyzed differently. For example, radiology services provided in the office would be calculated using the total non-facility RVU amount because the service provided outside the physician office would not generate any revenue for the provider. The facility component would be paid to the hospital and the professional component would be paid to the radiologist. However, if the complete radiology service was provided in the physician's office, the complete procedure reimbursement amount would be paid to the provider.)

7. Identify those payers (Medicare, Medicaid, private sector payers) that recognize the different PE RVUs and pay based on site-of-service and their respective conversion factors. Determine the average conversion factor. (Note: If the payer has

tracked the frequency of services you may wish to use actual experience rather than an average conversion factor to determine additional revenue.)

Medicare CF	Medicaid CF	Private Payer 1 CF	Private Payer 2 CF	AVG CF
36.1992	20.8389	43.5000	45.75	36.5720

(Medicare CF + Medicaid CF + Private Payer 1 CF + Private Payer 2 CF) / 4 = Average CF

8. Determine the total additional reimbursements expected from these payers for each service by multiplying the difference (Non-Fac PE RVU - Fac PE RVU) by the average conversion factor

CPT Code	Code Description	Frequency	Percent of services which can be moved to office setting	Non-Fac PE RVU	Facility PE RVU	Difference (Non-Fac PE RVU - Fac PE RVU)	AVG CF	Additional Revenue
25500	Closed treatment radial shaft fx w/o manip	40	75%	4.27	2.94	1.33	36.5720	$1,459.00
25505	Closed treatment radial shaft fx w/manip	20	50%	7.87	5.65	2.22	36.5720	$ 812.00
25530	Closed treatment ulnar shaft fx w/o manip	20	75%	4.21	2.87	1.34	36.5720	$ 735.00
25535	Closed treatment ulnar shaft fx w/manip	10	50%	7.74	5.72	2.02	36.5720	$ 369.00
73090[1]	Xray exam; forearm, 2 view	100	75%	0.50	0	0.50	36.5720	$1,371.00

[1]As noted on page 15, radiology services provided in the office are calculated using the total non-facility RVU amount because the service provided outside the physician office would not generate any revenue for the provider. When the complete radiology service is provided in the physician's office, the complete procedure reimbursement is paid to the provider.

Steps to analyze additional costs include:

1. Identify and calculate all direct costs. Direct costs include non-physician labor, medical equipment, and medical supplies. (Do not include the cost of equipment or supplies that can be billed separately. For example, treatment of radial shaft fracture with manipulation (25505) would require casting supplies, but those supplies are reported separately with HCPCS Level II codes

Direct Costs

CPT Code	Code Description	Additional Non-physician Cost/Proc	Additional Supply Costs/Proc	Additional Equipment Costs/Proc	Frequency	Percent of services which can be moved to office setting	Total Additional Costs
25500	Closed treatment radial shaft fx w/o manip	$ 3.00	$ -	$ -	40	75%	$ 90.00
25505	Closed treatment radial shaft fx w/manip	$ 4.00	$ -	$ -	20	50%	$ 40.00
25530	Closed treatment ulnar shaft fx w/o manip	$ 3.00	$ -	$ -	20	75%	$ 45.00
25535	Closed treatment ulnar shaft fx w/manip	$ 4.00	$ -	$ -	10	50%	$ 20.00
73090	Xray exam; forearm, 2 view	$ 5.00	$ 3.00	$ 22.00	100	75%	$2,250.00

2. Estimate indirect costs, which include rent, utilities, and general office supplies. Indirect costs should be allocated using standard accounting techniques. One approach might be to use the additional office time required per procedure. If each of these procedures requires an additional 15 minutes to perform, and indirect costs are $25/hour, then the indirect cost of each procedure would be $6.25

Indirect Costs

CPT Code	Code Description	Indirect Costs	Frequency	Percent of services which can be moved to office setting	Total Indirect Costs
25500	Closed treatment radial shaft fx w/o manip	$ 6.25	40	75%	$ 187.50
25505	Closed treatment radial shaft fx w/manip	$ 6.25	20	50%	$ 62.50
25530	Closed treatment ulnar shaft fx w/o manip	$ 6.25	20	75%	$ 93.75
25535	Closed treatment ulnar shaft fx w/manip	$ 6.25	10	50%	$ 31.25
73090	Xray exam; forearm, 2 view	$ 6.25	100	75%	$ 468.75

3. Total direct and indirect costs to determine total additional costs for each procedure

4. Identify additional factors. These factors may positively or negatively impact the decision to provide additional services and may include such things as:

   a. Increased patient satisfaction. For example, when considering the possible purchase of laboratory equipment, one additional benefit may be that patients no longer need to go to the hospital for more frequently performed laboratory services. This will save them time and generally increase satisfaction

   b. Increased physician liability. For example, when evaluating the costs of performing office radiology services, any increased physician liability for this additional service should be considered

   c. Space requirements. For example, the physician may decide that adding an x-ray room is not feasible due to space limitations

The table above identifies additional revenue that could be generated by moving specific services from a facility to a non-facility site. This must be weighed against the additional cost of providing the service in the physician's office. Using the above example, the physician may decide to move much of the fracture care to the office because moving these services provides significant additional revenue with little added cost. However, the forearm x-ray would not provide sufficient added revenue to offset the added equipment, supply costs, and staffing requirements.

This type of cost/benefit analysis should be performed on an annual basis for several reasons. First, since RVUs are evaluated on an ongoing basis and are subject to change, services that were previously not valued at a level high enough to be profitable in an office setting may be revalued, making them profitable enough to justify moving them to the office. Likewise, the opposite could occur. Services that were profitable may no longer generate the same profits if the RVUs are significantly decreased. In addition, costs of supplies and equipment are subject to change which also affects the profitability of performing services in the office.

Five-Year Review Process

Since January 1992, Medicare services have been valued using a resource-based relative value scale (RBRVS). Legislation contained in the Social Security Act requires that RVUs be reviewed at least every five years. The Physician Fee Schedule was initiated January 1, 1992, and the first review of RVUs was initiated in December 1994 with changes implemented in the January 1, 1997 Physician Fee Schedule.

The second five-year review of the Physician Fee Schedule is now complete. It was initiated in November 1999 by soliciting comments regarding potentially misvalued services. Comments were received from approximately 30 specialty groups, organizations, and individuals on over 900 CPT and HCPCS codes. In addition, comments were received related to the proposed process for the five-year review.

These comments were shared with the AMA Specialty Society Relative Value Update Committee (RUC). The RUC was formed in 1991 and is supported by the RUC Advisory Committee which is made up of over 100 specialty societies in the AMA's House of Delegates. The RUC currently makes recommendations to the CMS related to proposed RVUs for new and revised codes. Because the RUC is involved in the initial valuation of CPT codes and because they consult with specialty groups related to valuation of CPT codes, the CMS feels their recommendations related to revaluation of existing codes is also warranted. For codes used only by non-physician practitioners, the CMS consults the Health Care Professionals Advisory Committee (HCPAC), a companion to the RUC.

For the five-year review the RUC used the following process:

1. The RUC identified specialty societies interested in reviewing RVUs and making presentations related to potentially misvalued codes

2. The specialty societies used either a standard survey instrument or a mini-survey to value each CPT code being reviewed. The mini-surveys were used by those specialties where the number of codes being reviewed was exceptionally high

3. The specialty society selected a physician sample to be surveyed. A minimum of 30 responses was required for each code for the survey or mini-survey to be valid

4. Each specialty society reviewed and organized the surveys completed by the physicians participating in the review and then presented the results to the RUC

5. The RUC then divided into six workgroups to review and evaluate the recommendations of the specialty societies

6. Each workgroup submitted their reports to the full RUC who reviewed and evaluated the recommendations of the six work groups

7. RUC recommendations were then developed and sent to the CMS

The CMS analyzed the RUC recommendations. For each potentially misvalued code, the CMS evaluated both the RVU recommendation and the rationale for the recommendation. In addition, the CMS verified results using alternative methodologies as needed. The CMS then either accepted or rejected the RUC recommendation for each code. When the RUC recommendation was not accepted for a code, the CMS provided an explanation.

The RUC supplied recommendations on 857 services. CMS accepted the RUC recommendation on 792 services. This represents a 92 percent acceptance rate. Of the 65 codes where the CMS rejected the RUC recommendation, the value was increased for 37, decreased for 22, and six were left unchanged. The six that were not changed had been previously reviewed at the Multi-specialty Refinement Panel for Calendar Year 2000.

In addition, HCPAC reviewed 12 services. HCPAC did not offer an opinion on five services and these values were left unchanged by CMS. Recommended changes for the remaining seven services were accepted by CMS.

Many specialties will see significant changes to reimbursement rates for some services because of extensive changes to work RVUs. However, because of budget neutrality requirements these RVU changes have had to be offset by a reduction in the conversion factor for 2002. The RVU changes in conjunction with other factors affecting Medicare costs have resulted in a reduction in the conversion factor of 5.4 percent.

Medicare Sustainable Growth Rate (SGR)

The use of Sustainable Growth Rate (SGR) targets is intended to control the actual growth in aggregate Medicare expenditures for physicians' services. The SGR targets are not limits on expenditures. Payments for services are not withheld if the SGR target is exceeded by actual expenditures. Rather, the appropriate fee schedule update is adjusted to reflect the success or failure in meeting the SGR target. If expenditures exceed the target, the update is reduced. If expenditures are less than the target, the update is increased.

Several factors affect SGR. One significant factor for Calendar Year 2002 is the RVU changes that resulted from the completion of the transition to resource-based practice expense values and the five-year review of physician work values. Specifically, the legislation requires that increases or decreases in RVUs may not cause the amount of expenditures for the year to differ by more than $20 million from what expenditures would have been in the absence of these changes. If this threshold is exceeded, CMS makes across-the-board adjustments to preserve budget neutrality. Based on the proposed changes in RVUs, CMS indicated that budget-neutrality adjustments would be required. CMS proposed to reduce the conversion factor to meet the budget neutrality requirement, rather than applying an across-the-board reduction to all work RVUs.

Other factors affecting SGR include the estimated change in the average number of Medicare fee-for-service beneficiaries, the estimated projected growth in real gross domestic product (GDP) per capita, and the estimated change in expenditures due to changes in laws or regulations. As a result of the RVU changes as well as the additional budget-neutrality adjustments required by law, the conversion factor was reduced by 5.4 percent for Calendar Year 2002.

RBRVS Terminology

Base fee — The physician's current non-RBRVS fee for a specific service.

Cambridge Health Economics Group (CHEG) — Company founded in 1988 by members of the original Harvard University RBRVS studies team. CHEG is considered to be the expert in resource-based relative value scale methodology.

Capitation — Capitation is a system in which a fixed rate is paid, usually on a monthly basis, for each plan enrollee covered under the capitation agreement. All of the payer's membership may be capitated or only a portion of the membership (e.g., all those who live in a specific geographic area, all those who participate in a specific plan, or all Medicare enrollees). There are two basic methods used by payers to calculate the capitation payment. The more common method is to establish a fixed rate per member per month (PMPM). A newer method involves paying a fixed rate based on a percent of premium for each plan enrollee.

Centers for Medicare and Medicaid Services (CMS) — Government agency responsible for overseeing and administering the Medicare and Medicaid programs. (Formerly the Health Care Financing Administration or HCFA)

CF — *See Conversion Factor*

CHEG — *See Cambridge Health Economics Group*

CMS — *See Centers for Medicare and Medicaid Services*

Conversion Factor (CF) — The conversion factor represents the dollar value of each relative value unit. When this dollar amount is multiplied by the total relative value units (facility or non-facility) it will yield the reimbursement rate for the specific service.

CPR — *See Customary, Prevailing, and Reasonable Charge*

Customary, Prevailing, and Reasonable Charge (CPR) — The basis for Medicare's reimbursement rates prior to RBRVS. CPR reimbursement rates were based on historical physician charges rather than relative values, which allowed for wide variation in Medicare payments among physicians and specialties.

Diagnosis Related Group (DRG) — DRGs currently provide the basis for payment to hospitals for inpatient services for Medicare, Medicaid, and an increasing number of private sector payers. This system classifies patients based on their illness (diagnosis) and the treatment provided. It is assumed that patients with similar illnesses undergoing similar procedures will require similar resources. Therefore, this payment methodology reimburses a flat-rate based on the patient's diagnosis and treatment. DRGs for physician services were one of several proposed reimbursement methodologies considered along with RBRVS when it became apparent that the old CPR system was no longer an effective method for reimbursing physicians.

Direct Costs — Practice expense is composed of two types of costs: direct and indirect. Direct costs are directly associated with a specific service and include items such as non-physician labor, medical equipment, and medical supplies. *See Indirect Costs.*

DRG — *See Diagnosis Related Group*

Facility Practice Expense — One of the three components used to determine the relative value of physician services. Facility practice expense represents the physicians direct and indirect costs related to each service when that service is provided in a hospital, ambulatory surgery center (ASC), or skilled nursing facility (SNF). Direct expenses required for each procedure include non-physician labor, medical equipment, and medical supplies. Indirect expenses include the cost of general office supplies, rent, utilities, and other office overhead that cannot be directly tied to a specific procedure.

Facility Practice Expense Value — The relative value units assigned to the facility practice expense component for a specific service.

Facility Total Value — The sum of the three components (work value, facility practice expense, malpractice insurance) used to calculate Medicare fees for services provided in a facility setting. This would include services provided in a hospital, ambulatory surgery center (ASC), or skilled nursing facility (SNF).

Fee For Service (FFS) — Reimbursement methodology in which the physician is paid a fixed amount on a service-by-service basis.

FFS — *See Fee For Service*

Frequency — Frequency reflects the number of times a given service is provided during a specified time period. Frequency is an important factor to consider in determining a conversion factor.

Frequency-Adjusted Conversion Factor — The conversion factor obtained when converting a provider's non-RBRVS-based fee schedule to an RBRVS fee schedule using both current fees and frequencies. A frequency-adjusted conversion factor is more accurate than the more commonly used gross conversion factor because the income generated by each service provided is tied not only to the fee but also to the number of times the service is performed. A frequency-adjusted conversion factor allows for the development of an RBRVS fee schedule, which will generate the same amount of income as was generated under a non-RBRVS fee schedule.

Gap — Services not covered by Medicare and not represented on the MFS.

Gap Code — Any Level I (CPT) or Level II (HCPCS) code that is not found on the MFS.

Geographical Practice Cost Indices (GPCI) — GPCIs are indices used to adjust for cost differences among geographic areas. There are separate GPCIs for each of the three components (work value, practice expense, malpractice insurance), which comprise the total value of each service for each geographic area identified by Medicare. Therefore, prior to calculating the Medicare reimbursement rate, each of the three components must be adjusted by locality using the GPCI. GPCIs were developed according to statute and are revised every three years according to statute. The revisions are implemented in a step fashion over a three-year period in order to reduce the overall impact of any changes.

GPCI — *See Geographical Practice Cost Indices*

Gross Conversion Factor — The conversion factor obtained when converting a provider's non-RBRVS-based fees to a RBRVS fee schedule using only the current fee schedule. A gross conversion factor will give only a rough approximation of the conversion factor required to maintain income at the level currently generated using a non-RBRVS-based fee schedule. This is because a gross conversion factor does not take into account the frequencies of the services provided. Since income is tied not only to the fee for each service but also to the frequencies of each service, a more accurate conversion factor is one that is frequency-adjusted.

HCFA — *See Health Care Financing Administration*

HCPCS — HCPCS is an acronym for Health Care Procedure Coding System. It is a three-tier medical coding system composed of Level I CPT codes, Level II national codes, and Level III local codes.

Health Care Financing Administration (HCFA) — Former name of the government agency responsible for overseeing and administering the Medicare and Medicaid programs. Now called the Centers for Medicare and Medicaid Services (CMS).

Indirect Costs — Practice expense is composed of two types of costs: direct and indirect. Indirect expenses include the cost of services that cannot be directly tied to a specific service. These types of cost include general office supplies, rent, utilities, and other office overhead. *See Direct Costs.*

Level I Codes — The first level of the three-tier HCPCS system is the American Medical Association's CPT codes. This code set, known universally as CPT, reports a broad spectrum of medical procedures and services.

Level II Codes — This is the second level of the three-tier HCPCS system developed by CMS to report services and supplies not found in CPT. These Level II national codes are sometimes referred to collectively as HCPCS.

Level III Codes — The third tier of HCPCS codes are assigned by individual state and regional Medicare carriers and are sometimes referred to as local codes or carrier codes. These codes are generally used to report new and emerging services and procedures not yet available nationwide.

Malpractice Value — The relative value units assigned to the malpractice insurance component for a specific service.

Medicare Fee Schedule (MFS) — The allowed fees paid for Medicare services. These fees are based on a resource-based relative value scale (RBRVS), with the value of each service determined by three components: physician work, practice expense, and malpractice insurance. These three components are geographically adjusted using Geographic Practice Cost Indices (GPCIs) and then multiplied by the Medicare conversion factor to determine the locality specific Medicare fee.

MFS — *See Medicare Fee Schedule*

Non-facility Practice Expense — One of the three components used to determine the relative value of physician services. Non-facility practice expense represents the physicians direct and indirect costs related to each service when that service is provided in the physician's office, patient's home, or other non-hospital setting, such as a residential care facility. Direct expenses required for each procedure include non-physician labor, medical equipment, and medical supplies. Indirect expenses include the cost of general office supplies, rent, utilities, and other office overhead that cannot be directly tied to a specific procedure.

Non-facility Practice Expense Value — The relative value units assigned to the non-facility practice expense component for a specific service.

Non-facility Total Value — The sum of the three components (work value, non-facility practice expense, malpractice insurance) used to calculate Medicare fees for services provided in a non-facility setting. These would include services provided in the physician's office, patient's home, or other non-hospital setting such as a residential care facility.

PE — *See Practice Expense*

Per Member Per Month (PMPM) — One of two basic methods used by payers to calculate a capitation payment. PMPM is the fixed rate paid for each covered member each month. For example, the payer may contract with a group of orthopedic surgeons at a rate of $1.25/PMPM for all necessary orthopedic services. This PMPM is paid regardless of the actual services provided to the covered membership.

Percent of Premium — One of two basic methods used by payers to calculate a capitation payment. When a percent of premium is paid, a fixed rate is calculated as a percentage of the average monthly premium paid by each plan enrollee. For example, the payer may contract with a group of orthopedic surgeons at a rate of 1.25 percent (0.0125) of the average monthly premiums for a defined membership. If the average monthly premium per member is $100, then the group is paid $1.25 for each member. Any increases or decreases in the average monthly premium will affect the rate paid.

PMPM — *See Per Member Per Month*

Practice Expense (PE) — One of the three components used to determine the relative value of physician services. Practice expense represents the physician's direct and indirect costs related to each service. Direct expenses required for each procedure include non-physician labor, medical equipment, and medical supplies. Indirect expenses include the cost of general office supplies, rent, utilities, and other office overhead that cannot be directly tied to a specific procedure.

Practice Expense Value — The relative value units assigned to the practice expense component for a specific service.

Physician Work — One of the three components used to determine the relative value of physician services. The physician work component reflects the cost of the physician's time and skill for each service provided.

RBRVS — *See Resource-Based Relative Value Scale*

Relative Value (RV) — RBRVS ranks services based on the relative costs required to provide them. A relative value reflects the cost or value of a specific physician service as compared to all other physician services.

Relative Value Unit (RVU) — Relative values are expressed in numeric units that represent the unit of measure for physician services. Those services that have greater costs or value have higher relative value units than those services with lower costs or value.

Resource-Based Relative Value Scale (RBRVS) — Payment schedule based on the relative values of services provided. The current RBRVS system ranks services according to the relative costs required to provide them. These costs are defined in terms of units, with more complex, more time-consuming services having higher unit values than less complex, less time-consuming services. Furthermore, each service is compared to all other physician services so that each service is given a value that reflects its cost or value when compared to all other physician services.

Site-of-Service Reduction — Prior to 1999, a 50 percent site-of-service reduction was applied to those services that were determined by Medicare as being performed in the physician office at least 50 percent of the time. This site-of-service reduction affected approximately 675 codes. However, in 1999, the site-of-service reduction was eliminated when Medicare began the phase-in of resource-based practice expense units, which adjust for site-of-service using the new facility and non-facility practice expense values.

Total Value — The sum of the values of the three components of each Medicare fee, which includes physician work, practice expense, and malpractice insurance. Prior to 1999, each Medicare fee had a single total value. However, with the introduction of resource-based measurements to the practice expense component, each service now has two total values, a non-facility total value for services provided in the physician's office, patient's home, or other non-hospital setting and a facility total value for services provided in a hospital, ambulatory surgery center, or skilled nursing facility.

UCR — *See Usual, Customary, and Reasonable Charge*

Usual, Customary, and Reasonable Charge (UCR) — Reimbursement methodology used by some private sector payers, which bases payment on historical charges rather than on the relative value of services provided. More than 75 percent of all payers have replaced UCR with some type of relative value methodology with RBRVS being the most commonly used relative value scale.

Work Value — The relative value units assigned to the physician work component for a specific service.

Description of Columns in RBRVS Table

Code Column

The Code column lists the current numeric or alpha-numeric code designated in the Medicare Fee Schedule corresponding to the description in Physicians' Current Procedural Terminology (CPT) developed by the American Medical Association (AMA) or the HCPCS Level II short description for the alpha-numeric codes developed by the Centers for Medicare and Medicaid Services (CMS).

Note on starred procedures: Certain relatively small surgical procedures are characterized by variable pre- and postoperative services. Because of these indefinite parameters, the usual package concept for surgical services cannot be applied. Such procedures are identified by a star (*) following the procedure code.

When a star follows a surgical procedure code, the service listed includes only the surgical procedure, not any associated pre- and postoperative services. See your CPT book for further information regarding starred procedures.

Modifier Column (abbreviated as M)

The modifier column is listed to further describe the services rendered.

For CPT codes, no modifier indicates the total component value. It is the sum of the professional and technical components. This modifier indicates that both the professional services and the technical services (including the facility and personnel) are administered by the same physician group.

Modifier -26 is used to describe the professional or physician services required for the performance of that service.

Modifier -TC is used to describe the personnel, equipment, and facility costs related to providing that particular service.

For modifiers associated with HCPCS Level II codes, see the HCPCS guidelines immediately preceding that table.

Status Column (abbreviated as S)

The status column denotes the payment methodology regardless of whether or not Medicare will pay for a particular code. This indicator shows whether the CPT/HCPCS code is in the Medicare Fee Schedule and whether the service is separately payable if covered.

(A) An (A) in this column indicates that the corresponding code is an active code. These codes are separately payable under the Medicare Fee Schedule if covered. The relative value units for these codes are developed by the CMS process. An (A) status does not mean that Medicare has made a national decision regarding the coverage of the service. Carriers remain responsible for coverage decisions in the absence of a national Medicare policy.

(B) A (B) in this column indicates that the service is always bundled in a payment for another service. If RVUs are shown, they are not used for Medicare payment. If these services are covered, payment for them is subsumed by the payment for the services to which they are incident (e.g., a telephone call from a hospital nurse regarding care of a patient). Relative values assigned to a code with (B) status may be imputed using the Ingenix gap methodology. Gap values are indicated with a ■ in the Gap column.

(C) A (C) in this column indicates that Medicare allows the carrier to determine the payment level for these codes. Relative values assigned to a code with (C) status may be imputed using the Ingenix gap methodology. Gap values are indicated with a ■ in the Gap column.

(D) A (D) in this column indicates that the codes have been deleted and are no longer effective with beginning of the calendar year. Relative values assigned to a code with (D) status may be imputed using the Ingenix gap methodology. Gap values are indicated with a ■ in the Gap column.

(E) An (E) in this column indicates that these are excluded, by regulation, from the Medicare Fee Schedule. These codes may not be billed to Medicare. Relative values assigned to a code with (E) status may be imputed using the Ingenix gap methodology. Gap values are indicated with a ■ in the Gap column.

(G) A (G) or (I) in this column indicates that this code is not valued for Medicare purposes. Medicare does not recognize codes assigned this status. Medicare uses another code for reporting of, and payment for, these services. Relative values assigned to a code with (G) or (I) status may be imputed using the Ingenix gap methodology. Gap values are indicated with a ■ in the Gap column.

(N) An (N) in this column indicates that this is a non-covered service. Medicare payment may not be made for these codes. If RVUs are shown, they are not used for Medicare payment. Relative values assigned to a code with (N) status are imputed using the Ingenix gap methodology. Gap values are indicated with a ■ in the Gap column.

(P) A (P) in this column indicates codes that are considered to be bundled or excluded by Medicare. They may not be used to bill Medicare for these services.

- If the item or service is covered as incident to a physician service and is furnished on the same day as a physician service, payment for it is bundled into the payment for the physician service to which it is incident (e.g., an elastic bandage furnished by a physician is incident to a physician service).
- If the item or service is covered as other than incident to a physician service, it is excluded from the Medicare Fee Schedule (e.g., colostomy supplies) and is paid under the other payment provisions of the Act.
- Relative values assigned to a code with (P) status are imputed using the Ingenix gap methodology. Gap values are indicated with a ■ in the Gap column.

(R) An (R) in this column indicates codes that have restricted coverage. Medicare will apply special rules for payment and the codes are carrier priced. Relative values assigned to a code with (R) status may be imputed using the Ingenix gap methodology. Gap values are indicated with a ■ in the Gap column.

(T) A (T) in this column indicates an injection code. The relative value units and codes may be reported to Medicare if no other services are payable under the Medicare Fee Schedule or billed on the same date by the same provider. If any other services, payable under the Medicare Fee Schedule, are billed on the same date, these services are bundled into the services for which payment is made. The values for these codes are established by the Medicare Fee Schedule.

(X) An (X) in this column indicates that these codes are excluded by law. Codes indicated as status (X) may not be billed to Medicare. Relative values assigned to a code with (X) status are imputed using the Ingenix gap methodology. Gap values are indicated with a ■ in the Gap column.

Description Column

The description column includes the full CPT description for each code as it appears in the American Medical Association's *Physicians' Current Procedural Terminology* for 2002 (published in 2001).

Work RVU Column

Work relative value units were either: a) developed and determined by CMS for the physician work for this service, or b) imputed using the Ingenix gap methodology.

Non-facility Practice Expense RVU

There are two different levels (facility and non-facility) of practice expense RVUs for each procedure code depending on the site-of-service.

Some services are performed only in certain settings and will have only one level of practice expense RVU per code. Many of these are evaluation and management codes with code descriptions specific to the site-of-service. Other services, such as most major surgical services with 90-day global periods, are performed entirely or almost entirely in the hospital. Under the new system, CMS is providing a single practice expense RVU for these services and listing the same value in both the non-facility and facility column. When services can be provided in either a non-facility or facility setting, different values will be listed in the respective columns.

The higher non-facility practice expense RVUs are used to calculate payments for services performed in a physician's office and for services furnished to a patient in the patient's home, or facility or institution other than a hospital, skilled nursing facility

(SNF), or ambulatory surgical center (ASC). For these services, the physician typically bears the cost of resources, such as labor, medical supplies, and medical equipment associated with the physician's service.

Facility Practice Expense RVU

The lower facility practice expense RVUs are used to calculate payments for physicians' services furnished to hospital, SNF, and ASC patients. The cost for non-physician services and other items, including medical equipment and supplies, are typically borne by the hospital, by the SNF, or the ASC.

Malpractice Expense Column

This column indicates the malpractice expense relative value units for services calculated by final evaluation of CMS for the 2002 fiscal year.

Non-facility Total Value Column

The non-facility total value in this column reflects the sum of the work, non-facility practice expense, and malpractice values.

Facility Total Value Column

The facility total value in this column reflects the sum of the work, facility practice expense, and malpractice values.

Global Period Column

This column indicates the number of days in the global period for which services directly related to the procedure are included. The majority of codes have a numerical designation (i.e., 0, 10, or 90).

MMM codes describe services furnished in uncomplicated maternity care. This includes antepartum, delivery, and postpartum care. The usual global surgical concept does not apply.

XXX codes indicate that the global surgery concept does not apply.

YYY codes indicate that the global period is to be set by the local carrier.

ZZZ codes indicate that the code is an add-on service and therefore is treated in the global period of the other procedure billed in conjunction with a ZZZ code. Do not bill these codes with modifier -51. They should not be reduced.

Medicare Conversion Factors

Medicare has elected to eliminate the three conversion factor calculation. Consequently the update indicator for each code has been eliminated.

The 2002 conversion factor for all Medicare services (except Anesthesia) is $36.1992.

The 2002 national Medicare conversion factor for Anesthesia codes is $16.60.

Note: Adjustments to these conversion factors may be made for each area by the carrier.

Introduction

GPCI Tables

Carrier	Locality	Locality name	Work	Practice expense	Malpractice
00510	00	ALABAMA	0.978	0.870	0.807
00831	01	ALASKA	1.064	1.172	1.223
00832	00	ARIZONA	0.994	0.978	1.111
00520	13	ARKANSAS	0.953	0.847	0.340
02050	26	ANAHEIM/SANTA ANA, CA	1.037	1.184	0.955
02050	18	LOS ANGELES, CA	1.056	1.139	0.955
31140	03	MARIN/NAPA/SOLANO, CA	1.015	1.248	0.687
31140	07	OAKLAND/BERKELEY, CA	1.041	1.235	0.687
31140	05	SAN FRANCISCO, CA	1.068	1.458	0.687
31140	06	SAN MATEO, CA	1.048	1.432	0.687
31140	09	SANTA CLARA, CA	1.063	1.380	0.639
02050	17	VENTURA, CA	1.028	1.125	0.783
02050	99	REST OF CALIFORNIA*	1.007	1.034	0.748
31140	99	REST OF CALIFORNIA*	1.007	1.034	0.748
00824	01	COLORADO	0.985	0.992	0.840
10230	00	CONNECTICUT	1.050	1.156	0.966
00902	01	DELAWARE	1.019	1.035	0.712
00903	01	DC + MD/VA SUBURBS	1.050	1.166	0.909
00590	03	FORT LAUDERDALE, FL	0.996	1.018	1.877
00590	04	MIAMI, FL	1.015	1.052	2.528
00590	99	REST OF FLORIDA	0.975	0.946	1.265
00511	01	ATLANTA, GA	1.006	1.059	0.935
00511	99	REST OF GEORGIA	0.970	0.892	0.935
00833	01	HAWAII/GUAM	0.997	1.124	0.834
05130	00	IDAHO	0.960	0.881	0.497
00952	16	CHICAGO, IL	1.028	1.092	1.797
00952	12	EAST ST. LOUIS, IL	0.988	0.924	1.691
00952	15	SUBURBAN CHICAGO, IL	1.006	1.071	1.645
00952	99	REST OF ILLINOIS	0.964	0.889	1.157
00630	00	INDIANA	0.981	0.922	0.481
00826	00	IOWA	0.959	0.876	0.596
00650	00	KANSAS*	0.963	0.895	0.756

Carrier	Locality	Locality name	Work	Practice expense	Malpractice
00740	04	KANSAS*	0.963	0.895	0.756
00660	00	KENTUCKY	0.970	0.866	0.877
00528	01	NEW ORLEANS, LA	0.998	0.945	1.283
00528	99	REST OF LOUISIANA	0.968	0.870	1.073
31142	03	SOUTHERN MAINE	0.979	0.999	0.666
31142	99	REST OF MAINE	0.961	0.910	0.666
00901	01	BALTIMORE/SURR. CNTYS, MD	1.021	1.038	0.916
00901	99	REST OF MARYLAND	0.984	0.972	0.774
31143	01	METROPOLITAN BOSTON	1.041	1.239	0.784
31143	99	REST OF MASSACHUSETTS	1.010	1.129	0.784
00953	01	DETROIT, MI	1.043	1.038	2.738
00953	99	REST OF MICHIGAN	0.997	0.938	1.571
10240	00	MINNESOTA	0.990	0.974	0.452
10250	00	MISSISSIPPI	0.957	0.837	0.779
00740	02	METROPOLITAN KANSAS CITY, MO	0.988	0.967	0.846
00523	01	METROPOLITAN ST. LOUIS, MO	0.994	0.938	0.846
00523	99	REST OF MISSOURI*	0.946	0.825	0.793
00740	99	REST OF MISSOURI*	0.946	0.825	0.793
00751	01	MONTANA	0.950	0.876	0.727
00655	00	NEBRASKA	0.948	0.877	0.430
00834	00	NEVADA	1.005	1.039	1.209
31144	40	NEW HAMPSHIRE	0.986	1.030	0.825
00805	01	NORTHERN NJ	1.058	1.193	0.860
00805	99	REST OF NEW JERSEY	1.029	1.110	0.860
00521	05	NEW MEXICO	0.973	0.900	0.902
00803	01	MANHATTAN, NY	1.094	1.351	1.668
00803	02	NYC SUBURBS/LONG I., NY	1.068	1.251	1.952
00803	03	POUGHKPSIE/N NYC SUBURBS, NY	1.011	1.075	1.275
14330	04	QUEENS, NY	1.058	1.228	1.871
00801	99	REST OF NEW YORK	0.998	0.944	0.764
05535	00	NORTH CAROLINA	0.970	0.931	0.595
00820	01	NORTH DAKOTA	0.950	0.880	0.657

Introduction

Carrier	Locality	Locality name	Work	Practice expense	Malpractice
16360	00	OHIO	0.988	0.944	0.957
00522	00	OKLAHOMA	0.968	0.876	0.444
00835	01	PORTLAND, OR	0.996	1.049	0.436
00835	99	REST OF OREGON	0.961	0.933	0.436
00865	01	METROPOLITAN PHILADELPHIA, PA	1.023	1.092	1.413
00865	99	REST OF PENNSYLVANIA	0.989	0.929	0.774
00973	20	PUERTO RICO	0.881	0.712	0.275
00870	01	RHODE ISLAND	1.017	1.065	0.883
00880	01	SOUTH CAROLINA	0.974	0.904	0.279
00820	02	SOUTH DAKOTA	0.935	0.878	0.406
05440	35	TENNESSEE	0.975	0.900	0.592
00900	31	AUSTIN, TX	0.986	0.996	0.859
00900	20	BEAUMONT, TX	0.992	0.890	1.338
00900	09	BRAZORIA, TX	0.992	0.978	1.338
00900	11	DALLAS, TX	1.010	1.065	0.931
00900	28	FORT WORTH, TX	0.987	0.981	0.931
00900	15	GALVESTON, TX	0.988	0.969	1.338
00900	18	HOUSTON, TX	1.020	1.007	1.336
00900	99	REST OF TEXAS	0.966	0.880	0.956
00910	09	UTAH	0.976	0.941	0.644
31145	50	VERMONT	0.973	0.986	0.539
00973	50	VIRGIN ISLANDS	0.965	1.023	1.002
10490	00	VIRGINIA	0.984	0.938	0.500
00836	02	SEATTLE (KING CNTY), WA	1.005	1.100	0.788
00836	99	REST OF WASHINGTON	0.981	0.972	0.788
16510	16	WEST VIRGINIA	0.963	0.850	1.378
00951	00	WISCONSIN	0.981	0.929	0.939
00825	21	WYOMING	0.967	0.895	1.005
		* Payment locality is serviced by two carriers			

CPT and HCPCS Level II Modifier Codes

Listed values may be modified under certain circumstances. Two sources for modifiers are available. One source is the CPT book, which contains the AMA's modifiers for use with CPT codes. The other source is CMS which has developed additional modifiers for use with both CPT and HCPCS Level II codes. Medicare carriers vary on the use and acceptance of modifiers. Some carriers will accept all modifiers listed in the CPT book and HCPCS. Others may accept only select modifier codes. Determine which carriers will accept modifiers and which do not. The same is true for commercial payers. Some commercial payers require CMS modifiers because they are often more specific than CPT modifiers, but others accept only CPT modifiers. Check with individual payers regarding their requirements.

AMA CPT modifiers are two-digit numeric codes listed after the procedure code and separated from the procedure by a hyphen. When applicable, the modifying circumstance should be identified by the addition of the appropriate "modifier code number" (including the hyphen) after the usual procedure number (e.g., 47600-22). The modifier may also be listed using the modifier code along with 099 in front of the modifier (e.g., 09922 for -22). No hyphen is needed in this case. The fee should be listed as a single modified total for the procedure. Modifier descriptions should be carefully reviewed because in recent years, significant revisions have been made to modifier descriptions. In addition, some modifiers are specific for certain types of service.

CMS modifiers consist of either two alpha characters (e.g., -QB) or one alpha and one numeric character (e.g., -T1). They are listed after the CPT or HCPCS Level II procedure code and separated from these codes by a hyphen (e.g., 28112-T1).

Modifier codes listing additional value show customary increases, when available. However, it should be noted that actual reimbursement values may vary for both Medicare carriers and commercial payers. **Additional guidelines regarding the use of some modifiers are also provided. This supplemental information is not part of the official descriptions. It is listed in italics so that it can be differentiated from the official information.**

When multiple modifiers are used, see modifier -99.

CPT Modifier Codes

Listed below are CPT modifiers for physician services. Select HCPCS Level II modifiers are described in the introductions to the various sections. For a complete listing of current HCPCS modifiers, consult a current HCPCS Level II resource.

-21 **Prolonged Evaluation and Management Services:** When the face-to-face or floor/unit service(s) provided is prolonged or otherwise greater than that usually required for the highest level of evaluation and management service within a given category, it may be identified by adding modifier '-21' to the evaluation and management code number or by use of the separate five-digit modifier code 09921. A report may also be appropriate.

-22 **Unusual Procedural Services:** When the service(s) provided is greater than that usually provided for the listed procedure, it may be identified by adding modifier '-22' to the usual procedure number or by use of the separate five-digit modifier code 09922. A report may also be appropriate.

-23 **Unusual Anesthesia:** Occasionally, a procedure, which usually requires either no anesthesia *(e.g., proctoscopy)* or local anesthesia *(e.g., skin biopsy or excision of subcutaneous tumor)*, must be done under general anesthesia because of unusual circumstances *(e.g., age, non-cooperation of patient)*. This circumstance is reported by adding the modifier '-23' to the procedure code of the basic service or by use of the separate five-digit modifier code 09923.

-24 **Unrelated Evaluation and Management Service by the Same Physician During a Postoperative Period:** The physician may need to indicate that an evaluation and management service was performed during a post-operative period for reason(s) unrelated to the original procedure. This circumstance may be reported by adding the modifier '-24' to the appropriate level of E/M service or the separate five-digit modifier 09924 may be used. *Service should be substantiated by report and listed value should be allowed 100 percent. Most payers will require a new diagnosis when modifier '-24' is used.*

-25 **Significant, Separately Identifiable Evaluation and Management Service by the Same Physician on the Same Day of Procedure or Other Service:** The physician may need to indicate that on the day a procedure or service identified by a CPT code was performed, the patient's condition required a significant, separately identifiable E/M service above and beyond the other service provided or beyond the usual pre-operative and post-operative care associated with the procedure that was performed. The E/M service may be prompted by the symptom or condition for which the procedure and/or service provided. As such, different diagnoses are not required for reporting the E/M services on the same date. This circumstance may be reported by appending the modifier '-25' to the appropriate level of E/M service, or the separate five-digit modifier 009925 may be used. **Note:** This modifier is not used to report an E/M service that resulted in a decision to perform surgery. See modifier '-57.' *Listed value should be allowed at 100 percent. Medicare will accept this modifier for E/M services provided on the same day as a procedure with a 0- or 10-day global period only.*

-26 **Professional Component:** Certain procedures are a combination of a physician component and a technical component. When the physician component is reported separately, the service may be identified by adding the modifier '-26' to the usual procedure number or the service may be reported by use of the five-digit modifier code 09926.

-32 **Mandated Services:** Services related to mandated consultation and/or related services (e.g., PRO, third party payer, governmental, legislative, or regulatory requirement) may be identified by adding the modifier '-32' to the basic procedure or the service may be reported by use of the five-digit modifier 09932.

-47 **Anesthesia by Surgeon:** Regional or general anesthesia provided by the surgeon may be reported by adding the modifier '-47' to the basic service or by use of the separate five digit modifier code 09947. (This does not include local anesthesia.) **Note:** Modifier '-47' or 09947 would not be used as a modifier for the anesthesia procedures 00100-01999. *Medicare will not pay for anesthesia provided by the physician.*

-50 **Bilateral Procedure:** Unless otherwise identified in the listings, bilateral procedures that are performed at the same operative session should be identified by adding the modifier '-50' or by use of the separate five-digit modifier code 09950. *Bill Medicare on one line of the HCFA-1500 form by listing the code used and modifier '-50'. Bill at 150 percent of allowable. Some payers may require billing such that the first procedure and second procedure are valued the same and subsequently discounted. Other payers may require billing for the first procedure at 100 percent and the second procedure valued at a discounted rate. Also see Surgery Value Guidelines.*

-51 **Multiple Procedures:** When multiple procedures, other than Evaluation and Management Services, are performed on the same day or at the same session by the same provider, the primary procedure or service may be reported as listed. The additional procedure(s) or service(s) may be identified by appending the modifier '-51' to the additional procedure or service code(s) or by use of the separate five-digit modifier 09951. **Note:** This modifier should not be appended to designated "add-on" codes (see CPT Appendix E). *See Surgery Value Guidelines for rules.*

-52 **Reduced Services:** Under certain circumstances a service or procedure is partially reduced or eliminated at the physician's discretion. Under these circumstances the services provided can be identified by its usual procedure number and the addition of the modifier '-52', signifying that the service is reduced. This provides a means of reporting reduced services without disturbing the identification of the basic service. Modifier code 09952 may be used as an alternative to modifier '-52.'

-53 **Discontinued Procedure:** Under certain circumstances the physician may elect to terminate a surgical or diagnostic procedure Due to extenuating circumstances or those that threaten the well being of the patient, it may be necessary to indicate that a surgical or diagnostic procedure was started but discontinued. This circumstance may be reported by adding the modifier '-53' to the code reported by the physician for the discontinued procedure or by use of the separate five-digit modifier code 09953. **Note:** This modifier is not used to report the elective cancellation of a procedure prior to the patient's anesthesia induction and/or surgical preparation in the operating suite. *Value for a discontinued procedure should be based on actual work performed. A report may be required for value approval.*

-54 **Surgical Care Only:** When one physician performs the surgical procedure and another provides the preoperative and/or postoperative management, surgical services may be identified by adding the modifier '-54' to the usual procedure number or by use of the separate five-digit modifier code 09954. *The customary value should be listed at 70 percent of the value listed. Medicare payment is dependent upon pre-established percentages. See Surgery Value Guidelines for allowable payment rules.*

-55 **Post-operative Management Only:** When one physician performed the post-operative management and another physician performed the surgical procedure, the postoperative component may be identified by adding the modifier '-55' to the usual procedure number or by use of the separate five-digit modifier code 09955. *The customary value should be listed at 20 percent of the value listed. Medicare payment is dependent upon pre-established percentages. See Surgery Value Guidelines for allowable payment rules.*

-56 **Pre-operative Management Only:** When one physician performed the pre-operative care and evaluation and another physician performed the surgical procedure, the pre-operative component may be identified by adding the modifier '-56' to the usual procedure number or by use of the separate five-digit modifier code 09956. *If the physician* *provides the total preoperative care (no pre-op by surgeon), the provider may bill using this code and is entitled to 10 percent of listed value. Medicare will not reimburse for this modifier.*

-57 **Decision for Surgery:** An evaluation and management service that resulted in the initial decision to perform the surgery may be identified by adding the modifier '-57' to the appropriate level of E/M service, or the separate five-digit modifier 09957 may be used. *The E/M service should be allowed at 100 percent of the listed value. Medicare will accept this modifier for E/M services provided the day before or the day of surgeries with a 90-day global period.*

-58 **Staged or Related Procedure or Service by the Same Physician During the Post-operative Period:** The physician may need to indicate that the performance of a procedure or service during the post-operative period was: a) planned prospectively at the time of the original procedure (staged); b) more extensive than the original procedure; or c) for therapy following a diagnostic surgical procedure. These circumstances may be reported by adding the modifier '-58' to the staged or related procedure, or the separate five-digit modifier 09958. **Note:** This modifier is not used to report the treatment of a problem that requires a return to the operating room. See modifier '-78'. *Use of this modifier should be substantiated by a report and allowed at 100 percent of the listed value.*

-59 **Distinct Procedural Service:** Under certain circumstances, the physician may need to indicate that a procedure or service was distinct or independent from other services performed on the same day. Modifier '-59' is used to identify procedures/services that are not normally reported together, but are appropriate under the circumstances. This may represent a different session or patient encounter, different procedure or surgery, different site or organ system, separate incision/excision, separate lesion, or separate injury (or area of injury in extensive injuries) not ordinarily encountered or performed on the same day by the same physician. However, when another already established modifier is appropriate it should be used rather than modifier '-59.' Only if no more descriptive modifier is available, and the use of modifier '-59' best explains the circumstances, should modifier '-59' be used. Modifier code 09959 may be used as an alternative to modifier '-59'. *This modifier should not decrease or increase payment.*

-62 **Two Surgeons:** When two surgeons work together as primary surgeons performing distinct part(s) of a procedure, each surgeon should report his/her distinct operative work by adding the modifier '-62' to the procedure code and any associated add-on code(s) for that procedure as long as both surgeons continue to work together as primary surgeons. Each surgeon should report the co-surgery once using the same procedure code. If additional procedure(s) (including add-on procedure(s) are performed during the same surgical session, separate code(s) may also be reported with the modifier '-62' added. Modifier 09962 may be used as an alternative to modifier '-62.' **Note:** If a co-surgeon acts as an assistant in the performance of additional procedure(s) during the same surgical session, those services may be reported using separate procedure code(s) with the modifier '-80' or modifier '-82' added as appropriate. *Modifier '-62' is used primarily when two surgeons with different skills are required in the management of a specific surgical problem (i.e., a urologist and a general surgeon in the creation of an ileal conduit). The value of the procedure should be 125 percent of the customary value listed. The adjusted value (125 percent of customary) should be apportioned in relation to the responsibility and work done. The patient should be informed of the billing arrangement. Medicare will split the fee evenly between the co-surgeons.*

-66 **Surgical Team:** Under some circumstances, highly complex procedures (requiring the services of several physicians, often of different specialties, plus other highly skilled, specially trained personnel, and various types of complex equipment) are carried out under the "surgical team" concept. Such circumstances may be identified by each participating physician with the addition of the modifier '-66' to the basic procedure number used for reporting services. Modifier code 09966 may be used as an alternative to modifier '-66.' *The value should be supported by a report to include itemization of the services, personnel, and equipment included in a "global" value.*

-76 **Repeat Procedure by Same Physician:** The physician may need to indicate that a procedure or service was repeated subsequent to the original procedure or service. This circumstance may be reported by adding the modifier '-76' to the repeated procedure/service or the separate five-digit modifier code 09976 may be used.

-77 **Repeat Procedure by Another Physician:** The physician may need to indicate that a basic procedure or service performed by another physician had to be repeated. This situation may be reported by adding modifier '-77' to the repeated procedure/service or the separate five-digit modifier code 09977 may be used. *Use of this modifier should allow 100 percent of listed value.*

-78 **Return to the Operating Room for a Related Procedure During the Post-operative Period:** The physician may need to indicate that another procedure was performed during the post-operative period of the initial procedure. When this subsequent procedure is related to the first, and requires the use of the operating room, it may be reported by adding the modifier '-78' to the related procedure, or by using the separate five-digit modifier 09978. (For repeat procedures on the same day, see '-76'.) *Use of modifier '-78' should allow 70 percent of the listed value. Medicare payment is determined by use of the work value only.*

-79 **Unrelated Procedure or Service by the Same Physician During the Post-operative Period:** The physician may need to indicate that the performance of a procedure or service during the post-operative period was unrelated to the original procedure. This circumstance may be reported by using the modifier '-79' or by using the separate five-digit modifier 09979. (For repeat procedures on the same day, see '-76.') *An unrelated procedure or service should be allowed at 100 percent of the listed value and should be substantiated by a different diagnosis and/or by report.*

-80 **Assistant Surgeon:** Surgical assistant services may be identified by adding the modifier '-80' to the usual procedure number(s) or by use of the separate five-digit modifier code 09980. *A procedure with this modifier customarily warrants 20 percent of the value listed. Medicare will pay 16 percent.*

-81 **Minimum Assistant Surgeon:** Minimum surgical assistant services are identified by adding the modifier '-81' to the usual procedure number or by use of the separate five-digit modifier code 09980. *This modifier is frequently used to identify surgical assistant services provided by non-physicians (e.g., RN, LPN, PA). For non-physician surgical assistant services, it is recommended that this modifier be allowed at 10 percent of the value listed. For physician surgical assistant services, this modifier customarily warrants 20 percent of the value listed. Medicare will pay up to 16 percent.*

-82 **Assistant Surgeon (when a qualified resident surgeon is not available):** The unavailability of a qualified resident surgeon is a prerequisite for use of modifier '-82' appended to the usual procedure code number(s) or for use of the separate five-digit modifier code 09982. *It is recommended that the physician receive 20 percent of the value listed. Medicare will pay 16 percent.*

-90 **Reference (Outside) Laboratory:** When laboratory procedures are performed by a party other than the treating or reporting physician, the procedure(s) may be identified by adding modifier '-90' to the usual procedure number or by use of the separate five-digit modifier code 09990.

-91 **Repeat Clinical Diagnostic Laboratory Test:** In the course of patient treatment it may be necessary to repeat the same laboratory test on the same day to obtain subsequent (multiple) test results. Under these circumstances, the laboratory test performed can be identified by its usual procedure number and the addition of the modifier '-91' or by use of the separate five-digit modifier code 09991. **Note:** This modifier may not be used when tests are rerun to confirm initial results due to testing problems with the specimens or equipment or for any other reason when a normal, one-time, reportable result is all that is required. This modifier may not be used when other code(s) describe a series of test results (e.g., glucose tolerance tests, evocative/suppression testing). This modifier may only be used for laboratory test(s) performed more than once on the same day on the same patient.

-99 **Multiple Modifiers:** Under certain circumstances two or more modifiers may be necessary to completely delineate a service. In such situations, modifier '-99' should be added to the basic procedure, and other applicable modifiers may be listed as part of the description of the service. Modifier code 09999 may be used as an alternative to modifier '-99.'

Anesthesia

I. **General:** Values for anesthesia services are listed by CPT code in the Anesthesia section. These values are to be used only when the anesthesia is legally administered by or under the responsible supervision of a licensed physician. These values include usual pre- and post-operative visits, the administration of the anesthetic and administration of fluids and/or blood incident to the anesthesia or surgery. Discussion of calculated values as derived from the base unit and time increments are discussed under *Calculations of Total Anesthesia Values.*

II. **Unlisted Service or Procedure:** When an unlisted service or procedure is provided, the value should be substantiated "by report" (BR).

III. **Materials Supplied By Physician:** Identify as 99070 or by specific HCPCS Level II code(s). The codes identify supplies and materials provided by the physician (e.g., dressings, casting supplies, drugs, etc.) over and above those usually included with the office visit or other services.

Note: Medicare requires HCPCS codes for identifying supplies.

IV. **Stand-by Anesthesia:** When an anesthesiologist is requested by the attending physician to be present in the operating room to monitor vital signs and manage the patient from an anesthesia standpoint, even though the actual surgery is being done under local anesthesia, calculation will be the same as if the general anesthesia had been administered (time + base value). Medicare may not pay for stand-by anesthesia.

Stand-by anesthesia is generally accepted without justifying documentation for the following:

A. Deliveries

B. Subdural hematomas

C. Femoral or brachial arterial embolectomies

D. Patients with physical status 4 or 5—the physician must document the patient's condition (e.g., severe systemic disease, moribund patient). *See next page for Physical Status Modifiers*

E. Insertion of a cardiac pacemaker

F. Cataract extraction and/or lens implant

G. Stand-by anesthesia for other than the above generally requires documentation

V. **More Than One Anesthesiologist:** When it is necessary to have a second anesthesiologist, the necessity should be substantiated "by report" (BR). It is recommended that the second anesthesiologist receive 5.0 base units plus time units (calculation of total anesthesia value). Medicare may not pay for more than one anesthesiologist.

VI. **Modifiers:** All anesthesia services are reported by use of the anesthesia five-digit procedure code (00100–01999) plus the addition of a physical status modifier. These modifying units may be added to the basic values. The use of other modifiers may be used if appropriate. A comprehensive listing of CPT compatible modifiers is provided in the introduction.

Physical status modifiers are represented by the letter P followed by a single digit defined below:

Physical Status		Unit Values
1	Healthy patient	0
2	Patient with mild systemic disease	0
3	Patient with severe systemic disease	1
4	Patient with severe systemic disease that is a constant threat to life	2
5	A moribund patient who is not expected to survive without the operation	3
6	A declared brain-dead patient whose organs are being removed for donor purposes	0

Example: 00100-P1

VII. **Qualifying Circumstances:** Some circumstances warrant additional value due to unusual events. The following list of CPT codes and the corresponding anesthesia unit values may be listed if appropriate. More than one code may be necessary. The value listed is added to the existing anesthesia base.

CPT		Unit Values
99100	Anesthesia for patient of extreme age, under one year and over seventy	1
99116	Anesthesia complicated by utilization of total body hypothermia	5
99135	Anesthesia complicated by utilization of controlled hypotension	5
99140	Anesthesia complicated by emergency conditions (specify)	2
An emergency is defined as existing when delay in treatment of a patient would lead to a significant increase in the threat to life or body part.		

Calculations of Total Anesthesia Values

The total anesthesia value is calculated by adding the separately listed basic value and time value.

A basic value is listed for most procedures. This includes the value of all anesthesia services except the value of the actual time spent administering the anesthesia or in unusual detention with the patient. When multiple surgical procedures are performed during the same period of anesthesia, only the greater basic anesthesia value of the various surgical procedures should be used as the base.

The time value is computed by allowing 1.0 unit for each 15 minutes of anesthesia time. Five (5) minutes or greater is considered a significant portion of a time unit.

Anesthesia time begins when the anesthesiologist physically starts to prepare the patient for the induction of anesthesia in the operating room (or its equivalent) and ends when the anesthesiologist is no longer in constant attendance (when the patient may be safely placed under post-operative supervision).

The following examples illustrate the calculation of total anesthesia values:

1. Procedure Number + Anesthesia Modifier or Anesthesia Code

   Basic Value
   + Time Value

   Total Anesthesia Value (sum of basic value and time value)

2. For a needle thyroid biopsy performed in 48 minutes (3 time units):

00322	Basic Value	=	3
	+ Time Value	=	3
	Total Anesthesia Value	=	6

Note: Modifiers and additional or reduced values should be used when appropriate.

Anesthesia Values

Code	Description	Base Units
00100	Anesthesia for procedures on salivary glands, including biopsy	5.0
00102	Anesthesia for procedures on plastic repair of cleft lip	6.0
00103	Anesthesia for reconstructive procedures of eyelid (e.g., blepharoplasty, ptosis surgery)	5.0
00104	Anesthesia for electroconvulsive therapy	4.0
00120	Anesthesia for procedures on external, middle, and inner ear including biopsy; not otherwise specified	5.0
00124	Anesthesia for procedures on external, middle, and inner ear including biopsy; otoscopy	4.0
00126	Anesthesia for procedures on external, middle, and inner ear including biopsy; tympanotomy	4.0
00140	Anesthesia for procedures on eye; not otherwise specified	5.0
00142	Anesthesia for procedures on eye; lens surgery	6.0
00144	Anesthesia for procedures on eye; corneal transplant	6.0
00145	Anesthesia for procedures on eye; vitreoretinal surgery	6.0
00147	Anesthesia for procedures on eye; iridectomy	6.0
00148	Anesthesia for procedures on eye; ophthalmoscopy	4.0
00160	Anesthesia for procedures on nose and accessory sinuses; not otherwise specified	5.0
00162	Anesthesia for procedures on nose and accessory sinuses; radical surgery	7.0
00164	Anesthesia for procedures on nose and accessory sinuses; biopsy, soft tissue	4.0
00170	Anesthesia for intraoral procedures, including biopsy; not otherwise specified	5.0
00172	Anesthesia for intraoral procedures, including biopsy; repair of cleft palate	6.0
00174	Anesthesia for intraoral procedures, including biopsy; excision of retropharyngeal tumor	6.0
00176	Anesthesia for intraoral procedures, including biopsy; radical surgery	7.0
00190	Anesthesia for procedures on facial bones or skull; not otherwise specified	5.0
00192	Anesthesia for procedures on facial bones or skull; radical surgery (including prognathism)	7.0
00210	Anesthesia for intracranial procedures; not otherwise specified	11.0
00212	Anesthesia for intracranial procedures; subdural taps	5.0
00214	Anesthesia for intracranial procedures; burr holes, including ventriculography	9.0

Code	Description	Base Units
00215	Anesthesia for intracranial procedures; cranioplasty or elevation of depressed skull fracture, extradural (simple or compound)	9.0
00216	Anesthesia for intracranial procedures; vascular procedures	15.0
00218	Anesthesia for intracranial procedures; procedures in sitting position	13.0
00220	Anesthesia for intracranial procedures; spinal fluid shunting procedures	10.0
00222	Anesthesia for intracranial procedures; electrocoagulation of intracranial nerve	6.0
00300	Anesthesia for all procedures on the integumentary system, muscles and nerves of head, neck, and posterior trunk, not otherwise specified	5.0
00320	Anesthesia for all procedures on esophagus, thyroid, larynx, trachea and lymphatic system of neck; not otherwise specified	6.0
00322	Anesthesia for all procedures on esophagus, thyroid, larynx, trachea and lymphatic system of neck; needle biopsy of thyroid	3.0
00350	Anesthesia for procedures on major vessels of neck; not otherwise specified	10.0
00352	Anesthesia for procedures on major vessels of neck; simple ligation	5.0
00400	Anesthesia for procedures on the integumentary system on the extremities, anterior trunk and perineum; not otherwise specified	3.0
00402	Anesthesia for procedures on the integumentary system on the extremities, anterior trunk and perineum; reconstructive procedures on breast (e.g., reduction or augmentation mammoplasty, muscle flaps)	5.0
00404	Anesthesia for procedures on the integumentary system on the extremities, anterior trunk and perineum; radical or modified radical procedures on breast	5.0
00406	Anesthesia for procedures on the integumentary system on the extremities, anterior trunk and perineum; radical or modified radical procedures on breast with internal mammary node dissection	13.0
00410	Anesthesia for procedures on the integumentary system on the extremities, anterior trunk and perineum; electrical conversion of arrhythmias	4.0
00450	Anesthesia for procedures on clavicle and scapula; not otherwise specified	5.0
00452	Anesthesia for procedures on clavicle and scapula; radical surgery	6.0
00454	Anesthesia for procedures on clavicle and scapula; biopsy of clavicle	3.0
00470	Anesthesia for partial rib resection; not otherwise specified	6.0
00472	Anesthesia for partial rib resection; thoracoplasty (any type)	10.0
00474	Anesthesia for partial rib resection; radical procedures (e.g., pectus excavatum)	13.0
00500	Anesthesia for all procedures on esophagus	15.0

Code	Description	Base Units
00520	Anesthesia for closed chest procedures; (including bronchoscopy) not otherwise specified	6.0
00522	Anesthesia for closed chest procedures; needle biopsy of pleura	4.0
00524	Anesthesia for closed chest procedures; pneumocentesis	4.0
00528	Anesthesia for closed chest procedures; mediastinoscopy and diagnostic thoracoscopy	8.0
00530	Anesthesia for permanent transvenous pacemaker insertion	4.0
00532	Anesthesia for access to central venous circulation	4.0
00534	Anesthesia for transvenous insertion or replacement of pacing cardioverter-defibrillator	7.0
00537	Anesthesia for cardiac electrophysiologic procedures including radiofrequency ablation	10.0
00540	Anesthesia for thoracotomy procedures involving lungs, pleura, diaphragm, and mediastinum (including surgical thoracoscopy); not otherwise specified	13.0
00542	Anesthesia for thoracotomy procedures involving lungs, pleura, diaphragm, and mediastinum (including surgical thoracoscopy); decortication	15.0
00544	Anesthesia for thoracotomy procedures involving lungs, pleura, diaphragm, and mediastinum (including surgical thoracoscopy); pleurectomy	15.0
00546	Anesthesia for thoracotomy procedures involving lungs, pleura, diaphragm, and mediastinum (including surgical thoracoscopy); pulmonary resection with thoracoplasty	15.0
00548	Anesthesia for thoracotomy procedures involving lungs, pleura, diaphragm, and mediastinum (including surgical thoracoscopy); intrathoracic procedures on the trachea and bronchi	15.0
00550	Anesthesia for sternal debridement	10.0
00560	Anesthesia for procedures on heart, pericardium, and great vessels of chest; without pump oxygenator	15.0
00562	Anesthesia for procedures on heart, pericardium, and great vessels of chest; with pump oxygenator	20.0
00563	Anesthesia for procedures on heart, pericardium, and great vessels of chest; with pump oxygenator with hypothermic circulatory arrest	25.0
00566	Anesthesia for direct coronary artery bypass grafting without pump oxygenator	25.0
00580	Anesthesia for heart transplant or heart/lung transplant	20.0
00600	Anesthesia for procedures on cervical spine and cord; not otherwise specified	10.0
00604	Anesthesia for procedures on cervical spine and cord; procedures with patient in the sitting position	13.0
00620	Anesthesia for procedures on thoracic spine and cord; not otherwise specified	10.0
00622	Anesthesia for procedures on thoracic spine and cord; thoracolumbar sympathectomy	13.0
00630	Anesthesia for procedures in lumbar region; not otherwise specified	8.0

Code	Description	Base Units
00632	Anesthesia for procedures in lumbar region; lumbar sympathectomy	7.0
00634	Anesthesia for procedures in lumbar region; chemonucleolysis	10.0
00635	Anesthesia for procedures in lumbar region; diagnostic or therapeutic lumbar puncture	4.0
00670	Anesthesia for extensive spine and spinal cord procedures (e.g., spinal instrumentation or vascular procedures)	13.0
00700	Anesthesia for procedures on upper anterior abdominal wall; not otherwise specified	4.0
00702	Anesthesia for procedures on upper anterior abdominal wall; percutaneous liver biopsy	4.0
00730	Anesthesia for procedures on upper posterior abdominal wall	5.0
00740	Anesthesia for upper gastrointestinal endoscopic procedures, endoscope introduced proximal to duodenum	5.0
00750	Anesthesia for hernia repairs in upper abdomen; not otherwise specified	4.0
00752	Anesthesia for hernia repairs in upper abdomen; lumbar and ventral (incisional) hernias and/or wound dehiscence	6.0
00754	Anesthesia for hernia repairs in upper abdomen; omphalocele	7.0
00756	Anesthesia for hernia repairs in upper abdomen; transabdominal repair of diaphragmatic hernia	7.0
00770	Anesthesia for all procedures on major abdominal blood vessels	15.0
00790	Anesthesia for intraperitoneal procedures in upper abdomen including laparoscopy; not otherwise specified	7.0
00792	Anesthesia for intraperitoneal procedures in upper abdomen including laparoscopy; partial hepatectomy or management of liver hemorrhage (excluding liver biopsy)	13.0
00794	Anesthesia for intraperitoneal procedures in upper abdomen including laparoscopy; pancreatectomy, partial or total (e.g., Whipple procedure)	8.0
00796	Anesthesia for intraperitoneal procedures in upper abdomen including laparoscopy; liver transplant (recipient)	30.0
00797	Anesthesia for intraperitoneal procedures in upper abdomen including laparoscopy; gastric restrictive procedure for morbid obesity	10.0
00800	Anesthesia for procedures on lower anterior abdominal wall; not otherwise specified	4.0
00802	Anesthesia for procedures on lower anterior abdominal wall; panniculectomy	5.0
00810	Anesthesia for lower intestinal endoscopic procedures, endoscope introduced distal to duodenum	5.0
00820	Anesthesia for procedures on lower posterior abdominal wall	5.0
00830	Anesthesia for hernia repairs in lower abdomen; not otherwise specified	4.0
00832	Anesthesia for hernia repairs in lower abdomen; ventral and incisional hernias	6.0

Code	Description	Base Units
00840	Anesthesia for intraperitoneal procedures in lower abdomen including laparoscopy; not otherwise specified	6.0
00842	Anesthesia for intraperitoneal procedures in lower abdomen including laparoscopy; amniocentesis	4.0
00844	Anesthesia for intraperitoneal procedures in lower abdomen including laparoscopy; abdominoperineal resection	7.0
00846	Anesthesia for intraperitoneal procedures in lower abdomen including laparoscopy; radical hysterectomy	8.0
00848	Anesthesia for intraperitoneal procedures in lower abdomen including laparoscopy; pelvic exenteration	8.0
00851	Anesthesia for intraperitoneal procedures in lower abdomen including laparoscopy; tubal ligation/transection	6.0
00860	Anesthesia for extraperitoneal procedures in lower abdomen, including urinary tract; not otherwise specified	6.0
00862	Anesthesia for extraperitoneal procedures in lower abdomen, including urinary tract; renal procedures, including upper 1/3 of ureter, or donor nephrectomy	7.0
00864	Anesthesia for extraperitoneal procedures in lower abdomen, including urinary tract; total cystectomy	8.0
00865	Anesthesia for extraperitoneal procedures in lower abdomen, including urinary tract; radical prostatectomy (suprapubic, retropubic)	7.0
00866	Anesthesia for extraperitoneal procedures in lower abdomen, including urinary tract; adrenalectomy	10.0
00868	Anesthesia for extraperitoneal procedures in lower abdomen, including urinary tract; renal transplant (recipient)	10.0
00869	Anesthesia for extraperitoneal procedures in lower abdomen, including urinary tract; vasectomy, unilateral/ bilateral	6.0
00870	Anesthesia for extraperitoneal procedures in lower abdomen, including urinary tract; cystolithotomy	5.0
00872	Anesthesia for lithotripsy, extracorporeal shock wave; with water bath	7.0
00873	Anesthesia for lithotripsy, extracorporeal shock wave; without water bath	5.0
00880	Anesthesia for procedures on major lower abdominal vessels; not otherwise specified	15.0
00882	Anesthesia for procedures on major lower abdominal vessels; inferior vena cava ligation	10.0
00902	Anesthesia for; anorectal procedure	5.0
00904	Anesthesia for; radical perineal procedure	7.0
00906	Anesthesia for; vulvectomy	4.0
00908	Anesthesia for; perineal prostatectomy	6.0
00910	Anesthesia for transurethral procedures (including urethrocystoscopy); not otherwise specified	3.0
00912	Anesthesia for transurethral procedures (including urethrocystoscopy); transurethral resection of bladder tumor(s)	5.0

Code	Description	Base Units
00914	Anesthesia for transurethral procedures (including urethrocystoscopy); transurethral resection of prostate	5.0
00916	Anesthesia for transurethral procedures (including urethrocystoscopy); post-transurethral resection bleeding	5.0
00918	Anesthesia for transurethral procedures (including urethrocystoscopy); with fragmentation, manipulation and/or removal of ureteral calculus	5.0
00920	Anesthesia for procedures on male genitalia (including open urethral procedures); not otherwise specified	3.0
00922	Anesthesia for procedures on male genitalia (including open urethral procedures); seminal vesicles	6.0
00924	Anesthesia for procedures on male genitalia (including open urethral procedures); undescended testis, unilateral or bilateral	4.0
00926	Anesthesia for procedures on male genitalia (including open urethral procedures); radical orchiectomy, inguinal	4.0
00928	Anesthesia for procedures on male genitalia (including open urethral procedures); radical orchiectomy, abdominal	6.0
00930	Anesthesia for procedures on male genitalia (including open urethral procedures); orchiopexy, unilateral or bilateral	4.0
00932	Anesthesia for procedures on male genitalia (including open urethral procedures); complete amputation of penis	4.0
00934	Anesthesia for procedures on male genitalia (including open urethral procedures); radical amputation of penis with bilateral inguinal lymphadenectomy	6.0
00936	Anesthesia for procedures on male genitalia (including open urethral procedures); radical amputation of penis with bilateral inguinal and iliac lymphadenectomy	8.0
00938	Anesthesia for procedures on male genitalia (including open urethral procedures); insertion of penile prosthesis (perineal approach)	4.0
00940	Anesthesia for vaginal procedures (including biopsy of labia, vagina, cervix or endometrium); not otherwise specified	3.0
00942	Anesthesia for vaginal procedures (including biopsy of labia, vagina, cervix or endometrium); colpotomy, colpectomy, colporrhaphy, and open urethral procedures	4.0
00944	Anesthesia for vaginal procedures (including biopsy of labia, vagina, cervix or endometrium); vaginal hysterectomy	6.0
00948	Anesthesia for vaginal procedures (including biopsy of labia, vagina, cervix or endometrium); cervical cerclage	4.0
00950	Anesthesia for vaginal procedures (including biopsy of labia, vagina, cervix or endometrium); culdoscopy	5.0
00952	Anesthesia for vaginal procedures (including biopsy of labia, vagina, cervix or endometrium); hysteroscopy and/or hysterosalpingography	4.0
01112	Anesthesia for bone marrow aspiration and/or biopsy, anterior or posterior iliac crest	5.0
01120	Anesthesia for procedures on bony pelvis	6.0

Code	Description	Base Units
01130	Anesthesia for body cast application or revision	3.0
01140	Anesthesia for interpelviabdominal (hindquarter) amputation	15.0
01150	Anesthesia for radical procedures for tumor of pelvis, except hindquarter amputation	10.0
01160	Anesthesia for closed procedures involving symphysis pubis or sacroiliac joint	4.0
01170	Anesthesia for open procedures involving symphysis pubis or sacroiliac joint	8.0
01180	Anesthesia for obturator neurectomy; extrapelvic	3.0
01190	Anesthesia for obturator neurectomy; intrapelvic	4.0
01200	Anesthesia for all closed procedures involving hip joint	4.0
01202	Anesthesia for arthroscopic procedures of hip joint	4.0
01210	Anesthesia for open procedures involving hip joint; not otherwise specified	6.0
01212	Anesthesia for open procedures involving hip joint; hip disarticulation	10.0
01214	Anesthesia for open procedures involving hip joint; total hip replacement	8.0
01215	Anesthesia for open procedures involving hip joint; revision of total hip arthroplasty	10.0
01220	Anesthesia for all closed procedures involving upper 2/3 of femur	4.0
01230	Anesthesia for open procedures involving upper 2/3 of femur; not otherwise specified	6.0
01232	Anesthesia for open procedures involving upper 2/3 of femur; amputation	5.0
01234	Anesthesia for open procedures involving upper 2/3 of femur; radical resection	8.0
01250	Anesthesia for all procedures on nerves, muscles, tendons, fascia, and bursae of upper leg	4.0
01260	Anesthesia for all procedures involving veins of upper leg, including exploration	3.0
01270	Anesthesia for procedures involving arteries of upper leg, including bypass graft; not otherwise specified	8.0
01272	Anesthesia for procedures involving arteries of upper leg, including bypass graft; femoral artery ligation	4.0
01274	Anesthesia for procedures involving arteries of upper leg, including bypass graft; femoral artery embolectomy	6.0
01320	Anesthesia for all procedures on nerves, muscles, tendons, fascia, and bursae of knee and/or popliteal area	4.0
01340	Anesthesia for all closed procedures on lower 1/3 of femur	4.0
01360	Anesthesia for all open procedures on lower 1/3 of femur	5.0
01380	Anesthesia for all closed procedures on knee joint	3.0

Code	Description	Base Units
01382	Anesthesia for arthroscopic procedures of knee joint	3.0
01390	Anesthesia for all closed procedures on upper ends of tibia, fibula, and/or patella	3.0
01392	Anesthesia for all open procedures on upper ends of tibia, fibula, and/or patella	4.0
01400	Anesthesia for open procedures on knee joint; not otherwise specified	4.0
01402	Anesthesia for open procedures on knee joint; total knee replacement	7.0
01404	Anesthesia for open procedures on knee joint; disarticulation at knee	5.0
01420	Anesthesia for all cast applications, removal, or repair involving knee joint	3.0
01430	Anesthesia for procedures on veins of knee and popliteal area; not otherwise specified	3.0
01432	Anesthesia for procedures on veins of knee and popliteal area; arteriovenous fistula	6.0
01440	Anesthesia for procedures on arteries of knee and popliteal area; not otherwise specified	8.0
01442	Anesthesia for procedures on arteries of knee and popliteal area; popliteal thromboendarterectomy, with or without patch graft	8.0
01444	Anesthesia for procedures on arteries of knee and popliteal area; popliteal excision and graft or repair for occlusion or aneurysm	8.0
01462	Anesthesia for all closed procedures on lower leg, ankle, and foot	3.0
01464	Anesthesia for arthroscopic procedures of ankle joint	3.0
01470	Anesthesia for procedures on nerves, muscles, tendons, and fascia of lower leg, ankle, and foot; not otherwise specified	3.0
01472	Anesthesia for procedures on nerves, muscles, tendons, and fascia of lower leg, ankle, and foot; repair of ruptured Achilles tendon, with or without graft	5.0
01474	Anesthesia for procedures on nerves, muscles, tendons, and fascia of lower leg, ankle, and foot; gastrocnemius recession (e.g., Strayer procedure)	5.0
01480	Anesthesia for open procedures on bones of lower leg, ankle, and foot; not otherwise specified	3.0
01482	Anesthesia for open procedures on bones of lower leg, ankle, and foot; radical resection (including below knee amputation)	4.0
01484	Anesthesia for open procedures on bones of lower leg, ankle, and foot; osteotomy or osteoplasty of tibia and/or fibula	4.0
01486	Anesthesia for open procedures on bones of lower leg, ankle, and foot; total ankle replacement	7.0
01490	Anesthesia for lower leg cast application, removal, or repair	3.0
01500	Anesthesia for procedures on arteries of lower leg, including bypass graft; not otherwise specified	8.0

Code	Description	Base Units
01502	Anesthesia for procedures on arteries of lower leg, including bypass graft; embolectomy, direct or with catheter	6.0
01520	Anesthesia for procedures on veins of lower leg; not otherwise specified	3.0
01522	Anesthesia for procedures on veins of lower leg; venous thrombectomy, direct or with catheter	5.0
01610	Anesthesia for all procedures on nerves, muscles, tendons, fascia, and bursae of shoulder and axilla	5.0
01620	Anesthesia for all closed procedures on humeral head and neck, sternoclavicular joint, acromioclavicular joint, and shoulder joint	4.0
01622	Anesthesia for arthroscopic procedures of shoulder joint	4.0
01630	Anesthesia for open procedures on humeral head and neck, sternoclavicular joint, acromioclavicular joint, and shoulder joint; not otherwise specified	5.0
01632	Anesthesia for open procedures on humeral head and neck, sternoclavicular joint, acromioclavicular joint, and shoulder joint; radical resection	6.0
01634	Anesthesia for open procedures on humeral head and neck, sternoclavicular joint, acromioclavicular joint, and shoulder joint; shoulder disarticulation	9.0
01636	Anesthesia for open procedures on humeral head and neck, sternoclavicular joint, acromioclavicular joint, and shoulder joint; interthoracoscapular (forequarter) amputation	15.0
01638	Anesthesia for open procedures on humeral head and neck, sternoclavicular joint, acromioclavicular joint, and shoulder joint; total shoulder replacement	10.0
01650	Anesthesia for procedures on arteries of shoulder and axilla; not otherwise specified	6.0
01652	Anesthesia for procedures on arteries of shoulder and axilla; axillary-brachial aneurysm	10.0
01654	Anesthesia for procedures on arteries of shoulder and axilla; bypass graft	8.0
01656	Anesthesia for procedures on arteries of shoulder and axilla; axillary-femoral bypass graft	10.0
01670	Anesthesia for all procedures on veins of shoulder and axilla	4.0
01680	Anesthesia for shoulder cast application, removal or repair; not otherwise specified	3.0
01682	Anesthesia for shoulder cast application, removal or repair; shoulder spica	4.0
01710	Anesthesia for procedures on nerves, muscles, tendons, fascia, and bursae of upper arm and elbow; not otherwise specified	3.0
01712	Anesthesia for procedures on nerves, muscles, tendons, fascia, and bursae of upper arm and elbow; tenotomy, elbow to shoulder, open	5.0
01714	Anesthesia for procedures on nerves, muscles, tendons, fascia, and bursae of upper arm and elbow; tenoplasty, elbow to shoulder	5.0
01716	Anesthesia for procedures on nerves, muscles, tendons, fascia, and bursae of upper arm and elbow; tenodesis, rupture of long tendon of biceps	5.0

Code	Description	Base Units
01730	Anesthesia for all closed procedures on humerus and elbow	3.0
01732	Anesthesia for arthroscopic procedures of elbow joint	3.0
01740	Anesthesia for open procedures on humerus and elbow; not otherwise specified	4.0
01742	Anesthesia for open procedures on humerus and elbow; osteotomy of humerus	5.0
01744	Anesthesia for open procedures on humerus and elbow; repair of nonunion or malunion of humerus	5.0
01756	Anesthesia for open procedures on humerus and elbow; radical procedures	6.0
01758	Anesthesia for open procedures on humerus and elbow; excision of cyst or tumor of humerus	5.0
01760	Anesthesia for open procedures on humerus and elbow; total elbow replacement	7.0
01770	Anesthesia for procedures on arteries of upper arm and elbow; not otherwise specified	6.0
01772	Anesthesia for procedures on arteries of upper arm and elbow; embolectomy	6.0
01780	Anesthesia for procedures on veins of upper arm and elbow; not otherwise specified	3.0
01782	Anesthesia for procedures on veins of upper arm and elbow; phleborrhaphy	4.0
01810	Anesthesia for all procedures on nerves, muscles, tendons, fascia, and bursae of forearm, wrist, and hand	3.0
01820	Anesthesia for all closed procedures on radius, ulna, wrist, or hand bones	3.0
01830	Anesthesia for open procedures on radius, ulna, wrist, or hand bones; not otherwise specified	3.0
01832	Anesthesia for open procedures on radius, ulna, wrist, or hand bones; total wrist replacement	6.0
01840	Anesthesia for procedures on arteries of forearm, wrist, and hand; not otherwise specified	6.0
01842	Anesthesia for procedures on arteries of forearm, wrist, and hand; embolectomy	6.0
01844	Anesthesia for vascular shunt, or shunt revision, any type (e.g., dialysis)	6.0
01850	Anesthesia for procedures on veins of forearm, wrist, and hand; not otherwise specified	3.0
01852	Anesthesia for procedures on veins of forearm, wrist, and hand; phleborrhaphy	4.0
01860	Anesthesia for forearm, wrist, or hand cast application, removal, or repair	3.0
01916	Anesthesia for arteriograms, needle; carotid or vertebral	6.0
01920	Anesthesia for cardiac catheterization including coronary arteriography and ventriculography (not to include Swan-Ganz catheter)	7.0
01922	Anesthesia for non-invasive imaging or radiation therapy	7.0

Code	Description	Base Units
01924	Anesthesia for therapeutic interventional radiologic procedures involving the arterial system; not otherwise specified	6.0
01925	Anesthesia for therapeutic interventional radiologic procedures involving the arterial system; carotid or coronary	8.0
01926	Anesthesia for therapeutic interventional radiologic procedures involving the arterial system; intracranial, intracardiac, or aortic	10.0
01930	Anesthesia for therapeutic interventional radiologic procedures involving the venous/lymphatic system (not to include access to the central circulation); not otherwise specified	5.0
01931	Anesthesia for therapeutic interventional radiologic procedures involving the venous/lymphatic system (not to include access to the central circulation); intrahepatic or portal circulation (e.g., transcutaneous porto-caval shunt (TIPS))	7.0
01932	Anesthesia for therapeutic interventional radiologic procedures involving the venous/lymphatic system (not to include access to the central circulation); intrathoracic or jugular	7.0
01933	Anesthesia for therapeutic interventional radiologic procedures involving the venous/lymphatic system (not to include access to the central circulation); intracranial	8.0
01951	Anesthesia for second and third degree burn excision or debridement with or without skin grafting, any site, for total body surface area (TBSA) treated during anesthesia and surgery; less than one percent total body surface area	3.0
01952	Anesthesia for second and third degree burn excision or debridement with or without skin grafting, any site, for total body surface area (TBSA) treated during anesthesia and surgery; one percent to nine percent total body surface area	5.0
01953	Anesthesia for second and third degree burn excision or debridement with or without skin grafting, any site, for total body surface area (TBSA) treated during anesthesia and surgery; each additional nine percent total body surface area or part thereof (List separately in addition to code for primary procedure)	1.0
01960	Anesthesia for; vaginal delivery only	5.0
01961	Anesthesia for; cesarean delivery only	7.0
01962	Anesthesia for; urgent hysterectomy following delivery	8.0
01963	Anesthesia for; cesarean hysterectomy without any labor analgesia/anesthesia care	8.0
01964	Anesthesia for; abortion procedures	3.0
01967	Neuraxial labor analgesia/anesthesia for planned vaginal delivery (this includes any repeat subarachnoid needle placement and drug injection and/or any necessary replacement of an epidural catheter during labor)	5.0
01968	Cesarean delivery following neuraxial labor analgesia/anesthesia (List separately in addition to code for primary procedure)	1.0
01969	Cesarean hysterectomy following neuraxial labor analgesia/anesthesia (List separately in addition to code for primary procedure)	1.0
01990	Physiological support for harvesting of organ(s) from brain-dead patient	7.0

Code	Description	Base Units
01995	Regional IV administration of local anesthetic agent or other medication (upper or lower extremity)	5.0
01996	Daily management of epidural or subarachnoid drug administration	3.0
01999	Unlisted anesthesia procedure(s)	BR

Surgery

The Introduction provides complete descriptions for the status column (abbreviated as S). If a relative value is not available for a procedure, it is indicated with a "0.00" in the individual units column.

I. **Global Values:**

A. The relative values for CMS therapeutic surgical procedures are considered global and include:

1. The immediate pre-operative care which starts after the decision for surgery has been made. [Modifiers must be used when E/M services are provided prior to immediate pre-operative care, under certain circumstances. These circumstances include decisions made either: a) the day of surgery for procedures in which the global period is 0 or 10 days, modifier -25; or b) the day before or the day of surgery for procedures in which the global period is 90 days, modifier -57].

a. Additional value is warranted for pre-operative services under the following circumstances:

(1) Evaluation and Management services unrelated to the primary procedure

(2) Services required to stabilize the patient for the primary procedure

(3) When procedures not usually part of the basic surgical procedure (e.g., bronchoscopy prior to chest surgery) are provided during the immediate pre-operative period

b. The following is included in the surgical package and additional value is not warranted:

(1) A single E/M encounter subsequent to the decision for surgery immediately prior to or the day of surgery, including history and physical exam.

2. The surgical procedure, including local infiltration, metacarpal/metatarsal/digital block, or topical anesthesia (when used).

3. Normal uncomplicated follow-up care for the period indicated "global."

Some circumstances warrant additional value when care is rendered during the follow-up period, including repeat services (-76, -77), related procedure (-78), unrelated care (-79, -24), or staged procedures (-58). *See also "Modifiers" listed in the introduction.*

B. Diagnostic procedures (e.g., endoscopy, injection procedures for radiography, etc.) include only that care related to the diagnostic procedure itself. The condition for which the diagnostic procedure was performed or other concomitant conditions are not included and may be listed separately.

C. **Note on starred procedures:** Certain relatively small surgical procedures are characterized by variable pre- and postoperative services. Because of these indefinite parameters, the usual package concept for surgical services cannot be applied. Such procedures are identified by a star (*) following the procedure code.

When a star follows a surgical procedure code, the service listed includes only the surgical procedure, not any associated pre- and postoperative services. See your CPT book for further information regarding starred procedures.

Follow-up periods and special circumstances are listed under "Global:"

MMM codes describe services furnished in uncomplicated maternity care. This includes antepartum, delivery, and postpartum care. The usual global surgical concept does not apply.

XXX codes indicate that the global surgery concept does not apply.

YYY codes indicate that the global period is to be set by the local carrier.

ZZZ codes indicate that the code is an add-on service and therefore is treated in the global period of the other procedure which is billed in conjunction with a ZZZ code. Do not bill these codes with modifier -51. They should not be reduced.

II. **Separate Procedures:** Procedures identified as "separate procedures" are frequently included in the global value of other procedures. Listing of separate codes is not appropriate when a procedure is included in the global value of another (e.g., code 29870 is not appropriate to list in conjunction with 29874 when performed on the same side).

III. **Unusual Service Or Procedures:** A service may necessitate use of the skills and time of the physician over and above listed services and values. If substantiated "by report" (BR), additional values may be warranted. Use modifier -22 to indicate greater complexity.

IV. **Unlisted Procedural Services:** When a service or procedure provided is not adequately identified, use of the unlisted procedure code for the related anatomical area is appropriate. Unlisted codes have "9" for the last digit, with a few exceptions.

V. **"By Report" (BR):** Value of a procedure should be established for any "by report" circumstance by identifying a similar service and justifying value difference. When a report is indicated, the report should include the following:

A. Accurate procedure definition or description

B. Operative report

C. Justification for procedural variance, when appropriate

D. Similar procedure and value comparisons

E. Justification for value difference

VI. **Reduced Services:** Under some circumstances, value for a procedure may be reduced or eliminated. Use the modifier -52 to identify reduced value services.

VII. **Operating Microscope:** When an operating microscope is used to perform a procedure, the use of code 69990 is appropriate. An additional value of 25 percent is customarily added if the use of the microscope is medically beneficial and appropriate and it requires increased skill and time. Medicare will not reimburse for this code.

VIII. **Anesthesia By Surgeon:** Regional or general anesthesia provided by surgeon should be indicated using modifier -47. The surgeon may receive a value for the procedure equal to the base anesthesia value listed in the anesthesia section. **Note:** Anesthesia and surgery relative value units are based on different scales and conversion factors may vary significantly.

IX. **Pre-operative, Surgery, and/or Post-operative Care Provided By Different Physicians:** Medicare will pay for post-operative and surgical care modifiers based on the following percentages:

Percent of Total RVUs by Procedure Applied After Post-Hospital Discharge

Family	Procedure Codes	Surgery Percentage	Post-op Percentage
Integumentary	10000-19499	81	19
Musculoskeletal	20000-29909	79	21
Respiratory	30000-32999	86	14
Cardiovascular	33010-37799	93	7
Hemic and Lymphatic	38100-38999	93	7
Mediastinum	39000-39599	93	7
Digestive	40490-49999	90	10
Urinary	50010-53899	91	9
Male Genital	54000-55980	90	10
Female Genital	56000-58999	86	14
Maternity	590100-59899	77	23
Endocrine	60000-60699	91	9
Nervous	61000-64999	87	13
Eye	65091-68899	80	20
Auditory	69000-69979	86	14

A. **Surgical Care Only:** When a physician provides only the surgical care and another physician provides pre-operative and post-operative care, this circumstance should be indicated by the use of modifier -54. A customary 70 percent of the listed value is allowed for this circumstance.

B. **Post-operative Management Only:** If a physician provides the post-operative care only, the use of modifier -55 is warranted. A customary value of 20 percent of the listed value is appropriate.

C. **Pre-operative Management Only:** If a physician provides the pre-operative care only, the use of modifier -56 is warranted. A customary value of 10 percent of the listed value is appropriate. Medicare will not reimburse for this modifier.

X. **Two Surgeons:** When two surgeons work together as primary surgeons performing distinct part(s) of a procedure, each surgeon should report his/her distinct operative work by adding the modifier -62 to the procedure code and any associated add-on code(s) for that procedure as long as both surgeons continue to work together as primary surgeons. Each surgeon should report the co-surgery once using the same procedure code. If additional procedure(s) (including add-on procedure(s) are performed during the same surgical session, separate code(s) may also be reported with the modifier -62 added. Modifier 09962 may be used as an alternative to modifier -62. **Note:** If a co-surgeon acts as an assistant in the performance of additional procedure(s) during the same surgical session, those services may be reported using separate procedure code(s) with the modifier -80 or modifier -82 added as appropriate. *Modifier -62 is used primarily when two surgeons with different skills are required in the management of a specific surgical problem (i.e., a urologist and a general surgeon in the creation of an ileal conduit). The value of the procedure should be 125 percent of the customary value listed. The adjusted value (125 percent of customary) should be apportioned in relation to the responsibility and work done. The patient should be informed of the billing arrangement. Medicare will split the fee evenly between the co-surgeons.*

XI. **Surgical Team:** Under some circumstances, highly complex procedures (requiring the services of several physicians, often of different specialties, plus other highly skilled, specially trained personnel, and various types of complex equipment) are carried out under the "surgical team" concept. Such circumstances may be identified by each participating physician with the addition of the modifier -66 to the basic procedure number used for reporting services. Modifier code 09966 may be used as an alternative to modifier -66. *The value should be supported by a report to include itemization of the services, personnel, and equipment included in a "global" value. See Concurrent Care and Multiple Procedures for help in determining the global value.*

XII. **Surgical Assistants:**

A. **Assistant Surgeon:** Surgical assistant services may be identified by adding the modifier -80 to the usual procedure number(s) or by use of the separate five-digit modifier code 09980. *A procedure with this modifier customarily warrants 20 percent of the value listed. Medicare will pay 16 percent.*

B. **Minimum Assistant Surgeon:** Minimum surgical assistant services are identified by adding the modifier -81 to the usual procedure number or by use of the separate five-digit modifier code 09980. *This modifier is frequently used to identify surgical assistant services provided by non-physicians (e.g., RN, LPN, PA). For non-physician surgical assistant services, it is recommended that this modifier be allowed at 10 percent of the value listed. For physician surgical assistant services, this modifier customarily warrants 20 percent of the value listed. Medicare will pay up to 16 percent.*

C. **Assistant Surgeon (when a qualified resident surgeon is not available):** The unavailability of a qualified resident surgeon is a prerequisite for use of modifier -82 appended to the usual procedure code number(s) or for use of the separate five-digit modifier code 09982. *It is recommended that the physician receive 20 percent of the value listed. Medicare will pay 16 percent.*

XIII. **Concurrent Care:** When separate procedures or services are provided by two or more physicians on the same date, each physician should indicate his or her service(s) by appropriate procedure code(s). This circumstance does not warrant any increase or reduction in value. This circumstance can only be used if the procedures performed do not qualify for the use of modifiers -62 or -66. Medicare will pay only one service, per diagnosis, per day provided it is not a multiple or bilateral procedure. Consults are the exception.

XIV. **Multiple Procedures (Same Surgeon):**

A. **Single Surgeon:** Procedures performed on the same date which significantly increase time and skill warrant the use of modifier -51. Modifier -51 should be added to the secondary, tertiary, etc. procedure code(s). Multiple procedures should be listed according to value in descending order. (Multiple Procedure Guidelines do not apply to codes specifically identified as Add-on/Additional Procedures, Global indicator "ZZZ"). The primary procedure should reflect the greatest value and should not be reported with modifier -51. All other procedures should be listed in decreasing value order with modifier -51 appended. The values appropriate for each procedure are as follows:

Primary procedure	100 percent of listed value
Second, third, and fourth procedure	50 percent of listed value
Beyond fifth procedure and each additional	BR

XV. **Bilateral Procedures:** Some procedures which are performed on both the left and right (bilateral procedures) warrant the use of modifier -50 for the second procedure. Follow appropriate rules of valuation listed under Multiple Procedures. Bill Medicare on one line of HCFA-1500 by listing the procedure code and appending modifier -50. Bill at 150 percent of allowable.

XVI. **Multiple Modifiers:** If circumstances require the use of more than one modifier with any one procedure code, modifier -99 should be added to the procedure code. Other modifiers are then attached to the procedure code and listed separately with appropriate values for each.

XVII. **Materials Supplied By Physician:** CPT code 99070 or the specific HCPCS Level II code may be used to identify materials provided by the physician (e.g, dressings, casting supplies, drugs, etc.) over and above those usually indicated with the office visit. Medicare no longer provides separate payment for a sterile supply tray when the service is provided in the physician's office as the value of these types of supplies is now included in the non-facility practice expense component.

Surgery Values

Code	M	S	Description	Work Value	Non-Fac PE	Fac PE	Mal-prac-tice	Non-Fac Total	Fac Total	Global	Gap
10021		A	Fine needle aspiration; without imaging guidance	1.27	1.02	1.02	0.10	2.39	2.39	XXX	
	26	A		1.27	0.55	0.55	0.07	1.89	1.89	XXX	
	TC	A		0.00	0.47	0.47	0.03	0.50	0.50	XXX	
10022		A	with imaging guidance	1.27	1.11	1.11	0.08	2.46	2.46	XXX	
	26	A		1.27	0.48	0.48	0.05	1.80	1.80	XXX	
	TC	A		0.00	0.63	0.63	0.03	0.66	0.66	XXX	
10040*		A	Acne surgery (eg, marsupialization, opening or removal of multiple milia, comedones, cysts, pustules)	1.18	1.00	0.54	0.05	2.23	1.77	010	
10060*		A	Incision and drainage of abscess (eg, carbuncle, suppurative hidradenitis, cutaneous or subcutaneous abscess, cyst, furuncle, or paronychia); simple or single	1.17	1.51	0.70	0.08	2.76	1.95	010	
10061		A	complicated or multiple	2.40	1.88	1.48	0.17	4.45	4.05	010	
10080*		A	Incision and drainage of pilonidal cyst; simple	1.17	2.18	0.75	0.09	3.44	2.01	010	
10081		A	complicated	2.45	3.02	1.61	0.19	5.66	4.25	010	
10120*		A	Incision and removal of foreign body, subcutaneous tissues; simple	1.22	1.52	0.36	0.10	2.84	1.68	010	
10121		A	complicated	2.69	2.99	1.83	0.25	5.93	4.77	010	
10140*		A	Incision and drainage of hematoma, seroma or fluid collection	1.53	1.54	0.90	0.15	3.22	2.58	010	
10160*		A	Puncture aspiration of abscess, hematoma, bulla, or cyst	1.20	0.74	0.43	0.11	2.05	1.74	010	
10180		A	Incision and drainage, complex, post-operative wound infection	2.25	1.51	1.33	0.25	4.01	3.83	010	
11000*		A	Debridement of extensive eczematous or infected skin; up to 10% of body surface	0.60	0.66	0.24	0.05	1.31	0.89	000	
11001		A	each additional 10% of the body surface (List separately in addition to code for primary procedure)	0.30	0.37	0.11	0.02	0.69	0.43	ZZZ	
11010		A	Debridement including removal of foreign material associated with open fracture(s) and/or dislocation(s); skin and subcutaneous tissues	4.20	2.53	2.10	0.45	7.18	6.75	010	
11011		A	skin, subcutaneous tissue, muscle fascia, and muscle	4.95	3.90	2.69	0.53	9.38	8.17	000	
11012		A	skin, subcutaneous tissue, muscle fascia, muscle, and bone	6.88	5.52	4.35	0.89	13.29	12.12	000	
11040		A	Debridement; skin, partial thickness	0.50	0.55	0.22	0.05	1.10	0.77	000	
11041		A	skin, full thickness	0.82	0.69	0.34	0.08	1.59	1.24	000	

■ RVU not developed by CMS. Gap-filled RVUs developed by Ingenix/CHEG.

Code	M	S	Description	Work Value	Non-Fac PE	Fac PE	Mal-practice	Non-Fac Total	Fac Total	Global	Gap
11042		A	skin, and subcutaneous tissue	1.12	1.04	0.47	0.11	2.27	1.70	000	
11043		A	skin, subcutaneous tissue, and muscle	2.38	2.72	1.42	0.24	5.34	4.04	010	
11044		A	subcutaneous tissue, muscle, and bone	3.06	3.3	1.86	0.34	6.70	5.26	010	
11055		R	Paring or cutting of benign hyperkeratotic lesion (eg, corn or callus); single lesion	0.43	0.52	0.19	0.02	0.97	0.64	000	
11056		R	two to four lesions	0.61	0.59	0.26	0.03	1.23	0.90	000	
11057		R	more than four lesions	0.79	0.66	0.34	0.04	1.49	1.17	000	
11100		A	Biopsy of skin, subcutaneous tissue and/or mucous membrane (including simple closure), unless otherwise listed (separate procedure); single lesion	0.81	1.49	0.38	0.04	2.34	1.23	000	
11101		A	each separate/additional lesion (List separately in addition to code for primary procedure)	0.41	0.71	0.20	0.02	1.14	0.63	ZZZ	
11200*		A	Removal of skin tags, multiple fibrocutaneous tags, any area; up to and including 15 lesions	0.77	1.20	0.32	0.04	2.01	1.13	010	
11201		A	each additional ten lesions (List separately in addition to code for primary procedure)	0.29	0.53	0.12	0.02	0.84	0.43	ZZZ	
11300*		A	Shaving of epidermal or dermal lesion, single lesion, trunk, arms or legs; lesion diameter 0.5 cm or less	0.51	1.05	0.22	0.03	1.59	0.76	000	
11301		A	lesion diameter 0.6 to 1.0 cm	0.85	1.12	0.39	0.04	2.01	1.28	000	
11302		A	lesion diameter 1.1 to 2.0 cm	1.05	1.21	0.49	0.05	2.31	1.59	000	
11303		A	lesion diameter over 2.0 cm	1.24	1.36	0.55	0.06	2.66	1.85	000	
11305*		A	Shaving of epidermal or dermal lesion, single lesion, scalp, neck, hands, feet, genitalia; lesion diameter 0.5 cm or less	0.67	0.77	0.29	0.04	1.48	1.00	000	
11306		A	lesion diameter 0.6 to 1.0 cm	0.99	1.02	0.44	0.05	2.06	1.48	000	
11307		A	lesion diameter 1.1 to 2.0 cm	1.14	1.15	0.51	0.05	2.34	1.70	000	
11308		A	lesion diameter over 2.0 cm	1.41	1.29	0.62	0.07	2.77	2.10	000	
11310*		A	Shaving of epidermal or dermal lesion, single lesion, face, ears, eyelids, nose, lips, mucous membrane; lesion diameter 0.5 cm or less	0.73	1.15	0.34	0.04	1.92	1.11	000	
11311		A	lesion diameter 0.6 to 1.0 cm	1.05	1.24	0.51	0.05	2.34	1.61	000	
11312		A	lesion diameter 1.1 to 2.0 cm	1.20	1.32	0.58	0.06	2.58	1.84	000	
11313		A	lesion diameter over 2.0 cm	1.62	1.63	0.74	0.09	3.34	2.45	000	
11400		A	Excision, benign lesion, except skin tag (unless listed elsewhere), trunk, arms or legs; lesion diameter 0.5 cm or less	0.91	1.68	0.36	0.06	2.65	1.33	010	

■ RVU not developed by CMS. Gap-filled RVUs developed by Ingenix/CHEG.

Code	M	S	Description	Work Value	Non-Fac PE	Fac PE	Mal-prac-tice	Non-Fac Total	Fac Total	Global	Gap
11401		A	lesion diameter 0.6 to 1.0 cm	1.32	1.83	0.53	0.09	3.24	1.94	010	
11402		A	lesion diameter 1.1 to 2.0 cm	1.61	2.61	0.98	0.12	4.34	2.71	010	
11403		A	lesion diameter 2.1 to 3.0 cm	1.92	2.84	1.12	0.16	4.92	3.2	010	
11404		A	lesion diameter 3.1 to 4.0 cm	2.20	3.02	1.19	0.18	5.40	3.57	010	
11406		A	lesion diameter over 4.0 cm	2.76	3.33	1.41	0.25	6.34	4.42	010	
11420		A	Excision, benign lesion, except skin tag (unless listed elsewhere), scalp, neck, hands, feet, genitalia; lesion diameter 0.5 cm or less	1.06	1.52	0.44	0.08	2.66	1.58	010	
11421		A	lesion diameter 0.6 to 1.0 cm	1.53	1.84	0.64	0.11	3.48	2.28	010	
11422		A	lesion diameter 1.1 to 2.0 cm	1.76	2.60	1.08	0.14	4.50	2.98	010	
11423		A	lesion diameter 2.1 to 3.0 cm	2.17	3.02	1.26	0.17	5.36	3.60	010	
11424		A	lesion diameter 3.1 to 4.0 cm	2.62	3.20	1.43	0.21	6.03	4.26	010	
11426		A	lesion diameter over 4.0 cm	3.78	3.81	1.89	0.34	7.93	6.01	010	
11440		A	Excision, other benign lesion (unless listed elsewhere), face, ears, eyelids, nose, lips, mucous membrane; lesion diameter 0.5 cm or less	1.15	2.26	0.53	0.08	3.49	1.76	010	
11441		A	lesion diameter 0.6 to 1.0 cm	1.61	2.48	0.74	0.11	4.20	2.46	010	
11442		A	lesion diameter 1.1 to 2.0 cm	1.87	2.91	1.30	0.14	4.92	3.31	010	
11443		A	lesion diameter 2.1 to 3.0 cm	2.49	3.41	1.64	0.18	6.08	4.31	010	
11444		A	lesion diameter 3.1 to 4.0 cm	3.42	3.92	2.08	0.25	7.59	5.75	010	
11446		A	lesion diameter over 4.0 cm	4.49	4.37	2.58	0.30	9.16	7.37	010	
11450		A	Excision of skin and subcutaneous tissue for hidradenitis, axillary; with simple or intermediate repair	2.73	4.20	1.03	0.26	7.19	4.02	090	
11451		A	with complex repair	3.95	5.23	1.33	0.39	9.57	5.67	090	
11462		A	Excision of skin and subcutaneous tissue for hidradenitis, inguinal; with simple or intermediate repair	2.51	4.32	0.98	0.23	7.06	3.72	090	
11463		A	with complex repair	3.95	5.67	1.67	0.40	10.02	6.02	090	
11470		A	Excision of skin and subcutaneous tissue for hidradenitis, perianal, perineal, or umbilical; with simple or intermediate repair	3.25	4.97	1.26	0.30	8.52	4.81	090	
11471		A	with complex repair	4.41	5.54	1.74	0.40	10.35	6.55	090	
11600		A	Excision, malignant lesion, trunk, arms, or legs; lesion diameter 0.5 cm or less	1.41	2.48	1.08	0.09	3.98	2.58	010	
11601		A	lesion diameter 0.6 to 1.0 cm	1.93	2.52	1.36	0.12	4.57	3.41	010	

■ RVU not developed by CMS. Gap-filled RVUs developed by Ingenix/CHEG.

Code	M	S	Description	Work Value	Non-Fac PE	Fac PE	Mal-practice	Non-Fac Total	Fac Total	Global	Gap
11602		A	lesion diameter 1.1 to 2.0 cm	2.09	2.66	1.40	0.13	4.88	3.62	010	
11603		A	lesion diameter 2.1 to 3.0 cm	2.35	2.93	1.49	0.16	5.44	4.00	010	
11604		A	lesion diameter 3.1 to 4.0 cm	2.58	3.27	1.56	0.18	6.03	4.32	010	
11606		A	lesion diameter over 4.0 cm	3.43	3.88	1.85	0.28	7.59	5.56	010	
11620		A	Excision, malignant lesion, scalp, neck, hands, feet, genitalia; lesion diameter 0.5 cm or less	1.34	2.47	1.09	0.09	3.90	2.52	010	
11621		A	lesion diameter 0.6 to 1.0 cm	1.97	2.56	1.41	0.12	4.65	3.50	010	
11622		A	lesion diameter 1.1 to 2.0 cm	2.34	2.87	1.60	0.15	5.36	4.09	010	
11623		A	lesion diameter 2.1 to 3.0 cm	2.93	3.30	1.86	0.20	6.43	4.99	010	
11624		A	lesion diameter 3.1 to 4.0 cm	3.43	3.72	2.08	0.25	7.40	5.76	010	
11626		A	lesion diameter over 4.0 cm	4.3	4.48	2.57	0.35	9.13	7.22	010	
11640		A	Excision, malignant lesion, face, ears, eyelids, nose, lips; lesion diameter 0.5 cm or less	1.53	2.51	1.29	0.10	4.14	2.92	010	
11641		A	lesion diameter 0.6 to 1.0 cm	2.44	2.94	1.78	0.15	5.53	4.37	010	
11642		A	lesion diameter 1.1 to 2.0 cm	2.93	3.37	2.03	0.18	6.48	5.14	010	
11643		A	lesion diameter 2.1 to 3.0 cm	3.50	3.83	2.32	0.24	7.57	6.06	010	
11644		A	lesion diameter 3.1 to 4.0 cm	4.55	4.81	2.95	0.33	9.69	7.83	010	
11646		A	lesion diameter over 4.0 cm	5.95	5.68	3.77	0.46	12.09	10.18	010	
11719		R	Trimming of nondystrophic nails, any number	0.17	0.25	0.07	0.01	0.43	0.25	000	
11720		A	Debridement of nail(s) by any method(s); one to five	0.32	0.34	0.13	0.02	0.68	0.47	000	
11721		A	six or more	0.54	0.44	0.22	0.04	1.02	0.80	000	
11730*		A	Avulsion of nail plate, partial or complete, simple; single	1.13	0.83	0.46	0.09	2.05	1.68	000	
11732		A	each additional nail plate (List separately in addition to code for primary procedure)	0.57	0.30	0.24	0.05	0.92	0.86	ZZZ	
11740		A	Evacuation of subungual hematoma	0.37	0.81	0.14	0.03	1.21	0.54	000	
11750		A	Excision of nail and nail matrix, partial or complete, (eg, ingrown or deformed nail) for permanent removal;	1.86	1.75	0.78	0.16	3.77	2.80	010	
11752		A	with amputation of tuft of distal phalanx	2.67	2.20	1.77	0.33	5.20	4.77	010	
11755		A	Biopsy of nail unit (eg, plate, bed, matrix, hyponychium, proximal and lateral nail folds) (separate procedure)	1.31	1.10	0.60	0.06	2.47	1.97	000	
11760		A	Repair of nail bed	1.58	1.80	1.28	0.17	3.55	3.03	010	

■ RVU not developed by CMS. Gap-filled RVUs developed by Ingenix/CHEG.

Code	M	S	Description	Work Value	Non-Fac PE	Fac PE	Mal-prac-tice	Non-Fac Total	Fac Total	Global	Gap
11762		A	Reconstruction of nail bed with graft	2.89	2.28	1.95	0.32	5.49	5.16	010	
11765		A	Wedge excision of skin of nail fold (eg, for ingrown toenail)	0.69	1.14	0.51	0.05	1.88	1.25	010	
11770		A	Excision of pilonidal cyst or sinus; simple	2.61	3.11	1.26	0.24	5.96	4.11	010	
11771		A	extensive	5.74	5.80	4.01	0.56	12.1	10.31	090	
11772		A	complicated	6.98	6.95	4.44	0.68	14.61	12.10	090	
11900*		A	Injection, intralesional; up to and including seven lesions	0.52	0.77	0.23	0.02	1.31	0.77	000	
11901*		A	more than seven lesions	0.8	0.89	0.38	0.03	1.72	1.21	000	
11920		R	Tattooing, intradermal introduction of insoluble opaque pigments to correct color defects of skin, including micropigmentation; 6.0 sq cm or less	1.61	2.25	0.81	0.17	4.03	2.59	000	
11921		R	6.1 to 20.0 sq cm	1.93	2.78	1.02	0.21	4.92	3.16	000	
11922		R	each additional 20.0 sq cm (List separately in addition to code for primary procedure)	0.49	0.40	0.26	0.05	0.94	0.80	ZZZ	
11950		R	Subcutaneous injection of filling material (eg, collagen); 1 cc or less	0.84	1.23	0.47	0.06	2.13	1.37	000	
11951		R	1.1 to 5.0 cc	1.19	1.47	0.49	0.10	2.76	1.78	000	
11952		R	5.1 to 10.0 cc	1.69	1.65	0.64	0.17	3.51	2.50	000	
11954		R	over 10.0 cc	1.85	2.62	0.97	0.19	4.66	3.01	000	
11960		A	Insertion of tissue expander(s) for other than breast, including subsequent expansion	9.08	11.54	11.54	0.88	21.50	21.50	090	
11970		A	Replacement of tissue expander with permanent prosthesis	7.06	5.15	5.15	0.77	12.98	12.98	090	
11971		A	Removal of tissue expander(s) without insertion of prosthesis	2.13	6.10	4.07	0.21	8.44	6.41	090	
11975		N	Insertion, implantable contraceptive capsules	1.48	1.58	0.59	0.14	3.20	2.21	XXX	
11976		R	Removal, implantable contraceptive capsules	1.78	1.72	0.69	0.17	3.67	2.64	000	
11977		N	Removal with reinsertion, implantable contraceptive capsules	3.30	2.31	1.32	0.31	5.92	4.93	XXX	
11980		A	Subcutaneous hormone pellet implantation (implantation of estradiol and/or testosterone pellets beneath the skin)	1.48	1.14	0.58	0.10	2.72	2.16	000	
11981		A	Insertion, non-biodegradable drug delivery implant	1.48	1.58	0.59	0.14	3.20	2.21	XXX	
11982		A	Removal, non-biodegradable drug delivery implant	1.78	1.70	0.71	0.17	3.65	2.66	XXX	

Surgery

■ RVU not developed by CMS. Gap-filled RVUs developed by Ingenix/CHEG.

Code	M	S	Description	Work Value	Non-Fac PE	Fac PE	Mal-practice	Non-Fac Total	Fac Total	Global	Gap
11983		A	Removal with reinsertion, non-biodegradable drug delivery implant	3.30	2.31	1.32	0.31	5.92	4.93	XXX	
12001*		A	Simple repair of superficial wounds of scalp, neck, axillae, external genitalia, trunk and/or extremities (including hands and feet); 2.5 cm or less	1.70	2.13	0.44	0.13	3.96	2.27	010	
12002*		A	2.6 cm to 7.5 cm	1.86	2.21	0.95	0.15	4.22	2.96	010	
12004*		A	7.6 cm to 12.5 cm	2.24	2.47	1.07	0.17	4.88	3.48	010	
12005		A	12.6 cm to 20.0 cm	2.86	3.04	1.25	0.23	6.13	4.34	010	
12006		A	20.1 cm to 30.0 cm	3.67	3.59	1.59	0.31	7.57	5.57	010	
12007		A	over 30.0 cm	4.12	4.26	1.85	0.37	8.75	6.34	010	
12011*		A	Simple repair of superficial wounds of face, ears, eyelids, nose, lips and/or mucous membranes; 2.5 cm or less	1.76	2.30	0.45	0.14	4.20	2.35	010	
12013*		A	2.6 cm to 5.0 cm	1.99	2.45	0.99	0.16	4.60	3.14	010	
12014		A	5.1 cm to 7.5 cm	2.46	2.72	1.11	0.18	5.36	3.75	010	
12015		A	7.6 cm to 12.5 cm	3.19	3.38	1.31	0.24	6.81	4.74	010	
12016		A	12.6 cm to 20.0 cm	3.93	3.89	1.58	0.32	8.14	5.83	010	
12017		A	20.1 cm to 30.0 cm	4.71	1.93	1.93	0.39	7.03	7.03	010	
12018		A	over 30.0 cm	5.53	2.18	2.18	0.46	8.17	8.17	010	
12020		A	Treatment of superficial wound dehiscence; simple closure	2.62	2.51	1.44	0.24	5.37	4.30	010	
12021		A	with packing	1.84	1.65	1.02	0.19	3.68	3.05	010	
12031*		A	Layer closure of wounds of scalp, axillae, trunk and/or extremities (excluding hands and feet); 2.5 cm or less	2.15	2.21	0.81	0.15	4.51	3.11	010	
12032*		A	2.6 cm to 7.5 cm	2.47	2.84	1.36	0.15	5.46	3.98	010	
12034		A	7.6 cm to 12.5 cm	2.92	3.12	1.51	0.21	6.25	4.64	010	
12035		A	12.6 cm to 20.0 cm	3.43	3.20	1.73	0.30	6.93	5.46	010	
12036		A	20.1 cm to 30.0 cm	4.05	5.33	2.50	0.41	9.79	6.96	010	
12037		A	over 30.0 cm	4.67	5.57	2.86	0.49	10.73	8.02	010	
12041*		A	Layer closure of wounds of neck, hands, feet and/or external genitalia; 2.5 cm or less	2.37	2.41	0.87	0.17	4.95	3.41	010	
12042		A	2.6 cm to 7.5 cm	2.74	3.03	1.49	0.17	5.94	4.40	010	
12044		A	7.6 cm to 12.5 cm	3.14	3.22	1.67	0.24	6.60	5.05	010	
12045		A	12.6 cm to 20.0 cm	3.64	3.54	1.93	0.34	7.52	5.91	010	

■ RVU not developed by CMS. Gap-filled RVUs developed by Ingenix/CHEG.

Code	M	S	Description	Work Value	Non-Fac PE	Fac PE	Mal-practice	Non-Fac Total	Fac Total	Global	Gap
12046		A	20.1 cm to 30.0 cm	4.25	6.24	2.62	0.40	10.89	7.27	010	
12047		A	over 30.0 cm	4.65	7.21	2.86	0.41	12.27	7.92	010	
12051*		A	Layer closure of wounds of face, ears, eyelids, nose, lips and/or mucous membranes; 2.5 cm or less	2.47	3.11	1.49	0.16	5.74	4.12	010	
12052		A	2.6 cm to 5.0 cm	2.77	3.00	1.47	0.17	5.94	4.41	010	
12053		A	5.1 cm to 7.5 cm	3.12	3.20	1.63	0.20	6.52	4.95	010	
12054		A	7.6 cm to 12.5 cm	3.46	3.52	1.72	0.25	7.23	5.43	010	
12055		A	12.6 cm to 20.0 cm	4.43	4.49	2.27	0.35	9.27	7.05	010	
12056		A	20.1 cm to 30.0 cm	5.24	7.31	3.26	0.43	12.98	8.93	010	
12057		A	over 30.0 cm	5.96	6.31	3.66	0.50	12.77	10.12	010	
13100		A	Repair, complex, trunk; 1.1 cm to 2.5 cm	3.12	3.39	1.93	0.21	6.72	5.26	010	
13101		A	2.6 cm to 7.5 cm	3.92	3.59	2.39	0.22	7.73	6.53	010	
13102		A	each additional 5 cm or less (List separately in addition to code for primary procedure)	1.24	0.75	0.60	0.10	2.09	1.94	ZZZ	
13120		A	Repair, complex, scalp, arms, and/or legs; 1.1 cm to 2.5 cm	3.30	3.48	1.95	0.23	7.01	5.48	010	
13121		A	2.6 cm to 7.5 cm	4.33	3.84	2.52	0.25	8.42	7.10	010	
13122		A	each additional 5 cm or less (List separately in addition to code for primary procedure)	1.44	0.89	0.67	0.12	2.45	2.23	ZZZ	
13131		A	Repair, complex, forehead, cheeks, chin, mouth, neck, axillae, genitalia, hands and/or feet; 1.1 cm to 2.5 cm	3.79	3.75	2.30	0.25	7.79	6.34	010	
13132		A	2.6 cm to 7.5 cm	5.95	4.57	3.38	0.32	10.84	9.65	010	
13133		A	each additional 5 cm or less (List separately in addition to code for primary procedure)	2.19	1.23	1.08	0.17	3.59	3.44	ZZZ	
13150		A	Repair, complex, eyelids, nose, ears and/or lips; 1.0 cm or less	3.81	5.19	2.75	0.29	9.29	6.85	010	
13151		A	1.1 cm to 2.5 cm	4.45	5.07	3.19	0.28	9.80	7.92	010	
13152		A	2.6 cm to 7.5 cm	6.33	5.78	4.14	0.38	12.49	10.85	010	
13153		A	each additional 5 cm or less (List separately in addition to code for primary procedure)	2.38	1.38	1.20	0.18	3.94	3.76	ZZZ	
13160		A	Secondary closure of surgical wound or dehiscence, extensive or complicated	10.48	6.47	6.47	1.19	18.14	18.14	090	

Surgery

■ RVU not developed by CMS. Gap-filled RVUs developed by Ingenix/CHEG.

Code	M	S	Description	Work Value	Non-Fac PE	Fac PE	Mal-practice	Non-Fac Total	Fac Total	Global	Gap
14000		A	Adjacent tissue transfer or rearrangement, trunk; defect 10 sq cm or less	5.89	7.58	4.83	0.46	13.93	11.18	090	
14001		A	defect 10.1 sq cm to 30.0 sq cm	8.47	8.72	6.18	0.65	17.84	15.30	090	
14020		A	Adjacent tissue transfer or rearrangement, scalp, arms and/or legs; defect 10 sq cm or less	6.59	8.05	5.56	0.50	15.14	12.65	090	
14021		A	defect 10.1 sq cm to 30.0 sq cm	10.06	9.29	7.38	0.69	20.04	18.13	090	
14040		A	Adjacent tissue transfer or rearrangement, forehead, cheeks, chin, mouth, neck, axillae, genitalia, hands and/or feet; defect 10 sq cm or less	7.87	8.19	6.27	0.53	16.59	14.67	090	
14041		A	defect 10.1 sq cm to 30.0 sq cm	11.49	9.90	8.17	0.68	22.07	20.34	090	
14060		A	Adjacent tissue transfer or rearrangement, eyelids, nose, ears and/or lips; defect 10 sq cm or less	8.50	8.64	7.13	0.59	17.73	16.22	090	
14061		A	defect 10.1 sq cm to 30.0 sq cm	12.29	10.85	9.08	0.75	23.89	22.12	090	
14300		A	Adjacent tissue transfer or rearrangement, more than 30 sq cm, unusual or complicated, any area	11.76	10.11	8.68	0.88	22.75	21.32	090	
14350		A	Filleted finger or toe flap, including preparation of recipient site	9.61	6.48	6.48	1.09	17.18	17.18	090	
15000		A	Surgical preparation or creation of recipient site by excision of open wounds, burn eschar, or scar (including subcutaneous tissues); first 100 sq cm or one percent of body area of infants and children	4.00	2.51	1.91	0.37	6.88	6.28	000	
15001		A	each additional 100 sq cm or each additional one percent of body area of infants and children (List separately in addition to code for primary procedure)	1.00	0.64	0.43	0.11	1.75	1.54	ZZZ	
15050		A	Pinch graft, single or multiple, to cover small ulcer, tip of digit, or other minimal open area (except on face), up to defect size 2 cm diameter	4.30	4.98	4.12	0.46	9.74	8.88	090	
15100		A	Split graft, trunk, arms, legs; first 100 sq cm or less, or one percent of body area of infants and children (except 15050)	9.05	6.27	6.26	0.94	16.26	16.25	090	
15101		A	each additional 100 sq cm, or each additional one percent of body area of infants and children, or part thereof (List separately in addition to code for primary procedure)	1.72	1.40	0.76	0.18	3.30	2.66	ZZZ	
15120		A	Split graft, face, scalp, eyelids, mouth, neck, ears, orbits, genitalia, hands, feet and/or multiple digits; first 100 sq cm or less, or one percent of body area of infants and children (except 15050)	9.83	8.62	6.97	0.87	19.32	17.67	090	

■ RVU not developed by CMS. Gap-filled RVUs developed by Ingenix/CHEG.

Code	M	S	Description	Work Value	Non-Fac PE	Fac PE	Mal-practice	Non-Fac Total	Fac Total	Global	Gap
15121		A	each additional 100 sq cm, or each additional one percent of body area of infants and children, or part thereof (List separately in addition to code for primary procedure)	2.67	1.83	1.23	0.27	4.77	4.17	ZZZ	
15200		A	Full thickness graft, free, including direct closure of donor site, trunk; 20 sq cm or less	8.03	9.90	5.64	0.73	18.66	14.4	090	
15201		A	each additional 20 sq cm (List separately in addition to code for primary procedure)	1.32	1.00	0.68	0.14	2.46	2.14	ZZZ	
15220		A	Full thickness graft, free, including direct closure of donor site, scalp, arms, and/or legs; 20 sq cm or less	7.87	9.38	6.47	0.68	17.93	15.02	090	
15221		A	each additional 20 sq cm (List separately in addition to code for primary procedure)	1.19	0.92	0.60	0.12	2.23	1.91	ZZZ	
15240		A	Full thickness graft, free, including direct closure of donor site, forehead, cheeks, chin, mouth, neck, axillae, genitalia, hands, and/or feet; 20 sq cm or less	9.04	9.01	7.27	0.77	18.82	17.08	090	
15241		A	each additional 20 sq cm (List separately in addition to code for primary procedure)	1.86	1.47	0.95	0.17	3.50	2.98	ZZZ	
15260		A	Full thickness graft, free, including direct closure of donor site, nose, ears, eyelids, and/or lips; 20 sq cm or less	10.06	9.01	7.74	0.63	19.7	18.43	090	
15261		A	each additional 20 sq cm (List separately in addition to code for primary procedure)	2.23	1.59	1.16	0.17	3.99	3.56	ZZZ	
15342		A	Application of bilaminate skin substitute/ neodermis; 25 sq cm	1.00	2.18	1.04	0.09	3.27	2.13	010	
15343		A	each additional 25 sq cm (List separately in addition to code for primary procedure)	0.25	0.42	0.10	0.02	0.69	0.37	ZZZ	
15350		A	Application of allograft, skin; 100 sq cm or less	4.00	7.78	4.23	0.42	12.2	8.65	090	
15351		A	each additional 100 sq cm (List separately in addition to code for primary procedure)	1.00	0.85	0.42	0.11	1.96	1.53	ZZZ	
15400		A	Application of xenograft, skin; 100 sq cm or less	4.00	4.89	4.89	0.40	9.29	9.29	090	
15401		A	each additional 100 sq cm (List separately in addition to code for primary procedure)	1.00	1.59	0.47	0.11	2.70	1.58	ZZZ	
15570		A	Formation of direct or tubed pedicle, with or without transfer; trunk	9.21	7.80	6.37	0.96	17.97	16.54	090	
15572		A	scalp, arms, or legs	9.27	8.08	6.34	0.93	18.28	16.54	090	
15574		A	forehead, cheeks, chin, mouth, neck, axillae, genitalia, hands or feet	9.88	8.61	7.14	0.92	19.41	17.94	090	
15576		A	eyelids, nose, ears, lips, or intraoral	8.69	8.89	6.55	0.72	18.30	15.96	090	

Surgery

■ RVU not developed by CMS. Gap-filled RVUs developed by Ingenix/CHEG.

Code	M	S	Description	Work Value	Non-Fac PE	Fac PE	Mal-practice	Non-Fac Total	Fac Total	Global	Gap
15600		A	Delay of flap or sectioning of flap (division and inset); at trunk	1.91	6.66	2.51	0.19	8.76	4.61	090	
15610		A	at scalp, arms, or legs	2.42	5.90	2.67	0.25	8.57	5.34	090	
15620		A	at forehead, cheeks, chin, neck, axillae, genitalia, hands (except 15625), or feet	2.94	7.04	3.54	0.28	10.26	6.76	090	
15630		A	at eyelids, nose, ears, or lips	3.27	6.09	3.83	0.28	9.64	7.38	090	
15650		A	Transfer, intermediate, of any pedicle flap (eg, abdomen to wrist, Walking tube), any location	3.97	5.69	3.99	0.36	10.02	8.32	090	
15732		A	Muscle, myocutaneous, or fasciocutaneous flap; head and neck (eg, temporalis, masseter muscle, sternocleidomastoid, levator scapulae)	17.84	11.63	11.63	1.50	30.97	30.97	090	
15734		A	trunk	17.79	11.49	11.49	1.91	31.19	31.19	090	
15736		A	upper extremity	16.27	11.14	11.14	1.78	29.19	29.19	090	
15738		A	lower extremity	17.92	11.47	11.47	1.95	31.34	31.34	090	
15740		A	Flap; island pedicle	10.25	8.74	7.20	0.62	19.61	18.07	090	
15750		A	neurovascular pedicle	11.41	8.45	8.45	1.12	20.98	20.98	090	
15756		A	Free muscle flap with or without skin with microvascular anastomosis	35.23	22.50	22.50	3.11	60.84	60.84	090	
15757		A	Free skin flap with microvascular anastomosis	35.23	22.54	22.54	3.37	61.14	61.14	090	
15758		A	Free fascial flap with microvascular anastomosis	35.10	22.75	22.75	3.52	61.37	61.37	090	
15760		A	Graft; composite (eg, full thickness of external ear or nasal ala), including primary closure, donor area	8.74	9.27	6.93	0.72	18.73	16.39	090	
15770		A	derma-fat-fascia	7.52	6.14	6.14	0.78	14.44	14.44	090	
15775		R	Punch graft for hair transplant; 1 to 15 punch grafts	3.96	3.12	1.60	0.43	7.51	5.99	000	
15776		R	more than 15 punch grafts	5.54	3.97	2.97	0.60	10.11	9.11	000	
15780		A	Dermabrasion; total face (eg, for acne scarring, fine wrinkling, rhytids, general keratosis)	7.29	6.41	6.13	0.41	14.11	13.83	090	
15781		A	segmental, face	4.85	5.17	4.83	0.27	10.29	9.95	090	
15782		A	regional, other than face	4.32	4.37	4.09	0.21	8.90	8.62	090	
15783		A	superficial, any site, (eg, tattoo removal)	4.29	5.02	3.51	0.26	9.57	8.06	090	
15786*		A	Abrasion; single lesion (eg, keratosis, scar)	2.03	1.73	1.29	0.11	3.87	3.43	010	
15787		A	each additional four lesions or less (List separately in addition to code for primary procedure)	0.33	0.39	0.18	0.02	0.74	0.53	ZZZ	

■ RVU not developed by CMS. Gap-filled RVUs developed by Ingenix/CHEG.

Code	M	S	Description	Work Value	Non-Fac PE	Fac PE	Mal-practice	Non-Fac Total	Fac Total	Global	Gap
15788		R	Chemical peel, facial; epidermal	2.09	3.15	1.07	0.11	5.35	3.27	090	
15789		R	dermal	4.92	5.65	3.32	0.27	10.84	8.51	090	
15792		R	Chemical peel, nonfacial; epidermal	1.86	2.87	1.63	0.10	4.83	3.59	090	
15793		A	dermal	3.74	3.81	3.81	0.17	7.72	7.72	090	
15810		A	Salabrasion; 20 sq cm or less	4.74	4.04	4.04	0.42	9.20	9.20	090	
15811		A	over 20 sq cm	5.39	5.85	5.06	0.52	11.76	10.97	090	
15819		A	Cervicoplasty	9.38	6.24	6.24	0.77	16.39	16.39	090	
15820		A	Blepharoplasty, lower eyelid;	5.15	10.34	7.13	0.30	15.79	12.58	090	
15821		A	with extensive herniated fat pad	5.72	11.87	7.34	0.31	17.90	13.37	090	
15822		A	Blepharoplasty, upper eyelid;	4.45	10.58	6.58	0.22	15.25	11.25	090	
15823		A	with excessive skin weighting down lid	7.05	11.38	7.60	0.32	18.75	14.97	090	
15824		R	Rhytidectomy; forehead	10.30	8.19	8.19	1.10	19.59	19.59	000	■
15825		R	neck with platysmal tightening (platysmal flap, P-flap)	11.78	9.36	9.36	1.25	22.39	22.39	000	■
15826		R	glabellar frown lines	10.30	8.19	8.19	1.10	19.59	19.59	000	■
15828		R	cheek, chin, and neck	27.24	21.64	21.64	2.90	51.78	51.78	000	■
15829		R	superficial musculoaponeurotic system (SMAS) flap	30.18	23.98	23.98	3.21	57.37	57.37	000	■
15831		A	Excision, excessive skin and subcutaneous tissue (including lipectomy); abdomen (abdominoplasty)	12.40	8.14	8.14	1.30	21.84	21.84	090	
15832		A	thigh	11.59	8.04	8.04	1.21	20.84	20.84	090	
15833		A	leg	10.64	7.34	7.34	1.17	19.15	19.15	090	
15834		A	hip	10.85	7.59	7.59	1.18	19.62	19.62	090	
15835		A	buttock	11.67	7.94	7.94	1.13	20.74	20.74	090	
15836		A	arm	9.34	6.51	6.51	0.95	16.80	16.80	090	
15837		A	forearm or hand	8.43	7.30	6.38	0.78	16.51	15.59	090	
15838		A	submental fat pad	7.13	5.70	5.70	0.58	13.41	13.41	090	
15839		A	other area	9.38	7.64	5.97	0.88	17.90	16.23	090	
15840		A	Graft for facial nerve paralysis; free fascia graft (including obtaining fascia)	13.26	10.10	10.10	1.15	24.51	24.51	090	
15841		A	free muscle graft (including obtaining graft)	23.26	14.68	14.68	2.65	40.59	40.59	090	

■ RVU not developed by CMS. Gap-filled RVUs developed by Ingenix/CHEG.

Code	M	S	Description	Work Value	Non-Fac PE	Fac PE	Mal-practice	Non-Fac Total	Fac Total	Global	Gap
15842		A	free muscle flap by microsurgical technique	37.96	22.81	22.81	3.99	64.76	64.76	090	
15845		A	regional muscle transfer	12.57	8.81	8.81	0.80	22.18	22.18	090	
15850		B	Removal of sutures under anesthesia (other than local), same surgeon	0.78	1.43	0.31	0.04	2.25	1.13	XXX	
15851		A	Removal of sutures under anesthesia (other than local), other surgeon	0.86	1.64	0.35	0.05	2.55	1.26	000	
15852		A	Dressing change (for other than burns) under anesthesia (other than local)	0.86	1.93	0.36	0.07	2.86	1.29	000	
15860		A	Intravenous injection of agent (eg, fluorescein) to test vascular flow in flap or graft	1.95	1.35	0.84	0.13	3.43	2.92	000	
15876		R	Suction assisted lipectomy; head and neck	0.00	0.00	0.00	0.00	0.00	0.00	000	
15877		R	trunk	0.00	0.00	0.00	0.00	0.00	0.00	000	
15878		R	upper extremity	0.00	0.00	0.00	0.00	0.00	0.00	000	
15879		R	lower extremity	0.00	0.00	0.00	0.00	0.00	0.00	000	
15920		A	Excision, coccygeal pressure ulcer, with coccygectomy; with primary suture	7.95	5.90	5.90	0.83	14.68	14.68	090	
15922		A	with flap closure	9.90	7.78	7.78	1.06	18.74	18.74	090	
15931		A	Excision, sacral pressure ulcer, with primary suture;	9.24	5.89	5.89	0.95	16.08	16.08	090	
15933		A	with ostectomy	10.85	8.32	8.32	1.14	20.31	20.31	090	
15934		A	Excision, sacral pressure ulcer, with skin flap closure;	12.69	8.48	8.48	1.35	22.52	22.52	090	
15935		A	with ostectomy	14.57	10.12	10.12	1.56	26.25	26.25	090	
15936		A	Excision, sacral pressure ulcer, in preparation for muscle or myocutaneous flap or skin graft closure;	12.38	8.81	8.81	1.32	22.51	22.51	090	
15937		A	with ostectomy	14.21	10.75	10.75	1.51	26.47	26.47	090	
15940		A	Excision, ischial pressure ulcer, with primary suture;	9.34	6.17	6.17	0.98	16.49	16.49	090	
15941		A	with ostectomy (ischiectomy)	11.43	10.44	10.44	1.23	23.10	23.10	090	
15944		A	Excision, ischial pressure ulcer, with skin flap closure;	11.46	8.77	8.77	1.21	21.44	21.44	090	
15945		A	with ostectomy	12.69	9.73	9.73	1.38	23.80	23.80	090	
15946		A	Excision, ischial pressure ulcer, with ostectomy, in preparation for muscle or myocutaneous flap or skin graft closure	21.57	14.65	14.65	2.32	38.54	38.54	090	
15950		A	Excision, trochanteric pressure ulcer, with primary suture;	7.54	5.43	5.43	0.80	13.77	13.77	090	

■ RVU not developed by CMS. Gap-filled RVUs developed by Ingenix/CHEG.

Code	M	S	Description	Work Value	Non-Fac PE	Fac PE	Mal-practice	Non-Fac Total	Fac Total	Global	Gap
15951		A	with ostectomy	10.72	8.07	8.07	1.14	19.93	19.93	090	
15952		A	Excision, trochanteric pressure ulcer, with skin flap closure;	11.39	7.86	7.86	1.19	20.44	20.44	090	
15953		A	with ostectomy	12.63	9.24	9.24	1.38	23.25	23.25	090	
15956		A	Excision, trochanteric pressure ulcer, in preparation for muscle or myocutaneous flap or skin graft closure;	15.52	10.71	10.71	1.64	27.87	27.87	090	
15958		A	with ostectomy	15.48	11.20	11.20	1.66	28.34	28.34	090	
15999		C	Unlisted procedure, excision pressure ulcer	0.00	0.00	0.00	0.00	0.00	0.00	YYY	
16000		A	Initial treatment, first degree burn, when no more than local treatment is required	0.89	1.09	0.27	0.06	2.04	1.22	000	
16010		A	Dressings and/or debridement, initial or subsequent; under anesthesia, small	0.87	1.21	0.37	0.07	2.15	1.31	000	
16015		A	under anesthesia, medium or large, or with major debridement	2.35	2.01	1.03	0.22	4.58	3.60	000	
16020*		A	without anesthesia, office or hospital, small	0.80	1.20	0.27	0.06	2.06	1.13	000	
16025*		A	without anesthesia, medium (eg, whole face or whole extremity)	1.85	1.94	0.69	0.16	3.95	2.70	000	
16030		A	without anesthesia, large (eg, more than one extremity)	2.08	3.36	0.97	0.18	5.62	3.23	000	
16035		A	Escharotomy; initial incision	3.75	1.56	1.56	0.36	5.67	5.67	090	
16036		A	each additional incision (List separately in addition to code for primary procedure)	1.50	0.62	0.62	0.11	2.23	2.23	ZZZ	
17000*		A	Destruction (eg, laser surgery, electrosurgery, cryosurgery, chemosurgery, surgical curettement), all benign or premalignant lesions (eg, actinic keratoses) other than skin tags or cutaneous vascular proliferative lesions; first lesion	0.60	1.10	0.28	0.03	1.73	0.91	010	
17003		A	second through 14 lesions, each (List separately in addition to code for first lesion)	0.15	0.24	0.07	0.01	0.40	0.23	ZZZ	
17004		A	Destruction (eg, laser surgery, electrosurgery, cryosurgery, chemosurgery, surgical curettement), all benign or premalignant lesions (eg, actinic keratoses) other than skin tags or cutaneous vascular proliferative lesions; 15 or more lesions	2.79	2.56	1.30	0.12	5.47	4.21	010	
17106		A	Destruction of cutaneous vascular proliferative lesions (eg, laser technique); less than 10 sq cm	4.59	4.88	2.88	0.28	9.75	7.75	090	
17107		A	10.0 - 50.0 sq cm	9.16	6.92	5.28	0.53	16.61	14.97	090	
17108		A	over 50.0 sq cm	13.20	8.87	7.26	0.89	22.96	21.35	090	

■ RVU not developed by CMS. Gap-filled RVUs developed by Ingenix/CHEG.

Code	M	S	Description	Work Value	Non-Fac PE	Fac PE	Mal-practice	Non-Fac Total	Fac Total	Global	Gap
17110*		A	Destruction (eg, laser surgery, electrosurgery, cryosurgery, chemosurgery, surgical curettement), of flat warts, molluscum contagiosum, or milia; up to 14 lesions	0.65	1.11	0.26	0.04	1.80	0.95	010	
17111		A	15 or more lesions	0.92	1.13	0.41	0.04	2.09	1.37	010	
17250*		A	Chemical cauterization of granulation tissue (proud flesh, sinus or fistula)	0.50	0.76	0.21	0.04	1.30	0.75	000	
17260*		A	Destruction, malignant lesion (eg, laser surgery, electrosurgery, cryosurgery, chemosurgery, surgical curettement), trunk, arms or legs; lesion diameter 0.5 cm or less	0.91	1.37	0.39	0.04	2.32	1.34	010	
17261		A	lesion diameter 0.6 to 1.0 cm	1.17	1.48	0.56	0.05	2.70	1.78	010	
17262		A	lesion diameter 1.1 to 2.0 cm	1.58	1.69	0.76	0.07	3.34	2.41	010	
17263		A	lesion diameter 2.1 to 3.0 cm	1.79	1.80	0.83	0.08	3.67	2.70	010	
17264		A	lesion diameter 3.1 to 4.0 cm	1.94	1.87	0.87	0.08	3.89	2.89	010	
17266		A	lesion diameter over 4.0 cm	2.34	2.08	1.05	0.11	4.53	3.50	010	
17270*		A	Destruction, malignant lesion (eg, laser surgery, electrosurgery, cryosurgery, chemosurgery, surgical curettement), scalp, neck, hands, feet, genitalia; lesion diameter 0.5 cm or less	1.32	1.57	0.60	0.06	2.95	1.98	010	
17271		A	lesion diameter 0.6 to 1.0 cm	1.49	1.65	0.72	0.06	3.20	2.27	010	
17272		A	lesion diameter 1.1 to 2.0 cm	1.77	1.79	0.86	0.07	3.63	2.70	010	
17273		A	lesion diameter 2.1 to 3.0 cm	2.05	1.93	0.97	0.09	4.07	3.11	010	
17274		A	lesion diameter 3.1 to 4.0 cm	2.59	2.21	1.20	0.11	4.91	3.90	010	
17276		A	lesion diameter over 4.0 cm	3.20	2.52	1.84	0.15	5.87	5.19	010	
17280*		A	Destruction, malignant lesion (eg, laser surgery, electrosurgery, cryosurgery, chemosurgery, surgical curettement), face, ears, eyelids, nose, lips, mucous membrane; lesion diameter 0.5 cm or less	1.17	1.41	0.54	0.05	2.63	1.76	010	
17281		A	lesion diameter 0.6 to 1.0 cm	1.72	1.77	0.83	0.07	3.56	2.62	010	
17282		A	lesion diameter 1.1 to 2.0 cm	2.04	1.93	0.99	0.09	4.06	3.12	010	
17283		A	lesion diameter 2.1 to 3.0 cm	2.64	2.23	1.24	0.11	4.98	3.99	010	
17284		A	lesion diameter 3.1 to 4.0 cm	3.21	2.52	1.51	0.14	5.87	4.86	010	
17286		A	lesion diameter over 4.0 cm	4.44	3.23	2.52	0.22	7.89	7.18	010	

Surgery

■ RVU not developed by CMS. Gap-filled RVUs developed by Ingenix/CHEG.

Code	M	S	Description	Work Value	Non-Fac PE	Fac PE	Mal-practice	Non-Fac Total	Fac Total	Global	Gap
17304		A	Chemosurgery (Mohs' micrographic technique), including removal of all gross tumor, surgical excision of tissue specimens, mapping, color coding of specimens, microscopic examination of specimens by the surgeon, and complete histopathologic preparation; first stage, fresh tissue technique, up to 5 specimens	7.60	7.76	3.74	0.31	15.67	11.65	000	
17305		A	second stage, fixed or fresh tissue, up to 5 specimens	2.85	3.60	1.40	0.12	6.57	4.37	000	
17306		A	third stage, fixed or fresh tissue, up to 5 specimens	2.85	3.64	1.41	0.12	6.61	4.38	000	
17307		A	additional stage(s), up to 5 specimens, each stage	2.85	3.62	1.43	0.12	6.59	4.40	000	
17310		A	more than 5 specimens, fixed or fresh tissue, any stage	0.95	1.54	0.48	0.05	2.54	1.48	000	
17340*		A	Cryotherapy (CO2 slush, liquid N2) for acne	0.76	0.39	0.27	0.04	1.19	1.07	010	
17360*		A	Chemical exfoliation for acne (eg, acne paste, acid)	1.43	1.46	0.73	0.06	2.95	2.22	010	
17380*		R	Electrolysis epilation, each 1/2 hour	0.75	0.59	0.59	0.08	1.42	1.42	000	■
17999		C	Unlisted procedure, skin, mucous membrane and subcutaneous tissue	0.00	0.00	0.00	0.00	0.00	0.00	YYY	
19000*		A	Puncture aspiration of cyst of breast;	0.84	1.27	0.30	0.07	2.18	1.21	000	
19001		A	each additional cyst (List separately in addition to code for primary procedure)	0.42	0.86	0.15	0.03	1.31	0.60	ZZZ	
19020		A	Mastotomy with exploration or drainage of abscess, deep	3.57	7.13	3.51	0.35	11.05	7.43	090	
19030		A	Injection procedure only for mammary ductogram or galactogram	1.53	3.70	0.54	0.07	5.30	2.14	000	
19100		A	Biopsy of breast; percutaneous, needle core, not using imaging guidance (separate procedure)	1.27	1.50	0.45	0.10	2.87	1.82	000	
19101		A	open, incisional	3.18	5.27	1.97	0.20	8.65	5.35	010	
19102		A	percutaneous, needle core, using imaging guidance	2.00	5.13	0.71	0.13	7.26	2.84	000	
19103		A	percutaneous, automated vacuum assisted or rotating biopsy device, using imaging guidance	3.70	12.73	1.31	0.16	16.59	5.17	000	
19110		A	Nipple exploration, with or without excision of a solitary lactiferous duct or a papilloma lactiferous duct	4.30	9.79	4.56	0.44	14.53	9.30	090	
19112		A	Excision of lactiferous duct fistula	3.67	10.91	3.19	0.38	14.96	7.24	090	

■ RVU not developed by CMS. Gap-filled RVUs developed by Ingenix/CHEG.

Code	M	S	Description	Work Value	Non-Fac PE	Fac PE	Mal-practice	Non-Fac Total	Fac Total	Global	Gap
19120		A	Excision of cyst, fibroadenoma, or other benign or malignant tumor aberrant breast tissue, duct lesion, nipple or areolar lesion (except 19140), open, male or female, one or more lesions	5.56	5.18	3.20	0.56	11.30	9.32	090	
19125		A	Excision of breast lesion identified by pre-operative placement of radiological marker, open; single lesion	6.06	5.36	3.36	0.61	12.03	10.03	090	
19126		A	each additional lesion separately identified by a pre-operative radiological marker (List separately in addition to code for primary procedure)	2.93	1.06	1.06	0.30	4.29	4.29	ZZZ	
19140		A	Mastectomy for gynecomastia	5.14	10.26	3.79	0.52	15.92	9.45	090	
19160		A	Mastectomy, partial;	5.99	4.62	4.62	0.61	11.22	11.22	090	
19162		A	with axillary lymphadenectomy	13.53	8.07	8.07	1.38	22.98	22.98	090	
19180		A	Mastectomy, simple, complete	8.80	6.08	6.08	0.88	15.76	15.76	090	
19182		A	Mastectomy, subcutaneous	7.73	5.06	5.06	0.79	13.58	13.58	090	
19200		A	Mastectomy, radical, including pectoral muscles, axillary lymph nodes	15.49	9.33	9.33	1.51	26.33	26.33	090	
19220		A	Mastectomy, radical, including pectoral muscles, axillary and internal mammary lymph nodes (Urban type operation)	15.72	9.52	9.52	1.56	26.80	26.80	090	
19240		A	Mastectomy, modified radical, including axillary lymph nodes, with or without pectoralis minor muscle, but excluding pectoralis major muscle	16.00	8.94	8.94	1.62	26.56	26.56	090	
19260		A	Excision of chest wall tumor including ribs	15.44	9.12	9.12	1.64	26.20	26.20	090	
19271		A	Excision of chest wall tumor involving ribs, with plastic reconstruction; without mediastinal lymphadenectomy	18.90	11.13	11.13	2.27	32.30	32.30	090	
19272		A	with mediastinal lymphadenectomy	21.55	12.36	12.36	2.54	36.45	36.45	090	
19290		A	Pre-operative placement of needle localization wire, breast;	1.27	2.95	0.45	0.06	4.28	1.78	000	
19291		A	each additional lesion (List separately in addition to code for primary procedure)	0.63	1.74	0.22	0.03	2.40	0.88	ZZZ	
19295		A	Image guided placement, metallic localization clip, percutaneous, during breast biopsy (List separately in addition to code for primary procedure)	0.00	2.83	2.83	0.01	2.84	2.84	ZZZ	
19316		A	Mastopexy	10.69	8.00	8.00	1.15	19.84	19.84	090	
19318		A	Reduction mammaplasty	15.62	10.64	10.64	1.69	27.95	27.95	090	
19324		A	Mammaplasty, augmentation; without prosthetic implant	5.85	4.41	4.41	0.63	10.89	10.89	090	

■ RVU not developed by CMS. Gap-filled RVUs developed by Ingenix/CHEG.

Code	M	S	Description	Work Value	Non-Fac PE	Fac PE	Mal-practice	Non-Fac Total	Fac Total	Global	Gap
19325		**A**	with prosthetic implant	8.45	7.00	7.00	0.90	16.35	16.35	090	
19328		**A**	Removal of intact mammary implant	5.68	4.73	4.73	0.61	11.02	11.02	090	
19330		**A**	Removal of mammary implant material	7.59	5.41	5.41	0.81	13.81	13.81	090	
19340		**A**	Immediate insertion of breast prosthesis following mastopexy, mastectomy or in reconstruction	6.33	3.30	3.30	0.68	10.31	10.31	ZZZ	
19342		**A**	Delayed insertion of breast prosthesis following mastopexy, mastectomy or in reconstruction	11.20	8.15	8.15	1.21	20.56	20.56	090	
19350		**A**	Nipple/areola reconstruction	8.92	14.55	7.09	0.95	24.42	16.96	090	
19355		**A**	Correction of inverted nipples	7.57	12.42	5.93	0.80	20.79	14.30	090	
19357		**A**	Breast reconstruction, immediate or delayed, with tissue expander, including subsequent expansion	18.16	14.4	14.4	1.96	34.52	34.52	090	
19361		**A**	Breast reconstruction with latissimus dorsi flap, with or without prosthetic implant	19.26	12.45	12.45	2.08	33.79	33.79	090	
19364		**A**	Breast reconstruction with free flap	41.00	25.45	25.45	3.91	70.36	70.36	090	
19366		**A**	Breast reconstruction with other technique	21.28	12.02	12.02	2.27	35.57	35.57	090	
19367		**A**	Breast reconstruction with transverse rectus abdominis myocutaneous flap (TRAM), single pedicle, including closure of donor site;	25.73	15.77	15.77	2.78	44.28	44.28	090	
19368		**A**	with microvascular anastomosis (supercharging)	32.42	19.04	19.04	3.51	54.97	54.97	090	
19369		**A**	Breast reconstruction with transverse rectus abdominis myocutaneous flap (TRAM), double pedicle, including closure of donor site	29.82	18.29	18.29	3.24	51.35	51.35	090	
19370		**A**	Open periprosthetic capsulotomy, breast	8.05	6.39	6.39	0.86	15.3	15.30	090	
19371		**A**	Periprosthetic capsulectomy, breast	9.35	7.46	7.46	1.01	17.82	17.82	090	
19380		**A**	Revision of reconstructed breast	9.14	7.35	7.35	0.98	17.47	17.47	090	
19396		**A**	Preparation of moulage for custom breast implant	2.17	7.08	0.87	0.23	9.48	3.27	000	
19499		**C**	Unlisted procedure, breast	0.00	0.00	0.00	0.00	0.00	0.00	YYY	

Surgery

■ RVU not developed by CMS. Gap-filled RVUs developed by Ingenix/CHEG.

Code	M	S	Description	Work Value	Non-Fac PE	Fac PE	Mal-prac-tice	Non-Fac Total	Fac Total	Global	Gap
20000*		A	Incision of soft tissue abscess (eg, secondary to osteomyelitis); superficial	2.12	2.23	1.20	0.17	4.52	3.49	010	
20005		A	deep or complicated	3.42	3.07	2.22	0.34	6.83	5.98	010	
20100		A	Exploration of penetrating wound (separate procedure); neck	10.08	6.49	4.12	0.99	17.56	15.19	010	
20101		A	chest	3.22	3.03	1.64	0.24	6.49	5.10	010	
20102		A	abdomen/flank/back	3.94	3.43	1.85	0.35	7.72	6.14	010	
20103		A	extremity	5.30	4.41	3.01	0.57	10.28	8.88	010	
20150		A	Excision of epiphyseal bar, with or without autogenous soft tissue graft obtained through same fascial incision	13.69	9.72	9.72	0.96	24.37	24.37	090	
20200		A	Biopsy, muscle; superficial	1.46	1.72	0.62	0.17	3.35	2.25	000	
20205		A	deep	2.35	4.04	0.98	0.23	6.62	3.56	000	
20206*		A	Biopsy, muscle, percutaneous needle	0.99	3.27	0.36	0.06	4.32	1.41	000	
20220		A	Biopsy, bone, trocar, or needle; superficial (eg, ilium, sternum, spinous process, ribs)	1.27	4.96	2.98	0.06	6.29	4.31	000	
20225		A	deep (eg, vertebral body, femur)	1.87	4.47	3.06	0.11	6.45	5.04	000	
20240		A	Biopsy, bone, excisional; superficial (eg, ilium, sternum, spinous process, ribs, trochanter of femur)	3.23	4.15	4.15	0.33	7.71	7.71	010	
20245		A	deep (eg, humerus, ischium, femur)	7.78	6.91	6.91	0.44	15.13	15.13	010	
20250		A	Biopsy, vertebral body, open; thoracic	5.03	4.37	4.37	0.50	9.90	9.90	010	
20251		A	lumbar or cervical	5.56	4.86	4.86	0.79	11.21	11.21	010	
20500*		A	Injection of sinus tract; therapeutic (separate procedure)	1.23	5.34	3.91	0.10	6.67	5.24	010	
20501*		A	diagnostic (sinogram)	0.76	3.32	0.27	0.03	4.11	1.06	000	
20520*		A	Removal of foreign body in muscle or tendon sheath; simple	1.85	5.62	3.62	0.17	7.64	5.64	010	
20525		A	deep or complicated	3.50	7.26	4.40	0.40	11.16	8.30	010	
20526		A	Injection, therapeutic (eg, local anesthetic, corticosteroid), carpal tunnel	0.86	0.78	0.39	0.06	1.70	1.31	000	
20550*		A	Injection; tendon sheath, ligament, ganglion cyst	0.86	0.85	0.28	0.06	1.77	1.20	000	
20551		A	tendon origin/insertion	0.86	0.78	0.39	0.06	1.70	1.31	000	
20552		A	single or multiple trigger point(s), one or two muscle group(s)	0.86	0.78	0.39	0.06	1.70	1.31	000	

■ RVU not developed by CMS. Gap-filled RVUs developed by Ingenix/CHEG.

Code	M	S	Description	Work Value	Non-Fac PE	Fac PE	Mal-practice	Non-Fac Total	Fac Total	Global	Gap
20553		A	single or multiple trigger point(s), three or more muscle groups	0.86	0.78	0.39	0.06	1.7	1.31	000	
20600*		A	Arthrocentesis, aspiration and/or injection; small joint, bursa or ganglion cyst (eg, fingers, toes)	0.66	0.67	0.37	0.06	1.39	1.09	000	
20605*		A	intermediate joint, bursa or ganglion cyst (eg, temporomandibular, acromioclavicular, wrist, elbow or ankle, olecranon bursa)	0.68	0.78	0.38	0.06	1.52	1.12	000	
20610*		A	major joint or bursa (eg, shoulder, hip, knee joint, subacromial bursa)	0.79	0.96	0.44	0.08	1.83	1.31	000	
20615		A	Aspiration and injection for treatment of bone cyst	2.28	4.89	2.52	0.19	7.36	4.99	010	
20650*		A	Insertion of wire or pin with application of skeletal traction, including removal (separate procedure)	2.23	5.06	3.19	0.28	7.57	5.70	010	
20660		A	Application of cranial tongs, caliper, or stereotactic frame, including removal (separate procedure)	2.51	1.49	1.49	0.48	4.48	4.48	000	
20661		A	Application of halo, including removal; cranial	4.89	6.74	6.74	0.92	12.55	12.55	090	
20662		A	pelvic	6.07	5.12	5.12	0.81	12.00	12.00	090	
20663		A	femoral	5.43	4.94	4.94	0.77	11.14	11.14	090	
20664		A	Application of halo, including removal, cranial, 6 or more pins placed, for thin skull osteology (eg, pediatric patients, hydrocephalus, osteogenesis imperfecta), requiring general anesthesia	8.06	8.55	8.55	1.49	18.10	18.10	090	
20665*		A	Removal of tongs or halo applied by another physician	1.31	2.33	1.25	0.17	3.81	2.73	010	
20670*		A	Removal of implant; superficial, (eg, buried wire, pin or rod) (separate procedure)	1.74	5.73	3.42	0.23	7.70	5.39	010	
20680		A	deep (eg, buried wire, pin, screw, metal band, nail, rod or plate)	3.35	5.04	5.04	0.46	8.85	8.85	090	
20690		A	Application of a uniplane (pins or wires in one plane), unilateral, external fixation system	3.52	1.91	1.91	0.47	5.90	5.90	090	
20692		A	Application of a multiplane (pins or wires in more than one plane), unilateral, external fixation system (eg, Ilizarov, Monticelli type)	6.41	3.57	3.57	0.60	10.58	10.58	090	
20693		A	Adjustment or revision of external fixation system requiring anesthesia (eg, new pin(s) or wire(s) and/or new ring(s) or bar(s))	5.86	12.98	12.98	0.85	19.69	19.69	090	
20694		A	Removal, under anesthesia, of external fixation system	4.16	8.96	6.30	0.57	13.69	11.03	090	

■ RVU not developed by CMS. Gap-filled RVUs developed by Ingenix/CHEG.

Code	M	S	Description	Work Value	Non-Fac PE	Fac PE	Mal-practice	Non-Fac Total	Fac Total	Global	Gap
20802		A	Replantation, arm (includes surgical neck of humerus through elbow joint), complete amputation	41.15	28.95	28.95	5.81	75.91	75.91	090	
20805		A	Replantation, forearm (includes radius and ulna to radial carpal joint), complete amputation	50.00	38.72	38.72	3.95	92.67	92.67	090	
20808		A	Replantation, hand (includes hand through metacarpophalangeal joints), complete amputation	61.65	56.41	56.41	6.49	124.55	124.55	090	
20816		A	Replantation, digit, excluding thumb (includes metacarpophalangeal joint to insertion of flexor sublimis tendon), complete amputation	30.94	49.50	49.50	3.01	83.45	83.45	090	
20822		A	Replantation, digit, excluding thumb (includes distal tip to sublimis tendon insertion), complete amputation	25.59	45.97	45.97	3.07	74.63	74.63	090	
20824		A	Replantation, thumb (includes carpometacarpal joint to MP joint), complete amputation	30.94	49.10	49.10	3.48	83.52	83.52	090	
20827		A	Replantation, thumb (includes distal tip to MP joint), complete amputation	26.41	45.65	45.65	3.21	75.27	75.27	090	
20838		A	Replantation, foot, complete amputation	41.41	25.82	25.82	5.85	73.08	73.08	090	
20900		A	Bone graft, any donor area; minor or small (eg, dowel or button)	5.58	5.97	5.97	0.77	12.32	12.32	090	
20902		A	major or large	7.55	8.91	8.91	1.06	17.52	17.52	090	
20910		A	Cartilage graft; costochondral	5.34	9.09	6.94	0.50	14.93	12.78	090	
20912		A	nasal septum	6.35	7.68	7.68	0.55	14.58	14.58	090	
20920		A	Fascia lata graft; by stripper	5.31	5.44	5.44	0.54	11.29	11.29	090	
20922		A	by incision and area exposure, complex or sheet	6.61	8.50	6.28	0.88	15.99	13.77	090	
20924		A	Tendon graft, from a distance (eg, palmaris, toe extensor, plantaris)	6.48	7.03	7.03	0.82	14.33	14.33	090	
20926		A	Tissue grafts, other (eg, paratenon, fat, dermis)	5.53	6.54	6.54	0.73	12.80	12.80	090	
20930		B	Allograft for spine surgery only; morselized	1.35	1.07	1.07	0.14	2.56	2.56	XXX	■
20931		A	structural	1.81	0.98	0.98	0.34	3.13	3.13	ZZZ	
20936		B	Autograft for spine surgery only (includes harvesting the graft); local (eg, ribs, spinous process, or laminar fragments) obtained from same incision	1.40	1.11	1.11	0.15	2.66	2.66	XXX	■
20937		A	morselized (through separate skin or fascial incision)	2.79	1.54	1.54	0.43	4.76	4.76	ZZZ	
20938		A	structural, bicortical or tricortical (through separate skin or fascial incision)	3.02	1.64	1.64	0.52	5.18	5.18	ZZZ	

■ RVU not developed by CMS. Gap-filled RVUs developed by Ingenix/CHEG.

Surgery

Code	M	S	Description	Work Value	Non-Fac PE	Fac PE	Mal-practice	Non-Fac Total	Fac Total	Global	Gap
20950		A	Monitoring of interstitial fluid pressure (includes insertion of device, eg, wick catheter technique, needle manometer technique) in detection of muscle compartment syndrome	1.26	2.15	2.15	0.16	3.57	3.57	000	
20955		A	Bone graft with microvascular anastomosis; fibula	39.21	30.52	30.52	4.35	74.08	74.08	090	
20956		A	iliac crest	39.27	28.18	28.18	5.77	73.22	73.22	090	
20957		A	metatarsal	40.65	21.71	21.71	5.74	68.10	68.10	090	
20962		A	other than fibula, iliac crest, or metatarsal	39.27	28.54	28.54	5.19	73.00	73.00	090	
20969		A	Free osteocutaneous flap with microvascular anastomosis; other than iliac crest, metatarsal, or great toe	43.92	33.31	33.31	4.34	81.57	81.57	090	
20970		A	iliac crest	43.06	30.08	30.08	4.64	77.78	77.78	090	
20972		A	metatarsal	42.99	18.23	18.23	6.07	67.29	67.29	090	
20973		A	great toe with web space	45.76	30.52	30.52	4.65	80.93	80.93	090	
20974		A	Electrical stimulation to aid bone healing; noninvasive (nonoperative)	0.62	0.47	0.34	0.09	1.18	1.05	000	
20975		A	invasive (operative)	2.60	1.42	1.42	0.42	4.44	4.44	000	
20979		A	Low intensity ultrasound stimulation to aid bone healing, noninvasive (nonoperative)	0.62	0.58	0.25	0.04	1.24	0.91	000	
20999		C	Unlisted procedure, musculoskeletal system, general	0.00	0.00	0.00	0.00	0.00	0.00	YYY	
21010		A	Arthrotomy, temporomandibular joint	10.14	7.24	7.24	0.54	17.92	17.92	090	
21015		A	Radical resection of tumor (eg, malignant neoplasm), soft tissue of face or scalp	5.29	7.38	7.38	0.52	13.19	13.19	090	
21025		A	Excision of bone (eg, for osteomyelitis or bone abscess); mandible	10.06	7.40	7.00	0.79	18.25	17.85	090	
21026		A	facial bone(s)	4.85	5.23	5.12	0.4	10.48	10.37	090	
21029		A	Removal by contouring of benign tumor of facial bone (eg, fibrous dysplasia)	7.71	7.18	6.73	0.74	15.63	15.18	090	
21030		A	Excision of benign tumor or cyst of facial bone other than mandible	6.46	5.47	4.94	0.6	12.53	12.00	090	
21031		A	Excision of torus mandibularis	3.24	3.39	2.19	0.28	6.91	5.71	090	
21032		A	Excision of maxillary torus palatinus	3.24	3.38	2.47	0.27	6.89	5.98	090	
21034		A	Excision of malignant tumor of facial bone other than mandible	16.17	10.59	10.59	1.37	28.13	28.13	090	
21040		A	Excision of benign cyst or tumor of mandible; simple	2.11	3.03	1.81	0.19	5.33	4.11	090	
21041		A	complex	6.71	5.68	4.46	0.56	12.95	11.73	090	

■ RVU not developed by CMS. Gap-filled RVUs developed by Ingenix/CHEG.

Code	M	S	Description	Work Value	Non-Fac PE	Fac PE	Mal-practice	Non-Fac Total	Fac Total	Global	Gap
21044		A	Excision of malignant tumor of mandible;	11.86	8.33	8.33	0.87	21.06	21.06	090	
21045		A	radical resection	16.17	10.63	10.63	1.20	28.00	28.00	090	
21050		A	Condylectomy, temporomandibular joint (separate procedure)	10.77	11.93	11.93	0.84	23.54	23.54	090	
21060		A	Meniscectomy, partial or complete, temporomandibular joint (separate procedure)	10.23	10.59	10.59	1.16	21.98	21.98	090	
21070		A	Coronoidectomy (separate procedure)	8.20	6.36	6.36	0.67	15.23	15.23	090	
21076		A	Impression and custom preparation; surgical obturator prosthesis	13.42	9.87	7.41	1.36	24.65	22.19	010	
21077		A	orbital prosthesis	33.75	24.83	18.64	3.43	62.01	55.82	090	
21079		A	interim obturator prosthesis	22.34	17.55	12.90	1.59	41.48	36.83	090	
21080		A	definitive obturator prosthesis	25.10	19.72	14.49	2.55	47.37	42.14	090	
21081		A	mandibular resection prosthesis	22.88	17.97	13.21	1.87	42.72	37.96	090	
21082		A	palatal augmentation prosthesis	20.87	15.35	11.53	1.46	37.68	33.86	090	
21083		A	palatal lift prosthesis	19.30	15.16	11.14	1.96	36.42	32.40	090	
21084		A	speech aid prosthesis	22.51	17.68	12.99	1.57	41.76	37.07	090	
21085		A	oral surgical splint	9.00	6.62	4.97	0.65	16.27	14.62	010	
21086		A	auricular prosthesis	24.92	19.58	14.39	1.86	46.36	41.17	090	
21087		A	nasal prosthesis	24.92	18.33	13.76	2.22	45.47	40.90	090	
21088		C	facial prosthesis	0.00	0.00	0.00	0.00	0.00	0.00	090	
21089		C	Unlisted maxillofacial prosthetic procedure	0.00	0.00	0.00	0.00	0.00	0.00	090	
21100*		A	Application of halo type appliance for maxillofacial fixation, includes removal (separate procedure)	4.22	5.66	3.70	0.18	10.06	8.10	090	
21110		A	Application of interdental fixation device for conditions other than fracture or dislocation, includes removal	5.21	5.25	4.48	0.28	10.74	9.97	090	
21116		A	Injection procedure for temporomandibular joint arthrography	0.81	7.88	0.30	0.05	8.74	1.16	000	
21120		A	Genioplasty; augmentation (autograft, allograft, prosthetic material)	4.93	7.96	4.98	0.29	13.18	10.20	090	
21121		A	sliding osteotomy, single piece	7.64	7.68	6.65	0.56	15.88	14.85	090	
21122		A	sliding osteotomies, two or more osteotomies (eg, wedge excision or bone wedge reversal for asymmetrical chin)	8.52	7.95	7.95	0.59	17.06	17.06	090	
21123		A	sliding, augmentation with interpositional bone grafts (includes obtaining autografts)	11.16	7.68	7.68	1.16	20.00	20.00	090	

■ RVU not developed by CMS. Gap-filled RVUs developed by Ingenix/CHEG.

Code	M	S	Description	Work Value	Non-Fac PE	Fac PE	Mal-practice	Non-Fac Total	Fac Total	Global	Gap
21125		A	Augmentation, mandibular body or angle; prosthetic material	10.62	9.56	7.84	0.72	20.9	19.18	090	
21127		A	with bone graft, onlay or interpositional (includes obtaining autograft)	11.12	10.66	7.33	0.76	22.54	19.21	090	
21137		A	Reduction forehead; contouring only	9.82	8.20	8.20	0.53	18.55	18.55	090	
21138		A	contouring and application of prosthetic material or bone graft (includes obtaining autograft)	12.19	8.82	8.82	1.47	22.48	22.48	090	
21139		A	contouring and setback of anterior frontal sinus wall	14.61	8.23	8.23	1.02	23.86	23.86	090	
21141		A	Reconstruction midface, LeFort 1; single piece, segment movement in any direction (eg, for Long Face Syndrome), without bone graft	18.10	10.69	10.69	1.63	30.42	30.42	090	
21142		A	two pieces, segment movement in any direction, without bone graft	18.81	13.80	13.80	1.16	33.77	33.77	090	
21143		A	three or more pieces, segment movement in any direction, without bone graft	19.58	11.21	11.21	0.90	31.69	31.69	090	
21145		A	single piece, segment movement in any direction, requiring bone grafts (includes obtaining autografts)	19.94	11.69	11.69	2.09	33.72	33.72	090	
21146		A	two pieces, segment movement in any direction, requiring bone grafts (includes obtaining autografts) (eg, ungrafted unilateral alveolar cleft)	20.71	11.61	11.61	2.13	34.45	34.45	090	
21147		A	three or more pieces, segment movement in any direction, requiring bone grafts (includes obtaining autografts) (eg, ungrafted bilateral alveolar cleft or multiple osteotomies)	21.77	12.07	12.07	1.52	35.36	35.36	090	
21150		A	Reconstruction midface, LeFort II; anterior intrusion (eg, Treacher-Collins Syndrome)	25.24	17.20	17.20	1.09	43.53	43.53	090	
21151		A	any direction, requiring bone grafts (includes obtaining autografts)	28.30	21.35	21.35	1.98	51.63	51.63	090	
21154		A	Reconstruction midface, LeFort III (extracranial), any type, requiring bone grafts (includes obtaining autografts); without LeFort I	30.52	21.03	21.03	4.86	56.41	56.41	090	
21155		A	with LeFort I	34.45	23.20	23.20	5.48	63.13	63.13	090	
21159		A	Reconstruction midface, LeFort III (extra and intracranial) with forehead advancement (eg, mono bloc), requiring bone grafts (includes obtaining autografts); without LeFort I	42.38	21.72	21.72	6.74	70.84	70.84	090	
21160		A	with LeFort I	46.44	30.39	30.39	4.39	81.22	81.22	090	

■ RVU not developed by CMS. Gap-filled RVUs developed by Ingenix/CHEG.

Code	M	S	Description	Work Value	Non-Fac PE	Fac PE	Mal-practice	Non-Fac Total	Fac Total	Global	Gap
21172		A	Reconstruction superior-lateral orbital rim and lower forehead, advancement or alteration, with or without grafts (includes obtaining autografts)	27.80	16.39	16.39	1.91	46.10	46.10	090	
21175		A	Reconstruction, bifrontal, superior-lateral orbital rims and lower forehead, advancement or alteration (eg, plagiocephaly, trigonocephaly, brachycephaly), with or without grafts (includes obtaining autografts)	33.17	19.79	19.79	5.16	58.12	58.12	090	
21179		A	Reconstruction, entire or majority of forehead and/or supraorbital rims; with grafts (allograft or prosthetic material)	22.25	18.94	18.94	2.48	43.67	43.67	090	
21180		A	with autograft (includes obtaining grafts)	25.19	18.33	18.33	2.15	45.67	45.67	090	
21181		A	Reconstruction by contouring of benign tumor of cranial bones (eg, fibrous dysplasia), extracranial	9.90	8.46	8.46	0.97	19.33	19.33	090	
21182		A	Reconstruction of orbital walls, rims, forehead, nasoethmoid complex following intra- and extracranial excision of benign tumor of cranial bone (eg, fibrous dysplasia), with multiple autografts (includes obtaining grafts); total area of bone grafting less than 40 sq cm	32.19	21.97	21.97	2.53	56.69	56.69	090	
21183		A	total area of bone grafting greater than 40 sq cm but less than 80 sq cm	35.31	22.93	22.93	2.75	60.99	60.99	090	
21184		A	total area of bone grafting greater than 80 sq cm	38.24	19.54	19.54	4.12	61.90	61.90	090	
21188		A	Reconstruction midface, osteotomies (other than LeFort type) and bone grafts (includes obtaining autografts)	22.46	15.86	15.86	1.85	40.17	40.17	090	
21193		A	Reconstruction of mandibular rami, horizontal, vertical, C, or L osteotomy; without bone graft	17.15	10.77	10.77	1.53	29.45	29.45	090	
21194		A	with bone graft (includes obtaining graft)	19.84	12.44	12.44	1.39	33.67	33.67	090	
21195		A	Reconstruction of mandibular rami and/or body, sagittal split; without internal rigid fixation	17.24	12.36	12.36	1.20	30.80	30.80	090	
21196		A	with internal rigid fixation	18.91	12.83	12.83	1.62	33.36	33.36	090	
21198		A	Osteotomy, mandible, segmental;	14.16	12.30	12.30	1.05	27.51	27.51	090	
21199		A	with genioglossus advancement	16.00	10.85	10.85	1.26	28.11	28.11	090	
21206		A	Osteotomy, maxilla, segmental (eg, Wassmund or Schuchard)	14.10	9.39	9.39	1.01	24.50	24.50	090	
21208		A	Osteoplasty, facial bones; augmentation (autograft, allograft, or prosthetic implant)	10.23	8.95	8.62	0.92	20.10	19.77	090	
21209		A	reduction	6.72	8.05	6.54	0.60	15.37	13.86	090	

Surgery

■ RVU not developed by CMS. Gap-filled RVUs developed by Ingenix/CHEG.

Code	M	S	Description	Work Value	Non-Fac PE	Fac PE	Mal-practice	Non-Fac Total	Fac Total	Global	Gap
21210		A	Graft, bone; nasal, maxillary or malar areas (includes obtaining graft)	10.23	8.82	8.28	0.88	19.93	19.39	090	
21215		A	mandible (includes obtaining graft)	10.77	8.95	7.48	1.04	20.76	19.29	090	
21230		A	Graft; rib cartilage, autogenous, to face, chin, nose or ear (includes obtaining graft)	10.77	10.85	10.85	0.96	22.58	22.58	090	
21235		A	ear cartilage, autogenous, to nose or ear (includes obtaining graft)	6.72	11.90	8.36	0.52	19.14	15.60	090	
21240		A	Arthroplasty, temporomandibular joint, with or without autograft (includes obtaining graft)	14.05	11.79	11.79	1.15	26.99	26.99	090	
21242		A	Arthroplasty, temporomandibular joint, with allograft	12.95	10.85	10.85	1.40	25.20	25.20	090	
21243		A	Arthroplasty, temporomandibular joint, with prosthetic joint replacement	20.79	13.97	13.97	1.85	36.61	36.61	090	
21244		A	Reconstruction of mandible, extraoral, with transosteal bone plate (eg, mandibular staple bone plate)	11.86	9.56	9.56	0.95	22.37	22.37	090	
21245		A	Reconstruction of mandible or maxilla, subperiosteal implant; partial	11.86	24.85	10.25	0.88	37.59	22.99	090	
21246		A	complete	12.47	10.20	10.20	1.21	23.88	23.88	090	
21247		A	Reconstruction of mandibular condyle with bone and cartilage autografts (includes obtaining grafts) (eg, for hemifacial microsomia)	22.63	20.17	20.17	2.21	45.01	45.01	090	
21248		A	Reconstruction of mandible or maxilla, endosteal implant (eg, blade, cylinder); partial	11.48	8.91	7.86	1.01	21.40	20.35	090	
21249		A	complete	17.52	11.44	10.35	1.39	30.35	29.26	090	
21255		A	Reconstruction of zygomatic arch and glenoid fossa with bone and cartilage (includes obtaining autografts)	16.72	13.16	13.16	1.13	31.01	31.01	090	
21256		A	Reconstruction of orbit with osteotomies (extracranial) and with bone grafts (includes obtaining autografts) (eg, micro-ophthalmia)	16.19	13.87	13.87	1.04	31.10	31.10	090	
21260		A	Periorbital osteotomies for orbital hypertelorism, with bone grafts; extracranial approach	16.52	13.54	13.54	1.25	31.31	31.31	090	
21261		A	combined intra- and extracranial approach	31.49	20.04	20.04	2.20	53.73	53.73	090	
21263		A	with forehead advancement	28.42	15.09	15.09	2.16	45.67	45.67	090	
21267		A	Orbital repositioning, periorbital osteotomies, unilateral, with bone grafts; extracranial approach	18.90	14.75	14.75	1.35	35.00	35.00	090	
21268		A	combined intra- and extracranial approach	24.48	15.15	15.15	0.79	40.42	40.42	090	
21270		A	Malar augmentation, prosthetic material	10.23	10.39	9.99	0.73	21.35	20.95	090	

■ RVU not developed by CMS. Gap-filled RVUs developed by Ingenix/CHEG.

Code	M	S	Description	Work Value	Non-Fac PE	Fac PE	Mal-practice	Non-Fac Total	Fac Total	Global	Gap
21275		A	Secondary revision of orbitocraniofacial reconstruction	11.24	11.02	11.02	1.03	23.29	23.29	090	
21280		A	Medial canthopexy (separate procedure)	6.03	6.27	6.27	0.27	12.57	12.57	090	
21282		A	Lateral canthopexy	3.49	5.38	5.38	0.21	9.08	9.08	090	
21295		A	Reduction of masseter muscle and bone (eg, for treatment of benign masseteric hypertrophy); extraoral approach	1.53	4.34	4.34	0.13	6.00	6.00	090	
21296		A	intraoral approach	4.25	4.09	4.09	0.30	8.64	8.64	090	
21299		C	Unlisted craniofacial and maxillofacial procedure	0.00	0.00	0.00	0.00	0.00	0.00	YYY	
21300		A	Closed treatment of skull fracture without operation	0.72	2.77	0.30	0.09	3.58	1.11	000	
21310		A	Closed treatment of nasal bone fracture without manipulation	0.58	2.70	0.15	0.05	3.33	0.78	000	
21315*		A	Closed treatment of nasal bone fracture; without stabilization	1.51	3.49	1.27	0.12	5.12	2.90	010	
21320		A	with stabilization	1.85	4.96	2.10	0.15	6.96	4.10	010	
21325		A	Open treatment of nasal fracture; uncomplicated	3.77	3.73	3.73	0.31	7.81	7.81	090	
21330		A	complicated, with internal and/or external skeletal fixation	5.38	5.67	5.67	0.48	11.53	11.53	090	
21335		A	with concomitant open treatment of fractured septum	8.61	7.34	7.34	0.64	16.59	16.59	090	
21336		A	Open treatment of nasal septal fracture, with or without stabilization	5.72	5.74	5.74	0.45	11.91	11.91	090	
21337		A	Closed treatment of nasal septal fracture, with or without stabilization	2.70	5.24	3.42	0.22	8.16	6.34	090	
21338		A	Open treatment of nasoethmoid fracture; without external fixation	6.46	5.75	5.75	0.53	12.74	12.74	090	
21339		A	with external fixation	8.09	6.97	6.97	0.76	15.82	15.82	090	
21340		A	Percutaneous treatment of nasoethmoid complex fracture, with splint, wire or headcap fixation, including repair of canthal ligaments and/or the nasolacrimal apparatus	10.77	8.78	8.78	0.85	20.40	20.40	090	
21343		A	Open treatment of depressed frontal sinus fracture	12.95	9.48	9.48	1.06	23.49	23.49	090	
21344		A	Open treatment of complicated (eg, comminuted or involving posterior wall) frontal sinus fracture, via coronal or multiple approaches	19.72	13.82	13.82	1.72	35.26	35.26	090	

Surgery

■ RVU not developed by CMS. Gap-filled RVUs developed by Ingenix/CHEG.

Code	M	S	Description	Work Value	Non-Fac PE	Fac PE	Mal-practice	Non-Fac Total	Fac Total	Global	Gap
21345		A	Closed treatment of nasomaxillary complex fracture (LeFort II type), with interdental wire fixation or fixation of denture or splint	8.16	10.36	7.91	0.60	19.12	16.67	090	
21346		A	Open treatment of nasomaxillary complex fracture (LeFort II type); with wiring and/or local fixation	10.61	10.12	10.12	0.85	21.58	21.58	090	
21347		A	requiring multiple open approaches	12.69	9.68	9.68	1.14	23.51	23.51	090	
21348		A	with bone grafting (includes obtaining graft)	16.69	11.57	11.57	1.50	29.76	29.76	090	
21355*		A	Percutaneous treatment of fracture of malar area, including zygomatic arch and malar tripod, with manipulation	3.77	3.89	2.54	0.29	7.95	6.60	010	
21356		A	Open treatment of depressed zygomatic arch fracture (eg, Gilles approach)	4.15	3.31	3.31	0.36	7.82	7.82	010	
21360		A	Open treatment of depressed malar fracture, including zygomatic arch and malar tripod	6.46	5.74	5.74	0.52	12.72	12.72	090	
21365		A	Open treatment of complicated (eg, comminuted or involving cranial nerve foramina) fracture(s) of malar area, including zygomatic arch and malar tripod; with internal fixation and multiple surgical approaches	14.95	11.72	11.72	1.30	27.97	27.97	090	
21366		A	with bone grafting (includes obtaining graft)	17.77	14.28	14.28	1.41	33.46	33.46	090	
21385		A	Open treatment of orbital floor blowout fracture; transantral approach (Caldwell-Luc type operation)	9.16	8.04	8.04	0.64	17.84	17.84	090	
21386		A	periorbital approach	9.16	8.43	8.43	0.76	18.35	18.35	090	
21387		A	combined approach	9.70	8.55	8.55	0.78	19.03	19.03	090	
21390		A	periorbital approach, with alloplastic or other implant	10.13	8.73	8.73	0.70	19.56	19.56	090	
21395		A	periorbital approach with bone graft (includes obtaining graft)	12.68	9.24	9.24	1.09	23.01	23.01	090	
21400		A	Closed treatment of fracture of orbit, except blowout; without manipulation	1.40	3.29	1.05	0.12	4.81	2.57	090	
21401		A	with manipulation	3.26	4.34	3.65	0.34	7.94	7.25	090	
21406		A	Open treatment of fracture of orbit, except blowout; without implant	7.01	7.20	7.20	0.59	14.80	14.80	090	
21407		A	with implant	8.61	7.99	7.99	0.67	17.27	17.27	090	
21408		A	with bone grafting (includes obtaining graft)	12.38	10.29	10.29	1.24	23.91	23.91	090	
21421		A	Closed treatment of palatal or maxillary fracture (LeFort I type), with interdental wire fixation or fixation of denture or splint	5.14	7.23	6.84	0.42	12.79	12.40	090	

■ RVU not developed by CMS. Gap-filled RVUs developed by Ingenix/CHEG.

Code	M	S	Description	Work Value	Non-Fac PE	Fac PE	Mal-practice	Non-Fac Total	Fac Total	Global	Gap
21422		A	Open treatment of palatal or maxillary fracture (LeFort I type);	8.32	7.93	7.93	0.69	16.94	16.94	090	
21423		A	complicated (comminuted or involving cranial nerve foramina), multiple approaches	10.40	8.63	8.63	0.95	19.98	19.98	090	
21431		A	Closed treatment of craniofacial separation (LeFort III type) using interdental wire fixation of denture or splint	7.05	8.44	8.44	0.58	16.07	16.07	090	
21432		A	Open treatment of craniofacial separation (LeFort III type); with wiring and/or internal fixation	8.61	8.06	8.06	0.55	17.22	17.22	090	
21433		A	complicated (eg, comminuted or involving cranial nerve foramina), multiple surgical approaches	25.35	17.29	17.29	2.46	45.1	45.1	090	
21435		A	complicated, utilizing internal and/or external fixation techniques (eg, head cap, halo device, and/or intermaxillary fixation)	17.25	12.97	12.97	1.66	31.88	31.88	090	
21436		A	complicated, multiple surgical approaches, internal fixation, with bone grafting (includes obtaining graft)	28.04	16.02	16.02	2.32	46.38	46.38	090	
21440		A	Closed treatment of mandibular or maxillary alveolar ridge fracture (separate procedure)	2.70	5.44	3.73	0.22	8.36	6.65	090	
21445		A	Open treatment of mandibular or maxillary alveolar ridge fracture (separate procedure)	5.38	7.14	5.04	0.55	13.07	10.97	090	
21450		A	Closed treatment of mandibular fracture; without manipulation	2.97	6.45	2.90	0.23	9.65	6.10	090	
21451		A	with manipulation	4.87	6.46	6.11	0.39	11.72	11.37	090	
21452		A	Percutaneous treatment of mandibular fracture, with external fixation	1.98	13.44	4.35	0.14	15.56	6.47	090	
21453		A	Closed treatment of mandibular fracture with interdental fixation	5.54	7.32	6.69	0.49	13.35	12.72	090	
21454		A	Open treatment of mandibular fracture with external fixation	6.46	5.72	5.72	0.55	12.73	12.73	090	
21461		A	Open treatment of mandibular fracture; without interdental fixation	8.09	8.40	8.26	0.73	17.22	17.08	090	
21462		A	with interdental fixation	9.79	10.06	8.18	0.80	20.65	18.77	090	
21465		A	Open treatment of mandibular condylar fracture	11.91	8.42	8.42	0.84	21.17	21.17	090	
21470		A	Open treatment of complicated mandibular fracture by multiple surgical approaches including internal fixation, interdental fixation, and/or wiring of dentures or splints	15.34	10.31	10.31	1.36	27.01	27.01	090	
21480		A	Closed treatment of temporomandibular dislocation; initial or subsequent	0.61	1.62	0.18	0.05	2.28	0.84	000	

■ RVU not developed by CMS. Gap-filled RVUs developed by Ingenix/CHEG.

Surgery

Code	M	S	Description	Work Value	Non-Fac PE	Fac PE	Mal-practice	Non-Fac Total	Fac Total	Global	Gap
21485		A	complicated (eg, recurrent requiring intermaxillary fixation or splinting), initial or subsequent	3.99	3.82	3.34	0.31	8.12	7.64	090	
21490		A	Open treatment of temporomandibular dislocation	11.86	7.69	7.69	1.31	20.86	20.86	090	
21493		A	Closed treatment of hyoid fracture; without manipulation	1.27	3.68	3.68	0.10	5.05	5.05	090	
21494		A	with manipulation	6.28	4.21	4.21	0.44	10.93	10.93	090	
21495		A	Open treatment of hyoid fracture	5.69	5.28	5.28	0.41	11.38	11.38	090	
21497		A	Interdental wiring, for condition other than fracture	3.86	4.68	3.81	0.31	8.85	7.98	090	
21499		C	Unlisted musculoskeletal procedure, head	0.00	0.00	0.00	0.00	0.00	0.00	YYY	
21501		A	Incision and drainage, deep abscess or hematoma, soft tissues of neck or thorax;	3.81	4.50	3.64	0.36	8.67	7.81	090	
21502		A	with partial rib ostectomy	7.12	7.05	7.05	0.79	14.96	14.96	090	
21510		A	Incision, deep, with opening of bone cortex (eg, for osteomyelitis or bone abscess), thorax	5.74	7.47	7.47	0.67	13.88	13.88	090	
21550		A	Biopsy, soft tissue of neck or thorax	2.06	2.32	1.25	0.13	4.51	3.44	010	
21555		A	Excision tumor, soft tissue of neck or thorax; subcutaneous	4.35	4.25	2.43	0.41	9.01	7.19	090	
21556		A	deep, subfascial, intramuscular	5.57	3.29	3.29	0.51	9.37	9.37	090	
21557		A	Radical resection of tumor (eg, malignant neoplasm), soft tissue of neck or thorax	8.88	7.87	7.87	0.85	17.60	17.60	090	
21600		A	Excision of rib, partial	6.89	7.80	7.80	0.81	15.50	15.50	090	
21610		A	Costotransversectomy (separate procedure)	14.61	11.26	11.26	1.85	27.72	27.72	090	
21615		A	Excision first and/or cervical rib;	9.87	7.90	7.90	1.20	18.97	18.97	090	
21616		A	with sympathectomy	12.04	8.94	8.94	1.31	22.29	22.29	090	
21620		A	Ostectomy of sternum, partial	6.79	8.13	8.13	0.77	15.69	15.69	090	
21627		A	Sternal debridement	6.81	12.16	12.16	0.82	19.79	19.79	090	
21630		A	Radical resection of sternum;	17.38	14.03	14.03	1.95	33.36	33.36	090	
21632		A	with mediastinal lymphadenectomy	18.14	12.35	12.35	2.16	32.65	32.65	090	
21700		A	Division of scalenus anticus; without resection of cervical rib	6.19	8.63	7.19	0.31	15.13	13.69	090	
21705		A	with resection of cervical rib	9.60	7.87	7.87	0.92	18.39	18.39	090	
21720		A	Division of sternocleidomastoid for torticollis, open operation; without cast application	5.68	8.71	5.93	0.80	15.19	12.41	090	

■ RVU not developed by CMS. Gap-filled RVUs developed by Ingenix/CHEG.

Code	M	S	Description	Work Value	Non-Fac PE	Fac PE	Mal-practice	Non-Fac Total	Fac Total	Global	Gap
21725		A	with cast application	6.99	7.28	7.28	0.90	15.17	15.17	090	
21740		A	Reconstructive repair of pectus excavatum or carinatum	16.50	12.85	12.85	2.03	31.38	31.38	090	
21750		A	Closure of median sternotomy separation with or without debridement (separate procedure)	10.77	9.41	9.41	1.35	21.53	21.53	090	
21800		A	Closed treatment of rib fracture, uncomplicated, each	0.96	2.31	1.11	0.09	3.36	2.16	090	
21805		A	Open treatment of rib fracture without fixation, each	2.75	4.08	4.08	0.29	7.12	7.12	090	
21810		A	Treatment of rib fracture requiring external fixation (flail chest)	6.86	7.49	7.49	0.60	14.95	14.95	090	
21820		A	Closed treatment of sternum fracture	1.28	2.80	1.58	0.15	4.23	3.01	090	
21825		A	Open treatment of sternum fracture with or without skeletal fixation	7.41	9.90	9.90	0.84	18.15	18.15	090	
21899		C	Unlisted procedure, neck or thorax	0.00	0.00	0.00	0.00	0.00	0.00	YYY	
21920		A	Biopsy, soft tissue of back or flank; superficial	2.06	2.40	0.77	0.12	4.58	2.95	010	
21925		A	deep	4.49	10.19	4.79	0.44	15.12	9.72	090	
21930		A	Excision, tumor, soft tissue of back or flank	5.00	4.55	2.66	0.49	10.04	8.15	090	
21935		A	Radical resection of tumor (eg, malignant neoplasm), soft tissue of back or flank	17.96	13.53	13.53	1.87	33.36	33.36	090	
22100		A	Partial excision of posterior vertebral component (eg, spinous process, lamina or facet) for intrinsic bony lesion, single vertebral segment; cervical	9.73	8.36	8.36	1.55	19.64	19.64	090	
22101		A	thoracic	9.81	9.04	9.04	1.51	20.36	20.36	090	
22102		A	lumbar	9.81	9.18	9.18	1.46	20.45	20.45	090	
22103		A	each additional segment (List separately in addition to code for primary procedure)	2.34	1.27	1.27	0.37	3.98	3.98	ZZZ	
22110		A	Partial excision of vertebral body for intrinsic bony lesion, without decompression of spinal cord or nerve root(s), single vertebral segment; cervical	12.74	11.06	11.06	2.20	26.00	26.00	090	
22112		A	thoracic	12.81	10.95	10.95	1.96	25.72	25.72	090	
22114		A	lumbar	12.81	10.71	10.71	1.98	25.50	25.50	090	
22116		A	each additional vertebral segment (List separately in addition to code for primary procedure)	2.32	1.26	1.26	0.40	3.98	3.98	ZZZ	
22210		A	Osteotomy of spine, posterior or posterolateral approach, one vertebral segment; cervical	23.82	17.42	17.42	4.23	45.47	45.47	090	
22212		A	thoracic	19.42	14.60	14.60	2.78	36.80	36.80	090	

■ RVU not developed by CMS. Gap-filled RVUs developed by Ingenix/CHEG.

Code	M	S	Description	Work Value	Non-Fac PE	Fac PE	Mal-practice	Non-Fac Total	Fac Total	Global	Gap
22214		A	lumbar	19.45	15.32	15.32	2.78	37.55	37.55	090	
22216		A	each additional vertebral segment (List separately in addition to primary procedure)	6.04	3.31	3.31	0.98	10.33	10.33	ZZZ	
22220		A	Osteotomy of spine, including diskectomy, anterior approach, single vertebral segment; cervical	21.37	15.61	15.61	3.65	40.63	40.63	090	
22222		A	thoracic	21.52	15.08	15.08	3.08	39.68	39.68	090	
22224		A	lumbar	21.52	15.70	15.70	3.20	40.42	40.42	090	
22226		A	each additional vertebral segment (List separately in addition to code for primary procedure)	6.04	3.22	3.22	1.01	10.27	10.27	ZZZ	
22305		A	Closed treatment of vertebral process fracture(s)	2.05	3.25	2.01	0.29	5.59	4.35	090	
22310		A	Closed treatment of vertebral body fracture(s), without manipulation, requiring and including casting or bracing	2.61	4.77	3.54	0.37	7.75	6.52	090	
22315		A	Closed treatment of vertebral fracture(s) and/or dislocations(s) requiring casting or bracing, with and including casting and/or bracing, with or without anesthesia, by manipulation or traction	8.84	9.32	9.32	1.37	19.53	19.53	090	
22318		A	Open treatment and/or reduction of odontoid fracture(s) and or dislocation(s) (including os odontoideum), anterior approach, including placement of internal fixation; without grafting	21.5	15.02	15.02	4.26	40.78	40.78	090	
22319		A	with grafting	24.00	17.42	17.42	4.76	46.18	46.18	090	
22325		A	Open treatment and/or reduction of vertebral fracture(s) and/or dislocation(s); posterior approach, one fractured vertebrae or dislocated segment; lumbar	18.30	14.94	14.94	2.61	35.85	35.85	090	
22326		A	cervical	19.59	15.67	15.67	3.54	38.80	38.80	090	
22327		A	thoracic	19.20	15.43	15.43	2.75	37.38	37.38	090	
22328		A	each additional fractured vertebrae or dislocated segment (List separately in addition to code for primary procedure)	4.61	2.43	2.43	0.66	7.70	7.70	ZZZ	
22505		A	Manipulation of spine requiring anesthesia, any region	1.87	4.58	3.20	0.27	6.72	5.34	010	
22520		A	Percutaneous vertebroplasty, one vertebral body, unilateral or bilateral injection; thoracic	8.91	4.15	4.15	0.99	14.05	14.05	010	
22521		A	lumbar	8.34	3.92	3.92	0.93	13.19	13.19	010	
22522		A	each additional thoracic or lumbar vertebral body (List separately in addition to code for primary procedure)	4.31	1.75	1.75	0.33	6.39	6.39	ZZZ	

■ RVU not developed by CMS. Gap-filled RVUs developed by Ingenix/CHEG.

Code	M	S	Description	Work Value	Non-Fac PE	Fac PE	Mal-prac-tice	Non-Fac Total	Fac Total	Global	Gap
22548		A	Arthrodesis, anterior transoral or extraoral technique, clivus-C1-C2 (atlas-axis), with or without excision of odontoid process	25.82	18.08	18.08	4.98	48.88	48.88	090	
22554		A	Arthrodesis, anterior interbody technique, including minimal diskectomy to prepare interspace (other than for decompression); cervical below C2	18.62	13.94	13.94	3.51	36.07	36.07	090	
22556		A	thoracic	23.46	16.80	16.80	3.78	44.04	44.04	090	
22558		A	lumbar	22.28	15.27	15.27	3.18	40.73	40.73	090	
22585		A	each additional interspace (List separately in addition to code for primary procedure)	5.53	2.94	2.94	0.98	9.45	9.45	ZZZ	
22590		A	Arthrodesis, posterior technique, craniocervical (occiput-C2)	20.51	15.56	15.56	3.81	39.88	39.88	090	
22595		A	Arthrodesis, posterior technique, atlas-axis (C1-C2)	19.39	14.58	14.58	3.62	37.59	37.59	090	
22600		A	Arthrodesis, posterior or posterolateral technique, single level; cervical below C2 segment	16.14	12.66	12.66	2.89	31.69	31.69	090	
22610		A	thoracic (with or without lateral transverse technique)	16.02	12.98	12.98	2.66	31.66	31.66	090	
22612		A	lumbar (with or without lateral transverse technique)	21.00	15.75	15.75	3.28	40.03	40.03	090	
22614		A	each additional vertebral segment (List separately in addition to code for primary procedure)	6.44	3.54	3.54	1.04	11.02	11.02	ZZZ	
22630		A	Arthrodesis, posterior interbody technique, including laminectomy and/or diskectomy to prepare interspace (other than for decompression), single interspace; lumbar	20.84	16.01	16.01	3.79	40.64	40.64	090	
22632		A	each additional interspace (List separately in addition to code for primary procedure)	5.23	2.75	2.75	0.90	8.88	8.88	ZZZ	
22800		A	Arthrodesis, posterior, for spinal deformity, with or without cast; up to 6 vertebral segments	18.25	14.30	14.30	2.71	35.26	35.26	090	
22802		A	7 to 12 vertebral segments	30.88	21.88	21.88	4.42	57.18	57.18	090	
22804		A	13 or more vertebral segments	36.27	24.48	24.48	5.23	65.98	65.98	090	
22808		A	Arthrodesis, anterior, for spinal deformity, with or without cast; 2 to 3 vertebral segments	26.27	18.27	18.27	4.36	48.90	48.90	090	
22810		A	4 to 7 vertebral segments	30.27	19.63	19.63	4.49	54.39	54.39	090	
22812		A	8 or more vertebral segments	32.70	21.89	21.89	4.67	59.26	59.26	090	
22818		A	Kyphectomy, circumferential exposure of spine and resection of vertebral segment(s) (including body and posterior elements); single or 2 segments	31.83	21.69	21.69	5.01	58.53	58.53	090	

■ RVU not developed by CMS. Gap-filled RVUs developed by Ingenix/CHEG.

Code	M	S	Description	Work Value	Non-Fac PE	Fac PE	Mal-practice	Non-Fac Total	Fac Total	Global	Gap
22819		A	3 or more segments	36.44	22.19	22.19	5.20	63.83	63.83	090	
22830		A	Exploration of spinal fusion	10.85	10.05	10.05	1.73	22.63	22.63	090	
22840		A	Posterior non-segmental instrumentation (eg, Harrington rod technique, pedicle fixation across one interspace, atlantoaxial transarticular screw fixation, sublaminar wiring at C1, facet screw fixation)	12.54	6.84	6.84	2.03	21.41	21.41	ZZZ	
22841		B	Internal spinal fixation by wiring of spinous processes	3.57	2.84	2.84	0.38	6.79	6.79	XXX	■
22842		A	Posterior segmental instrumentation (eg, pedicle fixation, dual rods with multiple hooks and sublaminal wires); 3 to 6 vertebral segments	12.58	6.83	6.83	2.04	21.45	21.45	ZZZ	
22843		A	7 to 12 vertebral segments	13.46	7.39	7.39	2.10	22.95	22.95	ZZZ	
22844		A	13 or more vertebral segments	16.44	9.26	9.26	2.42	28.12	28.12	ZZZ	
22845		A	Anterior instrumentation; 2 to 3 vertebral segments	11.96	6.38	6.38	2.22	20.56	20.56	ZZZ	
22846		A	4 to 7 vertebral segments	12.42	6.70	6.70	2.26	21.38	21.38	ZZZ	
22847		A	8 or more vertebral segments	13.8	7.08	7.08	2.36	23.24	23.24	ZZZ	
22848		A	Pelvic fixation (attachment of caudal end of instrumentation to pelvic bony structures) other than sacrum	6.00	3.38	3.38	0.88	10.26	10.26	ZZZ	
22849		A	Reinsertion of spinal fixation device	18.51	14.22	14.22	2.87	35.60	35.60	090	
22850		A	Removal of posterior nonsegmental instrumentation (eg, Harrington rod)	9.52	8.89	8.89	1.51	19.92	19.92	090	
22851		A	Application of intervertebral biomechanical device(s) (eg, synthetic cage(s), threaded bone dowel(s), methylmethacrylate) to vertebral defect or interspace	6.71	3.54	3.54	1.11	11.36	11.36	ZZZ	
22852		A	Removal of posterior segmental instrumentation	9.01	8.60	8.60	1.40	19.01	19.01	090	
22855		A	Removal of anterior instrumentation	15.13	11.67	11.67	2.74	29.54	29.54	090	
22899		C	Unlisted procedure, spine	0.00	0.00	0.00	0.00	0.00	0.00	YYY	
22900		A	Excision, abdominal wall tumor, subfascial (eg, desmoid)	5.80	4.42	4.42	0.58	10.80	10.80	090	
22999		C	Unlisted procedure, abdomen, musculoskeletal system	0.00	0.00	0.00	0.00	0.00	0.00	YYY	
23000		A	Removal of subdeltoid calcareous deposits, open	4.36	9.04	6.97	0.50	13.9	11.83	090	
23020		A	Capsular contracture release (eg, Sever type procedure)	8.93	10.53	10.53	1.23	20.69	20.69	090	

■ RVU not developed by CMS. Gap-filled RVUs developed by Ingenix/CHEG.

Code	M	S	Description	Work Value	Non-Fac PE	Fac PE	Mal-practice	Non-Fac Total	Fac Total	Global	Gap
23030		A	Incision and drainage, shoulder area; deep abscess or hematoma	3.43	6.40	4.44	0.42	10.25	8.29	010	
23031		A	infected bursa	2.74	5.80	4.16	0.33	8.87	7.23	010	
23035		A	Incision, bone cortex (eg, osteomyelitis or bone abscess), shoulder area	8.61	16.13	16.13	1.19	25.93	25.93	090	
23040		A	Arthrotomy, glenohumeral joint, including exploration, drainage, or removal of foreign body	9.20	11.71	11.71	1.28	22.19	22.19	090	
23044		A	Arthrotomy, acromioclavicular, sternoclavicular joint, including exploration, drainage, or removal of foreign body	7.12	10.73	10.73	0.97	18.82	18.82	090	
23065		A	Biopsy, soft tissue of shoulder area; superficial	2.27	2.61	1.34	0.14	5.02	3.75	010	
23066		A	deep	4.16	8.34	6.16	0.50	13.00	10.82	090	
23075		A	Excision, soft tissue tumor, shoulder area; subcutaneous	2.39	5.40	3.17	0.25	8.04	5.81	010	
23076		A	deep, subfascial or intramuscular	7.63	8.36	8.36	0.87	16.86	16.86	090	
23077		A	Radical resection of tumor (eg, malignant neoplasm), soft tissue of shoulder area	16.09	14.41	14.41	1.81	32.31	32.31	090	
23100		A	Arthrotomy, glenohumeral joint, including biopsy	6.03	8.73	8.73	0.81	15.57	15.57	090	
23101		A	Arthrotomy, acromioclavicular joint or sternoclavicular joint, including biopsy and/or excision of torn cartilage	5.58	8.63	8.63	0.77	14.98	14.98	090	
23105		A	Arthrotomy; glenohumeral joint, with synovectomy, with or without biopsy	8.23	10.18	10.18	1.13	19.54	19.54	090	
23106		A	sternoclavicular joint, with synovectomy, with or without biopsy	5.96	9.27	9.27	0.82	16.05	16.05	090	
23107		A	Arthrotomy, glenohumeral joint, with joint exploration, with or without removal of loose or foreign body	8.62	10.41	10.41	1.19	20.22	20.22	090	
23120		A	Claviculectomy; partial	7.11	9.55	9.55	0.99	17.65	17.65	090	
23125		A	total	9.39	10.78	10.78	1.27	21.44	21.44	090	
23130		A	Acromioplasty or acromionectomy, partial, with or without coracoacromial ligament release	7.55	9.82	9.82	1.06	18.43	18.43	090	
23140		A	Excision or curettage of bone cyst or benign tumor of clavicle or scapula;	6.89	8.31	8.31	0.82	16.02	16.02	090	
23145		A	with autograft (includes obtaining graft)	9.09	10.87	10.87	1.24	21.20	21.20	090	
23146		A	with allograft	7.83	10.70	10.70	1.11	19.64	19.64	090	
23150		A	Excision or curettage of bone cyst or benign tumor of proximal humerus;	8.48	10.14	10.14	1.14	19.76	19.76	090	

■ RVU not developed by CMS. Gap-filled RVUs developed by Ingenix/CHEG.

Code	M	S	Description	Work Value	Non-Fac PE	Fac PE	Mal-practice	Non-Fac Total	Fac Total	Global	Gap
23155		A	with autograft (includes obtaining graft)	10.35	12.33	12.33	1.20	23.88	23.88	090	
23156		A	with allograft	8.68	10.45	10.45	1.18	20.31	20.31	090	
23170		A	Sequestrectomy (eg, for osteomyelitis or bone abscess), clavicle	6.86	11.33	11.33	0.84	19.03	19.03	090	
23172		A	Sequestrectomy (eg, for osteomyelitis or bone abscess), scapula	6.90	9.59	9.59	0.95	17.44	17.44	090	
23174		A	Sequestrectomy (eg, for osteomyelitis or bone abscess), humeral head to surgical neck	9.51	11.74	11.74	1.03	22.55	22.55	090	
23180		A	Partial excision (craterization, saucerization, or diaphysectomy) bone (eg, osteomyelitis), clavicle	8.53	16.16	16.16	1.18	25.87	25.87	090	
23182		A	Partial excision (craterization, saucerization, or diaphysectomy) bone (eg, osteomyelitis), scapula	8.15	16.18	16.18	1.08	25.41	25.41	090	
23184		A	Partial excision (craterization, saucerization, or diaphysectomy) bone (eg, osteomyelitis), proximal humerus	9.38	16.43	16.43	1.24	27.05	27.05	090	
23190		A	Ostectomy of scapula, partial (eg, superior medial angle)	7.24	8.74	8.74	0.97	16.95	16.95	090	
23195		A	Resection humeral head	9.81	10.03	10.03	1.38	21.22	21.22	090	
23200		A	Radical resection for tumor; clavicle	12.08	14.39	14.39	1.48	27.95	27.95	090	
23210		A	scapula	12.49	13.96	13.96	1.61	28.06	28.06	090	
23220		A	Radical resection of bone tumor, proximal humerus;	14.56	15.57	15.57	2.03	32.16	32.16	090	
23221		A	with autograft (includes obtaining graft)	17.74	16.93	16.93	2.51	37.18	37.18	090	
23222		A	with prosthetic replacement	23.92	20.66	20.66	3.37	47.95	47.95	090	
23330		A	Removal of foreign body, shoulder; subcutaneous	1.85	6.15	3.49	0.18	8.18	5.52	010	
23331		A	deep (eg, Neer hemiarthroplasty removal)	7.38	9.70	9.70	1.02	18.10	18.10	090	
23332		A	complicated (eg, total shoulder)	11.62	12.12	12.12	1.62	25.36	25.36	090	
23350		A	Injection procedure for shoulder arthrography or enhanced CT/MRI shoulder arthrography	1.00	7.22	0.35	0.05	8.27	1.40	000	
23395		A	Muscle transfer, any type, shoulder or upper arm; single	16.85	14.09	14.09	2.29	33.23	33.23	090	
23397		A	multiple	16.13	13.86	13.86	2.24	32.23	32.23	090	
23400		A	Scapulopexy (eg, Sprengel's deformity or for paralysis)	13.54	14.52	14.52	1.91	29.97	29.97	090	
23405		A	Tenotomy, shoulder area; single tendon	8.37	9.66	9.66	1.12	19.15	19.15	090	
23406		A	multiple tendons through same incision	10.79	11.55	11.55	1.48	23.82	23.82	090	

■ RVU not developed by CMS. Gap-filled RVUs developed by Ingenix/CHEG.

Code	M	S	Description	Work Value	Non-Fac PE	Fac PE	Mal-practice	Non-Fac Total	Fac Total	Global	Gap
23410		A	Repair of ruptured musculotendinous cuff (eg, rotator cuff); acute	12.45	12.55	12.55	1.72	26.72	26.72	090	
23412		A	chronic	13.31	13.05	13.05	1.86	28.22	28.22	090	
23415		A	Coracoacromial ligament release, with or without acromioplasty	9.97	10.22	10.22	1.39	21.58	21.58	090	
23420		A	Reconstruction of complete shoulder (rotator) cuff avulsion, chronic (includes acromioplasty)	13.30	13.94	13.94	1.86	29.1	29.10	090	
23430		A	Tenodesis of long tendon of biceps	9.98	11.15	11.15	1.40	22.53	22.53	090	
23440		A	Resection or transplantation of long tendon of biceps	10.48	11.54	11.54	1.47	23.49	23.49	090	
23450		A	Capsulorrhaphy, anterior; Putti-Platt procedure or Magnuson type operation	13.40	13.02	13.02	1.86	28.28	28.28	090	
23455		A	with labral repair (eg, Bankart procedure)	14.37	13.62	13.62	2.01	30.00	30.00	090	
23460		A	Capsulorrhaphy, anterior, any type; with bone block	15.37	14.21	14.21	2.17	31.75	31.75	090	
23462		A	with coracoid process transfer	15.30	13.68	13.68	2.16	31.14	31.14	090	
23465		A	Capsulorrhaphy, glenohumeral joint, posterior, with or without bone block	15.85	14.47	14.47	1.61	31.93	31.93	090	
23466		A	Capsulorrhaphy, glenohumeral joint, any type multi-directional instability	14.22	13.63	13.63	2.00	29.85	29.85	090	
23470		A	Arthroplasty, glenohumeral joint; hemiarthroplasty	17.15	15.16	15.16	2.40	34.71	34.71	090	
23472		A	total shoulder (glenoid and proximal humeral replacement (eg, total shoulder))	21.10	17.40	17.40	2.37	40.87	40.87	090	
23480		A	Osteotomy, clavicle, with or without internal fixation;	11.18	11.94	11.94	1.56	24.68	24.68	090	
23485		A	with bone graft for nonunion or malunion (includes obtaining graft and/or necessary fixation)	13.43	13.10	13.10	1.84	28.37	28.37	090	
23490		A	Prophylactic treatment (nailing, pinning, plating or wiring) with or without methylmethacrylate; clavicle	11.86	13.74	13.74	1.11	26.71	26.71	090	
23491		A	proximal humerus	14.21	13.54	13.54	2.00	29.75	29.75	090	
23500		A	Closed treatment of clavicular fracture; without manipulation	2.08	3.87	2.60	0.26	6.21	4.94	090	
23505		A	with manipulation	3.69	5.98	4.02	0.50	10.17	8.21	090	
23515		A	Open treatment of clavicular fracture, with or without internal or external fixation	7.41	8.24	8.24	1.03	16.68	16.68	090	
23520		A	Closed treatment of sternoclavicular dislocation; without manipulation	2.16	3.91	2.67	0.26	6.33	5.09	090	

■ RVU not developed by CMS. Gap-filled RVUs developed by Ingenix/CHEG.

Code	M	S	Description	Work Value	Non-Fac PE	Fac PE	Mal-practice	Non-Fac Total	Fac Total	Global	Gap
23525		A	with manipulation	3.60	7.16	4.08	0.44	11.20	8.12	090	
23530		A	Open treatment of sternoclavicular dislocation, acute or chronic;	7.31	7.94	7.94	0.85	16.10	16.10	090	
23532		A	with fascial graft (includes obtaining graft)	8.01	8.67	8.67	1.13	17.81	17.81	090	
23540		A	Closed treatment of acromioclavicular dislocation; without manipulation	2.23	4.56	2.63	0.24	7.03	5.10	090	
23545		A	with manipulation	3.25	4.99	3.65	0.39	8.63	7.29	090	
23550		A	Open treatment of acromioclavicular dislocation, acute or chronic;	7.24	8.29	8.29	0.94	16.47	16.47	090	
23552		A	with fascial graft (includes obtaining graft)	8.45	8.82	8.82	1.18	18.45	18.45	090	
23570		A	Closed treatment of scapular fracture; without manipulation	2.23	3.84	2.70	0.29	6.36	5.22	090	
23575		A	with manipulation, with or without skeletal traction (with or without shoulder joint involvement)	4.06	6.22	4.18	0.53	10.81	8.77	090	
23585		A	Open treatment of scapular fracture (body, glenoid or acromion) with or without internal fixation	8.96	9.31	9.31	1.25	19.52	19.52	090	
23600		A	Closed treatment of proximal humeral (surgical or anatomical neck) fracture; without manipulation	2.93	5.65	3.71	0.39	8.97	7.03	090	
23605		A	with manipulation, with or without skeletal traction	4.87	8.32	6.55	0.67	13.86	12.09	090	
23615		A	Open treatment of proximal humeral (surgical or anatomical neck) fracture, with or without internal or external fixation, with or without repair of tuberosity(s);	9.35	10.19	10.19	1.31	20.85	20.85	090	
23616		A	with proximal humeral prosthetic replacement	21.27	16.26	16.26	2.98	40.51	40.51	090	
23620		A	Closed treatment of greater humeral tuberosity fracture; without manipulation	2.40	5.35	3.43	0.32	8.07	6.15	090	
23625		A	with manipulation	3.93	7.35	5.57	0.53	11.81	10.03	090	
23630		A	Open treatment of greater humeral tuberosity fracture, with or without internal or external fixation	7.35	8.20	8.20	1.03	16.58	16.58	090	
23650		A	Closed treatment of shoulder dislocation, with manipulation; without anesthesia	3.39	5.58	3.67	0.31	9.28	7.37	090	
23655		A	requiring anesthesia	4.57	4.39	4.39	0.52	9.48	9.48	090	
23660		A	Open treatment of acute shoulder dislocation	7.49	8.27	8.27	1.01	16.77	16.77	090	
23665		A	Closed treatment of shoulder dislocation, with fracture of greater humeral tuberosity, with manipulation	4.47	7.68	5.81	0.60	12.75	10.88	090	

■ RVU not developed by CMS. Gap-filled RVUs developed by Ingenix/CHEG.

Code	M	S	Description	Work Value	Non-Fac PE	Fac PE	Mal-practice	Non-Fac Total	Fac Total	Global	Gap
23670		A	Open treatment of shoulder dislocation, with fracture of greater humeral tuberosity, with or without internal or external fixation	7.90	8.72	8.72	1.1	17.72	17.72	090	
23675		A	Closed treatment of shoulder dislocation, with surgical or anatomical neck fracture, with manipulation	6.05	8.22	6.71	0.83	15.1	13.59	090	
23680		A	Open treatment of shoulder dislocation, with surgical or anatomical neck fracture, with or without internal or external fixation	10.06	9.89	9.89	1.39	21.34	21.34	090	
23700*		A	Manipulation under anesthesia, shoulder joint, including application of fixation apparatus (dislocation excluded)	2.52	3.48	3.48	0.35	6.35	6.35	010	
23800		A	Arthrodesis, glenohumeral joint;	14.16	14.28	14.28	1.97	30.41	30.41	090	
23802		A	with autogenous graft (includes obtaining graft)	16.60	15.83	15.83	2.34	34.77	34.77	090	
23900		A	Interthoracoscapular amputation (forequarter)	19.72	16.35	16.35	2.47	38.54	38.54	090	
23920		A	Disarticulation of shoulder;	14.61	13.70	13.70	1.92	30.23	30.23	090	
23921		A	secondary closure or scar revision	5.49	6.67	6.67	0.78	12.94	12.94	090	
23929		C	Unlisted procedure, shoulder	0.00	0.00	0.00	0.00	0.00	0.00	YYY	
23930		A	Incision and drainage, upper arm or elbow area; deep abscess or hematoma	2.94	6.10	4.01	0.32	9.36	7.27	010	
23931		A	bursa	1.79	5.76	3.74	0.21	7.76	5.74	010	
23935		A	Incision, deep, with opening of bone cortex (eg, for osteomyelitis or bone abscess), humerus or elbow	6.09	12.9	12.9	0.84	19.83	19.83	090	
24000		A	Arthrotomy, elbow, including exploration, drainage, or removal of foreign body	5.82	6.06	6.06	0.77	12.65	12.65	090	
24006		A	Arthrotomy of the elbow, with capsular excision for capsular release (separate procedure)	9.31	8.64	8.64	1.27	19.22	19.22	090	
24065		A	Biopsy, soft tissue of upper arm or elbow area; superficial	2.08	5.50	3.25	0.14	7.72	5.47	010	
24066		A	deep (subfascial or intramuscular)	5.21	8.48	6.40	0.61	14.30	12.22	090	
24075		A	Excision, tumor, soft tissue of upper arm or elbow area; subcutaneous	3.92	7.80	5.91	0.43	12.15	10.26	090	
24076		A	deep, subfascial or intramuscular	6.30	7.39	7.39	0.70	14.39	14.39	090	
24077		A	Radical resection of tumor (eg, malignant neoplasm), soft tissue of upper arm or elbow area	11.76	14.23	14.23	1.32	27.31	27.31	090	
24100		A	Arthrotomy, elbow; with synovial biopsy only	4.93	5.83	5.83	0.62	11.38	11.38	090	

Surgery

■ RVU not developed by CMS. Gap-filled RVUs developed by Ingenix/CHEG.

Code	M	S	Description	Work Value	Non-Fac PE	Fac PE	Mal-prac-tice	Non-Fac Total	Fac Total	Global	Gap
24101		A	with joint exploration, with or without biopsy, with or without removal of loose or foreign body	6.13	6.82	6.82	0.84	13.79	13.79	090	
24102		A	with synovectomy	8.03	7.81	7.81	1.09	16.93	16.93	090	
24105		A	Excision, olecranon bursa	3.61	5.26	5.26	0.49	9.36	9.36	090	
24110		A	Excision or curettage of bone cyst or benign tumor, humerus;	7.39	9.75	9.75	0.99	18.13	18.13	090	
24115		A	with autograft (includes obtaining graft)	9.63	10.80	10.80	1.15	21.58	21.58	090	
24116		A	with allograft	11.81	12.20	12.20	1.66	25.67	25.67	090	
24120		A	Excision or curettage of bone cyst or benign tumor of head or neck of radius or olecranon process;	6.65	6.96	6.96	0.87	14.48	14.48	090	
24125		A	with autograft (includes obtaining graft)	7.89	6.67	6.67	0.88	15.44	15.44	090	
24126		A	with allograft	8.31	7.79	7.79	0.90	17.00	17.00	090	
24130		A	Excision, radial head	6.25	6.91	6.91	0.87	14.03	14.03	090	
24134		A	Sequestrectomy (eg, for osteomyelitis or bone abscess), shaft or distal humerus	9.73	16.50	16.50	1.31	27.54	27.54	090	
24136		A	Sequestrectomy (eg, for osteomyelitis or bone abscess), radial head or neck	7.99	7.09	7.09	0.85	15.93	15.93	090	
24138		A	Sequestrectomy (eg, for osteomyelitis or bone abscess), olecranon process	8.05	8.06	8.06	1.12	17.23	17.23	090	
24140		A	Partial excision (craterization, saucerization, or diaphysectomy) bone (eg, osteomyelitis), humerus	9.18	16.67	16.67	1.23	27.08	27.08	090	
24145		A	Partial excision (craterization, saucerization, or diaphysectomy) bone (eg, osteomyelitis), radial head or neck	7.58	11.43	11.43	1.01	20.02	20.02	090	
24147		A	Partial excision (craterization, saucerization, or diaphysectomy) bone (eg, osteomyelitis), olecranon process	7.54	11.40	11.40	1.04	19.98	19.98	090	
24149		A	Radical resection of capsule, soft tissue, and heterotopic bone, elbow, with contracture release (separate procedure)	14.20	11.28	11.28	1.90	27.38	27.38	090	
24150		A	Radical resection for tumor, shaft or distal humerus;	13.27	14.92	14.92	1.81	30.00	30.00	090	
24151		A	with autograft (includes obtaining graft)	15.58	16.64	16.64	2.19	34.41	34.41	090	
24152		A	Radical resection for tumor, radial head or neck;	10.06	9.96	9.96	1.19	21.21	21.21	090	
24153		A	with autograft (includes obtaining graft)	11.54	7.55	7.55	0.64	19.73	19.73	090	
24155		A	Resection of elbow joint (arthrectomy)	11.73	9.66	9.66	1.42	22.81	22.81	090	

■ RVU not developed by CMS. Gap-filled RVUs developed by Ingenix/CHEG.

Code	M	S	Description	Work Value	Non-Fac PE	Fac PE	Mal-practice	Non-Fac Total	Fac Total	Global	Gap
24160		A	Implant removal; elbow joint	7.83	7.77	7.77	1.07	16.67	16.67	090	
24164		A	radial head	6.23	6.93	6.93	0.84	14.00	14.00	090	
24200		A	Removal of foreign body, upper arm or elbow area; subcutaneous	1.76	5.80	3.25	0.15	7.71	5.16	010	
24201		A	deep (subfascial or intramuscular)	4.56	8.42	6.97	0.56	13.54	12.09	090	
24220		A	Injection procedure for elbow arthrography	1.31	11.16	0.47	0.07	12.54	1.85	000	
24300		A	Manipulation, elbow, under anesthesia	3.75	5.46	5.46	0.52	9.73	9.73	090	
24301		A	Muscle or tendon transfer, any type, upper arm or elbow, single (excluding 24320-24331)	10.20	9.11	9.11	1.30	20.61	20.61	090	
24305		A	Tendon lengthening, upper arm or elbow, each tendon	7.45	7.70	7.70	0.98	16.13	16.13	090	
24310		A	Tenotomy, open, elbow to shoulder, each tendon	5.98	8.43	8.43	0.74	15.15	15.15	090	
24320		A	Tenoplasty, with muscle transfer, with or without free graft, elbow to shoulder, single (Seddon-Brookes type procedure)	10.56	11.29	11.29	1.00	22.85	22.85	090	
24330		A	Flexor-plasty, elbow (eg, Steindler type advancement);	9.60	8.79	8.79	1.21	19.60	19.60	090	
24331		A	with extensor advancement	10.65	9.25	9.25	1.41	21.31	21.31	090	
24332		A	Tenolysis, triceps	7.45	5.23	5.23	0.77	13.45	13.45	090	
24340		A	Tenodesis of biceps tendon at elbow (separate procedure)	7.89	7.74	7.74	1.08	16.71	16.71	090	
24341		A	Repair, tendon or muscle, upper arm or elbow, each tendon or muscle, primary or secondary (excludes rotator cuff)	7.90	7.85	7.85	1.08	16.83	16.83	090	
24342		A	Reinsertion of ruptured biceps or triceps tendon, distal, with or without tendon graft	10.62	9.37	9.37	1.48	21.47	21.47	090	
24343		A	Repair lateral collateral ligament, elbow, with local tissue	8.65	7.91	7.91	1.21	17.77	17.77	090	
24344		A	Reconstruction lateral collateral ligament, elbow, with tendon graft (includes harvesting of graft)	14.00	10.87	10.87	1.95	26.82	26.82	090	
24345		A	Repair medial collateral ligament, elbow, with local tissue	8.65	7.91	7.91	1.21	17.77	17.77	090	
24346		A	Reconstruction medial collateral ligament, elbow, with tendon graft (includes harvesting of graft)	14.00	10.87	10.87	1.95	26.82	26.82	090	
24350		A	Fasciotomy, lateral or medial (eg, tennis elbow or epicondylitis);	5.25	6.25	6.25	0.72	12.22	12.22	090	
24351		A	with extensor origin detachment	5.91	6.72	6.72	0.82	13.45	13.45	090	

Surgery

■ RVU not developed by CMS. Gap-filled RVUs developed by Ingenix/CHEG.

Code	M	S	Description	Work Value	Non-Fac PE	Fac PE	Mal-prac-tice	Non-Fac Total	Fac Total	Global	Gap
24352		A	with annular ligament resection	6.43	7.01	7.01	0.90	14.34	14.34	090	
24354		A	with stripping	6.48	6.85	6.85	0.88	14.21	14.21	090	
24356		A	with partial ostectomy	6.68	7.21	7.21	0.90	14.79	14.79	090	
24360		A	Arthroplasty, elbow; with membrane (eg, fascial)	12.34	10.26	10.26	1.69	24.29	24.29	090	
24361		A	with distal humeral prosthetic replacement	14.08	11.30	11.30	1.95	27.33	27.33	090	
24362		A	with implant and fascia lata ligament reconstruction	14.99	11.30	11.30	1.92	28.21	28.21	090	
24363		A	with distal humerus and proximal ulnar prosthetic replacement (eg, total elbow)	18.49	13.80	13.80	2.52	34.81	34.81	090	
24365		A	Arthroplasty, radial head;	8.39	7.96	7.96	1.11	17.46	17.46	090	
24366		A	with implant	9.13	8.48	8.48	1.28	18.89	18.89	090	
24400		A	Osteotomy, humerus, with or without internal fixation	11.06	12.48	12.48	1.53	25.07	25.07	090	
24410		A	Multiple osteotomies with realignment on intramedullary rod, humeral shaft (Sofield type procedure)	14.82	13.75	13.75	1.89	30.46	30.46	090	
24420		A	Osteoplasty, humerus (eg, shortening or lengthening) (excluding 64876)	13.44	16.08	16.08	1.82	31.34	31.34	090	
24430		A	Repair of nonunion or malunion, humerus; without graft (eg, compression technique)	12.81	12.88	12.88	1.80	27.49	27.49	090	
24435		A	with iliac or other autograft (includes obtaining graft)	13.17	13.98	13.98	1.84	28.99	28.99	090	
24470		A	Hemiepiphyseal arrest (eg, cubitus varus or valgus, distal humerus)	8.74	6.59	6.59	1.23	16.56	16.56	090	
24495		A	Decompression fasciotomy, forearm, with brachial artery exploration	8.12	10.33	10.33	0.92	19.37	19.37	090	
24498		A	Prophylactic treatment (nailing, pinning, plating or wiring), with or without methylmethacrylate, humeral shaft	11.92	12.31	12.31	1.67	25.90	25.90	090	
24500		A	Closed treatment of humeral shaft fracture; without manipulation	3.21	5.09	3.38	0.41	8.71	7.00	090	
24505		A	with manipulation, with or without skeletal traction	5.17	8.88	6.81	0.72	14.77	12.70	090	
24515		A	Open treatment of humeral shaft fracture with plate/screws, with or without cerclage	11.65	11.40	11.40	1.63	24.68	24.68	090	
24516		A	Open treatment of humeral shaft fracture, with insertion of intramedullary implant, with or without cerclage and/or locking screws	11.65	11.85	11.85	1.63	25.13	25.13	090	

■ RVU not developed by CMS. Gap-filled RVUs developed by Ingenix/CHEG.

Code	M	S	Description	Work Value	Non-Fac PE	Fac PE	Mal-prac-tice	Non-Fac Total	Fac Total	Global	Gap
24530		A	Closed treatment of supracondylar or transcondylar humeral fracture, with or without intercondylar extension; without manipulation	3.50	6.19	4.86	0.47	10.16	8.83	090	
24535		A	with manipulation, with or without skin or skeletal traction	6.87	8.81	6.72	0.96	16.64	14.55	090	
24538		A	Percutaneous skeletal fixation of supracondylar or transcondylar humeral fracture, with or without intercondylar extension	9.43	10.61	10.61	1.25	21.29	21.29	090	
24545		A	Open treatment of humeral supracondylar or transcondylar fracture, with or without internal or external fixation; without intercondylar extension	10.46	10.18	10.18	1.47	22.11	22.11	090	
24546		A	with intercondylar extension	15.69	13.69	13.69	2.18	31.56	31.56	090	
24560		A	Closed treatment of humeral epicondylar fracture, medial or lateral; without manipulation	2.80	4.87	3.23	0.35	8.02	6.38	090	
24565		A	with manipulation	5.56	8.09	5.82	0.74	14.39	12.12	090	
24566		A	Percutaneous skeletal fixation of humeral epicondylar fracture, medial or lateral, with manipulation	7.79	9.96	9.96	1.10	18.85	18.85	090	
24575		A	Open treatment of humeral epicondylar fracture, medial or lateral, with or without internal or external fixation	10.66	8.49	8.49	1.44	20.59	20.59	090	
24576		A	Closed treatment of humeral condylar fracture, medial or lateral; without manipulation	2.86	4.62	3.26	0.38	7.86	6.50	090	
24577		A	with manipulation	5.79	8.22	6.13	0.81	14.82	12.73	090	
24579		A	Open treatment of humeral condylar fracture, medial or lateral, with or without internal or external fixation	11.60	11.32	11.32	1.62	24.54	24.54	090	
24582		A	Percutaneous skeletal fixation of humeral condylar fracture, medial or lateral, with manipulation	8.55	10.46	10.46	1.20	20.21	20.21	090	
24586		A	Open treatment of periarticular fracture and/or dislocation of the elbow (fracture distal humerus and proximal ulna and/or proximal radius);	15.21	11.23	11.23	2.12	28.56	28.56	090	
24587		A	with implant arthroplasty	15.16	11.13	11.13	2.14	28.43	28.43	090	
24600		A	Treatment of closed elbow dislocation; without anesthesia	4.23	6.82	5.12	0.49	11.54	9.84	090	
24605		A	requiring anesthesia	5.42	5.02	5.02	0.72	11.16	11.16	090	
24615		A	Open treatment of acute or chronic elbow dislocation	9.42	7.94	7.94	1.31	18.67	18.67	090	

Surgery

■ RVU not developed by CMS. Gap-filled RVUs developed by Ingenix/CHEG.

Code	M	S	Description	Work Value	Non-Fac PE	Fac PE	Mal-prac-tice	Non-Fac Total	Fac Total	Global	Gap
24620		A	Closed treatment of Monteggia type of fracture dislocation at elbow (fracture proximal end of ulna with dislocation of radial head), with manipulation	6.98	6.63	6.63	0.90	14.51	14.51	090	
24635		A	Open treatment of Monteggia type of fracture dislocation at elbow (fracture proximal end of ulna with dislocation of radial head), with or without internal or external fixation	13.19	16.55	16.55	1.84	31.58	31.58	090	
24640*		A	Closed treatment of radial head subluxation in child, nursemaid elbow, with manipulation	1.20	3.35	1.88	0.11	4.66	3.19	010	
24650		A	Closed treatment of radial head or neck fracture; without manipulation	2.16	4.55	2.92	0.28	6.99	5.36	090	
24655		A	with manipulation	4.40	7.33	5.22	0.58	12.31	10.20	090	
24665		A	Open treatment of radial head or neck fracture, with or without internal fixation or radial head excision;	8.14	9.40	9.40	1.13	18.67	18.67	090	
24666		A	with radial head prosthetic replacement	9.49	10.18	10.18	1.32	20.99	20.99	090	
24670		A	Closed treatment of ulnar fracture, proximal end (olecranon process); without manipulation	2.54	4.49	3.10	0.33	7.36	5.97	090	
24675		A	with manipulation	4.72	7.55	5.49	0.65	12.92	10.86	090	
24685		A	Open treatment of ulnar fracture proximal end (olecranon process), with or without internal or external fixation	8.80	9.79	9.79	1.23	19.82	19.82	090	
24800		A	Arthrodesis, elbow joint; local	11.2	9.90	9.90	1.41	22.51	22.51	090	
24802		A	with autogenous graft (includes obtaining graft)	13.69	11.5	11.5	1.89	27.08	27.08	090	
24900		A	Amputation, arm through humerus; with primary closure	9.60	11.37	11.37	1.18	22.15	22.15	090	
24920		A	open, circular (guillotine)	9.54	13.96	13.96	1.22	24.72	24.72	090	
24925		A	secondary closure or scar revision	7.07	9.64	9.64	0.95	17.66	17.66	090	
24930		A	re-amputation	10.25	10.86	10.86	1.23	22.34	22.34	090	
24931		A	with implant	12.72	11.63	11.63	1.56	25.91	25.91	090	
24935		A	Stump elongation, upper extremity	15.56	13.22	13.22	1.58	30.36	30.36	090	
24940		C	Cineplasty, upper extremity, complete procedure	16.06	12.77	12.77	1.71	30.54	30.54	090	■
24999		C	Unlisted procedure, humerus or elbow	0.00	0.00	0.00	0.00	0.00	0.00	YYY	
25000		A	Incision, extensor tendon sheath, wrist (eg, deQuervain's disease)	3.38	7.49	7.49	0.45	11.32	11.32	090	
25001		A	Incision, flexor tendon sheath, wrist (eg, flexor carpi radialis)	3.38	4.30	4.30	0.45	8.13	8.13	090	

■ RVU not developed by CMS. Gap-filled RVUs developed by Ingenix/CHEG.

Code	M	S	Description	Work Value	Non-Fac PE	Fac PE	Mal-prac-tice	Non-Fac Total	Fac Total	Global	Gap
25020		A	Decompression fasciotomy, forearm and/or wrist, flexor OR extensor compartment; without debridement of nonviable muscle and/or nerve	5.92	11.49	11.49	0.75	18.16	18.16	090	
25023		A	with debridement of nonviable muscle and/or nerve	12.96	17.5	17.5	1.50	31.96	31.96	090	
25024		A	Decompression fasciotomy, forearm and/or wrist, flexor AND extensor compartment; without debridement of nonviable muscle and/or nerve	9.50	8.17	8.17	1.20	18.87	18.87	090	
25025		A	with debridement of nonviable muscle and/or nerve	16.54	12.05	12.05	1.91	30.50	30.50	090	
25028		A	Incision and drainage, forearm and/or wrist; deep abscess or hematoma	5.25	10.20	10.20	0.61	16.06	16.06	090	
25031		A	bursa	4.14	10.24	10.24	0.50	14.88	14.88	090	
25035		A	Incision, deep, bone cortex, forearm and/or wrist (eg, osteomyelitis or bone abscess)	7.36	16.18	16.18	0.98	24.52	24.52	090	
25040		A	Arthrotomy, radiocarpal or midcarpal joint, with exploration, drainage, or removal of foreign body	7.18	9.40	9.40	0.96	17.54	17.54	090	
25065		A	Biopsy, soft tissue of forearm and/or wrist; superficial	1.99	2.53	2.53	0.12	4.64	4.64	010	
25066		A	deep (subfascial or intramuscular)	4.13	8.40	8.40	0.49	13.02	13.02	090	
25075		A	Excision, tumor, soft tissue of forearm and/or wrist area; subcutaneous	3.74	7.13	7.13	0.40	11.27	11.27	090	
25076		A	deep, subfascial or intramuscular	4.92	12.68	12.68	0.59	18.19	18.19	090	
25077		A	Radical resection of tumor (eg, malignant neoplasm), soft tissue of forearm and/or wrist area	9.76	15.66	15.66	1.10	26.52	26.52	090	
25085		A	Capsulotomy, wrist (eg, contracture)	5.50	11.29	11.29	0.71	17.50	17.50	090	
25100		A	Arthrotomy, wrist joint; with biopsy	3.90	7.99	7.99	0.50	12.39	12.39	090	
25101		A	with joint exploration, with or without biopsy, with or without removal of loose or foreign body	4.69	7.75	7.75	0.60	13.04	13.04	090	
25105		A	with synovectomy	5.85	11.22	11.22	0.77	17.84	17.84	090	
25107		A	Arthrotomy, distal radioulnar joint including repair of triangular cartilage, complex	6.43	11.41	11.41	0.82	18.66	18.66	090	
25110		A	Excision, lesion of tendon sheath, forearm and/or wrist	3.92	8.94	8.94	0.48	13.34	13.34	090	
25111		A	Excision of ganglion, wrist (dorsal or volar); primary	3.39	6.70	6.70	0.42	10.51	10.51	090	
25112		A	recurrent	4.53	7.43	7.43	0.54	12.50	12.50	090	

■ RVU not developed by CMS. Gap-filled RVUs developed by Ingenix/CHEG.

Surgery

Code	M	S	Description	Work Value	Non-Fac PE	Fac PE	Mal-practice	Non-Fac Total	Fac Total	Global	Gap
25115		A	Radical excision of bursa, synovia of wrist, or forearm tendon sheaths (eg, tenosynovitis, fungus, Tbc, or other granulomas, rheumatoid arthritis); flexors	8.82	17.19	17.19	1.11	27.12	27.12	090	
25116		A	extensors, with or without transposition of dorsal retinaculum	7.11	16.20	16.20	0.90	24.21	24.21	090	
25118		A	Synovectomy, extensor tendon sheath, wrist, single compartment;	4.37	7.93	7.93	0.55	12.85	12.85	090	
25119		A	with resection of distal ulna	6.04	11.45	11.45	0.80	18.29	18.29	090	
25120		A	Excision or curettage of bone cyst or benign tumor of radius or ulna (excluding head or neck of radius and olecranon process);	6.10	14.87	14.87	0.81	21.78	21.78	090	
25125		A	with autograft (includes obtaining graft)	7.48	16.11	16.11	1.02	24.61	24.61	090	
25126		A	with allograft	7.55	15.76	15.76	1.00	24.31	24.31	090	
25130		A	Excision or curettage of bone cyst or benign tumor of carpal bones;	5.26	8.33	8.33	0.66	14.25	14.25	090	
25135		A	with autograft (includes obtaining graft)	6.89	9.00	9.00	0.89	16.78	16.78	090	
25136		A	with allograft	5.97	9.26	9.26	0.58	15.81	15.81	090	
25145		A	Sequestrectomy (eg, for osteomyelitis or bone abscess), forearm and/or wrist	6.37	15.43	15.43	0.82	22.62	22.62	090	
25150		A	Partial excision (craterization, saucerization or diaphysectomy) of bone (eg, for osteomyelitis); ulna	7.09	12.00	12.00	0.96	20.05	20.05	090	
25151		A	radius	7.39	16.22	16.22	0.93	24.54	24.54	090	
25170		A	Radical resection for tumor, radius or ulna	11.09	17.56	17.56	1.52	30.17	30.17	090	
25210		A	Carpectomy; one bone	5.95	8.71	8.71	0.73	15.39	15.39	090	
25215		A	all bones of proximal row	7.89	12.27	12.27	1.02	21.18	21.18	090	
25230		A	Radial styloidectomy (separate procedure)	5.23	8.23	8.23	0.66	14.12	14.12	090	
25240		A	Excision distal ulna partial or complete (eg, Darrach type or matched resection)	5.17	10.78	10.78	0.69	16.64	16.64	090	
25246		A	Injection procedure for wrist arthrography	1.45	10.20	0.52	0.07	11.72	2.04	000	
25248		A	Exploration with removal of deep foreign body, forearm or wrist	5.14	10.66	10.66	0.54	16.34	16.34	090	
25250		A	Removal of wrist prosthesis; (separate procedure)	6.60	8.91	8.91	0.84	16.35	16.35	090	
25251		A	complicated, including total wrist	9.57	12.52	12.52	1.15	23.24	23.24	090	
25259		A	Manipulation, wrist, under anesthesia	3.75	5.35	5.35	0.52	9.62	9.62	090	

■ RVU not developed by CMS. Gap-filled RVUs developed by Ingenix/CHEG.

Code	M	S	Description	Work Value	Non-Fac PE	Fac PE	Mal-practice	Non-Fac Total	Fac Total	Global	Gap
25260		A	Repair, tendon or muscle, flexor, forearm and/or wrist; primary, single, each tendon or muscle	7.80	17.11	17.11	0.97	25.88	25.88	090	
25263		A	secondary, single, each tendon or muscle	7.82	15.65	15.65	0.94	24.41	24.41	090	
25265		A	secondary, with free graft (includes obtaining graft), each tendon or muscle	9.88	17.11	17.11	1.19	28.18	28.18	090	
25270		A	Repair, tendon or muscle, extensor, forearm and/or wrist; primary, single, each tendon or muscle	6.00	16.04	16.04	0.76	22.80	22.80	090	
25272		A	secondary, single, each tendon or muscle	7.04	16.50	16.50	0.89	24.43	24.43	090	
25274		A	secondary, with free graft (includes obtaining graft), each tendon or muscle	8.75	17.36	17.36	1.11	27.22	27.22	090	
25275		A	Repair, tendon sheath, extensor, forearm and/or wrist, with free graft (includes obtaining graft) (eg, for extensor carpi ulnaris subluxation)	8.50	7.53	7.53	1.11	17.14	17.14	090	
25280		A	Lengthening or shortening of flexor or extensor tendon, forearm and/or wrist, single, each tendon	7.22	15.80	15.80	0.91	23.93	23.93	090	
25290		A	Tenotomy, open, flexor or extensor tendon, forearm and/or wrist, single, each tendon	5.29	18.17	18.17	0.66	24.12	24.12	090	
25295		A	Tenolysis, flexor or extensor tendon, forearm and/or wrist, single, each tendon	6.55	15.16	15.16	0.84	22.55	22.55	090	
25300		A	Tenodesis at wrist; flexors of fingers	8.80	10.02	10.02	1.07	19.89	19.89	090	
25301		A	extensors of fingers	8.40	10.15	10.15	1.08	19.63	19.63	090	
25310		A	Tendon transplantation or transfer, flexor or extensor, forearm and/or wrist, single; each tendon	8.14	16.47	16.47	1.01	25.62	25.62	090	
25312		A	with tendon graft(s) (includes obtaining graft), each tendon	9.57	17.24	17.24	1.22	28.03	28.03	090	
25315		A	Flexor origin slide (eg, for cerebral palsy, Volkmann contracture), forearm and/or wrist;	10.20	18.59	18.59	1.26	30.05	30.05	090	
25316		A	with tendon(s) transfer	12.33	18.40	18.40	1.74	32.47	32.47	090	
25320		A	Capsulorrhaphy or reconstruction, wrist, any method (eg, capsulodesis, ligament repair, tendon transfer or graft) (includes synovectomy, capsulotomy and open reduction) for carpal instability	10.77	11.53	11.53	1.32	23.62	23.62	090	
25332		A	Arthroplasty, wrist, with or without interposition, with or without external or internal fixation	11.41	11.89	11.89	1.46	24.76	24.76	090	
25335		A	Centralization of wrist on ulna (eg, radial club hand)	12.88	13.60	13.60	1.66	28.14	28.14	090	

Surgery

■ RVU not developed by CMS. Gap-filled RVUs developed by Ingenix/CHEG.

Code	M	S	Description	Work Value	Non-Fac PE	Fac PE	Mal-practice	Non-Fac Total	Fac Total	Global	Gap
25337		A	Reconstruction for stabilization of unstable distal ulna or distal radioulnar joint, secondary by soft tissue stabilization (eg, tendon transfer, tendon graft or weave, or tenodesis) with or without open reduction of distal radioulnar joint	10.17	13.80	13.80	1.31	25.28	25.28	090	
25350		A	Osteotomy, radius; distal third	8.78	16.68	16.68	1.17	26.63	26.63	090	
25355		A	middle or proximal third	10.17	17.17	17.17	1.44	28.78	28.78	090	
25360		A	Osteotomy; ulna	8.43	16.86	16.86	1.17	26.46	26.46	090	
25365		A	radius AND ulna	12.40	18.74	18.74	1.67	32.81	32.81	090	
25370		A	Multiple osteotomies, with realignment on intramedullary rod (Sofield type procedure); radius OR ulna	13.36	17.84	17.84	1.88	33.08	33.08	090	
25375		A	radius AND ulna	13.04	16.44	16.44	1.84	31.32	31.32	090	
25390		A	Osteoplasty, radius OR ulna; shortening	10.40	17.38	17.38	1.38	29.16	29.16	090	
25391		A	lengthening with autograft	13.65	19.01	19.01	1.73	34.39	34.39	090	
25392		A	Osteoplasty, radius AND ulna; shortening (excluding 64876)	13.95	15.59	15.59	1.73	31.27	31.27	090	
25393		A	lengthening with autograft	15.87	21.72	21.72	1.87	39.46	39.46	090	
25394		A	Osteoplasty, carpal bone, shortening	10.40	8.43	8.43	1.15	19.98	19.98	090	
25400		A	Repair of nonunion or malunion, radius OR ulna; without graft (eg, compression technique)	10.92	17.98	17.98	1.50	30.40	30.40	090	
25405		A	with autograft (includes obtaining graft)v	14.38	20.38	20.38	1.95	36.71	36.71	090	
25415		A	Repair of nonunion or malunion, radius AND ulna; without graft (eg, compression technique)	13.35	19.14	19.14	1.87	34.36	34.36	090	
25420		A	with autograft (includes obtaining graft)	16.33	21.72	21.72	2.20	40.25	40.25	090	
25425		A	Repair of defect with autograft; radius OR ulna	13.21	24.75	24.75	1.61	39.57	39.57	090	
25426		A	radius AND ulna	15.82	18.15	18.15	2.23	36.20	36.20	090	
25430		A	Insertion of vascular pedicle into carpal bone (eg, Harii procedure)	9.25	7.82	7.82	0.56	17.63	17.63	090	
25431		A	Repair of nonunion of carpal bone (excluding carpal scaphoid (navicular)) (includes obtaining graft and necessary fixation), each bone	10.44	6.42	6.42	0.56	17.42	17.42	090	
25440		A	Repair of nonunion, scaphoid carpal (navicular) bone, with or without radial styloidectomy (includes obtaining graft and necessary fixation)	10.44	11.05	11.05	1.41	22.90	22.90	090	
25441		A	Arthroplasty with prosthetic replacement; distal radius	12.90	12.24	12.24	1.83	26.97	26.97	090	

■ RVU not developed by CMS. Gap-filled RVUs developed by Ingenix/CHEG.

Code	M	S	Description	Work Value	Non-Fac PE	Fac PE	Mal-practice	Non-Fac Total	Fac Total	Global	Gap
25442		A	distal ulna	10.85	11.46	11.46	1.24	23.55	23.55	090	
25443		A	scaphoid carpal (navicular)	10.39	13.29	13.29	1.30	24.98	24.98	090	
25444		A	lunate	11.15	14.29	14.29	1.43	26.87	26.87	090	
25445		A	trapezium	9.69	13.50	13.50	1.26	24.45	24.45	090	
25446		A	distal radius and partial or entire carpus (total wrist)	16.55	14.45	14.45	2.20	33.2	33.20	090	
25447		A	Arthroplasty, interposition, intercarpal or carpometacarpal joints	10.37	11.27	11.27	1.34	22.98	22.98	090	
25449		A	Revision of arthroplasty, including removal of implant, wrist joint	14.49	16.20	16.20	1.77	32.46	32.46	090	
25450		A	Epiphyseal arrest by epiphysiodesis or stapling; distal radius OR ulna	7.87	13.91	13.91	0.88	22.66	22.66	090	
25455		A	distal radius AND ulna	9.49	15.22	15.22	1.07	25.78	25.78	090	
25490		A	Prophylactic treatment (nailing, pinning, plating or wiring) with or without methylmethacrylate; radius	9.54	16.70	16.70	1.19	27.43	27.43	090	
25491		A	ulna	9.96	16.98	16.98	1.41	28.35	28.35	090	
25492		A	radius AND ulna	12.33	16.09	16.09	1.62	30.04	30.04	090	
25500		A	Closed treatment of radial shaft fracture; without manipulation	2.45	4.27	2.94	0.28	7.00	5.67	090	
25505		A	with manipulation	5.21	7.87	5.65	0.69	13.77	11.55	090	
25515		A	Open treatment of radial shaft fracture, with or without internal or external fixation	9.18	10.00	10.00	1.22	20.40	20.40	090	
25520		A	Closed treatment of radial shaft fracture and closed treatment of dislocation of distal radioulnar joint (Galeazzi fracture/dislocation)	6.26	8.00	6.28	0.85	15.11	13.39	090	
25525		A	Open treatment of radial shaft fracture, with internal and/ or external fixation and closed treatment of dislocation of distal radioulnar joint (Galeazzi fracture/dislocation), with or without percutaneous skeletal fixation	12.24	11.65	11.65	1.68	25.57	25.57	090	
25526		A	Open treatment of radial shaft fracture, with internal and/or external fixation and open treatment, with or without internal or external fixation of distal radioulnar joint (Galeazzi fracture/dislocation), includes repair of triangular fibrocartilage complex	12.98	15.01	15.01	1.80	29.79	29.79	090	
25530		A	Closed treatment of ulnar shaft fracture; without manipulation	2.09	4.21	2.87	0.27	6.57	5.23	090	
25535		A	with manipulation	5.14	7.74	5.72	0.68	13.56	11.54	090	
25545		A	Open treatment of ulnar shaft fracture, with or without internal or external fixation	8.90	9.88	9.88	1.23	20.01	20.01	090	

■ RVU not developed by CMS. Gap-filled RVUs developed by Ingenix/CHEG.

Code	M	S	Description	Work Value	Non-Fac PE	Fac PE	Mal-practice	Non-Fac Total	Fac Total	Global	Gap
25560		A	Closed treatment of radial and ulnar shaft fractures; without manipulation	2.44	4.28	2.93	0.27	6.99	5.64	090	
25565		A	with manipulation	5.63	8.02	5.94	0.76	14.41	12.33	090	
25574		A	Open treatment of radial AND ulnar shaft fractures, with internal or external fixation; of radius OR ulna	7.01	8.72	8.72	0.96	16.69	16.69	090	
25575		A	of radius AND ulna	10.45	10.74	10.74	1.46	22.65	22.65	090	
25600		A	Closed treatment of distal radial fracture (eg, Colles or Smith type) or epiphyseal separation, with or without fracture of ulnar styloid; without manipulation	2.63	4.53	3.10	0.34	7.50	6.07	090	
25605		A	with manipulation	5.81	8.18	6.11	0.81	14.8	12.73	090	
25611		A	Percutaneous skeletal fixation of distal radial fracture (eg, Colles or Smith type) or epiphyseal separation, with or without fracture of ulnar styloid, requiring manipulation, with or without external fixation	7.77	10.04	10.04	1.08	18.89	18.89	090	
25620		A	Open treatment of distal radial fracture (eg, Colles or Smith type) or epiphyseal separation, with or without fracture of ulnar styloid, with or without internal or external fixation	8.55	9.67	9.67	1.17	19.39	19.39	090	
25622		A	Closed treatment of carpal scaphoid (navicular) fracture; without manipulation	2.61	4.48	3.10	0.33	7.42	6.04	090	
25624		A	with manipulation	4.53	7.40	5.34	0.61	12.54	10.48	090	
25628		A	Open treatment of carpal scaphoid (navicular) fracture, with or without internal or external fixation	8.43	9.68	9.68	1.14	19.25	19.25	090	
25630		A	Closed treatment of carpal bone fracture (excluding carpal scaphoid (navicular)); without manipulation, each bone	2.88	4.66	3.20	0.37	7.91	6.45	090	
25635		A	with manipulation, each bone	4.39	7.45	5.11	0.39	12.23	9.89	090	
25645		A	Open treatment of carpal bone fracture (other than carpal scaphoid (navicular)), each bone	7.25	9.56	9.56	0.93	17.74	17.74	090	
25650		A	Closed treatment of ulnar styloid fracture	3.05	4.75	3.24	0.37	8.17	6.66	090	
25651		A	Percutaneous skeletal fixation of ulnar styloid fracture	5.36	4.39	4.39	0.73	10.48	10.48	090	
25652		A	Open treatment of ulnar styloid fracture	7.60	6.90	6.90	0.97	15.47	15.47	090	
25660		A	Closed treatment of radiocarpal or intercarpal dislocation, one or more bones, with manipulation	4.76	5.45	5.45	0.59	10.80	10.80	090	
25670		A	Open treatment of radiocarpal or intercarpal dislocation, one or more bones	7.92	9.54	9.54	1.07	18.53	18.53	090	

■ RVU not developed by CMS. Gap-filled RVUs developed by Ingenix/CHEG.

Code	M	S	Description	Work Value	Non-Fac PE	Fac PE	Mal-prac-tice	Non-Fac Total	Fac Total	Global	Gap
25671		A	Percutaneous skeletal fixation of distal radioulnar dislocation	6.00	6.02	6.02	0.75	12.77	12.77	090	
25675		A	Closed treatment of distal radioulnar dislocation with manipulation	4.67	7.57	5.39	0.57	12.81	10.63	090	
25676		A	Open treatment of distal radioulnar dislocation, acute or chronic	8.04	9.52	9.52	1.10	18.66	18.66	090	
25680		A	Closed treatment of trans-scaphoperilunar type of fracture dislocation, with manipulation	5.99	6.45	6.45	0.61	13.05	13.05	090	
25685		A	Open treatment of trans-scaphoperilunar type of fracture dislocation	9.78	10.20	10.20	1.25	21.23	21.23	090	
25690		A	Closed treatment of lunate dislocation, with manipulation	5.50	7.00	7.00	0.78	13.28	13.28	090	
25695		A	Open treatment of lunate dislocation	8.34	9.68	9.68	1.07	19.09	19.09	090	
25800		A	Arthrodesis, wrist; complete, without bone graft (includes radiocarpal and/or intercarpal and/or carpometacarpal joints)	9.76	10.87	10.87	1.30	21.93	21.93	090	
25805		A	with sliding graft	11.28	11.61	11.61	1.51	24.4	24.40	090	
25810		A	with iliac or other autograft (includes obtaining graft)	10.57	11.33	11.33	1.37	23.27	23.27	090	
25820		A	Arthrodesis, wrist; limited, without bone graft (eg, intercarpal or radiocarpal)	7.45	9.54	9.54	0.96	17.95	17.95	090	
25825		A	with autograft (includes obtaining graft)	9.27	10.51	10.51	1.20	20.98	20.98	090	
25830		A	Arthrodesis, distal radioulnar joint with segmental resection of ulna, with or without bone graft (eg, Sauve-Kapandji procedure)	10.06	16.99	16.99	1.27	28.32	28.32	090	
25900		A	Amputation, forearm, through radius and ulna;	9.01	15.04	15.04	1.08	25.13	25.13	090	
25905		A	open, circular (guillotine)	9.12	14.25	14.25	1.06	24.43	24.43	090	
25907		A	secondary closure or scar revision	7.80	15.26	15.26	1.01	24.07	24.07	090	
25909		A	re-amputation	8.96	14.51	14.51	1.07	24.54	24.54	090	
25915		A	Krukenberg procedure	17.08	15.11	15.11	2.41	34.60	34.60	090	
25920		A	Disarticulation through wrist;	8.68	10.12	10.12	1.06	19.86	19.86	090	
25922		A	secondary closure or scar revision	7.42	7.58	7.58	0.93	15.93	15.93	090	
25924		A	re-amputation	8.46	10.19	10.19	1.07	19.72	19.72	090	
25927		A	Transmetacarpal amputation;	8.80	14.11	14.11	1.02	23.93	23.93	090	
25929		A	secondary closure or scar revision	7.59	7.42	7.42	0.89	15.90	15.90	090	
25931		A	re-amputation	7.81	15.79	15.79	0.88	24.48	24.48	090	
25999		C	Unlisted procedure, forearm or wrist	0.00	0.00	0.00	0.00	0.00	0.00	YYY	

■ RVU not developed by CMS. Gap-filled RVUs developed by Ingenix/CHEG.

Surgery

Code	M	S	Description	Work Value	Non-Fac PE	Fac PE	Mal-practice	Non-Fac Total	Fac Total	Global	Gap
26010*		A	Drainage of finger abscess; simple	1.54	5.24	3.94	0.14	6.92	5.62	010	
26011*		A	complicated (eg, felon)	2.19	7.48	6.50	0.25	9.92	8.94	010	
26020		A	Drainage of tendon sheath, digit and/or palm, each	4.67	13.10	13.10	0.59	18.36	18.36	090	
26025		A	Drainage of palmar bursa; single, bursa	4.82	13.26	13.26	0.60	18.68	18.68	090	
26030		A	multiple bursa	5.93	14.02	14.02	0.72	20.67	20.67	090	
26034		A	Incision, bone cortex, hand or finger (eg, osteomyelitis or bone abscess)	6.23	14.84	14.84	0.79	21.86	21.86	090	
26035		A	Decompression fingers and/or hand, injection injury (eg, grease gun)	9.51	15.17	15.17	1.12	25.80	25.80	090	
26037		A	Decompressive fasciotomy, hand (excludes 26035)	7.25	12.67	12.67	0.87	20.79	20.79	090	
26040		A	Fasciotomy, palmar (eg, Dupuytrens contracture); percutaneous	3.33	12.87	12.87	0.45	16.65	16.65	090	
26045		A	open, partial	5.56	14.17	14.17	0.74	20.47	20.47	090	
26055		A	Tendon sheath incision (eg, for trigger finger)	2.69	8.12	7.69	0.36	11.17	10.74	090	
26060		A	Tenotomy, percutaneous, single, each digit	2.81	7.57	7.57	0.35	10.73	10.73	090	
26070		A	Arthrotomy, with exploration, drainage, or removal of loose or foreign body; carpometacarpal joint	3.69	11.69	11.69	0.35	15.73	15.73	090	
26075		A	metacarpophalangeal joint, each	3.79	12.47	12.47	0.40	16.66	16.66	090	
26080		A	interphalangeal joint, each	4.24	13.09	13.09	0.52	17.85	17.85	090	
26100		A	Arthrotomy with biopsy; carpometacarpal joint, each	3.67	8.43	8.43	0.45	12.55	12.55	090	
26105		A	metacarpophalangeal joint, each	3.71	12.95	12.95	0.45	17.11	17.11	090	
26110		A	interphalangeal joint, each	3.53	12.46	12.46	0.44	16.43	16.43	090	
26115		A	Excision, tumor or vascular malformation, soft tissue of hand or finger; subcutaneous	3.86	7.66	7.66	0.48	12.00	12.00	090	
26116		A	deep (subfascial or intramuscular)	5.53	13.91	13.91	0.69	20.13	20.13	090	
26117		A	Radical resection of tumor (eg, malignant neoplasm), soft tissue of hand or finger	8.55	15.41	15.41	1.01	24.97	24.97	090	
26121		A	Fasciectomy, palm only, with or without Z-plasty, other local tissue rearrangement, or skin grafting (includes obtaining graft)	7.54	15.80	15.80	0.94	24.28	24.28	090	
26123		A	Fasciectomy, partial palmar with release of single digit including proximal interphalangeal joint, with or without Z-plasty, other local tissue rearrangement, or skin grafting (includes obtaining graft);	9.29	16.73	16.73	1.17	27.19	27.19	090	

■ RVU not developed by CMS. Gap-filled RVUs developed by Ingenix/CHEG.

Code	M	S	Description	Work Value	Non-Fac PE	Fac PE	Mal-prac-tice	Non-Fac Total	Fac Total	Global	Gap
26125		A	each additional digit (List separately in addition to code for primary procedure)	4.61	2.60	2.60	0.57	7.78	7.78	ZZZ	
26130		A	Synovectomy, carpometacarpal joint	5.42	15.62	15.62	0.65	21.69	21.69	090	
26135		A	Synovectomy, metacarpophalangeal joint including intrinsic release and extensor hood reconstruction, each digit	6.96	17.04	17.04	0.87	24.87	24.87	090	
26140		A	Synovectomy, proximal interphalangeal joint, including extensor reconstruction, each interphalangeal joint	6.17	16.33	16.33	0.76	23.26	23.26	090	
26145		A	Synovectomy, tendon sheath, radical (tenosynovectomy), flexor tendon, palm and/or finger, each tendon	6.32	16.86	16.86	0.77	23.95	23.95	090	
26160		A	Excision of lesion of tendon sheath or joint capsule (eg, cyst, mucous cyst, or ganglion), hand or finger	3.15	7.93	7.88	0.39	11.47	11.42	090	
26170		A	Excision of tendon, palm, flexor, single (separate procedure), each	4.77	8.53	8.53	0.60	13.90	13.90	090	
26180		A	Excision of tendon, finger, flexor (separate procedure), each tendon	5.18	9.19	9.19	0.64	15.01	15.01	090	
26185		A	Sesamoidectomy, thumb or finger (separate procedure)	5.25	8.76	8.76	0.67	14.68	14.68	090	
26200		A	Excision or curettage of bone cyst or benign tumor of metacarpal;	5.51	13.97	13.97	0.71	20.19	20.19	090	
26205		A	with autograft (includes obtaining graft)	7.70	15.35	15.35	0.95	24.00	24.00	090	
26210		A	Excision or curettage of bone cyst or benign tumor of proximal, middle or distal phalanx of finger;	5.15	14.32	14.32	0.64	20.11	20.11	090	
26215		A	with autograft (includes obtaining graft)	7.10	14.89	14.89	0.77	22.76	22.76	090	
26230		A	Partial excision (craterization, saucerization, or diaphysectomy) bone (eg, osteomyelitis); metacarpal	6.33	12.87	12.87	0.84	20.04	20.04	090	
26235		A	proximal or middle phalanx of finger	6.19	12.56	12.56	0.78	19.53	19.53	090	
26236		A	distal phalanx of finger	5.32	12.62	12.62	0.66	18.60	18.60	090	
26250		A	Radical resection, metacarpal (eg, tumor);	7.55	17.33	17.33	0.92	25.80	25.80	090	
26255		A	with autograft (includes obtaining graft)	12.43	18.74	18.74	1.05	32.22	32.22	090	
26260		A	Radical resection, proximal or middle phalanx of finger (eg, tumor);	7.03	16.39	16.39	0.83	24.25	24.25	090	
26261		A	with autograft (includes obtaining graft)	9.09	16.10	16.10	0.84	26.03	26.03	090	
26262		A	Radical resection, distal phalanx of finger (eg, tumor)	5.67	14.81	14.81	0.70	21.18	21.18	090	
26320		A	Removal of implant from finger or hand	3.98	13.08	13.08	0.49	17.55	17.55	090	

■ RVU not developed by CMS. Gap-filled RVUs developed by Ingenix/CHEG.

Code	M	S	Description	Work Value	Non-Fac PE	Fac PE	Mal-practice	Non-Fac Total	Fac Total	Global	Gap
26340		A	Manipulation, finger joint, under anesthesia, each joint	2.50	4.53	4.53	0.32	7.35	7.35	090	
26350		A	Repair or advancement, flexor tendon, not in zone 2 digital flexor tendon sheath (eg, no man's land); primary or secondary without free graft, each tendon	5.99	20.24	20.24	0.73	26.96	26.96	090	
26352		A	secondary with free graft (includes obtaining graft), each tendon	7.68	19.74	19.74	0.93	28.35	28.35	090	
26356		A	Repair or advancement, flexor tendon, in zone 2 digital flexor tendon sheath (eg, no man's land); primary or secondary without free graft, each tendon	8.07	21.55	21.55	0.99	30.61	30.61	090	
26357		A	secondary, each tendon	8.58	21.30	21.30	1.02	30.90	30.90	090	
26358		A	secondary with free graft (includes obtaining graft), each tendon	9.14	22.43	22.43	1.07	32.64	32.64	090	
26370		A	Repair or advancement of profundus tendon, with intact superficialis tendon; primary, each tendon	7.11	20.61	20.61	0.90	28.62	28.62	090	
26372		A	secondary with free graft (includes obtaining graft), each tendon	8.76	20.46	20.46	1.06	30.28	30.28	090	
26373		A	secondary without free graft, each tendon	8.16	22.61	22.61	0.98	31.75	31.75	090	
26390		A	Excision flexor tendon, with implantation of synthetic rod for delayed tendon graft, hand or finger, each rod	9.19	16.93	16.93	1.09	27.21	27.21	090	
26392		A	Removal of synthetic rod and insertion of flexor tendon graft, hand or finger (includes obtaining graft), each rod	10.26	23.05	23.05	1.26	34.57	34.57	090	
26410		A	Repair, extensor tendon, hand, primary or secondary; without free graft, each tendon	4.63	16.26	16.26	0.57	21.46	21.46	090	
26412		A	with free graft (includes obtaining graft), each tendon	6.31	16.83	16.83	0.80	23.94	23.94	090	
26415		A	Excision of extensor tendon, with implantation of synthetic rod for delayed tendon graft, hand or finger, each rod	8.34	18.14	18.14	0.77	27.25	27.25	090	
26416		A	Removal of synthetic rod and insertion of extensor tendon graft (includes obtaining graft), hand or finger, each rod	9.37	18.95	18.95	1.20	29.52	29.52	090	
26418		A	Repair, extensor tendon, finger, primary or secondary; without free graft, each tendon	4.25	16.34	16.34	0.50	21.09	21.09	090	
26420		A	with free graft (includes obtaining graft) each tendon	6.77	17.92	17.92	0.83	25.52	25.52	090	
26426		A	Repair of extensor tendon, central slip, secondary (eg, boutonniere deformity); using local tissue(s), including lateral band(s), each finger	6.15	17.05	17.05	0.77	23.97	23.97	090	

■ RVU not developed by CMS. Gap-filled RVUs developed by Ingenix/CHEG.

Code	M	S	Description	Work Value	Non-Fac PE	Fac PE	Mal-practice	Non-Fac Total	Fac Total	Global	Gap
26428		A	with free graft (includes obtaining graft), each finger	7.21	16.05	16.05	0.84	24.1	24.10	090	
26432		A	Closed treatment of distal extensor tendon insertion, with or without percutaneous pinning (eg, mallet finger)	4.02	13.49	13.49	0.48	17.99	17.99	090	
26433		A	Repair of extensor tendon, distal insertion, primary or secondary; without graft (eg, mallet finger)	4.56	14.42	14.42	0.56	19.54	19.54	090	
26434		A	with free graft (includes obtaining graft)	6.09	15.34	15.34	0.71	22.14	22.14	090	
26437		A	Realignment of extensor tendon, hand, each tendon	5.82	14.16	14.16	0.74	20.72	20.72	090	
26440		A	Tenolysis, flexor tendon; palm OR finger; each tendon	5.02	18.48	18.48	0.62	24.12	24.12	090	
26442		A	palm AND finger, each tendon	8.16	19.40	19.40	0.94	28.50	28.50	090	
26445		A	Tenolysis, extensor tendon, hand OR finger; each tendon	4.31	18.27	18.27	0.54	23.12	23.12	090	
26449		A	Tenolysis, complex, extensor tendon, finger, including forearm, each tendon	7.00	20.16	20.16	0.84	28.00	28.00	090	
26450		A	Tenotomy, flexor, palm, open, each tendon	3.67	8.71	8.71	0.46	12.84	12.84	090	
26455		A	Tenotomy, flexor, finger, open, each tendon	3.64	8.38	8.38	0.47	12.49	12.49	090	
26460		A	Tenotomy, extensor, hand or finger, open, each tendon	3.46	8.06	8.06	0.44	11.96	11.96	090	
26471		A	Tenodesis; of proximal interphalangeal joint, each joint	5.73	13.93	13.93	0.73	20.39	20.39	090	
26474		A	of distal joint, each joint	5.32	13.30	13.30	0.69	19.31	19.31	090	
26476		A	Lengthening of tendon, extensor, hand or finger, each tendon	5.18	12.72	12.72	0.62	18.52	18.52	090	
26477		A	Shortening of tendon, extensor, hand or finger, each tendon	5.15	13.73	13.73	0.60	19.48	19.48	090	
26478		A	Lengthening of tendon, flexor, hand or finger, each tendon	5.80	14.73	14.73	0.77	21.30	21.30	090	
26479		A	Shortening of tendon, flexor, hand or finger, each tendon	5.74	13.71	13.71	0.76	20.21	20.21	090	
26480		A	Transfer or transplant of tendon, carpometacarpal area or dorsum of hand; without free graft, each tendon	6.69	19.63	19.63	0.84	27.16	27.16	090	
26483		A	with free tendon graft (includes obtaining graft), each tendon	8.29	19.79	19.79	1.03	29.11	29.11	090	
26485		A	Transfer or transplant of tendon, palmar; without free tendon graft, each tendon	7.70	20.08	20.08	0.94	28.72	28.72	090	

Surgery

■ RVU not developed by CMS. Gap-filled RVUs developed by Ingenix/CHEG.

Code	M	S	Description	Work Value	Non-Fac PE	Fac PE	Mal-practice	Non-Fac Total	Fac Total	Global	Gap
26489		A	with free tendon graft (includes obtaining graft), each tendon	9.55	17.34	17.34	0.98	27.87	27.87	090	
26490		A	Opponensplasty; superficialis tendon transfer type, each tendon	8.41	14.87	14.87	1.05	24.33	24.33	090	
26492		A	tendon transfer with graft (includes obtaining graft), each tendon	9.62	15.84	15.84	1.19	26.65	26.65	090	
26494		A	hypothenar muscle transfer	8.47	13.52	13.52	1.13	23.12	23.12	090	
26496		A	other methods	9.59	15.53	15.53	1.17	26.29	26.29	090	
26497		A	Transfer of tendon to restore intrinsic function; ring and small finger	9.57	16.42	16.42	1.17	27.16	27.16	090	
26498		A	all four fingers	14.00	18.19	18.19	1.74	33.93	33.93	090	
26499		A	Correction claw finger, other methods	8.98	14.61	14.61	0.94	24.53	24.53	090	
26500		A	Reconstruction of tendon pulley, each tendon; with local tissues (separate procedure)	5.96	15.16	15.16	0.66	21.78	21.78	090	
26502		A	with tendon or fascial graft (includes obtaining graft) (separate procedure)	7.14	15.14	15.14	0.87	23.15	23.15	090	
26504		A	with tendon prosthesis (separate procedure)	7.47	14.31	14.31	0.84	22.62	22.62	090	
26508		A	Release of thenar muscle(s) (eg, thumb contracture)	6.01	14.11	14.11	0.76	20.88	20.88	090	
26510		A	Cross intrinsic transfer, each tendon	5.43	14.18	14.18	0.71	20.32	20.32	090	
26516		A	Capsulodesis, metacarpophalangeal joint; single digit	7.15	15.06	15.06	0.90	23.11	23.11	090	
26517		A	two digits	8.83	15.89	15.89	0.96	25.68	25.68	090	
26518		A	three or four digits	9.02	15.91	15.91	1.13	26.06	26.06	090	
26520		A	Capsulectomy or capsulotomy; metacarpophalangeal joint, each joint	5.30	18.59	18.59	0.65	24.54	24.54	090	
26525		A	interphalangeal joint, each joint	5.33	18.67	18.67	0.66	24.66	24.66	090	
26530		A	Arthroplasty, metacarpophalangeal joint; each joint	6.69	19.35	19.35	0.86	26.90	26.90	090	
26531		A	with prosthetic implant, each joint	7.91	19.41	19.41	1.01	28.33	28.33	090	
26535		A	Arthroplasty, interphalangeal joint; each joint	5.24	11.10	11.10	0.66	17.00	17.00	090	
26536		A	with prosthetic implant, each joint	6.37	17.97	17.97	0.80	25.14	25.14	090	
26540		A	Repair of collateral ligament, metacarpophalangeal or interphalangeal joint	6.43	14.54	14.54	0.81	21.78	21.78	090	
26541		A	Reconstruction, collateral ligament, metacarpophalangeal joint, single, with tendon or fascial graft (includes obtaining graft)	8.62	16.36	16.36	1.12	26.10	26.10	090	

■ RVU not developed by CMS. Gap-filled RVUs developed by Ingenix/CHEG.

Code	M	S	Description	Work Value	Non-Fac PE	Fac PE	Mal-practice	Non-Fac Total	Fac Total	Global	Gap
26542		A	with local tissue (eg, adductor advancement)	6.78	14.51	14.51	0.87	22.16	22.16	090	
26545		A	Reconstruction, collateral ligament, interphalangeal joint, single, including graft, each joint	6.92	16.16	16.16	0.79	23.87	23.87	090	
26546		A	Repair non-union, metacarpal or phalanx, (includes obtaining bone graft with or without external or internal fixation)	8.92	15.95	15.95	1.14	26.01	26.01	090	
26548		A	Repair and reconstruction, finger, volar plate, interphalangeal joint	8.03	16.13	16.13	0.98	25.14	25.14	090	
26550		A	Pollicization of a digit	21.24	30.36	30.36	1.80	53.40	53.40	090	
26551		A	Transfer, toe-to-hand with microvascular anastomosis; great toe wrap-around with bone graft	46.58	29.35	29.35	6.57	82.50	82.50	090	
26553		A	other than great toe, single	46.27	29.23	29.23	1.99	77.49	77.49	090	
26554		A	other than great toe, double	54.95	32.69	32.69	7.76	95.40	95.40	090	
26555		A	Transfer, finger to another position without microvascular anastomosis	16.63	24.00	24.00	2.13	42.76	42.76	090	
26556		A	Transfer, free toe joint, with microvascular anastomosis	47.26	29.62	29.62	6.67	83.55	83.55	090	
26560		A	Repair of syndactyly (web finger) each web space; with skin flaps	5.38	12.55	12.55	0.60	18.53	18.53	090	
26561		A	with skin flaps and grafts	10.92	18.61	18.61	0.69	30.22	30.22	090	
26562		A	complex (eg, involving bone, nails)	15.00	13.44	13.44	0.98	29.42	29.42	090	
26565		A	Osteotomy; metacarpal, each	6.74	14.77	14.77	0.84	22.35	22.35	090	
26567		A	phalanx of finger, each	6.82	15.10	15.10	0.84	22.76	22.76	090	
26568		A	Osteoplasty, lengthening, metacarpal or phalanx	9.08	19.48	19.48	1.10	29.66	29.66	090	
26580		A	Repair cleft hand	18.18	17.22	17.22	1.46	36.86	36.86	090	
26587		A	Reconstruction of polydactylous digit, soft tissue and bone	14.05	4.67	4.67	1.08	19.80	19.80	090	
26590		A	Repair macrodactylia, each digit	17.96	14.62	14.62	1.32	33.90	33.90	090	
26591		A	Repair, intrinsic muscles of hand, each muscle	3.25	14.22	14.22	0.37	17.84	17.84	090	
26593		A	Release, intrinsic muscles of hand, each muscle	5.31	13.33	13.33	0.64	19.28	19.28	090	
26596		A	Excision of constricting ring of finger, with multiple Z-plasties	8.95	10.26	10.26	0.87	20.08	20.08	090	
26600		A	Closed treatment of metacarpal fracture, single; without manipulation, each bone	1.96	4.15	2.83	0.25	6.36	5.04	090	
26605		A	with manipulation, each bone	2.85	6.05	4.29	0.38	9.28	7.52	090	

■ RVU not developed by CMS. Gap-filled RVUs developed by Ingenix/CHEG.

Surgery

Code	M	S	Description	Work Value	Non-Fac PE	Fac PE	Mal-prac-tice	Non-Fac Total	Fac Total	Global	Gap
26607		A	Closed treatment of metacarpal fracture, with manipulation, with external fixation, each bone	5.36	8.33	8.33	0.70	14.39	14.39	090	
26608		A	Percutaneous skeletal fixation of metacarpal fracture, each bone	5.36	8.85	8.85	0.73	14.94	14.94	090	
26615		A	Open treatment of metacarpal fracture, single, with or without internal or external fixation, each bone	5.33	8.43	8.43	0.70	14.46	14.46	090	
26641		A	Closed treatment of carpometacarpal dislocation, thumb, with manipulation	3.94	6.58	4.99	0.42	10.94	9.35	090	
26645		A	Closed treatment of carpometacarpal fracture dislocation, thumb (Bennett fracture), with manipulation	4.41	7.33	5.30	0.54	12.28	10.25	090	
26650		A	Percutaneous skeletal fixation of carpometacarpal fracture dislocation, thumb (Bennett fracture), with manipulation, with or without external fixation	5.72	9.02	9.02	0.77	15.51	15.51	090	
26665		A	Open treatment of carpometacarpal fracture dislocation, thumb (Bennett fracture), with or without internal or external fixation	7.60	9.24	9.24	0.97	17.81	17.81	090	
26670		A	Closed treatment of carpometacarpal dislocation, other than thumb, with manipulation, each joint; without anesthesia	3.69	6.46	4.93	0.36	10.51	8.98	090	
26675		A	requiring anesthesia	4.64	6.82	4.71	0.56	12.02	9.91	090	
26676		A	Percutaneous skeletal fixation of carpometacarpal dislocation, other than thumb, with manipulation, each joint	5.52	9.36	9.36	0.76	15.64	15.64	090	
26685		A	Open treatment of carpometacarpal dislocation, other than thumb; with or without internal or external fixation, each joint	6.98	8.88	8.88	0.95	16.81	16.81	090	
26686		A	complex, multiple or delayed reduction	7.94	9.84	9.84	1.05	18.83	18.83	090	
26700		A	Closed treatment of metacarpophalangeal dislocation, single, with manipulation; without anesthesia	3.69	5.01	3.02	0.35	9.05	7.06	090	
26705		A	requiring anesthesia	4.19	6.26	4.33	0.50	10.95	9.02	090	
26706		A	Percutaneous skeletal fixation of metacarpophalangeal dislocation, single, with manipulation	5.12	5.87	5.87	0.64	11.63	11.63	090	
26715		A	Open treatment of metacarpophalangeal dislocation, single, with or without internal or external fixation	5.74	8.62	8.62	0.75	15.11	15.11	090	
26720		A	Closed treatment of phalangeal shaft fracture, proximal or middle phalanx, finger or thumb; without manipulation, each	1.66	3.06	1.72	0.20	4.92	3.58	090	
26725		A	with manipulation, with or without skin or skeletal traction, each	3.33	5.27	3.26	0.43	9.03	7.02	090	

■ RVU not developed by CMS. Gap-filled RVUs developed by Ingenix/CHEG.

Code	M	S	Description	Work Value	Non-Fac PE	Fac PE	Mal-practice	Non-Fac Total	Fac Total	Global	Gap
26727		A	Percutaneous skeletal fixation of unstable phalangeal shaft fracture, proximal or middle phalanx, finger or thumb, with manipulation, each	5.23	8.88	8.88	0.69	14.80	14.80	090	
26735		A	Open treatment of phalangeal shaft fracture, proximal or middle phalanx, finger or thumb, with or without internal or external fixation, each	5.98	8.99	8.99	0.77	15.74	15.74	090	
26740		A	Closed treatment of articular fracture, involving metacarpophalangeal or interphalangeal joint; without manipulation, each	1.94	3.86	2.67	0.24	6.04	4.85	090	
26742		A	with manipulation, each	3.85	7.21	5.13	0.49	11.55	9.47	090	
26746		A	Open treatment of articular fracture, involving metacarpophalangeal or interphalangeal joint, with or without internal or external fixation, each	5.81	8.93	8.93	0.74	15.48	15.48	090	
26750		A	Closed treatment of distal phalangeal fracture, finger or thumb; without manipulation, each	1.70	3.66	2.47	0.19	5.55	4.36	090	
26755		A	with manipulation, each	3.10	5.08	3.27	0.37	8.55	6.74	090	
26756		A	Percutaneous skeletal fixation of distal phalangeal fracture, finger or thumb, each	4.39	8.74	8.74	0.56	13.69	13.69	090	
26765		A	Open treatment of distal phalangeal fracture, finger or thumb, with or without internal or external fixation, each	4.17	8.02	8.02	0.51	12.7	12.70	090	
26770		A	Closed treatment of interphalangeal joint dislocation, single, with manipulation; without anesthesia	3.02	4.87	2.80	0.27	8.16	6.09	090	
26775		A	requiring anesthesia	3.71	6.07	4.09	0.43	10.21	8.23	090	
26776		A	Percutaneous skeletal fixation of interphalangeal joint dislocation, single, with manipulation	4.80	8.61	8.61	0.63	14.04	14.04	090	
26785		A	Open treatment of interphalangeal joint dislocation, with or without internal or external fixation, single	4.21	7.95	7.95	0.54	12.70	12.70	090	
26820		A	Fusion in opposition, thumb, with autogenous graft (includes obtaining graft)	8.26	15.80	15.80	1.11	25.17	25.17	090	
26841		A	Arthrodesis, carpometacarpal joint, thumb, with or without internal fixation;	7.13	15.37	15.37	0.97	23.47	23.47	090	
26842		A	with autograft (includes obtaining graft)	8.24	15.49	15.49	1.10	24.83	24.83	090	
26843		A	Arthrodesis, carpometacarpal joint, digit, other than thumb, each;	7.61	13.91	13.91	0.99	22.51	22.51	090	
26844		A	with autograft (includes obtaining graft)	8.73	15.63	15.63	1.12	25.48	25.48	090	
26850		A	Arthrodesis, metacarpophalangeal joint, with or without internal fixation;	6.97	14.63	14.63	0.89	22.49	22.49	090	

■ RVU not developed by CMS. Gap-filled RVUs developed by Ingenix/CHEG.

Code	M	S	Description	Work Value	Non-Fac PE	Fac PE	Mal-practice	Non-Fac Total	Fac Total	Global	Gap
26852		A	with autograft (includes obtaining graft)	8.46	15.19	15.19	1.05	24.70	24.70	090	
26860		A	Arthrodesis, interphalangeal joint, with or without internal fixation;	4.69	13.45	13.45	0.60	18.74	18.74	090	
26861		A	each additional interphalangeal joint (List separately in addition to code for primary procedure)	1.74	0.99	0.99	0.22	2.95	2.95	ZZZ	
26862		A	with autograft (includes obtaining graft)	7.37	15.18	15.18	0.92	23.47	23.47	090	
26863		A	with autograft (includes obtaining graft), each additional joint (List separately in addition to code for primary procedure)	3.90	2.25	2.25	0.51	6.66	6.66	ZZZ	
26910		A	Amputation, metacarpal, with finger or thumb (ray amputation), single, with or without interosseous transfer	7.60	13.98	13.98	0.90	22.48	22.48	090	
26951		A	Amputation, finger or thumb, primary or secondary, any joint or phalanx, single, including neurectomies; with direct closure	4.59	13.06	13.06	0.56	18.21	18.21	090	
26952		A	with local advancement flaps (V-Y, hood)	6.31	14.47	14.47	0.74	21.52	21.52	090	
26989		C	Unlisted procedure, hands or fingers	0.00	0.00	0.00	0.00	0.00	0.00	YYY	
26990		A	Incision and drainage, pelvis or hip joint area; deep abscess or hematoma	7.48	15.92	15.92	0.92	24.32	24.32	090	
26991		A	infected bursa	6.68	11.32	9.39	0.85	18.85	16.92	090	
26992		A	Incision, bone cortex, pelvis and/or hip joint (eg, osteomyelitis or bone abscess)	13.02	19.95	19.95	1.75	34.72	34.72	090	
27000		A	Tenotomy, adductor of hip, percutaneous (separate procedure)	5.62	7.48	7.48	0.76	13.86	13.86	090	
27001		A	Tenotomy, adductor of hip, open	6.94	8.42	8.42	0.95	16.31	16.31	090	
27003		A	Tenotomy, adductor, subcutaneous, open, with obturator neurectomy	7.34	9.01	9.01	0.93	17.28	17.28	090	
27005		A	Tenotomy, hip flexor(s), open (separate procedure)	9.66	10.50	10.50	1.36	21.52	21.52	090	
27006		A	Tenotomy, abductors and/or extensor(s) of hip, open (separate procedure)	9.68	10.59	10.59	1.33	21.60	21.60	090	
27025		A	Fasciotomy, hip or thigh, any type	11.16	10.53	10.53	1.38	23.07	23.07	090	
27030		A	Arthrotomy, hip, with drainage (eg, infection)	13.01	12.45	12.45	1.81	27.27	27.27	090	
27033		A	Arthrotomy, hip, including exploration or removal of loose or foreign body	13.39	12.62	12.62	1.87	27.88	27.88	090	
27035		A	Denervation, hip joint, intrapelvic or extrapelvic intra-articular branches of sciatic, femoral, or obturator nerves	16.69	19.67	19.67	1.70	38.06	38.06	090	

■ RVU not developed by CMS. Gap-filled RVUs developed by Ingenix/CHEG.

Code	M	S	Description	Work Value	Non-Fac PE	Fac PE	Mal-practice	Non-Fac Total	Fac Total	Global	Gap
27036		A	Capsulectomy or capsulotomy, hip, with or without excision of heterotopic bone, with release of hip flexor muscles (ie, gluteus medius, gluteus minimus, tensor fascia latae, rectus femoris, sartorius, iliopsoas)	12.88	14.03	14.03	1.80	28.71	28.71	090	
27040		A	Biopsy, soft tissue of pelvis and hip area; superficial	2.87	6.23	4.00	0.21	9.31	7.08	010	
27041		A	deep, subfascial or intramuscular	9.89	8.60	8.60	1.01	19.50	19.50	090	
27047		A	Excision, tumor, pelvis and hip area; subcutaneous tissue	7.45	9.26	7.03	0.79	17.5	15.27	090	
27048		A	deep, subfascial, intramuscular	6.25	7.94	7.94	0.73	14.92	14.92	090	
27049		A	Radical resection of tumor, soft tissue of pelvis and hip area (eg, malignant neoplasm)	13.66	13.77	13.77	1.60	29.03	29.03	090	
27050		A	Arthrotomy, with biopsy; sacroiliac joint	4.36	7.52	7.52	0.53	12.41	12.41	090	
27052		A	hip joint	6.23	8.24	8.24	0.85	15.32	15.32	090	
27054		A	Arthrotomy with synovectomy, hip joint	8.54	10.67	10.67	1.17	20.38	20.38	090	
27060		A	Excision; ischial bursa	5.43	7.21	7.21	0.60	13.24	13.24	090	
27062		A	trochanteric bursa or calcification	5.37	7.32	7.32	0.74	13.43	13.43	090	
27065		A	Excision of bone cyst or benign tumor; superficial (wing of ilium, symphysis pubis, or greater trochanter of femur) with or without autograft	5.90	8.65	8.65	0.76	15.31	15.31	090	
27066		A	deep, with or without autograft	10.33	12.53	12.53	1.42	24.28	24.28	090	
27067		A	with autograft requiring separate incision	13.83	14.54	14.54	1.95	30.32	30.32	090	
27070		A	Partial excision (craterization, saucerization) (eg, osteomyelitis or bone abscess); superficial (eg, wing of ilium, symphysis pubis, or greater trochanter of femur)	10.72	17.71	17.71	1.36	29.79	29.79	090	
27071		A	deep (subfascial or intramuscular)	11.46	18.67	18.67	1.51	31.64	31.64	090	
27075		A	Radical resection of tumor or infection; wing of ilium, one pubic or ischial ramus or symphysis pubis	35.00	25.75	25.75	2.22	62.97	62.97	090	
27076		A	ilium, including acetabulum, both pubic rami, or ischium and acetabulum	22.12	20.08	20.08	2.86	45.06	45.06	090	
27077		A	innominate bone, total	40.00	30.55	30.55	3.18	73.73	73.73	090	
27078		A	ischial tuberosity and greater trochanter of femur	13.44	16.30	16.30	1.67	31.41	31.41	090	
27079		A	ischial tuberosity and greater trochanter of femur, with skin flaps	13.75	13.43	13.43	1.86	29.04	29.04	090	
27080		A	Coccygectomy, primary	6.39	7.64	7.64	0.80	14.83	14.83	090	

■ RVU not developed by CMS. Gap-filled RVUs developed by Ingenix/CHEG.

Surgery

Code	M	S	Description	Work Value	Non-Fac PE	Fac PE	Mal-practice	Non-Fac Total	Fac Total	Global	Gap
27086*		A	Removal of foreign body, pelvis or hip; subcutaneous tissue	1.87	5.85	3.70	0.17	7.89	5.74	010	
27087		A	deep (subfascial or intramuscular)	8.54	9.04	9.04	1.09	18.67	18.67	090	
27090		A	Removal of hip prosthesis; (separate procedure)	11.15	11.37	11.37	1.55	24.07	24.07	090	
27091		A	complicated, including total hip prosthesis, methylmethacrylate with or without insertion of spacer	22.14	15.14	15.14	3.11	40.39	40.39	090	
27093		A	Injection procedure for hip arthrography; without anesthesia	1.30	13.59	0.53	0.09	14.98	1.92	000	
27095		A	with anesthesia	1.50	11.00	0.60	0.10	12.60	2.20	000	
27096		A	Injection procedure for sacroiliac joint, arthrography and/or anesthetic/steroid	1.40	8.86	0.35	0.08	10.34	1.83	000	
27097		A	Release or recession, hamstring, proximal	8.80	8.13	8.13	1.22	18.15	18.15	090	
27098		A	Transfer, adductor to ischium	8.83	9.18	9.18	1.24	19.25	19.25	090	
27100		A	Transfer external oblique muscle to greater trochanter including fascial or tendon extension (graft)	11.08	13.03	13.03	1.57	25.68	25.68	090	
27105		A	Transfer paraspinal muscle to hip (includes fascial or tendon extension graft)	11.77	12.14	12.14	1.66	25.57	25.57	090	
27110		A	Transfer iliopsoas; to greater trochanter of femur	13.26	12.99	12.99	1.38	27.63	27.63	090	
27111		A	to femoral neck	12.15	11.77	11.77	1.48	25.4	25.40	090	
27120		A	Acetabuloplasty; (eg, Whitman, Colonna, Haygroves, or cup type)	18.01	14.28	14.28	2.45	34.74	34.74	090	
27122		A	resection, femoral head (eg, Girdlestone procedure)	14.98	14.48	14.48	2.08	31.54	31.54	090	
27125		A	Hemiarthroplasty, hip, partial (eg, femoral stem prosthesis, bipolar arthroplasty)	14.69	14.02	14.02	2.05	30.76	30.76	090	
27130		A	Arthroplasty, acetabular and proximal femoral prosthetic replacement (total hip arthroplasty), with or without autograft or allograft	20.12	17.18	17.18	2.82	40.12	40.12	090	
27132		A	Conversion of previous hip surgery to total hip arthroplasty, with or without autograft or allograft	23.30	19.00	19.00	3.26	45.56	45.56	090	
27134		A	Revision of total hip arthroplasty; both components, with or without autograft or allograft	28.52	21.82	21.82	3.97	54.31	54.31	090	
27137		A	acetabular component only, with or without autograft or allograft	21.17	17.54	17.54	2.97	41.68	41.68	090	
27138		A	femoral component only, with or without allograft	22.17	17.94	17.94	3.11	43.22	43.22	090	

■ RVU not developed by CMS. Gap-filled RVUs developed by Ingenix/CHEG.

Code	M	S	Description	Work Value	Non-Fac PE	Fac PE	Mal-practice	Non-Fac Total	Fac Total	Global	Gap
27140		A	Osteotomy and transfer of greater trochanter of femur (separate procedure)	12.24	11.98	11.98	1.67	25.89	25.89	090	
27146		A	Osteotomy, iliac, acetabular or innominate bone;	17.43	15.87	15.87	2.27	35.57	35.57	090	
27147		A	with open reduction of hip	20.58	17.87	17.87	2.61	41.06	41.06	090	
27151		A	with femoral osteotomy	22.51	18.97	18.97	3.12	44.60	44.60	090	
27156		A	with femoral osteotomy and with open reduction of hip	24.63	19.84	19.84	3.48	47.95	47.95	090	
27158		A	Osteotomy, pelvis, bilateral (eg, congenital malformation)	19.74	15.58	15.58	2.60	37.92	37.92	090	
27161		A	Osteotomy, femoral neck (separate procedure)	16.71	14.47	14.47	2.32	33.50	33.50	090	
27165		A	Osteotomy, intertrochanteric or subtrochanteric including internal or external fixation and/or cast	17.91	14.92	14.92	2.51	35.34	35.34	090	
27170		A	Bone graft, femoral head, neck, intertrochanteric or subtrochanteric area (includes obtaining bone graft)	16.07	14.16	14.16	2.20	32.43	32.43	090	
27175		A	Treatment of slipped femoral epiphysis; by traction, without reduction	8.46	7.26	7.26	1.19	16.91	16.91	090	
27176		A	by single or multiple pinning, in situ	12.05	10.23	10.23	1.68	23.96	23.96	090	
27177		A	Open treatment of slipped femoral epiphysis; single or multiple pinning or bone graft (includes obtaining graft)	15.08	12.22	12.22	2.11	29.41	29.41	090	
27178		A	closed manipulation with single or multiple pinning	11.99	10.13	10.13	1.68	23.80	23.80	090	
27179		A	osteoplasty of femoral neck (Heyman type procedure)	12.98	10.90	10.90	1.84	25.72	25.72	090	
27181		A	osteotomy and internal fixation	14.68	11.92	11.92	1.74	28.34	28.34	090	
27185		A	Epiphyseal arrest by epiphysiodesis or stapling, greater trochanter of femur	9.18	10.04	10.04	1.29	20.51	20.51	090	
27187		A	Prophylactic treatment (nailing, pinning, plating or wiring) with or without methylmethacrylate, femoral neck and proximal femur	13.54	13.53	13.53	1.89	28.96	28.96	090	
27193		A	Closed treatment of pelvic ring fracture, dislocation, diastasis or subluxation; without manipulation	5.56	7.14	5.36	0.77	13.47	11.69	090	
27194		A	with manipulation, requiring more than local anesthesia	9.65	9.20	7.69	1.32	20.17	18.66	090	
27200		A	Closed treatment of coccygeal fracture	1.84	3.13	1.84	0.22	5.19	3.90	090	
27202		A	Open treatment of coccygeal fracture	7.04	21.62	21.62	0.69	29.35	29.35	090	

■ RVU not developed by CMS. Gap-filled RVUs developed by Ingenix/CHEG.

Code	M	S	Description	Work Value	Non-Fac PE	Fac PE	Mal-practice	Non-Fac Total	Fac Total	Global	Gap
27215		A	Open treatment of iliac spine(s), tuberosity avulsion, or iliac wing fracture(s) (eg, pelvic fracture(s) which do not disrupt the pelvic ring), with internal fixation	10.05	10.60	10.60	1.37	22.02	22.02	090	
27216		A	Percutaneous skeletal fixation of posterior pelvic ring fracture and/or dislocation (includes ilium, sacroiliac joint and/or sacrum)	15.19	15.51	15.51	2.15	32.85	32.85	090	
27217		A	Open treatment of anterior ring fracture and/or dislocation with internal fixation, (includes pubic symphysis and/or rami)	14.11	12.83	12.83	1.95	28.89	28.89	090	
27218		A	Open treatment of posterior ring fracture and/or dislocation with internal fixation (includes ilium, sacroiliac joint and/or sacrum)	20.15	16.68	16.68	2.85	39.68	39.68	090	
27220		A	Closed treatment of acetabulum (hip socket) fracture(s); without manipulation	6.18	7.48	5.72	0.85	14.51	12.75	090	
27222		A	with manipulation, with or without skeletal traction	12.70	10.37	10.37	1.77	24.84	24.84	090	
27226		A	Open treatment of posterior or anterior acetabular wall fracture, with internal fixation	14.91	10.36	10.36	2.07	27.34	27.34	090	
27227		A	Open treatment of acetabular fracture(s) involving anterior or posterior (one) column, or a fracture running transversely across the acetabulum, with internal fixation	23.45	17.22	17.22	3.24	43.91	43.91	090	
27228		A	Open treatment of acetabular fracture(s) involving anterior and posterior (two) columns, includes T-fracture and both column fracture with complete articular detachment, or single column or transverse fracture with associated acetabular wall fracture, with internal fixation	27.16	19.67	19.67	3.77	50.60	50.60	090	
27230		A	Closed treatment of femoral fracture, proximal end, neck; without manipulation	5.50	7.62	6.30	0.73	13.85	12.53	090	
27232		A	with manipulation, with or without skeletal traction	10.68	9.31	9.31	1.45	21.44	21.44	090	
27235		A	Percutaneous skeletal fixation of femoral fracture, proximal end, neck, undisplaced, mildly displaced, or impacted fracture	12.16	11.24	11.24	1.71	25.11	25.11	090	
27236		A	Open treatment of femoral fracture, proximal end, neck, internal fixation or prosthetic replacement	15.6	12.99	12.99	2.18	30.77	30.77	090	
27238		A	Closed treatment of intertrochanteric, pertrochanteric, or subtrochanteric femoral fracture; without manipulation	5.52	6.36	6.36	0.76	12.64	12.64	090	
27240		A	with manipulation, with or without skin or skeletal traction	12.5	10.38	10.38	1.69	24.57	24.57	090	

■ RVU not developed by CMS. Gap-filled RVUs developed by Ingenix/CHEG.

Code	M	S	Description	Work Value	Non-Fac PE	Fac PE	Mal-prac-tice	Non-Fac Total	Fac Total	Global	Gap
27244		A	Open treatment of intertrochanteric, pertrochanteric or subtrochanteric femoral fracture; with plate/screw type implant, with or without cerclage	15.94	13.25	13.25	2.23	31.42	31.42	090	
27245		A	with intramedullary implant, with or without interlocking screws and/or cerclage	20.31	15.61	15.61	2.85	38.77	38.77	090	
27246		A	Closed treatment of greater trochanteric fracture, without manipulation	4.71	7.31	5.93	0.66	12.68	11.30	090	
27248		A	Open treatment of greater trochanteric fracture, with or without internal or external fixation	10.45	10.20	10.20	1.45	22.10	22.10	090	
27250		A	Closed treatment of hip dislocation, traumatic; without anesthesia	6.95	6.55	6.55	0.68	14.18	14.18	090	
27252		A	requiring anesthesia	10.39	8.31	8.31	1.37	20.07	20.07	090	
27253		A	Open treatment of hip dislocation, traumatic, without internal fixation	12.92	11.10	11.10	1.81	25.83	25.83	090	
27254		A	Open treatment of hip dislocation, traumatic, with acetabular wall and femoral head fracture, with or without internal or external fixation	18.26	14.29	14.29	2.52	35.07	35.07	090	
27256*		A	Treatment of spontaneous hip dislocation (developmental, including congenital or pathological), by abduction, splint or traction; without anesthesia, without manipulation	4.12	4.31	4.31	0.49	8.92	8.92	010	
27257*		A	with manipulation, requiring anesthesia	5.22	4.59	4.59	0.56	10.37	10.37	010	
27258		A	Open treatment of spontaneous hip dislocation (developmental, including congenital or pathological), replacement of femoral head in acetabulum (including tenotomy, etc);	15.43	13.93	13.93	2.06	31.42	31.42	090	
27259		A	with femoral shaft shortening	21.55	18.02	18.02	2.99	42.56	42.56	090	
27265		A	Closed treatment of post hip arthroplasty dislocation; without anesthesia	5.05	6.09	6.09	0.65	11.79	11.79	090	
27266		A	requiring regional or general anesthesia	7.49	7.50	7.50	1.04	16.03	16.03	090	
27275*		A	Manipulation, hip joint, requiring general anesthesia	2.27	3.62	3.62	0.31	6.20	6.20	010	
27280		A	Arthrodesis, sacroiliac joint (including obtaining graft)	13.39	13.95	13.95	1.98	29.32	29.32	090	
27282		A	Arthrodesis, symphysis pubis (including obtaining graft)	11.34	12.33	12.33	1.14	24.81	24.81	090	
27284		A	Arthrodesis, hip joint (including obtaining graft);	23.45	18.86	18.86	2.36	44.67	44.67	090	
27286		A	with subtrochanteric osteotomy	23.45	19.13	19.13	2.37	44.95	44.95	090	
27290		A	Interpelviabdominal amputation (hindquarter amputation)	23.28	17.37	17.37	2.94	43.59	43.59	090	

■ RVU not developed by CMS. Gap-filled RVUs developed by Ingenix/CHEG.

Code	M	S	Description	Work Value	Non-Fac PE	Fac PE	Mal-practice	Non-Fac Total	Fac Total	Global	Gap
27295		A	Disarticulation of hip	18.65	14.65	14.65	2.35	35.65	35.65	090	
27299		C	Unlisted procedure, pelvis or hip joint	0.00	0.00	0.00	0.00	0.00	0.00	YYY	
27301		A	Incision and drainage, deep abscess, bursa, or hematoma, thigh or knee region	6.49	15.30	14.04	0.80	22.59	21.33	090	
27303		A	Incision, deep, with opening of bone cortex, femur or knee (eg, osteomyelitis or bone abscess)	8.28	14.63	14.63	1.14	24.05	24.05	090	
27305		A	Fasciotomy, iliotibial (tenotomy), open	5.92	8.88	8.88	0.77	15.57	15.57	090	
27306		A	Tenotomy, percutaneous, adductor or hamstring; single tendon (separate procedure)	4.62	7.54	7.54	0.62	12.78	12.78	090	
27307		A	multiple tendons	5.80	8.15	8.15	0.78	14.73	14.73	090	
27310		A	Arthrotomy, knee, with exploration, drainage, or removal of foreign body (eg, infection)	9.27	10.14	10.14	1.29	20.70	20.70	090	
27315		A	Neurectomy, hamstring muscle	6.97	4.04	4.04	0.79	11.80	11.80	090	
27320		A	Neurectomy, popliteal (gastrocnemius)	6.30	5.07	5.07	0.78	12.15	12.15	090	
27323		A	Biopsy, soft tissue of thigh or knee area; superficial	2.28	5.57	3.49	0.17	8.02	5.94	010	
27324		A	deep (subfascial or intramuscular)	4.90	6.79	6.79	0.59	12.28	12.28	090	
27327		A	Excision, tumor, thigh or knee area; subcutaneous	4.47	8.47	6.35	0.50	13.44	11.32	090	
27328		A	deep, subfascial, or intramuscular	5.57	7.19	7.19	0.66	13.42	13.42	090	
27329		A	Radical resection of tumor (eg, malignant neoplasm), soft tissue of thigh or knee area	14.14	15.02	15.02	1.68	30.84	30.84	090	
27330		A	Arthrotomy, knee; with synovial biopsy only	4.97	6.42	6.42	0.66	12.05	12.05	090	
27331		A	including joint exploration, biopsy, or removal of loose or foreign bodies	5.88	7.56	7.56	0.81	14.25	14.25	090	
27332		A	Arthrotomy, with excision of semilunar cartilage (meniscectomy) knee; medial OR lateral	8.27	8.84	8.84	1.15	18.26	18.26	090	
27333		A	medial AND lateral	7.30	8.49	8.49	1.03	16.82	16.82	090	
27334		A	Arthrotomy, with synovectomy, knee; anterior OR posterior	8.70	9.80	9.80	1.21	19.71	19.71	090	
27335		A	anterior AND posterior including popliteal area	10.00	10.58	10.58	1.41	21.99	21.99	090	
27340		A	Excision, prepatellar bursa	4.18	6.03	6.03	0.58	10.79	10.79	090	
27345		A	Excision of synovial cyst of popliteal space (eg, Bakers cyst)	5.92	7.49	7.49	0.81	14.22	14.22	090	
27347		A	Excision of lesion of meniscus or capsule (eg, cyst, ganglion), knee	5.78	2.64	2.64	0.76	9.18	9.18	090	

■ RVU not developed by CMS. Gap-filled RVUs developed by Ingenix/CHEG.

Code	M	S	Description	Work Value	Non-Fac PE	Fac PE	Mal-practice	Non-Fac Total	Fac Total	Global	Gap
27350		A	Patellectomy or hemipatellectomy	8.17	8.95	8.95	1.15	18.27	18.27	090	
27355		A	Excision or curettage of bone cyst or benign tumor of femur;	7.65	10.36	10.36	1.07	19.08	19.08	090	
27356		A	with allograft	9.48	11.32	11.32	1.29	22.09	22.09	090	
27357		A	with autograft (includes obtaining graft)	10.53	11.75	11.75	1.48	23.76	23.76	090	
27358		A	Excision or curettage of bone cyst or benign tumor of femur; with internal fixation (List in addition to code for primary procedure)	4.74	2.69	2.69	0.67	8.10	8.10	ZZZ	
27360		A	Partial excision (craterization, saucerization, or diaphysectomy) bone, femur, proximal tibia and/or fibula (eg, osteomyelitis or bone abscess)	10.50	18.43	18.43	1.42	30.35	30.35	090	
27365		A	Radical resection of tumor, bone, femur or knee	16.27	14.69	14.69	2.26	33.22	33.22	090	
27370		A	Injection procedure for knee arthrography	0.96	11.10	0.35	0.06	12.12	1.37	000	
27372		A	Removal of foreign body, deep, thigh region or knee area	5.07	8.66	6.28	0.62	14.35	11.97	090	
27380		A	Suture of infrapatellar tendon; primary	7.16	8.57	8.57	1.00	16.73	16.73	090	
27381		A	secondary reconstruction, including fascial or tendon graft	10.34	10.34	10.34	1.44	22.12	22.12	090	
27385		A	Suture of quadriceps or hamstring muscle rupture; primary	7.76	8.93	8.93	1.09	17.78	17.78	090	
27386		A	secondary reconstruction, including fascial or tendon graft	10.56	11.12	11.12	1.49	23.17	23.17	090	
27390		A	Tenotomy, open, hamstring, knee to hip; single tendon	5.33	8.22	8.22	0.69	14.24	14.24	090	
27391		A	multiple tendons, one leg	7.20	9.08	9.08	0.99	17.27	17.27	090	
27392		A	multiple tendons, bilateral	9.20	11.15	11.15	1.23	21.58	21.58	090	
27393		A	Lengthening of hamstring tendon; single tendon	6.39	8.45	8.45	0.90	15.74	15.74	090	
27394		A	multiple tendons, one leg	8.50	10.51	10.51	1.17	20.18	20.18	090	
27395		A	multiple tendons, bilateral	11.73	13.19	13.19	1.63	26.55	26.55	090	
27396		A	Transplant, hamstring tendon to patella; single tendon	7.86	9.65	9.65	1.11	18.62	18.62	090	
27397		A	multiple tendons	11.28	11.71	11.71	1.58	24.57	24.57	090	
27400		A	Transfer, tendon or muscle, hamstrings to femur (eg, Egger's type procedure)	9.02	10.67	10.67	1.18	20.87	20.87	090	
27403		A	Arthrotomy with meniscus repair, knee	8.33	8.88	8.88	1.16	18.37	18.37	090	
27405		A	Repair, primary, torn ligament and/or capsule, knee; collateral	8.65	9.81	9.81	1.21	19.67	19.67	090	

■ RVU not developed by CMS. Gap-filled RVUs developed by Ingenix/CHEG.

Surgery

Code	M	S	Description	Work Value	Non-Fac PE	Fac PE	Mal-practice	Non-Fac Total	Fac Total	Global	Gap
27407		A	cruciate	10.28	10.67	10.67	1.38	22.33	22.33	090	
27409		A	collateral and cruciate ligaments	12.90	12.11	12.11	1.75	26.76	26.76	090	
27418		A	Anterior tibial tubercleplasty (eg, Maquet type procedure)	10.85	10.99	10.99	1.51	23.35	23.35	090	
27420		A	Reconstruction of dislocating patella; (eg, Hauser type procedure)	9.83	9.87	9.87	1.38	21.08	21.08	090	
27422		A	with extensor realignment and/or muscle advancement or release (eg, Campbell, Goldwaite type procedure)	9.78	9.83	9.83	1.37	20.98	20.98	090	
27424		A	with patellectomy	9.81	9.75	9.75	1.38	20.94	20.94	090	
27425		A	Lateral retinacular release (any method)	5.22	7.29	7.29	0.73	13.24	13.24	090	
27427		A	Ligamentous reconstruction (augmentation), knee; extra-articular	9.36	9.57	9.57	1.29	20.22	20.22	090	
27428		A	intra-articular (open)	14.00	12.85	12.85	1.95	28.80	28.80	090	
27429		A	intra-articular (open) and extra-articular	15.52	13.69	13.69	2.18	31.39	31.39	090	
27430		A	Quadricepsplasty (eg, Bennett or Thompson type)	9.67	9.90	9.90	1.35	20.92	20.92	090	
27435		A	Capsulotomy, posterior capsular release, knee	9.49	9.68	9.68	1.33	20.50	20.50	090	
27437		A	Arthroplasty, patella; without prosthesis	8.46	10.06	10.06	1.18	19.70	19.70	090	
27438		A	with prosthesis	11.23	11.34	11.34	1.56	24.13	24.13	090	
27440		A	Arthroplasty, knee, tibial plateau;	10.43	10.92	10.92	1.42	22.77	22.77	090	
27441		A	with debridement and partial synovectomy	10.82	11.24	11.24	1.49	23.55	23.55	090	
27442		A	Arthroplasty, femoral condyles or tibial plateau(s), knee;	11.89	11.77	11.77	1.68	25.34	25.34	090	
27443		A	with debridement and partial synovectomy	10.93	11.56	11.56	1.52	24.01	24.01	090	
27445		A	Arthroplasty, knee, hinge prosthesis (eg, Walldius type)	17.68	14.98	14.98	2.49	35.15	35.15	090	
27446		A	Arthroplasty, knee, condyle and plateau; medial OR lateral compartment	15.84	14.26	14.26	2.22	32.32	32.32	090	
27447		A	medial AND lateral compartments with or without patella resurfacing (total knee arthroplasty)	21.48	17.35	17.35	3.00	41.83	41.83	090	
27448		A	Osteotomy, femur, shaft or supracondylar; without fixation	11.06	11.98	11.98	1.51	24.55	24.55	090	
27450		A	with fixation	13.98	13.83	13.83	1.96	29.77	29.77	090	
27454		A	Osteotomy, multiple, with realignment on intramedullary rod, femoral shaft (eg, Sofield type procedure)	17.56	15.83	15.83	2.46	35.85	35.85	090	

■ RVU not developed by CMS. Gap-filled RVUs developed by Ingenix/CHEG.

Code	M	S	Description	Work Value	Non-Fac PE	Fac PE	Mal-practice	Non-Fac Total	Fac Total	Global	Gap
27455		A	Osteotomy, proximal tibia, including fibular excision or osteotomy (includes correction of genu varus (bowleg) or genu valgus (knock-knee)); before epiphyseal closure	12.82	12.57	12.57	1.78	27.17	27.17	090	
27457		A	after epiphyseal closure	13.45	11.73	11.73	1.88	27.06	27.06	090	
27465		A	Osteoplasty, femur; shortening (excluding 64876)	13.87	14.09	14.09	1.86	29.82	29.82	090	
27466		A	lengthening	16.33	16.19	16.19	1.92	34.44	34.44	090	
27468		A	combined, lengthening and shortening with femoral segment transfer	18.97	14.57	14.57	2.68	36.22	36.22	090	
27470		A	Repair, nonunion or malunion, femur, distal to head and neck; without graft (eg, compression technique)	16.07	16.07	16.07	2.24	34.38	34.38	090	
27472		A	with iliac or other autogenous bone graft (includes obtaining graft)	17.72	16.98	16.98	2.49	37.19	37.19	090	
27475		A	Arrest, epiphyseal, any method (eg, epiphysiodesis); distal femur	8.64	9.51	9.51	1.13	19.28	19.28	090	
27477		A	tibia and fibula, proximal	9.85	10.10	10.10	1.31	21.26	21.26	090	
27479		A	combined distal femur, proximal tibia and fibula	12.80	12.09	12.09	1.81	26.70	26.70	090	
27485		A	Arrest, hemiepiphyseal, distal femur or proximal tibia or fibula (eg, genu varus or valgus)	8.84	9.40	9.40	1.24	19.48	19.48	090	
27486		A	Revision of total knee arthroplasty, with or without allograft; one component	19.27	16.13	16.13	2.70	38.10	38.10	090	
27487		A	femoral and entire tibial component	25.27	19.26	19.26	3.54	48.07	48.07	090	
27488		A	Removal of prosthesis, including total knee prosthesis, methylmethacrylate with or without insertion of spacer, knee	15.74	14.21	14.21	2.21	32.16	32.16	090	
27495		A	Prophylactic treatment (nailing, pinning, plating or wiring) with or without methylmethacrylate, femur	15.55	15.78	15.78	2.18	33.51	33.51	090	
27496		A	Decompression fasciotomy, thigh and/or knee, one compartment (flexor or extensor or adductor);	6.11	7.96	7.96	0.77	14.84	14.84	090	
27497		A	with debridement of nonviable muscle and/or nerve	7.17	8.16	8.16	0.84	16.17	16.17	090	
27498		A	Decompression fasciotomy, thigh and/or knee, multiple compartments;	7.99	8.37	8.37	0.97	17.33	17.33	090	
27499		A	with debridement of nonviable muscle and/or nerve	9.00	9.42	9.42	1.18	19.60	19.60	090	
27500		A	Closed treatment of femoral shaft fracture, without manipulation	5.92	9.84	7.57	0.80	16.56	14.29	090	

■ RVU not developed by CMS. Gap-filled RVUs developed by Ingenix/CHEG.

Code	M	S	Description	Work Value	Non-Fac PE	Fac PE	Mal-practice	Non-Fac Total	Fac Total	Global	Gap
27501		A	Closed treatment of supracondylar or transcondylar femoral fracture with or without intercondylar extension, without manipulation	5.92	10.92	8.62	0.83	17.67	15.37	090	
27502		A	Closed treatment of femoral shaft fracture, with manipulation, with or without skin or skeletal traction	10.58	11.27	11.27	1.49	23.34	23.34	090	
27503		A	Closed treatment of supracondylar or transcondylar femoral fracture with or without intercondylar extension, with manipulation, with or without skin or skeletal traction	10.58	11.26	11.26	1.49	23.33	23.33	090	
27506		A	Open treatment of femoral shaft fracture, with or without external fixation, with insertion of intramedullary implant, with or without cerclage and/or locking screws	17.45	14.57	14.57	2.33	34.35	34.35	090	
27507		A	Open treatment of femoral shaft fracture with plate/screws, with or without cerclage	13.99	12.58	12.58	1.95	28.52	28.52	090	
27508		A	Closed treatment of femoral fracture, distal end, medial or lateral condyle, without manipulation	5.83	7.17	5.43	0.80	13.80	12.06	090	
27509		A	Percutaneous skeletal fixation of femoral fracture, distal end, medial or lateral condyle, or supracondylar or transcondylar, with or without intercondylar extension, or distal femoral epiphyseal separation	7.71	9.44	9.44	1.08	18.23	18.23	090	
27510		A	Closed treatment of femoral fracture, distal end, medial or lateral condyle, with manipulation	9.13	7.37	7.37	1.26	17.76	17.76	090	
27511		A	Open treatment of femoral supracondylar or transcondylar fracture without intercondylar extension, with or without internal or external fixation	13.64	13.38	13.38	1.91	28.93	28.93	090	
27513		A	Open treatment of femoral supracondylar or transcondylar fracture with intercondylar extension, with or without internal or external fixation	17.92	15.8	15.8	2.51	36.23	36.23	090	
27514		A	Open treatment of femoral fracture, distal end, medial or lateral condyle, with or without internal or external fixation	17.3	14.55	14.55	2.41	34.26	34.26	090	
27516		A	Closed treatment of distal femoral epiphyseal separation; without manipulation	5.37	7.98	5.85	0.74	14.09	11.96	090	
27517		A	with manipulation, with or without skin or skeletal traction	8.78	9.94	7.90	1.22	19.94	17.90	090	
27519		A	Open treatment of distal femoral epiphyseal separation, with or without internal or external fixation	15.02	13.11	13.11	2.09	30.22	30.22	090	
27520		A	Closed treatment of patellar fracture, without manipulation	2.86	5.48	3.82	0.38	8.72	7.06	090	

Surgery

■ RVU not developed by CMS. Gap-filled RVUs developed by Ingenix/CHEG.

Code	M	S	Description	Work Value	Non-Fac PE	Fac PE	Mal-prac-tice	Non-Fac Total	Fac Total	Global	Gap
27524		A	Open treatment of patellar fracture, with internal fixation and/or partial or complete patellectomy and soft tissue repair	10.00	8.98	8.98	1.40	20.38	20.38	090	
27530		A	Closed treatment of tibial fracture, proximal (plateau); without manipulation	3.78	6.00	4.33	0.51	10.29	8.62	090	
27532		A	with or without manipulation, with skeletal traction	7.30	7.65	5.84	1.02	15.97	14.16	090	
27535		A	Open treatment of tibial fracture, proximal (plateau); unicondylar, with or without internal or external fixation	11.50	12.15	12.15	1.61	25.26	25.26	090	
27536		A	bicondylar, with or without internal fixation	15.65	12.16	12.16	2.19	30.00	30.00	090	
27538		A	Closed treatment of intercondylar spine(s) and/or tuberosity fracture(s) of knee, with or without manipulation	4.87	7.64	5.60	0.67	13.18	11.14	090	
27540		A	Open treatment of intercondylar spine(s) and/or tuberosity fracture(s) of the knee, with or without internal or external fixation	13.10	10.75	10.75	1.80	25.65	25.65	090	
27550		A	Closed treatment of knee dislocation; without anesthesia	5.76	7.60	5.79	0.68	14.04	12.23	090	
27552		A	requiring anesthesia	7.90	8.04	8.04	1.10	17.04	17.04	090	
27556		A	Open treatment of knee dislocation, with or without internal or external fixation; without primary ligamentous repair or augmentation/reconstruction	14.41	14.45	14.45	2.01	30.87	30.87	090	
27557		A	with primary ligamentous repair	16.77	15.78	15.78	2.37	34.92	34.92	090	
27558		A	with primary ligamentous repair, with augmentation/reconstruction	17.72	15.91	15.91	2.51	36.14	36.14	090	
27560		A	Closed treatment of patellar dislocation; without anesthesia	3.82	5.89	4.04	0.40	10.11	8.26	090	
27562		A	requiring anesthesia	5.79	5.67	5.67	0.69	12.15	12.15	090	
27566		A	Open treatment of patellar dislocation, with or without partial or total patellectomy	12.23	10.09	10.09	1.73	24.05	24.05	090	
27570*		A	Manipulation of knee joint under general anesthesia (includes application of traction or other fixation devices)	1.74	3.24	3.24	0.24	5.22	5.22	010	
27580		A	Arthrodesis, knee, any technique	19.37	16.63	16.63	2.70	38.70	38.70	090	
27590		A	Amputation, thigh, through femur, any level;	12.03	12.67	12.67	1.35	26.05	26.05	090	
27591		A	immediate fitting technique including first cast	12.68	14.01	14.01	1.63	28.32	28.32	090	
27592		A	open, circular (guillotine)	10.02	12.55	12.55	1.17	23.74	23.74	090	
27594		A	secondary closure or scar revision	6.92	9.05	9.05	0.82	16.79	16.79	090	

■ RVU not developed by CMS. Gap-filled RVUs developed by Ingenix/CHEG.

Surgery

Code	M	S	Description	Work Value	Non-Fac PE	Fac PE	Mal-practice	Non-Fac Total	Fac Total	Global	Gap
27596		A	re-amputation	10.60	12.64	12.64	1.24	24.48	24.48	090	
27598		A	Disarticulation at knee	10.53	11.69	11.69	1.24	23.46	23.46	090	
27599		C	Unlisted procedure, femur or knee	0.00	0.00	0.00	0.00	0.00	0.00	YYY	
27600		A	Decompression fasciotomy, leg; anterior and/or lateral compartments only	5.65	7.67	7.67	0.68	14.00	14.00	090	
27601		A	posterior compartment(s) only	5.64	7.68	7.68	0.69	14.01	14.01	090	
27602		A	anterior and/or lateral, and posterior compartment(s)	7.35	8.08	8.08	0.85	16.28	16.28	090	
27603		A	Incision and drainage, leg or ankle; deep abscess or hematoma	4.94	16.03	10.54	0.56	21.53	16.04	090	
27604		A	infected bursa	4.47	11.01	8.47	0.54	16.02	13.48	090	
27605*		A	Tenotomy, percutaneous, Achilles tendon (separate procedure); local anesthesia	2.87	9.81	3.67	0.38	13.06	6.92	010	
27606		A	general anesthesia	4.14	13.19	5.08	0.57	17.90	9.79	010	
27607		A	Incision (eg, osteomyelitis or bone abscess), leg or ankle	7.97	12.78	12.78	1.08	21.83	21.83	090	
27610		A	Arthrotomy, ankle, including exploration, drainage, or removal of foreign body	8.34	10.43	10.43	1.15	19.92	19.92	090	
27612		A	Arthrotomy, posterior capsular release, ankle, with or without Achilles tendon lengthening	7.33	8.32	8.32	1.01	16.66	16.66	090	
27613		A	Biopsy, soft tissue of leg or ankle area; superficial	2.17	5.38	2.96	0.16	7.71	5.29	010	
27614		A	deep (subfascial or intramuscular)	5.66	10.88	7.17	0.62	17.16	13.45	090	
27615		A	Radical resection of tumor (eg, malignant neoplasm), soft tissue of leg or ankle area	12.56	17.07	17.07	1.39	31.02	31.02	090	
27618		A	Excision, tumor, leg or ankle area; subcutaneous tissue	5.09	11.72	6.72	0.54	17.35	12.35	090	
27619		A	deep (subfascial or intramuscular)	8.40	12.63	9.55	1.01	22.04	18.96	090	
27620		A	Arthrotomy, ankle, with joint exploration, with or without biopsy, with or without removal of loose or foreign body	5.98	8.20	8.20	0.83	15.01	15.01	090	
27625		A	Arthrotomy, with synovectomy, ankle;	8.30	9.57	9.57	1.16	19.03	19.03	090	
27626		A	including tenosynovectomy	8.91	10.39	10.39	1.23	20.53	20.53	090	
27630		A	Excision of lesion of tendon sheath or capsule (eg, cyst or ganglion), leg and/or ankle	4.80	10.70	6.87	0.60	16.10	12.27	090	
27635		A	Excision or curettage of bone cyst or benign tumor, tibia or fibula;	7.78	11.13	11.13	1.06	19.97	19.97	090	
27637		A	with autograft (includes obtaining graft)	9.85	12.36	12.36	1.38	23.59	23.59	090	

■ RVU not developed by CMS. Gap-filled RVUs developed by Ingenix/CHEG.

Code	M	S	Description	Work Value	Non-Fac PE	Fac PE	Mal-practice	Non-Fac Total	Fac Total	Global	Gap
27638		A	with allograft	10.57	12.55	12.55	1.47	24.59	24.59	090	
27640		A	Partial excision (craterization, saucerization, or diaphysectomy) bone (eg, osteomyelitis or exostosis); tibia	11.37	18.46	18.46	1.54	31.37	31.37	090	
27641		A	fibula	9.24	16.52	16.52	1.22	26.98	26.98	090	
27645		A	Radical resection of tumor, bone; tibia	14.17	18.78	18.78	1.98	34.93	34.93	090	
27646		A	fibula	12.66	18.50	18.50	1.55	32.71	32.71	090	
27647		A	talus or calcaneus	12.24	11.31	11.31	1.64	25.19	25.19	090	
27648		A	Injection procedure for ankle arthrography	0.96	9.49	0.36	0.05	10.50	1.37	000	
27650		A	Repair, primary, open or percutaneous, ruptured Achilles tendon;	9.69	9.60	9.60	1.35	20.64	20.64	090	
27652		A	with graft (includes obtaining graft)	10.33	9.90	9.90	1.45	21.68	21.68	090	
27654		A	Repair, secondary, Achilles tendon, with or without graft	10.02	10.34	10.34	1.41	21.77	21.77	090	
27656		A	Repair, fascial defect of leg	4.57	11.38	7.06	0.48	16.43	12.11	090	
27658		A	Repair, flexor tendon, leg; primary, without graft, each tendon	4.98	10.63	9.14	0.68	16.29	14.80	090	
27659		A	secondary, with or without graft, each tendon	6.81	12.77	9.97	0.96	20.54	17.74	090	
27664		A	Repair, extensor tendon, leg; primary, without graft, each tendon	4.59	17.85	9.17	0.63	23.07	14.39	090	
27665		A	secondary, with or without graft, each tendon	5.40	8.95	8.95	0.75	15.10	15.10	090	
27675		A	Repair, dislocating peroneal tendons; without fibular osteotomy	7.18	8.48	8.48	1.01	16.67	16.67	090	
27676		A	with fibular osteotomy	8.42	9.72	9.72	1.15	19.29	19.29	090	
27680		A	Tenolysis, flexor or extensor tendon, leg and/or ankle; single, each tendon	5.74	8.27	8.27	0.80	14.81	14.81	090	
27681		A	multiple tendons (through separate incision(s))	6.82	8.88	8.88	0.92	16.62	16.62	090	
27685		A	Lengthening or shortening of tendon, leg or ankle; single tendon (separate procedure)	6.50	10.37	8.45	0.91	17.78	15.86	090	
27686		A	multiple tendons (through same incision), each	7.46	15.30	9.89	1.05	23.81	18.40	090	
27687		A	Gastrocnemius recession (eg, Strayer procedure)	6.24	8.70	8.70	0.88	15.82	15.82	090	
27690		A	Transfer or transplant of single tendon (with muscle redirection or rerouting); superficial (eg, anterior tibial extensors into midfoot)	8.71	9.61	9.61	1.22	19.54	19.54	090	

Surgery

■ RVU not developed by CMS. Gap-filled RVUs developed by Ingenix/CHEG.

Code	M	S	Description	Work Value	Non-Fac PE	Fac PE	Mal-prac-tice	Non-Fac Total	Fac Total	Global	Gap
27691		A	deep (eg, anterior tibial or posterior tibial through interosseous space, flexor digitorum longus, flexor hallicus longus, or peroneal tendon to midfoot or hindfoot)	9.96	11.10	11.10	1.40	22.46	22.46	090	
27692		A	each additional tendon (List in addition to code for primary procedure)	1.87	0.99	0.99	0.26	3.12	3.12	ZZZ	
27695		A	Repair, primary, disrupted ligament, ankle; collateral	6.51	9.20	9.20	0.90	16.61	16.61	090	
27696		A	both collateral ligaments	8.27	9.54	9.54	1.16	18.97	18.97	090	
27698		A	Repair, secondary, disrupted ligament, ankle, collateral (eg, Watson-Jones procedure)	9.36	9.72	9.72	1.31	20.39	20.39	090	
27700		A	Arthroplasty, ankle;	9.29	7.95	7.95	1.24	18.48	18.48	090	
27702		A	with implant (total ankle)	13.67	13.02	13.02	1.92	28.61	28.61	090	
27703		A	revision, total ankle	15.87	13.31	13.31	2.24	31.42	31.42	090	
27704		A	Removal of ankle implant	7.62	9.40	9.40	0.61	17.63	17.63	090	
27705		A	Osteotomy; tibia	10.38	11.55	11.55	1.44	23.37	23.37	090	
27707		A	fibula	4.37	8.48	8.48	0.60	13.45	13.45	090	
27709		A	tibia and fibula	9.95	11.48	11.48	1.39	22.82	22.82	090	
27712		A	multiple, with realignment on intramedullary rod (eg, Sofield type procedure)	14.25	13.92	13.92	2.00	30.17	30.17	090	
27715		A	Osteoplasty, tibia and fibula, lengthening or shortening	14.39	15.22	15.22	2.00	31.61	31.61	090	
27720		A	Repair of nonunion or malunion, tibia; without graft, (eg, compression technique)	11.79	13.67	13.67	1.66	27.12	27.12	090	
27722		A	with sliding graft	11.82	13.46	13.46	1.65	26.93	26.93	090	
27724		A	with iliac or other autograft (includes obtaining graft)	18.20	17.28	17.28	2.10	37.58	37.58	090	
27725		A	by synostosis, with fibula, any method	15.59	15.62	15.62	2.20	33.41	33.41	090	
27727		A	Repair of congenital pseudarthrosis, tibia	14.01	14.43	14.43	1.84	30.28	30.28	090	
27730		A	Arrest, epiphyseal (epiphysiodesis), any method; distal tibia	7.41	21.54	10.22	0.75	29.70	18.38	090	
27732		A	distal fibula	5.32	14.45	7.22	0.63	20.40	13.17	090	
27734		A	distal tibia and fibula	8.48	10.84	10.84	0.85	20.17	20.17	090	
27740		A	Arrest, epiphyseal (epiphysiodesis), any method, combined, proximal and distal tibia and fibula;	9.30	16.04	9.72	1.31	26.65	20.33	090	
27742		A	and distal femur	10.3	16.44	9.27	1.55	28.29	21.12	090	

■ RVU not developed by CMS. Gap-filled RVUs developed by Ingenix/CHEG.

Code	M	S	Description	Work Value	Non-Fac PE	Fac PE	Mal-practice	Non-Fac Total	Fac Total	Global	Gap
27745		A	Prophylactic treatment (nailing, pinning, plating or wiring) with or without methylmethacrylate, tibia	10.07	11.60	11.60	1.38	23.05	23.05	090	
27750		A	Closed treatment of tibial shaft fracture (with or without fibular fracture); without manipulation	3.19	5.65	4.00	0.43	9.27	7.62	090	
27752		A	with manipulation, with or without skeletal traction	5.84	8.20	6.17	0.82	14.86	12.83	090	
27756		A	Percutaneous skeletal fixation of tibial shaft fracture (with or without fibular fracture) (eg, pins or screws)	6.78	10.84	10.84	0.94	18.56	18.56	090	
27758		A	Open treatment of tibial shaft fracture, (with or without fibular fracture) with plate/screws, with or without cerclage	11.67	12.22	12.22	1.52	25.41	25.41	090	
27759		A	Open treatment of tibial shaft fracture (with or without fibular fracture) by intramedullary implant, with or without interlocking screws and/or cerclage	13.76	13.46	13.46	1.93	29.15	29.15	090	
27760		A	Closed treatment of medial malleolus fracture; without manipulation	3.01	5.42	3.87	0.39	8.82	7.27	090	
27762		A	with manipulation, with or without skin or skeletal traction	5.25	7.57	5.75	0.71	13.53	11.71	090	
27766		A	Open treatment of medial malleolus fracture, with or without internal or external fixation	8.36	8.26	8.26	1.17	17.79	17.79	090	
27780		A	Closed treatment of proximal fibula or shaft fracture; without manipulation	2.65	5.37	3.69	0.33	8.35	6.67	090	
27781		A	with manipulation	4.40	6.38	4.62	0.57	11.35	9.59	090	
27784		A	Open treatment of proximal fibula or shaft fracture, with or without internal or external fixation	7.11	8.63	8.63	0.98	16.72	16.72	090	
27786		A	Closed treatment of distal fibular fracture (lateral malleolus); without manipulation	2.84	5.38	3.78	0.37	8.59	6.99	090	
27788		A	with manipulation	4.45	6.65	4.62	0.61	11.71	9.68	090	
27792		A	Open treatment of distal fibular fracture (lateral malleolus), with or without internal or external fixation	7.66	8.18	8.18	1.07	16.91	16.91	090	
27808		A	Closed treatment of bimalleolar ankle fracture, (including Potts); without manipulation	2.83	6.44	4.50	0.38	9.65	7.71	090	
27810		A	with manipulation	5.13	7.77	5.71	0.71	13.61	11.55	090	
27814		A	Open treatment of bimalleolar ankle fracture, with or without internal or external fixation	10.68	10.93	10.93	1.50	23.11	23.11	090	
27816		A	Closed treatment of trimalleolar ankle fracture; without manipulation	2.89	5.97	4.55	0.37	9.23	7.81	090	
27818		A	with manipulation	5.50	7.89	5.88	0.74	14.13	12.12	090	

■ RVU not developed by CMS. Gap-filled RVUs developed by Ingenix/CHEG.

Code	M	S	Description	Work Value	Non-Fac PE	Fac PE	Mal-practice	Non-Fac Total	Fac Total	Global	Gap
27822		A	Open treatment of trimalleolar ankle fracture, with or without internal or external fixation, medial and/or lateral malleolus; without fixation of posterior lip	11.00	13.18	13.18	1.29	25.47	25.47	090	
27823		A	with fixation of posterior lip	13.00	14.39	14.39	1.65	29.04	29.04	090	
27824		A	Closed treatment of fracture of weight bearing articular portion of distal tibia (eg, pilon or tibial plafond), with or without anesthesia; without manipulation	2.89	6.43	4.50	0.39	9.71	7.78	090	
27825		A	with skeletal traction and/or requiring manipulation	6.19	8.30	6.32	0.85	15.34	13.36	090	
27826		A	Open treatment of fracture of weight bearing articular surface/portion of distal tibia (eg, pilon or tibial plafond), with internal or external fixation; of fibula only	8.54	11.88	11.88	1.19	21.61	21.61	090	
27827		A	of tibia only	14.06	15.00	15.00	1.96	31.02	31.02	090	
27828		A	of both tibia and fibula	16.23	15.03	15.03	2.27	33.53	33.53	090	
27829		A	Open treatment of distal tibiofibular joint (syndesmosis) disruption, with or without internal or external fixation	5.49	8.67	8.67	0.77	14.93	14.93	090	
27830		A	Closed treatment of proximal tibiofibular joint dislocation; without anesthesia	3.79	5.82	4.36	0.44	10.05	8.59	090	
27831		A	requiring anesthesia	4.56	4.94	4.94	0.61	10.11	10.11	090	
27832		A	Open treatment of proximal tibiofibular joint dislocation, with or without internal or external fixation, or with excision of proximal fibula	6.49	8.06	8.06	0.91	15.46	15.46	090	
27840		A	Closed treatment of ankle dislocation; without anesthesia	4.58	6.21	6.21	0.47	11.26	11.26	090	
27842		A	requiring anesthesia, with or without percutaneous skeletal fixation	6.21	5.25	5.25	0.76	12.22	12.22	090	
27846		A	Open treatment of ankle dislocation, with or without percutaneous skeletal fixation; without repair or internal fixation	9.79	10.46	10.46	1.36	21.61	21.61	090	
27848		A	with repair or internal or external fixation	11.20	11.70	11.70	1.55	24.45	24.45	090	
27860*		A	Manipulation of ankle under general anesthesia (includes application of traction or other fixation apparatus)	2.34	3.78	3.78	0.31	6.43	6.43	010	
27870		A	Arthrodesis, ankle, any method	13.91	13.76	13.76	1.95	29.62	29.62	090	
27871		A	Arthrodesis, tibiofibular joint, proximal or distal	9.17	11.03	11.03	1.29	21.49	21.49	090	
27880		A	Amputation, leg, through tibia and fibula;	11.85	11.95	11.95	1.38	25.18	25.18	090	
27881		A	with immediate fitting technique including application of first cast	12.34	13.44	13.44	1.59	27.37	27.37	090	

■ RVU not developed by CMS. Gap-filled RVUs developed by Ingenix/CHEG.

Code	M	S	Description	Work Value	Non-Fac PE	Fac PE	Mal-prac-tice	Non-Fac Total	Fac Total	Global	Gap
27882		A	open, circular (guillotine)	8.94	13.13	13.13	1.03	23.10	23.10	090	
27884		A	secondary closure or scar revision	8.21	10.78	10.78	0.95	19.94	19.94	090	
27886		A	re-amputation	9.32	11.26	11.26	1.13	21.71	21.71	090	
27888		A	Amputation, ankle, through malleoli of tibia and fibula (eg, Syme, Pirogoff type procedures), with plastic closure and resection of nerves	9.67	11.11	11.11	1.26	22.04	22.04	090	
27889		A	Ankle disarticulation	9.98	10.45	10.45	1.19	21.62	21.62	090	
27892		A	Decompression fasciotomy, leg; anterior and/or lateral compartments only, with debridement of nonviable muscle and/or nerve	7.39	8.41	8.41	0.86	16.66	16.66	090	
27893		A	posterior compartment(s) only, with debridement of nonviable muscle and/or nerve	7.35	8.58	8.58	0.90	16.83	16.83	090	
27894		A	anterior and/or lateral, and posterior compartment(s), with debridement of nonviable muscle and/or nerve	10.49	10.09	10.09	1.25	21.83	21.83	090	
27899		C	Unlisted procedure, leg or ankle	0.00	0.00	0.00	0.00	0.00	0.00	YYY	
28001*		A	Incision and drainage, bursa, foot	2.73	5.62	3.09	0.31	8.66	6.13	010	
28002*		A	Incision and drainage below fascia, with or without tendon sheath involvement, foot; single bursal space	4.62	6.78	4.22	0.56	11.96	9.40	010	
28003		A	multiple areas	8.41	11.40	10.63	1.03	20.84	20.07	090	
28005		A	Incision, bone cortex (eg, osteomyelitis or bone abscess), foot	8.68	10.26	10.26	1.14	20.08	20.08	090	
28008		A	Fasciotomy, foot and/or toe	4.45	8.17	6.38	0.56	13.18	11.39	090	
28010		A	Tenotomy, percutaneous, toe; single tendon	2.84	7.64	5.37	0.39	10.87	8.60	090	
28011		A	multiple tendons	4.14	9.36	6.79	0.58	14.08	11.51	090	
28020		A	Arthrotomy, including exploration, drainage, or removal of loose or foreign body; intertarsal or tarsometatarsal joint	5.01	8.12	6.81	0.64	13.77	12.46	090	
28022		A	metatarsophalangeal joint	4.67	7.90	6.26	0.62	13.19	11.55	090	
28024		A	interphalangeal joint	4.38	8.55	6.64	0.50	13.43	11.52	090	
28030		A	Neurectomy, intrinsic musculature of foot	6.15	3.50	3.50	0.85	10.50	10.50	090	
28035		A	Release, tarsal tunnel (posterior tibial nerve decompression)	5.09	8.80	5.35	0.71	14.60	11.15	090	
28043		A	Excision, tumor, foot; subcutaneous tissue	3.54	7.47	4.96	0.45	11.46	8.95	090	
28045		A	deep, subfascial, intramuscular	4.72	8.18	5.81	0.62	13.52	11.15	090	

■ RVU not developed by CMS. Gap-filled RVUs developed by Ingenix/CHEG.

Code	M	S	Description	Work Value	Non-Fac PE	Fac PE	Mal-practice	Non-Fac Total	Fac Total	Global	Gap
28046		A	Radical resection of tumor (eg, malignant neoplasm), soft tissue of foot	10.18	13.58	11.38	1.13	24.89	22.69	090	
28050		A	Arthrotomy with biopsy; intertarsal or tarsometatarsal joint	4.25	9.52	6.11	0.55	14.32	10.91	090	
28052		A	metatarsophalangeal joint	3.94	8.01	5.76	0.51	12.46	10.21	090	
28054		A	interphalangeal joint	3.45	7.70	5.50	0.45	11.60	9.40	090	
28060		A	Fasciectomy, plantar fascia; partial (separate procedure)	5.23	8.72	6.51	0.69	14.64	12.43	090	
28062		A	radical (separate procedure)	6.52	9.27	6.87	0.85	16.64	14.24	090	
28070		A	Synovectomy; intertarsal or tarsometatarsal joint, each	5.10	7.98	6.12	0.68	13.76	11.90	090	
28072		A	metatarsophalangeal joint, each	4.58	8.84	6.67	0.64	14.06	11.89	090	
28080		A	Excision, interdigital (Morton) neuroma, single, each	3.58	7.82	5.51	0.50	11.90	9.59	090	
28086		A	Synovectomy, tendon sheath, foot; flexor	4.78	11.87	7.11	0.66	17.31	12.55	090	
28088		A	extensor	3.86	9.97	6.62	0.52	14.35	11.00	090	
28090		A	Excision of lesion, tendon, tendon sheath, or capsule (including synovectomy) (eg, cyst or ganglion); foot	4.41	8.12	5.64	0.57	13.10	10.62	090	
28092		A	toe(s), each	3.64	8.17	6.08	0.46	12.27	10.18	090	
28100		A	Excision or curettage of bone cyst or benign tumor, talus or calcaneus;	5.66	13.07	7.70	0.76	19.49	14.12	090	
28102		A	with iliac or other autograft (includes obtaining graft)	7.73	9.00	9.00	0.97	17.70	17.70	090	
28103		A	with allograft	6.50	8.76	6.93	0.89	16.15	14.32	090	
28104		A	Excision or curettage of bone cyst or benign tumor, tarsal or metatarsal, except talus or calcaneus;	5.12	8.49	6.76	0.69	14.30	12.57	090	
28106		A	with iliac or other autograft (includes obtaining graft)	7.16	6.97	6.97	1.01	15.14	15.14	090	
28107		A	with allograft	5.56	9.96	7.13	0.74	16.26	13.43	090	
28108		A	Excision or curettage of bone cyst or benign tumor, phalanges of foot	4.16	7.49	5.36	0.52	12.17	10.04	090	
28110		A	Ostectomy, partial excision, fifth metatarsal head (bunionette) (separate procedure)	4.08	8.80	6.87	0.49	13.37	11.44	090	
28111		A	Ostectomy, complete excision; first metatarsal head	5.01	9.09	7.69	0.63	14.73	13.33	090	
28112		A	other metatarsal head (second, third or fourth)	4.49	8.89	7.47	0.60	13.98	12.56	090	

■ RVU not developed by CMS. Gap-filled RVUs developed by Ingenix/CHEG.

Code	M	S	Description	Work Value	Non-Fac PE	Fac PE	Mal-practice	Non-Fac Total	Fac Total	Global	Gap
28113		A	fifth metatarsal head	4.79	8.92	7.13	0.63	14.34	12.55	090	
28114		A	all metatarsal heads, with partial proximal phalangectomy, excluding first metatarsal (eg, Clayton type procedure)	9.79	12.36	10.85	1.36	23.51	22.00	090	
28116		A	Ostectomy, excision of tarsal coalition	7.75	9.27	6.38	1.03	18.05	15.16	090	
28118		A	Ostectomy, calcaneus;	5.96	9.37	7.24	0.79	16.12	13.99	090	
28119		A	for spur, with or without plantar fascial release	5.39	8.58	6.15	0.74	14.71	12.28	090	
28120		A	Partial excision (craterization, saucerization, sequestrectomy, or diaphysectomy) bone (eg, osteomyelitis or bossing); talus or calcaneus	5.40	11.28	9.83	0.69	17.37	15.92	090	
28122		A	tarsal or metatarsal bone, except talus or calcaneus	7.29	10.94	9.50	0.96	19.19	17.75	090	
28124		A	phalanx of toe	4.81	9.61	7.61	0.65	15.07	13.07	090	
28126		A	Resection, partial or complete, phalangeal base, each toe	3.52	8.37	6.76	0.49	12.38	10.77	090	
28130		A	Talectomy (astragalectomy)	8.11	8.77	8.77	1.11	17.99	17.99	090	
28140		A	Metatarsectomy	6.91	10.40	7.92	0.84	18.15	15.67	090	
28150		A	Phalangectomy, toe, each toe	4.09	8.75	7.07	0.52	13.36	11.68	090	
28153		A	Resection, condyle(s), distal end of phalanx, each toe	3.66	8.39	6.22	0.49	12.54	10.37	090	
28160		A	Hemiphalangectomy or interphalangeal joint excision, toe, proximal end of phalanx, each	3.74	8.55	7.22	0.51	12.80	11.47	090	
28171		A	Radical resection of tumor, bone; tarsal (except talus or calcaneus)	9.60	8.27	8.27	1.13	19.00	19.00	090	
28173		A	metatarsal	8.80	10.83	8.88	1.04	20.67	18.72	090	
28175		A	phalanx of toe	6.05	9.54	6.99	0.75	16.34	13.79	090	
28190*		A	Removal of foreign body, foot; subcutaneous	1.96	6.54	3.53	0.16	8.66	5.65	010	
28192		A	deep	4.64	8.20	5.44	0.52	13.36	10.60	090	
28193		A	complicated	5.73	8.94	6.67	0.63	15.30	13.03	090	
28200		A	Repair, tendon, flexor, foot; primary or secondary, without free graft, each tendon	4.60	8.47	6.32	0.59	13.66	11.51	090	
28202		A	secondary with free graft, each tendon (includes obtaining graft)	6.84	12.63	6.83	0.86	20.33	14.53	090	
28208		A	Repair, tendon, extensor, foot; primary or secondary, each tendon	4.37	8.17	6.03	0.59	13.13	10.99	090	
28210		A	secondary with free graft, each tendon (includes obtaining graft)	6.35	9.83	6.38	0.77	16.95	13.50	090	

■ RVU not developed by CMS. Gap-filled RVUs developed by Ingenix/CHEG.

Code	M	S	Description	Work Value	Non-Fac PE	Fac PE	Mal-practice	Non-Fac Total	Fac Total	Global	Gap
28220		A	Tenolysis, flexor, foot; single tendon	4.53	8.12	6.41	0.63	13.28	11.57	090	
28222		A	multiple tendons	5.62	8.40	6.77	0.77	14.79	13.16	090	
28225		A	Tenolysis, extensor, foot; single tendon	3.66	7.76	5.57	0.50	11.92	9.73	090	
28226		A	multiple tendons	4.53	8.30	6.66	0.62	13.45	11.81	090	
28230		A	Tenotomy, open, tendon flexor; foot, single or multiple tendon(s) (separate procedure)	4.24	8.26	6.83	0.59	13.09	11.66	090	
28232		A	toe, single tendon (separate procedure)	3.39	8.12	6.53	0.48	11.99	10.40	090	
28234		A	Tenotomy, open, extensor, foot or toe, each tendon	3.37	7.98	6.11	0.46	11.81	9.94	090	
28238		A	Reconstruction (advancement), posterior tibial tendon with excision of accessory tarsal navicular bone (eg, Kidner type procedure)	7.73	9.77	7.60	1.08	18.58	16.41	090	
28240		A	Tenotomy, lengthening, or release, abductor hallucis muscle	4.36	8.17	6.40	0.61	13.14	11.37	090	
28250		A	Division of plantar fascia and muscle (eg, Steindler stripping) (separate procedure)	5.92	9.05	7.12	0.81	15.78	13.85	090	
28260		A	Capsulotomy, midfoot; medial release only (separate procedure)	7.96	11.04	8.08	1.08	20.08	17.12	090	
28261		A	with tendon lengthening	11.73	11.16	9.64	1.66	24.55	23.03	090	
28262		A	extensive, including posterior talotibial capsulotomy and tendon(s) lengthening (eg, resistant clubfoot deformity)	15.83	15.66	15.09	2.22	33.71	33.14	090	
28264		A	Capsulotomy, midtarsal (eg, Heyman type procedure)	10.35	10.98	10.98	1.46	22.79	22.79	090	
28270		A	Capsulotomy; metatarsophalangeal joint, with or without tenorrhaphy, each joint (separate procedure)	4.76	8.75	7.43	0.67	14.18	12.86	090	
28272		A	interphalangeal joint, each joint (separate procedure)	3.80	7.70	5.50	0.52	12.02	9.82	090	
28280		A	Syndactylization, toes (eg, webbing or Kelikian type procedure)	5.19	8.39	6.77	0.72	14.30	12.68	090	
28285		A	Correction, hammertoe (eg, interphalangeal fusion, partial or total phalangectomy)	4.59	8.79	6.76	0.64	14.02	11.99	090	
28286		A	Correction, cock-up fifth toe, with plastic skin closure (eg, Ruiz-Mora type procedure)	4.56	8.78	6.75	0.64	13.98	11.95	090	
28288		A	Ostectomy, partial, exostectomy or condylectomy, metatarsal head, each metatarsal head	4.74	9.00	8.02	0.65	14.39	13.41	090	
28289		A	Hallux rigidus correction with cheilectomy, debridement and capsular release of the first metatarsophalangeal joint	7.04	10.54	9.75	0.96	18.54	17.75	090	

■ RVU not developed by CMS. Gap-filled RVUs developed by Ingenix/CHEG.

Code	M	S	Description	Work Value	Non-Fac PE	Fac PE	Mal-prac-tice	Non-Fac Total	Fac Total	Global	Gap
28290		A	Correction, hallux valgus (bunion), with or without sesamoidectomy; simple exostectomy (eg, Silver type procedure)	5.66	9.55	8.81	0.79	16.00	15.26	090	
28292		A	Keller, McBride or Mayo type procedure	7.04	9.82	7.69	0.98	17.84	15.71	090	
28293		A	resection of joint with implant	9.15	10.67	8.02	1.28	21.1	18.45	090	
28294		A	with tendon transplants (eg, Joplin type procedure)	8.56	10.52	8.30	1.16	20.24	18.02	090	
28296		A	with metatarsal osteotomy (eg, Mitchell, Chevron, or concentric type procedures)	9.18	10.84	8.65	1.28	21.30	19.11	090	
28297		A	Lapidus type procedure	9.18	12.80	10.25	1.31	23.29	20.74	090	
28298		A	by phalanx osteotomy	7.94	10.10	8.48	1.12	19.16	17.54	090	
28299		A	by double osteotomy	10.58	11.55	9.21	1.24	23.37	21.03	090	
28300		A	Osteotomy; calcaneus (eg, Dwyer or Chambers type procedure), with or without internal fixation	9.54	14.15	9.43	1.31	25.00	20.28	090	
28302		A	talus	9.55	9.55	9.22	1.15	20.25	19.92	090	
28304		A	Osteotomy, tarsal bones, other than calcaneus or talus;	9.16	9.53	7.88	1.00	19.69	18.04	090	
28305		A	with autograft (includes obtaining graft) (eg, Fowler type)	10.5	14.52	10.07	0.55	25.57	21.12	090	
28306		A	Osteotomy, with or without lengthening, shortening or angular correction, metatarsal; first metatarsal	5.86	8.84	6.51	0.81	15.51	13.18	090	
28307		A	first metatarsal with autograft (other than first toe)	6.33	13.70	7.74	0.71	20.74	14.78	090	
28308		A	other than first metatarsal, each	5.29	7.97	5.60	0.74	14.00	11.63	090	
28309		A	multiple (eg, Swanson type cavus foot procedure)	12.78	11.08	11.08	1.64	25.50	25.50	090	
28310		A	Osteotomy, shortening, angular or rotational correction; proximal phalanx, first toe (separate procedure)	5.43	9.00	6.93	0.76	15.19	13.12	090	
28312		A	other phalanges, any toe	4.55	8.66	7.87	0.62	13.83	13.04	090	
28313		A	Reconstruction, angular deformity of toe, soft tissue procedures only (eg, overlapping second toe, fifth toe, curly toes)	5.01	9.06	9.06	0.68	14.75	14.75	090	
28315		A	Sesamoidectomy, first toe (separate procedure)	4.86	7.95	5.82	0.66	13.47	11.34	090	
28320		A	Repair, nonunion or malunion; tarsal bones	9.18	9.02	9.02	1.27	19.47	19.47	090	
28322		A	metatarsal, with or without bone graft (includes obtaining graft)	8.34	11.71	8.38	1.17	21.22	17.89	090	

■ RVU not developed by CMS. Gap-filled RVUs developed by Ingenix/CHEG.

Code	M	S	Description	Work Value	Non-Fac PE	Fac PE	Mal-practice	Non-Fac Total	Fac Total	Global	Gap
28340		A	Reconstruction, toe, macrodactyly; soft tissue resection	6.98	8.96	6.28	0.98	16.92	14.24	090	
28341		A	requiring bone resection	8.41	9.55	6.88	1.18	19.14	16.47	090	
28344		A	Reconstruction, toe(s); polydactyly	4.26	7.38	4.86	0.60	12.24	9.72	090	
28345		A	syndactyly, with or without skin graft(s), each web	5.92	9.48	7.58	0.84	16.24	14.34	090	
28360		A	Reconstruction, cleft foot	13.34	12.22	12.22	1.88	27.44	27.44	090	
28400		A	Closed treatment of calcaneal fracture; without manipulation	2.16	5.76	4.74	0.29	8.21	7.19	090	
28405		A	with manipulation	4.57	6.66	5.87	0.63	11.86	11.07	090	
28406		A	Percutaneous skeletal fixation of calcaneal fracture, with manipulation	6.31	8.69	8.69	0.87	15.87	15.87	090	
28415		A	Open treatment of calcaneal fracture, with or without internal or external fixation;	15.97	15.72	15.72	2.24	33.93	33.93	090	
28420		A	with primary iliac or other autogenous bone graft (includes obtaining graft)	16.64	15.95	15.95	2.29	34.88	34.88	090	
28430		A	Closed treatment of talus fracture; without manipulation	2.09	5.25	4.26	0.27	7.61	6.62	090	
28435		A	with manipulation	3.40	5.41	4.57	0.47	9.28	8.44	090	
28436		A	Percutaneous skeletal fixation of talus fracture, with manipulation	4.71	7.86	7.86	0.66	13.23	13.23	090	
28445		A	Open treatment of talus fracture, with or without internal or external fixation	15.62	13.94	13.94	1.29	30.85	30.85	090	
28450		A	Treatment of tarsal bone fracture (except talus and calcaneus); without manipulation, each	1.90	5.28	4.07	0.25	7.43	6.22	090	
28455		A	with manipulation, each	3.09	5.51	4.94	0.43	9.03	8.46	090	
28456		A	Percutaneous skeletal fixation of tarsal bone fracture (except talus and calcaneus), with manipulation, each	2.68	6.27	6.27	0.36	9.31	9.31	090	
28465		A	Open treatment of tarsal bone fracture (except talus and calcaneus), with or without internal or external fixation, each	7.01	8.25	8.25	0.87	16.13	16.13	090	
28470		A	Closed treatment of metatarsal fracture; without manipulation, each	1.99	4.52	3.41	0.26	6.77	5.66	090	
28475		A	with manipulation, each	2.97	5.18	4.38	0.41	8.56	7.76	090	
28476		A	Percutaneous skeletal fixation of metatarsal fracture, with manipulation, each	3.38	6.71	6.71	0.46	10.55	10.55	090	
28485		A	Open treatment of metatarsal fracture, with or without internal or external fixation, each	5.71	8.16	8.16	0.80	14.67	14.67	090	

■ RVU not developed by CMS. Gap-filled RVUs developed by Ingenix/CHEG.

Code	M	S	Description	Work Value	Non-Fac PE	Fac PE	Mal-practice	Non-Fac Total	Fac Total	Global	Gap
28490		A	Closed treatment of fracture great toe, phalanx or phalanges; without manipulation	1.09	2.76	2.21	0.13	3.98	3.43	090	
28495		A	with manipulation	1.58	2.82	2.31	0.19	4.59	4.08	090	
28496		A	Percutaneous skeletal fixation of fracture great toe, phalanx or phalanges, with manipulation	2.33	11.10	4.58	0.32	13.75	7.23	090	
28505		A	Open treatment of fracture great toe, phalanx or phalanges, with or without internal or external fixation	3.81	11.46	6.74	0.50	15.77	11.05	090	
28510		A	Closed treatment of fracture, phalanx or phalanges, other than great toe; without manipulation, each	1.09	2.51	2.23	0.13	3.73	3.45	090	
28515		A	with manipulation, each	1.46	2.83	2.30	0.17	4.46	3.93	090	
28525		A	Open treatment of fracture, phalanx or phalanges, other than great toe, with or without internal or external fixation, each	3.32	10.82	6.16	0.44	14.58	9.92	090	
28530		A	Closed treatment of sesamoid fracture	1.06	2.91	2.91	0.13	4.10	4.10	090	
28531		A	Open treatment of sesamoid fracture, with or without internal fixation	2.35	11.91	4.73	0.33	14.59	7.41	090	
28540		A	Closed treatment of tarsal bone dislocation, other than talotarsal; without anesthesia	2.04	3.75	3.75	0.24	6.03	6.03	090	
28545		A	requiring anesthesia	2.45	4.76	4.76	0.33	7.54	7.54	090	
28546		A	Percutaneous skeletal fixation of tarsal bone dislocation, other than talotarsal, with manipulation	3.20	12.55	6.31	0.46	16.21	9.97	090	
28555		A	Open treatment of tarsal bone dislocation, with or without internal or external fixation	6.30	13.49	8.36	0.88	20.67	15.54	090	
28570		A	Closed treatment of talotarsal joint dislocation; without anesthesia	1.66	3.67	3.67	0.22	5.55	5.55	090	
28575		A	requiring anesthesia	3.31	5.19	5.19	0.45	8.95	8.95	090	
28576		A	Percutaneous skeletal fixation of talotarsal joint dislocation, with manipulation	4.17	12.06	6.85	0.56	16.79	11.58	090	
28585		A	Open treatment of talotarsal joint dislocation, with or without internal or external fixation	7.99	8.75	8.32	1.13	17.87	17.44	090	
28600		A	Closed treatment of tarsometatarsal joint dislocation; without anesthesia	1.89	4.32	3.89	0.24	6.45	6.02	090	
28605		A	requiring anesthesia	2.71	4.40	4.40	0.35	7.46	7.46	090	
28606		A	Percutaneous skeletal fixation of tarsometatarsal joint dislocation, with manipulation	4.90	16.14	7.09	0.68	21.72	12.67	090	
28615		A	Open treatment of tarsometatarsal joint dislocation, with or without internal or external fixation	7.77	9.45	9.45	1.09	18.31	18.31	090	

■ RVU not developed by CMS. Gap-filled RVUs developed by Ingenix/CHEG.

Code	M	S	Description	Work Value	Non-Fac PE	Fac PE	Mal-practice	Non-Fac Total	Fac Total	Global	Gap
28630*		A	Closed treatment of metatarsophalangeal joint dislocation; without anesthesia	1.70	2.35	2.35	0.17	4.22	4.22	010	
28635*		A	requiring anesthesia	1.91	2.49	2.49	0.24	4.64	4.64	010	
28636		A	Percutaneous skeletal fixation of metatarsophalangeal joint dislocation, with manipulation	2.77	4.81	3.22	0.39	7.97	6.38	010	
28645		A	Open treatment of metatarsophalangeal joint dislocation, with or without internal or external fixation	4.22	6.69	4.34	0.58	11.49	9.14	090	
28660*		A	Closed treatment of interphalangeal joint dislocation; without anesthesia	1.23	3.11	2.60	0.11	4.45	3.94	010	
28665*		A	requiring anesthesia	1.92	2.47	2.47	0.24	4.63	4.63	010	
28666		A	Percutaneous skeletal fixation of interphalangeal joint dislocation, with manipulation	2.66	13.30	3.00	0.38	16.34	6.04	010	
28675		A	Open treatment of interphalangeal joint dislocation, with or without internal or external fixation	2.92	9.48	4.90	0.41	12.81	8.23	090	
28705		A	Arthrodesis; pantalar	18.80	15.67	15.67	2.13	36.60	36.60	090	
28715		A	triple	13.10	12.57	12.57	1.84	27.51	27.51	090	
28725		A	subtalar	11.61	11.48	11.48	1.63	24.72	24.72	090	
28730		A	Arthrodesis, midtarsal or tarsometatarsal, multiple or transverse;	10.76	10.76	10.76	1.51	23.03	23.03	090	
28735		A	with osteotomy (eg, flatfoot correction)	10.85	10.45	10.45	1.51	22.81	22.81	090	
28737		A	Arthrodesis, with tendon lengthening and advancement, midtarsal, tarsal navicular-cuneiform (eg, Miller type procedure)	9.64	9.04	9.04	1.36	20.04	20.04	090	
28740		A	Arthrodesis, midtarsal or tarsometatarsal, single joint	8.02	13.03	8.94	1.13	22.18	18.09	090	
28750		A	Arthrodesis, great toe; metatarsophalangeal joint	7.30	12.48	9.13	1.03	20.81	17.46	090	
28755		A	interphalangeal joint	4.74	8.52	6.42	0.66	13.92	11.82	090	
28760		A	Arthrodesis, with extensor hallucis longus transfer to first metatarsal neck, great toe, interphalangeal joint (eg, Jones type procedure)	7.75	10.39	7.82	1.07	19.21	16.64	090	
28800		A	Amputation, foot; midtarsal (eg, Chopart type procedure)	8.21	8.90	8.90	0.98	18.09	18.09	090	
28805		A	transmetatarsal	8.39	9.00	9.00	0.97	18.36	18.36	090	
28810		A	Amputation, metatarsal, with toe, single	6.21	7.97	7.97	0.70	14.88	14.88	090	
28820		A	Amputation, toe; metatarsophalangeal joint	4.41	9.91	7.16	0.51	14.83	12.08	090	

■ RVU not developed by CMS. Gap-filled RVUs developed by Ingenix/CHEG.

Surgery

Code	M	S	Description	Work Value	Non-Fac PE	Fac PE	Mal-practice	Non-Fac Total	Fac Total	Global	Gap
28825		A	interphalangeal joint	3.59	10.12	6.95	0.43	14.14	10.97	090	
28899		C	Unlisted procedure, foot or toes	0.00	0.00	0.00	0.00	0.00	0.00	YYY	
29000		A	Application of halo type body cast (see 20661-20663 for insertion)	2.25	2.71	1.67	0.30	5.26	4.22	000	
29010		A	Application of Risser jacket, localizer, body; only	2.06	2.98	1.72	0.27	5.31	4.05	000	
29015		A	including head	2.41	3.17	1.93	0.21	5.79	4.55	000	
29020		A	Application of turnbuckle jacket, body; only	2.11	3.33	1.47	0.16	5.60	3.74	000	
29025		A	including head	2.40	3.32	1.86	0.26	5.98	4.52	000	
29035		A	Application of body cast, shoulder to hips;	1.77	3.05	1.56	0.24	5.06	3.57	000	
29040		A	including head, Minerva type	2.22	2.54	1.49	0.35	5.11	4.06	000	
29044		A	including one thigh	2.12	3.20	1.81	0.29	5.61	4.22	000	
29046		A	including both thighs	2.41	3.31	2.04	0.34	6.06	4.79	000	
29049		A	Application, cast; figure-of-eight	0.89	1.07	0.57	0.12	2.08	1.58	000	
29055		A	shoulder spica	1.78	2.40	1.42	0.24	4.42	3.44	000	
29058		A	plaster Velpeau	1.31	1.33	0.73	0.14	2.78	2.18	000	
29065		A	shoulder to hand (long arm)	0.87	1.10	0.69	0.12	2.09	1.68	000	
29075		A	elbow to finger (short arm)	0.77	1.05	0.63	0.11	1.93	1.51	000	
29085		A	hand and lower forearm (gauntlet)	0.87	1.10	0.62	0.11	2.08	1.60	000	
29086		A	finger (eg, contracture)	0.62	0.81	0.50	0.07	1.50	1.19	000	
29105		A	Application of long arm splint (shoulder to hand)	0.87	1.05	0.52	0.11	2.03	1.50	000	
29125		A	Application of short arm splint (forearm to hand); static	0.59	0.88	0.41	0.06	1.53	1.06	000	
29126		A	dynamic	0.77	1.21	0.47	0.06	2.04	1.30	000	
29130		A	Application of finger splint; static	0.50	0.44	0.18	0.05	0.99	0.73	000	
29131		A	dynamic	0.55	0.71	0.23	0.03	1.29	0.81	000	
29200		A	Strapping; thorax	0.65	0.85	0.37	0.04	1.54	1.06	000	
29220		A	low back	0.64	0.96	0.41	0.07	1.67	1.12	000	
29240		A	shoulder (eg, Velpeau)	0.71	0.92	0.39	0.05	1.68	1.15	000	
29260		A	elbow or wrist	0.55	0.85	0.35	0.04	1.44	0.94	000	
29280		A	hand or finger	0.51	0.91	0.39	0.04	1.46	0.94	000	
29305		A	Application of hip spica cast; one leg	2.03	2.74	1.60	0.29	5.06	3.92	000	

■ RVU not developed by CMS. Gap-filled RVUs developed by Ingenix/CHEG.

Code	M	S	Description	Work Value	Non-Fac PE	Fac PE	Mal-practice	Non-Fac Total	Fac Total	Global	Gap
29325		A	one and one-half spica or both legs	2.32	3.05	1.79	0.31	5.68	4.42	000	
29345		A	Application of long leg cast (thigh to toes);	1.40	1.51	1.02	0.19	3.10	2.61	000	
29355		A	walker or ambulatory type	1.53	1.47	1.11	0.20	3.20	2.84	000	
29358		A	Application of long leg cast brace	1.43	1.72	1.07	0.19	3.34	2.69	000	
29365		A	Application of cylinder cast (thigh to ankle)	1.18	1.38	0.90	0.17	2.73	2.25	000	
29405		A	Application of short leg cast (below knee to toes);	0.86	1.03	0.66	0.12	2.01	1.64	000	
29425		A	walking or ambulatory type	1.01	1.05	0.68	0.14	2.20	1.83	000	
29435		A	Application of patellar tendon bearing (PTB) cast	1.18	1.35	0.88	0.17	2.70	2.23	000	
29440		A	Adding walker to previously applied cast	0.57	0.61	0.26	0.07	1.25	0.90	000	
29445		A	Application of rigid total contact leg cast	1.78	1.58	0.96	0.24	3.60	2.98	000	
29450		A	Application of clubfoot cast with molding or manipulation, long or short leg	2.08	1.40	1.11	0.13	3.61	3.32	000	
29505		A	Application of long leg splint (thigh to ankle or toes)	0.69	1.10	0.48	0.06	1.85	1.23	000	
29515		A	Application of short leg splint (calf to foot)	0.73	0.78	0.48	0.07	1.58	1.28	000	
29520		A	Strapping; hip	0.54	0.93	0.44	0.02	1.49	1.00	000	
29530		A	knee	0.57	0.83	0.36	0.04	1.44	0.97	000	
29540		A	ankle	0.51	0.40	0.32	0.04	0.95	0.87	000	
29550		A	toes	0.47	0.40	0.29	0.05	0.92	0.81	000	
29580		A	Unna boot	0.57	0.61	0.36	0.05	1.23	0.98	000	
29590		A	Denis-Browne splint strapping	0.76	0.50	0.30	0.06	1.32	1.12	000	
29700		A	Removal or bivalving; gauntlet, boot or body cast	0.57	0.81	0.28	0.07	1.45	0.92	000	
29705		A	full arm or full leg cast	0.76	0.73	0.39	0.10	1.59	1.25	000	
29710		A	shoulder or hip spica, Minerva, or Risser jacket, etc.	1.34	1.50	0.66	0.17	3.01	2.17	000	
29715		A	turnbuckle jacket	0.94	0.98	0.29	0.08	2.00	1.31	000	
29720		A	Repair of spica, body cast or jacket	0.68	0.95	0.36	0.10	1.73	1.14	000	
29730		A	Windowing of cast	0.75	0.71	0.36	0.10	1.56	1.21	000	
29740		A	Wedging of cast (except clubfoot casts)	1.12	1.02	0.46	0.15	2.29	1.73	000	
29750		A	Wedging of clubfoot cast	1.26	1.13	0.62	0.16	2.55	2.04	000	
29799		C	Unlisted procedure, casting or strapping	0.00	0.00	0.00	0.00	0.00	0.00	YYY	

■ RVU not developed by CMS. Gap-filled RVUs developed by Ingenix/CHEG.

Code	M	S	Description	Work Value	Non-Fac PE	Fac PE	Mal-practice	Non-Fac Total	Fac Total	Global	Gap
29800		A	Arthroscopy, temporomandibular joint, diagnostic, with or without synovial biopsy (separate procedure)	6.43	9.15	9.15	0.84	16.42	16.42	090	
29804		A	Arthroscopy, temporomandibular joint, surgical	8.14	8.73	8.73	0.66	17.53	17.53	090	
29805		A	Arthroscopy, shoulder, diagnostic, with or without synovial biopsy (separate procedure)	5.89	3.23	3.23	0.83	9.95	9.95	090	
29806		A	Arthroscopy, shoulder, surgical; capsulorrhaphy	14.37	11.33	11.33	2.01	27.71	27.71	090	
29807		A	repair of slap lesion	13.90	11.06	11.06	2.01	26.97	26.97	090	
29819		A	Arthroscopy, shoulder, surgical; with removal of loose body or foreign body	7.62	9.82	9.82	1.07	18.51	18.51	090	
29820		A	synovectomy, partial	7.07	9.55	9.55	0.99	17.61	17.61	090	
29821		A	synovectomy, complete	7.72	9.84	9.84	1.08	18.64	18.64	090	
29822		A	debridement, limited	7.43	9.75	9.75	1.04	18.22	18.22	090	
29823		A	debridement, extensive	8.17	10.14	10.14	1.15	19.46	19.46	090	
29824		A	distal claviculectomy including distal articular surface (Mumford procedure)	8.25	7.48	7.48	1.16	16.89	16.89	090	
29825		A	with lysis and resection of adhesions, with or without manipulation	7.62	9.80	9.80	1.06	18.48	18.48	090	
29826		A	decompression of subacromial space with partial acromioplasty, with or without coracoacromial release	8.99	10.65	10.65	1.26	20.90	20.90	090	
29830		A	Arthroscopy, elbow, diagnostic, with or without synovial biopsy (separate procedure)	5.76	6.14	6.14	0.79	12.69	12.69	090	
29834		A	Arthroscopy, elbow, surgical; with removal of loose body or foreign body	6.28	6.94	6.94	0.86	14.08	14.08	090	
29835		A	synovectomy, partial	6.48	6.95	6.95	0.88	14.31	14.31	090	
29836		A	synovectomy, complete	7.55	7.62	7.62	1.06	16.23	16.23	090	
29837		A	debridement, limited	6.87	7.30	7.30	0.96	15.13	15.13	090	
29838		A	debridement, extensive	7.71	7.73	7.73	1.07	16.51	16.51	090	
29840		A	Arthroscopy, wrist, diagnostic, with or without synovial biopsy (separate procedure)	5.54	8.38	8.38	0.69	14.61	14.61	090	
29843		A	Arthroscopy, wrist, surgical; for infection, lavage and drainage	6.01	8.70	8.70	0.82	15.53	15.53	090	
29844		A	synovectomy, partial	6.37	8.96	8.96	0.86	16.19	16.19	090	
29845		A	synovectomy, complete	7.52	9.56	9.56	0.84	17.92	17.92	090	
29846		A	excision and/or repair of triangular fibrocartilage and/or joint debridement	6.75	11.67	11.67	0.89	19.31	19.31	090	

■ RVU not developed by CMS. Gap-filled RVUs developed by Ingenix/CHEG.

Code	M	S	Description	Work Value	Non-Fac PE	Fac PE	Mal-practice	Non-Fac Total	Fac Total	Global	Gap
29847		A	internal fixation for fracture or instability	7.08	11.85	11.85	0.91	19.84	19.84	090	
29848		A	Endoscopy, wrist, surgical, with release of transverse carpal ligament	5.44	8.46	8.46	0.72	14.62	14.62	090	
29850		A	Arthroscopically aided treatment of intercondylar spine(s) and/or tuberosity fracture(s) of the knee, with or without manipulation; without internal or external fixation (includes arthroscopy)	8.19	7.49	7.49	0.74	16.42	16.42	090	
29851		A	with internal or external fixation (includes arthroscopy)	13.10	12.00	12.00	1.81	26.91	26.91	090	
29855		A	Arthroscopically aided treatment of tibial fracture, proximal (plateau); unicondylar, with or without internal or external fixation (includes arthroscopy)	10.62	10.55	10.55	1.50	22.67	22.67	090	
29856		A	bicondylar, with or without internal or external fixation (includes arthroscopy)	14.14	12.49	12.49	2.00	28.63	28.63	090	
29860		A	Arthroscopy, hip, diagnostic with or without synovial biopsy (separate procedure)	8.05	8.05	8.05	1.14	17.24	17.24	090	
29861		A	Arthroscopy, hip, surgical; with removal of loose body or foreign body	9.15	8.71	8.71	1.29	19.15	19.15	090	
29862		A	Arthroscopy, hip, surgical; with debridement/shaving of articular cartilage (chondroplasty), abrasion arthroplasty, and/or resection of labrum	9.90	9.75	9.75	1.39	21.04	21.04	090	
29863		A	Arthroscopy, hip, surgical; with synovectomy	9.90	10.31	10.31	1.40	21.61	21.61	090	
29870		A	Arthroscopy, knee, diagnostic, with or without synovial biopsy (separate procedure)	5.07	6.27	6.27	0.67	12.01	12.01	090	
29871		A	Arthroscopy, knee, surgical; for infection, lavage and drainage	6.55	8.38	8.38	0.88	15.81	15.81	090	
29874		A	for removal of loose body or foreign body (eg, osteochondritis dissecans fragmentation, chondral fragmentation)	7.05	8.15	8.15	0.87	16.07	16.07	090	
29875		A	synovectomy, limited (eg, plica or shelf resection) (separate procedure)	6.31	7.69	7.69	0.88	14.88	14.88	090	
29876		A	synovectomy, major, two or more compartments (eg, medial or lateral)	7.92	9.19	9.19	1.11	18.22	18.22	090	
29877		A	debridement/shaving of articular cartilage (chondroplasty)	7.35	8.29	8.29	1.03	16.67	16.67	090	
29879		A	abrasion arthroplasty (includes chondroplasty where necessary) or multiple drilling or microfracture	8.04	8.68	8.68	1.13	17.85	17.85	090	
29880		A	with meniscectomy (medial AND lateral, including any meniscal shaving)	8.50	8.95	8.95	1.19	18.64	18.64	090	

■ RVU not developed by CMS. Gap-filled RVUs developed by Ingenix/CHEG.

Code	M	S	Description	Work Value	Non-Fac PE	Fac PE	Mal-prac-tice	Non-Fac Total	Fac Total	Global	Gap
29881		A	with meniscectomy (medial OR lateral, including any meniscal shaving)	7.76	8.53	8.53	1.09	17.38	17.38	090	
29882		A	with meniscus repair (medial OR lateral)	8.65	9.01	9.01	1.09	18.75	18.75	090	
29883		A	with meniscus repair (medial AND lateral)	11.05	10.41	10.41	1.33	22.79	22.79	090	
29884		A	with lysis of adhesions, with or without manipulation (separate procedure)	7.33	8.87	8.87	1.03	17.23	17.23	090	
29885		A	drilling for osteochondritis dissecans with bone grafting, with or without internal fixation (including debridement of base of lesion)	9.09	9.85	9.85	1.27	20.21	20.21	090	
29886		A	drilling for intact osteochondritis dissecans lesion	7.54	8.99	8.99	1.06	17.59	17.59	090	
29887		A	drilling for intact osteochondritis dissecans lesion with internal fixation	9.04	9.83	9.83	1.27	20.14	20.14	090	
29888		A	Arthroscopically aided anterior cruciate ligament repair/augmentation or reconstruction	13.90	12.50	12.50	1.95	28.35	28.35	090	
29889		A	Arthroscopically aided posterior cruciate ligament repair/augmentation or reconstruction	16.00	13.71	13.71	2.11	31.82	31.82	090	
29891		A	Arthroscopy, ankle, surgical; excision of osteochondral defect of talus and/or tibia, including drilling of the defect	8.40	8.92	8.92	1.17	18.49	18.49	090	
29892		A	Arthroscopically aided repair of large osteochondritis dissecans lesion, talar dome fracture, or tibial plafond fracture, with or without internal fixation (includes arthroscopy)	9.00	9.04	9.04	1.26	19.30	19.30	090	
29893		A	Endoscopic plantar fasciotomy	5.22	5.56	5.56	0.74	11.52	11.52	090	
29894		A	Arthroscopy, ankle (tibiotalar and fibulotalar joints), surgical; with removal of loose body or foreign body	7.21	8.04	8.04	1.01	16.26	16.26	090	
29895		A	synovectomy, partial	6.99	8.01	8.01	0.97	15.97	15.97	090	
29897		A	debridement, limited	7.18	8.73	8.73	1.01	16.92	16.92	090	
29898		A	debridement, extensive	8.32	8.79	8.79	1.14	18.25	18.25	090	
29900		A	Arthroscopy, metacarpophalangeal joint, diagnostic, includes synovial biopsy	5.42	5.88	5.88	0.69	11.99	11.99	090	
29901		A	Arthroscopy, metacarpophalangeal joint, surgical; with debridement	6.13	6.28	6.28	0.81	13.22	13.22	090	
29902		A	with reduction of displaced ulnar collateral ligament (eg, Stenar lesion)	6.70	6.60	6.60	0.89	14.19	14.19	090	
29999		C	Unlisted procedure, arthroscopy	0.00	0.00	0.00	0.00	0.00	0.00	YYY	

Surgery

■ RVU not developed by CMS. Gap-filled RVUs developed by Ingenix/CHEG.

Code	M	S	Description	Work Value	Non-Fac PE	Fac PE	Mal-practice	Non-Fac Total	Fac Total	Global	Gap
30000		A	Drainage abscess or hematoma, nasal, internal approach	1.43	2.53	1.51	0.10	4.06	3.04	010	
30020		A	Drainage abscess or hematoma, nasal septum	1.43	2.64	1.57	0.08	4.15	3.08	010	
30100		A	Biopsy, intranasal	0.94	1.34	0.53	0.06	2.34	1.53	000	
30110		A	Excision, nasal polyp(s), simple	1.63	2.80	0.88	0.12	4.55	2.63	010	
30115		A	Excision, nasal polyp(s), extensive	4.35	4.54	4.54	0.31	9.20	9.20	090	
30117		A	Excision or destruction (eg, laser), intranasal lesion; internal approach	3.16	4.95	3.20	0.22	8.33	6.58	090	
30118		A	external approach (lateral rhinotomy)	9.69	8.55	8.55	0.66	18.90	18.90	090	
30120		A	Excision or surgical planing of skin of nose for rhinophyma	5.27	5.71	5.71	0.41	11.39	11.39	090	
30124		A	Excision dermoid cyst, nose; simple, skin, subcutaneous	3.10	3.31	3.31	0.20	6.61	6.61	090	
30125		A	complex, under bone or cartilage	7.16	6.61	6.61	0.54	14.31	14.31	090	
30130		A	Excision turbinate, partial or complete, any method	3.38	3.99	3.99	0.22	7.59	7.59	090	
30140		A	Submucous resection turbinate, partial or complete, any method	3.43	4.61	4.61	0.24	8.28	8.28	090	
30150		A	Rhinectomy; partial	9.14	8.83	8.83	0.76	18.73	18.73	090	
30160		A	total	9.58	8.79	8.79	0.78	19.15	19.15	090	
30200		A	Injection into turbinate(s), therapeutic	0.78	1.23	0.46	0.06	2.07	1.30	000	
30210		A	Displacement therapy (Proetz type)	1.08	2.15	0.61	0.08	3.31	1.77	010	
30220		A	Insertion, nasal septal prosthesis (button)	1.54	2.52	0.84	0.11	4.17	2.49	010	
30300		A	Removal foreign body, intranasal; office type procedure	1.04	2.62	0.37	0.07	3.73	1.48	010	
30310		A	requiring general anesthesia	1.96	1.92	1.92	0.14	4.02	4.02	010	
30320		A	by lateral rhinotomy	4.52	5.26	5.26	0.36	10.14	10.14	090	
30400		R	Rhinoplasty, primary; lateral and alar cartilages and/or elevation of nasal tip	9.83	8.95	8.95	0.80	19.58	19.58	090	
30410		R	complete, external parts including bony pyramid, lateral and alar cartilages, and/or elevation of nasal tip	12.98	10.45	10.45	1.08	24.51	24.51	090	
30420		R	including major septal repair	15.88	12.50	12.50	1.24	29.62	29.62	090	
30430		R	Rhinoplasty, secondary; minor revision (small amount of nasal tip work)	7.21	7.40	7.40	0.62	15.23	15.23	090	

Surgery

■ RVU not developed by CMS. Gap-filled RVUs developed by Ingenix/CHEG.

Code	M	S	Description	Work Value	Non-Fac PE	Fac PE	Mal-practice	Non-Fac Total	Fac Total	Global	Gap
30435		R	intermediate revision (bony work with osteotomies)	11.71	10.68	10.68	1.10	23.49	23.49	090	
30450		R	major revision (nasal tip work and osteotomies)	18.65	14.37	14.37	1.53	34.55	34.55	090	
30460		A	Rhinoplasty for nasal deformity secondary to congenital cleft lip and/or palate, including columellar lengthening; tip only	9.96	9.16	9.16	0.85	19.97	19.97	090	
30462		A	tip, septum, osteotomies	19.57	14.30	14.30	1.92	35.79	35.79	090	
30465		A	Repair of nasal vestibular stenosis (eg, spreader grafting, lateral nasal wall reconstruction)	11.64	9.58	9.58	0.97	22.19	22.19	090	
30520		A	Septoplasty or submucous resection, with or without cartilage scoring, contouring or replacement with graft	5.70	5.93	5.93	0.41	12.04	12.04	090	
30540		A	Repair choanal atresia; intranasal	7.75	6.71	6.71	0.53	14.99	14.99	090	
30545		A	transpalatine	11.38	9.19	9.19	0.80	21.37	21.37	090	
30560		A	Lysis intranasal synechia	1.26	2.37	1.52	0.09	3.72	2.87	010	
30580		A	Repair fistula; oromaxillary (combine with 31030 if antrotomy is included)	6.69	5.00	5.00	0.50	12.19	12.19	090	
30600		A	oronasal	6.02	4.90	4.90	0.70	11.62	11.62	090	
30620		A	Septal or other intranasal dermatoplasty (does not include obtaining graft)	5.97	6.69	6.69	0.45	13.11	13.11	090	
30630		A	Repair nasal septal perforations	7.12	7.23	7.23	0.51	14.86	14.86	090	
30801		A	Cautery and/or ablation, mucosa of turbinates, unilateral or bilateral, any method, (separate procedure); superficial	1.09	2.57	2.31	0.08	3.74	3.48	010	
30802		A	intramural	2.03	3.14	2.87	0.15	5.32	5.05	010	
30901		A	Control nasal hemorrhage, anterior, simple (limited cautery and/or packing) any method	1.21	1.43	0.34	0.09	2.73	1.64	000	
30903		A	Control nasal hemorrhage, anterior, complex (extensive cautery and/or packing) any method	1.54	3.20	0.53	0.12	4.86	2.19	000	
30905		A	Control nasal hemorrhage, posterior, with posterior nasal packs and/or cautery, any method; initial	1.97	3.85	0.80	0.15	5.97	2.92	000	
30906		A	subsequent	2.45	4.27	1.27	0.17	6.89	3.89	000	
30915		A	Ligation arteries; ethmoidal	7.20	7.13	7.13	0.50	14.83	14.83	090	
30920		A	internal maxillary artery, transantral	9.83	8.64	8.64	0.69	19.16	19.16	090	
30930		A	Fracture nasal turbinate(s), therapeutic	1.26	2.17	2.17	0.09	3.52	3.52	010	
30999		C	Unlisted procedure, nose	0.00	0.00	0.00	0.00	0.00	0.00	YYY	

■ RVU not developed by CMS. Gap-filled RVUs developed by Ingenix/CHEG.

Code	M	S	Description	Work Value	Non-Fac PE	Fac PE	Mal-practice	Non-Fac Total	Fac Total	Global	Gap
31000		A	Lavage by cannulation; maxillary sinus (antrum puncture or natural ostium)	1.15	2.43	0.66	0.08	3.66	1.89	010	
31002		A	sphenoid sinus	1.91	2.07	2.07	0.14	4.12	4.12	010	
31020		A	Sinusotomy, maxillary (antrotomy); intranasal	2.94	4.20	3.68	0.20	7.34	6.82	090	
31030		A	radical (Caldwell-Luc) without removal of antrochoanal polyps	5.92	4.85	4.68	0.42	11.19	11.02	090	
31032		A	radical (Caldwell-Luc) with removal of antrochoanal polyps	6.57	6.16	6.16	0.47	13.20	13.20	090	
31040		A	Pterygomaxillary fossa surgery, any approach	9.42	7.34	7.34	0.71	17.47	17.47	090	
31050		A	Sinusotomy, sphenoid, with or without biopsy;	5.28	5.12	5.12	0.39	10.79	10.79	090	
31051		A	with mucosal stripping or removal of polyp(s)	7.11	6.66	6.66	0.55	14.32	14.32	090	
31070		A	Sinusotomy frontal; external, simple (trephine operation)	4.28	5.04	5.04	0.30	9.62	9.62	090	
31075		A	transorbital, unilateral (for mucocele or osteoma, Lynch type)	9.16	8.38	8.38	0.64	18.18	18.18	090	
31080		A	obliterative without osteoplastic flap, brow incision (includes ablation)	11.42	9.13	9.13	0.78	21.33	21.33	090	
31081		A	obliterative, without osteoplastic flap, coronal incision (includes ablation)	12.75	9.97	9.97	1.84	24.56	24.56	090	
31084		A	obliterative, with osteoplastic flap, brow incision	13.51	10.76	10.76	0.96	25.23	25.23	090	
31085		A	obliterative, with osteoplastic flap, coronal incision	14.20	11.12	11.12	1.18	26.50	26.50	090	
31086		A	nonobliterative, with osteoplastic flap, brow incision	12.86	10.50	10.50	0.90	24.26	24.26	090	
31087		A	nonobliterative, with osteoplastic flap, coronal incision	13.10	10.32	10.32	1.15	24.57	24.57	090	
31090		A	Sinusotomy, unilateral, three or more paranasal sinuses (frontal, maxillary, ethmoid, sphenoid)	9.53	9.05	9.05	0.66	19.24	19.24	090	
31200		A	Ethmoidectomy; intranasal, anterior	4.97	5.86	5.86	0.25	11.08	11.08	090	
31201		A	intranasal, total	8.37	7.91	7.91	0.58	16.86	16.86	090	
31205		A	extranasal, total	10.24	8.66	8.66	0.58	19.48	19.48	090	
31225		A	Maxillectomy; without orbital exenteration	19.23	15.42	15.42	1.38	36.03	36.03	090	
31230		A	with orbital exenteration (en bloc)	21.94	17.21	17.21	1.57	40.72	40.72	090	
31231		A	Nasal endoscopy, diagnostic, unilateral or bilateral (separate procedure)	1.10	2.01	0.61	0.08	3.19	1.79	000	

Surgery

■ RVU not developed by CMS. Gap-filled RVUs developed by Ingenix/CHEG.

Code	M	S	Description	Work Value	Non-Fac PE	Fac PE	Mal-prac-tice	Non-Fac Total	Fac Total	Global	Gap
31233		A	Nasal/sinus endoscopy, diagnostic with maxillary sinusoscopy (via inferior meatus or canine fossa puncture)	2.18	2.66	1.24	0.16	5.00	3.58	000	
31235		A	Nasal/sinus endoscopy, diagnostic with sphenoid sinusoscopy (via puncture of sphenoidal face or cannulation of ostium)	2.64	2.93	1.49	0.18	5.75	4.31	000	
31237		A	Nasal/sinus endoscopy, surgical; with biopsy, polypectomy or debridement (separate procedure)	2.98	3.22	1.66	0.21	6.41	4.85	000	
31238		A	with control of nasal hemorrhage	3.26	3.75	1.89	0.23	7.24	5.38	000	
31239		A	with dacryocystorhinostomy	8.70	6.72	6.72	0.46	15.88	15.88	010	
31240		A	with concha bullosa resection	2.61	1.62	1.62	0.18	4.41	4.41	000	
31254		A	Nasal/sinus endoscopy, surgical; with ethmoidectomy, partial (anterior)	4.65	2.79	2.79	0.32	7.76	7.76	000	
31255		A	with ethmoidectomy, total (anterior and posterior)	6.96	4.14	4.14	0.49	11.59	11.59	000	
31256		A	Nasal/sinus endoscopy, surgical, with maxillary antrostomy;	3.29	2.01	2.01	0.23	5.53	5.53	000	
31267		A	with removal of tissue from maxillary sinus	5.46	3.27	3.27	0.38	9.11	9.11	000	
31276		A	Nasal/sinus endoscopy, surgical with frontal sinus exploration, with or without removal of tissue from frontal sinus	8.85	5.24	5.24	0.62	14.71	14.71	000	
31287		A	Nasal/sinus endoscopy, surgical, with sphenoidotomy;	3.92	2.37	2.37	0.27	6.56	6.56	000	
31288		A	with removal of tissue from the sphenoid sinus	4.58	2.75	2.75	0.32	7.65	7.65	000	
31290		A	Nasal/sinus endoscopy, surgical, with repair of cerebrospinal fluid leak; ethmoid region	17.24	11.86	11.86	1.20	30.30	30.30	010	
31291		A	sphenoid region	18.19	12.28	12.28	1.73	32.20	32.20	010	
31292		A	Nasal/sinus endoscopy, surgical; with medial or inferior orbital wall decompression	14.76	10.36	10.36	0.99	26.11	26.11	010	
31293		A	with medial orbital wall and inferior orbital wall decompression	16.21	11.16	11.16	0.97	28.34	28.34	010	
31294		A	with optic nerve decompression	19.06	12.46	12.46	1.04	32.56	32.56	010	
31299		C	Unlisted procedure, accessory sinuses	0.00	0.00	0.00	0.00	0.00	0.00	YYY	
31300		A	Laryngotomy (thyrotomy, laryngofissure); with removal of tumor or laryngocele, cordectomy	14.29	17.46	17.46	0.99	32.74	32.74	090	
31320		A	diagnostic	5.26	12.54	12.54	0.40	18.20	18.20	090	
31360		A	Laryngectomy; total, without radical neck dissection	17.08	19.24	19.24	1.20	37.52	37.52	090	

■ RVU not developed by CMS. Gap-filled RVUs developed by Ingenix/CHEG.

Code	M	S	Description	Work Value	Non-Fac PE	Fac PE	Mal-practice	Non-Fac Total	Fac Total	Global	Gap
31365		A	total, with radical neck dissection	24.16	23.20	23.20	1.72	49.08	49.08	090	
31367		A	subtotal supraglottic, without radical neck dissection	21.86	23.92	23.92	1.57	47.35	47.35	090	
31368		A	subtotal supraglottic, with radical neck dissection	27.09	28.64	28.64	1.90	57.63	57.63	090	
31370		A	Partial laryngectomy (hemilaryngectomy); horizontal	21.38	23.46	23.46	1.51	46.35	46.35	090	
31375		A	laterovertical	20.21	21.16	21.16	1.43	42.80	42.80	090	
31380		A	anterovertical	20.21	21.41	21.41	1.40	43.02	43.02	090	
31382		A	antero-latero-vertical	20.52	23.06	23.06	1.44	45.02	45.02	090	
31390		A	Pharyngolaryngectomy, with radical neck dissection; without reconstruction	27.53	28.90	28.90	1.95	58.38	58.38	090	
31395		A	with reconstruction	31.09	35.02	35.02	2.27	68.38	68.38	090	
31400		A	Arytenoidectomy or arytenoidopexy, external approach	10.31	15.75	15.75	0.72	26.78	26.78	090	
31420		A	Epiglottidectomy	10.22	15.60	15.60	0.71	26.53	26.53	090	
31500		A	Intubation, endotracheal, emergency procedure	2.33	0.69	0.69	0.15	3.17	3.17	000	
31502		A	Tracheotomy tube change prior to establishment of fistula tract	0.65	1.97	0.27	0.04	2.66	0.96	000	
31505		A	Laryngoscopy, indirect; diagnostic (separate procedure)	0.61	1.85	0.35	0.04	2.50	1.00	000	
31510		A	with biopsy	1.92	2.86	1.04	0.15	4.93	3.11	000	
31511		A	with removal of foreign body	2.16	3.15	0.75	0.16	5.47	3.07	000	
31512		A	with removal of lesion	2.07	3.00	1.10	0.16	5.23	3.33	000	
31513		A	with vocal cord injection	2.10	1.32	1.32	0.15	3.57	3.57	000	
31515		A	Laryngoscopy direct, with or without tracheoscopy; for aspiration	1.80	2.30	0.90	0.12	4.22	2.82	000	
31520		A	diagnostic, newborn	2.56	1.41	1.41	0.17	4.14	4.14	000	
31525		A	diagnostic, except newborn	2.63	2.94	1.53	0.18	5.75	4.34	000	
31526		A	diagnostic, with operating microscope	2.57	1.59	1.59	0.18	4.34	4.34	000	
31527		A	with insertion of obturator	3.27	1.77	1.77	0.21	5.25	5.25	000	
31528		A	with dilation, initial	2.37	1.24	1.24	0.16	3.77	3.77	000	
31529		A	with dilation, subsequent	2.68	1.62	1.62	0.18	4.48	4.48	000	
31530		A	Laryngoscopy, direct, operative, with foreign body removal;	3.39	1.89	1.89	0.24	5.52	5.52	000	

■ RVU not developed by CMS. Gap-filled RVUs developed by Ingenix/CHEG.

Code	M	S	Description	Work Value	Non-Fac PE	Fac PE	Mal-practice	Non-Fac Total	Fac Total	Global	Gap
31531		A	with operating microscope	3.59	2.18	2.18	0.25	6.02	6.02	000	
31535		A	Laryngoscopy, direct, operative, with biopsy;	3.16	1.88	1.88	0.22	5.26	5.26	000	
31536		A	with operating microscope	3.56	2.16	2.16	0.25	5.97	5.97	000	
31540		A	Laryngoscopy, direct, operative, with excision of tumor and/or stripping of vocal cords or epiglottis;	4.13	2.48	2.48	0.29	6.90	6.90	000	
31541		A	with operating microscope	4.53	2.72	2.72	0.32	7.57	7.57	000	
31560		A	Laryngoscopy, direct, operative, with arytenoidectomy;	5.46	3.11	3.11	0.38	8.95	8.95	000	
31561		A	with operating microscope	6.00	2.96	2.96	0.42	9.38	9.38	000	
31570		A	Laryngoscopy, direct, with injection into vocal cord(s), therapeutic;	3.87	3.97	2.31	0.24	8.08	6.42	000	
31571		A	with operating microscope	4.27	2.46	2.46	0.30	7.03	7.03	000	
31575		A	Laryngoscopy, flexible fiberoptic; diagnostic	1.10	2.08	0.59	0.08	3.26	1.77	000	
31576		A	with biopsy	1.97	2.26	1.08	0.13	4.36	3.18	000	
31577		A	with removal of foreign body	2.47	2.90	1.31	0.17	5.54	3.95	000	
31578		A	with removal of lesion	2.84	3.13	1.62	0.20	6.17	4.66	000	
31579		A	Laryngoscopy, flexible or rigid fiberoptic, with stroboscopy	2.26	2.97	1.27	0.16	5.39	3.69	000	
31580		A	Laryngoplasty; for laryngeal web, two stage, with keel insertion and removal	12.38	16.85	16.85	0.87	30.10	30.10	090	
31582		A	for laryngeal stenosis, with graft or core mold, including tracheotomy	21.62	22.06	22.06	1.52	45.20	45.20	090	
31584		A	with open reduction of fracture	19.64	19.05	19.05	1.42	40.11	40.11	090	
31585		A	Treatment of closed laryngeal fracture; without manipulation	4.64	8.92	8.92	0.30	13.86	13.86	090	
31586		A	with closed manipulative reduction	8.03	12.71	12.71	0.56	21.30	21.30	090	
31587		A	Laryngoplasty, cricoid split	11.99	14.77	14.77	0.88	27.64	27.64	090	
31588		A	Laryngoplasty, not otherwise specified (eg, for burns, reconstruction after partial laryngectomy)	13.11	17.21	17.21	0.92	31.24	31.24	090	
31590		A	Laryngeal reinnervation by neuromuscular pedicle	6.97	12.63	12.63	0.50	20.10	20.10	090	
31595		A	Section recurrent laryngeal nerve, therapeutic (separate procedure), unilateral	8.34	11.90	11.90	0.62	20.86	20.86	090	
31599		C	Unlisted procedure, larynx	0.00	0.00	0.00	0.00	0.00	0.00	YYY	
31600		A	Tracheostomy, planned (separate procedure);	7.18	3.15	3.15	0.34	10.67	10.67	000	

■ RVU not developed by CMS. Gap-filled RVUs developed by Ingenix/CHEG.

Surgery

Code	M	S	Description	Work Value	Non-Fac PE	Fac PE	Mal-practice	Non-Fac Total	Fac Total	Global	Gap
31601		A	under two years	4.45	2.20	2.20	0.39	7.04	7.04	000	
31603		A	Tracheostomy, emergency procedure; transtracheal	4.15	1.88	1.88	0.35	6.38	6.38	000	
31605		A	cricothyroid membrane	3.58	1.24	1.24	0.33	5.15	5.15	000	
31610		A	Tracheostomy, fenestration procedure with skin flaps	8.76	10.98	10.98	0.69	20.43	20.43	090	
31611		A	Construction of tracheoesophageal fistula and subsequent insertion of an alaryngeal speech prosthesis (eg, voice button, Blom-Singer prosthesis)	5.64	10.28	10.28	0.40	16.32	16.32	090	
31612		A	Tracheal puncture, percutaneous with transtracheal aspiration and/or injection	0.91	1.53	0.48	0.06	2.50	1.45	000	
31613		A	Tracheostoma revision; simple, without flap rotation	4.59	8.94	8.94	0.37	13.90	13.90	090	
31614		A	complex, with flap rotation	7.12	12.47	12.47	0.51	20.10	20.10	090	
31615		A	Tracheobronchoscopy through established tracheostomy incision	2.09	3.76	1.20	0.14	5.99	3.43	000	
31622		A	Bronchoscopy (rigid or flexible); diagnostic, with or without cell washing (separate procedure)	2.78	3.69	1.20	0.14	6.61	4.12	000	
31623		A	with brushing or protected brushings	2.88	2.97	1.17	0.14	5.99	4.19	000	
31624		A	with bronchial alveolar lavage	2.88	2.75	1.17	0.13	5.76	4.18	000	
31625		A	with biopsy	3.37	2.96	1.34	0.16	6.49	4.87	000	
31628		A	with transbronchial lung biopsy, with or without fluoroscopic guidance	3.81	3.38	1.45	0.14	7.33	5.40	000	
31629		A	with transbronchial needle aspiration biopsy	3.37	1.32	1.32	0.13	4.82	4.82	000	
31630		A	with tracheal or bronchial dilation or closed reduction of fracture	3.82	1.99	1.99	0.30	6.11	6.11	000	
31631		A	with tracheal dilation and placement of tracheal stent	4.37	2.04	2.04	0.31	6.72	6.72	000	
31635		A	with removal of foreign body	3.68	1.70	1.70	0.21	5.59	5.59	000	
31640		A	with excision of tumor	4.94	2.36	2.36	0.37	7.67	7.67	000	
31641		A	Bronchoscopy, (rigid or flexible); with destruction of tumor or relief of stenosis by any method other than excision (eg, laser therapy, cryotherapy)	5.03	2.20	2.20	0.30	7.53	7.53	000	
31643		A	with placement of catheter(s) for intracavitary radioelement application	3.50	1.17	1.17	0.15	4.82	4.82	000	

Surgery

■ RVU not developed by CMS. Gap-filled RVUs developed by Ingenix/CHEG.

Code	M	S	Description	Work Value	Non-Fac PE	Fac PE	Mal-practice	Non-Fac Total	Fac Total	Global	Gap
31645		A	with therapeutic aspiration of tracheobronchial tree, initial (eg, drainage of lung abscess)	3.16	1.27	1.27	0.13	4.56	4.56	000	
31646		A	with therapeutic aspiration of tracheobronchial tree, subsequent	2.72	1.12	1.12	0.12	3.96	3.96	000	
31656		A	with injection of contrast material for segmental bronchography (fiberscope only)	2.17	1.05	1.05	0.10	3.32	3.32	000	
31700		A	Catheterization, transglottic (separate procedure)	1.34	3.44	0.68	0.07	4.85	2.09	000	
31708		A	Instillation of contrast material for laryngography or bronchography, without catheterization	1.41	0.64	0.64	0.06	2.11	2.11	000	
31710		A	Catheterization for bronchography, with or without instillation of contrast material	1.30	0.75	0.75	0.06	2.11	2.11	000	
31715		A	Transtracheal injection for bronchography	1.11	0.73	0.73	0.06	1.90	1.90	000	
31717		A	Catheterization with bronchial brush biopsy	2.12	3.25	0.89	0.09	5.46	3.10	000	
31720		A	Catheter aspiration (separate procedure); nasotracheal	1.06	1.90	0.35	0.06	3.02	1.47	000	
31725		A	tracheobronchial with fiberscope, bedside	1.96	0.61	0.61	0.10	2.67	2.67	000	
31730		A	Transtracheal (percutaneous) introduction of needle wire dilator/stent or indwelling tube for oxygen therapy	2.85	2.54	1.13	0.15	5.54	4.13	000	
31750		A	Tracheoplasty; cervical	13.02	16.22	16.22	1.02	30.26	30.26	090	
31755		A	tracheopharyngeal fistulization, each stage	15.93	19.27	19.27	1.15	36.35	36.35	090	
31760		A	intrathoracic	22.35	12.79	12.79	1.48	36.62	36.62	090	
31766		A	Carinal reconstruction	30.43	15.03	15.03	3.16	48.62	48.62	090	
31770		A	Bronchoplasty; graft repair	22.51	15.67	15.67	2.27	40.45	40.45	090	
31775		A	excision stenosis and anastomosis	23.54	15.14	15.14	2.91	41.59	41.59	090	
31780		A	Excision tracheal stenosis and anastomosis; cervical	17.72	12.97	12.97	1.55	32.24	32.24	090	
31781		A	cervicothoracic	23.53	15.49	15.49	2.04	41.06	41.06	090	
31785		A	Excision of tracheal tumor or carcinoma; cervical	17.23	13.05	13.05	1.36	31.64	31.64	090	
31786		A	thoracic	23.98	14.41	14.41	2.20	40.59	40.59	090	
31800		A	Suture of tracheal wound or injury; cervical	7.43	6.81	6.81	0.67	14.91	14.91	090	
31805		A	intrathoracic	13.13	10.72	10.72	1.45	25.30	25.30	090	

■ RVU not developed by CMS. Gap-filled RVUs developed by Ingenix/CHEG.

Code	M	S	Description	Work Value	Non-Fac PE	Fac PE	Mal-prac-tice	Non-Fac Total	Fac Total	Global	Gap
31820		A	Surgical closure tracheostomy or fistula; without plastic repair	4.49	8.24	8.07	0.35	13.08	12.91	090	
31825		A	with plastic repair	6.81	10.86	10.86	0.50	18.17	18.17	090	
31830		A	Revision of tracheostomy scar	4.50	7.82	7.82	0.36	12.68	12.68	090	
31899		C	Unlisted procedure, trachea, bronchi	0.00	0.00	0.00	0.00	0.00	0.00	YYY	
32000		A	Thoracentesis, puncture of pleural cavity for aspiration, initial or subsequent	1.54	3.10	0.51	0.07	4.71	2.12	000	
32002		A	Thoracentesis with insertion of tube with or without water seal (eg, for pneumothorax) (separate procedure)	2.19	0.87	0.87	0.11	3.17	3.17	000	
32005		A	Chemical pleurodesis (eg, for recurrent or persistent pneumothorax)	2.19	0.88	0.88	0.17	3.24	3.24	000	
32020		A	Tube thoracostomy with or without water seal (eg, for abscess, hemothorax, empyema) (separate procedure)	3.98	1.48	1.48	0.36	5.82	5.82	000	
32035		A	Thoracostomy; with rib resection for empyema	8.67	7.83	7.83	1.02	17.52	17.52	090	
32036		A	with open flap drainage for empyema	9.68	8.39	8.39	1.20	19.27	19.27	090	
32095		A	Thoracotomy, limited, for biopsy of lung or pleura	8.36	8.05	8.05	0.99	17.40	17.40	090	
32100		A	Thoracotomy, major; with exploration and biopsy	15.24	10.30	10.30	1.45	26.99	26.99	090	
32110		A	with control of traumatic hemorrhage and/or repair of lung tear	23.00	12.72	12.72	1.63	37.35	37.35	090	
32120		A	for postoperative complications	11.54	9.34	9.34	1.42	22.30	22.30	090	
32124		A	with open intrapleural pneumonolysis	12.72	9.53	9.53	1.51	23.76	23.76	090	
32140		A	with cyst(s) removal, with or without a pleural procedure	13.93	9.79	9.79	1.68	25.40	25.40	090	
32141		A	with excision-plication of bullae, with or without any pleural procedure	14.00	9.98	9.98	1.72	25.70	25.70	090	
32150		A	with removal of intrapleural foreign body or fibrin deposit	14.15	9.70	9.70	1.60	25.45	25.45	090	
32151		A	with removal of intrapulmonary foreign body	14.21	10.20	10.20	1.49	25.90	25.90	090	
32160		A	with cardiac massage	9.30	6.34	6.34	1.01	16.65	16.65	090	
32200		A	Pneumonostomy; with open drainage of abscess or cyst	15.29	10.08	10.08	1.46	26.83	26.83	090	
32201		A	with percutaneous drainage of abscess or cyst	4.00	5.67	5.67	0.18	9.85	9.85	000	
32215		A	Pleural scarification for repeat pneumothorax	11.33	9.16	9.16	1.34	21.83	21.83	090	

■ RVU not developed by CMS. Gap-filled RVUs developed by Ingenix/CHEG.

Code	M	S	Description	Work Value	Non-Fac PE	Fac PE	Mal-practice	Non-Fac Total	Fac Total	Global	Gap
32220		A	Decortication, pulmonary, (separate procedure); total	24.00	13.56	13.56	2.39	39.95	39.95	090	
32225		A	Decortication, pulmonary (separate procedure); partial	13.96	9.95	9.95	1.70	25.61	25.61	090	
32310		A	Pleurectomy, parietal (separate procedure)	13.44	9.86	9.86	1.65	24.95	24.95	090	
32320		A	Decortication and parietal pleurectomy	24.00	13.21	13.21	2.50	39.71	39.71	090	
32400		A	Biopsy, pleura; percutaneous needle	1.76	1.89	0.59	0.07	3.72	2.42	000	
32402		A	open	7.56	7.76	7.76	0.91	16.23	16.23	090	
32405		A	Biopsy, lung or mediastinum, percutaneous needle	1.93	2.33	0.67	0.09	4.35	2.69	000	
32420		A	Pneumocentesis, puncture of lung for aspiration	2.18	0.88	0.88	0.11	3.17	3.17	000	
32440		A	Removal of lung, total pneumonectomy;	25.00	13.57	13.57	2.56	41.13	41.13	090	
32442		A	Removal of lung, total pneumonectomy; with resection of segment of trachea followed by broncho-tracheal anastomosis (sleeve pneumonectomy)	26.24	14.35	14.35	3.12	43.71	43.71	090	
32445		A	Removal of lung, total pneumonectomy; extrapleural	25.09	13.83	13.83	3.11	42.03	42.03	090	
32480		A	Removal of lung, other than total pneumonectomy; single lobe (lobectomy)	23.75	12.78	12.78	2.24	38.77	38.77	090	
32482		A	two lobes (bilobectomy)	25.00	13.39	13.39	2.35	40.74	40.74	090	
32484		A	single segment (segmentectomy)	20.69	11.97	11.97	2.54	35.20	35.20	090	
32486		A	with circumferential resection of segment of bronchus followed by broncho-bronchial anastomosis (sleeve lobectomy)	23.92	13.32	13.32	3.00	40.24	40.24	090	
32488		A	all remaining lung following previous removal of a portion of lung (completion pneumonectomy)	25.71	13.89	13.89	3.18	42.78	42.78	090	
32491		R	excision-plication of emphysematous lung(s) (bullous or non-bullous) for lung volume reduction, sternal split or transthoracic approach, with or without any pleural procedure	21.25	12.67	12.67	2.66	36.58	36.58	090	
32500		A	wedge resection, single or multiple	22.00	12.70	12.70	1.77	36.47	36.47	090	
32501		A	Resection and repair of portion of bronchus (bronchoplasty) when performed at time of lobectomy or segmentectomy (List separately in addition to code for primary procedure)	4.69	1.59	1.59	0.56	6.84	6.84	ZZZ	
32520		A	Resection of lung; with resection of chest wall	21.68	12.56	12.56	2.71	36.95	36.95	090	
32522		A	with reconstruction of chest wall, without prosthesis	24.20	13.63	13.63	2.84	40.67	40.67	090	

■ RVU not developed by CMS. Gap-filled RVUs developed by Ingenix/CHEG.

Code	M	S	Description	Work Value	Non-Fac PE	Fac PE	Mal-practice	Non-Fac Total	Fac Total	Global	Gap
32525		A	with major reconstruction of chest wall, with prosthesis	26.50	14.22	14.22	3.25	43.97	43.97	090	
32540		A	Extrapleural enucleation of empyema (empyemectomy)	14.64	9.99	9.99	1.84	26.47	26.47	090	
32601		A	Thoracoscopy, diagnostic (separate procedure); lungs and pleural space, without biopsy	5.46	3.60	3.60	0.63	9.69	9.69	000	
32602		A	lungs and pleural space, with biopsy	5.96	3.72	3.72	0.70	10.38	10.38	000	
32603		A	pericardial sac, without biopsy	7.81	4.33	4.33	0.76	12.90	12.90	000	
32604		A	pericardial sac, with biopsy	8.78	4.79	4.79	0.97	14.54	14.54	000	
32605		A	mediastinal space, without biopsy	6.93	4.19	4.19	0.86	11.98	11.98	000	
32606		A	mediastinal space, with biopsy	8.40	4.55	4.55	0.99	13.94	13.94	000	
32650		A	Thoracoscopy, surgical; with pleurodesis (eg, mechanical or chemical)	10.75	8.47	8.47	1.25	20.47	20.47	090	
32651		A	with partial pulmonary decortication	12.91	8.84	8.84	1.50	23.25	23.25	090	
32652		A	with total pulmonary decortication, including intrapleural pneumonolysis	18.66	11.16	11.16	2.30	32.12	32.12	090	
32653		A	with removal of intrapleural foreign body or fibrin deposit	12.87	9.15	9.15	1.55	23.57	23.57	090	
32654		A	with control of traumatic hemorrhage	12.44	7.53	7.53	1.51	21.48	21.48	090	
32655		A	with excision-plication of bullae, including any pleural procedure	13.10	8.86	8.86	1.53	23.49	23.49	090	
32656		A	with parietal pleurectomy	12.91	9.53	9.53	1.61	24.05	24.05	090	
32657		A	with wedge resection of lung, single or multiple	13.65	9.36	9.36	1.64	24.65	24.65	090	
32658		A	with removal of clot or foreign body from pericardial sac	11.63	9.05	9.05	1.47	22.15	22.15	090	
32659		A	with creation of pericardial window or partial resection of pericardial sac for drainage	11.59	9.10	9.10	1.39	22.08	22.08	090	
32660		A	with total pericardiectomy	17.43	10.53	10.53	2.09	30.05	30.05	090	
32661		A	with excision of pericardial cyst, tumor, or mass	13.25	9.15	9.15	1.66	24.06	24.06	090	
32662		A	with excision of mediastinal cyst, tumor, or mass	16.44	10.59	10.59	2.01	29.04	29.04	090	
32663		A	with lobectomy, total or segmental	18.47	11.22	11.22	2.28	31.97	31.97	090	
32664		A	with thoracic sympathectomy	14.20	9.43	9.43	1.70	25.33	25.33	090	
32665		A	with esophagomyotomy (Heller type)	15.54	9.18	9.18	1.79	26.51	26.51	090	
32800		A	Repair lung hernia through chest wall	13.69	10.05	10.05	1.51	25.25	25.25	090	

■ RVU not developed by CMS. Gap-filled RVUs developed by Ingenix/CHEG.

Surgery

Code	M	S	Description	Work Value	Non-Fac PE	Fac PE	Mal-practice	Non-Fac Total	Fac Total	Global	Gap
32810		A	Closure of chest wall following open flap drainage for empyema (Clagett type procedure)	13.05	10.05	10.05	1.55	24.65	24.65	090	
32815		A	Open closure of major bronchial fistula	23.15	13.32	13.32	2.84	39.31	39.31	090	
32820		A	Major reconstruction, chest wall (post-traumatic)	21.48	13.99	13.99	2.31	37.78	37.78	090	
32850		X	Donor pneumonectomy(ies) with preparation and maintenance of allograft (cadaver)	0.00	0.00	0.00	0.00	0.00	0.00	XXX	
32851		A	Lung transplant, single; without cardiopulmonary bypass	38.63	19.94	19.94	4.90	63.47	63.47	090	
32852		A	with cardiopulmonary bypass	41.80	21.40	21.40	5.17	68.37	68.37	090	
32853		A	Lung transplant, double (bilateral sequential or en bloc); without cardiopulmonary bypass	47.81	23.49	23.49	6.13	77.43	77.43	090	
32854		A	with cardiopulmonary bypass	50.98	24.35	24.35	6.41	81.74	81.74	090	
32900		A	Resection of ribs, extrapleural, all stages	20.27	12.27	12.27	2.42	34.96	34.96	090	
32905		A	Thoracoplasty, Schede type or extrapleural (all stages);	20.75	12.77	12.77	2.54	36.06	36.06	090	
32906		A	with closure of bronchopleural fistula	26.77	14.12	14.12	3.30	44.19	44.19	090	
32940		A	Pneumonolysis, extraperiosteal, including filling or packing procedures	19.43	11.96	11.96	2.47	33.86	33.86	090	
32960		A	Pneumothorax, therapeutic, intrapleural injection of air	1.84	2.16	0.70	0.12	4.12	2.66	000	
32997		A	Total lung lavage (unilateral)	6.00	2.00	2.00	0.55	8.55	8.55	000	
32999		C	Unlisted procedure, lungs and pleura	0.00	0.00	0.00	0.00	0.00	0.00	YYY	
33010		A	Pericardiocentesis; initial	2.24	1.01	1.01	0.13	3.38	3.38	000	
33011		A	subsequent	2.24	1.05	1.05	0.13	3.42	3.42	000	
33015		A	Tube pericardiostomy	6.80	4.41	4.41	0.64	11.85	11.85	090	
33020		A	Pericardiotomy for removal of clot or foreign body (primary procedure)	12.61	7.91	7.91	1.50	22.02	22.02	090	
33025		A	Creation of pericardial window or partial resection for drainage	12.09	7.77	7.77	1.50	21.36	21.36	090	
33030		A	Pericardiectomy, subtotal or complete; without cardiopulmonary bypass	18.71	12.12	12.12	2.40	33.23	33.23	090	
33031		A	with cardiopulmonary bypass	21.79	13.20	13.20	2.78	37.77	37.77	090	
33050		A	Excision of pericardial cyst or tumor	14.36	10.24	10.24	1.73	26.33	26.33	090	
33120		A	Excision of intracardiac tumor, resection with cardiopulmonary bypass	24.56	15.68	15.68	3.06	43.30	43.30	090	
33130		A	Resection of external cardiac tumor	21.39	12.40	12.40	2.51	36.30	36.30	090	

■ RVU not developed by CMS. Gap-filled RVUs developed by Ingenix/CHEG.

Code	M	S	Description	Work Value	Non-Fac PE	Fac PE	Mal-practice	Non-Fac Total	Fac Total	Global	Gap
33140		A	Transmyocardial laser revascularization, by thoracotomy (separate procedure)	20.00	10.57	10.57	2.27	32.84	32.84	090	
33141		A	performed at the time of other open cardiac procedure(s) (List separately in addition to code for primary procedure)	4.84	1.63	1.63	0.55	7.02	7.02	ZZZ	
33200		A	Insertion of permanent pacemaker with epicardial electrode(s); by thoracotomy	12.48	9.59	9.59	1.17	23.24	23.24	090	
33201		A	by xiphoid approach	10.18	9.39	9.39	1.21	20.78	20.78	090	
33206		A	Insertion or replacement of permanent pacemaker with transvenous electrode(s); atrial	6.67	5.35	5.35	0.50	12.52	12.52	090	
33207		A	ventricular	8.04	6.00	6.00	0.57	14.61	14.61	090	
33208		A	atrial and ventricular	8.13	6.14	6.14	0.54	14.81	14.81	090	
33210		A	Insertion or replacement of temporary transvenous single chamber cardiac electrode transvenous single chamber cardiac electrode or pacemaker catheter (separate procedure)	3.30	1.34	1.34	0.17	4.81	4.81	000	
33211		A	Insertion or replacement of temporary transvenous dual chamber pacing electrodes (separate procedure)	3.40	1.41	1.41	0.17	4.98	4.98	000	
33212		A	Insertion or replacement of pacemaker pulse generator only; single chamber, atrial or ventricular	5.52	4.44	4.44	0.44	10.40	10.40	090	
33213		A	dual chamber	6.37	4.85	4.85	0.46	11.68	11.68	090	
33214		A	Upgrade of implanted pacemaker system, conversion of single chamber system to dual chamber system (includes removal of previously placed pulse generator, testing of existing lead, insertion of new lead, insertion of new pulse generator)	7.75	5.95	5.95	0.52	14.22	14.22	090	
33216		A	Insertion or repositioning of a transvenous electrode (15 days or more after initial insertion); single chamber (one electrode) permanent pacemaker or single chamber pacing cardioverter-defibrillator	5.39	4.95	4.95	0.36	10.70	10.70	090	
33217		A	dual chamber (two electrodes) permanent pacemaker or dual chamber pacing cardioverter-defibrillator	5.75	5.26	5.26	0.36	11.37	11.37	090	
33218		A	Repair of single transvenous electrode for a single chamber, permanent pacemaker or single chamber pacing cardioverter-defibrillator	5.44	4.51	4.51	0.40	10.35	10.35	090	
33220		A	Repair of two transvenous electrodes for a dual chamber permanent pacemaker or dual chamber pacing cardioverter-defibrillator	5.52	4.45	4.45	0.39	10.36	10.36	090	
33222		A	Revision or relocation of skin pocket for pacemaker	4.96	3.93	3.93	0.39	9.28	9.28	090	

Surgery

■ RVU not developed by CMS. Gap-filled RVUs developed by Ingenix/CHEG.

Code	M	S	Description	Work Value	Non-Fac PE	Fac PE	Mal-practice	Non-Fac Total	Fac Total	Global	Gap
33223		A	Revision of skin pocket for single or dual chamber pacing cardioverter-defibrillator	6.46	5.06	5.06	0.44	11.96	11.96	090	
33233		A	Removal of permanent pacemaker pulse generator	3.29	3.80	3.80	0.22	7.31	7.31	090	
33234		A	Removal of transvenous pacemaker electrode(s); single lead system, atrial or ventricular	7.82	5.03	5.03	0.56	13.41	13.41	090	
33235		A	dual lead system	9.40	6.26	6.26	0.68	16.34	16.34	090	
33236		A	Removal of permanent epicardial pacemaker and electrodes by thoracotomy; single lead system, atrial or ventricular	12.60	9.35	9.35	1.49	23.44	23.44	090	
33237		A	dual lead system	13.71	9.51	9.51	1.57	24.79	24.79	090	
33238		A	Removal of permanent transvenous electrode(s) by thoracotomy	15.22	9.24	9.24	1.56	26.02	26.02	090	
33240		A	Insertion of single or dual chamber pacing cardioverter-defibrillator pulse generator	7.60	5.49	5.49	0.53	13.62	13.62	090	
33241		A	Subcutaneous removal of single or dual chamber pacing cardioverter-defibrillator pulse generator	3.24	3.39	3.39	0.21	6.84	6.84	090	
33243		A	Removal of single or dual chamber pacing cardioverter-defibrillator electrode(s); by thoracotomy	22.64	10.88	10.88	2.53	36.05	36.05	090	
33244		A	by transvenous extraction	13.76	8.22	8.22	1.05	23.03	23.03	090	
33245		A	Insertion of epicardial single or dual chamber pacing cardioverter-defibrillator electrodes by thoracotomy;	14.30	10.79	10.79	1.28	26.37	26.37	090	
33246		A	with insertion of pulse generator	20.71	14.16	14.16	2.22	37.09	37.09	090	
33249		A	Insertion or repositioning of electrode lead(s) for single or dual chamber pacing cardioverter-defibrillator and insertion of pulse generator	14.23	8.98	8.98	0.80	24.01	24.01	090	
33250		A	Operative ablation of supraventricular arrhythmogenic focus or pathway (eg, Wolff-Parkinson-White, atrioventricular node re-entry), tract(s) and/or focus (foci); without cardiopulmonary bypass	21.85	13.65	13.65	1.01	36.51	36.51	090	
33251		A	with cardiopulmonary bypass	24.88	14.06	14.06	2.41	41.35	41.35	090	
33253		A	Operative incisions and reconstruction of atria for treatment of atrial fibrillation or atrial flutter (eg, maze procedure)	31.06	16.58	16.58	3.68	51.32	51.32	090	
33261		A	Operative ablation of ventricular arrhythmogenic focus with cardiopulmonary bypass	24.88	14.47	14.47	2.82	42.17	42.17	090	
33282		A	Implantation of patient-activated cardiac event recorder	4.17	4.42	4.42	0.39	8.98	8.98	090	

■ RVU not developed by CMS. Gap-filled RVUs developed by Ingenix/CHEG.

Code	M	S	Description	Work Value	Non-Fac PE	Fac PE	Mal-practice	Non-Fac Total	Fac Total	Global	Gap
33284		A	Removal of an implantable, patient-activated cardiac event recorder	2.50	3.94	3.94	0.23	6.67	6.67	090	
33300		A	Repair of cardiac wound; without bypass	17.92	11.56	11.56	1.91	31.39	31.39	090	
33305		A	with cardiopulmonary bypass	21.44	13.24	13.24	2.68	37.36	37.36	090	
33310		A	Cardiotomy, exploratory (includes removal of foreign body); without bypass	18.51	11.85	11.85	2.26	32.62	32.62	090	
33315		A	with cardiopulmonary bypass	22.37	13.43	13.43	2.90	38.70	38.70	090	
33320		A	Suture repair of aorta or great vessels; without shunt or cardiopulmonary bypass	16.79	11.06	11.06	1.66	29.51	29.51	090	
33321		A	with shunt bypass	20.20	13.15	13.15	2.70	36.05	36.05	090	
33322		A	with cardiopulmonary bypass	20.62	13.02	13.02	2.51	36.15	36.15	090	
33330		A	Insertion of graft, aorta or great vessels; without shunt, or cardiopulmonary bypass	21.43	12.35	12.35	2.49	36.27	36.27	090	
33332		A	with shunt bypass	23.96	12.94	12.94	2.45	39.35	39.35	090	
33335		A	with cardiopulmonary bypass	30.01	16.15	16.15	3.79	49.95	49.95	090	
33400		A	Valvuloplasty, aortic valve; open, with cardiopulmonary bypass	28.50	17.04	17.04	3.09	48.63	48.63	090	
33401		A	open, with inflow occlusion	23.91	14.85	14.85	2.71	41.47	41.47	090	
33403		A	using transventricular dilation, with cardiopulmonary bypass	24.89	15.99	15.99	2.48	43.36	43.36	090	
33404		A	Construction of apical-aortic conduit	28.54	17.22	17.22	3.31	49.07	49.07	090	
33405		A	Replacement, aortic valve, with cardiopulmonary bypass; with prosthetic valve other than homograft or stentless valve	35.00	17.69	17.69	3.86	56.55	56.55	090	
33406		A	with allograft valve (freehand)	37.50	18.53	18.53	4.07	60.10	60.10	090	
33410		A	with stentless tissue valve	32.46	16.93	16.93	4.11	53.50	53.50	090	
33411		A	Replacement, aortic valve; with aortic annulus enlargement, noncoronary cusp	36.25	18.07	18.07	4.16	58.48	58.48	090	
33412		A	with transventricular aortic annulus enlargement (Konno procedure)	42.00	21.90	21.90	4.66	68.56	68.56	090	
33413		A	by translocation of autologous pulmonary valve with allograft replacement of pulmonary valve (Ross procedure)	43.50	23.05	23.05	4.26	70.81	70.81	090	
33414		A	Repair of left ventricular outflow tract obstruction by patch enlargement of the outflow tract	30.35	17.67	17.67	3.79	51.81	51.81	090	
33415		A	Resection or incision of subvalvular tissue for discrete subvalvular aortic stenosis	27.15	16.53	16.53	3.25	46.93	46.93	090	

■ RVU not developed by CMS. Gap-filled RVUs developed by Ingenix/CHEG.

Code	M	S	Description	Work Value	Non-Fac PE	Fac PE	Mal-practice	Non-Fac Total	Fac Total	Global	Gap
33416		A	Ventriculomyotomy (-myectomy) for idiopathic hypertrophic subaortic stenosis (eg, asymmetric septal hypertrophy)	30.35	16.06	16.06	3.85	50.26	50.26	090	
33417		A	Aortoplasty (gusset) for supravalvular stenosis	28.53	17.09	17.09	3.58	49.20	49.20	090	
33420		A	Valvotomy, mitral valve; closed heart	22.70	11.77	11.77	1.48	35.95	35.95	090	
33422		A	open heart, with cardiopulmonary bypass	25.94	14.74	14.74	3.30	43.98	43.98	090	
33425		A	Valvuloplasty, mitral valve, with cardiopulmonary bypass;	27.00	14.98	14.98	3.00	44.98	44.98	090	
33426		A	with prosthetic ring	33.00	17.14	17.14	3.87	54.01	54.01	090	
33427		A	radical reconstruction, with or without ring	40.00	19.42	19.42	4.30	63.72	63.72	090	
33430		A	Replacement, mitral valve, with cardiopulmonary bypass	33.50	17.26	17.26	3.95	54.71	54.71	090	
33460		A	Valvectomy, tricuspid valve, with cardiopulmonary bypass	23.60	13.83	13.83	3.02	40.45	40.45	090	
33463		A	Valvuloplasty, tricuspid valve; without ring insertion	25.62	14.60	14.60	3.17	43.39	43.39	090	
33464		A	with ring insertion	27.33	15.22	15.22	3.47	46.02	46.02	090	
33465		A	Replacement, tricuspid valve, with cardiopulmonary bypass	28.79	15.67	15.67	3.61	48.07	48.07	090	
33468		A	Tricuspid valve repositioning and plication for Ebstein anomaly	30.12	19.06	19.06	4.00	53.18	53.18	090	
33470		A	Valvotomy, pulmonary valve, closed heart; transventricular	20.81	14.20	14.20	2.81	37.82	37.82	090	
33471		A	via pulmonary artery	22.25	13.13	13.13	3.00	38.38	38.38	090	
33472		A	Valvotomy, pulmonary valve, open heart; with inflow occlusion	22.25	13.13	13.13	2.92	38.30	38.30	090	
33474		A	with cardiopulmonary bypass	23.04	13.45	13.45	2.84	39.33	39.33	090	
33475		A	Replacement, pulmonary valve	33.00	18.28	18.28	2.64	53.92	53.92	090	
33476		A	Right ventricular resection for infundibular stenosis, with or without commissurotomy	25.77	14.23	14.23	2.40	42.40	42.40	090	
33478		A	Outflow tract augmentation (gusset), with or without commissurotomy or infundibular resection	26.74	14.43	14.43	3.56	44.73	44.73	090	
33496		A	Repair of non-structural prosthetic valve dysfunction with cardiopulmonary bypass (separate procedure)	27.25	16.84	16.84	3.44	47.53	47.53	090	
33500		A	Repair of coronary arteriovenous or arteriocardiac chamber fistula; with cardiopulmonary bypass	25.55	13.99	13.99	2.80	42.34	42.34	090	

■ RVU not developed by CMS. Gap-filled RVUs developed by Ingenix/CHEG.

Code	M	S	Description	Work Value	Non-Fac PE	Fac PE	Mal-practice	Non-Fac Total	Fac Total	Global	Gap
33501		A	without cardiopulmonary bypass	17.78	10.24	10.24	2.05	30.07	30.07	090	
33502		A	Repair of anomalous coronary artery; by ligation	21.04	16.64	16.64	2.51	40.19	40.19	090	
33503		A	by graft, without cardiopulmonary bypass	21.78	13.90	13.90	1.42	37.10	37.10	090	
33504		A	by graft, with cardiopulmonary bypass	24.66	16.55	16.55	3.04	44.25	44.25	090	
33505		A	with construction of intrapulmonary artery tunnel (Takeuchi procedure)	26.84	18.16	18.16	1.52	46.52	46.52	090	
33506		A	by translocation from pulmonary artery to aorta	35.50	19.27	19.27	3.19	57.96	57.96	090	
33510		A	Coronary artery bypass, vein only; single coronary venous graft	29.00	15.53	15.53	3.13	47.66	47.66	090	
33511		A	two coronary venous grafts	30.00	16.05	16.05	3.34	49.39	49.39	090	
33512		A	three coronary venous grafts	31.80	16.65	16.65	3.70	52.15	52.15	090	
33513		A	four coronary venous grafts	32.00	16.77	16.77	3.99	52.76	52.76	090	
33514		A	five coronary venous grafts	32.75	17.00	17.00	4.37	54.12	54.12	090	
33516		A	six or more coronary venous grafts	35.00	17.74	17.74	4.62	57.36	57.36	090	
33517		A	Coronary artery bypass, using venous graft(s) and arterial graft(s); single vein graft (list separately in addition to code for arterial graft)	2.57	0.86	0.86	0.32	3.75	3.75	ZZZ	
33518		A	two venous grafts (list separately in addition to code for arterial graft)	4.85	1.62	1.62	0.61	7.08	7.08	ZZZ	
33519		A	three venous grafts (list separately in addition to code for arterial graft)	7.12	2.38	2.38	0.89	10.39	10.39	ZZZ	
33521		A	four venous grafts (list separately in addition to code for arterial graft)	9.40	3.15	3.15	1.18	13.73	13.73	ZZZ	
33522		A	five venous grafts (list separately in addition to code for arterial graft)	11.67	3.91	3.91	1.48	17.06	17.06	ZZZ	
33523		A	six or more venous grafts (list separately in addition to code for arterial graft)	13.95	4.63	4.63	1.78	20.36	20.36	ZZZ	
33530		A	Reoperation, coronary artery bypass procedure or valve procedure, more than one month after original operation (list separately in addition to code for primary procedure)	5.86	1.96	1.96	0.73	8.55	8.55	ZZZ	
33533		A	Coronary artery bypass, using arterial graft(s); single arterial graft	30.00	17.24	17.24	3.24	50.48	50.48	090	
33534		A	two coronary arterial grafts	32.20	17.45	17.45	3.63	53.28	53.28	090	
33535		A	three coronary arterial grafts	34.50	17.77	17.77	3.97	56.24	56.24	090	
33536		A	four or more coronary arterial grafts	37.50	19.27	19.27	3.29	60.06	60.06	090	

■ RVU not developed by CMS. Gap-filled RVUs developed by Ingenix/CHEG.

Code	M	S	Description	Work Value	Non-Fac PE	Fac PE	Mal-practice	Non-Fac Total	Fac Total	Global	Gap
33542		A	Myocardial resection (eg, ventricular aneurysmectomy)	28.85	17.05	17.05	3.61	49.51	49.51	090	
33545		A	Repair of postinfarction ventricular septal defect, with or without myocardial resection	36.78	19.79	19.79	4.40	60.97	60.97	090	
33572		A	Coronary endarterectomy, open, any method, of left anterior descending, circumflex, or right coronary artery performed in conjunction with coronary artery bypass graft procedure, each vessel (list separately in addition to primary procedure)	4.45	1.48	1.48	0.55	6.48	6.48	ZZZ	
33600		A	Closure of atrioventricular valve (mitral or tricuspid) by suture or patch	29.51	17.79	17.79	2.30	49.60	49.60	090	
33602		A	Closure of semilunar valve (aortic or pulmonary) by suture or patch	28.54	16.65	16.65	2.90	48.09	48.09	090	
33606		A	Anastomosis of pulmonary artery to aorta (Damus-Kaye-Stansel procedure)	30.74	17.53	17.53	3.59	51.86	51.86	090	
33608		A	Repair of complex cardiac anomaly other than pulmonary atresia with ventricular septal defect by construction or replacement of conduit from right or left ventricle to pulmonary artery	31.09	16.38	16.38	4.17	51.64	51.64	090	
33610		A	Repair of complex cardiac anomalies (eg, single ventricle with subaortic obstruction) by surgical enlargement of ventricular septal defect	30.61	18.89	18.89	4.02	53.52	53.52	090	
33611		A	Repair of double outlet right ventricle with intraventricular tunnel repair;	34.00	19.08	19.08	3.28	56.36	56.36	090	
33612		A	with repair of right ventricular outflow tract obstruction	35.00	20.17	20.17	4.44	59.61	59.61	090	
33615		A	Repair of complex cardiac anomalies (eg, tricuspid atresia) by closure of atrial septal defect and anastomosis of atria or vena cava to pulmonary artery (simple Fontan procedure)	34.00	19.33	19.33	3.15	56.48	56.48	090	
33617		A	Repair of complex cardiac anomalies (eg, single ventricle) by modified Fontan procedure	37.00	21.25	21.25	4.09	62.34	62.34	090	
33619		A	Repair of single ventricle with aortic outflow obstruction and aortic arch hypoplasia (hypoplastic left heart syndrome) (eg, Norwood procedure)	45.00	26.49	26.49	4.71	76.20	76.20	090	
33641		A	Repair atrial septal defect, secundum, with cardiopulmonary bypass, with or without patch	21.39	11.82	11.82	2.67	35.88	35.88	090	
33645		A	Direct or patch closure, sinus venosus, with or without anomalous pulmonary venous drainage	24.82	13.92	13.92	3.27	42.01	42.01	090	
33647		A	Repair of atrial septal defect and ventricular septal defect, with direct or patch closure	28.73	17.08	17.08	3.37	49.18	49.18	090	
33660		A	Repair of incomplete or partial atrioventricular canal (ostium primum atrial septal defect), with or without atrioventricular valve repair	30.00	17.09	17.09	2.82	49.91	49.91	090	

■ RVU not developed by CMS. Gap-filled RVUs developed by Ingenix/CHEG.

Code	M	S	Description	Work Value	Non-Fac PE	Fac PE	Mal-practice	Non-Fac Total	Fac Total	Global	Gap
33665		A	Repair of intermediate or transitional atrioventricular canal, with or without atrioventricular valve repair	28.60	16.87	16.87	3.81	49.28	49.28	090	
33670		A	Repair of complete atrioventricular canal, with or without prosthetic valve	35.00	16.68	16.68	2.18	53.86	53.86	090	
33681		A	Closure of ventricular septal defect, with or without patch	30.61	17.83	17.83	3.53	51.97	51.97	090	
33684		A	with pulmonary valvotomy or infundibular resection (acyanotic)	29.65	17.82	17.82	3.77	51.24	51.24	090	
33688		A	with removal of pulmonary artery band, with or without gusset	30.62	16.70	16.70	3.89	51.21	51.21	090	
33690		A	Banding of pulmonary artery	19.55	13.55	13.55	2.56	35.66	35.66	090	
33692		A	Complete repair tetralogy of Fallot without pulmonary atresia;	30.75	17.52	17.52	3.77	52.04	52.04	090	
33694		A	with transannular patch	34.00	17.82	17.82	4.27	56.09	56.09	090	
33697		A	Complete repair tetralogy of Fallot with pulmonary atresia including construction of conduit from right ventricle to pulmonary artery and closure of ventricular septal defect	36.00	18.62	18.62	4.54	59.16	59.16	090	
33702		A	Repair sinus of Valsalva fistula, with cardiopulmonary bypass;	26.54	16.53	16.53	3.45	46.52	46.52	090	
33710		A	with repair of ventricular septal defect	29.71	16.82	16.82	3.85	50.38	50.38	090	
33720		A	Repair sinus of Valsalva aneurysm, with cardiopulmonary bypass	26.56	16.51	16.51	3.21	46.28	46.28	090	
33722		A	Closure of aortico-left ventricular tunnel	28.41	17.05	17.05	3.80	49.26	49.26	090	
33730		A	Complete repair of anomalous venous return (supracardiac, intracardiac, or infracardiac types)	34.25	18.35	18.35	2.85	55.45	55.45	090	
33732		A	Repair of cor triatriatum or supravalvular mitral ring by resection of left atrial membrane	28.16	17.95	17.95	2.78	48.89	48.89	090	
33735		A	Atrial septectomy or septostomy; closed heart (Blalock-Hanlon type operation)	21.39	13.00	13.00	1.12	35.51	35.51	090	
33736		A	open heart with cardiopulmonary bypass	23.52	14.06	14.06	2.70	40.28	40.28	090	
33737		A	open heart, with inflow occlusion	21.76	15.22	15.22	2.93	39.91	39.91	090	
33750		A	Shunt; subclavian to pulmonary artery (Blalock-Taussig type operation)	21.41	12.83	12.83	1.74	35.98	35.98	090	
33755		A	ascending aorta to pulmonary artery (Waterston type operation)	21.79	12.94	12.94	2.93	37.66	37.66	090	
33762		A	descending aorta to pulmonary artery (Potts-Smith type operation)	21.79	13.32	13.32	1.59	36.70	36.70	090	
33764		A	central, with prosthetic graft	21.79	14.22	14.22	1.93	37.94	37.94	090	

■ RVU not developed by CMS. Gap-filled RVUs developed by Ingenix/CHEG.

Code	M	S	Description	Work Value	Non-Fac PE	Fac PE	Mal-practice	Non-Fac Total	Fac Total	Global	Gap
33766		A	superior vena cava to pulmonary artery for flow to one lung (classical Glenn procedure)	22.76	15.16	15.16	3.04	40.96	40.96	090	
33767		A	superior vena cava to pulmonary artery for flow to both lungs (bidirectional Glenn procedure)	24.50	14.92	14.92	3.14	42.56	42.56	090	
33770		A	Repair of transposition of the great arteries with ventricular septal defect and subpulmonary stenosis; without surgical enlargement of ventricular septal defect	37.00	19.01	19.01	4.49	60.50	60.50	090	
33771		A	with surgical enlargement of ventricular septal defect	34.65	18.08	18.08	4.67	57.40	57.40	090	
33774		A	Repair of transposition of the great arteries, atrial baffle procedure (eg, Mustard or Senning type) with cardiopulmonary bypass;	30.98	16.61	16.61	4.18	51.77	51.77	090	
33775		A	with removal of pulmonary band	32.20	17.10	17.10	4.34	53.64	53.64	090	
33776		A	with closure of ventricular septal defect	34.04	17.83	17.83	4.58	56.45	56.45	090	
33777		A	with repair of subpulmonic obstruction	33.46	17.60	17.60	4.51	55.57	55.57	090	
33778		A	Repair of transposition of the great arteries, aortic pulmonary artery reconstruction (eg, Jatene type);	40.00	20.21	20.21	4.83	65.04	65.04	090	
33779		A	with removal of pulmonary band	36.21	17.93	17.93	2.40	56.54	56.54	090	
33780		A	with closure of ventricular septal defect	41.75	20.98	20.98	5.21	67.94	67.94	090	
33781		A	with repair of subpulmonic obstruction	36.45	18.80	18.80	4.91	60.16	60.16	090	
33786		A	Total repair, truncus arteriosus (Rastelli type operation)	39.00	19.81	19.81	4.69	63.50	63.50	090	
33788		A	Reimplantation of an anomalous pulmonary artery	26.62	14.87	14.87	3.32	44.81	44.81	090	
33800		A	Aortic suspension (aortopexy) for tracheal decompression (eg, for tracheomalacia) (separate procedure)	16.24	13.12	13.12	1.11	30.47	30.47	090	
33802		A	Division of aberrant vessel (vascular ring);	17.66	12.22	12.22	1.56	31.44	31.44	090	
33803		A	with reanastomosis	19.60	13.53	13.53	2.63	35.76	35.76	090	
33813		A	Obliteration of aortopulmonary septal defect; without cardiopulmonary bypass	20.65	14.12	14.12	2.78	37.55	37.55	090	
33814		A	with cardiopulmonary bypass	25.77	15.61	15.61	2.52	43.90	43.90	090	
33820		A	Repair of patent ductus arteriosus; by ligation	16.29	10.95	10.95	2.10	29.34	29.34	090	
33822		A	by division, under 18 years	17.32	11.16	11.16	2.33	30.81	30.81	090	
33824		A	by division, 18 years and older	19.52	11.97	11.97	2.61	34.10	34.10	090	

■ RVU not developed by CMS. Gap-filled RVUs developed by Ingenix/CHEG.

Code	M	S	Description	Work Value	Non-Fac PE	Fac PE	Mal-practice	Non-Fac Total	Fac Total	Global	Gap
33840		**A**	Excision of coarctation of aorta, with or without associated patent ductus arteriosus; with direct anastomosis	20.63	14.11	14.11	2.36	37.10	37.10	090	
33845		**A**	with graft	22.12	14.85	14.85	2.90	39.87	39.87	090	
33851		**A**	repair using either left subclavian artery or prosthetic material as gusset for enlargement	21.27	12.98	12.98	2.86	37.11	37.11	090	
33852		**A**	Repair of hypoplastic or interrupted aortic arch using autogenous or prosthetic material; without cardiopulmonary bypass	23.71	14.14	14.14	3.19	41.04	41.04	090	
33853		**A**	with cardiopulmonary bypass	31.72	18.25	18.25	4.23	54.20	54.20	090	
33860		**A**	Ascending aorta graft, with cardiopulmonary bypass, with or without valve suspension;	38.00	18.74	18.74	4.30	61.04	61.04	090	
33861		**A**	with coronary reconstruction	42.00	20.15	20.15	4.24	66.39	66.39	090	
33863		**A**	with aortic root replacement using composite prosthesis and coronary reconstruction	45.00	21.10	21.10	4.60	70.70	70.70	090	
33870		**A**	Transverse arch graft, with cardiopulmonary bypass	44.00	20.69	20.69	5.09	69.78	69.78	090	
33875		**A**	Descending thoracic aorta graft, with or without bypass	33.06	17.01	17.01	4.08	54.15	54.15	090	
33877		**A**	Repair of thoracoabdominal aortic aneurysm with graft, with or without cardiopulmonary bypass	42.60	19.96	19.96	5.07	67.63	67.63	090	
33910		**A**	Pulmonary artery embolectomy; with cardiopulmonary bypass	24.59	14.16	14.16	3.06	41.81	41.81	090	
33915		**A**	without cardiopulmonary bypass	21.02	12.31	12.31	1.20	34.53	34.53	090	
33916		**A**	Pulmonary endarterectomy, with or without embolectomy, with cardiopulmonary bypass	25.83	15.49	15.49	3.04	44.36	44.36	090	
33917		**A**	Repair of pulmonary artery stenosis by reconstruction with patch or graft	24.50	15.36	15.36	3.17	43.03	43.03	090	
33918		**A**	Repair of pulmonary atresia with ventricular septal defect, by unifocalization of pulmonary arteries; without cardiopulmonary bypass	26.45	14.80	14.80	3.42	44.67	44.67	090	
33919		**A**	with cardiopulmonary bypass	40.00	21.02	21.02	3.48	64.50	64.50	090	
33920		**A**	Repair of pulmonary atresia with ventricular septal defect, by construction or replacement of conduit from right or left ventricle to pulmonary artery	31.95	17.28	17.28	3.61	52.84	52.84	090	
33922		**A**	Transection of pulmonary artery with cardiopulmonary bypass	23.52	13.79	13.79	2.30	39.61	39.61	090	

Surgery

■ RVU not developed by CMS. Gap-filled RVUs developed by Ingenix/CHEG.

Code	M	S	Description	Work Value	Non-Fac PE	Fac PE	Mal-prac-tice	Non-Fac Total	Fac Total	Global	Gap
33924		A	Ligation and takedown of a systemic-to-pulmonary artery shunt, performed in conjunction with a congenital heart procedure (List separately in addition to code for primary procedure)	5.50	2.05	2.05	0.74	8.29	8.29	ZZZ	
33930		X	Donor cardiectomy-pneumonectomy, with preparation and maintenance of allograft	0.00	0.00	0.00	0.00	0.00	0.00	XXX	
33935		R	Heart-lung transplant with recipient cardiectomy-pneumonectomy	60.96	27.93	27.93	8.15	97.04	97.04	090	
33940		X	Donor cardiectomy, with preparation and maintenance of allograft	0.00	0.00	0.00	0.00	0.00	0.00	XXX	
33945		R	Heart transplant, with or without recipient cardiectomy	42.10	21.67	21.67	5.42	69.19	69.19	090	
33960		A	Prolonged extracorporeal circulation for cardiopulmonary insufficiency; initial 24 hours	19.36	6.06	6.06	2.14	27.56	27.56	000	
33961		A	each additional 24 hours (List separately in addition to code for primary procedure)	10.93	3.79	3.79	1.47	16.19	16.19	ZZZ	
33967		A	Insertion of intra-aortic balloon assist device, percutaneous	4.85	2.01	1.96	0.27	7.13	7.08	000	
33968		A	Removal of intra-aortic balloon assist device, percutaneous	0.64	0.24	0.24	0.07	0.95	0.95	000	
33970		A	Insertion of intra-aortic balloon assist device through the femoral artery, open approach	6.75	2.37	2.37	0.70	9.82	9.82	000	
33971		A	Removal of intra-aortic balloon assist device including repair of femoral artery, with or without graft	9.69	7.82	7.82	0.97	18.48	18.48	090	
33973		A	Insertion of intra-aortic balloon assist device through the ascending aorta	9.76	3.44	3.44	1.01	14.21	14.21	000	
33974		A	Removal of intra-aortic balloon assist device from the ascending aorta, including repair of the ascending aorta, with or without graft	14.41	10.69	10.69	1.48	26.58	26.58	090	
33975		A	Insertion of ventricular assist device; extracorporeal, single ventricle	21.00	7.04	7.04	1.72	29.76	29.76	XXX	
33976		A	extracorporeal, biventricular	23.00	7.78	7.78	2.82	33.60	33.60	XXX	
33977		A	Removal of ventricular assist device; extracorporeal, single ventricle	19.29	10.46	10.46	2.44	32.19	32.19	090	
33978		A	extracorporeal, biventricular	21.73	11.27	11.27	2.66	35.66	35.66	090	
33979		C	Insertion of ventricular assist device, implantable intracorporeal, single ventricle	18.38	14.61	14.61	1.96	34.95	34.95	XXX	■
33980		C	Removal of ventricular assist device, implantable intracorporeal, single ventricle	16.12	12.81	12.81	1.72	30.65	30.65	090	■
33999		C	Unlisted procedure, cardiac surgery	0.00	0.00	0.00	0.00	0.00	0.00	YYY	

■ RVU not developed by CMS. Gap-filled RVUs developed by Ingenix/CHEG.

Code	M	S	Description	Work Value	Non-Fac PE	Fac PE	Mal-practice	Non-Fac Total	Fac Total	Global	Gap
34001		A	Embolectomy or thrombectomy, with or without catheter; carotid, subclavian or innominate artery, by neck incision	12.91	5.97	5.97	1.46	20.34	20.34	090	
34051		A	innominate, subclavian artery, by thoracic incision	15.21	7.07	7.07	1.90	24.18	24.18	090	
34101		A	axillary, brachial, innominate, subclavian artery, by arm incision	10.00	4.84	4.84	1.11	15.95	15.95	090	
34111		A	radial or ulnar artery, by arm incision	10.00	4.88	4.88	0.85	15.73	15.73	090	
34151		A	renal, celiac, mesentery, aortoiliac artery, by abdominal incision	25.00	10.54	10.54	1.84	37.38	37.38	090	
34201		A	femoropopliteal, aortoiliac artery, by leg incision	10.03	5.12	5.12	1.02	16.17	16.17	090	
34203		A	popliteal-tibio-peroneal artery, by leg incision	16.50	7.65	7.65	1.37	25.52	25.52	090	
34401		A	Thrombectomy, direct or with catheter; vena cava, iliac vein, by abdominal incision	25.00	10.47	10.47	1.20	36.67	36.67	090	
34421		A	vena cava, iliac, femoropopliteal vein, by leg incision	12.00	6.01	6.01	0.95	18.96	18.96	090	
34451		A	vena cava, iliac, femoropopliteal vein, by abdominal and leg incision	27.00	11.08	11.08	1.59	39.67	39.67	090	
34471		A	subclavian vein, by neck incision	10.18	5.18	5.18	0.90	16.26	16.26	090	
34490		A	axillary and subclavian vein, by arm incision	9.86	6.26	6.26	0.73	16.85	16.85	090	
34501		A	Valvuloplasty, femoral vein	16.00	8.98	8.98	1.37	26.35	26.35	090	
34502		A	Reconstruction of vena cava, any method	26.95	11.34	11.34	2.99	41.28	41.28	090	
34510		A	Venous valve transposition, any vein donor	18.95	10.23	10.23	1.60	30.78	30.78	090	
34520		A	Cross-over vein graft to venous system	17.95	9.59	9.59	1.41	28.95	28.95	090	
34530		A	Saphenopopliteal vein anastomosis	16.64	8.48	8.48	2.06	27.18	27.18	090	
34800		A	Endovascular repair of infrarenal abdominal aortic aneurysm or dissection; using aorto-aortic tube prosthesis	20.75	9.79	9.79	1.49	32.03	32.03	090	
34802		A	using modular bifurcated prosthesis (one docking limb)	23.00	10.69	10.69	1.65	35.34	35.34	090	
34804		A	using unibody bifurcated prosthesis	23.00	10.69	10.69	1.65	35.34	35.34	090	
34808		A	Endovascular placement of iliac artery occlusion device (List separately in addition to code for primary procedure)	4.13	1.65	1.65	0.29	6.07	6.07	ZZZ	
34812		A	Open femoral artery exposure for delivery of aortic endovascular prosthesis, by groin incision, unilateral	6.75	2.69	2.69	0.49	9.93	9.93	000	

■ RVU not developed by CMS. Gap-filled RVUs developed by Ingenix/CHEG.

Code	M	S	Description	Work Value	Non-Fac PE	Fac PE	Mal-practice	Non-Fac Total	Fac Total	Global	Gap
34813		A	Placement of femoral-femoral prosthetic graft during endovascular aortic aneurysm repair (List separately in addition to code for primary procedure)	4.80	1.92	1.92	0.34	7.06	7.06	ZZZ	
34820		A	Open iliac artery exposure for delivery of endovascular prosthesis or iliac occlusion during endovascular therapy, by abdominal or retroperitoneal incision, unilateral	9.75	3.89	3.89	0.70	14.34	14.34	000	
34825		A	Placement of proximal or distal extension prosthesis for endovascular repair of infrarenal abdominal aortic aneurysm; initial vessel	12.00	6.30	6.30	0.86	19.16	19.16	090	
34826		A	each additional vessel (List separately in addition to code for primary procedure)	4.13	1.65	1.65	0.29	6.07	6.07	ZZZ	
34830		A	Open repair of infrarenal aortic aneurysm or dissection, plus repair of associated arterial trauma, following unsuccessful endovascular repair; tube prosthesis	32.59	14.89	14.89	2.34	49.82	49.82	090	
34831		A	aorto-bi-iliac prosthesis	35.34	15.99	15.99	2.53	53.86	53.86	090	
34832		A	aorto-bifemoral prosthesis	35.34	15.99	15.99	2.53	53.86	53.86	090	
35001		A	Direct repair of aneurysm, pseudoaneurysm, or excision (partial or total) and graft insertion, with or without patch graft; for aneurysm and associated occlusive disease, carotid, subclavian artery, by neck incision	19.64	8.41	8.41	2.44	30.49	30.49	090	
35002		A	for ruptured aneurysm, carotid, subclavian artery, by neck incision	21.00	9.12	9.12	1.82	31.94	31.94	090	
35005		A	for aneurysm, pseudoaneurysm, and associated occlusive disease, vertebral artery	18.12	8.04	8.04	1.35	27.51	27.51	090	
35011		A	for aneurysm and associated occlusive disease, axillary-brachial artery, by arm incision	18.00	7.59	7.59	1.30	26.89	26.89	090	
35013		A	for ruptured aneurysm, axillary-brachial artery, by arm incision	22.00	8.98	8.98	1.91	32.89	32.89	090	
35021		A	for aneurysm, pseudoaneurysm, and associated occlusive disease, innominate, subclavian artery, by thoracic incision	19.65	8.64	8.64	1.93	30.22	30.22	090	
35022		A	for ruptured aneurysm, innominate, subclavian artery, by thoracic incision	23.18	9.57	9.57	1.99	34.74	34.74	090	
35045		A	for aneurysm, pseudoaneurysm, and associated occlusive disease, radial or ulnar artery	17.57	7.99	7.99	1.25	26.81	26.81	090	
35081		A	for aneurysm, pseudoaneurysm, and associated occlusive disease, abdominal aorta	28.01	11.69	11.69	3.20	42.90	42.90	090	
35082		A	for ruptured aneurysm, abdominal aorta	38.50	15.08	15.08	4.07	57.65	57.65	090	

■ RVU not developed by CMS. Gap-filled RVUs developed by Ingenix/CHEG.

Code	M	S	Description	Work Value	Non-Fac PE	Fac PE	Mal-practice	Non-Fac Total	Fac Total	Global	Gap
35091		A	for aneurysm, pseudoaneurysm, and associated occlusive disease, abdominal aorta involving visceral vessels (mesenteric, celiac, renal)	35.40	14.22	14.22	4.09	53.71	53.71	090	
35092		A	for ruptured aneurysm, abdominal aorta involving visceral vessels (mesenteric, celiac, renal)	45.00	17.35	17.35	4.31	66.66	66.66	090	
35102		A	for aneurysm, pseudoaneurysm, and associated occlusive disease, abdominal aorta involving iliac vessels (common, hypogastric, external)	30.76	12.67	12.67	3.44	46.87	46.87	090	
35103		A	for ruptured aneurysm, abdominal aorta involving iliac vessels (common, hypogastric, external)	40.50	15.81	15.81	3.79	60.10	60.10	090	
35111		A	for aneurysm, pseudoaneurysm, and associated occlusive disease, splenic artery	25.00	10.43	10.43	1.81	37.24	37.24	090	
35112		A	for ruptured aneurysm, splenic artery	30.00	12.06	12.06	1.95	44.01	44.01	090	
35121		A	for aneurysm, pseudoaneurysm, and associated occlusive disease, hepatic, celiac, renal, or mesenteric artery	30.00	12.39	12.39	2.93	45.32	45.32	090	
35122		A	for ruptured aneurysm, hepatic, celiac, renal, or mesenteric artery	35.00	13.73	13.73	3.54	52.27	52.27	090	
35131		A	for aneurysm, pseudoaneurysm, and associated occlusive disease, iliac artery (common, hypogastric, external)	25.00	10.64	10.64	2.11	37.75	37.75	090	
35132		A	for ruptured aneurysm, iliac artery (common, hypogastric, external)	30.00	12.14	12.14	2.48	44.62	44.62	090	
35141		A	for aneurysm, pseudoaneurysm, and associated occlusive disease, common femoral artery (profunda femoris, superficial femoral)	20.00	8.66	8.66	1.65	30.31	30.31	090	
35142		A	for ruptured aneurysm, common femoral artery (profunda femoris, superficial femoral)	23.30	9.76	9.76	1.75	34.81	34.81	090	
35151		A	for aneurysm, pseudoaneurysm, and associated occlusive disease, popliteal artery	22.64	9.72	9.72	1.93	34.29	34.29	090	
35152		A	for ruptured aneurysm, popliteal artery	25.62	10.50	10.50	1.93	38.05	38.05	090	
35161		A	for aneurysm, pseudoaneurysm, and associated occlusive disease, other arteries	18.76	8.96	8.96	2.21	29.93	29.93	090	
35162		A	for ruptured aneurysm, other arteries	19.78	9.05	9.05	2.21	31.04	31.04	090	
35180		A	Repair, congenital arteriovenous fistula; head and neck	13.62	6.49	6.49	1.44	21.55	21.55	090	
35182		A	thorax and abdomen	30.00	12.39	12.39	1.88	44.27	44.27	090	

■ RVU not developed by CMS. Gap-filled RVUs developed by Ingenix/CHEG.

Surgery

Code	M	S	Description	Work Value	Non-Fac PE	Fac PE	Mal-practice	Non-Fac Total	Fac Total	Global	Gap
35184		A	extremities	18.00	7.92	7.92	1.34	27.26	27.26	090	
35188		A	Repair, acquired or traumatic arteriovenous fistula; head and neck	14.28	6.70	6.70	1.53	22.51	22.51	090	
35189		A	thorax and abdomen	28.00	11.71	11.71	2.12	41.83	41.83	090	
35190		A	extremities	12.75	6.03	6.03	1.33	20.11	20.11	090	
35201		A	Repair blood vessel, direct; neck	16.14	7.18	7.18	1.17	24.49	24.49	090	
35206		A	upper extremity	13.25	7.60	7.60	1.04	21.89	21.89	090	
35207		A	hand, finger	10.15	9.91	9.91	1.15	21.21	21.21	090	
35211		A	intrathoracic, with bypass	22.12	13.55	13.55	2.83	38.50	38.50	090	
35216		A	intrathoracic, without bypass	18.75	11.83	11.83	2.17	32.75	32.75	090	
35221		A	intra-abdominal	24.39	10.31	10.31	1.79	36.49	36.49	090	
35226		A	lower extremity	14.50	8.54	8.54	0.84	23.88	23.88	090	
35231		A	Repair blood vessel with vein graft; neck	20.00	9.45	9.45	1.32	30.77	30.77	090	
35236		A	upper extremity	17.11	8.97	8.97	1.19	27.27	27.27	090	
35241		A	intrathoracic, with bypass	23.12	14.09	14.09	2.90	40.11	40.11	090	
35246		A	intrathoracic, without bypass	26.45	14.32	14.32	2.22	42.99	42.99	090	
35251		A	intra-abdominal	30.20	12.39	12.39	1.87	44.46	44.46	090	
35256		A	lower extremity	18.36	9.63	9.63	1.32	29.31	29.31	090	
35261		A	Repair blood vessel with graft other than vein; neck	17.80	7.56	7.56	1.34	26.70	26.70	090	
35266		A	upper extremity	14.91	8.12	8.12	1.16	24.19	24.19	090	
35271		A	intrathoracic, with bypass	22.12	13.43	13.43	2.77	38.32	38.32	090	
35276		A	intrathoracic, without bypass	24.25	13.56	13.56	2.37	40.18	40.18	090	
35281		A	intra-abdominal	28.00	11.66	11.66	1.82	41.48	41.48	090	
35286		A	lower extremity	16.16	8.88	8.88	1.36	26.40	26.40	090	
35301		A	Thromboendarterectomy, with or without patch graft; carotid, vertebral, subclavian, by neck incision	18.70	8.39	8.39	2.23	29.32	29.32	090	
35311		A	subclavian, innominate, by thoracic incision	27.00	11.10	11.10	2.75	40.85	40.85	090	
35321		A	axillary-brachial	16.00	6.87	6.87	1.36	24.23	24.23	090	
35331		A	abdominal aorta	26.20	11.11	11.11	2.71	40.02	40.02	090	
35341		A	mesenteric, celiac, or renal	25.11	10.70	10.70	2.87	38.68	38.68	090	

■ RVU not developed by CMS. Gap-filled RVUs developed by Ingenix/CHEG.

Code	M	S	Description	Work Value	Non-Fac PE	Fac PE	Mal-practice	Non-Fac Total	Fac Total	Global	Gap
35351		A	iliac	23.00	9.84	9.84	2.29	35.13	35.13	090	
35355		A	iliofemoral	18.50	8.33	8.33	1.80	28.63	28.63	090	
35361		A	combined aortoiliac	28.20	11.60	11.60	2.66	42.46	42.46	090	
35363		A	combined aortoiliofemoral	30.20	12.54	12.54	2.77	45.51	45.51	090	
35371		A	common femoral	14.72	6.75	6.75	1.32	22.79	22.79	090	
35372		A	deep (profunda) femoral	18.00	7.91	7.91	1.53	27.44	27.44	090	
35381		A	femoral and/or popliteal, and/or tibioperoneal	15.81	7.35	7.35	1.80	24.96	24.96	090	
35390		A	Reoperation, carotid, thromboendarterectomy, more than one month after original operation (List separately in addition to code for primary procedure)	3.19	1.11	1.11	0.38	4.68	4.68	ZZZ	
35400		A	Angioscopy (non-coronary vessels or grafts) during therapeutic intervention (List separately in addition to code for primary procedure)	3.00	1.05	1.05	0.34	4.39	4.39	ZZZ	
35450		A	Transluminal balloon angioplasty, open; renal or other visceral artery	10.07	4.22	4.22	0.84	15.13	15.13	000	
35452		A	aortic	6.91	3.11	3.11	0.76	10.78	10.78	000	
35454		A	iliac	6.04	2.83	2.83	0.67	9.54	9.54	000	
35456		A	femoral-popliteal	7.35	3.27	3.27	0.82	11.44	11.44	000	
35458		A	brachiocephalic trunk or branches, each vessel	9.49	4.03	4.03	1.09	14.61	14.61	000	
35459		A	tibioperoneal trunk and branches	8.63	3.69	3.69	0.96	13.28	13.28	000	
35460		A	venous	6.04	2.70	2.70	0.66	9.40	9.40	000	
35470		A	Transluminal balloon angioplasty, percutaneous; tibioperoneal trunk or branches, each vessel	8.63	3.98	3.98	0.50	13.11	13.11	000	
35471		A	renal or visceral artery	10.07	4.67	4.67	0.50	15.24	15.24	000	
35472		A	aortic	6.91	3.32	3.32	0.39	10.62	10.62	000	
35473		A	iliac	6.04	3.01	3.01	0.34	9.39	9.39	000	
35474		A	femoral-popliteal	7.36	3.52	3.52	0.40	11.28	11.28	000	
35475		R	brachiocephalic trunk or branches, each vessel	9.49	4.23	4.23	0.47	14.19	14.19	000	
35476		A	venous	6.04	2.94	2.94	0.27	9.25	9.25	000	
35480		A	Transluminal peripheral atherectomy, open; renal or other visceral artery	11.08	4.58	4.58	1.13	16.79	16.79	000	
35481		A	aortic	7.61	3.54	3.54	0.84	11.99	11.99	000	

■ RVU not developed by CMS. Gap-filled RVUs developed by Ingenix/CHEG.

Code	M	S	Description	Work Value	Non-Fac PE	Fac PE	Mal-practice	Non-Fac Total	Fac Total	Global	Gap
35482		A	iliac	6.65	3.16	3.16	0.75	10.56	10.56	000	
35483		A	femoral-popliteal	8.10	3.52	3.52	0.81	12.43	12.43	000	
35484		A	brachiocephalic trunk or branches, each vessel	10.44	4.21	4.21	1.13	15.78	15.78	000	
35485		A	tibioperoneal trunk and branches	9.49	4.05	4.05	1.06	14.60	14.60	000	
35490		A	Transluminal peripheral atherectomy, percutaneous; renal or other visceral artery	11.08	4.83	4.83	0.55	16.46	16.46	000	
35491		A	aortic	7.61	3.59	3.59	0.49	11.69	11.69	000	
35492		A	iliac	6.65	3.22	3.22	0.43	10.30	10.30	000	
35493		A	femoral-popliteal	8.10	3.90	3.90	0.47	12.47	12.47	000	
35494		A	brachiocephalic trunk or branches, each vessel	10.44	4.57	4.57	0.48	15.49	15.49	000	
35495		A	tibioperoneal trunk and branches	9.49	4.52	4.52	0.51	14.52	14.52	000	
35500		A	Harvest of upper extremity vein, one segment, for lower extremity or coronary artery bypass procedure (List separately in addition to code for primary procedure)	6.45	2.25	2.25	0.63	9.33	9.33	ZZZ	
35501		A	Bypass graft, with vein; carotid	19.19	8.14	8.14	2.33	29.66	29.66	090	
35506		A	carotid-subclavian	19.67	8.32	8.32	2.33	30.32	30.32	090	
35507		A	subclavian-carotid	19.67	8.29	8.29	2.27	30.23	30.23	090	
35508		A	carotid-vertebral	18.65	7.91	7.91	2.34	28.90	28.90	090	
35509		A	carotid-carotid	18.07	7.70	7.70	2.12	27.89	27.89	090	
35511		A	subclavian-subclavian	21.20	8.80	8.80	1.74	31.74	31.74	090	
35515		A	subclavian-vertebral	18.65	7.80	7.80	2.26	28.71	28.71	090	
35516		A	subclavian-axillary	16.32	4.94	4.94	1.88	23.14	23.14	090	
35518		A	axillary-axillary	21.20	8.80	8.80	1.78	31.78	31.78	090	
35521		A	axillary-femoral	22.20	9.53	9.53	1.82	33.55	33.55	090	
35526		A	aortosubclavian or carotid	29.95	12.19	12.19	2.18	44.32	44.32	090	
35531		A	aortoceliac or aortomesenteric	36.20	14.53	14.53	2.91	53.64	53.64	090	
35533		A	axillary-femoral-femoral	28.00	11.74	11.74	2.35	42.09	42.09	090	
35536		A	splenorenal	31.70	12.85	12.85	2.62	47.17	47.17	090	
35541		A	aortoiliac or bi-iliac	25.80	10.98	10.98	2.74	39.52	39.52	090	
35546		A	aortofemoral or bifemoral	25.54	10.75	10.75	2.84	39.13	39.13	090	
35548		A	aortoiliofemoral, unilateral	21.57	9.45	9.45	2.45	33.47	33.47	090	

■ RVU not developed by CMS. Gap-filled RVUs developed by Ingenix/CHEG.

Code	M	S	Description	Work Value	Non-Fac PE	Fac PE	Mal-practice	Non-Fac Total	Fac Total	Global	Gap
35549		A	aortoiliofemoral, bilateral	23.35	9.88	9.88	2.77	36.00	36.00	090	
35551		A	aortofemoral-popliteal	26.67	11.20	11.20	3.19	41.06	41.06	090	
35556		A	femoral-popliteal	21.76	9.45	9.45	2.48	33.69	33.69	090	
35558		A	femoral-femoral	21.20	9.11	9.11	1.58	31.89	31.89	090	
35560		A	aortorenal	32.00	13.12	13.12	2.73	47.85	47.85	090	
35563		A	ilioiliac	24.20	10.42	10.42	1.68	36.30	36.30	090	
35565		A	iliofemoral	23.20	9.99	9.99	1.71	34.90	34.90	090	
35566		A	femoral-anterior tibial, posterior tibial, peroneal artery or other distal vessels	26.92	11.77	11.77	3.02	41.71	41.71	090	
35571		A	popliteal-tibial, -peroneal artery or other distal vessels	24.06	12.13	12.13	2.14	38.33	38.33	090	
35582		A	In-situ vein bypass; aortofemoral-popliteal (only femoral-popliteal portion in-situ)	27.13	11.35	11.35	3.11	41.59	41.59	090	
35583		A	femoral-popliteal	22.37	10.62	10.62	2.53	35.52	35.52	090	
35585		A	femoral-anterior tibial, posterior tibial, or peroneal artery	28.39	14.53	14.53	3.21	46.13	46.13	090	
35587		A	popliteal-tibial, peroneal	24.75	12.79	12.79	2.17	39.71	39.71	090	
35600		A	Harvest of upper extremity artery, one segment, for coronary artery bypass procedure	4.95	1.98	1.98	0.60	7.53	7.53	ZZZ	
35601		A	Bypass graft, with other than vein; carotid	17.50	7.49	7.49	2.08	27.07	27.07	090	
35606		A	carotid-subclavian	18.71	7.93	7.93	2.17	28.81	28.81	090	
35612		A	subclavian-subclavian	15.76	6.70	6.70	1.72	24.18	24.18	090	
35616		A	subclavian-axillary	15.70	7.05	7.05	1.84	24.59	24.59	090	
35621		A	axillary-femoral	20.00	8.79	8.79	1.68	30.47	30.47	090	
35623		A	axillary-popliteal or -tibial	24.00	10.22	10.22	1.91	36.13	36.13	090	
35626		A	aortosubclavian or carotid	27.75	11.08	11.08	2.89	41.72	41.72	090	
35631		A	aortoceliac, aortomesenteric, aortorenal	34.00	13.74	13.74	2.83	50.57	50.57	090	
35636		A	splenorenal (splenic to renal arterial anastomosis)	29.50	12.26	12.26	2.37	44.13	44.13	090	
35641		A	aortoiliac or bi-iliac	24.57	10.47	10.47	2.83	37.87	37.87	090	
35642		A	carotid-vertebral	17.98	7.92	7.92	1.84	27.74	27.74	090	
35645		A	subclavian-vertebral	17.47	8.36	8.36	1.91	27.74	27.74	090	
35646		A	aortobifemoral	31.00	13.26	13.26	2.98	47.24	47.24	090	
35647		A	aortofemoral	28.00	11.97	11.97	2.98	42.95	42.95	090	

■ RVU not developed by CMS. Gap-filled RVUs developed by Ingenix/CHEG.

Surgery

Code	M	S	Description	Work Value	Non-Fac PE	Fac PE	Mal-practice	Non-Fac Total	Fac Total	Global	Gap
35650		A	axillary-axillary	19.00	7.93	7.93	1.64	28.57	28.57	090	
35651		A	aortofemoral-popliteal	25.04	10.70	10.70	2.53	38.27	38.27	090	
35654		A	axillary-femoral-femoral	25.00	10.60	10.60	2.10	37.70	37.70	090	
35656		A	femoral-popliteal	19.53	8.44	8.44	2.21	30.18	30.18	090	
35661		A	femoral-femoral	19.00	8.26	8.26	1.50	28.76	28.76	090	
35663		A	ilioiliac	22.00	9.65	9.65	1.55	33.20	33.20	090	
35665		A	iliofemoral	21.00	9.18	9.18	1.76	31.94	31.94	090	
35666		A	femoral-anterior tibial, posterior tibial, or peroneal artery	22.19	11.93	11.93	2.19	36.31	36.31	090	
35671		A	popliteal-tibial or -peroneal artery	19.33	10.53	10.53	1.68	31.54	31.54	090	
35681		A	Bypass graft; composite, prosthetic and vein (List separately in addition to code for primary procedure)	1.60	0.56	0.56	0.18	2.34	2.34	ZZZ	
35682		A	autogenous composite, two segments of veins from two locations (List separately in addition to code for primary procedure)	7.20	2.51	2.51	0.83	10.54	10.54	ZZZ	
35683		A	autogenous composite, three or more segments of vein from two or more locations (List separately in addition to code for primary procedure)	8.50	2.99	2.99	0.98	12.47	12.47	ZZZ	
35685		A	Placement of vein patch or cuff at distal anastomosis of bypass graft, synthetic conduit (List separately in addition to code for primary procedure)	4.05	1.50	1.50	0.41	5.96	5.96	ZZZ	
35686		A	Creation of distal arteriovenous fistula during lower extremity bypass surgery (non-hemodialysis) (List separately in addition to code for primary procedure)	3.35	1.24	1.24	0.34	4.93	4.93	ZZZ	
35691		A	Transposition and/or reimplantation; vertebral to carotid artery	18.05	7.65	7.65	2.06	27.76	27.76	090	
35693		A	vertebral to subclavian artery	15.36	6.66	6.66	1.80	23.82	23.82	090	
35694		A	subclavian to carotid artery	19.16	8.02	8.02	2.13	29.31	29.31	090	
35695		A	carotid to subclavian artery	19.16	7.92	7.92	2.19	29.27	29.27	090	
35700		A	Reoperation, femoral-popliteal or femoral (popliteal) -anterior tibial, posterior tibial, peroneal artery or other distal vessels, more than one month after original operation (List separately in addition to code for primary procedure)	3.08	1.07	1.07	0.36	4.51	4.51	ZZZ	
35701		A	Exploration (not followed by surgical repair), with or without lysis of artery; carotid artery	8.50	4.70	4.70	0.64	13.84	13.84	090	

■ RVU not developed by CMS. Gap-filled RVUs developed by Ingenix/CHEG.

Code	M	S	Description	Work Value	Non-Fac PE	Fac PE	Mal-prac-tice	Non-Fac Total	Fac Total	Global	Gap
35721		A	femoral artery	7.18	5.10	5.10	0.59	12.87	12.87	090	
35741		A	popliteal artery	8.00	5.47	5.47	0.60	14.07	14.07	090	
35761		A	other vessels	5.37	4.47	4.47	0.60	10.44	10.44	090	
35800		A	Exploration for postoperative hemorrhage, thrombosis or infection; neck	7.02	3.95	3.95	0.79	11.76	11.76	090	
35820		A	chest	12.88	4.32	4.32	1.61	18.81	18.81	090	
35840		A	abdomen	9.77	5.21	5.21	1.06	16.04	16.04	090	
35860		A	extremity	5.55	3.62	3.62	0.63	9.80	9.80	090	
35870		A	Repair of graft-enteric fistula	22.17	10.21	10.21	2.47	34.85	34.85	090	
35875		A	Thrombectomy of arterial or venous graft (other than hemodialysis graft or fistula);	10.13	6.63	6.63	0.97	17.73	17.73	090	
35876		A	with revision of arterial or venous graft	17.00	9.16	9.16	1.88	28.04	28.04	090	
35879		A	Revision, lower extremity arterial bypass, without thrombectomy, open; with vein patch angioplasty	16.00	7.77	7.77	1.35	25.12	25.12	090	
35881		A	with segmental vein interposition	18.00	8.65	8.65	1.44	28.09	28.09	090	
35901		A	Excision of infected graft; neck	8.19	5.85	5.85	0.90	14.94	14.94	090	
35903		A	extremity	9.39	8.20	8.20	1.03	18.62	18.62	090	
35905		A	thorax	31.25	15.39	15.39	2.15	48.79	48.79	090	
35907		A	abdomen	35.00	14.97	14.97	2.17	52.14	52.14	090	
36000		A	Introduction of needle or intracatheter, vein	0.18	0.65	0.05	0.01	0.84	0.24	XXX	
36002		A	Injection procedures (eg, thrombin) for percutaneous treatment of extremity pseudoaneurysm	1.96	2.95	1.03	0.08	4.99	3.07	000	
36005		A	Injection procedure for extremity venography (including introduction of needle or intracatheter)	0.95	7.29	0.34	0.04	8.28	1.33	000	
36010		A	Introduction of catheter, superior or inferior vena cava	2.43	0.84	0.84	0.16	3.43	3.43	XXX	
36011		A	Selective catheter placement, venous system; first order branch (eg, renal vein, jugular vein)	3.14	1.10	1.10	0.17	4.41	4.41	XXX	
36012		A	second order, or more selective, branch (eg, left adrenal vein, petrosal sinus)	3.52	1.23	1.23	0.17	4.92	4.92	XXX	
36013		A	Introduction of catheter, right heart or main pulmonary artery	2.52	0.61	0.61	0.17	3.30	3.30	XXX	
36014		A	Selective catheter placement, left or right pulmonary artery	3.02	1.06	1.06	0.14	4.22	4.22	XXX	

■ RVU not developed by CMS. Gap-filled RVUs developed by Ingenix/CHEG.

Surgery

Code	M	S	Description	Work Value	Non-Fac PE	Fac PE	Mal-practice	Non-Fac Total	Fac Total	Global	Gap
36015		A	Selective catheter placement, segmental or subsegmental pulmonary artery	3.52	1.24	1.24	0.16	4.92	4.92	XXX	
36100		A	Introduction of needle or intracatheter, carotid or vertebral artery	3.02	1.16	1.16	0.18	4.36	4.36	XXX	
36120		A	Introduction of needle or intracatheter; retrograde brachial artery	2.01	0.69	0.69	0.11	2.81	2.81	XXX	
36140		A	extremity artery	2.01	0.69	0.69	0.12	2.82	2.82	XXX	
36145		A	arteriovenous shunt created for dialysis (cannula, fistula, or graft)	2.01	0.70	0.70	0.10	2.81	2.81	XXX	
36160		A	Introduction of needle or intracatheter, aortic, translumbar	2.52	0.90	0.90	0.20	3.62	3.62	XXX	
36200		A	Introduction of catheter, aorta	3.02	1.09	1.09	0.15	4.26	4.26	XXX	
36215		A	Selective catheter placement, arterial system; each first order thoracic or brachiocephalic branch, within a vascular family	4.68	1.68	1.68	0.22	6.58	6.58	XXX	
36216		A	initial second order thoracic or brachiocephalic branch, within a vascular family	5.28	1.89	1.89	0.24	7.41	7.41	XXX	
36217		A	initial third order or more selective thoracic or brachiocephalic branch, within a vascular family	6.30	2.29	2.29	0.32	8.91	8.91	XXX	
36218		A	additional second order, third order, and beyond, thoracic or brachiocephalic branch, within a vascular family (List in addition to code for initial second or third order vessel as appropriate)	1.01	0.37	0.37	0.05	1.43	1.43	ZZZ	
36245		A	Selective catheter placement, arterial system; each first order abdominal, pelvic, or lower extremity artery branch, within a vascular family	4.68	1.78	1.78	0.23	6.69	6.69	XXX	
36246		A	initial second order abdominal, pelvic, or lower extremity artery branch, within a vascular family	5.28	1.91	1.91	0.26	7.45	7.45	XXX	
36247		A	initial third order or more selective abdominal, pelvic, or lower extremity artery branch, within a vascular family	6.30	2.25	2.25	0.32	8.87	8.87	XXX	
36248		A	additional second order, third order, and beyond, abdominal, pelvic, or lower extremity artery branch, within a vascular family (List in addition to code for initial second or third order vessel as appropriate)	1.01	0.37	0.37	0.06	1.44	1.44	ZZZ	
36260		A	Insertion of implantable intra-arterial infusion pump (eg, for chemotherapy of liver)	9.71	5.63	5.63	1.00	16.34	16.34	090	
36261		A	Revision of implanted intra-arterial infusion pump	5.45	3.47	3.47	0.50	9.42	9.42	090	

■ RVU not developed by CMS. Gap-filled RVUs developed by Ingenix/CHEG.

Code	M	S	Description	Work Value	Non-Fac PE	Fac PE	Mal-practice	Non-Fac Total	Fac Total	Global	Gap
36262		A	Removal of implanted intra-arterial infusion pump	4.02	2.59	2.59	0.43	7.04	7.04	090	
36299		C	Unlisted procedure, vascular injection	0.00	0.00	0.00	0.00	0.00	0.00	YYY	
36400		A	Venipuncture, under age 3 years; femoral or jugular	0.38	0.72	0.10	0.01	1.11	0.49	XXX	
36405		A	scalp vein	0.31	0.58	0.09	0.01	0.90	0.41	XXX	
36406		A	other vein	0.18	0.94	0.06	0.01	1.13	0.25	XXX	
36410		A	Venipuncture, child over age 3 years or adult, necessitating physician's skill (separate procedure), for diagnostic or therapeutic purposes. Not to be used for routine venipuncture.	0.18	0.50	0.05	0.01	0.69	0.24	XXX	
36415		I	Routine venipuncture or finger/heel/ear stick for collection of specimen(s)	0.10	0.08	0.08	0.01	0.19	0.19	XXX	■
36420		A	Venipuncture, cutdown; under age 1 year	1.01	0.33	0.33	0.09	1.43	1.43	XXX	
36425		A	age 1 or over	0.76	3.44	0.17	0.05	4.25	0.98	XXX	
36430		A	Transfusion, blood or blood components	0.00	0.95	0.95	0.05	1.00	1.00	XXX	
36440		A	Push transfusion, blood, 2 years or under	1.03	0.31	0.31	0.08	1.42	1.42	XXX	
36450		A	Exchange transfusion, blood; newborn	2.23	0.71	0.71	0.16	3.10	3.10	XXX	
36455		A	other than newborn	2.43	0.97	0.97	0.10	3.50	3.50	XXX	
36460		A	Transfusion, intrauterine, fetal	6.59	2.55	2.55	0.56	9.70	9.70	XXX	
36468		R	Single or multiple injections of sclerosing solutions, spider veins (telangiectasia); limb or trunk	0.00	0.00	0.00	0.00	0.00	0.00	000	
36469		R	face	0.00	0.00	0.00	0.00	0.00	0.00	000	
36470		A	Injection of sclerosing solution; single vein	1.09	2.60	0.40	0.10	3.79	1.59	010	
36471		A	multiple veins, same leg	1.57	2.65	0.58	0.15	4.37	2.30	010	
36481		A	Percutaneous portal vein catheterization by any method	6.99	2.86	2.86	0.40	10.25	10.25	000	
36488		A	Placement of central venous catheter (subclavian, jugular, or other vein) (eg, for central venous pressure, hyperalimentation, hemodialysis, or chemotherapy); percutaneous, age 2 years or under	1.35	0.76	0.76	0.09	2.20	2.20	000	
36489		A	percutaneous, over age 2	2.50	4.70	1.08	0.08	7.28	3.66	000	
36490		A	cutdown, age 2 years or under	1.67	0.86	0.86	0.17	2.70	2.70	000	
36491		A	cutdown, over age 2	1.43	0.75	0.75	0.13	2.31	2.31	000	

■ RVU not developed by CMS. Gap-filled RVUs developed by Ingenix/CHEG.

Code	M	S	Description	Work Value	Non-Fac PE	Fac PE	Mal-practice	Non-Fac Total	Fac Total	Global	Gap
36493		A	Repositioning of previously placed central venous catheter under fluoroscopic guidance	1.21	0.88	0.88	0.06	2.15	2.15	000	
36500		A	Venous catheterization for selective organ blood sampling	3.52	1.31	1.31	0.14	4.97	4.97	000	
36510		A	Catheterization of umbilical vein for diagnosis or therapy, newborn	1.09	0.73	0.73	0.06	1.88	1.88	000	
36520		A	Therapeutic apheresis; plasma and/or cell exchange	1.74	1.07	1.07	0.06	2.87	2.87	000	
36521		A	with extracorporeal affinity column adsorption and plasma reinfusion	1.74	1.07	1.07	0.06	2.87	2.87	000	
36522		A	Photopheresis, extracorporeal	1.67	6.03	1.16	0.07	7.77	2.90	000	
36530		R	Insertion of implantable intravenous infusion pump	6.20	4.17	4.17	0.56	10.93	10.93	010	
36531		R	Revision of implantable intravenous infusion pump	4.87	3.32	3.32	0.44	8.63	8.63	010	
36532		R	Removal of implantable intravenous infusion pump	3.30	1.57	1.57	0.34	5.21	5.21	010	
36533		A	Insertion of implantable venous access device, with or without subcutaneous reservoir	5.32	4.67	3.50	0.49	10.48	9.31	010	
36534		A	Revision of implantable venous access device, and/or subcutaneous reservoir	2.80	1.55	1.55	0.19	4.54	4.54	010	
36535		A	Removal of implantable venous access device, and/or subcutaneous reservoir	2.27	2.95	1.89	0.21	5.43	4.37	010	
36540		B	Collection of blood specimen from a partially or completely implantable venous access device	0.23	0.18	0.18	0.02	0.44	0.44	XXX	■
36550		A	Declotting by thrombolytic agent of implanted vascular access device or catheter	0.00	0.38	0.38	0.31	0.69	0.69	XXX	
36600		A	Arterial puncture, withdrawal of blood for diagnosis	0.32	0.43	0.09	0.02	0.77	0.43	XXX	
36620		A	Arterial catheterization or cannulation for sampling, monitoring or transfusion (separate procedure); percutaneous	1.15	0.25	0.25	0.06	1.46	1.46	000	
36625		A	cutdown	2.11	0.61	0.61	0.16	2.88	2.88	000	
36640		A	Arterial catheterization for prolonged infusion therapy (chemotherapy), cutdown	2.10	0.75	0.75	0.18	3.03	3.03	000	
36660		A	Catheterization, umbilical artery, newborn, for diagnosis or therapy	1.40	0.38	0.38	0.08	1.86	1.86	000	
36680		A	Placement of needle for intraosseous infusion	1.20	0.66	0.66	0.08	1.94	1.94	000	
36800		A	Insertion of cannula for hemodialysis, other purpose (separate procedure); vein to vein	2.43	1.59	1.59	0.17	4.19	4.19	000	
36810		A	arteriovenous, external (Scribner type)	3.97	2.22	2.22	0.40	6.59	6.59	000	

■ RVU not developed by CMS. Gap-filled RVUs developed by Ingenix/CHEG.

Code	M	S	Description	Work Value	Non-Fac PE	Fac PE	Mal-practice	Non-Fac Total	Fac Total	Global	Gap
36815		A	arteriovenous, external revision, or closure	2.62	1.28	1.28	0.26	4.16	4.16	000	
36819		A	Arteriovenous anastomosis, open; by upper arm basilic vein transposition	14.00	6.56	6.56	1.53	22.09	22.09	090	
36820		A	by forearm vein transposition	14.00	6.56	6.56	1.53	22.09	22.09	090	
36821		A	direct, any site (eg, Cimino type) (separate procedure)	8.93	5.03	5.03	0.97	14.93	14.93	090	
36822		A	Insertion of cannula(s) for prolonged extracorporeal circulation for cardiopulmonary insufficiency (ECMO) (separate procedure)	5.42	6.81	6.81	0.63	12.86	12.86	090	
36823		A	Insertion of arterial and venous cannula(s) for isolated extracorporeal circulation including regional chemotherapy perfusion to an extremity, with or without hyperthermia, with removal of cannula(s) and repair of arteriotomy and venotomy sites	21.00	10.63	10.63	2.18	33.81	33.81	090	
36825		A	Creation of arteriovenous fistula by other than direct arteriovenous anastomosis (separate procedure); autogenous graft	9.84	5.58	5.58	1.09	16.51	16.51	090	
36830		A	nonautogenous graft	12.00	6.14	6.14	1.32	19.46	19.46	090	
36831		A	Thrombectomy, open, arteriovenous fistula without revision, autogenous or nonautogenous dialysis graft (separate procedure)	8.00	3.99	3.99	0.79	12.78	12.78	090	
36832		A	Revision, open, arteriovenous fistula; without thrombectomy, autogenous or nonautogenous dialysis graft (separate procedure)	10.50	5.59	5.59	1.13	17.22	17.22	090	
36833		A	with thrombectomy, autogenous or nonautogenous dialysis graft (separate procedure)	11.95	6.11	6.11	1.29	19.35	19.35	090	
36834		A	Plastic repair of arteriovenous aneurysm (separate procedure)	9.93	3.93	3.93	1.06	14.92	14.92	090	
36835		A	Insertion of Thomas shunt (separate procedure)	7.15	4.50	4.50	0.80	12.45	12.45	090	
36860		A	External cannula declotting (separate procedure); without balloon catheter	2.01	2.52	1.33	0.10	4.63	3.44	000	
36861		A	with balloon catheter	2.52	1.50	1.50	0.14	4.16	4.16	000	
36870		A	Thrombectomy, percutaneous, arteriovenous fistula, autogenous or nonautogenous graft (includes mechanical thrombus extraction and intra-graft thrombolysis)	5.16	41.63	2.45	0.23	47.02	7.84	090	
37140		A	Venous anastomosis; portocaval	23.60	10.56	10.56	1.21	35.37	35.37	090	
37145		A	renoportal	24.61	12.97	12.97	2.48	40.06	40.06	090	
37160		A	caval-mesenteric	21.60	9.43	9.43	2.16	33.19	33.19	090	

■ RVU not developed by CMS. Gap-filled RVUs developed by Ingenix/CHEG.

Code	M	S	Description	Work Value	Non-Fac PE	Fac PE	Mal-practice	Non-Fac Total	Fac Total	Global	Gap
37180		A	splenorenal, proximal	24.61	10.66	10.66	2.63	37.90	37.90	090	
37181		A	splenorenal, distal (selective decompression of esophagogastric varices, any technique)	26.68	11.02	11.02	2.67	40.37	40.37	090	
37195		A	Thrombolysis, cerebral, by intravenous infusion	0.00	7.65	7.65	0.38	8.03	8.03	XXX	
37200		A	Transcatheter biopsy	4.56	1.60	1.60	0.19	6.35	6.35	000	
37201		A	Transcatheter therapy, infusion for thrombolysis other than coronary	5.00	2.59	2.59	0.24	7.83	7.83	000	
37202		A	Transcatheter therapy, infusion other than for thrombolysis, any type (eg, spasmolytic, vasoconstrictive)	5.68	3.33	3.33	0.38	9.39	9.39	000	
37203		A	Transcatheter retrieval, percutaneous, of intravascular foreign body (eg, fractured venous or arterial catheter)	5.03	2.62	2.62	0.23	7.88	7.88	000	
37204		A	Transcatheter occlusion or embolization (eg, for tumor destruction, to achieve hemostasis, to occlude a vascular malformation), percutaneous, any method, non-central nervous system, non-head or neck	18.14	6.36	6.36	0.85	25.35	25.35	000	
37205		A	Transcatheter placement of an intravascular stent(s), (non-coronary vessel), percutaneous; initial vessel	8.28	3.90	3.90	0.43	12.61	12.61	000	
37206		A	each additional vessel (List separately in addition to code for primary procedure)	4.13	1.54	1.54	0.22	5.89	5.89	ZZZ	
37207		A	Transcatheter placement of an intravascular stent(s), (non-coronary vessel), open; initial vessel	8.28	3.61	3.61	0.89	12.78	12.78	000	
37208		A	each additional vessel (List separately in addition to code for primary procedure)	4.13	1.45	1.45	0.44	6.02	6.02	ZZZ	
37209		A	Exchange of a previously placed arterial catheter during thrombolytic therapy	2.27	0.80	0.80	0.11	3.18	3.18	000	
37250		A	Intravascular ultrasound (non-coronary vessel) during diagnostic evaluation and/or therapeutic intervention; initial vessel (List separately in addition to code for primary procedure)	2.10	0.79	0.79	0.17	3.06	3.06	ZZZ	
37251		A	each additional vessel (List separately in addition to code for primary procedure)	1.60	0.58	0.58	0.14	2.32	2.32	ZZZ	
37565		A	Ligation, internal jugular vein	10.88	5.34	5.34	0.45	16.67	16.67	090	
37600		A	Ligation; external carotid artery	11.25	6.51	6.51	0.40	18.16	18.16	090	
37605		A	internal or common carotid artery	13.11	6.63	6.63	0.77	20.51	20.51	090	
37606		A	internal or common carotid artery, with gradual occlusion, as with Selverstone or Crutchfield clamp	6.28	3.85	3.85	0.79	10.92	10.92	090	

■ RVU not developed by CMS. Gap-filled RVUs developed by Ingenix/CHEG.

Code	M	S	Description	Work Value	Non-Fac PE	Fac PE	Mal-practice	Non-Fac Total	Fac Total	Global	Gap
37607		A	Ligation or banding of angioaccess arteriovenous fistula	6.16	3.71	3.71	0.67	10.54	10.54	090	
37609		A	Ligation or biopsy, temporal artery	3.00	7.25	2.58	0.21	10.46	5.79	010	
37615		A	Ligation, major artery (eg, post-traumatic, rupture); neck	5.73	3.61	3.61	0.57	9.91	9.91	090	
37616		A	chest	16.49	10.54	10.54	1.93	28.96	28.96	090	
37617		A	abdomen	22.06	9.81	9.81	1.69	33.56	33.56	090	
37618		A	extremity	4.84	3.56	3.56	0.54	8.94	8.94	090	
37620		A	Interruption, partial or complete, of inferior vena cava by suture, ligation, plication, clip, extravascular, intravascular (umbrella device)	10.56	5.53	5.53	0.75	16.84	16.84	090	
37650		A	Ligation of femoral vein	7.80	4.64	4.64	0.56	13.00	13.00	090	
37660		A	Ligation of common iliac vein	21.00	9.44	9.44	1.17	31.61	31.61	090	
37700		A	Ligation and division of long saphenous vein at saphenofemoral junction, or distal interruptions	3.73	3.20	3.20	0.40	7.33	7.33	090	
37720		A	Ligation and division and complete stripping of long or short saphenous veins	5.66	3.72	3.72	0.61	9.99	9.99	090	
37730		A	Ligation and division and complete stripping of long and short saphenous veins	7.33	4.59	4.59	0.77	12.69	12.69	090	
37735		A	Ligation and division and complete stripping of long or short saphenous veins with radical excision of ulcer and skin graft and/or interruption of communicating veins of lower leg, with excision of deep fascia	10.53	5.94	5.94	1.17	17.64	17.64	090	
37760		A	Ligation of perforators, subfascial, radical (Linton type), with or without skin graft	10.47	5.78	5.78	1.11	17.36	17.36	090	
37780		A	Ligation and division of short saphenous vein at saphenopopliteal junction (separate procedure)	3.84	2.89	2.89	0.41	7.14	7.14	090	
37785		A	Ligation, division, and/or excision of recurrent or secondary varicose veins (clusters), one leg	3.84	7.18	2.91	0.41	11.43	7.16	090	
37788		A	Penile revascularization, artery, with or without vein graft	22.01	14.08	14.08	1.35	37.44	37.44	090	
37790		A	Penile venous occlusive procedure	8.34	6.78	6.78	0.63	15.75	15.75	090	
37799		C	Unlisted procedure, vascular surgery	0.00	0.00	0.00	0.00	0.00	0.00	YYY	
38100		A	Splenectomy; total (separate procedure)	14.50	6.73	6.73	1.30	22.53	22.53	090	
38101		A	partial (separate procedure)	15.31	7.27	7.27	1.38	23.96	23.96	090	
38102		A	total, en bloc for extensive disease, in conjunction with other procedure (List in addition to code for primary procedure)	4.80	1.73	1.73	0.49	7.02	7.02	ZZZ	

■ RVU not developed by CMS. Gap-filled RVUs developed by Ingenix/CHEG.

Code	M	S	Description	Work Value	Non-Fac PE	Fac PE	Mal-practice	Non-Fac Total	Fac Total	Global	Gap
38115		A	Repair of ruptured spleen (splenorrhaphy) with or without partial splenectomy	15.82	7.23	7.23	1.40	24.45	24.45	090	
38120		A	Laparoscopy, surgical, splenectomy	17.00	7.58	7.58	1.73	26.31	26.31	090	
38129		C	Unlisted laparoscopy procedure, spleen	0.00	0.00	0.00	0.00	0.00	0.00	YYY	
38200		A	Injection procedure for splenoportography	2.64	0.93	0.93	0.12	3.69	3.69	000	
38220		A	Bone marrow aspiration	1.08	4.64	0.44	0.03	5.75	1.55	XXX	
38221		A	Bone marrow biopsy, needle or trocar	1.37	4.74	0.56	0.04	6.15	1.97	XXX	
38230		R	Bone marrow harvesting for transplantation	4.54	2.45	2.45	0.25	7.24	7.24	010	
38231		R	Blood-derived peripheral stem cell harvesting for transplantation, per collection	1.50	0.61	0.61	0.05	2.16	2.16	000	
38240		R	Bone marrow or blood-derived peripheral stem cell transplantation; allogenic	2.24	0.88	0.88	0.08	3.20	3.20	XXX	
38241		R	autologous	2.24	0.86	0.86	0.08	3.18	3.18	XXX	
38300		A	Drainage of lymph node abscess or lymphadenitis; simple	1.99	4.88	2.65	0.15	7.02	4.79	010	
38305		A	extensive	6.00	7.99	6.41	0.36	14.35	12.77	090	
38308		A	Lymphangiotomy or other operations on lymphatic channels	6.45	5.40	5.40	0.51	12.36	12.36	090	
38380		A	Suture and/or ligation of thoracic duct; cervical approach	7.46	7.61	7.61	0.68	15.75	15.75	090	
38381		A	thoracic approach	12.88	9.72	9.72	1.58	24.18	24.18	090	
38382		A	abdominal approach	10.08	8.81	8.81	1.08	19.97	19.97	090	
38500		A	Biopsy or excision of lymph node(s); open, superficial	3.75	3.15	2.63	0.28	7.18	6.66	010	
38505		A	by needle, superficial (eg, cervical, inguinal, axillary)	1.14	3.21	1.13	0.09	4.44	2.36	000	
38510		A	open, deep cervical node(s)	6.43	5.55	5.55	0.38	12.36	12.36	010	
38520		A	open, deep cervical node(s) with excision scalene fat pad	6.67	5.67	5.67	0.52	12.86	12.86	090	
38525		A	open, deep axillary node(s)	6.07	4.51	4.51	0.48	11.06	11.06	090	
38530		A	open, internal mammary node(s)	7.98	5.78	5.78	0.63	14.39	14.39	090	
38542		A	Dissection, deep jugular node(s)	5.91	6.09	6.09	0.50	12.50	12.50	090	
38550		A	Excision of cystic hygroma, axillary or cervical; without deep neurovascular dissection	6.92	5.01	5.01	0.69	12.62	12.62	090	
38555		A	with deep neurovascular dissection	14.14	9.47	9.47	1.46	25.07	25.07	090	

■ RVU not developed by CMS. Gap-filled RVUs developed by Ingenix/CHEG.

Code	M	S	Description	Work Value	Non-Fac PE	Fac PE	Mal-prac-tice	Non-Fac Total	Fac Total	Global	Gap
38562		A	Limited lymphadenectomy for staging (separate procedure); pelvic and para-aortic	10.49	6.79	6.79	0.97	18.25	18.25	090	
38564		A	retroperitoneal (aortic and/or splenic)	10.83	6.54	6.54	1.06	18.43	18.43	090	
38570		A	Laparoscopy, surgical; with retroperitoneal lymph node sampling (biopsy), single or multiple	9.25	4.63	4.63	0.89	14.77	14.77	010	
38571		A	with bilateral total pelvic lymphadenectomy	14.68	6.50	6.50	0.80	21.98	21.98	010	
38572		A	with bilateral total pelvic lymphadenectomy and peri-aortic lymph node sampling (biopsy), single or multiple	16.59	7.71	7.71	1.32	25.62	25.62	010	
38589		C	Unlisted laparoscopy procedure, lymphatic system	0.00	0.00	0.00	0.00	0.00	0.00	YYY	
38700		A	Suprahyoid lymphadenectomy	8.24	13.61	13.61	0.60	22.45	22.45	090	
38720		A	Cervical lymphadenectomy (complete)	13.61	16.25	16.25	1.03	30.89	30.89	090	
38724		A	Cervical lymphadenectomy (modified radical neck dissection)	14.54	16.82	16.82	1.10	32.46	32.46	090	
38740		A	Axillary lymphadenectomy; superficial	10.03	5.89	5.89	0.69	16.61	16.61	090	
38745		A	complete	13.10	8.47	8.47	0.90	22.47	22.47	090	
38746		A	Thoracic lymphadenectomy, regional, including mediastinal and peritracheal nodes (List in addition to code for primary procedure)	4.89	1.65	1.65	0.55	7.09	7.09	ZZZ	
38747		A	Abdominal lymphadenectomy, regional, including celiac, gastric, portal, peripancreatic, with or without para-aortic and vena caval nodes (List separately in addition to code for primary procedure)	4.89	1.75	1.75	0.50	7.14	7.14	ZZZ	
38760		A	Inguinofemoral lymphadenectomy, superficial, including Cloquet's node (separate procedure)	12.95	7.36	7.36	0.88	21.19	21.19	090	
38765		A	Inguinofemoral lymphadenectomy, superficial, in continuity with pelvic lymphadenectomy, including external iliac, hypogastric, and obturator nodes (separate procedure)	19.98	11.57	11.57	1.50	33.05	33.05	090	
38770		A	Pelvic lymphadenectomy, including external iliac, hypogastric, and obturator nodes (separate procedure)	13.23	7.18	7.18	0.94	21.35	21.35	090	
38780		A	Retroperitoneal transabdominal lymphadenectomy, extensive, including pelvic, aortic, and renal nodes (separate procedure)	16.59	9.67	9.67	1.60	27.86	27.86	090	
38790		A	Injection procedure; lymphangiography	1.29	14.77	0.46	0.09	16.15	1.84	000	
38792		A	for identification of sentinel node	0.52	0.19	0.19	0.04	0.75	0.75	000	
38794		A	Cannulation, thoracic duct	4.45	1.57	1.57	0.17	6.19	6.19	090	

■ RVU not developed by CMS. Gap-filled RVUs developed by Ingenix/CHEG.

Surgery

Code	M	S	Description	Work Value	Non-Fac PE	Fac PE	Mal-practice	Non-Fac Total	Fac Total	Global	Gap
38999		C	Unlisted procedure, hemic or lymphatic system	0.00	0.00	0.00	0.00	0.00	0.00	YYY	
39000		A	Mediastinotomy with exploration, drainage, removal of foreign body, or biopsy; cervical approach	6.10	7.41	7.41	0.73	14.24	14.24	090	
39010		A	transthoracic approach, including either transthoracic or median sternotomy	11.79	9.31	9.31	1.46	22.56	22.56	090	
39200		A	Excision of mediastinal cyst	13.62	10.10	10.10	1.65	25.37	25.37	090	
39220		A	Excision of mediastinal tumor	17.42	11.29	11.29	2.10	30.81	30.81	090	
39400		A	Mediastinoscopy, with or without biopsy	5.61	7.01	7.01	0.69	13.31	13.31	010	
39499		C	Unlisted procedure, mediastinum	0.00	0.00	0.00	0.00	0.00	0.00	YYY	
39501		A	Repair, laceration of diaphragm, any approach	13.19	7.82	7.82	1.38	22.39	22.39	090	
39502		A	Repair, paraesophageal hiatus hernia, transabdominal, with or without fundoplasty, vagotomy, and/or pyloroplasty, except neonatal	16.33	8.41	8.41	1.68	26.42	26.42	090	
39503		A	Repair, neonatal diaphragmatic hernia, with or without chest tube insertion and with or without creation of ventral hernia	95.00	37.24	37.24	3.52	135.76	135.76	090	
39520		A	Repair, diaphragmatic hernia (esophageal hiatal); transthoracic	16.10	9.59	9.59	1.83	27.52	27.52	090	
39530		A	combined, thoracoabdominal	15.41	8.69	8.69	1.66	25.76	25.76	090	
39531		A	combined, thoracoabdominal, with dilation of stricture (with or without gastroplasty)	16.42	8.45	8.45	1.83	26.70	26.70	090	
39540		A	Repair, diaphragmatic hernia (other than neonatal), traumatic; acute	13.32	7.79	7.79	1.38	22.49	22.49	090	
39541		A	chronic	14.41	7.97	7.97	1.52	23.90	23.90	090	
39545		A	Imbrication of diaphragm for eventration, transthoracic or transabdominal, paralytic or nonparalytic	13.37	9.32	9.32	1.55	24.24	24.24	090	
39560		A	Resection, diaphragm; with simple repair (eg, primary suture)	12.00	7.62	7.62	1.35	20.97	20.97	090	
39561		A	with complex repair (eg, prosthetic material, local muscle flap)	17.50	9.84	9.84	1.97	29.31	29.31	090	
39599		C	Unlisted procedure, diaphragm	0.00	0.00	0.00	0.00	0.00	0.00	YYY	

Surgery

■ RVU not developed by CMS. Gap-filled RVUs developed by Ingenix/CHEG.

Code	M	S	Description	Work Value	Non-Fac PE	Fac PE	Mal-prac-tice	Non-Fac Total	Fac Total	Global	Gap
40490		A	Biopsy of lip	1.22	1.63	0.63	0.06	2.91	1.91	000	
40500		A	Vermilionectomy (lip shave), with mucosal advancement	4.28	5.72	5.72	0.31	10.31	10.31	090	
40510		A	Excision of lip; transverse wedge excision with primary closure	4.70	6.75	6.52	0.38	11.83	11.60	090	
40520		A	V-excision with primary direct linear closure	4.67	7.97	7.15	0.42	13.06	12.24	090	
40525		A	full thickness, reconstruction with local flap (eg, Estlander or fan)	7.55	8.84	8.84	0.68	17.07	17.07	090	
40527		A	full thickness, reconstruction with cross lip flap (Abbe-Estlander)	9.13	9.60	9.60	0.82	19.55	19.55	090	
40530		A	Resection of lip, more than one-fourth, without reconstruction	5.40	7.35	6.56	0.47	13.22	12.43	090	
40650		A	Repair lip, full thickness; vermilion only	3.64	5.78	5.18	0.31	9.73	9.13	090	
40652		A	up to half vertical height	4.26	7.08	7.04	0.39	11.73	11.69	090	
40654		A	over one-half vertical height, or complex	5.31	7.95	7.95	0.48	13.74	13.74	090	
40700		A	Plastic repair of cleft lip/nasal deformity; primary, partial or complete, unilateral	12.79	10.88	10.88	0.93	24.60	24.60	090	
40701		A	primary bilateral, one stage procedure	15.85	14.66	14.66	1.36	31.87	31.87	090	
40702		A	primary bilateral, one of two stages	13.04	8.99	8.99	1.01	23.04	23.04	090	
40720		A	secondary, by recreation of defect and reclosure	13.55	12.89	12.89	1.31	27.75	27.75	090	
40761		A	with cross lip pedicle flap (Abbe-Estlander type), including sectioning and inserting of pedicle	14.72	12.76	12.76	1.41	28.89	28.89	090	
40799		C	Unlisted procedure, lips	0.00	0.00	0.00	0.00	0.00	0.00	YYY	
40800		A	Drainage of abscess, cyst, hematoma, vestibule of mouth; simple	1.17	2.01	0.48	0.09	3.27	1.74	010	
40801		A	complicated	2.53	2.52	1.98	0.18	5.23	4.69	010	
40804		A	Removal of embedded foreign body, vestibule of mouth; simple	1.24	2.59	2.03	0.09	3.92	3.36	010	
40805		A	complicated	2.69	3.27	2.85	0.17	6.13	5.71	010	
40806		A	Incision of labial frenum (frenotomy)	0.31	0.89	0.89	0.02	1.22	1.22	000	
40808		A	Biopsy, vestibule of mouth	0.96	2.11	2.11	0.07	3.14	3.14	010	
40810		A	Excision of lesion of mucosa and submucosa, vestibule of mouth; without repair	1.31	2.70	2.47	0.09	4.10	3.87	010	

Surgery

■ RVU not developed by CMS. Gap-filled RVUs developed by Ingenix/CHEG.

Code	M	S	Description	Work Value	Non-Fac PE	Fac PE	Mal-practice	Non-Fac Total	Fac Total	Global	Gap
40812		A	with simple repair	2.31	2.95	2.93	0.17	5.43	5.41	010	
40814		A	with complex repair	3.42	4.08	4.08	0.26	7.76	7.76	090	
40816		A	complex, with excision of underlying muscle	3.67	4.32	4.32	0.27	8.26	8.26	090	
40818		A	Excision of mucosa of vestibule of mouth as donor graft	2.41	4.05	4.05	0.14	6.60	6.60	090	
40819		A	Excision of frenum, labial or buccal (frenumectomy, frenulectomy, frenectomy)	2.41	3.67	3.48	0.17	6.25	6.06	090	
40820		A	Destruction of lesion or scar of vestibule of mouth by physical methods (eg, laser, thermal, cryo, chemical)	1.28	2.38	2.30	0.08	3.74	3.66	010	
40830		A	Closure of laceration, vestibule of mouth; 2.5 cm or less	1.76	2.48	2.48	0.14	4.38	4.38	010	
40831		A	over 2.5 cm or complex	2.46	2.72	2.72	0.21	5.39	5.39	010	
40840		R	Vestibuloplasty; anterior	8.73	5.93	5.93	0.79	15.45	15.45	090	
40842		R	posterior, unilateral	8.73	5.90	5.90	0.65	15.28	15.28	090	
40843		R	posterior, bilateral	12.10	7.35	7.35	0.84	20.29	20.29	090	
40844		R	entire arch	16.01	9.01	9.01	1.63	26.65	26.65	090	
40845		R	complex (including ridge extension, muscle repositioning)	18.58	12.25	12.25	1.47	32.30	32.30	090	
40899		C	Unlisted procedure, vestibule of mouth	0.00	0.00	0.00	0.00	0.00	0.00	YYY	
41000		A	Intraoral incision and drainage of abscess, cyst, or hematoma of tongue or floor of mouth; lingual	1.30	2.40	1.55	0.09	3.79	2.94	010	
41005		A	sublingual, superficial	1.26	2.33	1.62	0.09	3.68	2.97	010	
41006		A	sublingual, deep, supramylohyoid	3.24	3.58	3.28	0.25	7.07	6.77	090	
41007		A	submental space	3.10	3.78	3.33	0.22	7.10	6.65	090	
41008		A	submandibular space	3.37	3.69	3.22	0.24	7.30	6.83	090	
41009		A	masticator space	3.59	3.65	3.42	0.25	7.49	7.26	090	
41010		A	Incision of lingual frenum (frenotomy)	1.06	3.57	3.57	0.06	4.69	4.69	010	
41015		A	Extraoral incision and drainage of abscess, cyst, or hematoma of floor of mouth; sublingual	3.96	4.05	3.39	0.29	8.30	7.64	090	
41016		A	submental	4.07	4.31	3.61	0.28	8.66	7.96	090	
41017		A	submandibular	4.07	4.26	3.46	0.32	8.65	7.85	090	
41018		A	masticator space	5.10	4.39	3.87	0.35	9.84	9.32	090	
41100		A	Biopsy of tongue; anterior two-thirds	1.63	2.67	2.64	0.12	4.42	4.39	010	

■ RVU not developed by CMS. Gap-filled RVUs developed by Ingenix/CHEG.

Code	M	S	Description	Work Value	Non-Fac PE	Fac PE	Mal-practice	Non-Fac Total	Fac Total	Global	Gap
41105		A	posterior one-third	1.42	2.42	2.42	0.10	3.94	3.94	010	
41108		A	Biopsy of floor of mouth	1.05	2.38	2.38	0.08	3.51	3.51	010	
41110		A	Excision of lesion of tongue without closure	1.51	3.19	2.63	0.11	4.81	4.25	010	
41112		A	Excision of lesion of tongue with closure; anterior two-thirds	2.73	3.56	3.56	0.20	6.49	6.49	090	
41113		A	posterior one-third	3.19	3.50	3.50	0.23	6.92	6.92	090	
41114		A	with local tongue flap	8.47	6.59	6.59	0.64	15.70	15.70	090	
41115		A	Excision of lingual frenum (frenectomy)	1.74	2.69	2.53	0.13	4.56	4.40	010	
41116		A	Excision, lesion of floor of mouth	2.44	3.37	3.37	0.17	5.98	5.98	090	
41120		A	Glossectomy; less than one-half tongue	9.77	9.12	9.12	0.70	19.59	19.59	090	
41130		A	hemiglossectomy	11.15	9.76	9.76	0.81	21.72	21.72	090	
41135		A	partial, with unilateral radical neck dissection	23.09	16.63	16.63	1.66	41.38	41.38	090	
41140		A	complete or total, with or without tracheostomy, without radical neck dissection	25.50	17.39	17.39	1.85	44.74	44.74	090	
41145		A	complete or total, with or without tracheostomy, with unilateral radical neck dissection	30.06	21.36	21.36	2.11	53.53	53.53	090	
41150		A	composite procedure with resection floor of mouth and mandibular resection, without radical neck dissection	23.04	17.64	17.64	1.67	42.35	42.35	090	
41153		A	composite procedure with resection floor of mouth, with suprahyoid neck dissection	23.77	18.04	18.04	1.71	43.52	43.52	090	
41155		A	composite procedure with resection floor of mouth, mandibular resection, and radical neck dissection (Commando type)	27.72	20.44	20.44	2.02	50.18	50.18	090	
41250		A	Repair of laceration 2.5 cm or less; floor of mouth and/or anterior two-thirds of tongue	1.91	2.98	1.77	0.15	5.04	3.83	010	
41251		A	posterior one-third of tongue	2.27	3.12	1.88	0.18	5.57	4.33	010	
41252		A	Repair of laceration of tongue, floor of mouth, over 2.6 cm or complex	2.97	3.23	2.33	0.23	6.43	5.53	010	
41500		A	Fixation of tongue, mechanical, other than suture (eg, K-wire)	3.71	4.43	4.43	0.26	8.40	8.40	090	
41510		A	Suture of tongue to lip for micrognathia (Douglas type procedure)	3.42	5.39	5.39	0.24	9.05	9.05	090	
41520		A	Frenoplasty (surgical revision of frenum, eg, with Z-plasty)	2.73	3.06	3.06	0.19	5.98	5.98	090	
41599		C	Unlisted procedure, tongue, floor of mouth	0.00	0.00	0.00	0.00	0.00	0.00	YYY	

Surgery

■ RVU not developed by CMS. Gap-filled RVUs developed by Ingenix/CHEG.

Code	M	S	Description	Work Value	Non-Fac PE	Fac PE	Mal-practice	Non-Fac Total	Fac Total	Global	Gap
41800		A	Drainage of abscess, cyst, hematoma from dentoalveolar structures	1.17	1.96	1.43	0.09	3.22	2.69	010	
41805		A	Removal of embedded foreign body from dentoalveolar structures; soft tissues	1.24	2.08	2.08	0.09	3.41	3.41	010	
41806		A	bone	2.69	2.54	2.54	0.22	5.45	5.45	010	
41820		R	Gingivectomy, excision gingiva, each quadrant	2.81	2.23	2.23	0.30	5.34	5.34	000	■
41821		R	Operculectomy, excision pericoronal tissues	0.63	0.50	0.50	0.07	1.20	1.20	000	■
41822		R	Excision of fibrous tuberosities, dentoalveolar structures	2.31	2.82	0.98	0.24	5.37	3.53	010	
41823		R	Excision of osseous tuberosities, dentoalveolar structures	3.30	3.54	3.23	0.29	7.13	6.82	090	
41825		A	Excision of lesion or tumor (except listed above), dentoalveolar structures; without repair	1.31	2.43	2.41	0.10	3.84	3.82	010	
41826		A	with simple repair	2.31	2.66	2.66	0.17	5.14	5.14	010	
41827		A	with complex repair	3.42	3.63	3.63	0.25	7.30	7.30	090	
41828		R	Excision of hyperplastic alveolar mucosa, each quadrant (specify)	3.09	3.07	2.47	0.22	6.38	5.78	010	
41830		R	Alveolectomy, including curettage of osteitis or sequestrectomy	3.35	3.39	2.98	0.23	6.97	6.56	010	
41850		R	Destruction of lesion (except excision), dentoalveolar structures	1.40	1.12	1.12	0.15	2.67	2.67	000	■
41870		R	Periodontal mucosal grafting	3.51	2.79	2.79	0.37	6.67	6.67	000	■
41872		R	Gingivoplasty, each quadrant (specify)	2.59	2.93	2.93	0.18	5.70	5.70	090	
41874		R	Alveoloplasty, each quadrant (specify)	3.09	2.86	2.45	0.23	6.18	5.77	090	
41899		C	Unlisted procedure, dentoalveolar structures	0.00	0.00	0.00	0.00	0.00	0.00	YYY	
42000		A	Drainage of abscess of palate, uvula	1.23	2.52	1.51	0.10	3.85	2.84	010	
42100		A	Biopsy of palate, uvula	1.31	2.47	2.47	0.10	3.88	3.88	010	
42104		A	Excision, lesion of palate, uvula; without closure	1.64	2.58	2.58	0.12	4.34	4.34	010	
42106		A	with simple primary closure	2.10	2.66	2.66	0.16	4.92	4.92	010	
42107		A	with local flap closure	4.44	4.26	4.26	0.32	9.02	9.02	090	
42120		A	Resection of palate or extensive resection of lesion	6.17	6.19	6.19	0.44	12.80	12.80	090	
42140		A	Uvulectomy, excision of uvula	1.62	3.91	3.36	0.12	5.65	5.10	090	
42145		A	Palatopharyngoplasty (eg, uvulopalatopharyngoplasty, uvulopharyngoplasty)	8.05	7.59	7.59	0.56	16.20	16.20	090	

■ RVU not developed by CMS. Gap-filled RVUs developed by Ingenix/CHEG.

Surgery

Code	M	S	Description	Work Value	Non-Fac PE	Fac PE	Mal-practice	Non-Fac Total	Fac Total	Global	Gap
42160		A	Destruction of lesion, palate or uvula (thermal, cryo or chemical)	1.80	3.25	2.72	0.13	5.18	4.65	010	
42180		A	Repair, laceration of palate; up to 2 cm	2.50	3.29	2.25	0.19	5.98	4.94	010	
42182		A	over 2 cm or complex	3.83	3.10	3.10	0.27	7.20	7.20	010	
42200		A	Palatoplasty for cleft palate, soft and/or hard palate only	12.00	9.78	9.78	0.97	22.75	22.75	090	
42205		A	Palatoplasty for cleft palate, with closure of alveolar ridge; soft tissue only	13.29	9.76	9.76	0.82	23.87	23.87	090	
42210		A	with bone graft to alveolar ridge (includes obtaining graft)	14.50	11.47	11.47	1.24	27.21	27.21	090	
42215		A	Palatoplasty for cleft palate; major revision	8.82	9.72	9.72	0.96	19.50	19.50	090	
42220		A	secondary lengthening procedure	7.02	6.85	6.85	0.41	14.28	14.28	090	
42225		A	attachment pharyngeal flap	9.54	9.16	9.16	0.75	19.45	19.45	090	
42226		A	Lengthening of palate, and pharyngeal flap	10.01	9.96	9.96	0.73	20.70	20.70	090	
42227		A	Lengthening of palate, with island flap	9.52	9.09	9.09	0.70	19.31	19.31	090	
42235		A	Repair of anterior palate, including vomer flap	7.87	5.93	5.93	0.49	14.29	14.29	090	
42260		A	Repair of nasolabial fistula	9.80	6.43	6.43	0.85	17.08	17.08	090	
42280		A	Maxillary impression for palatal prosthesis	1.54	1.44	0.60	0.12	3.10	2.26	010	
42281		A	Insertion of pin-retained palatal prosthesis	1.93	1.57	0.92	0.14	3.64	2.99	010	
42299		C	Unlisted procedure, palate, uvula	0.00	0.00	0.00	0.00	0.00	0.00	YYY	
42300		A	Drainage of abscess; parotid, simple	1.93	2.65	1.98	0.15	4.73	4.06	010	
42305		A	parotid, complicated	6.07	5.38	5.38	0.46	11.91	11.91	090	
42310		A	Drainage of abscess; submaxillary or sublingual, intraoral	1.56	2.32	1.82	0.11	3.99	3.49	010	
42320		A	submaxillary, external	2.35	2.79	2.15	0.17	5.31	4.67	010	
42325		A	Fistulization of sublingual salivary cyst (ranula);	2.75	3.85	1.26	0.17	6.77	4.18	090	
42326		A	with prosthesis	3.78	3.33	1.51	0.34	7.45	5.63	090	
42330		A	Sialolithotomy; submandibular (submaxillary), sublingual or parotid, uncomplicated, intraoral	2.21	2.81	1.20	0.16	5.18	3.57	010	
42335		A	submandibular (submaxillary), complicated, intraoral	3.31	3.71	3.71	0.23	7.25	7.25	090	
42340		A	parotid, extraoral or complicated intraoral	4.60	5.07	5.07	0.34	10.01	10.01	090	
42400		A	Biopsy of salivary gland; needle	0.78	2.52	0.40	0.06	3.36	1.24	000	
42405		A	incisional	3.29	3.44	3.44	0.24	6.97	6.97	010	

Surgery

■ RVU not developed by CMS. Gap-filled RVUs developed by Ingenix/CHEG.

Code	M	S	Description	Work Value	Non-Fac PE	Fac PE	Mal-practice	Non-Fac Total	Fac Total	Global	Gap
42408		A	Excision of sublingual salivary cyst (ranula)	4.54	4.71	4.71	0.34	9.59	9.59	090	
42409		A	Marsupialization of sublingual salivary cyst (ranula)	2.81	3.34	3.34	0.20	6.35	6.35	090	
42410		A	Excision of parotid tumor or parotid gland; lateral lobe, without nerve dissection	9.34	8.20	8.20	0.77	18.31	18.31	090	
42415		A	lateral lobe, with dissection and preservation of facial nerve	16.89	12.82	12.82	1.26	30.97	30.97	090	
42420		A	total, with dissection and preservation of facial nerve	19.59	14.46	14.46	1.45	35.50	35.50	090	
42425		A	total, en bloc removal with sacrifice of facial nerve	13.02	10.70	10.70	0.98	24.70	24.70	090	
42426		A	total, with unilateral radical neck dissection	21.26	15.44	15.44	1.57	38.27	38.27	090	
42440		A	Excision of submandibular (submaxillary) gland	6.97	6.13	6.13	0.51	13.61	13.61	090	
42450		A	Excision of sublingual gland	4.62	4.38	4.38	0.34	9.34	9.34	090	
42500		A	Plastic repair of salivary duct, sialodochoplasty; primary or simple	4.30	5.14	5.10	0.30	9.74	9.70	090	
42505		A	secondary or complicated	6.18	6.02	6.02	0.44	12.64	12.64	090	
42507		A	Parotid duct diversion, bilateral (Wilke type procedure);	6.11	5.44	5.44	0.66	12.21	12.21	090	
42508		A	with excision of one submandibular gland	9.10	8.40	8.40	0.64	18.14	18.14	090	
42509		A	with excision of both submandibular glands	11.54	9.25	9.25	1.24	22.03	22.03	090	
42510		A	with ligation of both submandibular (Wharton's) ducts	8.15	7.27	7.27	0.57	15.99	15.99	090	
42550		A	Injection procedure for sialography	1.25	12.45	0.44	0.06	13.76	1.75	000	
42600		A	Closure salivary fistula	4.82	7.89	5.61	0.34	13.05	10.77	090	
42650		A	Dilation salivary duct	0.77	1.13	0.41	0.06	1.96	1.24	000	
42660		A	Dilation and catheterization of salivary duct, with or without injection	1.13	1.15	1.15	0.07	2.35	2.35	000	
42665		A	Ligation salivary duct, intraoral	2.53	3.03	3.03	0.17	5.73	5.73	090	
42699		C	Unlisted procedure, salivary glands or ducts	0.00	0.00	0.00	0.00	0.00	0.00	YYY	
42700		A	Incision and drainage abscess; peritonsillar	1.62	3.30	1.93	0.12	5.04	3.67	010	
42720		A	retropharyngeal or parapharyngeal, intraoral approach	5.42	4.77	4.77	0.39	10.58	10.58	010	
42725		A	retropharyngeal or parapharyngeal, external approach	10.72	8.70	8.70	0.80	20.22	20.22	090	

■ RVU not developed by CMS. Gap-filled RVUs developed by Ingenix/CHEG.

Code	M	S	Description	Work Value	Non-Fac PE	Fac PE	Mal-practice	Non-Fac Total	Fac Total	Global	Gap
42800		A	Biopsy; oropharynx	1.39	3.09	2.63	0.10	4.58	4.12	010	
42802		A	hypopharynx	1.54	3.24	2.72	0.11	4.89	4.37	010	
42804		A	nasopharynx, visible lesion, simple	1.24	3.04	2.56	0.09	4.37	3.89	010	
42806		A	nasopharynx, survey for unknown primary lesion	1.58	3.53	2.76	0.12	5.23	4.46	010	
42808		A	Excision or destruction of lesion of pharynx, any method	2.30	5.00	3.17	0.17	7.47	5.64	010	
42809		A	Removal of foreign body from pharynx	1.81	3.48	1.77	0.13	5.42	3.71	010	
42810		A	Excision branchial cleft cyst or vestige, confined to skin and subcutaneous tissues	3.25	5.66	4.61	0.25	9.16	8.11	090	
42815		A	Excision branchial cleft cyst, vestige, or fistula, extending beneath subcutaneous tissues and/or into pharynx	7.07	6.67	6.67	0.53	14.27	14.27	090	
42820		A	Tonsillectomy and adenoidectomy; under age 12	3.91	4.02	4.02	0.28	8.21	8.21	090	
42821		A	age 12 or over	4.29	4.30	4.30	0.30	8.89	8.89	090	
42825		A	Tonsillectomy, primary or secondary; under age 12	3.42	3.74	3.74	0.24	7.40	7.40	090	
42826		A	age 12 or over	3.38	3.81	3.81	0.23	7.42	7.42	090	
42830		A	Adenoidectomy, primary; under age 12	2.57	2.51	2.51	0.18	5.26	5.26	090	
42831		A	age 12 or over	2.71	2.59	2.59	0.19	5.49	5.49	090	
42835		A	Adenoidectomy, secondary; under age 12	2.30	3.20	3.20	0.17	5.67	5.67	090	
42836		A	age 12 or over	3.18	3.69	3.69	0.22	7.09	7.09	090	
42842		A	Radical resection of tonsil, tonsillar pillars, and/or retromolar trigone; without closure	8.76	7.96	7.96	0.61	17.33	17.33	090	
42844		A	closure with local flap (eg, tongue, buccal)	14.31	11.57	11.57	1.04	26.92	26.92	090	
42845		A	closure with other flap	24.29	18.00	18.00	1.76	44.05	44.05	090	
42860		A	Excision of tonsil tags	2.22	3.08	3.08	0.16	5.46	5.46	090	
42870		A	Excision or destruction lingual tonsil, any method (separate procedure)	5.40	6.18	6.18	0.38	11.96	11.96	090	
42890		A	Limited pharyngectomy	12.94	11.03	11.03	0.91	24.88	24.88	090	
42892		A	Resection of lateral pharyngeal wall or pyriform sinus, direct closure by advancement of lateral and posterior pharyngeal walls	15.83	12.68	12.68	1.14	29.65	29.65	090	
42894		A	Resection of pharyngeal wall requiring closure with myocutaneous flap	22.88	17.38	17.38	1.64	41.90	41.90	090	
42900		A	Suture pharynx for wound or injury	5.25	3.93	3.93	0.39	9.57	9.57	010	

■ RVU not developed by CMS. Gap-filled RVUs developed by Ingenix/CHEG.

Code	M	S	Description	Work Value	Non-Fac PE	Fac PE	Mal-practice	Non-Fac Total	Fac Total	Global	Gap
42950		A	Pharyngoplasty (plastic or reconstructive operation on pharynx)	8.10	7.60	7.60	0.58	16.28	16.28	090	
42953		A	Pharyngoesophageal repair	8.96	9.14	9.14	0.73	18.83	18.83	090	
42955		A	Pharyngostomy (fistulization of pharynx, external for feeding)	7.39	6.55	6.55	0.63	14.57	14.57	090	
42960		A	Control oropharyngeal hemorrhage, primary or secondary (eg, post-tonsillectomy); simple	2.33	2.13	2.13	0.17	4.63	4.63	010	
42961		A	complicated, requiring hospitalization	5.59	5.30	5.30	0.40	11.29	11.29	090	
42962		A	with secondary surgical intervention	7.14	6.35	6.35	0.51	14.00	14.00	090	
42970		A	Control of nasopharyngeal hemorrhage, primary or secondary (eg, postadenoidectomy); simple, with posterior nasal packs, with or without anterior packs and/or cautery	5.43	3.99	3.99	0.37	9.79	9.79	090	
42971		A	complicated, requiring hospitalization	6.21	5.99	5.99	0.45	12.65	12.65	090	
42972		A	with secondary surgical intervention	7.20	5.73	5.73	0.54	13.47	13.47	090	
42999		C	Unlisted procedure, pharynx, adenoids, or tonsils	0.00	0.00	0.00	0.00	0.00	0.00	YYY	
43020		A	Esophagotomy, cervical approach, with removal of foreign body	8.09	6.77	6.77	0.70	15.56	15.56	090	
43030		A	Cricopharyngeal myotomy	7.69	7.00	7.00	0.60	15.29	15.29	090	
43045		A	Esophagotomy, thoracic approach, with removal of foreign body	20.12	11.14	11.14	2.15	33.41	33.41	090	
43100		A	Excision of lesion, esophagus, with primary repair; cervical approach	9.19	7.58	7.58	0.79	17.56	17.56	090	
43101		A	thoracic or abdominal approach	16.24	8.84	8.84	1.81	26.89	26.89	090	
43107		A	Total or near total esophagectomy, without thoracotomy; with pharyngogastrostomy or cervical esophagogastrostomy, with or without pyloroplasty (transhiatal)	40.00	18.49	18.49	3.29	61.78	61.78	090	
43108		A	with colon interposition or small intestine reconstruction, including intestine mobilization, preparation and anastomosis(es)	34.19	16.39	16.39	3.78	54.36	54.36	090	
43112		A	Total or near total esophagectomy, with thoracotomy; with pharyngogastrostomy or cervical esophagogastrostomy, with or without pyloroplasty	43.50	20.06	20.06	3.67	67.23	67.23	090	
43113		A	with colon interposition or small intestine reconstruction, including intestine mobilization, preparation, and anastomosis(es)	35.27	16.38	16.38	4.33	55.98	55.98	090	

■ RVU not developed by CMS. Gap-filled RVUs developed by Ingenix/CHEG.

Code	M	S	Description	Work Value	Non-Fac PE	Fac PE	Mal-prac-tice	Non-Fac Total	Fac Total	Global	Gap
43116		A	Partial esophagectomy, cervical, with free intestinal graft, including microvascular anastomosis, obtaining the graft and intestinal reconstruction	31.22	18.49	18.49	2.62	52.33	52.33	090	
43117		A	Partial esophagectomy, distal two-thirds, with thoracotomy and separate abdominal incision, with or without proximal gastrectomy; with thoracic esophagogastrostomy, with or without pyloroplasty (Ivor Lewis)	40.00	18.51	18.51	3.51	62.02	62.02	090	
43118		A	with colon interposition or small intestine reconstruction, including intestine mobilization, preparation, and anastomosis(es)	33.20	15.76	15.76	3.56	52.52	52.52	090	
43121		A	Partial esophagectomy, distal two-thirds, with thoracotomy only, with or without proximal gastrectomy, with thoracic esophagogastrostomy, with or without pyloroplasty	29.19	15.08	15.08	3.44	47.71	47.71	090	
43122		A	Partial esophagectomy, thoracoabdominal or abdominal approach, with or without proximal gastrectomy; with esophagogastrostomy, with or without pyloroplasty	40.00	18.05	18.05	3.27	61.32	61.32	090	
43123		A	with colon interposition or small intestine reconstruction, including intestine mobilization, preparation, and anastomosis(es)	33.20	15.58	15.58	3.96	52.74	52.74	090	
43124		A	Total or partial esophagectomy, without reconstruction (any approach), with cervical esophagostomy	27.32	15.15	15.15	2.95	45.42	45.42	090	
43130		A	Diverticulectomy of hypopharynx or esophagus, with or without myotomy; cervical approach	11.75	9.05	9.05	1.06	21.86	21.86	090	
43135		A	thoracic approach	16.10	10.09	10.09	1.85	28.04	28.04	090	
43200		A	Esophagoscopy, rigid or flexible; diagnostic, with or without collection of specimen(s) by brushing or washing (separate procedure)	1.59	7.92	1.22	0.11	9.62	2.92	000	
43202		A	with biopsy, single or multiple	1.89	6.46	1.15	0.12	8.47	3.16	000	
43204		A	with injection sclerosis of esophageal varices	3.77	1.71	1.71	0.18	5.66	5.66	000	
43205		A	with band ligation of esophageal varices	3.79	1.71	1.71	0.17	5.67	5.67	000	
43215		A	with removal of foreign body	2.60	1.26	1.26	0.17	4.03	4.03	000	
43216		A	with removal of tumor(s), polyp(s), or other lesion(s) by hot biopsy forceps or bipolar cautery	2.40	1.20	1.20	0.15	3.75	3.75	000	
43217		A	with removal of tumor(s), polyp(s), or other lesion(s) by snare technique	2.90	1.35	1.35	0.17	4.42	4.42	000	

■ RVU not developed by CMS. Gap-filled RVUs developed by Ingenix/CHEG.

Code	M	S	Description	Work Value	Non-Fac PE	Fac PE	Mal-practice	Non-Fac Total	Fac Total	Global	Gap
43219		A	with insertion of plastic tube or stent	2.80	1.43	1.43	0.16	4.39	4.39	000	
43220		A	with balloon dilation (less than 30 mm diameter)	2.10	1.14	1.14	0.12	3.36	3.36	000	
43226		A	with insertion of guide wire followed by dilation over guide wire	2.34	1.21	1.21	0.12	3.67	3.67	000	
43227		A	with control of bleeding (eg, injection, bipolar cautery, unipolar cautery, laser, heater probe, stapler, plasma coagulator)	3.60	1.64	1.64	0.18	5.42	5.42	000	
43228		A	with ablation of tumor(s), polyp(s), or other lesion(s), not amenable to removal by hot biopsy forceps, bipolar cautery or snare technique	3.77	1.77	1.77	0.25	5.79	5.79	000	
43231		A	with endoscopic ultrasound examination	3.19	1.60	1.60	0.20	4.99	4.99	000	
43232		A	with transendoscopic ultrasound-guided intramural or transmural fine needle aspiration/biopsy(s)	4.48	2.15	2.15	0.26	6.89	6.89	000	
43234		A	Upper gastrointestinal endoscopy, simple primary examination (eg, with small diameter flexible endoscope) (separate procedure)	2.01	4.58	1.06	0.13	6.72	3.20	000	
43235		A	Upper gastrointestinal endoscopy including esophagus, stomach, and either the duodenum and/or jejunum as appropriate; diagnostic, with or without collection of specimen(s) by brushing or washing (separate procedure)	2.39	6.38	1.23	0.13	8.90	3.75	000	
43239		A	with biopsy, single or multiple	2.87	6.79	1.27	0.14	9.80	4.28	000	
43240		A	with transmural drainage of pseudocyst	6.86	2.97	2.97	0.36	10.19	10.19	000	
43241		A	with transendoscopic intraluminal tube or catheter placement	2.59	1.27	1.27	0.14	4.00	4.00	000	
43242		A	with transendoscopic ultrasound-guided intramural or transmural fine needle aspiration/biopsy(s)	7.31	2.64	2.64	0.29	10.24	10.24	000	
43243		A	with injection sclerosis of esophageal and/or gastric varices	4.57	2.00	2.00	0.21	6.78	6.78	000	
43244		A	with band ligation of esophageal and/or gastric varices	5.05	2.18	2.18	0.21	7.44	7.44	000	
43245		A	with dilation of gastric outlet for obstruction (eg, balloon, guide wire, bougie)	3.39	1.55	1.55	0.18	5.12	5.12	000	
43246		A	with directed placement of percutaneous gastrostomy tube	4.33	1.84	1.84	0.24	6.41	6.41	000	
43247		A	with removal of foreign body	3.39	1.56	1.56	0.17	5.12	5.12	000	
43248		A	with insertion of guide wire followed by dilation of esophagus over guide wire	3.15	1.49	1.49	0.15	4.79	4.79	000	

■ RVU not developed by CMS. Gap-filled RVUs developed by Ingenix/CHEG.

Code	M	S	Description	Work Value	Non-Fac PE	Fac PE	Mal-practice	Non-Fac Total	Fac Total	Global	Gap
43249		A	with balloon dilation of esophagus (less than 30 mm diameter)	2.90	1.39	1.39	0.15	4.44	4.44	000	
43250		A	with removal of tumor(s), polyp(s), or other lesion(s) by hot biopsy forceps or bipolar cautery	3.20	1.48	1.48	0.17	4.85	4.85	000	
43251		A	with removal of tumor(s), polyp(s), or other lesion(s) by snare technique	3.70	1.67	1.67	0.19	5.56	5.56	000	
43255		A	with control of bleeding, any method	4.82	1.97	1.97	0.20	6.99	6.99	000	
43256		A	with transendoscopic stent placement (includes predilation)	4.60	1.66	1.66	0.23	6.49	6.49	000	
43258		A	with ablation of tumor(s), polyp(s), or other lesion(s) not amenable to removal by hot biopsy forceps, bipolar cautery or snare technique	4.55	1.99	1.99	0.22	6.76	6.76	000	
43259		A	with endoscopic ultrasound examination	4.89	2.22	2.22	0.22	7.33	7.33	000	
43260		A	Endoscopic retrograde cholangiopancreatography (ERCP); diagnostic, with or without collection of specimen(s) by brushing or washing (separate procedure)	5.96	2.50	2.50	0.27	8.73	8.73	000	
43261		A	with biopsy, single or multiple	6.27	2.62	2.62	0.29	9.18	9.18	000	
43262		A	with sphincterotomy/papillotomy	7.39	3.03	3.03	0.34	10.76	10.76	000	
43263		A	with pressure measurement of sphincter of Oddi (pancreatic duct or common bile duct)	7.29	3.00	3.00	0.28	10.57	10.57	000	
43264		A	with endoscopic retrograde removal of calculus/calculi from biliary and/or pancreatic ducts	8.90	3.58	3.58	0.41	12.89	12.89	000	
43265		A	with endoscopic retrograde destruction, lithotripsy of calculus/calculi, any method	10.02	3.99	3.99	0.42	14.43	14.43	000	
43267		A	with endoscopic retrograde insertion of nasobiliary or nasopancreatic drainage tube	7.39	3.04	3.04	0.34	10.77	10.77	000	
43268		A	with endoscopic retrograde insertion of tube or stent into bile or pancreatic duct	7.39	3.03	3.03	0.34	10.76	10.76	000	
43269		A	with endoscopic retrograde removal of foreign body and/or change of tube or stent	8.21	3.33	3.33	0.28	11.82	11.82	000	
43271		A	with endoscopic retrograde balloon dilation of ampulla, biliary and/or pancreatic duct(s)	7.39	3.02	3.02	0.34	10.75	10.75	000	
43272		A	with ablation of tumor(s), polyp(s), or other lesion(s) not amenable to removal by hot biopsy forceps, bipolar cautery or snare technique	7.39	3.04	3.04	0.34	10.77	10.77	000	

Surgery

■ RVU not developed by CMS. Gap-filled RVUs developed by Ingenix/CHEG.

Code	M	S	Description	Work Value	Non-Fac PE	Fac PE	Mal-practice	Non-Fac Total	Fac Total	Global	Gap
43280		A	Laparoscopy, surgical, esophagogastric fundoplasty (eg, Nissen, Toupet procedures)	17.25	8.43	8.43	1.76	27.44	27.44	090	
43289		C	Unlisted laparoscopy procedure, esophagus	0.00	0.00	0.00	0.00	0.00	0.00	YYY	
43300		A	Esophagoplasty, (plastic repair or reconstruction), cervical approach; without repair of tracheoesophageal fistula	9.14	7.31	7.31	0.85	17.30	17.30	090	
43305		A	with repair of tracheoesophageal fistula	17.39	12.84	12.84	1.36	31.59	31.59	090	
43310		A	Esophagoplasty, (plastic repair or reconstruction), thoracic approach; without repair of tracheoesophageal fistula	25.39	14.51	14.51	3.18	43.08	43.08	090	
43312		A	with repair of tracheoesophageal fistula	28.42	17.45	17.45	3.38	49.25	49.25	090	
43313		A	Esophagoplasty for congenital defect, (plastic repair or reconstruction), thoracic approach; without repair of congenital tracheoesophageal fistula	45.28	22.01	22.01	5.43	72.72	72.72	090	
43314		A	with repair of congenital tracheoesophageal fistula	50.27	24.07	24.07	5.53	79.87	79.87	090	
43320		A	Esophagogastrostomy (cardioplasty), with or without vagotomy and pyloroplasty, transabdominal or transthoracic approach	19.93	10.67	10.67	1.59	32.19	32.19	090	
43324		A	Esophagogastric fundoplasty (eg, Nissen, Belsey IV, Hill procedures)	20.57	9.79	9.79	1.72	32.08	32.08	090	
43325		A	Esophagogastric fundoplasty; with fundic patch (Thal-Nissen procedure)	20.06	10.08	10.08	1.65	31.79	31.79	090	
43326		A	with gastroplasty (eg, Collis)	19.74	10.33	10.33	1.84	31.91	31.91	090	
43330		A	Esophagomyotomy (Heller type); abdominal approach	19.77	9.78	9.78	1.52	31.07	31.07	090	
43331		A	thoracic approach	20.13	11.41	11.41	1.93	33.47	33.47	090	
43340		A	Esophagojejunostomy (without total gastrectomy); abdominal approach	19.61	10.31	10.31	1.53	31.45	31.45	090	
43341		A	thoracic approach	20.85	11.17	11.17	2.14	34.16	34.16	090	
43350		A	Esophagostomy, fistulization of esophagus, external; abdominal approach	15.78	10.50	10.50	1.15	27.43	27.43	090	
43351		A	thoracic approach	18.35	10.91	10.91	1.51	30.77	30.77	090	
43352		A	cervical approach	15.26	9.59	9.59	1.28	26.13	26.13	090	
43360		A	Gastrointestinal reconstruction for previous esophagectomy, for obstructing esophageal lesion or fistula, or for previous esophageal exclusion; with stomach, with or without pyloroplasty	35.70	17.43	17.43	3.00	56.13	56.13	090	

Surgery

■ RVU not developed by CMS. Gap-filled RVUs developed by Ingenix/CHEG.

Code	M	S	Description	Work Value	Non-Fac PE	Fac PE	Mal-practice	Non-Fac Total	Fac Total	Global	Gap
43361		A	with colon interposition or small intestine reconstruction, including intestine mobilization, preparation, and anastomosis(es)	40.50	17.93	17.93	3.52	61.95	61.95	090	
43400		A	Ligation, direct, esophageal varices	21.20	10.46	10.46	0.99	32.65	32.65	090	
43401		A	Transection of esophagus with repair, for esophageal varices	22.09	10.34	10.34	1.73	34.16	34.16	090	
43405		A	Ligation or stapling at gastroesophageal junction for pre-existing esophageal perforation	20.01	9.45	9.45	1.63	31.09	31.09	090	
43410		A	Suture of esophageal wound or injury; cervical approach	13.47	9.35	9.35	1.15	23.97	23.97	090	
43415		A	transthoracic or transabdominal approach	25.00	12.50	12.50	1.92	39.42	39.42	090	
43420		A	Closure of esophagostomy or fistula; cervical approach	14.35	9.15	9.15	0.86	24.36	24.36	090	
43425		A	transthoracic or transabdominal approach	21.03	11.00	11.00	2.03	34.06	34.06	090	
43450		A	Dilation of esophagus, by unguided sound or bougie, single or multiple passes	1.38	1.47	0.63	0.07	2.92	2.08	000	
43453		A	Dilation of esophagus, over guide wire	1.51	0.68	0.68	0.08	2.27	2.27	000	
43456		A	Dilation of esophagus, by balloon or dilator, retrograde	2.57	1.07	1.07	0.14	3.78	3.78	000	
43458		A	Dilation of esophagus with balloon (30 mm diameter or larger) for achalasia	3.06	1.26	1.26	0.17	4.49	4.49	000	
43460		A	Esophagogastric tamponade, with balloon (Sengstaaken type)	3.80	1.54	1.54	0.21	5.55	5.55	000	
43496		C	Free jejunum transfer with microvascular anastomosis	0.00	0.00	0.00	0.00	0.00	0.00	090	
43499		C	Unlisted procedure, esophagus	0.00	0.00	0.00	0.00	0.00	0.00	YYY	
43500		A	Gastrotomy; with exploration or foreign body removal	11.05	5.23	5.23	0.84	17.12	17.12	090	
43501		A	with suture repair of bleeding ulcer	20.04	8.86	8.86	1.55	30.45	30.45	090	
43502		A	with suture repair of pre-existing esophagogastric laceration (eg, Mallory-Weiss)	23.13	10.16	10.16	1.83	35.12	35.12	090	
43510		A	with esophageal dilation and insertion of permanent intraluminal tube (eg, Celestin or Mousseaux-Barbin)	13.08	7.50	7.50	0.90	21.48	21.48	090	
43520		A	Pyloromyotomy, cutting of pyloric muscle (Fredet-Ramstedt type operation)	9.99	5.73	5.73	0.84	16.56	16.56	090	
43600		A	Biopsy of stomach; by capsule, tube, peroral (one or more specimens)	1.91	1.05	1.05	0.11	3.07	3.07	000	
43605		A	by laparotomy	11.98	5.55	5.55	0.93	18.46	18.46	090	

■ RVU not developed by CMS. Gap-filled RVUs developed by Ingenix/CHEG.

Surgery

Code	M	S	Description	Work Value	Non-Fac PE	Fac PE	Mal-practice	Non-Fac Total	Fac Total	Global	Gap
43610		A	Excision, local; ulcer or benign tumor of stomach	14.60	6.85	6.85	1.14	22.59	22.59	090	
43611		A	malignant tumor of stomach	17.84	8.12	8.12	1.38	27.34	27.34	090	
43620		A	Gastrectomy, total; with esophagoenterostomy	30.04	12.89	12.89	2.29	45.22	45.22	090	
43621		A	with Roux-en-Y reconstruction	30.73	13.21	13.21	2.36	46.30	46.30	090	
43622		A	with formation of intestinal pouch, any type	32.53	13.79	13.79	2.48	48.80	48.80	090	
43631		A	Gastrectomy, partial, distal; with gastroduodenostomy	22.59	9.72	9.72	1.99	34.30	34.30	090	
43632		A	with gastrojejunostomy	22.59	9.73	9.73	2.00	34.32	34.32	090	
43633		A	with Roux-en-Y reconstruction	23.10	9.87	9.87	2.05	35.02	35.02	090	
43634		A	with formation of intestinal pouch	25.12	10.84	10.84	2.18	38.14	38.14	090	
43635		A	Vagotomy when performed with partial distal gastrectomy (List separately in addition to code(s) for primary procedure)	2.06	0.74	0.74	0.21	3.01	3.01	ZZZ	
43638		A	Gastrectomy, partial, proximal, thoracic or abdominal approach including esophagogastrostomy, with vagotomy;	29.00	12.13	12.13	2.24	43.37	43.37	090	
43639		A	with pyloroplasty or pyloromyotomy	29.65	12.30	12.30	2.31	44.26	44.26	090	
43640		A	Vagotomy including pyloroplasty, with or without gastrostomy; truncal or selective	17.02	7.72	7.72	1.51	26.25	26.25	090	
43641		A	parietal cell (highly selective)	17.27	7.82	7.82	1.53	26.62	26.62	090	
43651		A	Laparoscopy, surgical; transection of vagus nerves, truncal	10.15	4.71	4.71	1.03	15.89	15.89	090	
43652		A	transection of vagus nerves, selective or highly selective	12.15	5.53	5.53	1.25	18.93	18.93	090	
43653		A	gastrostomy, without construction of gastric tube (eg, Stamm procedure) (separate procedure)	7.73	4.37	4.37	0.78	12.88	12.88	090	
43659		C	Unlisted laparoscopy procedure, stomach	0.00	0.00	0.00	0.00	0.00	0.00	YYY	
43750		A	Percutaneous placement of gastrostomy tube	4.49	2.72	2.72	0.33	7.54	7.54	010	
43752		B	Naso- or oro-gastric tube placement, necessitating physician's skill	0.63	0.50	0.50	0.07	1.20	1.20	XXX	■
43760		A	Change of gastrostomy tube	1.10	1.47	0.46	0.07	2.64	1.63	000	
43761		A	Repositioning of the gastric feeding tube, any method, through the duodenum for enteric nutrition	2.01	0.83	0.83	0.10	2.94	2.94	000	
43800		A	Pyloroplasty	13.69	6.60	6.60	1.07	21.36	21.36	090	

■ RVU not developed by CMS. Gap-filled RVUs developed by Ingenix/CHEG.

Code	M	S	Description	Work Value	Non-Fac PE	Fac PE	Mal-practice	Non-Fac Total	Fac Total	Global	Gap
43810		A	Gastroduodenostomy	14.65	6.94	6.94	1.10	22.69	22.69	090	
43820		A	Gastrojejunostomy; without vagotomy	15.37	7.15	7.15	1.18	23.70	23.70	090	
43825		A	with vagotomy, any type	19.22	8.56	8.56	1.50	29.28	29.28	090	
43830		A	Gastrostomy, open; without construction of gastric tube (eg, Stamm procedure) (separate procedure)	9.53	5.06	5.06	0.69	15.28	15.28	090	
43831		A	neonatal, for feeding	7.84	4.67	4.67	0.81	13.32	13.32	090	
43832		A	with construction of gastric tube (eg, Janeway procedure)	15.60	7.66	7.66	1.13	24.39	24.39	090	
43840		A	Gastrorrhaphy, suture of perforated duodenal or gastric ulcer, wound, or injury	15.56	7.21	7.21	1.20	23.97	23.97	090	
43842		A	Gastric restrictive procedure, without gastric bypass, for morbid obesity; vertical-banded gastroplasty	18.47	11.24	11.24	1.51	31.22	31.22	090	
43843		A	other than vertical-banded gastroplasty	18.65	11.25	11.25	1.53	31.43	31.43	090	
43846		A	Gastric restrictive procedure, with gastric bypass for morbid obesity; with short limb (less than 100 cm) Roux-en-Y gastroenterostomy	24.05	13.68	13.68	1.96	39.69	39.69	090	
43847		A	with small intestine reconstruction to limit absorption	26.92	15.28	15.28	2.14	44.34	44.34	090	
43848		A	Revision of gastric restrictive procedure for morbid obesity (separate procedure)	29.39	16.54	16.54	2.39	48.32	48.32	090	
43850		A	Revision of gastroduodenal anastomosis (gastroduodenostomy) with reconstruction; without vagotomy	24.72	10.42	10.42	1.97	37.11	37.11	090	
43855		A	with vagotomy	26.16	11.12	11.12	2.01	39.29	39.29	090	
43860		A	Revision of gastrojejunal anastomosis (gastrojejunostomy) with reconstruction, with or without partial gastrectomy or intestine resection; without vagotomy	25.00	10.58	10.58	2.03	37.61	37.61	090	
43865		A	with vagotomy	26.52	11.21	11.21	2.15	39.88	39.88	090	
43870		A	Closure of gastrostomy, surgical	9.69	5.22	5.22	0.71	15.62	15.62	090	
43880		A	Closure of gastrocolic fistula	24.65	10.87	10.87	1.94	37.46	37.46	090	
43999		C	Unlisted procedure, stomach	0.00	0.00	0.00	0.00	0.00	0.00	YYY	
44005		A	Enterolysis (freeing of intestinal adhesion) (separate procedure)	16.23	7.40	7.40	1.39	25.02	25.02	090	
44010		A	Duodenotomy, for exploration, biopsy(s), or foreign body removal	12.52	6.48	6.48	1.05	20.05	20.05	090	
44015		A	Tube or needle catheter jejunostomy for enteral alimentation, intraoperative, any method (List separately in addition to primary procedure)	2.62	0.93	0.93	0.25	3.80	3.80	ZZZ	

■ RVU not developed by CMS. Gap-filled RVUs developed by Ingenix/CHEG.

Code	M	S	Description	Work Value	Non-Fac PE	Fac PE	Mal-practice	Non-Fac Total	Fac Total	Global	Gap
44020		A	Enterotomy, small intestine, other than duodenum; for exploration, biopsy(s), or foreign body removal	13.99	6.56	6.56	1.20	21.75	21.75	090	
44021		A	for decompression (eg, Baker tube)	14.08	7.02	7.02	1.18	22.28	22.28	090	
44025		A	Colotomy, for exploration, biopsy(s), or foreign body removal	14.28	6.65	6.65	1.21	22.14	22.14	090	
44050		A	Reduction of volvulus, intussusception, internal hernia, by laparotomy	14.03	6.60	6.60	1.15	21.78	21.78	090	
44055		A	Correction of malrotation by lysis of duodenal bands and/or reduction of midgut volvulus (eg, Ladd procedure)	22.00	9.51	9.51	1.32	32.83	32.83	090	
44100		A	Biopsy of intestine by capsule, tube, peroral (one or more specimens)	2.01	1.09	1.09	0.12	3.22	3.22	000	
44110		A	Excision of one or more lesions of small or large intestine not requiring anastomosis, exteriorization, or fistulization; single enterotomy	11.81	5.84	5.84	1.00	18.65	18.65	090	
44111		A	multiple enterotomies	14.29	7.10	7.10	1.22	22.61	22.61	090	
44120		A	Enterectomy, resection of small intestine; single resection and anastomosis	17.00	7.67	7.67	1.46	26.13	26.13	090	
44121		A	each additional resection and anastomosis (List separately in addition to code for primary procedure)	4.45	1.60	1.60	0.45	6.50	6.50	ZZZ	
44125		A	with enterostomy	17.54	7.86	7.86	1.49	26.89	26.89	090	
44126		A	Enterectomy, resection of small intestine for congenital atresia, single resection and anastomosis of proximal segment of intestine; without tapering	35.50	18.03	18.03	0.36	53.89	53.89	090	
44127		A	with tapering	41.00	20.56	20.56	0.41	61.97	61.97	090	
44128		A	each additional resection and anastomosis (List separately in addition to code for primary procedure)	4.45	1.78	1.78	0.45	6.68	6.68	ZZZ	
44130		A	Enteroenterostomy, anastomosis of intestine, with or without cutaneous enterostomy (separate procedure)	14.49	6.78	6.78	1.23	22.50	22.50	090	
44132		R	Donor enterectomy, open, with preparation and maintenance of allograft; from cadaver donor	0.00	0.00	0.00	0.00	0.00	0.00	XXX	
44133		R	partial, from living donor	0.00	0.00	0.00	0.00	0.00	0.00	XXX	
44135		R	Intestinal allotransplantation; from cadaver donor	0.00	0.00	0.00	0.00	0.00	0.00	XXX	
44136		R	from living donor	0.00	0.00	0.00	0.00	0.00	0.00	XXX	

■ RVU not developed by CMS. Gap-filled RVUs developed by Ingenix/CHEG.

Code	M	S	Description	Work Value	Non-Fac PE	Fac PE	Mal-prac-tice	Non-Fac Total	Fac Total	Global	Gap
44139		A	Mobilization (take-down) of splenic flexure performed in conjunction with partial colectomy (List separately in addition to primary procedure)	2.23	0.80	0.80	0.21	3.24	3.24	ZZZ	
44140		A	Colectomy, partial; with anastomosis	21.00	9.53	9.53	1.83	32.36	32.36	090	
44141		A	with skin level cecostomy or colostomy	19.51	11.93	11.93	1.95	33.39	33.39	090	
44143		A	with end colostomy and closure of distal segment (Hartmann type procedure)	22.99	13.14	13.14	2.02	38.15	38.15	090	
44144		A	with resection, with colostomy or ileostomy and creation of mucofistula	21.53	11.75	11.75	1.89	35.17	35.17	090	
44145		A	with coloproctostomy (low pelvic anastomosis)	26.42	11.90	11.90	2.22	40.54	40.54	090	
44146		A	with coloproctostomy (low pelvic anastomosis), with colostomy	27.54	15.41	15.41	2.20	45.15	45.15	090	
44147		A	abdominal and transanal approach	20.71	10.15	10.15	1.74	32.60	32.60	090	
44150		A	Colectomy, total, abdominal, without proctectomy; with ileostomy or ileoproctostomy	23.95	14.08	14.08	2.05	40.08	40.08	090	
44151		A	with continent ileostomy	26.88	15.74	15.74	1.97	44.59	44.59	090	
44152		A	with rectal mucosectomy, ileoanal anastomosis, with or without loop ileostomy	27.83	17.01	17.01	2.36	47.20	47.20	090	
44153		A	with rectal mucosectomy, ileoanal anastomosis, creation of ileal reservoir (S or J), with or without loop ileostomy	30.59	16.64	16.64	2.33	49.56	49.56	090	
44155		A	Colectomy, total, abdominal, with proctectomy; with ileostomy	27.86	15.28	15.28	2.26	45.40	45.40	090	
44156		A	with continent ileostomy	30.79	17.86	17.86	2.19	50.84	50.84	090	
44160		A	Colectomy, partial, with removal of terminal ileum with ileocolostomy	18.62	8.65	8.65	1.55	28.82	28.82	090	
44200		A	Laparoscopy, surgical; enterolysis (freeing of intestinal adhesion) (separate procedure)	14.44	6.79	6.79	1.46	22.69	22.69	090	
44201		A	jejunostomy (eg, for decompression or feeding)	9.78	5.16	5.16	0.97	15.91	15.91	090	
44202		A	enterectomy, resection of small intestine, single resection and anastomosis	22.04	9.82	9.82	2.16	34.02	34.02	090	
44203		A	each additional small intestine resection and anastomosis (List separately in addition to code for primary procedure)	4.45	1.60	1.60	0.45	6.50	6.50	ZZZ	
44204		A	colectomy, partial, with anastomosis	25.08	10.46	10.46	1.83	37.37	37.37	090	
44205		A	colectomy, partial, with removal of terminal ileum with ileocolostomy	22.23	9.31	9.31	1.55	33.09	33.09	090	

■ RVU not developed by CMS. Gap-filled RVUs developed by Ingenix/CHEG.

Surgery

Code	M	S	Description	Work Value	Non-Fac PE	Fac PE	Mal-practice	Non-Fac Total	Fac Total	Global	Gap
44209		C	Unlisted laparoscopy procedure, intestine (except rectum)	0.00	0.00	0.00	0.00	0.00	0.00	YYY	
44300		A	Enterostomy or cecostomy, tube (eg, for decompression or feeding) (separate procedure)	12.11	6.79	6.79	0.88	19.78	19.78	090	
44310		A	Ileostomy or jejunostomy, non-tube (separate procedure)	15.95	10.50	10.50	1.13	27.58	27.58	090	
44312		A	Revision of ileostomy; simple (release of superficial scar) (separate procedure)	8.02	5.25	5.25	0.54	13.81	13.81	090	
44314		A	complicated (reconstruction in-depth) (separate procedure)	15.05	10.37	10.37	0.99	26.41	26.41	090	
44316		A	Continent ileostomy (Kock procedure) (separate procedure)	21.09	13.77	13.77	1.41	36.27	36.27	090	
44320		A	Colostomy or skin level cecostomy; (separate procedure)	17.64	12.13	12.13	1.28	31.05	31.05	090	
44322		A	with multiple biopsies (eg, for congenital megacolon) (separate procedure)	11.98	10.41	10.41	1.18	23.57	23.57	090	
44340		A	Revision of colostomy; simple (release of superficial scar) (separate procedure)	7.72	4.86	4.86	0.56	13.14	13.14	090	
44345		A	complicated (reconstruction in-depth) (separate procedure)	15.43	8.34	8.34	1.11	24.88	24.88	090	
44346		A	with repair of paracolostomy hernia (separate procedure)	16.99	8.91	8.91	1.20	27.10	27.10	090	
44360		A	Small intestinal endoscopy, enteroscopy beyond second portion of duodenum, not including ileum; diagnostic, with or without collection of specimen(s) by brushing or washing (separate procedure)	2.59	1.39	1.39	0.14	4.12	4.12	000	
44361		A	with biopsy, single or multiple	2.87	1.50	1.50	0.15	4.52	4.52	000	
44363		A	with removal of foreign body	3.50	1.71	1.71	0.19	5.40	5.40	000	
44364		A	with removal of tumor(s), polyp(s), or other lesion(s) by snare technique	3.74	1.80	1.80	0.21	5.75	5.75	000	
44365		A	with removal of tumor(s), polyp(s), or other lesion(s) by hot biopsy forceps or bipolar cautery	3.31	1.68	1.68	0.18	5.17	5.17	000	
44366		A	with control of bleeding (eg, injection, bipolar cautery, unipolar cautery, laser, heater probe, stapler, plasma coagulator)	4.41	2.05	2.05	0.22	6.68	6.68	000	
44369		A	with ablation of tumor(s), polyp(s), or other lesion(s) not amenable to removal by hot biopsy forceps, bipolar cautery or snare technique	4.52	2.05	2.05	0.23	6.80	6.80	000	
44370		A	with transendoscopic stent placement (includes predilation)	4.80	1.74	1.74	0.21	6.75	6.75	000	

■ RVU not developed by CMS. Gap-filled RVUs developed by Ingenix/CHEG.

Code	M	S	Description	Work Value	Non-Fac PE	Fac PE	Mal-practice	Non-Fac Total	Fac Total	Global	Gap
44372		A	with placement of percutaneous jejunostomy tube	4.41	2.04	2.04	0.27	6.72	6.72	000	
44373		A	with conversion of percutaneous gastrostomy tube to percutaneous jejunostomy tube	3.50	1.80	1.80	0.19	5.49	5.49	000	
44376		A	Small intestinal endoscopy, enteroscopy beyond second portion of duodenum, including ileum; diagnostic, with or without collection of specimen(s) by brushing or washing (separate procedure)	5.26	2.36	2.36	0.29	7.91	7.91	000	
44377		A	with biopsy, single or multiple	5.53	2.47	2.47	0.28	8.28	8.28	000	
44378		A	with control of bleeding (eg, injection, bipolar cautery, unipolar cautery, laser, heater probe, stapler, plasma coagulator)	7.13	3.06	3.06	0.37	10.56	10.56	000	
44379		A	with transendoscopic stent placement (includes predilation)	7.47	2.67	2.67	0.38	10.52	10.52	000	
44380		A	Ileoscopy, through stoma; diagnostic, with or without collection of specimen(s) by brushing or washing (separate procedure)	1.05	0.79	0.79	0.08	1.92	1.92	000	
44382		A	with biopsy, single or multiple	1.27	0.90	0.90	0.09	2.26	2.26	000	
44383		A	with transendoscopic stent placement (includes predilation)	3.26	1.16	1.16	0.13	4.55	4.55	000	
44385		A	Endoscopic evaluation of small intestinal (abdominal or pelvic) pouch; diagnostic, with or without collection of specimen(s) by brushing or washing (separate procedure)	1.82	5.26	0.95	0.12	7.20	2.89	000	
44386		A	with biopsy, single or multiple	2.12	6.98	1.09	0.15	9.25	3.36	000	
44388		A	Colonoscopy through stoma; diagnostic, with or without collection of specimen(s) by brushing or washing (separate procedure)	2.82	6.91	1.42	0.18	9.91	4.42	000	
44389		A	with biopsy, single or multiple	3.13	7.62	1.55	0.18	10.93	4.86	000	
44390		A	with removal of foreign body	3.83	6.68	1.80	0.22	10.73	5.85	000	
44391		A	with control of bleeding (eg, injection, bipolar cautery, unipolar cautery, laser, heater probe, stapler, plasma coagulator)	4.32	6.04	1.78	0.23	10.59	6.33	000	
44392		A	with removal of tumor(s), polyp(s), or other lesion(s) by hot biopsy forceps or bipolar cautery	3.82	8.21	1.79	0.23	12.26	5.84	000	
44393		A	with ablation of tumor(s), polyp(s), or other lesion(s) not amenable to removal by hot biopsy forceps, bipolar cautery or snare technique	4.84	8.45	2.19	0.27	13.56	7.30	000	
44394		A	with removal of tumor(s), polyp(s), or other lesion(s) by snare technique	4.43	7.71	2.04	0.26	12.40	6.73	000	

■ RVU not developed by CMS. Gap-filled RVUs developed by Ingenix/CHEG.

Surgery

Surgery

Code	M	S	Description	Work Value	Non-Fac PE	Fac PE	Mal-practice	Non-Fac Total	Fac Total	Global	Gap
44397		A	with transendoscopic stent placement (includes predilation)	4.71	2.10	2.10	0.28	7.09	7.09	000	
44500		A	Introduction of long gastrointestinal tube (eg, Miller-Abbott) (separate procedure)	0.49	0.37	0.37	0.02	0.88	0.88	000	
44602		A	Suture of small intestine (enterorrhaphy) for perforated ulcer, diverticulum, wound, injury or rupture; single perforation	16.03	7.34	7.34	1.07	24.44	24.44	090	
44603		A	multiple perforations	18.66	8.25	8.25	1.39	28.30	28.30	090	
44604		A	Suture of large intestine (colorrhaphy) for perforated ulcer, diverticulum, wound, injury or rupture (single or multiple perforations); without colostomy	16.03	7.35	7.35	1.42	24.80	24.80	090	
44605		A	with colostomy	19.53	8.94	8.94	1.54	30.01	30.01	090	
44615		A	Intestinal stricturoplasty (enterotomy and enterorrhaphy) with or without dilation, for intestinal obstruction	15.93	7.32	7.32	1.39	24.64	24.64	090	
44620		A	Closure of enterostomy, large or small intestine;	12.20	5.81	5.81	1.05	19.06	19.06	090	
44625		A	with resection and anastomosis other than colorectal	15.05	6.86	6.86	1.30	23.21	23.21	090	
44626		A	with resection and colorectal anastomosis (eg, closure of Hartmann type procedure)	25.36	10.60	10.60	2.19	38.15	38.15	090	
44640		A	Closure of intestinal cutaneous fistula	21.65	9.70	9.70	1.46	32.81	32.81	090	
44650		A	Closure of enteroenteric or enterocolic fistula	22.57	10.01	10.01	1.49	34.07	34.07	090	
44660		A	Closure of enterovesical fistula; without intestinal or bladder resection	21.36	9.51	9.51	1.14	32.01	32.01	090	
44661		A	with intestine and/or bladder resection	24.81	10.73	10.73	1.53	37.07	37.07	090	
44680		A	Intestinal plication (separate procedure)	15.40	7.47	7.47	1.37	24.24	24.24	090	
44700		A	Exclusion of small intestine from pelvis by mesh or other prosthesis, or native tissue (eg, bladder or omentum)	16.11	7.57	7.57	1.21	24.89	24.89	090	
44799		C	Unlisted procedure, intestine	0.00	0.00	0.00	0.00	0.00	0.00	YYY	
44800		A	Excision of Meckel's diverticulum (diverticulectomy) or omphalomesenteric duct	11.23	5.61	5.61	1.11	17.95	17.95	090	
44820		A	Excision of lesion of mesentery (separate procedure)	12.09	5.98	5.98	1.03	19.10	19.10	090	
44850		A	Suture of mesentery (separate procedure)	10.74	5.41	5.41	0.99	17.14	17.14	090	
44899		C	Unlisted procedure, Meckels diverticulum and the mesentery	0.00	0.00	0.00	0.00	0.00	0.00	YYY	
44900		A	Incision and drainage of appendiceal abscess; open	10.14	5.96	5.96	0.84	16.94	16.94	090	

■ RVU not developed by CMS. Gap-filled RVUs developed by Ingenix/CHEG.

Code	M	S	Description	Work Value	Non-Fac PE	Fac PE	Mal-practice	Non-Fac Total	Fac Total	Global	Gap
44901		A	percutaneous	3.38	5.01	5.01	0.17	8.56	8.56	000	
44950		A	Appendectomy;	10.00	5.31	5.31	0.88	16.19	16.19	090	
44955		A	when done for indicated purpose at time of other major procedure (not as separate procedure) (List separately in addition to code for primary procedure)	1.53	0.57	0.57	0.16	2.26	2.26	ZZZ	
44960		A	for ruptured appendix with abscess or generalized peritonitis	12.34	6.50	6.50	1.09	19.93	19.93	090	
44970		A	Laparoscopy, surgical, appendectomy	8.70	4.21	4.21	0.88	13.79	13.79	090	
44979		C	Unlisted laparoscopy procedure, appendix	0.00	0.00	0.00	0.00	0.00	0.00	YYY	
45000		A	Transrectal drainage of pelvic abscess	4.52	3.80	3.80	0.37	8.69	8.69	090	
45005		A	Incision and drainage of submucosal abscess, rectum	1.99	4.58	1.62	0.18	6.75	3.79	010	
45020		A	Incision and drainage of deep supralevator, pelvirectal, or retrorectal abscess	4.72	4.21	4.21	0.41	9.34	9.34	090	
45100		A	Biopsy of anorectal wall, anal approach (eg, congenital megacolon)	3.68	4.86	2.12	0.33	8.87	6.13	090	
45108		A	Anorectal myomectomy	4.76	6.40	2.95	0.46	11.62	8.17	090	
45110		A	Proctectomy; complete, combined abdominoperineal, with colostomy	28.00	13.26	13.26	2.26	43.52	43.52	090	
45111		A	partial resection of rectum, transabdominal approach	16.48	8.78	8.78	1.60	26.86	26.86	090	
45112		A	Proctectomy, combined abdominoperineal, pull-through procedure (eg, colo-anal anastomosis)	30.54	13.70	13.70	2.35	46.59	46.59	090	
45113		A	Proctectomy, partial, with rectal mucosectomy, ileoanal anastomosis, creation of ileal reservoir (S or J), with or without loop ileostomy	30.58	13.39	13.39	2.13	46.10	46.10	090	
45114		A	Proctectomy, partial, with anastomosis; abdominal and transsacral approach	27.32	12.61	12.61	2.28	42.21	42.21	090	
45116		A	transsacral approach only (Kraske type)	24.58	11.58	11.58	2.00	38.16	38.16	090	
45119		A	Proctectomy, combined abdominoperineal pull-through procedure (eg, colo-anal anastomosis), with creation of colonic reservoir (eg, J-pouch), with or without proximal diverting ostomy	30.84	13.25	13.25	2.13	46.22	46.22	090	
45120		A	Proctectomy, complete (for congenital megacolon), abdominal and perineal approach; with pull-through procedure and anastomosis (eg, Swenson, Duhamel, or Soave type operation)	24.60	11.63	11.63	2.28	38.51	38.51	090	
45121		A	with subtotal or total colectomy, with multiple biopsies	27.04	12.53	12.53	2.66	42.23	42.23	090	

■ RVU not developed by CMS. Gap-filled RVUs developed by Ingenix/CHEG.

Surgery

Code	M	S	Description	Work Value	Non-Fac PE	Fac PE	Mal-practice	Non-Fac Total	Fac Total	Global	Gap
45123		A	Proctectomy, partial, without anastomosis, perineal approach	16.71	8.21	8.21	1.04	25.96	25.96	090	
45126		A	Pelvic exenteration for colorectal malignancy, with proctectomy (with or without colostomy), with removal of bladder and ureteral transplantations, and/or hysterectomy, or cervicectomy, with or without removal of tube(s), with or without removal of ovary(s), or any combination thereof	45.16	19.12	19.12	3.23	67.51	67.51	090	
45130		A	Excision of rectal procidentia, with anastomosis; perineal approach	16.44	7.80	7.80	1.12	25.36	25.36	090	
45135		A	abdominal and perineal approach	19.28	9.10	9.10	1.52	29.90	29.90	090	
45136		A	Excision of ileoanal reservoir with ileostomy	27.30	12.66	12.66	2.19	42.15	42.15	090	
45150		A	Division of stricture of rectum	5.67	5.89	3.19	0.46	12.02	9.32	090	
45160		A	Excision of rectal tumor by proctotomy, transacral or transcoccygeal approach	15.32	7.14	7.14	1.07	23.53	23.53	090	
45170		A	Excision of rectal tumor, transanal approach	11.49	5.89	5.89	0.89	18.27	18.27	090	
45190		A	Destruction of rectal tumor (eg, electrodessication, electrosurgery, laser ablation, laser resection, cryosurgery) transanal approach	9.74	5.33	5.33	0.76	15.83	15.83	090	
45300		A	Proctosigmoidoscopy, rigid; diagnostic, with or without collection of specimen(s) by brushing or washing (separate procedure)	0.38	1.34	0.23	0.05	1.77	0.66	000	
45303		A	with dilation (eg, balloon, guide wire, bougie)	0.44	1.55	0.27	0.06	2.05	0.77	000	
45305		A	with biopsy, single or multiple	1.01	1.64	0.46	0.09	2.74	1.56	000	
45307		A	with removal of foreign body	0.94	2.68	0.44	0.15	3.77	1.53	000	
45308		A	with removal of single tumor, polyp, or other lesion by hot biopsy forceps or bipolar cautery	0.83	1.59	0.39	0.13	2.55	1.35	000	
45309		A	with removal of single tumor, polyp, or other lesion by snare technique	2.01	2.43	0.81	0.17	4.61	2.99	000	
45315		A	with removal of multiple tumors, polyps, or other lesions by hot biopsy forceps, bipolar cautery or snare technique	1.40	2.84	0.60	0.20	4.44	2.20	000	
45317		A	with control of bleeding (eg, injection, bipolar cautery, unipolar cautery, laser, heater probe, stapler, plasma coagulator)	1.50	1.94	0.63	0.20	3.64	2.33	000	
45320		A	with ablation of tumor(s), polyp(s), or other lesion(s) not amenable to removal by hot biopsy forceps, bipolar cautery or snare technique (eg, laser)	1.58	1.88	0.68	0.20	3.66	2.46	000	
45321		A	with decompression of volvulus	1.17	0.52	0.52	0.17	1.86	1.86	000	

■ RVU not developed by CMS. Gap-filled RVUs developed by Ingenix/CHEG.

Code	M	S	Description	Work Value	Non-Fac PE	Fac PE	Mal-practice	Non-Fac Total	Fac Total	Global	Gap
45327		A	with transendoscopic stent placement (includes predilation)	1.65	0.89	0.89	0.10	2.64	2.64	000	
45330		A	Sigmoidoscopy, flexible; diagnostic, with or without collection of specimen(s) by brushing or washing (separate procedure)	0.96	1.92	0.53	0.05	2.93	1.54	000	
45331		A	with biopsy, single or multiple	1.15	2.38	0.54	0.07	3.60	1.76	000	
45332		A	with removal of foreign body	1.79	4.36	0.76	0.11	6.26	2.66	000	
45333		A	with removal of tumor(s), polyp(s), or other lesion(s) by hot biopsy forceps or bipolar cautery	1.79	3.93	0.77	0.12	5.84	2.68	000	
45334		A	with control of bleeding (eg, injection, bipolar cautery, unipolar cautery, laser, heater probe, stapler, plasma coagulator)	2.73	1.12	1.12	0.16	4.01	4.01	000	
45337		A	with decompression of volvulus, any method	2.36	0.97	0.97	0.15	3.48	3.48	000	
45338		A	with removal of tumor(s), polyp(s), or other lesion(s) by snare technique	2.34	4.75	0.97	0.15	7.24	3.46	000	
45339		A	with ablation of tumor(s), polyp(s), or other lesion(s) not amenable to removal by hot biopsy forceps, bipolar cautery or snare technique	3.14	3.62	1.27	0.17	6.93	4.58	000	
45341		A	with endoscopic ultrasound examination	2.60	1.40	1.40	0.20	4.20	4.20	000	
45342		A	with transendoscopic ultrasound guided intramural or transmural fine needle aspiration/biopsy(s)	4.06	1.85	1.85	0.23	6.14	6.14	000	
45345		A	with transendoscopic stent placement (includes predilation)	2.92	1.44	1.44	0.15	4.51	4.51	000	
45355		A	Colonoscopy, rigid or flexible, transabdominal via colotomy, single or multiple	3.52	1.28	1.28	0.26	5.06	5.06	000	
45378		A	Colonoscopy, flexible, proximal to splenic flexure; diagnostic, with or without collection of specimen(s) by brushing or washing, with or without colon decompression (separate procedure)	3.70	8.79	1.77	0.20	12.69	5.67	000	
	53	A		0.96	1.92	0.53	0.05	2.93	1.54	000	
45379		A	with removal of foreign body	4.69	8.25	2.13	0.25	13.19	7.07	000	
45380		A	with biopsy, single or multiple	4.44	9.28	2.05	0.21	13.93	6.70	000	
45382		A	with control of bleeding (eg, injection, bipolar cautery, unipolar cautery, laser, heater probe, stapler, plasma coagulator)	5.69	10.32	2.29	0.27	16.28	8.25	000	
45383		A	with ablation of tumor(s), polyp(s), or other lesion(s) not amenable to removal by hot biopsy forceps, bipolar cautery or snare technique	5.87	10.01	2.56	0.32	16.20	8.75	000	

■ RVU not developed by CMS. Gap-filled RVUs developed by Ingenix/CHEG.

Surgery

Code	M	S	Description	Work Value	Non-Fac PE	Fac PE	Mal-practice	Non-Fac Total	Fac Total	Global	Gap
45384		A	with removal of tumor(s), polyp(s), or other lesion(s) by hot biopsy forceps or bipolar cautery	4.70	9.74	2.14	0.24	14.68	7.08	000	
45385		A	with removal of tumor(s), polyp(s), or other lesion(s) by snare technique	5.31	10.19	2.36	0.28	15.78	7.95	000	
45387		A	with transendoscopic stent placement (includes predilation)	5.91	2.57	2.57	0.33	8.81	8.81	000	
45500		A	Proctoplasty; for stenosis	7.29	4.24	4.24	0.56	12.09	12.09	090	
45505		A	for prolapse of mucous membrane	7.58	3.86	3.86	0.50	11.94	11.94	090	
45520		A	Perirectal injection of sclerosing solution for prolapse	0.55	0.77	0.20	0.04	1.36	0.79	000	
45540		A	Proctopexy for prolapse; abdominal approach	16.27	8.18	8.18	1.17	25.62	25.62	090	
45541		A	perineal approach	13.40	7.03	7.03	0.88	21.31	21.31	090	
45550		A	Proctopexy combined with sigmoid resection, abdominal approach	23.00	10.40	10.40	1.58	34.98	34.98	090	
45560		A	Repair of rectocele (separate procedure)	10.58	6.12	6.12	0.73	17.43	17.43	090	
45562		A	Exploration, repair, and presacral drainage for rectal injury;	15.38	7.52	7.52	1.15	24.05	24.05	090	
45563		A	with colostomy	23.47	11.34	11.34	1.84	36.65	36.65	090	
45800		A	Closure of rectovesical fistula;	17.77	8.23	8.23	1.14	27.14	27.14	090	
45805		A	with colostomy	20.78	10.72	10.72	1.47	32.97	32.97	090	
45820		A	Closure of rectourethral fistula;	18.48	8.55	8.55	1.17	28.20	28.20	090	
45825		A	with colostomy	21.25	10.57	10.57	0.97	32.79	32.79	090	
45900		A	Reduction of procidentia (separate procedure) under anesthesia	2.61	1.04	1.04	0.17	3.82	3.82	010	
45905		A	Dilation of anal sphincter (separate procedure) under anesthesia other than local	2.30	12.19	0.96	0.14	14.63	3.40	010	
45910		A	Dilation of rectal stricture (separate procedure) under anesthesia other than local	2.80	17.62	1.15	0.14	20.56	4.09	010	
45915		A	Removal of fecal impaction or foreign body (separate procedure) under anesthesia	3.14	4.89	1.16	0.17	8.20	4.47	010	
45999		C	Unlisted procedure, rectum	0.00	0.00	0.00	0.00	0.00	0.00	YYY	
46020		A	Placement of seton	2.90	3.09	2.36	0.22	6.21	5.48	010	
46030		A	Removal of anal seton, other marker	1.23	2.90	1.22	0.11	4.24	2.56	010	
46040		A	Incision and drainage of ischiorectal and/or perirectal abscess (separate procedure)	4.96	5.57	3.15	0.48	11.01	8.59	090	

Surgery

■ RVU not developed by CMS. Gap-filled RVUs developed by Ingenix/CHEG.

Code	M	S	Description	Work Value	Non-Fac PE	Fac PE	Mal-practice	Non-Fac Total	Fac Total	Global	Gap
46045		A	Incision and drainage of intramural, intramuscular or submucosal abscess, transanal, under anesthesia	4.32	2.88	2.88	0.40	7.60	7.60	090	
46050		A	Incision and drainage, perianal abscess, superficial	1.19	3.68	1.37	0.11	4.98	2.67	010	
46060		A	Incision and drainage of ischiorectal or intramural abscess, with fistulectomy or fistulotomy, submuscular, with or without placement of seton	5.69	3.83	3.83	0.52	10.04	10.04	090	
46070		A	Incision, anal septum (infant)	2.71	2.54	2.54	0.27	5.52	5.52	090	
46080		A	Sphincterotomy, anal, division of sphincter (separate procedure)	2.49	3.81	1.65	0.23	6.53	4.37	010	
46083		A	Incision of thrombosed hemorrhoid, external	1.40	4.78	1.59	0.12	6.30	3.11	010	
46200		A	Fissurectomy, with or without sphincterotomy	3.42	4.01	2.42	0.30	7.73	6.14	090	
46210		A	Cryptectomy; single	2.67	5.12	2.17	0.26	8.05	5.10	090	
46211		A	multiple (separate procedure)	4.25	4.97	3.10	0.37	9.59	7.72	090	
46220		A	Papillectomy or excision of single tag, anus (separate procedure)	1.56	1.32	0.56	0.14	3.02	2.26	010	
46221		A	Hemorrhoidectomy, by simple ligature (eg, rubber band)	2.04	1.80	1.12	0.12	3.96	3.28	010	
46230		A	Excision of external hemorrhoid tags and/or multiple papillae	2.57	4.38	1.69	0.22	7.17	4.48	010	
46250		A	Hemorrhoidectomy, external, complete	3.89	5.59	2.71	0.43	9.91	7.03	090	
46255		A	Hemorrhoidectomy, internal and external, simple;	4.60	6.45	2.96	0.51	11.56	8.07	090	
46257		A	with fissurectomy	5.40	3.12	3.12	0.59	9.11	9.11	090	
46258		A	with fistulectomy, with or without fissurectomy	5.73	3.30	3.30	0.64	9.67	9.67	090	
46260		A	Hemorrhoidectomy, internal and external, complex or extensive;	6.37	4.04	4.04	0.68	11.09	11.09	090	
46261		A	with fissurectomy	7.08	4.19	4.19	0.70	11.97	11.97	090	
46262		A	with fistulectomy, with or without fissurectomy	7.50	4.35	4.35	0.76	12.61	12.61	090	
46270		A	Surgical treatment of anal fistula (fistulectomy/ fistulotomy); subcutaneous	3.72	5.23	2.65	0.36	9.31	6.73	090	
46275		A	submuscular	4.56	4.65	2.85	0.40	9.61	7.81	090	
46280		A	complex or multiple, with or without placement of seton	5.98	3.83	3.83	0.50	10.31	10.31	090	
46285		A	second stage	4.09	4.28	2.69	0.34	8.71	7.12	090	

■ RVU not developed by CMS. Gap-filled RVUs developed by Ingenix/CHEG.

Code	M	S	Description	Work Value	Non-Fac PE	Fac PE	Mal-practice	Non-Fac Total	Fac Total	Global	Gap
46288		A	Closure of anal fistula with rectal advancement flap	7.13	4.25	4.25	0.60	11.98	11.98	090	
46320		A	Enucleation or excision of external thrombotic hemorrhoid	1.61	4.00	1.57	0.14	5.75	3.32	010	
46500		A	Injection of sclerosing solution, hemorrhoids	1.61	2.89	0.58	0.12	4.62	2.31	010	
46600		A	Anoscopy; diagnostic, with or without collection of specimen(s) by brushing or washing (separate procedure)	0.50	0.82	0.15	0.04	1.36	0.69	000	
46604		A	with dilation (eg, balloon, guide wire, bougie)	1.31	0.99	0.47	0.09	2.39	1.87	000	
46606		A	with biopsy, single or multiple	0.81	0.87	0.29	0.07	1.75	1.17	000	
46608		A	with removal of foreign body	1.51	1.81	0.49	0.13	3.45	2.13	000	
46610		A	with removal of single tumor, polyp, or other lesion by hot biopsy forceps or bipolar cautery	1.32	1.46	0.48	0.12	2.90	1.92	000	
46611		A	with removal of single tumor, polyp, or other lesion by snare technique	1.81	2.07	0.65	0.15	4.03	2.61	000	
46612		A	with removal of multiple tumors, polyps, or other lesions by hot biopsy forceps, bipolar cautery or snare technique	2.34	2.65	0.85	0.18	5.17	3.37	000	
46614		A	with control of bleeding (eg, injection, bipolar cautery, unipolar cautery, laser, heater probe, stapler, plasma coagulator)	2.01	1.90	0.71	0.14	4.05	2.86	000	
46615		A	with ablation of tumor(s), polyp(s), or other lesion(s) not amenable to removal by hot biopsy forceps, bipolar cautery or snare technique	2.68	1.76	0.96	0.23	4.67	3.87	000	
46700		A	Anoplasty, plastic operation for stricture; adult	9.13	4.78	4.78	0.56	14.47	14.47	090	
46705		A	infant	6.90	4.53	4.53	0.73	12.16	12.16	090	
46715		A	Repair of low imperforate anus; with anoperineal fistula (cut-back procedure)	7.20	4.46	4.46	0.76	12.42	12.42	090	
46716		A	with transposition of anoperineal or anovestibular fistula	15.07	8.05	8.05	1.30	24.42	24.42	090	
46730		A	Repair of high imperforate anus without fistula; perineal or sacroperineal approach	26.75	12.25	12.25	2.03	41.03	41.03	090	
46735		A	combined transabdominal and sacroperineal approaches	32.17	15.49	15.49	2.64	50.30	50.30	090	
46740		A	Repair of high imperforate anus with rectourethral or rectovaginal fistula; perineal or sacroperineal approach	30.00	14.61	14.61	1.99	46.60	46.60	090	
46742		A	combined transabdominal and sacroperineal approaches	35.80	18.31	18.31	2.63	56.74	56.74	090	

■ RVU not developed by CMS. Gap-filled RVUs developed by Ingenix/CHEG.

Code	M	S	Description	Work Value	Non-Fac PE	Fac PE	Mal-practice	Non-Fac Total	Fac Total	Global	Gap
46744		A	Repair of cloacal anomaly by anorectovaginoplasty and urethroplasty, sacroperineal approach	52.63	22.78	22.78	2.27	77.68	77.68	090	
46746		A	Repair of cloacal anomaly by anorectovaginoplasty and urethroplasty, combined abdominal and sacroperineal approach;	58.22	27.19	27.19	2.51	87.92	87.92	090	
46748		A	with vaginal lengthening by intestinal graft or pedicle flaps	64.21	29.58	29.58	2.77	96.56	96.56	090	
46750		A	Sphincteroplasty, anal, for incontinence or prolapse; adult	10.25	5.79	5.79	0.69	16.73	16.73	090	
46751		A	child	8.77	6.14	6.14	0.78	15.69	15.69	090	
46753		A	Graft (Thiersch operation) for rectal incontinence and/or prolapse	8.29	4.13	4.13	0.58	13.00	13.00	090	
46754		A	Removal of Thiersch wire or suture, anal canal	2.20	5.36	1.43	0.12	7.68	3.75	010	
46760		A	Sphincteroplasty, anal, for incontinence, adult; muscle transplant	14.43	7.07	7.07	0.86	22.36	22.36	090	
46761		A	levator muscle imbrication (Park posterior anal repair)	13.84	6.87	6.87	0.84	21.55	21.55	090	
46762		A	implantation artificial sphincter	12.71	6.08	6.08	0.71	19.50	19.50	090	
46900		A	Destruction of lesion(s), anus (eg, condyloma, papilloma, molluscum contagiosum, herpetic vesicle), simple; chemical	1.91	3.52	0.74	0.13	5.56	2.78	010	
46910		A	electrodesiccation	1.86	3.81	1.48	0.14	5.81	3.48	010	
46916		A	cryosurgery	1.86	3.24	1.68	0.09	5.19	3.63	010	
46917		A	laser surgery	1.86	5.32	1.62	0.16	7.34	3.64	010	
46922		A	surgical excision	1.86	3.96	1.46	0.17	5.99	3.49	010	
46924		A	Destruction of lesion(s), anus (eg, condyloma, papilloma, molluscum contagiosum, herpetic vesicle), extensive (eg, laser surgery, electrosurgery, cryosurgery, chemosurgery)	2.76	4.81	1.77	0.20	7.77	4.73	010	
46934		A	Destruction of hemorrhoids, any method; internal	3.51	6.62	3.77	0.26	10.39	7.54	090	
46935		A	external	2.43	4.60	0.87	0.17	7.20	3.47	010	
46936		A	internal and external	3.69	6.67	3.58	0.30	10.66	7.57	090	
46937		A	Cryosurgery of rectal tumor; benign	2.69	4.51	1.72	0.12	7.32	4.53	010	
46938		A	malignant	4.66	6.22	3.27	0.40	11.28	8.33	090	
46940		A	Curettage or cautery of anal fissure, including dilation of anal sphincter (separate procedure); initial	2.32	3.47	0.83	0.17	5.96	3.32	010	

Surgery

■ RVU not developed by CMS. Gap-filled RVUs developed by Ingenix/CHEG.

Code	M	S	Description	Work Value	Non-Fac PE	Fac PE	Mal-practice	Non-Fac Total	Fac Total	Global	Gap
46942		A	subsequent	2.04	2.84	0.71	0.14	5.02	2.89	010	
46945		A	Ligation of internal hemorrhoids; single procedure	1.84	4.04	2.29	0.17	6.05	4.30	090	
46946		A	multiple procedures	2.58	5.40	2.61	0.22	8.20	5.41	090	
46999		C	Unlisted procedure, anus	0.00	0.00	0.00	0.00	0.00	0.00	YYY	
47000		A	Biopsy of liver, needle; percutaneous	1.90	8.36	0.67	0.09	10.35	2.66	000	
47001		A	when done for indicated purpose at time of other major procedure (List separately in addition to code for primary procedure)	1.90	0.68	0.68	0.18	2.76	2.76	ZZZ	
47010		A	Hepatotomy; for open drainage of abscess or cyst, one or two stages	16.01	9.60	9.60	0.65	26.26	26.26	090	
47011		A	for percutaneous drainage of abscess or cyst, one or two stages	3.70	4.61	4.61	0.17	8.48	8.48	000	
47015		A	Laparotomy, with aspiration and/or injection of hepatic parasitic (eg, amoebic or echinococcal) cyst(s) or abscess(es)	15.11	8.23	8.23	0.86	24.20	24.20	090	
47100		A	Biopsy of liver, wedge	11.67	6.50	6.50	0.75	18.92	18.92	090	
47120		A	Hepatectomy, resection of liver; partial lobectomy	35.50	17.02	17.02	2.29	54.81	54.81	090	
47122		A	trisegmentectomy	55.13	24.11	24.11	3.60	82.84	82.84	090	
47125		A	total left lobectomy	49.19	22.12	22.12	3.18	74.49	74.49	090	
47130		A	total right lobectomy	53.35	23.49	23.49	3.47	80.31	80.31	090	
47133		X	Donor hepatectomy, with preparation and maintenance of allograft; from cadaver donor	0.00	0.00	0.00	0.00	0.00	0.00	XXX	
47134		R	partial, from living donor	39.15	13.91	13.91	3.98	57.04	57.04	XXX	
47135		R	Liver allotransplantation; orthotopic, partial or whole, from cadaver or living donor, any age	81.52	43.28	43.28	8.13	132.93	132.93	090	
47136		R	heterotopic, partial or whole, from cadaver or living donor, any age	68.60	47.00	47.00	6.93	122.53	122.53	090	
47300		A	Marsupialization of cyst or abscess of liver	15.08	7.75	7.75	0.97	23.80	23.80	090	
47350		A	Management of liver hemorrhage; simple suture of liver wound or injury	19.56	9.45	9.45	1.25	30.26	30.26	090	
47360		A	complex suture of liver wound or injury, with or without hepatic artery ligation	26.92	12.96	12.96	1.71	41.59	41.59	090	
47361		A	exploration of hepatic wound, extensive debridement, coagulation and/or suture, with or without packing of liver	47.12	19.94	19.94	3.11	70.17	70.17	090	
47362		A	re-exploration of hepatic wound for removal of packing	18.51	9.77	9.77	1.22	29.50	29.50	090	

■ RVU not developed by CMS. Gap-filled RVUs developed by Ingenix/CHEG.

Surgery

Code	M	S	Description	Work Value	Non-Fac PE	Fac PE	Mal-practice	Non-Fac Total	Fac Total	Global	Gap
47370		A	Laparoscopy, surgical, ablation of one or more liver tumor(s); radiofrequency	18.00	7.19	7.19	0.85	26.04	26.04	090	
47371		A	cryosurgical	16.94	6.76	6.76	0.85	24.55	24.55	090	
47379		C	Unlisted laparoscopic procedure, liver	0.00	0.00	0.00	0.00	0.00	0.00	YYY	
47380		A	Ablation, open, of one or more liver tumor(s); radiofrequency	21.25	8.48	8.48	0.85	30.58	30.58	090	
47381		A	cryosurgical	21.00	8.38	8.38	0.85	30.23	30.23	090	
47382		A	Ablation, one or more liver tumor(s), percutaneous, radiofrequency	12.00	5.37	5.37	0.85	18.22	18.22	010	
47399		C	Unlisted procedure, liver	0.00	0.00	0.00	0.00	0.00	0.00	YYY	
47400		A	Hepaticotomy or hepaticostomy with exploration, drainage, or removal of calculus	32.49	14.99	14.99	1.82	49.30	49.30	090	
47420		A	Choledochotomy or choledochostomy with exploration, drainage, or removal of calculus, with or without cholecystotomy; without transduodenal sphincterotomy or sphincteroplasty	19.88	9.46	9.46	1.70	31.04	31.04	090	
47425		A	with transduodenal sphincterotomy or sphincteroplasty	19.83	9.38	9.38	1.60	30.81	30.81	090	
47460		A	Transduodenal sphincterotomy or sphincteroplasty, with or without transduodenal extraction of calculus (separate procedure)	18.04	9.26	9.26	1.24	28.54	28.54	090	
47480		A	Cholecystotomy or cholecystostomy with exploration, drainage, or removal of calculus (separate procedure)	10.82	6.80	6.80	0.85	18.47	18.47	090	
47490		A	Percutaneous cholecystostomy	7.23	7.67	7.67	0.33	15.23	15.23	090	
47500		A	Injection procedure for percutaneous transhepatic cholangiography	1.96	0.68	0.68	0.09	2.73	2.73	000	
47505		A	Injection procedure for cholangiography through an existing catheter (eg, percutaneous transhepatic or T-tube)	0.76	2.88	0.26	0.03	3.67	1.05	000	
47510		A	Introduction of percutaneous transhepatic catheter for biliary drainage	7.83	9.46	9.46	0.36	17.65	17.65	090	
47511		A	Introduction of percutaneous transhepatic stent for internal and external biliary drainage	10.50	10.57	10.57	0.47	21.54	21.54	090	
47525		A	Change of percutaneous biliary drainage catheter	5.55	3.34	3.34	0.24	9.13	9.13	010	
47530		A	Revision and/or reinsertion of transhepatic tube	5.85	5.07	5.07	0.29	11.21	11.21	090	
47550		A	Biliary endoscopy, intraoperative (choledochoscopy) (List separately in addition to code for primary procedure)	3.02	1.08	1.08	0.30	4.40	4.40	ZZZ	

Surgery

■ RVU not developed by CMS. Gap-filled RVUs developed by Ingenix/CHEG.

Code	M	S	Description	Work Value	Non-Fac PE	Fac PE	Mal-practice	Non-Fac Total	Fac Total	Global	Gap
47552		A	Biliary endoscopy, percutaneous via T-tube or other tract; diagnostic, with or without collection of specimen(s) by brushing and/or washing (separate procedure)	6.04	2.52	2.52	0.42	8.98	8.98	000	
47553		A	with biopsy, single or multiple	6.35	2.70	2.70	0.30	9.35	9.35	000	
47554		A	with removal of calculus/calculi	9.06	3.55	3.55	0.74	13.35	13.35	000	
47555		A	with dilation of biliary duct stricture(s) without stent	7.56	3.15	3.15	0.35	11.06	11.06	000	
47556		A	with dilation of biliary duct stricture(s) with stent	8.56	3.49	3.49	0.38	12.43	12.43	000	
47560		A	Laparoscopy, surgical; with guided transhepatic cholangiography, without biopsy	4.89	1.89	1.89	0.49	7.27	7.27	000	
47561		A	with guided transhepatic cholangiography with biopsy	5.18	2.19	2.19	0.49	7.86	7.86	000	
47562		A	cholecystectomy	11.09	5.15	5.15	1.13	17.37	17.37	090	
47563		A	cholecystectomy with cholangiography	11.94	5.43	5.43	1.21	18.58	18.58	090	
47564		A	cholecystectomy with exploration of common duct	14.23	6.26	6.26	1.44	21.93	21.93	090	
47570		A	cholecystoenterostomy	12.58	5.67	5.67	1.28	19.53	19.53	090	
47579		C	Unlisted laparoscopy procedure, biliary tract	0.00	0.00	0.00	0.00	0.00	0.00	YYY	
47600		A	Cholecystectomy;	13.58	6.86	6.86	1.16	21.60	21.60	090	
47605		A	with cholangiography	14.69	7.23	7.23	1.25	23.17	23.17	090	
47610		A	Cholecystectomy with exploration of common duct;	18.82	8.80	8.80	1.61	29.23	29.23	090	
47612		A	with choledochoenterostomy	18.78	8.70	8.70	1.60	29.08	29.08	090	
47620		A	with transduodenal sphincterotomy or sphincteroplasty, with or without cholangiography	20.64	9.35	9.35	1.77	31.76	31.76	090	
47630		A	Biliary duct stone extraction, percutaneous via T-tube tract, basket or snare (eg, Burhenne technique)	9.11	3.20	3.20	0.46	12.77	12.77	090	
47700		A	Exploration for congenital atresia of bile ducts, without repair, with or without liver biopsy, with or without cholangiography	15.62	8.79	8.79	1.40	25.81	25.81	090	
47701		A	Portoenterostomy (eg, Kasai procedure)	27.81	13.60	13.60	3.00	44.41	44.41	090	
47711		A	Excision of bile duct tumor, with or without primary repair of bile duct; extrahepatic	23.03	11.34	11.34	1.98	36.35	36.35	090	
47712		A	intrahepatic	30.24	14.00	14.00	2.67	46.91	46.91	090	
47715		A	Excision of choledochal cyst	18.80	8.95	8.95	1.59	29.34	29.34	090	

■ RVU not developed by CMS. Gap-filled RVUs developed by Ingenix/CHEG.

Code	M	S	Description	Work Value	Non-Fac PE	Fac PE	Mal-prac-tice	Non-Fac Total	Fac Total	Global	Gap
47716		A	Anastomosis, choledochal cyst, without excision	16.44	8.19	8.19	1.41	26.04	26.04	090	
47720		A	Cholecystoenterostomy; direct	15.91	8.66	8.66	1.37	25.94	25.94	090	
47721		A	with gastroenterostomy	19.12	9.90	9.90	1.63	30.65	30.65	090	
47740		A	Roux-en-Y	18.48	9.64	9.64	1.59	29.71	29.71	090	
47741		A	Roux-en-Y with gastroenterostomy	21.34	10.62	10.62	1.82	33.78	33.78	090	
47760		A	Anastomosis, of extrahepatic biliary ducts and gastrointestinal tract	25.85	12.28	12.28	2.21	40.34	40.34	090	
47765		A	Anastomosis, of intrahepatic ducts and gastrointestinal tract	24.88	12.73	12.73	2.18	39.79	39.79	090	
47780		A	Anastomosis, Roux-en-Y, of extrahepatic biliary ducts and gastrointestinal tract	26.50	12.49	12.49	2.27	41.26	41.26	090	
47785		A	Anastomosis, Roux-en-Y, of intrahepatic biliary ducts and gastrointestinal tract	31.18	14.97	14.97	2.69	48.84	48.84	090	
47800		A	Reconstruction, plastic, of extrahepatic biliary ducts with end-to-end anastomosis	23.30	11.57	11.57	1.95	36.82	36.82	090	
47801		A	Placement of choledochal stent	15.17	10.21	10.21	0.69	26.07	26.07	090	
47802		A	U-tube hepaticoenterostomy	21.55	11.60	11.60	1.84	34.99	34.99	090	
47900		A	Suture of extrahepatic biliary duct for pre-existing injury (separate procedure)	19.90	10.25	10.25	1.65	31.80	31.80	090	
47999		C	Unlisted procedure, biliary tract	0.00	0.00	0.00	0.00	0.00	0.00	YYY	
48000		A	Placement of drains, peripancreatic, for acute pancreatitis;	28.07	12.59	12.59	1.32	41.98	41.98	090	
48001		A	with cholecystostomy, gastrostomy, and jejunostomy	35.45	15.04	15.04	1.90	52.39	52.39	090	
48005		A	Resection or debridement of pancreas and peripancreatic tissue for acute necrotizing pancreatitis	42.17	17.39	17.39	2.26	61.82	61.82	090	
48020		A	Removal of pancreatic calculus	15.70	7.44	7.44	1.36	24.50	24.50	090	
48100		A	Biopsy of pancreas, open (eg, fine needle aspiration, needle core biopsy, wedge biopsy)	12.23	7.03	7.03	1.08	20.34	20.34	090	
48102		A	Biopsy of pancreas, percutaneous needle	4.68	8.96	2.45	0.20	13.84	7.33	010	
48120		A	Excision of lesion of pancreas (eg, cyst, adenoma)	15.85	7.69	7.69	1.35	24.89	24.89	090	
48140		A	Pancreatectomy, distal subtotal, with or without splenectomy; without pancreaticojejunostomy	22.94	10.78	10.78	2.12	35.84	35.84	090	
48145		A	with pancreaticojejunostomy	24.02	11.48	11.48	2.25	37.75	37.75	090	

■ RVU not developed by CMS. Gap-filled RVUs developed by Ingenix/CHEG.

Code	M	S	Description	Work Value	Non-Fac PE	Fac PE	Mal-practice	Non-Fac Total	Fac Total	Global	Gap
48146		A	Pancreatectomy, distal, near-total with preservation of duodenum (Child-type procedure)	26.40	13.96	13.96	2.43	42.79	42.79	090	
48148		A	Excision of ampulla of Vater	17.34	9.15	9.15	1.61	28.10	28.10	090	
48150		A	Pancreatectomy, proximal subtotal with total duodenectomy, partial gastrectomy, choledochoenterostomy and gastrojejunostomy (Whipple-type procedure); with pancreatojejunostomy	48.00	21.29	21.29	4.43	73.72	73.72	090	
48152		A	without pancreatojejunostomy	43.75	20.74	20.74	4.07	68.56	68.56	090	
48153		A	Pancreatectomy, proximal subtotal with near-total duodenectomy, choledochoenterostomy and duodenojejunostomy (pylorus-sparing, Whipple-type procedure); with pancreatojejunostomy	47.89	22.18	22.18	4.40	74.47	74.47	090	
48154		A	without pancreatojejunostomy	44.10	20.82	20.82	4.10	69.02	69.02	090	
48155		A	Pancreatectomy, total	24.64	13.89	13.89	2.30	40.83	40.83	090	
48160		N	Pancreatectomy, total or subtotal, with autologous transplantation of pancreas or pancreatic islet cells	35.74	28.40	28.40	3.80	67.94	67.94	XXX	■
48180		A	Pancreaticojejunostomy, side-to-side anastomosis (Puestow-type operation)	24.72	11.16	11.16	2.24	38.12	38.12	090	
48400		A	Injection procedure for intraoperative pancreatography (List separately in addition to code for primary procedure)	1.95	0.69	0.69	0.10	2.74	2.74	ZZZ	
48500		A	Marsupialization of pancreatic cyst	15.28	7.74	7.74	1.35	24.37	24.37	090	
48510		A	External drainage, pseudocyst of pancreas; open	14.31	7.45	7.45	1.07	22.83	22.83	090	
48511		A	percutaneous	4.00	3.95	3.95	0.17	8.12	8.12	000	
48520		A	Internal anastomosis of pancreatic cyst to gastrointestinal tract; direct	15.59	7.49	7.49	1.41	24.49	24.49	090	
48540		A	Roux-en-Y	19.72	8.84	8.84	1.82	30.38	30.38	090	
48545		A	Pancreatorrhaphy for injury	18.18	8.88	8.88	1.61	28.67	28.67	090	
48547		A	Duodenal exclusion with gastrojejunostomy for pancreatic injury	25.83	11.04	11.04	2.30	39.17	39.17	090	
48550		X	Donor pancreatectomy, with preparation and maintenance of allograft from cadaver donor, with or without duodenal segment for transplantation	0.00	0.00	0.00	0.00	0.00	0.00	XXX	
48554		R	Transplantation of pancreatic allograft	34.17	12.27	12.27	3.30	49.74	49.74	090	
48556		A	Removal of transplanted pancreatic allograft	15.71	8.71	8.71	1.52	25.94	25.94	090	

■ RVU not developed by CMS. Gap-filled RVUs developed by Ingenix/CHEG.

Code	M	S	Description	Work Value	Non-Fac PE	Fac PE	Mal-practice	Non-Fac Total	Fac Total	Global	Gap
48999		C	Unlisted procedure, pancreas	0.00	0.00	0.00	0.00	0.00	0.00	YYY	
49000		A	Exploratory laparotomy, exploratory celiotomy with or without biopsy(s) (separate procedure)	11.68	6.22	6.22	1.17	19.07	19.07	090	
49002		A	Reopening of recent laparotomy	10.49	6.10	6.10	1.06	17.65	17.65	090	
49010		A	Exploration, retroperitoneal area with or without biopsy(s) (separate procedure)	12.28	7.05	7.05	1.22	20.55	20.55	090	
49020		A	Drainage of peritoneal abscess or localized peritonitis, exclusive of appendiceal abscess; open	22.84	11.41	11.41	1.31	35.56	35.56	090	
49021		A	percutaneous	3.38	5.84	5.84	0.16	9.38	9.38	000	
49040		A	Drainage of subdiaphragmatic or subphrenic abscess; open	13.52	8.02	8.02	0.84	22.38	22.38	090	
49041		A	percutaneous	4.00	6.07	6.07	0.18	10.25	10.25	000	
49060		A	Drainage of retroperitoneal abscess; open	15.86	9.62	9.62	0.77	26.25	26.25	090	
49061		A	percutaneous	3.70	5.99	5.99	0.17	9.86	9.86	000	
49062		A	Drainage of extraperitoneal lymphocele to peritoneal cavity, open	11.36	7.06	7.06	1.08	19.50	19.50	090	
49080		A	Peritoneocentesis, abdominal paracentesis, or peritoneal lavage (diagnostic or therapeutic); initial	1.35	4.56	0.48	0.07	5.98	1.90	000	
49081		A	subsequent	1.26	3.14	0.60	0.06	4.46	1.92	000	
49085		A	Removal of peritoneal foreign body from peritoneal cavity	12.14	6.72	6.72	0.88	19.74	19.74	090	
49180		A	Biopsy, abdominal or retroperitoneal mass, percutaneous needle	1.73	8.50	0.60	0.08	10.31	2.41	000	
49200		A	Excision or destruction by any method of intra-abdominal or retroperitoneal tumors or cysts or endometriomas;	10.25	6.59	6.59	0.89	17.73	17.73	090	
49201		A	extensive	14.84	8.90	8.90	1.44	25.18	25.18	090	
49215		A	Excision of presacral or sacrococcygeal tumor	33.50	15.52	15.52	2.48	51.50	51.50	090	
49220		A	Staging laparotomy for Hodgkins disease or lymphoma (includes splenectomy, needle or open biopsies of both liver lobes, possibly also removal of abdominal nodes, abdominal node and/or bone marrow biopsies, ovarian repositioning)	14.88	7.94	7.94	1.51	24.33	24.33	090	
49250		A	Umbilectomy, omphalectomy, excision of umbilicus (separate procedure)	8.35	5.26	5.26	0.84	14.45	14.45	090	
49255		A	Omentectomy, epiploectomy, resection of omentum (separate procedure)	11.14	6.66	6.66	1.12	18.92	18.92	090	

■ RVU not developed by CMS. Gap-filled RVUs developed by Ingenix/CHEG.

Code	M	S	Description	Work Value	Non-Fac PE	Fac PE	Mal-practice	Non-Fac Total	Fac Total	Global	Gap
49320		A	Laparoscopy, abdomen, peritoneum, and omentum, diagnostic, with or without collection of specimen(s) by brushing or washing (separate procedure)	5.10	3.08	3.08	0.50	8.68	8.68	010	
49321		A	Laparoscopy, surgical; with biopsy (single or multiple)	5.40	3.07	3.07	0.53	9.00	9.00	010	
49322		A	with aspiration of cavity or cyst (eg, ovarian cyst) (single or multiple)	5.70	3.53	3.53	0.57	9.80	9.80	010	
49323		A	with drainage of lymphocele to peritoneal cavity	9.48	4.18	4.18	0.88	14.54	14.54	090	
49329		C	Unlisted laparoscopy procedure, abdomen, peritoneum and omentum	0.00	0.00	0.00	0.00	0.00	0.00	YYY	
49400		A	Injection of air or contrast into peritoneal cavity (separate procedure)	1.88	0.82	0.82	0.11	2.81	2.81	000	
49420		A	Insertion of intraperitoneal cannula or catheter for drainage or dialysis; temporary	2.22	0.98	0.98	0.13	3.33	3.33	000	
49421		A	permanent	5.54	4.08	4.08	0.55	10.17	10.17	090	
49422		A	Removal of permanent intraperitoneal cannula or catheter	6.25	3.01	3.01	0.63	9.89	9.89	010	
49423		A	Exchange of previously placed abscess or cyst drainage catheter under radiological guidance (separate procedure)	1.46	0.70	0.70	0.07	2.23	2.23	000	
49424		A	Contrast injection for assessment of abscess or cyst via previously placed drainage catheter or tube (separate procedure)	0.76	0.45	0.45	0.03	1.24	1.24	000	
49425		A	Insertion of peritoneal-venous shunt	11.37	6.79	6.79	1.21	19.37	19.37	090	
49426		A	Revision of peritoneal-venous shunt	9.63	6.17	6.17	0.93	16.73	16.73	090	
49427		A	Injection procedure (eg, contrast media) for evaluation of previously placed peritoneal-venous shunt	0.89	0.50	0.50	0.05	1.44	1.44	000	
49428		A	Ligation of peritoneal-venous shunt	6.06	3.19	3.19	0.31	9.56	9.56	010	
49429		A	Removal of peritoneal-venous shunt	7.40	3.55	3.55	0.81	11.76	11.76	010	
49491		A	Repair, initial inguinal hernia, preterm infant (less than 37 weeks gestation at birth), performed from birth up to 50 weeks post-conceptual age, with or without hydrocelectomy; reducible	11.13	5.65	5.65	1.00	17.78	17.78	090	
49492		A	incarcerated or strangulated	14.03	6.40	6.40	1.42	21.85	21.85	090	
49495		A	Repair, initial inguinal hernia, full term infant under age 6 months, or preterm infant over 50 weeks postconceptual age and under age 6 months at the time of surgery, with or without hydrocelectomy; reducible	5.89	3.72	3.72	0.55	10.16	10.16	090	

■ RVU not developed by CMS. Gap-filled RVUs developed by Ingenix/CHEG.

Code	M	S	Description	Work Value	Non-Fac PE	Fac PE	Mal-practice	Non-Fac Total	Fac Total	Global	Gap
49496		A	incarcerated or strangulated	8.79	5.94	5.94	0.89	15.62	15.62	090	
49500		A	Repair initial inguinal hernia, age 6 months to under 5 years, with or without hydrocelectomy; reducible	5.48	3.48	3.48	0.46	9.42	9.42	090	
49501		A	incarcerated or strangulated	8.88	4.62	4.62	0.76	14.26	14.26	090	
49505		A	Repair initial inguinal hernia, age 5 years or over; reducible	7.60	4.58	4.13	0.65	12.83	12.38	090	
49507		A	incarcerated or strangulated	9.57	6.17	6.17	0.83	16.57	16.57	090	
49520		A	Repair recurrent inguinal hernia, any age; reducible	9.63	5.49	5.49	0.84	15.96	15.96	090	
49521		A	incarcerated or strangulated	11.97	5.85	5.85	1.04	18.86	18.86	090	
49525		A	Repair inguinal hernia, sliding, any age	8.57	4.97	4.97	0.74	14.28	14.28	090	
49540		A	Repair lumbar hernia	10.39	5.65	5.65	0.90	16.94	16.94	090	
49550		A	Repair initial femoral hernia, any age, reducible;	8.63	4.55	4.55	0.75	13.93	13.93	090	
49553		A	incarcerated or strangulated	9.44	4.95	4.95	0.83	15.22	15.22	090	
49555		A	Repair recurrent femoral hernia; reducible	9.03	5.30	5.30	0.79	15.12	15.12	090	
49557		A	incarcerated or strangulated	11.15	5.59	5.59	0.97	17.71	17.71	090	
49560		A	Repair initial incisional or ventral hernia; reducible	11.57	6.11	6.11	1.00	18.68	18.68	090	
49561		A	incarcerated or strangulated	14.25	6.71	6.71	1.23	22.19	22.19	090	
49565		A	Repair recurrent incisional or ventral hernia; reducible	11.57	6.27	6.27	1.00	18.84	18.84	090	
49566		A	incarcerated or strangulated	14.40	6.79	6.79	1.24	22.43	22.43	090	
49568		A	Implantation of mesh or other prosthesis for incisional or ventral hernia repair (List separately in addition to code for the incisional or ventral hernia repair)	4.89	1.76	1.76	0.50	7.15	7.15	ZZZ	
49570		A	Repair epigastric hernia (eg, preperitoneal fat); reducible (separate procedure)	5.69	3.54	3.54	0.50	9.73	9.73	090	
49572		A	incarcerated or strangulated	6.73	4.00	4.00	0.58	11.31	11.31	090	
49580		A	Repair umbilical hernia, under age 5 years; reducible	4.11	3.03	3.03	0.34	7.48	7.48	090	
49582		A	incarcerated or strangulated	6.65	5.02	5.02	0.57	12.24	12.24	090	
49585		A	Repair umbilical hernia, age 5 years or over; reducible	6.23	4.15	4.15	0.53	10.91	10.91	090	
49587		A	incarcerated or strangulated	7.56	4.27	4.27	0.65	12.48	12.48	090	

■ RVU not developed by CMS. Gap-filled RVUs developed by Ingenix/CHEG.

Code	M	S	Description	Work Value	Non-Fac PE	Fac PE	Mal-practice	Non-Fac Total	Fac Total	Global	Gap
49590		A	Repair spigelian hernia	8.54	4.96	4.96	0.74	14.24	14.24	090	
49600		A	Repair of small omphalocele, with primary closure	10.96	6.30	6.30	1.13	18.39	18.39	090	
49605		A	Repair of large omphalocele or gastroschisis; with or without prosthesis	76.00	30.79	30.79	2.57	109.36	109.36	090	
49606		A	with removal of prosthesis, final reduction and closure, in operating room	18.60	9.61	9.61	2.22	30.43	30.43	090	
49610		A	Repair of omphalocele (Gross type operation); first stage	10.50	6.87	6.87	0.77	18.14	18.14	090	
49611		A	second stage	8.92	6.56	6.56	0.65	16.13	16.13	090	
49650		A	Laparoscopy, surgical; repair initial inguinal hernia	6.27	3.33	3.33	0.64	10.24	10.24	090	
49651		A	repair recurrent inguinal hernia	8.24	4.40	4.40	0.84	13.48	13.48	090	
49659		C	Unlisted laparoscopy procedure, hernioplasty, herniorrhaphy, herniotomy	0.00	0.00	0.00	0.00	0.00	0.00	YYY	
49900		A	Suture, secondary, of abdominal wall for evisceration or dehiscence	12.28	6.80	6.80	1.23	20.31	20.31	090	
49905		A	Omental flap (eg, for reconstruction of sternal and chest wall defects) (list separately in addition to code for primary procedure)	6.55	2.44	2.44	0.61	9.60	9.60	ZZZ	
49906		C	Free omental flap with microvascular anastomosis	0.00	0.00	0.00	0.00	0.00	0.00	090	
49999		C	Unlisted procedure, abdomen, peritoneum and omentum	0.00	0.00	0.00	0.00	0.00	0.00	YYY	

■ RVU not developed by CMS. Gap-filled RVUs developed by Ingenix/CHEG.

Code	M	S	Description	Work Value	Non-Fac PE	Fac PE	Mal-practice	Non-Fac Total	Fac Total	Global	Gap
50010		A	Renal exploration, not necessitating other specific procedures	10.98	7.07	7.07	0.79	18.84	18.84	090	
50020		A	Drainage of perirenal or renal abscess; open	14.66	13.72	13.72	0.80	29.18	29.18	090	
50021		A	percutaneous	3.38	10.46	10.46	0.15	13.99	13.99	000	
50040		A	Nephrostomy, nephrotomy with drainage	14.94	11.56	11.56	0.82	27.32	27.32	090	
50045		A	Nephrotomy, with exploration	15.46	8.55	8.55	1.06	25.07	25.07	090	
50060		A	Nephrolithotomy; removal of calculus	19.30	10.03	10.03	1.14	30.47	30.47	090	
50065		A	secondary surgical operation for calculus	20.79	10.56	10.56	1.13	32.48	32.48	090	
50070		A	complicated by congenital kidney abnormality	20.32	10.70	10.70	1.20	32.22	32.22	090	
50075		A	removal of large staghorn calculus filling renal pelvis and calyces (including anatrophic pyelolithotomy)	25.34	12.65	12.65	1.51	39.50	39.50	090	
50080		A	Percutaneous nephrostolithotomy or pyelostolithotomy, with or without dilation, endoscopy, lithotripsy, stenting or basket extraction; up to 2 cm	14.71	11.03	11.03	0.86	26.60	26.60	090	
50081		A	over 2 cm	21.80	13.27	13.27	1.30	36.37	36.37	090	
50100		A	Transection or repositioning of aberrant renal vessels (separate procedure)	16.09	9.34	9.34	1.64	27.07	27.07	090	
50120		A	Pyelotomy; with exploration	15.91	8.93	8.93	1.04	25.88	25.88	090	
50125		A	with drainage, pyelostomy	16.52	9.48	9.48	1.07	27.07	27.07	090	
50130		A	with removal of calculus (pyelolithotomy, pelviolithotomy, including coagulum pyelolithotomy)	17.29	9.24	9.24	1.04	27.57	27.57	090	
50135		A	complicated (eg, secondary operation, congenital kidney abnormality)	19.18	9.93	9.93	1.18	30.29	30.29	090	
50200		A	Renal biopsy; percutaneous, by trocar or needle	2.63	0.96	0.96	0.12	3.71	3.71	000	
50205		A	by surgical exposure of kidney	11.31	6.52	6.52	0.94	18.77	18.77	090	
50220		A	Nephrectomy, including partial ureterectomy, any open approach including rib resection;	17.15	9.29	9.29	1.16	27.60	27.60	090	
50225		A	complicated because of previous surgery on same kidney	20.23	10.30	10.30	1.26	31.79	31.79	090	
50230		A	radical, with regional lymphadenectomy and/or vena caval thrombectomy	22.07	10.92	10.92	1.35	34.34	34.34	090	
50234		A	Nephrectomy with total ureterectomy and bladder cuff; through same incision	22.40	11.05	11.05	1.37	34.82	34.82	090	

■ RVU not developed by CMS. Gap-filled RVUs developed by Ingenix/CHEG.

Code	M	S	Description	Work Value	Non-Fac PE	Fac PE	Mal-practice	Non-Fac Total	Fac Total	Global	Gap
50236		A	through separate incision	24.86	14.27	14.27	1.50	40.63	40.63	090	
50240		A	Nephrectomy, partial	22.00	13.32	13.32	1.36	36.68	36.68	090	
50280		A	Excision or unroofing of cyst(s) of kidney	15.67	8.69	8.69	0.99	25.35	25.35	090	
50290		A	Excision of perinephric cyst	14.73	8.49	8.49	1.11	24.33	24.33	090	
50300		X	Donor nephrectomy, with preparation and maintenance of allograft, from cadaver donor, unilateral or bilateral	15.29	12.15	12.15	1.63	29.07	29.07	XXX	■
50320		A	Donor nephrectomy, open from living donor (excluding preparation and maintenance of allograft)	22.21	10.98	10.98	1.78	34.97	34.97	090	
50340		A	Recipient nephrectomy (separate procedure)	12.15	9.31	9.31	1.15	22.61	22.61	090	
50360		A	Renal allotransplantation, implantation of graft; excluding donor and recipient nephrectomy	31.53	17.87	17.87	2.97	52.37	52.37	090	
50365		A	with recipient nephrectomy	36.81	21.29	21.29	3.51	61.61	61.61	090	
50370		A	Removal of transplanted renal allograft	13.72	9.88	9.88	1.26	24.86	24.86	090	
50380		A	Renal autotransplantation, reimplantation of kidney	20.76	13.52	13.52	1.80	36.08	36.08	090	
50390		A	Aspiration and/or injection of renal cyst or pelvis by needle, percutaneous	1.96	0.68	0.68	0.09	2.73	2.73	000	
50392		A	Introduction of intracatheter or catheter into renal pelvis for drainage and/or injection, percutaneous	3.38	1.18	1.18	0.15	4.71	4.71	000	
50393		A	Introduction of ureteral catheter or stent into ureter through renal pelvis for drainage and/or injection, percutaneous	4.16	1.44	1.44	0.18	5.78	5.78	000	
50394		A	Injection procedure for pyelography (as nephrostogram, pyelostogram, antegrade pyeloureterograms) through nephrostomy or pyelostomy tube, or indwelling ureteral catheter	0.76	2.60	0.26	0.04	3.40	1.06	000	
50395		A	Introduction of guide into renal pelvis and/or ureter with dilation to establish nephrostomy tract, percutaneous	3.38	1.17	1.17	0.16	4.71	4.71	000	
50396		A	Manometric studies through nephrostomy or pyelostomy tube, or indwelling ureteral catheter	2.09	0.89	0.89	0.10	3.08	3.08	000	
50398		A	Change of nephrostomy or pyelostomy tube	1.46	1.06	0.51	0.07	2.59	2.04	000	
50400		A	Pyeloplasty (Foley Y-pyeloplasty), plastic operation on renal pelvis, with or without plastic operation on ureter, nephropexy, nephrostomy, pyelostomy, or ureteral splinting; simple	19.50	10.06	10.06	1.21	30.77	30.77	090	

■ RVU not developed by CMS. Gap-filled RVUs developed by Ingenix/CHEG.

Code	M	S	Description	Work Value	Non-Fac PE	Fac PE	Mal-practice	Non-Fac Total	Fac Total	Global	Gap
50405		A	complicated (congenital kidney abnormality, secondary pyeloplasty, solitary kidney, calycoplasty)	23.93	11.84	11.84	1.45	37.22	37.22	090	
50500		A	Nephrorrhaphy, suture of kidney wound or injury	19.57	11.37	11.37	1.45	32.39	32.39	090	
50520		A	Closure of nephrocutaneous or pyelocutaneous fistula	17.23	11.80	11.80	1.26	30.29	30.29	090	
50525		A	Closure of nephrovisceral fistula (eg, renocolic), including visceral repair; abdominal approach	22.27	13.30	13.30	1.51	37.08	37.08	090	
50526		A	thoracic approach	24.02	14.86	14.86	1.62	40.50	40.50	090	
50540		A	Symphysiotomy for horseshoe kidney with or without pyeloplasty and/or other plastic procedure, unilateral or bilateral (one operation)	19.93	10.42	10.42	1.28	31.63	31.63	090	
50541		A	Laparoscopy, surgical; ablation of renal cysts	16.00	6.79	6.79	0.99	23.78	23.78	090	
50544		A	pyeloplasty	22.40	9.04	9.04	1.41	32.85	32.85	090	
50545		A	radical nephrectomy (includes removal of Gerota's fascia and surrounding fatty tissue, removal of regional lymph nodes, and adrenalectomy)	24.00	9.65	9.65	1.53	35.18	35.18	090	
50546		A	nephrectomy, including partial ureterectomy	20.48	8.40	8.40	1.37	30.25	30.25	090	
50547		A	donor nephrectomy from living donor (excluding preparation and maintenance of allograft)	25.50	11.27	11.27	2.04	38.81	38.81	090	
50548		A	nephrectomy with total ureterectomy	24.40	9.70	9.70	1.49	35.59	35.59	090	
50549		C	Unlisted laparoscopy procedure, renal	0.00	0.00	0.00	0.00	0.00	0.00	YYY	
50551		A	Renal endoscopy through established nephrostomy or pyelostomy, with or without irrigation, instillation, or ureteropyelography, exclusive of radiologic service;	5.60	4.93	1.90	0.33	10.86	7.83	000	
50553		A	with ureteral catheterization, with or without dilation of ureter	5.99	16.25	2.05	0.35	22.59	8.39	000	
50555		A	with biopsy	6.53	20.11	2.25	0.38	27.02	9.16	000	
50557		A	with fulguration and/or incision, with or without biopsy	6.62	20.23	2.25	0.39	27.24	9.26	000	
50559		A	with insertion of radioactive substance with or without biopsy and/or fulguration	6.78	2.42	2.42	0.27	9.47	9.47	000	
50561		A	with removal of foreign body or calculus	7.59	18.31	2.58	0.44	26.34	10.61	000	

Surgery

■ RVU not developed by CMS. Gap-filled RVUs developed by Ingenix/CHEG.

Surgery

Code	M	S	Description	Work Value	Non-Fac PE	Fac PE	Mal-prac-tice	Non-Fac Total	Fac Total	Global	Gap
50570		A	Renal endoscopy through nephrotomy or pyelotomy, with or without irrigation, instillation, or ureteropyelography, exclusive of radiologic service;	9.54	3.24	3.24	0.56	13.34	13.34	000	
50572		A	with ureteral catheterization, with or without dilation of ureter	10.35	3.52	3.52	0.64	14.51	14.51	000	
50574		A	with biopsy	11.02	3.87	3.87	0.65	15.54	15.54	000	
50575		A	with endopyelotomy (includes cystoscopy, ureteroscopy, dilation of ureter and ureteral pelvic junction, incision of ureteral pelvic junction and insertion of endopyelotomy stent)	13.98	4.73	4.73	0.84	19.55	19.55	000	
50576		A	with fulguration and/or incision, with or without biopsy	10.99	3.74	3.74	0.66	15.39	15.39	000	
50578		A	with insertion of radioactive substance, with or without biopsy and/or fulguration	11.35	4.01	4.01	0.67	16.03	16.03	000	
50580		A	with removal of foreign body or calculus	11.86	4.03	4.03	0.70	16.59	16.59	000	
50590		A	Lithotripsy, extracorporeal shock wave	9.09	10.78	5.35	0.54	20.41	14.98	090	
50600		A	Ureterotomy with exploration or drainage (separate procedure)	15.84	9.07	9.07	0.99	25.90	25.90	090	
50605		A	Ureterotomy for insertion of indwelling stent, all types	15.46	8.88	8.88	1.13	25.47	25.47	090	
50610		A	Ureterolithotomy; upper one-third of ureter	15.92	9.09	9.09	1.08	26.09	26.09	090	
50620		A	middle one-third of ureter	15.16	8.55	8.55	0.91	24.62	24.62	090	
50630		A	lower one-third of ureter	14.94	8.48	8.48	0.90	24.32	24.32	090	
50650		A	Ureterectomy, with bladder cuff (separate procedure)	17.41	9.71	9.71	1.07	28.19	28.19	090	
50660		A	Ureterectomy, total, ectopic ureter, combination abdominal, vaginal and/or perineal approach	19.55	10.43	10.43	1.19	31.17	31.17	090	
50684		A	Injection procedure for ureterography or ureteropyelography through ureterostomy or indwelling ureteral catheter	0.76	15.02	0.26	0.04	15.82	1.06	000	
50686		A	Manometric studies through ureterostomy or indwelling ureteral catheter	1.51	5.08	0.65	0.09	6.68	2.25	000	
50688		A	Change of ureterostomy tube	1.17	1.76	1.76	0.06	2.99	2.99	010	
50690		A	Injection procedure for visualization of ileal conduit and/or ureteropyelography, exclusive of radiologic service	1.16	15.40	0.40	0.06	16.62	1.62	000	
50700		A	Ureteroplasty, plastic operation on ureter (eg, stricture)	15.21	9.09	9.09	0.86	25.16	25.16	090	
50715		A	Ureterolysis, with or without repositioning of ureter for retroperitoneal fibrosis	18.90	12.37	12.37	1.68	32.95	32.95	090	

■ RVU not developed by CMS. Gap-filled RVUs developed by Ingenix/CHEG.

Code	M	S	Description	Work Value	Non-Fac PE	Fac PE	Mal-practice	Non-Fac Total	Fac Total	Global	Gap
50722		A	Ureterolysis for ovarian vein syndrome	16.35	10.42	10.42	1.41	28.18	28.18	090	
50725		A	Ureterolysis for retrocaval ureter, with reanastomosis of upper urinary tract or vena cava	18.49	10.61	10.61	1.44	30.54	30.54	090	
50727		A	Revision of urinary-cutaneous anastomosis (any type urostomy);	8.18	6.54	6.54	0.51	15.23	15.23	090	
50728		A	with repair of fascial defect and hernia	12.02	8.18	8.18	0.88	21.08	21.08	090	
50740		A	Ureteropyelostomy, anastomosis of ureter and renal pelvis	18.42	9.66	9.66	1.49	29.57	29.57	090	
50750		A	Ureterocalycostomy, anastomosis of ureter to renal calyx	19.51	10.48	10.48	1.24	31.23	31.23	090	
50760		A	Ureteroureterostomy	18.42	10.11	10.11	1.25	29.78	29.78	090	
50770		A	Transureteroureterostomy, anastomosis of ureter to contralateral ureter	19.51	10.43	10.43	1.25	31.19	31.19	090	
50780		A	Ureteroneocystostomy; anastomosis of single ureter to bladder	18.36	10.01	10.01	1.20	29.57	29.57	090	
50782		A	anastomosis of duplicated ureter to bladder	19.54	11.91	11.91	1.13	32.58	32.58	090	
50783		A	with extensive ureteral tailoring	20.55	11.22	11.22	1.35	33.12	33.12	090	
50785		A	with vesico-psoas hitch or bladder flap	20.52	10.83	10.83	1.30	32.65	32.65	090	
50800		A	Ureteroenterostomy, direct anastomosis of ureter to intestine	14.52	10.02	10.02	0.92	25.46	25.46	090	
50810		A	Ureterosigmoidostomy, with creation of sigmoid bladder and establishment of abdominal or perineal colostomy, including intestine anastomosis	20.05	12.23	12.23	1.78	34.06	34.06	090	
50815		A	Ureterocolon conduit, including intestine anastomosis	19.93	11.71	11.71	1.31	32.95	32.95	090	
50820		A	Ureteroileal conduit (ileal bladder), including intestine anastomosis (Bricker operation)	21.89	12.38	12.38	1.38	35.65	35.65	090	
50825		A	Continent diversion, including intestine anastomosis using any segment of small and/or large intestine (Kock pouch or Camey enterocystoplasty)	28.18	15.30	15.30	1.81	45.29	45.29	090	
50830		A	Urinary undiversion (eg, taking down of ureteroileal conduit, ureterosigmoidostomy or ureteroenterostomy with ureteroureterostomy or ureteroneocystostomy)	31.28	15.96	15.96	2.20	49.44	49.44	090	
50840		A	Replacement of all or part of ureter by intestine segment, including intestine anastomosis	20.00	11.83	11.83	1.26	33.09	33.09	090	
50845		A	Cutaneous appendico-vesicostomy	20.89	10.20	10.20	1.26	32.35	32.35	090	
50860		A	Ureterostomy, transplantation of ureter to skin	15.36	8.93	8.93	1.01	25.30	25.30	090	

■ RVU not developed by CMS. Gap-filled RVUs developed by Ingenix/CHEG.

Surgery

Code	M	S	Description	Work Value	Non-Fac PE	Fac PE	Mal-practice	Non-Fac Total	Fac Total	Global	Gap
50900		A	Ureterorrhaphy, suture of ureter (separate procedure)	13.62	8.08	8.08	0.98	22.68	22.68	090	
50920		A	Closure of ureterocutaneous fistula	14.33	8.37	8.37	0.84	23.54	23.54	090	
50930		A	Closure of ureterovisceral fistula (including visceral repair)	18.72	10.80	10.80	1.57	31.09	31.09	090	
50940		A	Deligation of ureter	14.51	8.44	8.44	1.04	23.99	23.99	090	
50945		A	Laparoscopy, surgical; ureterolithotomy	17.00	7.42	7.42	1.15	25.57	25.57	090	
50947		A	ureteroneocystostomy with cystoscopy and ureteral stent placement	24.50	11.74	11.74	1.99	38.23	38.23	090	
50948		A	ureteroneocystostomy without cystoscopy and ureteral stent placement	22.50	10.61	10.61	1.83	34.94	34.94	090	
50949		C	Unlisted laparoscopy procedure, ureter	0.00	0.00	0.00	0.00	0.00	0.00	YYY	
50951		A	Ureteral endoscopy through established ureterostomy, with or without irrigation, instillation, or ureteropyelography, exclusive of radiologic service;	5.84	5.28	1.98	0.35	11.47	8.17	000	
50953		A	with ureteral catheterization, with or without dilation of ureter	6.24	16.55	2.12	0.37	23.16	8.73	000	
50955		A	with biopsy	6.75	21.11	2.38	0.38	28.24	9.51	000	
50957		A	with fulguration and/or incision, with or without biopsy	6.79	19.64	2.28	0.40	26.83	9.47	000	
50959		A	with insertion of radioactive substance, with or without biopsy and/or fulguration (not including provision of material)	4.40	1.58	1.58	0.18	6.16	6.16	000	
50961		A	with removal of foreign body or calculus	6.05	23.38	2.04	0.35	29.78	8.44	000	
50970		A	Ureteral endoscopy through ureterotomy, with or without irrigation, instillation, or ureteropyelography, exclusive of radiologic service;	7.14	2.43	2.43	0.43	10.00	10.00	000	
50972		A	with ureteral catheterization, with or without dilation of ureter	6.89	2.52	2.52	0.39	9.80	9.80	000	
50974		A	with biopsy	9.17	3.16	3.16	0.53	12.86	12.86	000	
50976		A	with fulguration and/or incision, with or without biopsy	9.04	3.09	3.09	0.53	12.66	12.66	000	
50978		A	with insertion of radioactive substance, with or without biopsy and/or fulguration (not including provision of material)	5.10	1.88	1.88	0.30	7.28	7.28	000	
50980		A	with removal of foreign body or calculus	6.85	2.34	2.34	0.41	9.60	9.60	000	
51000		A	Aspiration of bladder by needle	0.78	2.03	0.25	0.05	2.86	1.08	000	
51005		A	Aspiration of bladder; by trocar or intracatheter	1.02	3.37	0.35	0.08	4.47	1.45	000	

■ RVU not developed by CMS. Gap-filled RVUs developed by Ingenix/CHEG.

Code	M	S	Description	Work Value	Non-Fac PE	Fac PE	Mal-prac-tice	Non-Fac Total	Fac Total	Global	Gap
51010		A	with insertion of suprapubic catheter	3.53	4.42	2.37	0.23	8.18	6.13	010	
51020		A	Cystotomy or cystostomy; with fulguration and/or insertion of radioactive material	6.71	5.72	5.72	0.42	12.85	12.85	090	
51030		A	with cryosurgical destruction of intravesical lesion	6.77	6.01	6.01	0.42	13.20	13.20	090	
51040		A	Cystostomy, cystotomy with drainage	4.40	4.47	4.47	0.27	9.14	9.14	090	
51045		A	Cystotomy, with insertion of ureteral catheter or stent (separate procedure)	6.77	6.01	6.01	0.47	13.25	13.25	090	
51050		A	Cystolithotomy, cystotomy with removal of calculus, without vesical neck resection	6.92	5.27	5.27	0.42	12.61	12.61	090	
51060		A	Transvesical ureterolithotomy	8.85	6.53	6.53	0.54	15.92	15.92	090	
51065		A	Cystotomy, with calculus basket extraction and/or ultrasonic or electrohydraulic fragmentation of ureteral calculus	8.85	6.06	6.06	0.53	15.44	15.44	090	
51080		A	Drainage of perivesical or prevesical space abscess	5.96	5.67	5.67	0.35	11.98	11.98	090	
51500		A	Excision of urachal cyst or sinus, with or without umbilical hernia repair	10.14	6.13	6.13	0.88	17.15	17.15	090	
51520		A	Cystotomy; for simple excision of vesical neck (separate procedure)	9.29	6.66	6.66	0.58	16.53	16.53	090	
51525		A	for excision of bladder diverticulum, single or multiple (separate procedure)	13.97	8.15	8.15	0.85	22.97	22.97	090	
51530		A	for excision of bladder tumor	12.38	7.81	7.81	0.82	21.01	21.01	090	
51535		A	Cystotomy for excision, incision, or repair of ureterocele	12.57	8.23	8.23	0.90	21.70	21.70	090	
51550		A	Cystectomy, partial; simple	15.66	8.68	8.68	1.05	25.39	25.39	090	
51555		A	complicated (eg, postradiation, previous surgery, difficult location)	21.23	11.00	11.00	1.37	33.60	33.60	090	
51565		A	Cystectomy, partial, with reimplantation of ureter(s) into bladder (ureteroneocystostomy)	21.62	11.62	11.62	1.40	34.64	34.64	090	
51570		A	Cystectomy, complete; (separate procedure)	24.24	12.60	12.60	1.59	38.43	38.43	090	
51575		A	with bilateral pelvic lymphadenectomy, including external iliac, hypogastric, and obturator nodes	30.45	15.35	15.35	1.88	47.68	47.68	090	
51580		A	Cystectomy, complete, with ureterosigmoidostomy or ureterocutaneous transplantations;	31.08	16.01	16.01	1.94	49.03	49.03	090	
51585		A	with bilateral pelvic lymphadenectomy, including external iliac, hypogastric, and obturator nodes	35.23	17.34	17.34	2.18	54.75	54.75	090	

■ RVU not developed by CMS. Gap-filled RVUs developed by Ingenix/CHEG.

Code	M	S	Description	Work Value	Non-Fac PE	Fac PE	Mal-practice	Non-Fac Total	Fac Total	Global	Gap
51590		A	Cystectomy, complete, with ureteroileal conduit or sigmoid bladder, including intestine anastomosis;	32.66	16.01	16.01	2.01	50.68	50.68	090	
51595		A	with bilateral pelvic lymphadenectomy, including external iliac, hypogastric, and obturator nodes	37.14	17.55	17.55	2.23	56.92	56.92	090	
51596		A	Cystectomy, complete, with continent diversion, any open technique, using any segment of small and/or large intestine to construct neobladder	39.52	18.94	18.94	2.39	60.85	60.85	090	
51597		A	Pelvic exenteration, complete, for vesical, prostatic or urethral malignancy, with removal of bladder and ureteral transplantations, with or without hysterectomy and/or abdominoperineal resection of rectum and colon and colostomy, or any combination thereof	38.35	18.06	18.06	2.49	58.90	58.90	090	
51600		A	Injection procedure for cystography or voiding urethrocystography	0.88	5.51	0.30	0.04	6.43	1.22	000	
51605		A	Injection procedure and placement of chain for contrast and/or chain urethrocystography	0.64	16.73	0.22	0.04	17.41	0.90	000	
51610		A	Injection procedure for retrograde urethrocystography	1.05	16.20	0.36	0.05	17.30	1.46	000	
51700		A	Bladder irrigation, simple, lavage and/or instillation	0.88	1.32	0.30	0.05	2.25	1.23	000	
51705		A	Change of cystostomy tube; simple	1.02	2.15	0.65	0.06	3.23	1.73	010	
51710		A	complicated	1.49	5.11	1.47	0.09	6.69	3.05	010	
51715		A	Endoscopic injection of implant material into the submucosal tissues of the urethra and/or bladder neck	3.74	4.44	1.29	0.24	8.42	5.27	000	
51720		A	Bladder instillation of anticarcinogenic agent (including detention time)	1.96	1.68	0.74	0.12	3.76	2.82	000	
51725		A	Simple cystometrogram (CMG) (eg, spinal manometer)	1.51	5.92	5.92	0.13	7.56	7.56	000	
	26	A		1.51	0.52	0.52	0.10	2.13	2.13	000	
	TC	A		0.00	5.40	5.40	0.03	5.43	5.43	000	
51726		A	Complex cystometrogram (eg, calibrated electronic equipment)	1.71	4.65	4.65	0.15	6.51	6.51	000	
	26	A		1.71	0.59	0.59	0.11	2.41	2.41	000	
	TC	A		0.00	4.06	4.06	0.04	4.10	4.10	000	
51736		A	Simple uroflowmetry (UFR) (eg, stop-watch flow rate, mechanical uroflowmeter)	0.61	1.07	1.07	0.05	1.73	1.73	000	
	26	A		0.61	0.21	0.21	0.04	0.86	0.86	000	
	TC	A		0.00	0.86	0.86	0.01	0.87	0.87	000	
51741		A	Complex uroflowmetry (eg, calibrated electronic equipment)	1.14	1.93	1.93	0.09	3.16	3.16	000	
	26	A		1.14	0.40	0.40	0.07	1.61	1.61	000	
	TC	A		0.00	1.53	1.53	0.02	1.55	1.55	000	

■ RVU not developed by CMS. Gap-filled RVUs developed by Ingenix/CHEG.

Surgery

Code	M	S	Description	Work Value	Non-Fac PE	Fac PE	Mal-practice	Non-Fac Total	Fac Total	Global	Gap
51772		A	Urethral pressure profile studies (UPP) (urethral closure pressure profile), any technique	1.61	4.73	4.73	0.16	6.50	6.50	000	
	26	A		1.61	0.59	0.59	0.12	2.32	2.32	000	
	TC	A		0.00	4.14	4.14	0.04	4.18	4.18	000	
51784		A	Electromyography studies (EMG) of anal or urethral sphincter, other than needle, any technique	1.53	3.36	3.36	0.13	5.02	5.02	000	
	26	A		1.53	0.53	0.53	0.10	2.16	2.16	000	
	TC	A		0.00	2.83	2.83	0.03	2.86	2.86	000	
51785		A	Needle electromyography studies (EMG) of anal or urethral sphincter, any technique	1.53	3.46	3.46	0.12	5.11	5.11	000	
	26	A		1.53	0.53	0.53	0.09	2.15	2.15	000	
	TC	A		0.00	2.93	2.93	0.03	2.96	2.96	00	
51792		A	Stimulus evoked response (eg, measurement of bulbocavernosus reflex latency time)	1.10	3.33	3.33	0.20	4.63	4.63	000	
	26	A		1.10	0.43	0.43	0.09	1.62	1.62	000	
	TC	A		0.00	2.90	2.90	0.11	3.01	3.01	000	
51795		A	Voiding pressure studies (VP); bladder voiding pressure, any technique	1.53	4.84	4.84	0.18	6.55	6.55	000	
	26	A		1.53	0.53	0.53	0.10	2.16	2.16	000	
	TC	A		0.00	4.31	4.31	0.08	4.39	4.39	000	
51797		A	intra-abdominal voiding pressure (AP) (rectal, gastric, intraperitoneal)	1.60	4.87	4.87	0.14	6.61	6.61	000	
	26	A		1.60	0.56	0.56	0.10	2.26	2.26	000	
	TC	A		0.00	4.31	4.31	0.04	4.35	4.35	000	
51800		A	Cystoplasty or cystourethroplasty, plastic operation on bladder and/or vesical neck (anterior Y-plasty, vesical fundus resection), any procedure, with or without wedge resection of posterior vesical neck	17.42	9.59	9.59	1.17	28.18	28.18	090	
51820		A	Cystourethroplasty with unilateral or bilateral ureteroneocystostomy	17.89	10.91	10.91	1.45	30.25	30.25	090	
51840		A	Anterior vesicourethropexy, or urethropexy (eg, Marshall-Marchetti-Krantz, Burch); simple	10.71	6.88	6.88	0.87	18.46	18.46	090	
51841		A	complicated (eg, secondary repair)	13.03	8.57	8.57	1.04	22.64	22.64	090	
51845		A	Abdomino-vaginal vesical neck suspension, with or without endoscopic control (eg, Stamey, Raz, modified Pereyra)	9.73	6.90	6.90	0.62	17.25	17.25	090	
51860		A	Cystorrhaphy, suture of bladder wound, injury or rupture; simple	12.02	7.90	7.90	0.89	20.81	20.81	090	
51865		A	complicated	15.04	8.93	8.93	1.01	24.98	24.98	090	
51880		A	Closure of cystostomy (separate procedure)	7.66	5.98	5.98	0.54	14.18	14.18	090	
51900		A	Closure of vesicovaginal fistula, abdominal approach	12.97	8.29	8.29	0.87	22.13	22.13	090	
51920		A	Closure of vesicouterine fistula;	11.81	7.65	7.65	0.86	20.32	20.32	090	
51925		A	with hysterectomy	15.58	9.65	9.65	1.48	26.71	26.71	090	
51940		A	Closure, exstrophy of bladder	28.43	16.41	16.41	1.97	46.81	46.81	090	
51960		A	Enterocystoplasty, including intestinal anastomosis	23.01	13.39	13.39	1.41	37.81	37.81	090	

■ RVU not developed by CMS. Gap-filled RVUs developed by Ingenix/CHEG.

Code	M	S	Description	Work Value	Non-Fac PE	Fac PE	Mal-practice	Non-Fac Total	Fac Total	Global	Gap
51980		A	Cutaneous vesicostomy	11.36	7.30	7.30	0.74	19.40	19.40	090	
51990		A	Laparoscopy, surgical; urethral suspension for stress incontinence	12.50	6.79	6.79	1.02	20.31	20.31	090	
51992		A	sling operation for stress incontinence (eg, fascia or synthetic)	14.01	6.81	6.81	0.93	21.75	21.75	090	
52000		A	Cystourethroscopy (separate procedure)	2.01	3.45	0.69	0.12	5.58	2.82	000	
52001		A	Cystourethroscopy with irrigation and evacuation of clots	2.37	0.98	0.98	0.32	3.67	3.67	000	
52005		A	Cystourethroscopy, with ureteral catheterization, with or without irrigation, instillation, or ureteropyelography, exclusive of radiologic service;	2.37	13.40	0.91	0.15	15.92	3.43	000	
52007		A	with brush biopsy of ureter and/or renal pelvis	3.02	1.02	1.02	0.18	4.22	4.22	000	
52010		A	Cystourethroscopy, with ejaculatory duct catheterization, with or without irrigation, instillation, or duct radiography, exclusive of radiologic service	3.02	5.91	1.02	0.18	9.11	4.22	000	
52204		A	Cystourethroscopy, with biopsy	2.37	6.17	0.80	0.15	8.69	3.32	000	
52214		A	Cystourethroscopy, with fulguration (including cryosurgery or laser surgery) of trigone, bladder neck, prostatic fossa, urethra, or periurethral glands	3.71	6.53	1.26	0.22	10.46	5.19	000	
52224		A	Cystourethroscopy, with fulguration (including cryosurgery or laser surgery) or treatment of MINOR (less than 0.5 cm) lesion(s) with or without biopsy	3.14	6.41	1.07	0.18	9.73	4.39	000	
52234		A	Cystourethroscopy, with fulguration (including cryosurgery or laser surgery) and/or resection of; SMALL bladder tumor(s) (0.5 to 2.0 cm)	4.63	1.68	1.68	0.27	6.58	6.58	000	
52235		A	MEDIUM bladder tumor(s) (2.0 to 5.0 cm)	5.45	1.97	1.97	0.32	7.74	7.74	000	
52240		A	LARGE bladder tumor(s)	9.72	3.43	3.43	0.58	13.73	13.73	000	
52250		A	Cystourethroscopy with insertion of radioactive substance, with or without biopsy or fulguration	4.50	1.53	1.53	0.27	6.30	6.30	000	
52260		A	Cystourethroscopy, with dilation of bladder for interstitial cystitis; general or conduction (spinal) anesthesia	3.92	1.34	1.34	0.23	5.49	5.49	000	
52265		A	local anesthesia	2.94	3.77	1.00	0.18	6.89	4.12	000	
52270		A	Cystourethroscopy, with internal urethrotomy; female	3.37	6.88	1.14	0.20	10.45	4.71	000	
52275		A	male	4.70	7.42	1.59	0.28	12.40	6.57	000	

■ RVU not developed by CMS. Gap-filled RVUs developed by Ingenix/CHEG.

Code	M	S	Description	Work Value	Non-Fac PE	Fac PE	Mal-practice	Non-Fac Total	Fac Total	Global	Gap
52276		A	Cystourethroscopy with direct vision internal urethrotomy	5.00	7.55	1.70	0.30	12.85	7.00	000	
52277		A	Cystourethroscopy, with resection of external sphincter (sphincterotomy)	6.17	2.12	2.12	0.38	8.67	8.67	000	
52281		A	Cystourethroscopy, with calibration and/or dilation of urethral stricture or stenosis, with or without meatotomy, with or without injection procedure for cystography, male or female	2.80	14.54	1.08	0.17	17.51	4.05	000	
52282		A	Cystourethroscopy, with insertion of urethral stent	6.40	15.36	2.18	0.38	22.14	8.96	000	
52283		A	Cystourethroscopy, with steroid injection into stricture	3.74	6.58	1.27	0.22	10.54	5.23	000	
52285		A	Cystourethroscopy for treatment of the female urethral syndrome with any or all of the following: urethral meatotomy, urethral dilation, internal urethrotomy, lysis of urethrovaginal septal fibrosis, lateral incisions of the bladder neck, and fulguration of polyp(s) of urethra, bladder neck, and/or trigone	3.61	7.06	1.23	0.22	10.89	5.06	000	
52290		A	Cystourethroscopy; with ureteral meatotomy, unilateral or bilateral	4.59	1.56	1.56	0.27	6.42	6.42	000	
52300		A	with resection or fulguration of orthotopic ureterocele(s), unilateral or bilateral	5.31	1.80	1.80	0.32	7.43	7.43	000	
52301		A	with resection or fulguration of ectopic ureterocele(s), unilateral or bilateral	5.51	1.82	1.82	0.39	7.72	7.72	000	
52305		A	with incision or resection of orifice of bladder diverticulum, single or multiple	5.31	1.80	1.80	0.31	7.42	7.42	000	
52310		A	Cystourethroscopy, with removal of foreign body, calculus, or ureteral stent from urethra or bladder (separate procedure); simple	2.81	3.85	1.02	0.17	6.83	4.00	000	
52315		A	complicated	5.21	16.43	1.76	0.31	21.95	7.28	000	
52317		A	Litholapaxy: crushing or fragmentation of calculus by any means in bladder and removal of fragments; simple or small (less than 2.5 cm)	6.72	26.09	2.28	0.40	33.21	9.40	000	
52318		A	complicated or large (over 2.5 cm)	9.19	3.11	3.11	0.54	12.84	12.84	000	
52320		A	Cystourethroscopy (including ureteral catheterization); with removal of ureteral calculus	4.70	1.59	1.59	0.28	6.57	6.57	000	
52325		A	with fragmentation of ureteral calculus (eg, ultrasonic or electro-hydraulic technique)	6.16	2.08	2.08	0.37	8.61	8.61	000	
52327		A	with subureteric injection of implant material	5.19	1.77	1.77	0.32	7.28	7.28	000	
52330		A	with manipulation, without removal of ureteral calculus	5.04	20.79	1.71	0.30	26.13	7.05	000	

■ RVU not developed by CMS. Gap-filled RVUs developed by Ingenix/CHEG.

Surgery

Code	M	S	Description	Work Value	Non-Fac PE	Fac PE	Mal-practice	Non-Fac Total	Fac Total	Global	Gap
52332		A	Cystourethroscopy, with insertion of indwelling ureteral stent (eg, Gibbons or double-J type)	2.83	18.84	1.07	0.17	21.84	4.07	000	
52334		A	Cystourethroscopy with insertion of ureteral guide wire through kidney to establish a percutaneous nephrostomy, retrograde	4.83	1.63	1.63	0.28	6.74	6.74	000	
52341		A	Cystourethroscopy; with treatment of ureteral stricture (eg, balloon dilation, laser, electrocautery, and incision)	6.00	2.40	2.40	0.37	8.77	8.77	000	
52342		A	with treatment of ureteropelvic junction stricture (eg, balloon dilation, laser, electrocautery, and incision)	6.50	2.59	2.59	0.40	9.49	9.49	000	
52343		A	with treatment of intra-renal stricture (eg, balloon dilation, laser, electrocautery, and incision)	7.20	2.87	2.87	0.44	10.51	10.51	000	
52344		A	Cystourethroscopy with ureteroscopy; with treatment of ureteral stricture (eg, balloon dilation, laser, electrocautery, and incision)	7.70	3.07	3.07	0.47	11.24	11.24	000	
52345		A	with treatment of ureteropelvic junction stricture (eg, balloon dilation, laser, electrocautery, and incision)	8.20	3.27	3.27	0.50	11.97	11.97	000	
52346		A	with treatment of intra-renal stricture (eg, balloon dilation, laser, electrocautery, and incision)	9.23	3.68	3.68	0.57	13.48	13.48	000	
52347		A	Cystourethroscopy with transurethral resection or incision of ejaculatory ducts	5.28	2.14	2.14	0.33	7.75	7.75	000	
52351		A	Cystourethroscopy, with ureteroscopy and/or pyeloscopy; diagnostic	5.86	1.99	1.99	0.36	8.21	8.21	000	
52352		A	with removal or manipulation of calculus (ureteral catheterization is included)	6.88	2.33	2.33	0.42	9.63	9.63	000	
52353		A	with lithotripsy (ureteral catheterization is included)	7.97	2.69	2.69	0.49	11.15	11.15	000	
52354		A	with biopsy and/or fulguration of lesion	7.34	2.49	2.49	0.45	10.28	10.28	000	
52355		A	with resection of tumor	8.82	2.99	2.99	0.55	12.36	12.36	000	
52400		A	Cystourethroscopy with incision, fulguration, or resection of congenital posterior urethral valves, or congenital obstructive hypertrophic mucosal folds	9.68	5.75	5.75	0.60	16.03	16.03	090	
52450		A	Transurethral incision of prostate	7.64	6.56	6.56	0.46	14.66	14.66	090	
52500		A	Transurethral resection of bladder neck (separate procedure)	8.47	6.81	6.81	0.50	15.78	15.78	090	
52510		A	Transurethral balloon dilation of the prostatic urethra	6.72	5.80	5.80	0.40	12.92	12.92	090	

■ RVU not developed by CMS. Gap-filled RVUs developed by Ingenix/CHEG.

Code	M	S	Description	Work Value	Non-Fac PE	Fac PE	Mal-prac-tice	Non-Fac Total	Fac Total	Global	Gap
52601		A	Transurethral electrosurgical resection of prostate, including control of postoperative bleeding, complete (vasectomy, meatotomy, cystourethroscopy, urethral calibration and/or dilation, and internal urethrotomy are included)	12.37	8.16	8.16	0.74	21.27	21.27	090	
52606		A	Transurethral fulguration for postoperative bleeding occurring after the usual follow-up time	8.13	6.27	6.27	0.49	14.89	14.89	090	
52612		A	Transurethral resection of prostate; first stage of two-stage resection (partial resection)	7.98	6.72	6.72	0.48	15.18	15.18	090	
52614		A	second stage of two-stage resection (resection completed)	6.84	6.30	6.30	0.41	13.55	13.55	090	
52620		A	Transurethral resection; of residual obstructive tissue after 90 days postoperative	6.61	6.22	6.22	0.39	13.22	13.22	090	
52630		A	of regrowth of obstructive tissue longer than one year postoperative	7.26	6.44	6.44	0.43	14.13	14.13	090	
52640		A	of postoperative bladder neck contracture	6.62	5.73	5.73	0.39	12.74	12.74	090	
52647		A	Non-contact laser coagulation of prostate, including control of postoperative bleeding, complete (vasectomy, meatotomy, cystourethroscopy, urethral calibration and/or dilation, and internal urethrotomy are included)	10.36	59.33	4.85	0.61	70.30	15.82	090	
52648		A	Contact laser vaporization with or without transurethral resection of prostate, including control of postoperative bleeding, complete (vasectomy, meatotomy, cystourethroscopy, urethral calibration and/or dilation, and internal urethrotomy are included)	11.21	7.63	7.63	0.66	19.50	19.50	090	
52700		A	Transurethral drainage of prostatic abscess	6.80	6.32	6.32	0.41	13.53	13.53	090	
53000		A	Urethrotomy or urethrostomy, external (separate procedure); pendulous urethra	2.28	7.47	2.63	0.13	9.88	5.04	010	
53010		A	perineal urethra, external	3.64	4.12	4.12	0.20	7.96	7.96	090	
53020		A	Meatotomy, cutting of meatus (separate procedure); except infant	1.77	4.43	0.67	0.11	6.31	2.55	000	
53025		A	infant	1.13	4.81	0.45	0.07	6.01	1.65	000	
53040		A	Drainage of deep periurethral abscess	6.40	14.74	8.33	0.41	21.55	15.14	090	
53060		A	Drainage of Skene's gland abscess or cyst	2.63	6.21	2.91	0.23	9.07	5.77	010	
53080		A	Drainage of perineal urinary extravasation; uncomplicated (separate procedure)	6.29	8.37	8.37	0.42	15.08	15.08	090	
53085		A	complicated	10.27	10.29	10.29	0.67	21.23	21.23	090	
53200		A	Biopsy of urethra	2.59	5.63	0.97	0.17	8.39	3.73	000	

Surgery

■ RVU not developed by CMS. Gap-filled RVUs developed by Ingenix/CHEG.

Code	M	S	Description	Work Value	Non-Fac PE	Fac PE	Mal-prac-tice	Non-Fac Total	Fac Total	Global	Gap
53210		A	Urethrectomy, total, including cystostomy; female	12.57	8.00	8.00	0.81	21.38	21.38	090	
53215		A	male	15.58	8.81	8.81	0.93	25.32	25.32	090	
53220		A	Excision or fulguration of carcinoma of urethra	7.00	5.71	5.71	0.44	13.15	13.15	090	
53230		A	Excision of urethral diverticulum (separate procedure); female	9.58	6.36	6.36	0.60	16.54	16.54	090	
53235		A	male	10.14	6.49	6.49	0.60	17.23	17.23	090	
53240		A	Marsupialization of urethral diverticulum, male or female	6.45	5.32	5.32	0.42	12.19	12.19	090	
53250		A	Excision of bulbourethral gland (Cowper's gland)	5.89	4.74	4.74	0.35	10.98	10.98	090	
53260		A	Excision or fulguration; urethral polyp(s), distal urethra	2.98	6.11	2.44	0.23	9.32	5.65	010	
53265		A	urethral caruncle	3.12	6.60	2.42	0.20	9.92	5.74	010	
53270		A	Skene's glands	3.09	7.03	2.83	0.21	10.33	6.13	010	
53275		A	urethral prolapse	4.53	3.43	3.43	0.28	8.24	8.24	010	
53400		A	Urethroplasty; first stage, for fistula, diverticulum, or stricture (eg, Johannsen type)	12.77	8.31	8.31	0.85	21.93	21.93	090	
53405		A	second stage (formation of urethra), including urinary diversion	14.48	8.61	8.61	0.91	24.00	24.00	090	
53410		A	Urethroplasty, one-stage reconstruction of male anterior urethra	16.44	9.21	9.21	0.99	26.64	26.64	090	
53415		A	Urethroplasty, transpubic or perineal, one stage, for reconstruction or repair of prostatic or membranous urethra	19.41	10.16	10.16	1.16	30.73	30.73	090	
53420		A	Urethroplasty, two-stage reconstruction or repair of prostatic or membranous urethra; first stage	14.08	8.82	8.82	0.90	23.80	23.80	090	
53425		A	second stage	15.98	9.02	9.02	0.97	25.97	25.97	090	
53430		A	Urethroplasty, reconstruction of female urethra	16.34	9.34	9.34	1.01	26.69	26.69	090	
53431		A	Urethroplasty with tubularization of posterior urethra and/or lower bladder for incontinence (eg, Tenago, Leadbetter procedure)	19.89	7.94	7.94	1.25	29.08	29.08	090	
53440		A	Operation for correction of male urinary incontinence, with or without introduction of prosthesis	12.34	8.09	8.09	0.73	21.16	21.16	090	
53442		A	Removal of perineal prosthesis introduced for continence	8.27	6.08	6.08	0.55	14.90	14.90	090	
53444		A	Insertion of tandem cuff (dual cuff)	13.40	6.66	6.66	0.79	20.85	20.85	090	

■ RVU not developed by CMS. Gap-filled RVUs developed by Ingenix/CHEG.

Code	M	S	Description	Work Value	Non-Fac PE	Fac PE	Mal-practice	Non-Fac Total	Fac Total	Global	Gap
53445		A	Insertion of inflatable urethral/bladder neck sphincter, including placement of pump, reservoir, and cuff	14.06	8.72	8.72	0.84	23.62	23.62	090	
53446		A	Removal of inflatable urethral/bladder neck sphincter, including pump, reservoir, and cuff	10.23	8.46	8.46	0.61	19.30	19.30	090	
53447		A	Removal and replacement of inflatable urethral/ bladder neck sphincter including pump, reservoir, and cuff at the same operative session	13.49	7.90	7.90	0.79	22.18	22.18	090	
53448		A	Removal and replacement of inflatable urethral/ bladder neck sphincter including pump, reservoir, and cuff through an infected field at the same operative session including irrigation and debridement of infected tissue	21.15	12.35	12.35	1.27	34.77	34.77	090	
53449		A	Repair of inflatable urethral/bladder neck sphincter, including pump, reservoir, and cuff	9.70	6.73	6.73	0.57	17.00	17.00	090	
53450		A	Urethromeatoplasty, with mucosal advancement	6.14	5.16	5.16	0.37	11.67	11.67	090	
53460		A	Urethromeatoplasty, with partial excision of distal urethral segment (Richardson type procedure)	7.12	5.50	5.50	0.43	13.05	13.05	090	
53502		A	Urethrorrhaphy, suture of urethral wound or injury, female	7.63	5.80	5.80	0.50	13.93	13.93	090	
53505		A	Urethrorrhaphy, suture of urethral wound or injury; penile	7.63	5.62	5.62	0.46	13.71	13.71	090	
53510		A	perineal	10.11	6.58	6.58	0.60	17.29	17.29	090	
53515		A	prostatomembranous	13.31	7.81	7.81	0.83	21.95	21.95	090	
53520		A	Closure of urethrostomy or urethrocutaneous fistula, male (separate procedure)	8.68	6.12	6.12	0.53	15.33	15.33	090	
53600		A	Dilation of urethral stricture by passage of sound or urethral dilator, male; initial	1.21	1.19	0.46	0.07	2.47	1.74	000	
53601		A	subsequent	0.98	1.31	0.40	0.06	2.35	1.44	000	
53605		A	Dilation of urethral stricture or vesical neck by passage of sound or urethral dilator, male, general or conduction (spinal) anesthesia	1.28	0.44	0.44	0.08	1.80	1.80	000	
53620		A	Dilation of urethral stricture by passage of filiform and follower, male; initial	1.62	1.91	0.63	0.10	3.63	2.35	000	
53621		A	subsequent	1.35	2.00	0.52	0.08	3.43	1.95	000	
53660		A	Dilation of female urethra including suppository and/or instillation; initial	0.71	1.22	0.33	0.04	1.97	1.08	000	
53661		A	subsequent	0.72	1.21	0.31	0.04	1.97	1.07	000	
53665		A	Dilation of female urethra, general or conduction (spinal) anesthesia	0.76	0.27	0.27	0.05	1.08	1.08	000	

Surgery

■ RVU not developed by CMS. Gap-filled RVUs developed by Ingenix/CHEG.

Code	M	S	Description	Work Value	Non-Fac PE	Fac PE	Mal-practice	Non-Fac Total	Fac Total	Global	Gap
53670		A	Catheterization, urethra; simple	0.50	1.74	0.18	0.03	2.27	0.71	000	
53675		A	complicated (may include difficult removal of balloon catheter)	1.47	2.63	0.58	0.09	4.19	2.14	000	
53850		A	Transurethral destruction of prostate tissue; by microwave thermotherapy	9.45	87.54	4.50	0.56	97.55	14.51	090	
53852		A	by radiofrequency thermotherapy	9.88	75.53	4.68	0.58	85.99	15.14	090	
53853		A	by water-induced thermotherapy	4.14	52.75	2.55	0.38	57.27	7.07	090	
53899		C	Unlisted procedure, urinary system	0.00	0.00	0.00	0.00	0.00	0.00	YYY	
54000		A	Slitting of prepuce, dorsal or lateral (separate procedure); newborn	1.54	5.66	1.51	0.10	7.30	3.15	010	
54001		A	except newborn	2.19	6.56	2.15	0.14	8.89	4.48	010	
54015		A	Incision and drainage of penis, deep	5.32	7.95	3.21	0.33	13.60	8.86	010	
54050		A	Destruction of lesion(s), penis (eg, condyloma, papilloma, molluscum contagiosum, herpetic vesicle), simple; chemical	1.24	2.85	0.47	0.07	4.16	1.78	010	
54055		A	electrodesiccation	1.22	6.64	1.42	0.07	7.93	2.71	010	
54056		A	cryosurgery	1.24	2.96	0.58	0.06	4.26	1.88	010	
54057		A	laser surgery	1.24	2.97	1.41	0.08	4.29	2.73	010	
54060		A	surgical excision	1.93	5.65	1.66	0.12	7.70	3.71	010	
54065		A	Destruction of lesion(s), penis (eg, condyloma, papilloma, molluscum contagiosum, herpetic vesicle), extensive (eg, laser surgery, electrosurgery, cryosurgery, chemosurgery)	2.42	5.38	2.24	0.13	7.93	4.79	010	
54100		A	Biopsy of penis; (separate procedure)	1.90	3.54	0.77	0.10	5.54	2.77	000	
54105		A	deep structures	3.50	6.75	2.19	0.21	10.46	5.90	010	
54110		A	Excision of penile plaque (Peyronie disease);	10.13	8.20	8.20	0.60	18.93	18.93	090	
54111		A	with graft to 5 cm in length	13.57	9.37	9.37	0.79	23.73	23.73	090	
54112		A	with graft greater than 5 cm in length	15.86	10.08	10.08	0.94	26.88	26.88	090	
54115		A	Removal foreign body from deep penile tissue (eg, plastic implant)	6.15	11.63	6.77	0.39	18.17	13.31	090	
54120		A	Amputation of penis; partial	9.97	8.14	8.14	0.60	18.71	18.71	090	
54125		A	complete	13.53	9.37	9.37	0.81	23.71	23.71	090	
54130		A	Amputation of penis, radical; with bilateral inguinofemoral lymphadenectomy	20.14	12.00	12.00	1.19	33.33	33.33	090	
54135		A	in continuity with bilateral pelvic lymphadenectomy, including external iliac, hypogastric and obturator nodes	26.36	14.68	14.68	1.58	42.62	42.62	090	

■ RVU not developed by CMS. Gap-filled RVUs developed by Ingenix/CHEG.

Code	M	S	Description	Work Value	Non-Fac PE	Fac PE	Mal-practice	Non-Fac Total	Fac Total	Global	Gap
54150		A	Circumcision, using clamp or other device; newborn	1.81	6.04	1.87	0.17	8.02	3.85	010	
54152		A	except newborn	2.31	1.76	1.76	0.16	4.23	4.23	010	
54160		A	Circumcision, surgical excision other than clamp, device or dorsal slit; newborn	2.48	5.04	1.82	0.16	7.68	4.46	010	
54161		A	except newborn	3.27	2.10	2.10	0.20	5.57	5.57	010	
54162		A	Lysis or excision of penile post-circumcision adhesions	3.00	2.91	2.91	0.18	6.09	6.09	010	
54163		A	Repair incomplete circumcision	3.00	2.54	2.54	0.18	5.72	5.72	010	
54164		A	Frenulotomy of penis	2.50	2.37	2.37	0.15	5.02	5.02	010	
54200		A	Injection procedure for Peyronie disease;	1.06	2.87	0.38	0.06	3.99	1.50	010	
54205		A	with surgical exposure of plaque	7.93	7.50	7.50	0.47	15.90	15.90	090	
54220		A	Irrigation of corpora cavernosa for priapism	2.42	2.08	1.04	0.15	4.65	3.61	000	
54230		A	Injection procedure for corpora cavernosography	1.34	0.46	0.46	0.08	1.88	1.88	000	
54231		A	Dynamic cavernosometry, including intracavernosal injection of vasoactive drugs (eg, papaverine, phentolamine)	2.04	2.26	0.83	0.14	4.44	3.01	000	
54235		A	Injection of corpora cavernosa with pharmacologic agent(s) (eg, papaverine, phentolamine)	1.19	1.19	0.41	0.07	2.45	1.67	000	
54240		A	Penile plethysmography	1.31	1.59	1.59	0.13	3.03	3.03	000	
	26	A		1.31	0.45	0.45	0.08	1.84	1.84	000	
	TC	A		0.00	1.14	1.14	0.05	1.19	1.19	000	
54250		A	Nocturnal penile tumescence and/or rigidity test	2.22	2.90	2.90	0.16	5.28	5.28	000	
	26	A		2.22	0.75	0.75	0.14	3.11	3.11	000	
	TC	A		0.00	2.15	2.15	0.02	2.17	2.17	000	
54300		A	Plastic operation of penis for straightening of chordee (eg, hypospadias), with or without mobilization of urethra	10.41	8.89	8.89	0.64	19.94	19.94	090	
54304		A	Plastic operation on penis for correction of chordee or for first stage hypospadias repair with or without transplantation of prepuce and/or skin flaps	12.49	10.04	10.04	0.74	23.27	23.27	090	
54308		A	Urethroplasty for second stage hypospadias repair (including urinary diversion); less than 3 cm	11.83	9.94	9.94	0.70	22.47	22.47	090	
54312		A	greater than 3 cm	13.57	10.73	10.73	0.81	25.11	25.11	090	
54316		A	Urethroplasty for second stage hypospadias repair (including urinary diversion) with free skin graft obtained from site other than genitalia	16.82	11.67	11.67	1.00	29.49	29.49	090	

■ RVU not developed by CMS. Gap-filled RVUs developed by Ingenix/CHEG.

Surgery

Code	M	S	Description	Work Value	Non-Fac PE	Fac PE	Mal-prac-tice	Non-Fac Total	Fac Total	Global	Gap
54318		A	Urethroplasty for third stage hypospadias repair to release penis from scrotum (eg, third stage Cecil repair)	11.25	10.06	10.06	1.15	22.46	22.46	090	
54322		A	One stage distal hypospadias repair (with or without chordee or circumcision); with simple meatal advancement (eg, Magpi, V-flap)	13.01	9.56	9.56	0.77	23.34	23.34	090	
54324		A	with urethroplasty by local skin flaps (eg, flip-flap, prepucial flap)	16.31	12.02	12.02	1.03	29.36	29.36	090	
54326		A	with urethroplasty by local skin flaps and mobilization of urethra	15.72	11.17	11.17	0.93	27.82	27.82	090	
54328		A	with extensive dissection to correct chordee and urethroplasty with local skin flaps, skin graft patch, and/or island flap	15.65	11.59	11.59	0.92	28.16	28.16	090	
54332		A	One stage proximal penile or penoscrotal hypospadias repair requiring extensive dissection to correct chordee and urethroplasty by use of skin graft tube and/or island flap	17.08	11.87	11.87	1.01	29.96	29.96	090	
54336		A	One stage perineal hypospadias repair requiring extensive dissection to correct chordee and urethroplasty by use of skin graft tube and/or island flap	20.04	13.59	13.59	1.90	35.53	35.53	090	
54340		A	Repair of hypospadias complications (ie, fistula, stricture, diverticula); by closure, incision, or excision, simple	8.91	9.80	9.80	0.72	19.43	19.43	090	
54344		A	requiring mobilization of skin flaps and urethroplasty with flap or patch graft	15.94	10.91	10.91	1.10	27.95	27.95	090	
54348		A	requiring extensive dissection and urethroplasty with flap, patch or tubed graft (includes urinary diversion)	17.15	12.10	12.10	1.02	30.27	30.27	090	
54352		A	Repair of hypospadias cripple requiring extensive dissection and excision of previously constructed structures including re-release of chordee and reconstruction of urethra and penis by use of local skin as grafts and island flaps and skin brought in as flaps or grafts	24.74	16.53	16.53	1.62	42.89	42.89	090	
54360		A	Plastic operation on penis to correct angulation	11.93	8.82	8.82	0.72	21.47	21.47	090	
54380		A	Plastic operation on penis for epispadias distal to external sphincter;	13.18	10.79	10.79	1.16	25.13	25.13	090	
54385		A	with incontinence	15.39	12.20	12.20	0.71	28.30	28.30	090	
54390		A	with exstrophy of bladder	21.61	14.69	14.69	1.28	37.58	37.58	090	
54400		A	Insertion of penile prosthesis; non-inflatable (semi-rigid)	8.99	6.53	6.53	0.53	16.05	16.05	090	
54401		A	inflatable (self-contained)	10.28	7.37	7.37	0.61	18.26	18.26	090	

■ RVU not developed by CMS. Gap-filled RVUs developed by Ingenix/CHEG.

Code	M	S	Description	Work Value	Non-Fac PE	Fac PE	Mal-practice	Non-Fac Total	Fac Total	Global	Gap
54405		A	Insertion of multi-component, inflatable penile prosthesis, including placement of pump, cylinders, and reservoir	13.43	8.45	8.45	0.80	22.68	22.68	090	
54406		A	Removal of all components of a multi-component, inflatable penile prosthesis without replacement of prosthesis	12.10	6.09	6.09	0.80	18.99	18.99	090	
54408		A	Repair of component(s) of a multi-component, inflatable penile prosthesis	12.75	6.46	6.46	0.80	20.01	20.01	090	
54410		A	Removal and replacement of all component(s) of a multi-component, inflatable penile prosthesis at the same operative session	15.50	7.36	7.36	0.80	23.66	23.66	090	
54411		A	Removal and replacement of all components of a multi-component inflatable penile prosthesis through an infected field at the same operative session, including irrigation and debridement of infected tissue	16.00	8.98	8.98	0.80	25.78	25.78	090	
54415		A	Removal of non-inflatable (semi-rigid) or inflatable (self-contained) penile prosthesis, without replacement of prosthesis	8.20	5.35	5.35	0.55	14.10	14.10	090	
54416		A	Removal and replacement of non-inflatable (semi-rigid) or inflatable (self-contained) penile prosthesis at the same operative session	10.87	6.94	6.94	0.55	18.36	18.36	090	
54417		A	Removal and replacement of non-inflatable (semi-rigid) or inflatable (self-contained) penile prosthesis through an infected field at the same operative session, including irrigation and debridement of infected tissue	14.19	7.89	7.89	0.55	22.63	22.63	090	
54420		A	Corpora cavernosa-saphenous vein shunt (priapism operation), unilateral or bilateral	11.42	8.70	8.70	0.72	20.84	20.84	090	
54430		A	Corpora cavernosa-corpus spongiosum shunt (priapism operation), unilateral or bilateral	10.15	8.17	8.17	0.60	18.92	18.92	090	
54435		A	Corpora cavernosa-glans penis fistulization (eg, biopsy needle, Winter procedure, rongeur, or punch) for priapism	6.12	6.30	6.30	0.36	12.78	12.78	090	
54440		C	Plastic operation of penis for injury	9.18	7.30	7.30	0.98	17.46	17.46	090	■
54450		A	Foreskin manipulation including lysis of preputial adhesions and stretching	1.12	1.10	0.49	0.07	2.29	1.68	000	
54500		A	Biopsy of testis, needle (separate procedure)	1.31	6.26	0.45	0.08	7.65	1.84	000	
54505		A	Biopsy of testis, incisional (separate procedure)	3.46	2.75	2.75	0.21	6.42	6.42	010	
54512		A	Excision of extraparenchymal lesion of testis	8.58	5.19	5.19	0.56	14.33	14.33	090	
54520		A	Orchiectomy, simple (including subcapsular), with or without testicular prosthesis, scrotal or inguinal approach	5.23	3.75	3.75	0.33	9.31	9.31	090	
54522		A	Orchiectomy, partial	9.50	6.15	6.15	0.62	16.27	16.27	090	

■ RVU not developed by CMS. Gap-filled RVUs developed by Ingenix/CHEG.

Surgery

Code	M	S	Description	Work Value	Non-Fac PE	Fac PE	Mal-practice	Non-Fac Total	Fac Total	Global	Gap
54530		A	Orchiectomy, radical, for tumor; inguinal approach	8.58	5.46	5.46	0.53	14.57	14.57	090	
54535		A	with abdominal exploration	12.16	7.62	7.62	0.83	20.61	20.61	090	
54550		A	Exploration for undescended testis (inguinal or scrotal area)	7.78	4.97	4.97	0.49	13.24	13.24	090	
54560		A	Exploration for undescended testis with abdominal exploration	11.13	7.10	7.10	0.79	19.02	19.02	090	
54600		A	Reduction of torsion of testis, surgical, with or without fixation of contralateral testis	7.01	4.38	4.38	0.45	11.84	11.84	090	
54620		A	Fixation of contralateral testis (separate procedure)	4.90	3.26	3.26	0.31	8.47	8.47	010	
54640		A	Orchiopexy, inguinal approach, with or without hernia repair	6.90	4.40	4.40	0.49	11.79	11.79	090	
54650		A	Orchiopexy, abdominal approach, for intra-abdominal testis (eg, Fowler-Stephens)	11.45	7.29	7.29	0.81	19.55	19.55	090	
54660		A	Insertion of testicular prosthesis (separate procedure)	5.11	3.65	3.65	0.35	9.11	9.11	090	
54670		A	Suture or repair of testicular injury	6.41	4.30	4.30	0.41	11.12	11.12	090	
54680		A	Transplantation of testis(es) to thigh (because of scrotal destruction)	12.65	7.65	7.65	0.94	21.24	21.24	090	
54690		A	Laparoscopy, surgical; orchiectomy	10.96	7.08	7.08	0.99	19.03	19.03	090	
54692		A	orchiopexy for intra-abdominal testis	12.88	5.84	5.84	0.87	19.59	19.59	090	
54699		C	Unlisted laparoscopy procedure, testis	0.00	0.00	0.00	0.00	0.00	0.00	YYY	
54700		A	Incision and drainage of epididymis, testis and/ or scrotal space (eg, abscess or hematoma)	3.43	8.80	3.53	0.23	12.46	7.19	010	
54800		A	Biopsy of epididymis, needle	2.33	6.45	0.79	0.14	8.92	3.26	000	
54820		A	Exploration of epididymis, with or without biopsy	5.14	3.61	3.61	0.33	9.08	9.08	090	
54830		A	Excision of local lesion of epididymis	5.38	3.85	3.85	0.34	9.57	9.57	090	
54840		A	Excision of spermatocele, with or without epididymectomy	5.20	3.79	3.79	0.31	9.30	9.30	090	
54860		A	Epididymectomy; unilateral	6.32	4.40	4.40	0.38	11.10	11.10	090	
54861		A	bilateral	8.90	5.28	5.28	0.52	14.70	14.70	090	
54900		A	Epididymovasostomy, anastomosis of epididymis to vas deferens; unilateral	13.20	6.99	6.99	1.34	21.53	21.53	090	
54901		A	bilateral	17.94	9.27	9.27	1.83	29.04	29.04	090	
55000		A	Puncture aspiration of hydrocele, tunica vaginalis, with or without injection of medication	1.43	2.24	0.49	0.10	3.77	2.02	000	

■ RVU not developed by CMS. Gap-filled RVUs developed by Ingenix/CHEG.

Code	M	S	Description	Work Value	Non-Fac PE	Fac PE	Mal-prac-tice	Non-Fac Total	Fac Total	Global	Gap
55040		**A**	Excision of hydrocele; unilateral	5.36	3.56	3.56	0.35	9.27	9.27	090	
55041		**A**	bilateral	7.74	4.63	4.63	0.50	12.87	12.87	090	
55060		**A**	Repair of tunica vaginalis hydrocele (Bottle type)	5.52	3.64	3.64	0.37	9.53	9.53	090	
55100		**A**	Drainage of scrotal wall abscess	2.13	10.06	3.63	0.15	12.34	5.91	010	
55110		**A**	Scrotal exploration	5.70	3.71	3.71	0.36	9.77	9.77	090	
55120		**A**	Removal of foreign body in scrotum	5.09	3.52	3.52	0.33	8.94	8.94	090	
55150		**A**	Resection of scrotum	7.22	4.76	4.76	0.47	12.45	12.45	090	
55175		**A**	Scrotoplasty; simple	5.24	3.88	3.88	0.33	9.45	9.45	090	
55180		**A**	complicated	10.72	6.38	6.38	0.72	17.82	17.82	090	
55200		**A**	Vasotomy, cannulization with or without incision of vas, unilateral or bilateral (separate procedure)	4.24	3.10	3.10	0.25	7.59	7.59	090	
55250		**A**	Vasectomy, unilateral or bilateral (separate procedure), including postoperative semen examination(s)	3.29	9.72	3.28	0.21	13.22	6.78	090	
55300		**A**	Vasotomy for vasograms, seminal vesiculograms, or epididymograms, unilateral or bilateral	3.51	1.56	1.56	0.20	5.27	5.27	000	
55400		**A**	Vasovasostomy, vasovasorrhaphy	8.49	5.32	5.32	0.50	14.31	14.31	090	
55450		**A**	Ligation (percutaneous) of vas deferens, unilateral or bilateral (separate procedure)	4.12	8.08	2.62	0.24	12.44	6.98	010	
55500		**A**	Excision of hydrocele of spermatic cord, unilateral (separate procedure)	5.59	3.76	3.76	0.43	9.78	9.78	090	
55520		**A**	Excision of lesion of spermatic cord (separate procedure)	6.03	3.82	3.82	0.56	10.41	10.41	090	
55530		**A**	Excision of varicocele or ligation of spermatic veins for varicocele; (separate procedure)	5.66	3.92	3.92	0.36	9.94	9.94	090	
55535		**A**	abdominal approach	6.56	4.23	4.23	0.42	11.21	11.21	090	
55540		**A**	with hernia repair	7.67	4.37	4.37	0.74	12.78	12.78	090	
55550		**A**	Laparoscopy, surgical, with ligation of spermatic veins for varicocele	6.57	3.67	3.67	0.47	10.71	10.71	090	
55559		**C**	Unlisted laparoscopy procedure, spermatic cord	0.00	0.00	0.00	0.00	0.00	0.00	YYY	
55600		**A**	Vesiculotomy;	6.38	4.41	4.41	0.38	11.17	11.17	090	
55605		**A**	complicated	7.96	5.39	5.39	0.54	13.89	13.89	090	
55650		**A**	Vesiculectomy, any approach	11.80	6.44	6.44	0.72	18.96	18.96	090	
55680		**A**	Excision of Mullerian duct cyst	5.19	3.77	3.77	0.31	9.27	9.27	090	

■ RVU not developed by CMS. Gap-filled RVUs developed by Ingenix/CHEG.

Code	M	S	Description	Work Value	Non-Fac PE	Fac PE	Mal-practice	Non-Fac Total	Fac Total	Global	Gap
55700		A	Biopsy, prostate; needle or punch, single or multiple, any approach	1.57	4.68	0.73	0.10	6.35	2.40	000	
55705		A	incisional, any approach	4.57	3.92	3.92	0.26	8.75	8.75	010	
55720		A	Prostatotomy, external drainage of prostatic abscess, any approach; simple	7.64	5.88	5.88	0.44	13.96	13.96	090	
55725		A	complicated	8.68	6.58	6.58	0.51	15.77	15.77	090	
55801		A	Prostatectomy, perineal, subtotal (including control of postoperative bleeding, vasectomy, meatotomy, urethral calibration and/or dilation, and internal urethrotomy)	17.80	9.78	9.78	1.08	28.66	28.66	090	
55810		A	Prostatectomy, perineal radical;	22.58	11.85	11.85	1.35	35.78	35.78	090	
55812		A	with lymph node biopsy(s) (limited pelvic lymphadenectomy)	27.51	13.91	13.91	1.69	43.11	43.11	090	
55815		A	with bilateral pelvic lymphadenectomy, including external iliac, hypogastric and obturator nodes	30.46	15.01	15.01	1.84	47.31	47.31	090	
55821		A	Prostatectomy (including control of postoperative bleeding, vasectomy, meatotomy, urethral calibration and/or dilation, and internal urethrotomy); suprapubic, subtotal, one or two stages	14.25	8.20	8.20	0.85	23.30	23.30	090	
55831		A	retropubic, subtotal	15.62	8.67	8.67	0.94	25.23	25.23	090	
55840		A	Prostatectomy, retropubic radical, with or without nerve sparing;	22.69	12.32	12.32	1.37	36.38	36.38	090	
55842		A	with lymph node biopsy(s) (limited pelvic lymphadenectomy)	24.38	12.86	12.86	1.48	38.72	38.72	090	
55845		A	with bilateral pelvic lymphadenectomy, including external iliac, hypogastric, and obturator nodes	28.55	14.26	14.26	1.71	44.52	44.52	090	
55859		A	Transperineal placement of needles or catheters into prostate for interstitial radioelement application, with or without cystoscopy	12.52	7.71	7.71	0.74	20.97	20.97	090	
55860		A	Exposure of prostate, any approach, for insertion of radioactive substance;	14.45	7.93	7.93	0.82	23.20	23.20	090	
55862		A	with lymph node biopsy(s) (limited pelvic lymphadenectomy)	18.39	9.69	9.69	1.14	29.22	29.22	090	
55865		A	with bilateral pelvic lymphadenectomy, including external iliac, hypogastric and obturator nodes	22.87	11.49	11.49	1.37	35.73	35.73	090	
55870		A	Electroejaculation	2.58	1.96	0.98	0.14	4.68	3.70	000	
55873		A	Cryosurgical ablation of the prostate (includes ultrasonic guidance for interstitial cryosurgical probe placement)	19.47	10.65	10.65	1.02	31.14	31.14	090	

■ RVU not developed by CMS. Gap-filled RVUs developed by Ingenix/CHEG.

Code	M	S	Description	Work Value	Non-Fac PE	Fac PE	Mal-practice	Non-Fac Total	Fac Total	Global	Gap
55899		C	Unlisted procedure, male genital system	0.00	0.00	0.00	0.00	0.00	0.00	YYY	
55970		N	Intersex surgery; male to female	0.00	0.00	0.00	0.00	0.00	0.00	XXX	
55980		N	female to male	0.00	0.00	0.00	0.00	0.00	0.00	XXX	
56405		A	Incision and drainage of vulva or perineal abscess	1.44	2.50	1.33	0.14	4.08	2.91	010	
56420		A	Incision and drainage of Bartholin's gland abscess	1.39	2.48	1.33	0.13	4.00	2.85	010	
56440		A	Marsupialization of Bartholin's gland cyst	2.84	3.83	2.40	0.28	6.95	5.52	010	
56441		A	Lysis of labial adhesions	1.97	2.74	2.11	0.17	4.88	4.25	010	
56501		A	Destruction of lesion(s), vulva; simple (eg, laser surgery, electrosurgery, cryosurgery, chemosurgery)	1.53	2.42	1.42	0.15	4.10	3.10	010	
56515		A	extensive (eg, laser surgery, electrosurgery, cryosurgery, chemosurgery)	2.76	3.20	2.46	0.18	6.14	5.40	010	
56605		A	Biopsy of vulva or perineum (separate procedure); one lesion	1.10	1.90	0.50	0.11	3.11	1.71	000	
56606		A	each separate additional lesion (List separately in addition to code for primary procedure)	0.55	1.69	0.23	0.06	2.30	0.84	ZZZ	
56620		A	Vulvectomy simple; partial	7.47	5.13	5.13	0.76	13.36	13.36	090	
56625		A	complete	8.40	6.20	6.20	0.84	15.44	15.44	090	
56630		A	Vulvectomy, radical, partial;	12.36	7.93	7.93	1.23	21.52	21.52	090	
56631		A	with unilateral inguinofemoral lymphadenectomy	16.20	10.80	10.80	1.63	28.63	28.63	090	
56632		A	with bilateral inguinofemoral lymphadenectomy	20.29	12.42	12.42	2.03	34.74	34.74	090	
56633		A	Vulvectomy, radical, complete;	16.47	9.70	9.70	1.66	27.83	27.83	090	
56634		A	with unilateral inguinofemoral lymphadenectomy	17.88	11.25	11.25	1.78	30.91	30.91	090	
56637		A	with bilateral inguinofemoral lymphadenectomy	21.97	13.16	13.16	2.18	37.31	37.31	090	
56640		A	Vulvectomy, radical, complete, with inguinofemoral, iliac, and pelvic lymphadenectomy	22.17	12.58	12.58	2.26	37.01	37.01	090	
56700		A	Partial hymenectomy or revision of hymenal ring	2.52	3.18	2.16	0.24	5.94	4.92	010	
56720		A	Hymenotomy, simple incision	0.68	1.79	0.57	0.07	2.54	1.32	000	
56740		A	Excision of Bartholin's gland or cyst	4.57	4.08	3.08	0.37	9.02	8.02	010	
56800		A	Plastic repair of introitus	3.89	2.86	2.86	0.37	7.12	7.12	010	

■ RVU not developed by CMS. Gap-filled RVUs developed by Ingenix/CHEG.

Code	M	S	Description	Work Value	Non-Fac PE	Fac PE	Mal-practice	Non-Fac Total	Fac Total	Global	Gap
56805		A	Clitoroplasty for intersex state	18.86	9.69	9.69	1.82	30.37	30.37	090	
56810		A	Perineoplasty, repair of perineum, non-obstetrical (separate procedure)	4.13	2.91	2.91	0.41	7.45	7.45	010	
57000		A	Colpotomy; with exploration	2.97	2.49	2.49	0.28	5.74	5.74	010	
57010		A	with drainage of pelvic abscess	6.03	4.08	4.08	0.57	10.68	10.68	090	
57020		A	Colpocentesis (separate procedure)	1.50	1.63	0.66	0.15	3.28	2.31	000	
57022		A	Incision and drainage of vaginal hematoma; obstetrical/postpartum	2.56	2.14	2.14	0.24	4.94	4.94	010	
57023		A	non-obstetrical (eg, post-trauma, spontaneous bleeding)	4.75	3.01	3.01	0.24	8.00	8.00	010	
57061		A	Destruction of vaginal lesion(s); simple (eg, laser surgery, electrosurgery, cryosurgery, chemosurgery)	1.25	2.37	1.33	0.13	3.75	2.71	010	
57065		A	extensive (eg, laser surgery, electrosurgery, cryosurgery, chemosurgery)	2.61	3.09	2.41	0.26	5.96	5.28	010	
57100		A	Biopsy of vaginal mucosa; simple (separate procedure)	1.20	1.64	0.53	0.10	2.94	1.83	000	
57105		A	extensive, requiring suture (including cysts)	1.69	2.35	2.34	0.17	4.21	4.20	010	
57106		A	Vaginectomy, partial removal of vaginal wall;	6.36	2.67	2.67	0.58	9.61	9.61	090	
57107		A	with removal of paravaginal tissue (radical vaginectomy)	23.00	10.65	10.65	2.17	35.82	35.82	090	
57109		A	with removal of paravaginal tissue (radical vaginectomy) with bilateral total pelvic lymphadenectomy and para-aortic lymph node sampling (biopsy)	27.00	13.89	13.89	1.97	42.86	42.86	090	
57110		A	Vaginectomy, complete removal of vaginal wall;	14.29	7.56	7.56	1.43	23.28	23.28	090	
57111		A	with removal of paravaginal tissue (radical vaginectomy)	27.00	12.85	12.85	2.71	42.56	42.56	090	
57112		A	with removal of paravaginal tissue (radical vaginectomy) with bilateral total pelvic lymphadenectomy and para-aortic lymph node sampling (biopsy)	29.00	14.38	14.38	2.19	45.57	45.57	090	
57120		A	Colpocleisis (Le Fort type)	7.41	4.85	4.85	0.75	13.01	13.01	090	
57130		A	Excision of vaginal septum	2.43	2.25	2.25	0.23	4.91	4.91	010	
57135		A	Excision of vaginal cyst or tumor	2.67	3.09	2.35	0.26	6.02	5.28	010	
57150		A	Irrigation of vagina and/or application of medicament for treatment of bacterial, parasitic, or fungoid disease	0.55	1.04	0.22	0.06	1.65	0.83	000	
57155		A	Insertion of uterine tandems and/or vaginal ovoids for clinical brachytherapy	6.27	3.67	3.67	0.63	10.57	10.57	090	

■ RVU not developed by CMS. Gap-filled RVUs developed by Ingenix/CHEG.

Code	M	S	Description	Work Value	Non-Fac PE	Fac PE	Mal-prac-tice	Non-Fac Total	Fac Total	Global	Gap
57160		A	Fitting and insertion of pessary or other intravaginal support device	0.89	1.12	0.41	0.09	2.10	1.39	000	
57170		A	Diaphragm or cervical cap fitting with instructions	0.91	1.46	0.36	0.09	2.46	1.36	000	
57180		A	Introduction of any hemostatic agent or pack for spontaneous or traumatic nonobstetrical vaginal hemorrhage (separate procedure)	1.58	2.37	1.55	0.16	4.11	3.29	010	
57200		A	Colporrhaphy, suture of injury of vagina (nonobstetrical)	3.94	3.14	3.14	0.38	7.46	7.46	090	
57210		A	Colpoperineorrhaphy, suture of injury of vagina and/or perineum (nonobstetrical)	5.17	3.69	3.69	0.50	9.36	9.36	090	
57220		A	Plastic operation on urethral sphincter, vaginal approach (eg, Kelly urethral plication)	4.31	3.52	3.52	0.42	8.25	8.25	090	
57230		A	Plastic repair of urethrocele	5.64	4.49	4.49	0.50	10.63	10.63	090	
57240		A	Anterior colporrhaphy, repair of cystocele with or without repair of urethrocele	6.07	4.62	4.62	0.53	11.22	11.22	090	
57250		A	Posterior colporrhaphy, repair of rectocele with or without perineorrhaphy	5.53	4.01	4.01	0.54	10.08	10.08	090	
57260		A	Combined anteroposterior colporrhaphy;	8.27	5.17	5.17	0.83	14.27	14.27	090	
57265		A	with enterocele repair	11.34	7.22	7.22	1.14	19.70	19.70	090	
57268		A	Repair of enterocele, vaginal approach (separate procedure)	6.76	4.54	4.54	0.66	11.96	11.96	090	
57270		A	Repair of enterocele, abdominal approach (separate procedure)	12.11	6.58	6.58	1.17	19.86	19.86	090	
57280		A	Colpopexy, abdominal approach	15.04	7.74	7.74	1.44	24.22	24.22	090	
57282		A	Sacrospinous ligament fixation for prolapse of vagina	8.86	5.44	5.44	0.86	15.16	15.16	090	
57284		A	Paravaginal defect repair (including repair of cystocele, stress urinary incontinence, and/or incomplete vaginal prolapse)	12.70	7.45	7.45	1.17	21.32	21.32	090	
57287		A	Removal or revision of sling for stress incontinence (eg, fascia or synthetic)	10.71	7.47	7.47	0.74	18.92	18.92	090	
57288		A	Sling operation for stress incontinence (eg, fascia or synthetic)	13.02	7.24	7.24	0.86	21.12	21.12	090	
57289		A	Pereyra procedure, including anterior colporrhaphy	11.58	7.12	7.12	0.95	19.65	19.65	090	
57291		A	Construction of artificial vagina; without graft	7.95	5.93	5.93	0.78	14.66	14.66	090	
57292		A	with graft	13.09	7.20	7.20	1.29	21.58	21.58	090	
57300		A	Closure of rectovaginal fistula; vaginal or transanal approach	7.61	4.82	4.82	0.70	13.13	13.13	090	

■ RVU not developed by CMS. Gap-filled RVUs developed by Ingenix/CHEG.

Surgery

Code	M	S	Description	Work Value	Non-Fac PE	Fac PE	Mal-practice	Non-Fac Total	Fac Total	Global	Gap
57305		A	abdominal approach	13.77	7.00	7.00	1.33	22.10	22.10	090	
57307		A	abdominal approach, with concomitant colostomy	15.93	7.72	7.72	1.59	25.24	25.24	090	
57308		A	transperineal approach, with perineal body reconstruction, with or without levator plication	9.94	5.96	5.96	0.91	16.81	16.81	090	
57310		A	Closure of urethrovaginal fistula;	6.78	4.95	4.95	0.45	12.18	12.18	090	
57311		A	with bulbocavernosus transplant	7.98	5.45	5.45	0.51	13.94	13.94	090	
57320		A	Closure of vesicovaginal fistula; vaginal approach	8.01	5.68	5.68	0.60	14.29	14.29	090	
57330		A	transvesical and vaginal approach	12.35	6.96	6.96	0.86	20.17	20.17	090	
57335		A	Vaginoplasty for intersex state	18.73	9.84	9.84	1.66	30.23	30.23	090	
57400		A	Dilation of vagina under anesthesia	2.27	1.18	1.18	0.22	3.67	3.67	000	
57410		A	Pelvic examination under anesthesia	1.75	2.75	1.12	0.14	4.64	3.01	000	
57415		A	Removal of impacted vaginal foreign body (separate procedure) under anesthesia	2.17	3.71	2.18	0.19	6.07	4.54	010	
57452		A	Colposcopy (vaginoscopy); (separate procedure)	0.99	1.69	0.46	0.10	2.78	1.55	000	
57454		A	with biopsy(s) of the cervix and/or endocervical curettage	1.27	1.88	0.62	0.13	3.28	2.02	000	
57460		A	with loop electrode excision procedure of the cervix	2.83	2.17	1.19	0.28	5.28	4.30	000	
57500		A	Biopsy, single or multiple, or local excision of lesion, with or without fulguration (separate procedure)	0.97	2.29	0.50	0.10	3.36	1.57	000	
57505		A	Endocervical curettage (not done as part of a dilation and curettage)	1.14	2.05	1.36	0.12	3.31	2.62	010	
57510		A	Cautery of cervix; electro or thermal	1.90	3.39	1.66	0.18	5.47	3.74	010	
57511		A	cryocautery, initial or repeat	1.90	2.54	0.77	0.18	4.62	2.85	010	
57513		A	laser ablation	1.90	2.72	1.66	0.19	4.81	3.75	010	
57520		A	Conization of cervix, with or without fulguration, with or without dilation and curettage, with or without repair; cold knife or laser	4.04	4.43	2.93	0.41	8.88	7.38	090	
57522		A	loop electrode excision	3.36	4.02	2.68	0.34	7.72	6.38	090	
57530		A	Trachelectomy (cervicectomy), amputation of cervix (separate procedure)	4.79	3.78	3.78	0.48	9.05	9.05	090	

■ RVU not developed by CMS. Gap-filled RVUs developed by Ingenix/CHEG.

Code	M	S	Description	Work Value	Non-Fac PE	Fac PE	Mal-practice	Non-Fac Total	Fac Total	Global	Gap
57531		A	Radical trachelectomy, with bilateral total pelvic lymphadenectomy and para-aortic lymph node sampling biopsy, with or without removal of tube(s), with or without removal of ovary(s)	28.00	14.44	14.44	2.46	44.90	44.90	090	
57540		A	Excision of cervical stump, abdominal approach;	12.22	6.49	6.49	1.21	19.92	19.92	090	
57545		A	with pelvic floor repair	13.03	6.95	6.95	1.30	21.28	21.28	090	
57550		A	Excision of cervical stump, vaginal approach;	5.53	3.98	3.98	0.55	10.06	10.06	090	
57555		A	with anterior and/or posterior repair	8.95	5.90	5.90	0.89	15.74	15.74	090	
57556		A	with repair of enterocele	8.37	5.14	5.14	0.80	14.31	14.31	090	
57700		A	Cerclage of uterine cervix, nonobstetrical	3.55	2.71	2.71	0.33	6.59	6.59	090	
57720		A	Trachelorrhaphy, plastic repair of uterine cervix, vaginal approach	4.13	3.41	3.41	0.41	7.95	7.95	090	
57800		A	Dilation of cervical canal, instrumental (separate procedure)	0.77	1.22	0.36	0.08	2.07	1.21	000	
57820		A	Dilation and curettage of cervical stump	1.67	2.70	2.40	0.17	4.54	4.24	010	
58100		A	Endometrial sampling (biopsy) with or without endocervical sampling (biopsy), without cervical dilation, any method (separate procedure)	1.53	1.56	0.76	0.07	3.16	2.36	000	
58120		A	Dilation and curettage, diagnostic and/or therapeutic (nonobstetrical)	3.27	4.01	2.55	0.33	7.61	6.15	010	
58140		A	Myomectomy, excision of leiomyomata of uterus, single or multiple (separate procedure); abdominal approach	14.60	7.38	7.38	1.46	23.44	23.44	090	
58145		A	vaginal approach	8.04	5.11	5.11	0.80	13.95	13.95	090	
58150		A	Total abdominal hysterectomy (corpus and cervix), with or without removal of tube(s), with or without removal of ovary(s);	15.24	7.90	7.90	1.53	24.67	24.67	090	
58152		A	with colpo-urethrocystopexy (eg, Marshall-Marchetti-Krantz, Burch)	20.60	10.17	10.17	1.52	32.29	32.29	090	
58180		A	Supracervical abdominal hysterectomy (subtotal hysterectomy), with or without removal of tube(s), with or without removal of ovary(s)	15.29	7.90	7.90	1.54	24.73	24.73	090	
58200		A	Total abdominal hysterectomy, including partial vaginectomy, with para-aortic and pelvic lymph node sampling, with or without removal of tube(s), with or without removal of ovary(s)	21.59	11.62	11.62	2.15	35.36	35.36	090	
58210		A	Radical abdominal hysterectomy, with bilateral total pelvic lymphadenectomy and para-aortic lymph node sampling (biopsy), with or without removal of tube(s), with or without removal of ovary(s)	28.85	14.67	14.67	2.91	46.43	46.43	090	

■ RVU not developed by CMS. Gap-filled RVUs developed by Ingenix/CHEG.

Surgery

Code	M	S	Description	Work Value	Non-Fac PE	Fac PE	Mal-practice	Non-Fac Total	Fac Total	Global	Gap
58240		A	Pelvic exenteration for gynecologic malignancy, with total abdominal hysterectomy or cervicectomy, with or without removal of tube(s), with or without removal of ovary(s), with removal of bladder and ureteral transplantations, and/or abdominoperineal resection of rectum and colon and colostomy, or any combination thereof	38.39	19.71	19.71	3.76	61.86	61.86	090	
58260		A	Vaginal hysterectomy;	12.98	6.90	6.90	1.23	21.11	21.11	090	
58262		A	with removal of tube(s), and/or ovary(s)	14.77	7.66	7.66	1.42	23.85	23.85	090	
58263		A	with removal of tube(s), and/or ovary(s), with repair of enterocele	16.06	8.22	8.22	1.55	25.83	25.83	090	
58267		A	with colpo-urethrocystopexy (Marshall-Marchetti-Krantz type, Pereyra type, with or without endoscopic control)	17.04	8.81	8.81	1.51	27.36	27.36	090	
58270		A	with repair of enterocele	14.26	7.43	7.43	1.37	23.06	23.06	090	
58275		A	Vaginal hysterectomy, with total or partial vaginectomy;	15.76	7.94	7.94	1.51	25.21	25.21	090	
58280		A	with repair of enterocele	17.01	8.46	8.46	1.54	27.01	27.01	090	
58285		A	Vaginal hysterectomy, radical (Schauta type operation)	22.26	11.15	11.15	1.88	35.29	35.29	090	
58300		N	Insertion of intrauterine device (IUD)	1.01	1.42	0.40	0.10	2.53	1.51	XXX	
58301		A	Removal of intrauterine device (IUD)	1.27	1.62	0.51	0.13	3.02	1.91	000	
58321		A	Artificial insemination; intra-cervical	0.92	1.03	0.37	0.10	2.05	1.39	000	
58322		A	intra-uterine	1.10	1.05	0.42	0.11	2.26	1.63	000	
58323		A	Sperm washing for artificial insemination	0.23	0.53	0.10	0.02	0.78	0.35	000	
58340		A	Catheterization and introduction of saline or contrast material for hysterosonography or hysterosalpingography	0.88	12.42	0.33	0.08	13.38	1.29	000	
58345		A	Transcervical introduction of fallopian tube catheter for diagnosis and/or re-establishing patency (any method), with or without hysterosalpingography	4.66	1.73	1.73	0.36	6.75	6.75	010	
58346		A	Insertion of Heyman capsules for clinical brachytherapy	6.75	3.84	3.84	0.68	11.27	11.27	090	
58350		A	Chromotubation of oviduct, including materials	1.01	2.15	1.17	0.10	3.26	2.28	010	
58353		A	Endometrial ablation, thermal, without hysteroscopic guidance	3.56	2.28	2.28	0.37	6.21	6.21	010	
58400		A	Uterine suspension, with or without shortening of round ligaments, with or without shortening of sacrouterine ligaments; (separate procedure)	6.36	4.17	4.17	0.62	11.15	11.15	090	

■ RVU not developed by CMS. Gap-filled RVUs developed by Ingenix/CHEG.

Code	M	S	Description	Work Value	Non-Fac PE	Fac PE	Mal-practice	Non-Fac Total	Fac Total	Global	Gap
58410		A	with presacral sympathectomy	12.73	6.84	6.84	1.09	20.66	20.66	090	
58520		A	Hysterorrhaphy, repair of ruptured uterus (nonobstetrical)	11.92	6.24	6.24	1.17	19.33	19.33	090	
58540		A	Hysteroplasty, repair of uterine anomaly (Strassman type)	14.64	6.96	6.96	1.28	22.88	22.88	090	
58550		A	Laparoscopy, surgical; with vaginal hysterectomy with or without removal of tube(s), with or without removal of ovary(s) (laparoscopic assisted vaginal hysterectomy)	14.19	7.11	7.11	1.44	22.74	22.74	010	
58551		A	with removal of leiomyomata (single or multiple)	14.21	7.09	7.09	1.45	22.75	22.75	010	
58555		A	Hysteroscopy, diagnostic (separate procedure)	3.33	2.95	1.49	0.34	6.62	5.16	000	
58558		A	Hysteroscopy, surgical; with sampling (biopsy) of endometrium and/or polypectomy, with or without D & C	4.75	3.55	2.13	0.49	8.79	7.37	000	
58559		A	with lysis of intrauterine adhesions (any method)	6.17	2.59	2.59	0.62	9.38	9.38	000	
58560		A	with division or resection of intrauterine septum (any method)	7.00	3.01	3.01	0.71	10.72	10.72	000	
58561		A	with removal of leiomyomata	10.00	3.78	3.78	1.02	14.80	14.80	000	
58562		A	with removal of impacted foreign body	5.21	2.34	2.34	0.52	8.07	8.07	000	
58563		A	with endometrial ablation (eg, endometrial resection, electrosurgical ablation, thermoablation)	6.17	2.62	2.62	0.62	9.41	9.41	000	
58578		C	Unlisted laparoscopy procedure, uterus	0.00	0.00	0.00	0.00	0.00	0.00	YYY	
58579		C	Unlisted hysteroscopy procedure, uterus	0.00	0.00	0.00	0.00	0.00	0.00	YYY	
58600		A	Ligation or transection of fallopian tube(s), abdominal or vaginal approach, unilateral or bilateral	5.60	3.51	3.51	0.39	9.50	9.50	090	
58605		A	Ligation or transection of fallopian tube(s), abdominal or vaginal approach, postpartum, unilateral or bilateral, during same hospitalization (separate procedure)	5.00	3.32	3.32	0.33	8.65	8.65	090	
58611		A	Ligation or transection of fallopian tube(s) when done at the time of cesarean delivery or intra-abdominal surgery (not a separate procedure) (List separately in addition to code for primary procedure)	1.45	0.61	0.61	0.07	2.13	2.13	ZZZ	
58615		A	Occlusion of fallopian tube(s) by device (eg, band, clip, Falope ring) vaginal or suprapubic approach	3.90	3.35	3.35	0.40	7.65	7.65	010	
58660		A	Laparoscopy, surgical; with lysis of adhesions (salpingolysis, ovariolysis) (separate procedure)	11.29	5.78	5.78	1.14	18.21	18.21	090	

■ RVU not developed by CMS. Gap-filled RVUs developed by Ingenix/CHEG.

Code	M	S	Description	Work Value	Non-Fac PE	Fac PE	Mal-practice	Non-Fac Total	Fac Total	Global	Gap
58661		A	with removal of adnexal structures (partial or total oophorectomy and/or salpingectomy)	11.05	5.47	5.47	1.12	17.64	17.64	010	
58662		A	with fulguration or excision of lesions of the ovary, pelvic viscera, or peritoneal surface by any method	11.79	5.75	5.75	1.18	18.72	18.72	090	
58670		A	with fulguration of oviducts (with or without transection)	5.60	3.73	3.73	0.55	9.88	9.88	090	
58671		A	with occlusion of oviducts by device (eg, band, clip, or Falope ring)	5.60	3.74	3.74	0.56	9.90	9.90	090	
58672		A	with fimbrioplasty	12.88	6.81	6.81	1.22	20.91	20.91	090	
58673		A	with salpingostomy (salpingoneostomy)	13.74	7.16	7.16	1.40	22.30	22.30	090	
58679		C	Unlisted laparoscopy procedure, oviduct, ovary	0.00	0.00	0.00	0.00	0.00	0.00	YYY	
58700		A	Salpingectomy, complete or partial, unilateral or bilateral (separate procedure)	12.05	6.05	6.05	0.64	18.74	18.74	090	
58720		A	Salpingo-oophorectomy, complete or partial, unilateral or bilateral (separate procedure)	11.36	6.05	6.05	1.14	18.55	18.55	090	
58740		A	Lysis of adhesions (salpingolysis, ovariolysis)	14.00	7.34	7.34	0.59	21.93	21.93	090	
58750		A	Tubotubal anastomosis	14.84	7.60	7.60	1.52	23.96	23.96	090	
58752		A	Tubouterine implantation	14.84	7.92	7.92	1.51	24.27	24.27	090	
58760		A	Fimbrioplasty	13.13	7.00	7.00	1.34	21.47	21.47	090	
58770		A	Salpingostomy (salpingoneostomy)	13.97	7.24	7.24	1.42	22.63	22.63	090	
58800		A	Drainage of ovarian cyst(s), unilateral or bilateral, (separate procedure); vaginal approach	4.14	4.43	4.36	0.36	8.93	8.86	090	
58805		A	abdominal approach	5.88	3.66	3.66	0.56	10.10	10.10	090	
58820		A	Drainage of ovarian abscess; vaginal approach, open	4.22	3.38	3.38	0.29	7.89	7.89	090	
58822		A	abdominal approach	10.13	5.20	5.20	0.92	16.25	16.25	090	
58823		A	Drainage of pelvic abscess, transvaginal or transrectal approach, percutaneous (eg, ovarian, pericolic)	3.38	2.38	2.38	0.18	5.94	5.94	000	
58825		A	Transposition, ovary(s)	10.98	5.95	5.95	0.62	17.55	17.55	090	
58900		A	Biopsy of ovary, unilateral or bilateral (separate procedure)	5.99	3.64	3.64	0.56	10.19	10.19	090	
58920		A	Wedge resection or bisection of ovary, unilateral or bilateral	11.36	5.85	5.85	0.68	17.89	17.89	090	
58925		A	Ovarian cystectomy, unilateral or bilateral	11.36	5.79	5.79	1.14	18.29	18.29	090	

■ RVU not developed by CMS. Gap-filled RVUs developed by Ingenix/CHEG.

Code	M	S	Description	Work Value	Non-Fac PE	Fac PE	Mal-practice	Non-Fac Total	Fac Total	Global	Gap
58940		A	Oophorectomy, partial or total, unilateral or bilateral;	7.29	4.18	4.18	0.73	12.20	12.20	090	
58943		A	for ovarian, tubal or primary peritoneal malignancy, with para-aortic and pelvic lymph node biopsies, peritoneal washings, peritoneal biopsies, diaphragmatic assessments, with or without salpingectomy(s), with or without omentectomy	18.43	9.92	9.92	1.86	30.21	30.21	090	
58950		A	Resection of ovarian, tubal or primary peritoneal malignancy with bilateral salpingo-oophorectomy and omentectomy;	16.93	9.41	9.41	1.55	27.89	27.89	090	
58951		A	with total abdominal hysterectomy, pelvic and limited para-aortic lymphadenectomy	22.38	11.81	11.81	2.20	36.39	36.39	090	
58952		A	with radical dissection for debulking (ie, radical excision or destruction, intra-abdominal or retroperitoneal tumors)	25.01	12.99	12.99	2.50	40.50	40.50	090	
58953		A	Bilateral salpingo-oophorectomy with omentectomy, total abdominal hysterectomy and radical dissection for debulking;	32.00	15.59	15.59	3.20	50.79	50.79	090	
58954		A	with pelvic lymphadenectomy and limited para-aortic lymphadenectomy	35.00	16.71	16.71	3.50	55.21	55.21	090	
58960		A	Laparotomy, for staging or restaging of ovarian, tubal or primary peritoneal malignancy (second look), with or without omentectomy, peritoneal washing, biopsy of abdominal and pelvic peritoneum, diaphragmatic assessment with pelvic and limited para-aortic lymphadenectomy	14.65	8.52	8.52	1.47	24.64	24.64	090	
58970		A	Follicle puncture for oocyte retrieval, any method	3.53	8.56	1.92	0.36	12.45	5.81	000	
58974		C	Embryo transfer, intrauterine	1.94	1.54	1.54	0.21	3.69	3.69	000	■
58976		A	Gamete, zygote, or embryo intrafallopian transfer, any method	3.83	2.30	1.53	0.39	6.52	5.75	000	
58999		C	Unlisted procedure, female genital system (nonobstetrical)	0.00	0.00	0.00	0.00	0.00	0.00	YYY	
59000		A	Amniocentesis; diagnostic	1.30	2.05	0.72	0.23	3.58	2.25	000	
59001		A	therapeutic amniotic fluid reduction (includes ultrasound guidance)	3.00	1.37	1.37	0.23	4.60	4.60	000	
59012		A	Cordocentesis (intrauterine), any method	3.45	1.71	1.71	0.62	5.78	5.78	000	
59015		A	Chorionic villus sampling, any method	2.20	1.64	1.11	0.40	4.24	3.71	000	
59020		A	Fetal contraction stress test	0.66	0.78	0.78	0.20	1.64	1.64	000	
	26	A		0.66	0.28	0.28	0.12	1.06	1.06	000	
	TC	A		0.00	0.50	0.50	0.08	0.58	0.58	000	

Surgery

■ RVU not developed by CMS. Gap-filled RVUs developed by Ingenix/CHEG.

Code	M	S	Description	Work Value	Non-Fac PE	Fac PE	Mal-practice	Non-Fac Total	Fac Total	Global	Gap
59025		A	Fetal non-stress test	0.53	0.44	0.44	0.12	1.09	1.09	000	
	26	A		0.53	0.22	0.22	0.10	0.85	0.85	000	
	TC	A		0.00	0.22	0.22	0.02	0.24	0.24	000	
59030		A	Fetal scalp blood sampling	1.99	1.14	1.14	0.36	3.49	3.49	000	
59050		A	Fetal monitoring during labor by consulting physician (ie, non-attending physician) with written report; supervision and interpretation	0.89	0.38	0.38	0.16	1.43	1.43	XXX	
59051		A	interpretation only	0.74	0.31	0.31	0.14	1.19	1.19	XXX	
59100		A	Hysterotomy, abdominal (eg, for hydatidiform mole, abortion)	12.35	6.61	6.61	2.21	21.17	21.17	090	
59120		A	Surgical treatment of ectopic pregnancy; tubal or ovarian, requiring salpingectomy and/or oophorectomy, abdominal or vaginal approach	11.49	6.35	6.35	2.06	19.90	19.90	090	
59121		A	tubal or ovarian, without salpingectomy and/or oophorectomy	11.67	6.39	6.39	2.09	20.15	20.15	090	
59130		A	abdominal pregnancy	14.22	7.16	7.16	2.54	23.92	23.92	090	
59135		A	interstitial, uterine pregnancy requiring total hysterectomy	13.88	7.27	7.27	2.49	23.64	23.64	090	
59136		A	interstitial, uterine pregnancy with partial resection of uterus	13.18	6.36	6.36	2.36	21.90	21.90	090	
59140		A	cervical, with evacuation	5.46	3.70	3.70	0.98	10.14	10.14	090	
59150		A	Laparoscopic treatment of ectopic pregnancy; without salpingectomy and/or oophorectomy	11.67	6.69	6.69	1.23	19.59	19.59	090	
59151		A	with salpingectomy and/or oophorectomy	11.49	6.12	6.12	1.41	19.02	19.02	090	
59160		A	Curettage, postpartum	2.71	3.73	2.29	0.49	6.93	5.49	010	
59200		A	Insertion of cervical dilator (eg, laminaria, prostaglandin) (separate procedure)	0.79	1.41	0.32	0.15	2.35	1.26	000	
59300		A	Episiotomy or vaginal repair, by other than attending physician	2.41	2.01	1.01	0.43	4.85	3.85	000	
59320		A	Cerclage of cervix, during pregnancy; vaginal	2.48	1.31	1.31	0.45	4.24	4.24	000	
59325		A	abdominal	4.07	1.97	1.97	0.73	6.77	6.77	000	
59350		A	Hysterorrhaphy of ruptured uterus	4.95	2.19	2.19	0.88	8.02	8.02	000	
59400		A	Routine obstetric care including antepartum care, vaginal delivery (with or without episiotomy, and/or forceps) and postpartum care	23.06	15.41	15.41	4.14	42.61	42.61	MMM	
59409		A	Vaginal delivery only (with or without episiotomy and/or forceps);	13.50	5.57	5.57	2.42	21.49	21.49	MMM	
59410		A	including postpartum care	14.78	6.98	6.98	2.65	24.41	24.41	MMM	

■ RVU not developed by CMS. Gap-filled RVUs developed by Ingenix/CHEG.

Code	M	S	Description	Work Value	Non-Fac PE	Fac PE	Mal-practice	Non-Fac Total	Fac Total	Global	Gap
59412		A	External cephalic version, with or without tocolysis	1.71	1.38	0.72	0.31	3.40	2.74	MMM	
59414		A	Delivery of placenta (separate procedure)	1.61	1.34	1.34	0.29	3.24	3.24	MMM	
59425		A	Antepartum care only; 4-6 visits	4.81	5.36	5.32	0.86	11.03	10.99	MMM	
59426		A	7 or more visits	8.28	9.14	9.14	1.49	18.91	18.91	MMM	
59430		A	Postpartum care only (separate procedure)	2.13	1.29	1.29	0.38	3.80	3.80	MMM	
59510		A	Routine obstetric care including antepartum care, cesarean delivery, and postpartum care	26.22	17.61	17.61	4.70	48.53	48.53	MMM	
59514		A	Cesarean delivery only;	15.97	6.57	6.57	2.86	25.40	25.40	MMM	
59515		A	including postpartum care	17.37	8.52	8.52	3.12	29.01	29.01	MMM	
59525		A	Subtotal or total hysterectomy after cesarean delivery (List separately in addition to code for primary procedure)	8.54	3.52	3.52	1.53	13.59	13.59	ZZZ	
59610		A	Routine obstetric care including antepartum care, vaginal delivery (with or without episiotomy, and/or forceps) and postpartum care, after previous cesarean delivery	24.62	16.29	16.29	4.41	45.32	45.32	MMM	
59612		A	Vaginal delivery only, after previous cesarean delivery (with or without episiotomy and/or forceps);	15.06	6.43	6.43	2.70	24.19	24.19	MMM	
59614		A	including postpartum care	16.34	7.70	7.70	2.93	26.97	26.97	MMM	
59618		A	Routine obstetric care including antepartum care, cesarean delivery, and postpartum care, following attempted vaginal delivery after previous cesarean delivery	27.78	18.38	18.38	4.98	51.14	51.14	MMM	
59620		A	Cesarean delivery only, following attempted vaginal delivery after previous cesarean delivery;	17.53	6.87	6.87	3.15	27.55	27.55	MMM	
59622		A	including postpartum care	18.93	8.91	8.91	3.39	31.23	31.23	MMM	
59812		A	Treatment of incomplete abortion, any trimester, completed surgically	4.01	3.75	2.51	0.58	8.34	7.10	090	
59820		A	Treatment of missed abortion, completed surgically; first trimester	4.01	3.79	2.85	0.72	8.52	7.58	090	
59821		A	second trimester	4.47	3.79	3.01	0.80	9.06	8.28	090	
59830		A	Treatment of septic abortion, completed surgically	6.11	3.85	3.85	1.10	11.06	11.06	090	
59840		R	Induced abortion, by dilation and curettage	3.01	4.01	2.47	0.54	7.56	6.02	010	
59841		R	Induced abortion, by dilation and evacuation	5.24	5.78	3.72	0.94	11.96	9.90	010	

Surgery

■ RVU not developed by CMS. Gap-filled RVUs developed by Ingenix/CHEG.

Code	M	S	Description	Work Value	Non-Fac PE	Fac PE	Mal-practice	Non-Fac Total	Fac Total	Global	Gap
59850		R	Induced abortion, by one or more intra-amniotic injections (amniocentesis-injections), including hospital admission and visits, delivery of fetus and secundines;	5.91	2.75	2.75	1.06	9.72	9.72	090	
59851		R	with dilation and curettage and/or evacuation	5.93	3.22	3.22	1.06	10.21	10.21	090	
59852		R	with hysterotomy (failed intra-amniotic injection)	8.24	4.58	4.58	1.48	14.30	14.30	090	
59855		R	Induced abortion, by one or more vaginal suppositories (eg, prostaglandin) with or without cervical dilation (eg, laminaria), including hospital admission and visits, delivery of fetus and secundines;	6.12	3.38	3.38	1.10	10.60	10.60	090	
59856		R	with dilation and curettage and/or evacuation	7.48	3.74	3.74	1.34	12.56	12.56	090	
59857		R	with hysterotomy (failed medical evacuation)	9.29	4.46	4.46	1.66	15.41	15.41	090	
59866		R	Multifetal pregnancy reduction(s) (MPR)	4.00	1.60	1.60	0.72	6.32	6.32	000	
59870		A	Uterine evacuation and curettage for hydatidiform mole	6.01	3.83	3.83	0.77	10.61	10.61	090	
59871		A	Removal of cerclage suture under anesthesia (other than local)	2.13	2.19	0.93	0.38	4.70	3.44	000	
59898		C	Unlisted laparoscopy procedure, maternity care and delivery	0.00	0.00	0.00	0.00	0.00	0.00	YYY	
59899		C	Unlisted procedure, maternity care and delivery	0.00	0.00	0.00	0.00	0.00	0.00	YYY	

Surgery

■ RVU not developed by CMS. Gap-filled RVUs developed by Ingenix/CHEG.

Code	M	S	Description	Work Value	Non-Fac PE	Fac PE	Mal-practice	Non-Fac Total	Fac Total	Global	Gap
60000		A	Incision and drainage of thyroglossal duct cyst, infected	1.76	2.40	2.22	0.14	4.30	4.12	010	
60001		A	Aspiration and/or injection, thyroid cyst	0.97	1.77	0.35	0.06	2.80	1.38	000	
60100		A	Biopsy thyroid, percutaneous core needle	1.56	2.70	0.56	0.05	4.31	2.17	000	
60200		A	Excision of cyst or adenoma of thyroid, or transection of isthmus	9.55	6.88	6.88	0.84	17.27	17.27	090	
60210		A	Partial thyroid lobectomy, unilateral; with or without isthmusectomy	10.88	6.63	6.63	1.01	18.52	18.52	090	
60212		A	with contralateral subtotal lobectomy, including isthmusectomy	16.03	8.62	8.62	1.51	26.16	26.16	090	
60220		A	Total thyroid lobectomy, unilateral; with or without isthmusectomy	11.90	7.27	7.27	0.97	20.14	20.14	090	
60225		A	with contralateral subtotal lobectomy, including isthmusectomy	14.19	8.05	8.05	1.31	23.55	23.55	090	
60240		A	Thyroidectomy, total or complete	16.06	9.32	9.32	1.50	26.88	26.88	090	
60252		A	Thyroidectomy, total or subtotal for malignancy; with limited neck dissection	20.57	11.64	11.64	1.63	33.84	33.84	090	
60254		A	with radical neck dissection	26.99	16.39	16.39	1.96	45.34	45.34	090	
60260		A	Thyroidectomy, removal of all remaining thyroid tissue following previous removal of a portion of thyroid	17.47	10.66	10.66	1.39	29.52	29.52	090	
60270		A	Thyroidectomy, including substernal thyroid; sternal split or transthoracic approach	20.27	11.54	11.54	1.78	33.59	33.59	090	
60271		A	cervical approach	16.83	10.20	10.20	1.35	28.38	28.38	090	
60280		A	Excision of thyroglossal duct cyst or sinus;	5.87	5.29	5.29	0.45	11.61	11.61	090	
60281		A	recurrent	8.53	6.27	6.27	0.67	15.47	15.47	090	
60500		A	Parathyroidectomy or exploration of parathyroid(s);	16.23	7.99	7.99	1.61	25.83	25.83	090	
60502		A	re-exploration	20.35	9.97	9.97	2.00	32.32	32.32	090	
60505		A	with mediastinal exploration, sternal split or transthoracic approach	21.49	11.53	11.53	2.14	35.16	35.16	090	
60512		A	Parathyroid autotransplantation (List separately in addition to code for primary procedure)	4.45	1.72	1.72	0.44	6.61	6.61	ZZZ	
60520		A	Thymectomy, partial or total; transcervical approach (separate procedure)	16.81	9.55	9.55	1.84	28.20	28.20	090	
60521		A	sternal split or transthoracic approach, without radical mediastinal dissection (separate procedure)	18.87	11.57	11.57	2.34	32.78	32.78	090	

■ RVU not developed by CMS. Gap-filled RVUs developed by Ingenix/CHEG.

Code	M	S	Description	Work Value	Non-Fac PE	Fac PE	Mal-practice	Non-Fac Total	Fac Total	Global	Gap
60522		A	sternal split or transthoracic approach, with radical mediastinal dissection (separate procedure)	23.09	12.88	12.88	2.83	38.80	38.80	090	
60540		A	Adrenalectomy, partial or complete, or exploration of adrenal gland with or without biopsy, transabdominal, lumbar or dorsal (separate procedure);	17.03	8.09	8.09	1.42	26.54	26.54	090	
60545		A	with excision of adjacent retroperitoneal tumor	19.88	9.73	9.73	1.75	31.36	31.36	090	
60600		A	Excision of carotid body tumor; without excision of carotid artery	17.93	13.43	13.43	1.87	33.23	33.23	090	
60605		A	with excision of carotid artery	20.24	18.12	18.12	2.28	40.64	40.64	090	
60650		A	Laparoscopy, surgical, with adrenalectomy, partial or complete, or exploration of adrenal gland with or without biopsy, transabdominal, lumbar or dorsal	20.00	8.34	8.34	1.98	30.32	30.32	090	
60659		C	Unlisted laparoscopy procedure, endocrine system	0.00	0.00	0.00	0.00	0.00	0.00	YYY	
60699		C	Unlisted procedure, endocrine system	0.00	0.00	0.00	0.00	0.00	0.00	YYY	
61000		A	Subdural tap through fontanelle, or suture, infant, unilateral or bilateral; initial	1.58	1.79	1.53	0.13	3.50	3.24	000	
61001		A	subsequent taps	1.49	2.08	1.47	0.15	3.72	3.11	000	
61020		A	Ventricular puncture through previous burr hole, fontanelle, suture, or implanted ventricular catheter/reservoir; without injection	1.51	2.52	1.51	0.26	4.29	3.28	000	
61026		A	with injection of medication or other substance for diagnosis or treatment	1.69	2.28	1.73	0.21	4.18	3.63	000	
61050		A	Cisternal or lateral cervical (C1-C2) puncture; without injection (separate procedure)	1.51	1.56	1.56	0.13	3.20	3.20	000	
61055		A	with injection of medication or other substance for diagnosis or treatment (eg, C1-C2)	2.10	1.80	1.80	0.13	4.03	4.03	000	
61070		A	Puncture of shunt tubing or reservoir for aspiration or injection procedure	0.89	7.33	1.22	0.09	8.31	2.20	000	
61105		A	Twist drill hole for subdural or ventricular puncture;	5.14	3.67	3.67	1.05	9.86	9.86	090	
61107		A	for implanting ventricular catheter or pressure recording device	5.00	3.12	3.12	1.02	9.14	9.14	000	
61108		A	for evacuation and/or drainage of subdural hematoma	10.19	7.09	7.09	2.04	19.32	19.32	090	
61120		A	Burr hole(s) for ventricular puncture (including injection of gas, contrast media, dye, or radioactive material)	8.76	5.88	5.88	1.81	16.45	16.45	090	

■ RVU not developed by CMS. Gap-filled RVUs developed by Ingenix/CHEG.

Code	M	S	Description	Work Value	Non-Fac PE	Fac PE	Mal-practice	Non-Fac Total	Fac Total	Global	Gap
61140		A	Burr hole(s) or trephine; with biopsy of brain or intracranial lesion	15.90	10.00	10.00	3.15	29.05	29.05	090	
61150		A	with drainage of brain abscess or cyst	17.57	10.74	10.74	3.52	31.83	31.83	090	
61151		A	with subsequent tapping (aspiration) of intracranial abscess or cyst	12.42	8.16	8.16	2.45	23.03	23.03	090	
61154		A	Burr hole(s) with evacuation and/or drainage of hematoma, extradural or subdural	14.99	9.43	9.43	3.05	27.47	27.47	090	
61156		A	Burr hole(s); with aspiration of hematoma or cyst, intracerebral	16.32	10.30	10.30	3.42	30.04	30.04	090	
61210		A	for implanting ventricular catheter, reservoir, EEG electrode(s) or pressure recording device (separate procedure)	5.84	3.53	3.53	1.16	10.53	10.53	000	
61215		A	Insertion of subcutaneous reservoir, pump or continuous infusion system for connection to ventricular catheter	4.89	4.24	4.24	0.99	10.12	10.12	090	
61250		A	Burr hole(s) or trephine, supratentorial, exploratory, not followed by other surgery	10.42	6.73	6.73	2.02	19.17	19.17	090	
61253		A	Burr hole(s) or trephine, infratentorial, unilateral or bilateral	12.36	7.65	7.65	2.26	22.27	22.27	090	
61304		A	Craniectomy or craniotomy, exploratory; supratentorial	21.96	12.85	12.85	4.33	39.14	39.14	090	
61305		A	infratentorial (posterior fossa)	26.61	15.31	15.31	5.25	47.17	47.17	090	
61312		A	Craniectomy or craniotomy for evacuation of hematoma, supratentorial; extradural or subdural	24.57	14.57	14.57	4.99	44.13	44.13	090	
61313		A	intracerebral	24.93	14.76	14.76	5.07	44.76	44.76	090	
61314		A	Craniectomy or craniotomy for evacuation of hematoma, infratentorial; extradural or subdural	24.23	11.55	11.55	4.00	39.78	39.78	090	
61315		A	intracerebellar	27.68	16.22	16.22	5.62	49.52	49.52	090	
61320		A	Craniectomy or craniotomy, drainage of intracranial abscess; supratentorial	25.62	15.20	15.20	5.20	46.02	46.02	090	
61321		A	infratentorial	28.50	16.09	16.09	5.35	49.94	49.94	090	
61330		A	Decompression of orbit only, transcranial approach	23.32	19.43	19.43	2.58	45.33	45.33	090	
61332		A	Exploration of orbit (transcranial approach); with biopsy	27.28	20.43	20.43	4.15	51.86	51.86	090	
61333		A	with removal of lesion	27.95	16.45	16.45	2.24	46.64	46.64	090	
61334		A	with removal of foreign body	18.27	10.08	10.08	3.02	31.37	31.37	090	
61340		A	Other cranial decompression (eg, subtemporal), supratentorial	18.66	11.75	11.75	3.66	34.07	34.07	090	

■ RVU not developed by CMS. Gap-filled RVUs developed by Ingenix/CHEG.

Surgery

Code	M	S	Description	Work Value	Non-Fac PE	Fac PE	Mal-practice	Non-Fac Total	Fac Total	Global	Gap
61343		A	Craniectomy, suboccipital with cervical laminectomy for decompression of medulla and spinal cord, with or without dural graft (eg, Arnold-Chiari malformation)	29.77	17.96	17.96	6.04	53.77	53.77	090	
61345		A	Other cranial decompression, posterior fossa	27.20	16.17	16.17	5.23	48.60	48.60	090	
61440		A	Craniotomy for section of tentorium cerebelli (separate procedure)	26.63	12.14	12.14	5.57	44.34	44.34	090	
61450		A	Craniectomy, subtemporal, for section, compression, or decompression of sensory root of gasserian ganglion	25.95	14.46	14.46	5.11	45.52	45.52	090	
61458		A	Craniectomy, suboccipital; for exploration or decompression of cranial nerves	27.29	15.89	15.89	5.28	48.46	48.46	090	
61460		A	for section of one or more cranial nerves	28.39	16.77	16.77	5.13	50.29	50.29	090	
61470		A	for medullary tractotomy	26.06	13.74	13.74	4.65	44.45	44.45	090	
61480		A	for mesencephalic tractotomy or pedunculotomy	26.49	12.34	12.34	5.54	44.37	44.37	090	
61490		A	Craniotomy for lobotomy, including cingulotomy	25.66	15.18	15.18	5.37	46.21	46.21	090	
61500		A	Craniectomy; with excision of tumor or other bone lesion of skull	17.92	11.03	11.03	3.26	32.21	32.21	090	
61501		A	for osteomyelitis	14.84	9.62	9.62	2.63	27.09	27.09	090	
61510		A	Craniectomy, trephination, bone flap craniotomy; for excision of brain tumor, supratentorial, except meningioma	28.45	16.60	16.60	5.77	50.82	50.82	090	
61512		A	for excision of meningioma, supratentorial	35.09	20.18	20.18	7.14	62.41	62.41	090	
61514		A	for excision of brain abscess, supratentorial	25.26	14.91	14.91	5.12	45.29	45.29	090	
61516		A	for excision or fenestration of cyst, supratentorial	24.61	15.01	15.01	4.94	44.56	44.56	090	
61518		A	Craniectomy for excision of brain tumor, infratentorial or posterior fossa; except meningioma, cerebellopontine angle tumor, or midline tumor at base of skull	37.32	22.34	22.34	7.53	67.19	67.19	090	
61519		A	meningioma	41.39	24.42	24.42	8.15	73.96	73.96	090	
61520		A	cerebellopontine angle tumor	54.84	31.93	31.93	10.10	96.87	96.87	090	
61521		A	midline tumor at base of skull	44.48	26.22	26.22	8.85	79.55	79.55	090	
61522		A	Craniectomy, infratentorial or posterior fossa; for excision of brain abscess	29.45	17.20	17.20	5.30	51.95	51.95	090	
61524		A	for excision or fenestration of cyst	27.86	16.83	16.83	5.01	49.70	49.70	090	

■ RVU not developed by CMS. Gap-filled RVUs developed by Ingenix/CHEG.

Code	M	S	Description	Work Value	Non-Fac PE	Fac PE	Mal-practice	Non-Fac Total	Fac Total	Global	Gap
61526		A	Craniectomy, bone flap craniotomy, transtemporal (mastoid) for excision of cerebellopontine angle tumor;	52.17	31.55	31.55	6.72	90.44	90.44	090	
61530		A	combined with middle/posterior fossa craniotomy/craniectomy	43.86	27.43	27.43	6.17	77.46	77.46	090	
61531		A	Subdural implantation of strip electrodes through one or more burr or trephine hole(s) for long term seizure monitoring	14.63	9.56	9.56	2.84	27.03	27.03	090	
61533		A	Craniotomy with elevation of bone flap; for subdural implantation of an electrode array, for long term seizure monitoring	19.71	12.21	12.21	3.80	35.72	35.72	090	
61534		A	for excision of epileptogenic focus without electrocorticography during surgery	20.97	13.30	13.30	4.15	38.42	38.42	090	
61535		A	for removal of epidural or subdural electrode array, without excision of cerebral tissue (separate procedure)	11.63	8.16	8.16	2.29	22.08	22.08	090	
61536		A	for excision of cerebral epileptogenic focus, with electrocorticography during surgery (includes removal of electrode array)	35.52	21.18	21.18	6.68	63.38	63.38	090	
61538		A	for lobectomy with electrocorticography during surgery, temporal lobe	26.81	16.30	16.30	5.38	48.49	48.49	090	
61539		A	for lobectomy with electrocorticography during surgery, other than temporal lobe, partial or total	32.08	18.91	18.91	6.62	57.61	57.61	090	
61541		A	for transection of corpus callosum	28.85	16.89	16.89	5.50	51.24	51.24	090	
61542		A	for total hemispherectomy	31.02	18.00	18.00	6.49	55.51	55.51	090	
61543		A	for partial or subtotal hemispherectomy	29.22	17.42	17.42	6.11	52.75	52.75	090	
61544		A	for excision or coagulation of choroid plexus	25.50	15.21	15.21	4.91	45.62	45.62	090	
61545		A	for excision of craniopharyngioma	43.80	25.09	25.09	8.88	77.77	77.77	090	
61546		A	Craniotomy for hypophysectomy or excision of pituitary tumor, intracranial approach	31.30	18.74	18.74	6.06	56.10	56.10	090	
61548		A	Hypophysectomy or excision of pituitary tumor, transnasal or transseptal approach, nonstereotactic	21.53	13.74	13.74	3.63	38.90	38.90	090	
61550		A	Craniectomy for craniosynostosis; single cranial suture	14.65	4.89	4.89	1.14	20.68	20.68	090	
61552		A	multiple cranial sutures	19.56	9.87	9.87	0.88	30.31	30.31	090	
61556		A	Craniotomy for craniosynostosis; frontal or parietal bone flap	22.26	11.74	11.74	3.57	37.57	37.57	090	
61557		A	bifrontal bone flap	22.38	13.41	13.41	4.68	40.47	40.47	090	

Surgery

■ RVU not developed by CMS. Gap-filled RVUs developed by Ingenix/CHEG.

Code	M	S	Description	Work Value	Non-Fac PE	Fac PE	Mal-practice	Non-Fac Total	Fac Total	Global	Gap
61558		A	Extensive craniectomy for multiple cranial suture craniosynostosis (eg, cloverleaf skull); not requiring bone grafts	25.58	12.67	12.67	2.61	40.86	40.86	090	
61559		A	recontouring with multiple osteotomies and bone autografts (eg, barrel-stave procedure) (includes obtaining grafts)	32.79	18.89	18.89	6.86	58.54	58.54	090	
61563		A	Excision, intra and extracranial, benign tumor of cranial bone (eg, fibrous dysplasia); without optic nerve decompression	26.83	16.25	16.25	4.46	47.54	47.54	090	
61564		A	with optic nerve decompression	33.83	18.73	18.73	7.08	59.64	59.64	090	
61570		A	Craniectomy or craniotomy; with excision of foreign body from brain	24.60	13.80	13.80	4.60	43.00	43.00	090	
61571		A	with treatment of penetrating wound of brain	26.39	15.43	15.43	5.23	47.05	47.05	090	
61575		A	Transoral approach to skull base, brain stem or upper spinal cord for biopsy, decompression or excision of lesion;	34.36	21.38	21.38	5.02	60.76	60.76	090	
61576		A	requiring splitting of tongue and/or mandible (including tracheostomy)	52.43	28.89	28.89	4.68	86.00	86.00	090	
61580		A	Craniofacial approach to anterior cranial fossa; extradural, including lateral rhinotomy, ethmoidectomy, sphenoidectomy, without maxillectomy or orbital exenteration	30.35	19.96	19.96	2.75	53.06	53.06	090	
61581		A	extradural, including lateral rhinotomy, orbital exenteration, ethmoidectomy, sphenoidectomy and/or maxillectomy	34.60	22.57	22.57	3.37	60.54	60.54	090	
61582		A	extradural, including unilateral or bifrontal craniotomy, elevation of frontal lobe(s), osteotomy of base of anterior cranial fossa	31.66	19.56	19.56	6.30	57.52	57.52	090	
61583		A	intradural, including unilateral or bifrontal craniotomy, elevation or resection of frontal lobe, osteotomy of base of anterior cranial fossa	36.21	22.71	22.71	6.94	65.86	65.86	090	
61584		A	Orbitocranial approach to anterior cranial fossa, extradural, including supraorbital ridge osteotomy and elevation of frontal and/or temporal lobe(s); without orbital exenteration	34.65	20.99	20.99	6.53	62.17	62.17	090	
61585		A	with orbital exenteration	38.61	22.21	22.21	6.19	67.01	67.01	090	
61586		A	Bicoronal, transzygomatic and/or LeFort I osteotomy approach to anterior cranial fossa with or without internal fixation, without bone graft	25.10	16.39	16.39	3.52	45.01	45.01	090	

■ RVU not developed by CMS. Gap-filled RVUs developed by Ingenix/CHEG.

Code	M	S	Description	Work Value	Non-Fac PE	Fac PE	Mal-practice	Non-Fac Total	Fac Total	Global	Gap
61590		A	Infratemporal pre-auricular approach to middle cranial fossa (parapharyngeal space, infratemporal and midline skull base, nasopharynx), with or without disarticulation of the mandible, including parotidectomy, craniotomy, decompression and/or mobilization of the facial nerve and/or petrous carotid artery	41.78	26.12	26.12	4.28	72.18	72.18	090	
61591		A	Infratemporal post-auricular approach to middle cranial fossa (internal auditory meatus, petrous apex, tentorium, cavernous sinus, parasellar area, infratemporal fossa) including mastoidectomy, resection of sigmoid sinus, with or without decompression and/or mobilization of contents of auditory canal or petrous carotid artery	43.68	26.89	26.89	5.26	75.83	75.83	090	
61592		A	Orbitocranial zygomatic approach to middle cranial fossa (cavernous sinus and carotid artery, clivus, basilar artery or petrous apex) including osteotomy of zygoma, craniotomy, extra- or intradural elevation of temporal lobe	39.64	23.59	23.59	7.55	70.78	70.78	090	
61595		A	Transtemporal approach to posterior cranial fossa, jugular foramen or midline skull base, including mastoidectomy, decompression of sigmoid sinus and/or facial nerve, with or without mobilization	29.57	19.74	19.74	3.05	52.36	52.36	090	
61596		A	Transcochlear approach to posterior cranial fossa, jugular foramen or midline skull base, including labyrinthectomy, decompression, with or without mobilization of facial nerve and/or petrous carotid artery	35.63	21.88	21.88	4.25	61.76	61.76	090	
61597		A	Transcondylar (far lateral) approach to posterior cranial fossa, jugular foramen or midline skull base, including occipital condylectomy, mastoidectomy, resection of C1-C3 vertebral body(s), decompression of vertebral artery, with or without mobilization	37.96	22.41	22.41	6.65	67.02	67.02	090	
61598		A	Transpetrosal approach to posterior cranial fossa, clivus or foramen magnum, including ligation of superior petrosal sinus and/or sigmoid sinus	33.41	20.92	20.92	4.60	58.93	58.93	090	
61600		A	Resection or excision of neoplastic, vascular or infectious lesion of base of anterior cranial fossa; extradural	25.85	15.01	15.01	3.12	43.98	43.98	090	
61601		A	intradural, including dural repair, with or without graft	27.89	17.34	17.34	5.29	50.52	50.52	090	
61605		A	Resection or excision of neoplastic, vascular or infectious lesion of infratemporal fossa, parapharyngeal space, petrous apex; extradural	29.33	18.97	18.97	2.51	50.81	50.81	090	
61606		A	intradural, including dural repair, with or without graft	38.83	23.17	23.17	6.81	68.81	68.81	090	

■ RVU not developed by CMS. Gap-filled RVUs developed by Ingenix/CHEG.

Surgery

Code	M	S	Description	Work Value	Non-Fac PE	Fac PE	Mal-prac-tice	Non-Fac Total	Fac Total	Global	Gap
61607		A	Resection or excision of neoplastic, vascular or infectious lesion of parasellar area, cavernous sinus, clivus or midline skull base; extradural	36.27	22.17	22.17	5.69	64.13	64.13	090	
61608		A	intradural, including dural repair, with or without graft	42.10	24.89	24.89	8.31	75.30	75.30	090	
61609		A	Transection or ligation, carotid artery in cavernous sinus; without repair (List separately in addition to code for primary procedure)	9.89	5.11	5.11	2.07	17.07	17.07	ZZZ	
61610		A	with repair by anastomosis or graft (List separately in addition to code for primary procedure)	29.67	14.38	14.38	3.52	47.57	47.57	ZZZ	
61611		A	Transection or ligation, carotid artery in petrous canal; without repair (List separately in addition to code for primary procedure)	7.42	2.96	2.96	1.55	11.93	11.93	ZZZ	
61612		A	with repair by anastomosis or graft (List separately in addition to code for primary procedure)	27.88	14.30	14.30	3.55	45.73	45.73	ZZZ	
61613		A	Obliteration of carotid aneurysm, arteriovenous malformation, or carotid-cavernous fistula by dissection within cavernous sinus	40.86	23.34	23.34	8.32	72.52	72.52	090	
61615		A	Resection or excision of neoplastic, vascular or infectious lesion of base of posterior cranial fossa, jugular foramen, foramen magnum, or C1-C3 vertebral bodies; extradural	32.07	20.81	20.81	4.64	57.52	57.52	090	
61616		A	intradural, including dural repair, with or without graft	43.33	26.97	26.97	7.02	77.32	77.32	090	
61618		A	Secondary repair of dura for cerebrospinal fluid leak, anterior, middle or posterior cranial fossa following surgery of the skull base; by free tissue graft (eg, pericranium, fascia, tensor fascia lata, adipose tissue, homologous or synthetic grafts)	16.99	11.43	11.43	2.92	31.34	31.34	090	
61619		A	by local or regionalized vascularized pedicle flap or myocutaneous flap (including galea, temporalis, frontalis or occipitalis muscle)	20.71	13.67	13.67	3.42	37.80	37.80	090	
61624		A	Transcatheter occlusion or embolization (eg, for tumor destruction, to achieve hemostasis, to occlude a vascular malformation), percutaneous, any method; central nervous system (intracranial, spinal cord)	20.15	7.46	7.46	1.15	28.76	28.76	000	
61626		A	non-central nervous system, head or neck (extracranial, brachiocephalic branch)	16.62	5.88	5.88	0.84	23.34	23.34	000	
61680		A	Surgery of intracranial arteriovenous malformation; supratentorial, simple	30.71	18.38	18.38	6.04	55.13	55.13	090	
61682		A	supratentorial, complex	61.57	34.65	34.65	12.69	108.91	108.91	090	
61684		A	infratentorial, simple	39.81	22.60	22.60	7.87	70.28	70.28	090	

■ RVU not developed by CMS. Gap-filled RVUs developed by Ingenix/CHEG.

Code	M	S	Description	Work Value	Non-Fac PE	Fac PE	Mal-practice	Non-Fac Total	Fac Total	Global	Gap
61686		A	infratentorial, complex	64.49	36.70	36.70	13.20	114.39	114.39	090	
61690		A	dural, simple	29.31	17.64	17.64	5.51	52.46	52.46	090	
61692		A	dural, complex	51.87	29.51	29.51	10.17	91.55	91.55	090	
61697		A	Surgery of complex intracranial aneurysm, intracranial approach; carotid circulation	50.52	28.42	28.42	10.31	89.25	89.25	090	
61698		A	vertebrobasilar circulation	48.41	27.31	27.31	9.99	85.71	85.71	090	
61700		A	Surgery of simple intracranial aneurysm, intracranial approach; carotid circulation	50.52	28.42	28.42	10.18	89.12	89.12	090	
61702		A	vertebrobasilar circulation	48.41	27.31	27.31	9.75	85.47	85.47	090	
61703		A	Surgery of intracranial aneurysm, cervical approach by application of occluding clamp to cervical carotid artery (Selverstone-Crutchfield type)	17.47	11.13	11.13	3.62	32.22	32.22	090	
61705		A	Surgery of aneurysm, vascular malformation or carotid-cavernous fistula; by intracranial and cervical occlusion of carotid artery	36.20	19.89	19.89	6.67	62.76	62.76	090	
61708		A	by intracranial electrothrombosis	35.30	16.52	16.52	2.18	54.00	54.00	090	
61710		A	by intra-arterial embolization, injection procedure, or balloon catheter	29.67	14.68	14.68	2.42	46.77	46.77	090	
61711		A	Anastomosis, arterial, extracranial-intracranial (eg, middle cerebral/cortical) arteries	36.33	20.68	20.68	7.39	64.40	64.40	090	
61720		A	Creation of lesion by stereotactic method, including burr hole(s) and localizing and recording techniques, single or multiple stages; globus pallidus or thalamus	16.77	10.90	10.90	3.51	31.18	31.18	090	
61735		A	subcortical structure(s) other than globus pallidus or thalamus	20.43	12.77	12.77	4.16	37.36	37.36	090	
61750		A	Stereotactic biopsy, aspiration, or excision, including burr hole(s), for intracranial lesion;	18.20	11.08	11.08	3.71	32.99	32.99	090	
61751		A	with computerized axial tomography and/ or magnetic resonance guidance	17.62	10.92	10.92	3.57	32.11	32.11	090	
61760		A	Stereotactic implantation of depth electrodes into the cerebrum for long term seizure monitoring	22.27	12.85	12.85	4.59	39.71	39.71	090	
61770		A	Stereotactic localization, including burr hole(s), with insertion of catheter(s) or probe(s) for placement of radiation source	21.44	13.26	13.26	4.09	38.79	38.79	090	
61790		A	Creation of lesion by stereotactic method, percutaneous, by neurolytic agent (eg, alcohol, thermal, electrical, radiofrequency); gasserian ganglion	10.86	6.92	6.92	1.82	19.60	19.60	090	
61791		A	trigeminal medullary tract	14.61	9.39	9.39	3.03	27.03	27.03	090	

■ RVU not developed by CMS. Gap-filled RVUs developed by Ingenix/CHEG.

Code	M	S	Description	Work Value	Non-Fac PE	Fac PE	Mal-practice	Non-Fac Total	Fac Total	Global	Gap
61793		A	Stereotactic radiosurgery (particle beam, gamma ray or linear accelerator), one or more sessions	17.24	11.07	11.07	3.51	31.82	31.82	090	
61795		A	Stereotactic computer assisted volumetric (navigational) procedure, intracranial, extracranial, or spinal (List separately in addition to code for primary procedure)	4.04	2.14	2.14	0.81	6.99	6.99	ZZZ	
61850		A	Twist drill or burr hole(s) for implantation of neurostimulator electrodes, cortical	12.39	8.13	8.13	2.23	22.75	22.75	090	
61860		A	Craniectomy or craniotomy for implantation of neurostimulator electrodes, cerebral, cortical	20.87	12.59	12.59	4.04	37.50	37.50	090	
61862		A	Twist drill, burr hole, craniotomy, or craniectomy for stereotactic implantation of one neurostimulator array in subcortical site (eg, thalamus, globus pallidus, subthalamic nucleus, periventricular, periaqueductal gray)	19.34	12.16	12.16	3.97	35.47	35.47	090	
61870		A	Craniectomy for implantation of neurostimulator electrodes, cerebellar; cortical	14.94	9.97	9.97	1.70	26.61	26.61	090	
61875		A	subcortical	15.06	7.39	7.39	2.42	24.87	24.87	090	
61880		A	Revision or removal of intracranial neurostimulator electrodes	6.29	5.26	5.26	1.31	12.86	12.86	090	
61885		A	Incision and subcutaneous placement of cranial neurostimulator pulse generator or receiver, direct or inductive coupling; with connection to a single electrode array	5.85	4.36	4.36	1.22	11.43	11.43	090	
61886		A	with connection to two or more electrode arrays	8.00	6.13	6.13	1.64	15.77	15.77	090	
61888		A	Revision or removal of cranial neurostimulator pulse generator or receiver	5.07	3.90	3.90	1.04	10.01	10.01	010	
62000		A	Elevation of depressed skull fracture; simple, extradural	12.53	6.19	6.19	0.87	19.59	19.59	090	
62005		A	compound or comminuted, extradural	16.17	9.35	9.35	2.33	27.85	27.85	090	
62010		A	with repair of dura and/or debridement of brain	19.81	11.83	11.83	4.05	35.69	35.69	090	
62100		A	Craniotomy for repair of dural/cerebrospinal fluid leak, including surgery for rhinorrhea/otorrhea	22.03	13.97	13.97	4.07	40.07	40.07	090	
62115		A	Reduction of craniomegalic skull (eg, treated hydrocephalus); not requiring bone grafts or cranioplasty	21.66	11.03	11.03	4.53	37.22	37.22	090	
62116		A	with simple cranioplasty	23.59	14.04	14.04	4.85	42.48	42.48	090	
62117		A	requiring craniotomy and reconstruction with or without bone graft (includes obtaining grafts)	26.60	12.68	12.68	5.56	44.84	44.84	090	

■ RVU not developed by CMS. Gap-filled RVUs developed by Ingenix/CHEG.

Code	M	S	Description	Work Value	Non-Fac PE	Fac PE	Mal-prac-tice	Non-Fac Total	Fac Total	Global	Gap
62120		A	Repair of encephalocele, skull vault, including cranioplasty	23.35	15.14	15.14	3.07	41.56	41.56	090	
62121		A	Craniotomy for repair of encephalocele, skull base	21.58	13.52	13.52	2.47	37.57	37.57	090	
62140		A	Cranioplasty for skull defect; up to 5 cm diameter	13.51	8.72	8.72	2.60	24.83	24.83	090	
62141		A	larger than 5 cm diameter	14.91	9.89	9.89	2.85	27.65	27.65	090	
62142		A	Removal of bone flap or prosthetic plate of skull	10.79	7.31	7.31	2.10	20.20	20.20	090	
62143		A	Replacement of bone flap or prosthetic plate of skull	13.05	8.81	8.81	2.55	24.41	24.41	090	
62145		A	Cranioplasty for skull defect with reparative brain surgery	18.82	11.77	11.77	3.81	34.40	34.40	090	
62146		A	Cranioplasty with autograft (includes obtaining bone grafts); up to 5 cm diameter	16.12	10.63	10.63	2.94	29.69	29.69	090	
62147		A	larger than 5 cm diameter	19.34	12.38	12.38	3.64	35.36	35.36	090	
62180		A	Ventriculocisternostomy (Torkildsen type operation)	21.06	13.08	13.08	4.32	38.46	38.46	090	
62190		A	Creation of shunt; subarachnoid/subdural-atrial, -jugular, -auricular	11.07	7.77	7.77	2.18	21.02	21.02	090	
62192		A	subarachnoid/subdural-peritoneal, -pleural, other terminus	12.25	8.25	8.25	2.46	22.96	22.96	090	
62194		A	Replacement or irrigation, subarachnoid/ subdural catheter	5.03	2.25	2.25	0.50	7.78	7.78	010	
62200		A	Ventriculocisternostomy, third ventricle;	18.32	11.72	11.72	3.70	33.74	33.74	090	
62201		A	stereotactic method	14.86	9.76	9.76	2.52	27.14	27.14	090	
62220		A	Creation of shunt; ventriculo-atrial, -jugular, -auricular	13.00	8.60	8.60	2.53	24.13	24.13	090	
62223		A	ventriculo-peritoneal, -pleural, other terminus	12.87	8.54	8.54	2.58	23.99	23.99	090	
62225		A	Replacement or irrigation, ventricular catheter	5.41	4.11	4.11	1.09	10.61	10.61	090	
62230		A	Replacement or revision of cerebrospinal fluid shunt, obstructed valve, or distal catheter in shunt system	10.54	6.42	6.42	2.10	19.06	19.06	090	
62252		A	Reprogramming of programmable cerebrospinal shunt	0.74	1.35	1.35	0.18	2.27	2.27	XXX	
	26	A		0.74	0.30	0.30	0.16	1.20	1.20	XXX	
	TC	A		0.00	1.05	1.05	0.02	1.07	1.07	XXX	
62256		A	Removal of complete cerebrospinal fluid shunt system; without replacement	6.60	5.40	5.40	1.34	13.34	13.34	090	
62258		A	with replacement by similar or other shunt at same operation	14.54	8.82	8.82	2.91	26.27	26.27	090	

Surgery

■ RVU not developed by CMS. Gap-filled RVUs developed by Ingenix/CHEG.

Code	M	S	Description	Work Value	Non-Fac PE	Fac PE	Mal-practice	Non-Fac Total	Fac Total	Global	Gap
62263		A	Percutaneous lysis of epidural adhesions using solution injection (eg, hypertonic saline, enzyme) or mechanical means (eg, spring-wound catheter) including radiologic localization (includes contrast when administered)	6.14	5.15	2.07	0.42	11.71	8.63	010	
62268		A	Percutaneous aspiration, spinal cord cyst or syrinx	4.74	2.74	2.74	0.29	7.77	7.77	000	
62269		A	Biopsy of spinal cord, percutaneous needle	5.02	2.40	2.40	0.29	7.71	7.71	000	
62270		A	Spinal puncture, lumbar, diagnostic	1.13	4.08	0.48	0.06	5.27	1.67	000	
62272		A	Spinal puncture, therapeutic, for drainage of cerebrospinal fluid (by needle or catheter)	1.35	3.38	0.62	0.13	4.86	2.10	000	
62273		A	Injection, epidural, of blood or clot patch	2.15	1.57	1.27	0.14	3.86	3.56	000	
62280		A	Injection/infusion of neurolytic substance (eg, alcohol, phenol, iced saline solutions), with or without other therapeutic substance; subarachnoid	2.63	3.79	0.70	0.17	6.59	3.50	010	
62281		A	epidural, cervical or thoracic	2.66	4.50	0.62	0.16	7.32	3.44	010	
62282		A	epidural, lumbar, sacral (caudal)	2.33	5.57	0.62	0.14	8.04	3.09	010	
62284		A	Injection procedure for myelography and/or computerized axial tomography, spinal (other than C1-C2 and posterior fossa)	1.54	5.53	0.55	0.10	7.17	2.19	000	
62287		A	Aspiration or decompression procedure, percutaneous, of nucleus pulposus of intervertebral disk, any method, single or multiple levels, lumbar (eg, manual or automated percutaneous diskectomy, percutaneous laser diskectomy)	8.08	5.05	5.05	0.66	13.79	13.79	090	
62290		A	Injection procedure for diskography, each level; lumbar	3.00	5.68	1.30	0.20	8.88	4.50	000	
62291		A	cervical or thoracic	2.91	6.24	1.20	0.17	9.32	4.28	000	
62292		A	Injection procedure for chemonucleolysis, including diskography, intervertebral disk, single or multiple levels, lumbar	7.86	5.34	5.34	0.65	13.85	13.85	090	
62294		A	Injection procedure, arterial, for occlusion of arteriovenous malformation, spinal	11.83	7.37	7.37	0.85	20.05	20.05	090	
62310		A	Injection, single (not via indwelling catheter), not including neurolytic substances, with or without contrast (for either localization or epidurography), of diagnostic or therapeutic substance(s) (including anesthetic, antispasmodic, opioid, steroid, other solution), epidural or subarachnoid; cervical or thoracic	1.91	3.71	0.43	0.11	5.73	2.45	000	
62311		A	lumbar, sacral (caudal)	1.54	4.22	0.37	0.09	5.85	2.00	000	

■ RVU not developed by CMS. Gap-filled RVUs developed by Ingenix/CHEG.

Code	M	S	Description	Work Value	Non-Fac PE	Fac PE	Mal-practice	Non-Fac Total	Fac Total	Global	Gap
62318		A	Injection, including catheter placement, continuous infusion or intermittent bolus, not including neurolytic substances, with or without contrast (for either localization or epidurography), of diagnostic or therapeutic substance(s) (including anesthetic, antispasmodic, opioid, steroid, other solution), epidural or subarachnoid; cervical or thoracic	2.04	3.83	0.44	0.12	5.99	2.60	000	
62319		A	lumbar, sacral (caudal)	1.87	3.67	0.40	0.11	5.65	2.38	000	
62350		A	Implantation, revision or repositioning of tunneled intrathecal or epidural catheter, for long-term medication administration via an external pump or implantable reservoir/ infusion pump; without laminectomy	6.87	3.79	3.79	0.64	11.30	11.30	090	
62351		A	with laminectomy	10.00	6.90	6.90	1.79	18.69	18.69	090	
62355		A	Removal of previously implanted intrathecal or epidural catheter	5.45	3.02	3.02	0.47	8.94	8.94	090	
62360		A	Implantation or replacement of device for intrathecal or epidural drug infusion; subcutaneous reservoir	2.62	2.46	2.46	0.21	5.29	5.29	090	
62361		A	non-programmable pump	5.42	3.67	3.67	0.50	9.59	9.59	090	
62362		A	programmable pump, including preparation of pump, with or without programming	7.04	4.06	4.06	0.86	11.96	11.96	090	
62365		A	Removal of subcutaneous reservoir or pump, previously implanted for intrathecal or epidural infusion	5.42	3.99	3.99	0.58	9.99	9.99	090	
62367		C	Electronic analysis of programmable, implanted pump for intrathecal or epidural drug infusion (includes evaluation of reservoir status, alarm status, drug prescription status); without reprogramming	0.00	0.00	0.00	0.00	0.00	0.00	XXX	
	26	A		0.48	0.14	0.14	0.03	0.65	0.65	XXX	
	TC	C		0.00	0.00	0.00	0.00	0.00	0.00	XXX	
62368		C	with reprogramming	0.00	0.00	0.00	0.00	0.00	0.00	XXX	
	26	A		0.75	0.20	0.20	0.05	1.00	1.00	XXX	
	TC	C		0.00	0.00	0.00	0.00	0.00	0.00	XXX	
63001		A	Laminectomy with exploration and/or decompression of spinal cord and/or cauda equina, without facetectomy, foraminotomy or diskectomy, (eg, spinal stenosis), one or two vertebral segments; cervical	15.82	11.68	11.68	3.03	30.53	30.53	090	
63003		A	thoracic	15.95	11.95	11.95	2.98	30.88	30.88	090	
63005		A	lumbar, except for spondylolisthesis	14.92	11.49	11.49	2.62	29.03	29.03	090	
63011		A	sacral	14.52	11.29	11.29	1.43	27.24	27.24	090	

■ RVU not developed by CMS. Gap-filled RVUs developed by Ingenix/CHEG.

Surgery

Code	M	S	Description	Work Value	Non-Fac PE	Fac PE	Mal-practice	Non-Fac Total	Fac Total	Global	Gap
63012		A	Laminectomy with removal of abnormal facets and/or pars inter-articularis with decompression of cauda equina and nerve roots for spondylolisthesis, lumbar (Gill type procedure)	15.40	10.34	10.34	2.71	28.45	28.45	090	
63015		A	Laminectomy with exploration and/or decompression of spinal cord and/or cauda equina, without facetectomy, foraminotomy or diskectomy, (eg, spinal stenosis), more than 2 vertebral segments; cervical	19.35	13.68	13.68	3.84	36.87	36.87	090	
63016		A	thoracic	19.20	13.66	13.66	3.62	36.48	36.48	090	
63017		A	lumbar	15.94	12.00	12.00	2.91	30.85	30.85	090	
63020		A	Laminotomy (hemilaminectomy), with decompression of nerve root(s), including partial facetectomy, foraminotomy and/or excision of herniated intervertebral disk; one interspace, cervical	14.81	11.33	11.33	2.89	29.03	29.03	090	
63030		A	one interspace, lumbar (including open or endoscopically-assisted approach)	12.00	9.92	9.92	2.21	24.13	24.13	090	
63035		A	each additional interspace, cervical or lumbar (List separately in addition to code for primary procedure)	3.15	1.67	1.67	0.57	5.39	5.39	ZZZ	
63040		A	Laminotomy (hemilaminectomy), with decompression of nerve root(s), including partial facetectomy, foraminotomy and/or excision of herniated intervertebral disk, reexploration, single interspace; cervical	18.81	13.39	13.39	3.36	35.56	35.56	090	
63042		A	lumbar	17.47	12.95	12.95	3.11	33.53	33.53	090	
63043		C	each additional cervical interspace (List separately in addition to code for primary procedure)	7.65	6.08	6.08	0.81	14.54	14.54	ZZZ	■
63044		C	each additional lumbar interspace (List separately in addition to code for primary procedure)	7.26	5.77	5.77	0.77	13.81	13.81	ZZZ	■
63045		A	Laminectomy, facetectomy and foraminotomy (unilateral or bilateral with decompression of spinal cord, cauda equina and/or nerve root(s), (eg, spinal or lateral recess stenosis), single vertebral segment; cervical	16.50	12.22	12.22	3.19	31.91	31.91	090	
63046		A	thoracic	15.80	12.02	12.02	2.89	30.71	30.71	090	
63047		A	lumbar	14.61	11.42	11.42	2.61	28.64	28.64	090	
63048		A	each additional segment, cervical, thoracic, or lumbar (List separately in addition to code for primary procedure)	3.26	1.75	1.75	0.58	5.59	5.59	ZZZ	

■ RVU not developed by CMS. Gap-filled RVUs developed by Ingenix/CHEG.

Code	M	S	Description	Work Value	Non-Fac PE	Fac PE	Mal-practice	Non-Fac Total	Fac Total	Global	Gap
63055		A	Transpedicular approach with decompression of spinal cord, equina and/or nerve root(s) (eg, herniated intervertebral disk), single segment; thoracic	21.99	15.11	15.11	4.09	41.19	41.19	090	
63056		A	lumbar (including transfacet, or lateral extraforaminal approach) (eg, far lateral herniated intervertebral disk)	20.36	14.44	14.44	3.34	38.14	38.14	090	
63057		A	each additional segment, thoracic or lumbar (List separately in addition to code for primary procedure)	5.26	2.82	2.82	0.81	8.89	8.89	ZZZ	
63064		A	Costovertebral approach with decompression of spinal cord or nerve root(s), (eg, herniated intervertebral disk), thoracic; single segment	24.61	17.12	17.12	4.72	46.45	46.45	090	
63066		A	each additional segment (List separately in addition to code for primary procedure)	3.26	1.76	1.76	0.63	5.65	5.65	ZZZ	
63075		A	Diskectomy, anterior, with decompression of spinal cord and/or nerve root(s), including osteophytectomy; cervical, single interspace	19.41	13.83	13.83	3.73	36.97	36.97	090	
63076		A	cervical, each additional interspace (List separately in addition to code for primary procedure)	4.05	2.16	2.16	0.78	6.99	6.99	ZZZ	
63077		A	thoracic, single interspace	21.44	15.47	15.47	3.44	40.35	40.35	090	
63078		A	thoracic, each additional interspace (List separately in addition to code for primary procedure)	3.28	1.72	1.72	0.50	5.50	5.50	ZZZ	
63081		A	Vertebral corpectomy (vertebral body resection), partial or complete, anterior approach with decompression of spinal cord and/or nerve root(s); cervical, single segment	23.73	16.68	16.68	4.46	44.87	44.87	090	
63082		A	cervical, each additional segment (List separately in addition to code for primary procedure)	4.37	2.34	2.34	0.82	7.53	7.53	ZZZ	
63085		A	Vertebral corpectomy (vertebral body resection), partial or complete, transthoracic approach with decompression of spinal cord and/or nerve root(s); thoracic, single segment	26.92	17.89	17.89	4.70	49.51	49.51	090	
63086		A	thoracic, each additional segment (List separately in addition to code for primary procedure)	3.19	1.66	1.66	0.55	5.40	5.40	ZZZ	
63087		A	Vertebral corpectomy (vertebral body resection), partial or complete, combined thoracolumbar approach with decompression of spinal cord, cauda equina or nerve root(s), lower thoracic or lumbar; single segment	35.57	22.45	22.45	5.87	63.89	63.89	090	
63088		A	each additional segment (List separately in addition to code for primary procedure)	4.33	2.30	2.30	0.77	7.40	7.40	ZZZ	

Surgery

■ RVU not developed by CMS. Gap-filled RVUs developed by Ingenix/CHEG.

Code	M	S	Description	Work Value	Non-Fac PE	Fac PE	Mal-practice	Non-Fac Total	Fac Total	Global	Gap
63090		A	Vertebral corpectomy (vertebral body resection), partial or complete, transperitoneal or retroperitoneal approach with decompression of spinal cord, cauda equina or nerve root(s), lower thoracic, lumbar, or sacral; single segment	28.16	18.12	18.12	4.27	50.55	50.55	090	
63091		A	each additional segment (List separately in addition to code for primary procedure)	3.03	1.48	1.48	0.45	4.96	4.96	ZZZ	
63170		A	Laminectomy with myelotomy (eg, Bischof or DREZ type), cervical, thoracic or thoracolumbar	19.83	13.54	13.54	3.89	37.26	37.26	090	
63172		A	Laminectomy with drainage of intramedullary cyst/syrinx; to subarachnoid space	17.66	13.37	13.37	3.46	34.49	34.49	090	
63173		A	to peritoneal space	21.99	15.54	15.54	4.14	41.67	41.67	090	
63180		A	Laminectomy and section of dentate ligaments, with or without dural graft, cervical; one or two segments	18.27	13.04	13.04	3.83	35.14	35.14	090	
63182		A	more than two segments	20.50	13.61	13.61	3.48	37.59	37.59	090	
63185		A	Laminectomy with rhizotomy; one or two segments	15.04	9.70	9.70	2.08	26.82	26.82	090	
63190		A	more than two segments	17.45	11.68	11.68	2.88	32.01	32.01	090	
63191		A	Laminectomy with section of spinal accessory nerve	17.54	10.65	10.65	3.50	31.69	31.69	090	
63194		A	Laminectomy with cordotomy, with section of one spinothalamic tract, one stage; cervical	19.19	13.48	13.48	4.01	36.68	36.68	090	
63195		A	thoracic	18.84	13.02	13.02	3.44	35.30	35.30	090	
63196		A	Laminectomy with cordotomy, with section of both spinothalamic tracts, one stage; cervical	22.30	14.03	14.03	4.66	40.99	40.99	090	
63197		A	thoracic	21.11	13.49	13.49	4.42	39.02	39.02	090	
63198		A	Laminectomy with cordotomy with section of both spinothalamic tracts, two stages within 14 days; cervical	25.38	12.70	12.70	5.31	43.39	43.39	090	
63199		A	thoracic	26.89	14.38	14.38	5.62	46.89	46.89	090	
63200		A	Laminectomy, with release of tethered spinal cord, lumbar	19.18	13.42	13.42	3.61	36.21	36.21	090	
63250		A	Laminectomy for excision or occlusion of arteriovenous malformation of spinal cord; cervical	40.76	23.15	23.15	7.65	71.56	71.56	090	
63251		A	thoracic	41.20	23.51	23.51	7.98	72.69	72.69	090	
63252		A	thoracolumbar	41.19	23.36	23.36	7.75	72.30	72.30	090	

■ RVU not developed by CMS. Gap-filled RVUs developed by Ingenix/CHEG.

Code	M	S	Description	Work Value	Non-Fac PE	Fac PE	Mal-prac-tice	Non-Fac Total	Fac Total	Global	Gap
63265		A	Laminectomy for excision or evacuation of intraspinal lesion other than neoplasm, extradural; cervical	21.56	13.21	13.21	4.29	39.06	39.06	090	
63266		A	thoracic	22.30	13.70	13.70	4.47	40.47	40.47	090	
63267		A	lumbar	17.95	11.48	11.48	3.50	32.93	32.93	090	
63268		A	sacral	18.52	10.97	10.97	3.18	32.67	32.67	090	
63270		A	Laminectomy for excision of intraspinal lesion other than neoplasm, intradural; cervical	26.80	16.10	16.10	5.41	48.31	48.31	090	
63271		A	thoracic	26.92	16.17	16.17	5.56	48.65	48.65	090	
63272		A	lumbar	25.32	15.31	15.31	5.07	45.70	45.70	090	
63273		A	sacral	24.29	14.84	14.84	5.08	44.21	44.21	090	
63275		A	Laminectomy for biopsy/excision of intraspinal neoplasm; extradural, cervical	23.68	14.47	14.47	4.68	42.83	42.83	090	
63276		A	extradural, thoracic	23.45	14.27	14.27	4.63	42.35	42.35	090	
63277		A	extradural, lumbar	20.83	12.99	12.99	4.03	37.85	37.85	090	
63278		A	extradural, sacral	20.56	13.08	13.08	4.02	37.66	37.66	090	
63280		A	intradural, extramedullary, cervical	28.35	16.76	16.76	5.80	50.91	50.91	090	
63281		A	intradural, extramedullary, thoracic	28.05	16.73	16.73	5.67	50.45	50.45	090	
63282		A	intradural, extramedullary, lumbar	26.39	15.79	15.79	5.33	47.51	47.51	090	
63283		A	intradural, sacral	25.00	15.07	15.07	5.12	45.19	45.19	090	
63285		A	intradural, intramedullary, cervical	36.00	20.82	20.82	7.31	64.13	64.13	090	
63286		A	intradural, intramedullary, thoracic	35.63	20.51	20.51	7.07	63.21	63.21	090	
63287		A	intradural, intramedullary, thoracolumbar	36.70	21.03	21.03	7.48	65.21	65.21	090	
63290		A	combined extradural-intradural lesion, any level	37.38	21.58	21.58	7.65	66.61	66.61	090	
63300		A	Vertebral corpectomy (vertebral body resection), partial or complete, for excision of intraspinal lesion, single segment; extradural, cervical	24.43	14.63	14.63	4.78	43.84	43.84	090	
63301		A	extradural, thoracic by transthoracic approach	27.60	15.65	15.65	5.03	48.28	48.28	090	
63302		A	extradural, thoracic by thoracolumbar approach	27.81	16.45	16.45	5.25	49.51	49.51	090	
63303		A	extradural, lumbar or sacral by transperitoneal or retroperitoneal approach	30.50	17.71	17.71	5.21	53.42	53.42	090	
63304		A	intradural, cervical	30.33	17.80	17.80	4.72	52.85	52.85	090	

■ RVU not developed by CMS. Gap-filled RVUs developed by Ingenix/CHEG.

Surgery

Code	M	S	Description	Work Value	Non-Fac PE	Fac PE	Mal-practice	Non-Fac Total	Fac Total	Global	Gap
63305		A	intradural, thoracic by transthoracic approach	32.03	19.24	19.24	5.39	56.66	56.66	090	
63306		A	intradural, thoracic by thoracolumbar approach	32.22	18.19	18.19	2.39	52.80	52.80	090	
63307		A	intradural, lumbar or sacral by transperitoneal or retroperitoneal approach	31.63	17.29	17.29	4.23	53.15	53.15	090	
63308		A	each additional segment (List separately in addition to codes for single segment)	5.25	2.74	2.74	1.01	9.00	9.00	ZZZ	
63600		A	Creation of lesion of spinal cord by stereotactic method, percutaneous, any modality (including stimulation and/or recording)	14.02	6.38	6.38	1.22	21.62	21.62	090	
63610		A	Stereotactic stimulation of spinal cord, percutaneous, separate procedure not followed by other surgery	8.73	3.90	3.90	0.43	13.06	13.06	000	
63615		A	Stereotactic biopsy, aspiration, or excision of lesion, spinal cord	16.28	9.50	9.50	2.85	28.63	28.63	090	
63650		A	Percutaneous implantation of neurostimulator electrode array, epidural	6.74	2.97	2.97	0.48	10.19	10.19	090	
63655		A	Laminectomy for implantation of neurostimulator electrodes, plate/paddle, epidural	10.29	7.26	7.26	1.85	19.40	19.40	090	
63660		A	Revision or removal of spinal neurostimulator electrode percutaneous array(s) or plate/paddle(s)	6.16	3.67	3.67	0.65	10.48	10.48	090	
63685		A	Incision and subcutaneous placement of spinal neurostimulator pulse generator or receiver, direct or inductive coupling	7.04	4.15	4.15	0.96	12.15	12.15	090	
63688		A	Revision or removal of implanted spinal neurostimulator pulse generator or receiver	5.39	3.69	3.69	0.70	9.78	9.78	090	
63700		A	Repair of meningocele; less than 5 cm diameter	16.53	10.47	10.47	2.69	29.69	29.69	090	
63702		A	larger than 5 cm diameter	18.48	9.90	9.90	1.36	29.74	29.74	090	
63704		A	Repair of myelomeningocele; less than 5 cm diameter	21.18	12.37	12.37	3.84	37.39	37.39	090	
63706		A	larger than 5 cm diameter	24.11	13.60	13.60	4.73	42.44	42.44	090	
63707		A	Repair of dural/cerebrospinal fluid leak, not requiring laminectomy	11.26	8.06	8.06	1.96	21.28	21.28	090	
63709		A	Repair of dural/cerebrospinal fluid leak or pseudomeningocele, with laminectomy	14.32	9.79	9.79	2.49	26.60	26.60	090	
63710		A	Dural graft, spinal	14.07	9.54	9.54	2.61	26.22	26.22	090	
63740		A	Creation of shunt, lumbar, subarachnoid-peritoneal, -pleural, or other; including laminectomy	11.36	7.79	7.79	2.15	21.30	21.30	090	

■ RVU not developed by CMS. Gap-filled RVUs developed by Ingenix/CHEG.

Code	M	S	Description	Work Value	Non-Fac PE	Fac PE	Mal-practice	Non-Fac Total	Fac Total	Global	Gap
63741		A	percutaneous, not requiring laminectomy	8.25	4.72	4.72	1.05	14.02	14.02	090	
63744		A	Replacement, irrigation or revision of lumbosubarachnoid shunt	8.10	5.72	5.72	1.51	15.33	15.33	090	
63746		A	Removal of entire lumbosubarachnoid shunt system without replacement	6.43	4.96	4.96	1.15	12.54	12.54	090	
64400		A	Injection, anesthetic agent; trigeminal nerve, any division or branch	1.11	2.70	0.29	0.06	3.87	1.46	000	
64402		A	facial nerve	1.25	4.38	0.45	0.07	5.70	1.77	000	
64405		A	greater occipital nerve	1.32	1.34	0.37	0.08	2.74	1.77	000	
64408		A	vagus nerve	1.41	2.95	0.62	0.09	4.45	2.12	000	
64410		A	phrenic nerve	1.43	3.27	0.35	0.08	4.78	1.86	000	
64412		A	spinal accessory nerve	1.18	2.49	0.37	0.08	3.75	1.63	000	
64413		A	cervical plexus	1.40	2.81	0.34	0.09	4.30	1.83	000	
64415		A	brachial plexus	1.48	2.65	0.32	0.08	4.21	1.88	000	
64417		A	axillary nerve	1.44	3.21	0.38	0.09	4.74	1.91	000	
64418		A	suprascapular nerve	1.32	2.49	0.29	0.07	3.88	1.68	000	
64420		A	intercostal nerve, single	1.18	2.37	0.27	0.07	3.62	1.52	000	
64421		A	intercostal nerves, multiple, regional block	1.68	2.91	0.38	0.10	4.69	2.16	000	
64425		A	ilioinguinal, iliohypogastric nerves	1.75	2.33	0.41	0.11	4.19	2.27	000	
64430		A	pudendal nerve	1.46	2.89	0.47	0.11	4.46	2.04	000	
64435		A	paracervical (uterine) nerve	1.45	2.96	0.60	0.15	4.56	2.20	000	
64445		A	sciatic nerve	1.48	1.60	0.42	0.08	3.16	1.98	000	
64450		A	other peripheral nerve or branch	1.27	1.79	0.33	0.08	3.14	1.68	000	
64470		A	Injection, anesthetic agent and/or steroid, paravertebral facet joint or facet joint nerve; cervical or thoracic, single level	1.85	4.02	0.48	0.12	5.99	2.45	000	
64472		A	cervical or thoracic, each additional level (List separately in addition to code for primary procedure)	1.29	3.90	0.33	0.09	5.28	1.71	ZZZ	
64475		A	lumbar or sacral, single level	1.41	3.82	0.39	0.09	5.32	1.89	000	
64476		A	lumbar or sacral, each additional level (List separately in addition to code for primary procedure)	0.98	3.86	0.26	0.06	4.90	1.30	ZZZ	
64479		A	Injection, anesthetic agent and/or steroid, transforaminal epidural; cervical or thoracic, single level	2.20	4.40	0.64	0.14	6.74	2.98	000	

■ RVU not developed by CMS. Gap-filled RVUs developed by Ingenix/CHEG.

Code	M	S	Description	Work Value	Non-Fac PE	Fac PE	Mal-practice	Non-Fac Total	Fac Total	Global	Gap
64480		A	cervical or thoracic, each additional level (List separately in addition to code for primary procedure)	1.54	4.07	0.50	0.09	5.70	2.13	ZZZ	
64483		A	lumbar or sacral, single level	1.90	4.44	0.56	0.12	6.46	2.58	000	
64484		A	lumbar or sacral, each additional level (List separately in addition to code for primary procedure)	1.33	4.05	0.40	0.08	5.46	1.81	ZZZ	
64505		A	Injection, anesthetic agent; sphenopalatine ganglion	1.36	2.41	0.35	0.08	3.85	1.79	000	
64508		A	carotid sinus (separate procedure)	1.12	2.32	0.48	0.06	3.50	1.66	000	
64510		A	stellate ganglion (cervical sympathetic)	1.22	2.53	0.26	0.07	3.82	1.55	000	
64520		A	lumbar or thoracic (paravertebral sympathetic)	1.35	3.49	0.31	0.08	4.92	1.74	000	
64530		A	celiac plexus, with or without radiologic monitoring	1.58	3.07	0.37	0.09	4.74	2.04	000	
64550		A	Application of surface (transcutaneous) neurostimulator	0.18	0.56	0.07	0.01	0.75	0.26	000	
64553		A	Percutaneous implantation of neurostimulator electrodes; cranial nerve	2.31	4.25	1.33	0.17	6.73	3.81	010	
64555		A	peripheral nerve (excludes sacral nerve)	2.27	2.38	0.77	0.11	4.76	3.15	010	
64560		A	autonomic nerve	2.36	2.30	0.94	0.17	4.83	3.47	010	
64561		A	sacral nerve (transforaminal placement)	6.74	15.28	3.83	0.11	22.13	10.68	010	
64565		A	neuromuscular	1.76	3.41	0.69	0.08	5.25	2.53	010	
64573		A	Incision for implantation of neurostimulator electrodes; cranial nerve	7.50	5.40	5.40	1.48	14.38	14.38	090	
64575		A	peripheral nerve (excludes sacral nerve)	4.35	3.03	3.03	0.37	7.75	7.75	090	
64577		A	autonomic nerve	4.62	3.44	3.44	0.50	8.56	8.56	090	
64580		A	neuromuscular	4.12	3.94	3.94	0.21	8.27	8.27	090	
64581		A	sacral nerve (transforaminal placement)	13.50	6.72	6.72	0.37	20.59	20.59	090	
64585		A	Revision or removal of peripheral neurostimulator electrodes	2.06	2.82	2.20	0.29	5.17	4.55	010	
64590		A	Incision and subcutaneous placement of peripheral neurostimulator pulse generator or receiver, direct or inductive coupling	2.40	2.17	2.17	0.40	4.97	4.97	010	
64595		A	Revision or removal of peripheral neurostimulator pulse generator or receiver	1.73	2.08	2.08	0.22	4.03	4.03	010	
64600		A	Destruction by neurolytic agent, trigeminal nerve; supraorbital, infraorbital, mental, or inferior alveolar branch	3.45	2.98	2.06	0.28	6.71	5.79	010	

■ RVU not developed by CMS. Gap-filled RVUs developed by Ingenix/CHEG.

Code	M	S	Description	Work Value	Non-Fac PE	Fac PE	Mal-practice	Non-Fac Total	Fac Total	Global	Gap
64605		A	second and third division branches at foramen ovale	5.61	3.62	2.90	0.53	9.76	9.04	010	
64610		A	second and third division branches at foramen ovale under radiologic monitoring	7.16	4.18	4.18	1.12	12.46	12.46	010	
64612		A	Chemodenervation of muscle(s); muscle(s) innervated by facial nerve (eg, for blepharospasm, hemifacial spasm)	1.96	3.00	1.65	0.09	5.05	3.70	010	
64613		A	cervical spinal muscle(s) (eg, for spasmodic torticollis)	1.96	1.82	1.48	0.10	3.88	3.54	010	
64614		A	extremity(s) and/or trunk muscle(s) (eg, for dystonia, cerebral palsy, multiple sclerosis)	2.20	3.23	0.82	0.09	5.52	3.11	010	
64620		A	Destruction by neurolytic agent, intercostal nerve	2.84	2.98	0.67	0.17	5.99	3.68	010	
64622		A	Destruction by neurolytic agent, paravertebral facet joint nerve; lumbar or sacral, single level	3.00	4.77	0.74	0.17	7.94	3.91	010	
64623		A	lumbar or sacral, each additional level (List separately in addition to code for primary procedure)	0.99	3.85	0.24	0.06	4.90	1.29	ZZZ	
64626		A	cervical or thoracic, single level	3.28	4.34	0.80	0.22	7.84	4.30	010	
64627		A	cervical or thoracic, each additional level (List separately in addition to code for primary procedure)	1.16	3.74	0.29	0.08	4.98	1.53	ZZZ	
64630		A	Destruction by neurolytic agent; pudendal nerve	3.00	3.66	0.88	0.16	6.82	4.04	010	
64640		A	other peripheral nerve or branch	2.76	3.67	1.72	0.11	6.54	4.59	010	
64680		A	Destruction by neurolytic agent, celiac plexus, with or without radiologic monitoring	2.62	2.89	0.76	0.15	5.66	3.53	010	
64702		A	Neuroplasty; digital, one or both, same digit	4.23	4.05	4.05	0.51	8.79	8.79	090	
64704		A	nerve of hand or foot	4.57	3.23	3.23	0.59	8.39	8.39	090	
64708		A	Neuroplasty, major peripheral nerve, arm or leg; other than specified	6.12	5.19	5.19	0.82	12.13	12.13	090	
64712		A	sciatic nerve	7.75	5.61	5.61	0.54	13.90	13.90	090	
64713		A	brachial plexus	11.00	6.66	6.66	1.01	18.67	18.67	090	
64714		A	lumbar plexus	10.33	4.25	4.25	0.64	15.22	15.22	090	
64716		A	Neuroplasty and/or transposition; cranial nerve (specify)	6.31	5.18	5.18	0.59	12.08	12.08	090	
64718		A	ulnar nerve at elbow	5.99	5.29	5.29	0.87	12.15	12.15	090	
64719		A	ulnar nerve at wrist	4.85	4.78	4.78	0.63	10.26	10.26	090	

Surgery

■ RVU not developed by CMS. Gap-filled RVUs developed by Ingenix/CHEG.

Code	M	S	Description	Work Value	Non-Fac PE	Fac PE	Mal-practice	Non-Fac Total	Fac Total	Global	Gap
64721		A	median nerve at carpal tunnel	4.29	6.59	6.14	0.59	11.47	11.02	090	
64722		A	Decompression; unspecified nerve(s) (specify)	4.70	3.49	3.49	0.32	8.51	8.51	090	
64726		A	plantar digital nerve	4.18	3.14	3.14	0.57	7.89	7.89	090	
64727		A	Internal neurolysis, requiring use of operating microscope (list separately in addition to code for neuroplasty) (Neuroplasty includes external neurolysis)	3.10	1.68	1.68	0.40	5.18	5.18	ZZZ	
64732		A	Transection or avulsion of; supraorbital nerve	4.41	3.69	3.69	0.77	8.87	8.87	090	
64734		A	infraorbital nerve	4.92	3.80	3.80	0.83	9.55	9.55	090	
64736		A	mental nerve	4.60	2.98	2.98	0.71	8.29	8.29	090	
64738		A	inferior alveolar nerve by osteotomy	5.73	3.92	3.92	0.84	10.49	10.49	090	
64740		A	lingual nerve	5.59	4.11	4.11	0.43	10.13	10.13	090	
64742		A	facial nerve, differential or complete	6.22	4.96	4.96	0.69	11.87	11.87	090	
64744		A	greater occipital nerve	5.24	3.94	3.94	0.98	10.16	10.16	090	
64746		A	phrenic nerve	5.93	4.58	4.58	0.75	11.26	11.26	090	
64752		A	vagus nerve (vagotomy), transthoracic	7.06	4.96	4.96	0.83	12.85	12.85	090	
64755		A	vagus nerves limited to proximal stomach (selective proximal vagotomy, proximal gastric vagotomy, parietal cell vagotomy, supra- or highly selective vagotomy)	13.52	6.40	6.40	1.16	21.08	21.08	090	
64760		A	vagus nerve (vagotomy), abdominal	6.96	4.05	4.05	0.51	11.52	11.52	090	
64761		A	pudendal nerve	6.41	3.48	3.48	0.26	10.15	10.15	090	
64763		A	Transection or avulsion of obturator nerve, extrapelvic, with or without adductor tenotomy	6.93	6.21	6.21	0.77	13.91	13.91	090	
64766		A	Transection or avulsion of obturator nerve, intrapelvic, with or without adductor tenotomy	8.67	4.73	4.73	0.99	14.39	14.39	090	
64771		A	Transection or avulsion of other cranial nerve, extradural	7.35	5.44	5.44	1.32	14.11	14.11	090	
64772		A	Transection or avulsion of other spinal nerve, extradural	7.21	4.88	4.88	1.20	13.29	13.29	090	
64774		A	Excision of neuroma; cutaneous nerve, surgically identifiable	5.17	3.92	3.92	0.60	9.69	9.69	090	
64776		A	digital nerve, one or both, same digit	5.12	3.89	3.89	0.63	9.64	9.64	090	
64778		A	digital nerve, each additional digit (List separately in addition to code for primary procedure)	3.11	1.64	1.64	0.38	5.13	5.13	ZZZ	
64782		A	hand or foot, except digital nerve	6.23	3.93	3.93	0.79	10.95	10.95	090	

■ RVU not developed by CMS. Gap-filled RVUs developed by Ingenix/CHEG.

Code	M	S	Description	Work Value	Non-Fac PE	Fac PE	Mal-practice	Non-Fac Total	Fac Total	Global	Gap
64783		A	hand or foot, each additional nerve, except same digit (List separately in addition to code for primary procedure)	3.72	1.95	1.95	0.48	6.15	6.15	ZZZ	
64784		A	major peripheral nerve, except sciatic	9.82	6.99	6.99	1.17	17.98	17.98	090	
64786		A	sciatic nerve	15.46	10.41	10.41	2.22	28.09	28.09	090	
64787		A	Implantation of nerve end into bone or muscle (list separately in addition to neuroma excision)	4.30	2.28	2.28	0.56	7.14	7.14	ZZZ	
64788		A	Excision of neurofibroma or neurolemmoma; cutaneous nerve	4.61	3.50	3.50	0.54	8.65	8.65	090	
64790		A	major peripheral nerve	11.31	7.53	7.53	1.68	20.52	20.52	090	
64792		A	extensive (including malignant type)	14.92	9.13	9.13	1.88	25.93	25.93	090	
64795		A	Biopsy of nerve	3.01	1.81	1.81	0.40	5.22	5.22	000	
64802		A	Sympathectomy, cervical	9.15	5.17	5.17	0.87	15.19	15.19	090	
64804		A	Sympathectomy, cervicothoracic	14.64	6.83	6.83	1.79	23.26	23.26	090	
64809		A	Sympathectomy, thoracolumbar	13.67	6.04	6.04	0.96	20.67	20.67	090	
64818		A	Sympathectomy, lumbar	10.30	5.76	5.76	1.08	17.14	17.14	090	
64820		A	Sympathectomy; digital arteries, each digit	10.37	6.48	6.48	1.17	18.02	18.02	090	
64821		A	radial artery	8.75	7.09	7.09	0.99	16.83	16.83	090	
64822		A	ulnar artery	8.75	7.09	7.09	0.99	16.83	16.83	090	
64823		A	superficial palmar arch	10.37	7.89	7.89	1.17	19.43	19.43	090	
64831		A	Suture of digital nerve, hand or foot; one nerve	9.44	7.44	7.44	1.14	18.02	18.02	090	
64832		A	each additional digital nerve (List separately in addition to code for primary procedure)	5.66	3.11	3.11	0.68	9.45	9.45	ZZZ	
64834		A	Suture of one nerve, hand or foot; common sensory nerve	10.19	7.40	7.40	1.23	18.82	18.82	090	
64835		A	median motor thenar	10.94	8.06	8.06	1.36	20.36	20.36	090	
64836		A	ulnar motor	10.94	7.94	7.94	1.32	20.20	20.20	090	
64837		A	Suture of each additional nerve, hand or foot (List separately in addition to code for primary procedure)	6.26	3.47	3.47	0.80	10.53	10.53	ZZZ	
64840		A	Suture of posterior tibial nerve	13.02	7.79	7.79	0.86	21.67	21.67	090	
64856		A	Suture of major peripheral nerve, arm or leg, except sciatic; including transposition	13.80	9.66	9.66	1.71	25.17	25.17	090	
64857		A	without transposition	14.49	10.21	10.21	1.76	26.46	26.46	090	

■ RVU not developed by CMS. Gap-filled RVUs developed by Ingenix/CHEG.

Code	M	S	Description	Work Value	Non-Fac PE	Fac PE	Mal-prac-tice	Non-Fac Total	Fac Total	Global	Gap
64858		A	Suture of sciatic nerve	16.49	11.04	11.04	2.78	30.31	30.31	090	
64859		A	Suture of each additional major peripheral nerve (List separately in addition to code for primary procedure)	4.26	2.24	2.24	0.50	7.00	7.00	ZZZ	
64861		A	Suture of; brachial plexus	19.24	13.02	13.02	2.45	34.71	34.71	090	
64862		A	lumbar plexus	19.44	12.29	12.29	2.47	34.20	34.20	090	
64864		A	Suture of facial nerve; extracranial	12.55	8.63	8.63	1.13	22.31	22.31	090	
64865		A	infratemporal, with or without grafting	15.24	10.46	10.46	1.37	27.07	27.07	090	
64866		A	Anastomosis; facial-spinal accessory	15.74	9.84	9.84	1.06	26.64	26.64	090	
64868		A	facial-hypoglossal	14.04	9.57	9.57	1.40	25.01	25.01	090	
64870		A	facial-phrenic	15.99	9.65	9.65	1.08	26.72	26.72	090	
64872		A	Suture of nerve; requiring secondary or delayed suture (list separately in addition to code for primary neurorrhaphy)	1.99	1.08	1.08	0.24	3.31	3.31	ZZZ	
64874		A	requiring extensive mobilization, or transposition of nerve (list separately in addition to code for nerve suture)	2.98	1.64	1.64	0.34	4.96	4.96	ZZZ	
64876		A	requiring shortening of bone of extremity (list separately in addition to code for nerve suture)	3.38	1.35	1.35	0.39	5.12	5.12	ZZZ	
64885		A	Nerve graft (includes obtaining graft), head or neck; up to 4 cm in length	17.53	11.66	11.66	1.51	30.70	30.70	090	
64886		A	more than 4 cm in length	20.75	13.60	13.60	1.73	36.08	36.08	090	
64890		A	Nerve graft (includes obtaining graft), single strand, hand or foot; up to 4 cm length	15.15	10.27	10.27	1.74	27.16	27.16	090	
64891		A	more than 4 cm length	16.14	5.75	5.75	1.38	23.27	23.27	090	
64892		A	Nerve graft (includes obtaining graft), single strand, arm or leg; up to 4 cm length	14.65	8.96	8.96	1.65	25.26	25.26	090	
64893		A	more than 4 cm length	15.60	10.75	10.75	1.77	28.12	28.12	090	
64895		A	Nerve graft (includes obtaining graft), multiple strands (cable), hand or foot; up to 4 cm length	19.25	8.62	8.62	2.04	29.91	29.91	090	
64896		A	more than 4 cm length	20.49	11.75	11.75	1.85	34.09	34.09	090	
64897		A	Nerve graft (includes obtaining graft), multiple strands (cable), arm or leg; up to 4 cm length	18.24	10.92	10.92	2.64	31.80	31.80	090	
64898		A	more than 4 cm length	19.50	10.75	10.75	2.71	32.96	32.96	090	
64901		A	Nerve graft, each additional nerve; single strand (List separately in addition to code for primary procedure)	10.22	5.75	5.75	0.99	16.96	16.96	ZZZ	

■ RVU not developed by CMS. Gap-filled RVUs developed by Ingenix/CHEG.

Surgery

Code	M	S	Description	Work Value	Non-Fac PE	Fac PE	Mal-practice	Non-Fac Total	Fac Total	Global	Gap
64902		A	multiple strands (cable) (List separately in addition to code for primary procedure)	11.83	6.32	6.32	1.10	19.25	19.25	ZZZ	
64905		A	Nerve pedicle transfer; first stage	14.02	8.93	8.93	1.52	24.47	24.47	090	
64907		A	second stage	18.83	12.07	12.07	1.79	32.69	32.69	090	
64999		C	Unlisted procedure, nervous system	0.00	0.00	0.00	0.00	0.00	0.00	YYY	
65091		A	Evisceration of ocular contents; without implant	6.46	11.59	11.59	0.26	18.31	18.31	090	
65093		A	with implant	6.87	11.83	11.83	0.28	18.98	18.98	090	
65101		A	Enucleation of eye; without implant	7.03	12.04	12.04	0.28	19.35	19.35	090	
65103		A	with implant, muscles not attached to implant	7.57	12.17	12.17	0.30	20.04	20.04	090	
65105		A	with implant, muscles attached to implant	8.49	12.67	12.67	0.34	21.50	21.50	090	
65110		A	Exenteration of orbit (does not include skin graft), removal of orbital contents; only	13.95	15.90	15.90	0.68	30.53	30.53	090	
65112		A	with therapeutic removal of bone	16.38	17.26	17.26	0.96	34.60	34.60	090	
65114		A	with muscle or myocutaneous flap	17.53	18.54	18.54	0.94	37.01	37.01	090	
65125		A	Modification of ocular implant with placement or replacement of pegs (eg, drilling receptacle for prosthesis appendage) (separate procedure)	3.12	6.23	1.48	0.15	9.50	4.75	090	
65130		A	Insertion of ocular implant secondary; after evisceration, in scleral shell	7.15	11.46	11.46	0.28	18.89	18.89	090	
65135		A	after enucleation, muscles not attached to implant	7.33	12.37	12.37	0.29	19.99	19.99	090	
65140		A	after enucleation, muscles attached to implant	8.02	12.36	12.36	0.31	20.69	20.69	090	
65150		A	Reinsertion of ocular implant; with or without conjunctival graft	6.26	10.94	10.94	0.25	17.45	17.45	090	
65155		A	with use of foreign material for reinforcement and/or attachment of muscles to implant	8.66	12.59	12.59	0.40	21.65	21.65	090	
65175		A	Removal of ocular implant	6.28	11.35	11.35	0.26	17.89	17.89	090	
65205		A	Removal of foreign body, external eye; conjunctival superficial	0.71	0.63	0.20	0.03	1.37	0.94	000	
65210		A	conjunctival embedded (includes concretions), subconjunctival, or scleral nonperforating	0.84	0.78	0.32	0.03	1.65	1.19	000	
65220		A	corneal, without slit lamp	0.71	8.23	0.19	0.05	8.99	0.95	000	
65222		A	corneal, with slit lamp	0.93	0.80	0.29	0.04	1.77	1.26	000	

Surgery

■ RVU not developed by CMS. Gap-filled RVUs developed by Ingenix/CHEG.

Code	M	S	Description	Work Value	Non-Fac PE	Fac PE	Mal-practice	Non-Fac Total	Fac Total	Global	Gap
65235		A	Removal of foreign body, intraocular; from anterior chamber of eye or lens	7.57	7.04	7.04	0.30	14.91	14.91	090	
65260		A	from posterior segment, magnetic extraction, anterior or posterior route	10.96	12.66	12.66	0.43	24.05	24.05	090	
65265		A	from posterior segment, nonmagnetic extraction	12.59	14.38	14.38	0.50	27.47	27.47	090	
65270		A	Repair of laceration; conjunctiva, with or without nonperforating laceration sclera, direct closure	1.90	4.07	2.44	0.08	6.05	4.42	010	
65272		A	conjunctiva, by mobilization and rearrangement, without hospitalization	3.82	5.76	4.75	0.16	9.74	8.73	090	
65273		A	conjunctiva, by mobilization and rearrangement, with hospitalization	4.36	5.15	5.15	0.17	9.68	9.68	090	
65275		A	cornea, nonperforating, with or without removal foreign body	5.34	5.50	5.32	0.27	11.11	10.93	090	
65280		A	cornea and/or sclera, perforating, not involving uveal tissue	7.66	7.88	7.88	0.30	15.84	15.84	090	
65285		A	cornea and/or sclera, perforating, with reposition or resection of uveal tissue	12.90	13.86	13.86	0.51	27.27	27.27	090	
65286		A	application of tissue glue, wounds of cornea and/or sclera	5.51	9.12	7.85	0.21	14.84	13.57	090	
65290		A	Repair of wound, extraocular muscle, tendon and/or Tenon's capsule	5.41	6.60	6.60	0.26	12.27	12.27	090	
65400		A	Excision of lesion, cornea (keratectomy, lamellar, partial), except pterygium	6.06	8.61	7.13	0.24	14.91	13.43	090	
65410		A	Biopsy of cornea	1.47	1.76	0.71	0.06	3.29	2.24	000	
65420		A	Excision or transposition of pterygium; without graft	4.17	8.36	7.22	0.17	12.70	11.56	090	
65426		A	with graft	5.25	8.01	6.75	0.20	13.46	12.20	090	
65430		A	Scraping of cornea, diagnostic, for smear and/or culture	1.47	8.68	0.71	0.06	10.21	2.24	000	
65435		A	Removal of corneal epithelium; with or without chemocauterization (abrasion, curettage)	0.92	1.37	0.41	0.04	2.33	1.37	000	
65436		A	with application of chelating agent (eg, EDTA)	4.19	6.02	5.03	0.17	10.38	9.39	090	
65450		A	Destruction of lesion of cornea by cryotherapy, photocoagulation or thermocauterization	3.27	7.97	6.80	0.13	11.37	10.20	090	
65600		A	Multiple punctures of anterior cornea (eg, for corneal erosion, tattoo)	3.40	5.54	1.54	0.14	9.08	5.08	090	
65710		A	Keratoplasty (corneal transplant); lamellar	12.35	13.25	13.25	0.49	26.09	26.09	090	
65730		A	penetrating (except in aphakia)	14.25	12.16	12.16	0.56	26.97	26.97	090	

■ RVU not developed by CMS. Gap-filled RVUs developed by Ingenix/CHEG.

Code	M	S	Description	Work Value	Non-Fac PE	Fac PE	Mal-practice	Non-Fac Total	Fac Total	Global	Gap
65750		A	penetrating (in aphakia)	15.00	14.54	14.54	0.59	30.13	30.13	090	
65755		A	penetrating (in pseudophakia)	14.89	14.48	14.48	0.58	29.95	29.95	090	
65760		N	Keratomileusis	18.53	14.72	14.72	1.97	35.22	35.22	XXX	■
65765		N	Keratophakia	21.49	17.08	17.08	2.29	40.86	40.86	XXX	■
65767		N	Epikeratoplasty	20.01	15.90	15.90	2.13	38.04	38.04	XXX	■
65770		A	Keratoprosthesis	17.56	15.48	15.48	0.69	33.73	33.73	090	
65771		N	Radial keratotomy	10.89	8.66	8.66	1.16	20.71	20.71	XXX	■
65772		A	Corneal relaxing incision for correction of surgically induced astigmatism	4.29	7.51	6.47	0.17	11.97	10.93	090	
65775		A	Corneal wedge resection for correction of surgically induced astigmatism	5.79	8.63	8.63	0.22	14.64	14.64	090	
65800		A	Paracentesis of anterior chamber of eye (separate procedure); with diagnostic aspiration of aqueous	1.91	2.33	1.45	0.08	4.32	3.44	000	
65805		A	with therapeutic release of aqueous	1.91	2.34	1.46	0.08	4.33	3.45	000	
65810		A	with removal of vitreous and/or discission of anterior hyaloid membrane, with or without air injection	4.87	8.95	8.95	0.19	14.01	14.01	090	
65815		A	with removal of blood, with or without irrigation and/or air injection	5.05	9.40	8.16	0.20	14.65	13.41	090	
65820		A	Goniotomy	8.13	10.99	10.99	0.32	19.44	19.44	090	
65850		A	Trabeculotomy ab externo	10.52	10.35	10.35	0.41	21.28	21.28	090	
65855		A	Trabeculoplasty by laser surgery, one or more sessions (defined treatment series)	3.85	5.17	3.70	0.17	9.19	7.72	010	
65860		A	Severing adhesions of anterior segment, laser technique (separate procedure)	3.55	4.15	3.18	0.14	7.84	6.87	090	
65865		A	Severing adhesions of anterior segment of eye, incisional technique (with or without injection of air or liquid) (separate procedure); goniosynechiae	5.60	6.92	6.92	0.22	12.74	12.74	090	
65870		A	anterior synechiae, except goniosynechiae	6.27	7.25	7.25	0.24	13.76	13.76	090	
65875		A	posterior synechiae	6.54	7.37	7.37	0.25	14.16	14.16	090	
65880		A	corneovitreal adhesions	7.09	7.64	7.64	0.28	15.01	15.01	090	
65900		A	Removal of epithelial downgrowth, anterior chamber of eye	10.93	12.75	12.75	0.46	24.14	24.14	090	
65920		A	Removal of implanted material, anterior segment of eye	8.40	8.26	8.26	0.33	16.99	16.99	090	
65930		A	Removal of blood clot, anterior segment of eye	7.44	8.83	8.83	0.29	16.56	16.56	090	

■ RVU not developed by CMS. Gap-filled RVUs developed by Ingenix/CHEG.

Code	M	S	Description	Work Value	Non-Fac PE	Fac PE	Mal-practice	Non-Fac Total	Fac Total	Global	Gap
66020		A	Injection, anterior chamber of eye (separate procedure); air or liquid	1.59	2.43	1.57	0.07	4.09	3.23	010	
66030		A	medication	1.25	2.25	1.40	0.05	3.55	2.70	010	
66130		A	Excision of lesion, sclera	7.69	7.63	6.71	0.31	15.63	14.71	090	
66150		A	Fistulization of sclera for glaucoma; trephination with iridectomy	8.30	10.98	10.98	0.33	19.61	19.61	090	
66155		A	thermocauterization with iridectomy	8.29	10.94	10.94	0.32	19.55	19.55	090	
66160		A	sclerectomy with punch or scissors, with iridectomy	10.17	11.84	11.84	0.41	22.42	22.42	090	
66165		A	iridencleisis or iridotasis	8.01	10.72	10.72	0.31	19.04	19.04	090	
66170		A	trabeculectomy ab externo in absence of previous surgery	12.16	17.11	17.11	0.48	29.75	29.75	090	
66172		A	trabeculectomy ab externo with scarring from previous ocular surgery or trauma (includes injection of antifibrotic agents)	15.04	15.67	15.67	0.59	31.30	31.30	090	
66180		A	Aqueous shunt to extraocular reservoir (eg, Molteno, Schocket, Denver-Krupin)	14.55	12.44	12.44	0.57	27.56	27.56	090	
66185		A	Revision of aqueous shunt to extraocular reservoir	8.14	8.47	8.47	0.32	16.93	16.93	090	
66220		A	Repair of scleral staphyloma; without graft	7.77	9.99	9.99	0.32	18.08	18.08	090	
66225		A	with graft	11.05	9.65	9.65	0.44	21.14	21.14	090	
66250		A	Revision or repair of operative wound of anterior segment, any type, early or late, major or minor procedure	5.98	8.08	6.48	0.23	14.29	12.69	090	
66500		A	Iridotomy by stab incision (separate procedure); except transfixion	3.71	4.82	4.82	0.15	8.68	8.68	090	
66505		A	with transfixion as for iris bombe	4.08	5.01	5.01	0.17	9.26	9.26	090	
66600		A	Iridectomy, with corneoscleral or corneal section; for removal of lesion	8.68	8.90	8.90	0.34	17.92	17.92	090	
66605		A	with cyclectomy	12.79	12.54	12.54	0.61	25.94	25.94	090	
66625		A	peripheral for glaucoma (separate procedure)	5.13	7.90	6.81	0.20	13.23	12.14	090	
66630		A	sector for glaucoma (separate proedure)	6.16	7.76	7.76	0.24	14.16	14.16	090	
66635		A	optical (separate procedure)	6.25	6.65	6.65	0.24	13.14	13.14	090	
66680		A	Repair of iris, ciliary body (as for iridodialysis)	5.44	6.30	6.30	0.21	11.95	11.95	090	
66682		A	Suture of iris, ciliary body (separate procedure) with retrieval of suture through small incision (eg, McCannel suture)	6.21	7.75	7.75	0.24	14.20	14.20	090	
66700		A	Ciliary body destruction; diathermy	4.78	7.17	7.17	0.19	12.14	12.14	090	

■ RVU not developed by CMS. Gap-filled RVUs developed by Ingenix/CHEG.

Code	M	S	Description	Work Value	Non-Fac PE	Fac PE	Mal-practice	Non-Fac Total	Fac Total	Global	Gap
66710		A	cyclophotocoagulation	4.78	8.92	7.53	0.18	13.88	12.49	090	
66720		A	cryotherapy	4.78	8.40	7.53	0.19	13.37	12.50	090	
66740		A	cyclodialysis	4.78	6.53	6.53	0.18	11.49	11.49	090	
66761		A	Iridotomy/iridectomy by laser surgery (eg, for glaucoma) (one or more sessions)	4.07	5.66	4.38	0.16	9.89	8.61	090	
66762		A	Iridoplasty by photocoagulation (one or more sessions) (eg, for improvement of vision, for widening of anterior chamber angle)	4.58	5.65	4.45	0.18	10.41	9.21	090	
66770		A	Destruction of cyst or lesion iris or ciliary body (nonexcisional procedure)	5.18	5.94	4.68	0.20	11.32	10.06	090	
66820		A	Discission of secondary membranous cataract (opacified posterior lens capsule and/or anterior hyaloid); stab incision technique (Ziegler or Wheeler knife)	3.89	8.50	8.50	0.16	12.55	12.55	090	
66821		A	laser surgery (eg, YAG laser) (one or more stages)	2.35	3.89	3.46	0.10	6.34	5.91	090	
66825		A	Repositioning of intraocular lens prosthesis, requiring an incision (separate procedure)	8.23	10.56	10.56	0.32	19.11	19.11	090	
66830		A	Removal of secondary membranous cataract (opacified posterior lens capsule and/or anterior hyaloid) with corneo-scleral section, with or without iridectomy (iridocapsulotomy, iridocapsulectomy)	8.20	7.06	7.06	0.32	15.58	15.58	090	
66840		A	Removal of lens material; aspiration technique, one or more stages	7.91	6.92	6.92	0.31	15.14	15.14	090	
66850		A	phacofragmentation technique (mechanical or ultrasonic) (eg, phacoemulsification), with aspiration	9.11	7.52	7.52	0.36	16.99	16.99	090	
66852		A	pars plana approach, with or without vitrectomy	9.97	7.99	7.99	0.39	18.35	18.35	090	
66920		A	intracapsular	8.86	7.42	7.42	0.35	16.63	16.63	090	
66930		A	intracapsular, for dislocated lens	10.18	8.94	8.94	0.41	19.53	19.53	090	
66940		A	extracapsular (other than 66840, 66850, 66852)	8.93	8.39	8.39	0.35	17.67	17.67	090	
66982		A	Extracapsular cataract removal with insertion of intraocular lens prosthesis (one stage procedure), manual or mechanical technique (eg, irrigation and aspiration or phacoemulsification), complex, requiring devices or techniques not generally used in routine cataract surgery (eg, iris expansion device, suture support for intraocular lens, or primary posterior capsulorrhexis) or performed on patients in the amblyogenic developmental stage	13.50	9.31	9.31	0.56	23.37	23.37	090	

Surgery

■ RVU not developed by CMS. Gap-filled RVUs developed by Ingenix/CHEG.

Code	M	S	Description	Work Value	Non-Fac PE	Fac PE	Mal-prac-tice	Non-Fac Total	Fac Total	Global	Gap
66983		A	Intracapsular cataract extraction with insertion of intraocular lens prosthesis (one stage procedure)	8.99	6.34	6.34	0.37	15.70	15.70	090	
66984		A	Extracapsular cataract removal with insertion of intraocular lens prosthesis (one stage procedure), manual or mechanical technique (eg, irrigation and aspiration or phacoemulsification)	10.23	7.85	7.85	0.41	18.49	18.49	090	
66985		A	Insertion of intraocular lens prosthesis (secondary implant), not associated with concurrent cataract removal	8.39	7.05	7.05	0.33	15.77	15.77	090	
66986		A	Exchange of intraocular lens	12.28	8.86	8.86	0.49	21.63	21.63	090	
66999		C	Unlisted procedure, anterior segment of eye	0.00	0.00	0.00	0.00	0.00	0.00	YYY	
67005		A	Removal of vitreous, anterior approach (open sky technique or limbal incision); partial removal	5.70	2.75	2.75	0.22	8.67	8.67	090	
67010		A	subtotal removal with mechanical vitrectomy	6.87	3.32	3.32	0.27	10.46	10.46	090	
67015		A	Aspiration or release of vitreous, subretinal or choroidal fluid, pars plana approach (posterior sclerotomy)	6.92	8.38	8.38	0.27	15.57	15.57	090	
67025		A	Injection of vitreous substitute, pars plana or limbal approach, (fluid-gas exchange), with or without aspiration (separate procedure)	6.84	18.23	7.77	0.27	25.34	14.88	090	
67027		A	Implantation of intravitreal drug delivery system (eg, ganciclovir implant), includes concomitant removal of vitreous	10.85	15.12	9.26	0.46	26.43	20.57	090	
67028		A	Intravitreal injection of a pharmacologic agent (separate procedure)	2.52	11.92	1.21	0.11	14.55	3.84	000	
67030		A	Discission of vitreous strands (without removal), pars plana approach	4.84	6.96	6.96	0.19	11.99	11.99	090	
67031		A	Severing of vitreous strands, vitreous face adhesions, sheets, membranes or opacities, laser surgery (one or more stages)	3.67	4.22	3.24	0.15	8.04	7.06	090	
67036		A	Vitrectomy, mechanical, pars plana approach;	11.89	9.30	9.30	0.47	21.66	21.66	090	
67038		A	with epiretinal membrane stripping	21.24	16.01	16.01	0.84	38.09	38.09	090	
67039		A	with focal endolaser photocoagulation	14.52	12.74	12.74	0.57	27.83	27.83	090	
67040		A	with endolaser panretinal photocoagulation	17.23	14.08	14.08	0.68	31.99	31.99	090	
67101		A	Repair of retinal detachment, one or more sessions; cryotherapy or diathermy, with or without drainage of subretinal fluid	7.53	11.29	9.12	0.29	19.11	16.94	090	
67105		A	photocoagulation, with or without drainage of subretinal fluid	7.41	7.80	5.70	0.29	15.50	13.40	090	

■ RVU not developed by CMS. Gap-filled RVUs developed by Ingenix/CHEG.

Code	M	S	Description	Work Value	Non-Fac PE	Fac PE	Mal-practice	Non-Fac Total	Fac Total	Global	Gap
67107		A	Repair of retinal detachment; scleral buckling (such as lamellar scleral dissection, imbrication or encircling procedure), with or without implant, with or without cryotherapy, photocoagulation, and drainage of subretinal fluid	14.84	13.63	13.63	0.58	29.05	29.05	090	
67108		A	with vitrectomy, any method, with or without air or gas tamponade, focal endolaser photocoagulation, cryotherapy, drainage of subretinal fluid, scleral buckling, and/or removal of lens by same technique	20.82	18.30	18.30	0.82	39.94	39.94	090	
67110		A	by injection of air or other gas (eg, pneumatic retinopexy)	8.81	21.74	10.56	0.35	30.90	19.72	090	
67112		A	by scleral buckling or vitrectomy, on patient having previous ipsilateral retinal detachment repair(s) using scleral buckling or vitrectomy techniques	16.86	15.66	15.66	0.66	33.18	33.18	090	
67115		A	Release of encircling material (posterior segment)	4.99	7.02	7.02	0.19	12.20	12.20	090	
67120		A	Removal of implanted material, posterior segment; extraocular	5.98	17.57	7.36	0.23	23.78	13.57	090	
67121		A	intraocular	10.67	12.47	12.47	0.42	23.56	23.56	090	
67141		A	Prophylaxis of retinal detachment (eg, retinal break, lattice degeneration) without drainage, one or more sessions; cryotherapy, diathermy	5.20	8.29	7.16	0.20	13.69	12.56	090	
67145		A	photocoagulation (laser or xenon arc)	5.37	5.43	4.28	0.21	11.01	9.86	090	
67208		A	Destruction of localized lesion of retina (eg, macular edema, tumors), one or more sessions; cryotherapy, diathermy	6.70	8.62	7.26	0.26	15.58	14.22	090	
67210		A	photocoagulation	8.82	7.49	5.93	0.35	16.66	15.10	090	
67218		A	radiation by implantation of source (includes removal of source)	18.53	16.36	16.36	0.53	35.42	35.42	090	
67220		A	Destruction of localized lesion of choroid (eg, choroidal neovascularization); photocoagulation (eg, laser), one or more sessions	13.13	11.18	9.94	0.51	24.82	23.58	090	
67221		A	photodynamic therapy (includes intravenous infusion)	4.01	4.80	1.95	0.16	8.97	6.12	000	
67225		A	photodynamic therapy, second eye, at single session (List separately in addition to code for primary eye treatment)	0.47	0.24	0.19	0.50	1.21	1.16	ZZZ	
67227		A	Destruction of extensive or progressive retinopathy (eg, diabetic retinopathy), one or more sessions; cryotherapy, diathermy	6.58	9.29	7.40	0.26	16.13	14.24	090	
67228		A	photocoagulation (laser or xenon arc)	12.74	10.17	7.47	0.50	23.41	20.71	090	

■ RVU not developed by CMS. Gap-filled RVUs developed by Ingenix/CHEG.

Code	M	S	Description	Work Value	Non-Fac PE	Fac PE	Mal-practice	Non-Fac Total	Fac Total	Global	Gap
67250		A	Scleral reinforcement (separate procedure); without graft	8.66	12.10	12.10	0.36	21.12	21.12	090	
67255		A	with graft	8.90	12.11	12.11	0.35	21.36	21.36	090	
67299		C	Unlisted procedure, posterior segment	0.00	0.00	0.00	0.00	0.00	0.00	YYY	
67311		A	Strabismus surgery, recession or resection procedure; one horizontal muscle	6.65	6.36	6.36	0.27	13.28	13.28	090	
67312		A	two horizontal muscles	8.54	7.46	7.46	0.35	16.35	16.35	090	
67314		A	one vertical muscle (excluding superior oblique)	7.52	6.94	6.94	0.30	14.76	14.76	090	
67316		A	two or more vertical muscles (excluding superior oblique)	9.66	7.99	7.99	0.40	18.05	18.05	090	
67318		A	Strabismus surgery, any procedure, superior oblique muscle	7.85	7.37	7.37	0.31	15.53	15.53	090	
67320		A	Transposition procedure (eg, for paretic extraocular muscle), any extraocular muscle (specify) (List separately in addition to code for primary procedure)	4.33	2.09	2.09	0.17	6.59	6.59	ZZZ	
67331		A	Strabismus surgery on patient with previous eye surgery or injury that did not involve the extraocular muscles (List separately in addition to code for primary procedure)	4.06	2.02	2.02	0.17	6.25	6.25	ZZZ	
67332		A	Strabismus surgery on patient with scarring of extraocular muscles (eg, prior ocular injury, strabismus or retinal detachment surgery) or restrictive myopathy (eg, dysthyroid ophthalmopathy) (List separately in addition to code for primary procedure)	4.49	2.16	2.16	0.18	6.83	6.83	ZZZ	
67334		A	Strabismus surgery by posterior fixation suture technique, with or without muscle recession (List separately in addition to code for primary procedure)	3.98	1.90	1.90	0.16	6.04	6.04	ZZZ	
67335		A	Placement of adjustable suture(s) during strabismus surgery, including postoperative adjustment(s) of suture(s) (List separately in addition to code for specific strabismus surgery)	2.49	1.20	1.20	0.10	3.79	3.79	ZZZ	
67340		A	Strabismus surgery involving exploration and/or repair of detached extraocular muscle(s) (List separately in addition to code for primary procedure)	4.93	2.41	2.41	0.19	7.53	7.53	ZZZ	
67343		A	Release of extensive scar tissue without detaching extraocular muscle (separate procedure)	7.35	7.26	7.26	0.30	14.91	14.91	090	
67345		A	Chemodenervation of extraocular muscle	2.96	4.46	1.36	0.13	7.55	4.45	010	
67350		A	Biopsy of extraocular muscle	2.87	1.99	1.99	0.13	4.99	4.99	000	

■ RVU not developed by CMS. Gap-filled RVUs developed by Ingenix/CHEG.

Code	M	S	Description	Work Value	Non-Fac PE	Fac PE	Mal-prac-tice	Non-Fac Total	Fac Total	Global	Gap
67399		C	Unlisted procedure, ocular muscle	0.00	0.00	0.00	0.00	0.00	0.00	YYY	
67400		A	Orbitotomy without bone flap (frontal or transconjunctival approach); for exploration, with or without biopsy	9.76	13.85	13.85	0.43	24.04	24.04	090	
67405		A	with drainage only	7.93	12.56	12.56	0.36	20.85	20.85	090	
67412		A	with removal of lesion	9.50	16.02	16.02	0.41	25.93	25.93	090	
67413		A	with removal of foreign body	10.00	13.80	13.80	0.43	24.23	24.23	090	
67414		A	with removal of bone for decompression	11.13	16.90	16.90	0.48	28.51	28.51	090	
67415		A	Fine needle aspiration of orbital contents	1.76	0.80	0.80	0.09	2.65	2.65	000	
67420		A	Orbitotomy with bone flap or window, lateral approach (eg, Kroenlein); with removal of lesion	20.06	20.79	20.79	0.84	41.69	41.69	090	
67430		A	with removal of foreign body	13.39	18.38	18.38	0.97	32.74	32.74	090	
67440		A	with drainage	13.09	18.43	18.43	0.58	32.10	32.10	090	
67445		A	with removal of bone for decompression	14.42	18.19	18.19	0.63	33.24	33.24	090	
67450		A	for exploration, with or without biopsy	13.51	17.51	17.51	0.56	31.58	31.58	090	
67500		A	Retrobulbar injection; medication (separate procedure, does not include supply of medication)	0.79	0.95	0.20	0.04	1.78	1.03	000	
67505		A	alcohol	0.82	0.95	0.21	0.04	1.81	1.07	000	
67515		A	Injection of medication or other substance into Tenon's capsule	0.61	0.86	0.29	0.02	1.49	0.92	000	
67550		A	Orbital implant (implant outside muscle cone); insertion	10.19	13.57	13.57	0.50	24.26	24.26	090	
67560		A	removal or revision	10.60	13.50	13.50	0.47	24.57	24.57	090	
67570		A	Optic nerve decompression (eg, incision or fenestration of optic nerve sheath)	13.58	17.66	17.66	0.69	31.93	31.93	090	
67599		C	Unlisted procedure, orbit	0.00	0.00	0.00	0.00	0.00	0.00	YYY	
67700		A	Blepharotomy, drainage of abscess, eyelid	1.35	7.80	0.60	0.06	9.21	2.01	010	
67710		A	Severing of tarsorrhaphy	1.02	7.92	0.49	0.04	8.98	1.55	010	
67715		A	Canthotomy (separate procedure)	1.22	0.59	0.59	0.05	1.86	1.86	010	
67800		A	Excision of chalazion; single	1.38	2.67	0.66	0.06	4.11	2.10	010	
67801		A	multiple, same lid	1.88	8.23	0.91	0.08	10.19	2.87	010	
67805		A	multiple, different lids	2.22	8.41	1.06	0.09	10.72	3.37	010	
67808		A	under general anesthesia and/or requiring hospitalization, single or multiple	3.80	4.34	4.34	0.17	8.31	8.31	090	

Surgery

■ RVU not developed by CMS. Gap-filled RVUs developed by Ingenix/CHEG.

Code	M	S	Description	Work Value	Non-Fac PE	Fac PE	Mal-practice	Non-Fac Total	Fac Total	Global	Gap
67810		A	Biopsy of eyelid	1.48	5.26	0.72	0.06	6.80	2.26	000	
67820		A	Correction of trichiasis; epilation, by forceps only	0.89	2.02	0.39	0.04	2.95	1.32	000	
67825		A	epilation by other than forceps (eg, by electrosurgery, cryotherapy, laser surgery)	1.38	5.70	1.07	0.06	7.14	2.51	010	
67830		A	incision of lid margin	1.70	11.55	2.20	0.07	13.32	3.97	010	
67835		A	incision of lid margin, with free mucous membrane graft	5.56	4.90	4.90	0.22	10.68	10.68	090	
67840		A	Excision of lesion of eyelid (except chalazion) without closure or with simple direct closure	2.04	8.19	0.99	0.08	10.31	3.11	010	
67850		A	Destruction of lesion of lid margin (up to 1 cm)	1.69	8.79	2.07	0.07	10.55	3.83	010	
67875		A	Temporary closure of eyelids by suture (eg, Frost suture)	1.35	11.62	2.16	0.06	13.03	3.57	000	
67880		A	Construction of intermarginal adhesions, median tarsorrhaphy, or canthorrhaphy;	3.80	12.77	3.24	0.16	16.73	7.20	090	
67882		A	with transposition of tarsal plate	5.07	15.42	4.84	0.21	20.70	10.12	090	
67900		A	Repair of brow ptosis (supraciliary, mid-forehead or coronal approach)	6.14	11.29	6.69	0.30	17.73	13.13	090	
67901		A	Repair of blepharoptosis; frontalis muscle technique with suture or other material	6.97	7.22	7.22	0.32	14.51	14.51	090	
67902		A	frontalis muscle technique with fascial sling (includes obtaining fascia)	7.03	7.17	7.17	0.34	14.54	14.54	090	
67903		A	(tarso)levator resection or advancement, internal approach	6.37	10.72	6.80	0.39	17.48	13.56	090	
67904		A	(tarso)levator resection or advancement, external approach	6.26	14.97	8.57	0.26	21.49	15.09	090	
67906		A	superior rectus technique with fascial sling (includes obtaining fascia)	6.79	9.91	6.30	0.42	17.12	13.51	090	
67908		A	conjunctivo-tarso-Muller's muscle-levator resection (eg, Fasanella-Servat type)	5.13	9.65	6.36	0.20	14.98	11.69	090	
67909		A	Reduction of overcorrection of ptosis	5.40	10.20	6.87	0.25	15.85	12.52	090	
67911		A	Correction of lid retraction	5.27	6.92	6.92	0.23	12.42	12.42	090	
67914		A	Repair of ectropion; suture	3.68	13.22	3.70	0.16	17.06	7.54	090	
67915		A	thermocauterization	3.18	11.73	1.52	0.13	15.04	4.83	090	
67916		A	blepharoplasty, excision tarsal wedge	5.31	17.26	5.52	0.22	22.79	11.05	090	
67917		A	blepharoplasty, extensive (eg, Kuhnt-Szymanowski or tarsal strip operations)	6.02	10.63	6.86	0.25	16.90	13.13	090	
67921		A	Repair of entropion; suture	3.40	12.94	3.47	0.14	16.48	7.01	090	

■ RVU not developed by CMS. Gap-filled RVUs developed by Ingenix/CHEG.

Code	M	S	Description	Work Value	Non-Fac PE	Fac PE	Mal-practice	Non-Fac Total	Fac Total	Global	Gap
67922		A	thermocauterization	3.06	11.73	3.31	0.13	14.92	6.50	090	
67923		A	blepharoplasty, excision tarsal wedge	5.88	16.33	5.62	0.24	22.45	11.74	090	
67924		A	blepharoplasty, extensive (eg, Wheeler operation)	5.79	9.97	6.20	0.23	15.99	12.22	090	
67930		A	Suture of recent wound, eyelid, involving lid margin, tarsus, and/or palpebral conjunctiva direct closure; partial thickness	3.61	12.50	3.15	0.17	16.28	6.93	010	
67935		A	full thickness	6.22	16.12	5.60	0.29	22.63	12.11	090	
67938		A	Removal of embedded foreign body, eyelid	1.33	9.65	0.53	0.06	11.04	1.92	010	
67950		A	Canthoplasty (reconstruction of canthus)	5.82	9.01	7.67	0.30	15.13	13.79	090	
67961		A	Excision and repair of eyelid, involving lid margin, tarsus, conjunctiva, canthus, or full thickness, may include preparation for skin graft or pedicle flap with adjacent tissue transfer or rearrangement; up to one-fourth of lid margin	5.69	9.39	6.03	0.26	15.34	11.98	090	
67966		A	over one-fourth of lid margin	6.57	9.01	6.25	0.33	15.91	13.15	090	
67971		A	Reconstruction of eyelid, full thickness by transfer of tarsoconjunctival flap from opposing eyelid; up to two-thirds of eyelid, one stage or first stage	9.79	7.85	7.85	0.42	18.06	18.06	090	
67973		A	total eyelid, lower, one stage or first stage	12.87	9.95	9.95	0.59	23.41	23.41	090	
67974		A	total eyelid, upper, one stage or first stage	12.84	9.87	9.87	0.54	23.25	23.25	090	
67975		A	second stage	9.13	7.51	7.51	0.38	17.02	17.02	090	
67999		C	Unlisted procedure, eyelids	0.00	0.00	0.00	0.00	0.00	0.00	YYY	
68020		A	Incision of conjunctiva, drainage of cyst	1.37	7.79	0.65	0.06	9.22	2.08	010	
68040		A	Expression of conjunctival follicles, eg, for trachoma	0.85	7.68	0.41	0.03	8.56	1.29	000	
68100		A	Biopsy of conjunctiva	1.35	7.93	0.65	0.06	9.34	2.06	000	
68110		A	Excision of lesion, conjunctiva; up to 1 cm	1.77	8.98	1.41	0.07	10.82	3.25	010	
68115		A	over 1 cm	2.36	8.47	1.14	0.10	10.93	3.60	010	
68130		A	with adjacent sclera	4.93	2.38	2.38	0.19	7.50	7.50	090	
68135		A	Destruction of lesion, conjunctiva	1.84	8.23	0.89	0.07	10.14	2.80	010	
68200		A	Subconjunctival injection	0.49	0.76	0.24	0.02	1.27	0.75	000	
68320		A	Conjunctivoplasty; with conjunctival graft or extensive rearrangement	5.37	5.75	5.34	0.21	11.33	10.92	090	
68325		A	with buccal mucous membrane graft (includes obtaining graft)	7.36	6.33	6.33	0.30	13.99	13.99	090	

■ RVU not developed by CMS. Gap-filled RVUs developed by Ingenix/CHEG.

Code	M	S	Description	Work Value	Non-Fac PE	Fac PE	Mal-practice	Non-Fac Total	Fac Total	Global	Gap
68326		A	Conjunctivoplasty, reconstruction cul-de-sac; with conjunctival graft or extensive rearrangement	7.15	6.26	6.26	0.30	13.71	13.71	090	
68328		A	with buccal mucous membrane graft (includes obtaining graft)	8.18	7.07	7.07	0.40	15.65	15.65	090	
68330		A	Repair of symblepharon; conjunctivoplasty, without graft	4.83	7.34	5.82	0.19	12.36	10.84	090	
68335		A	with free graft conjunctiva or buccal mucous membrane (includes obtaining graft)	7.19	5.68	5.68	0.29	13.16	13.16	090	
68340		A	division of symblepharon, with or without insertion of conformer or contact lens	4.17	15.87	4.33	0.17	20.21	8.67	090	
68360		A	Conjunctival flap; bridge or partial (separate procedure)	4.37	6.77	5.42	0.17	11.31	9.96	090	
68362		A	total (such as Gunderson thin flap or purse string flap)	7.34	8.02	8.02	0.29	15.65	15.65	090	
68399		C	Unlisted procedure, conjunctiva	0.00	0.00	0.00	0.00	0.00	0.00	YYY	
68400		A	Incision, drainage of lacrimal gland	1.69	11.48	2.18	0.07	13.24	3.94	10	
68420		A	Incision, drainage of lacrimal sac (dacryocystotomy or dacryocystostomy)	2.30	11.89	2.52	0.10	14.29	4.92	010	
68440		A	Snip incision of lacrimal punctum	0.94	7.86	0.45	0.04	8.84	1.43	010	
68500		A	Excision of lacrimal gland (dacryoadenectomy), except for tumor; total	11.02	9.13	9.13	0.60	20.75	20.75	090	
68505		A	partial	10.94	10.31	10.31	0.57	21.82	21.82	090	
68510		A	Biopsy of lacrimal gland	4.61	13.09	2.22	0.19	17.89	7.02	000	
68520		A	Excision of lacrimal sac (dacryocystectomy)	7.51	7.47	7.47	0.33	15.31	15.31	090	
68525		A	Biopsy of lacrimal sac	4.43	2.15	2.15	0.18	6.76	6.76	000	
68530		A	Removal of foreign body or dacryolith, lacrimal passages	3.66	15.33	3.18	0.16	19.15	7.00	010	
68540		A	Excision of lacrimal gland tumor; frontal approach	10.60	9.73	9.73	0.46	20.79	20.79	090	
68550		A	involving osteotomy	13.26	10.50	10.50	0.66	24.42	24.42	090	
68700		A	Plastic repair of canaliculi	6.60	6.87	6.87	0.27	13.74	13.74	090	
68705		A	Correction of everted punctum, cautery	2.06	8.33	1.00	0.08	10.47	3.14	010	
68720		A	Dacryocystorhinostomy (fistulization of lacrimal sac to nasal cavity)	8.96	8.04	8.04	0.38	17.38	17.38	090	
68745		A	Conjunctivorhinostomy (fistulization of conjunctiva to nasal cavity); without tube	8.63	7.82	7.82	0.38	16.83	16.83	090	
68750		A	with insertion of tube or stent	8.66	8.46	8.46	0.37	17.49	17.49	090	

■ RVU not developed by CMS. Gap-filled RVUs developed by Ingenix/CHEG.

Code	M	S	Description	Work Value	Non-Fac PE	Fac PE	Mal-practice	Non-Fac Total	Fac Total	Global	Gap
68760		A	Closure of the lacrimal punctum; by thermocauterization, ligation, or laser surgery	1.73	6.77	1.25	0.07	8.57	3.05	010	
68761		A	by plug, each	1.36	3.09	1.03	0.06	4.51	2.45	010	
68770		A	Closure of lacrimal fistula (separate procedure)	7.02	17.74	6.15	0.28	25.04	13.45	090	
68801		A	Dilation of lacrimal punctum, with or without irrigation	0.94	0.88	0.57	0.04	1.86	1.55	010	
68810		A	Probing of nasolacrimal duct, with or without irrigation;	1.90	2.48	0.91	0.08	4.46	2.89	010	
68811		A	requiring general anesthesia	2.35	2.46	2.46	0.10	4.91	4.91	010	
68815		A	with insertion of tube or stent	3.20	14.08	2.92	0.14	17.42	6.26	010	
68840		A	Probing of lacrimal canaliculi, with or without irrigation	1.25	1.62	1.00	0.05	2.92	2.30	010	
68850		A	Injection of contrast medium for dacryocystography	0.80	15.29	0.32	0.03	16.12	1.15	000	
68899		C	Unlisted procedure, lacrimal system	0.00	0.00	0.00	0.00	0.00	0.00	YYY	
69000		A	Drainage external ear, abscess or hematoma; simple	1.45	2.14	0.59	0.10	3.69	2.14	010	
69005		A	complicated	2.11	2.55	2.11	0.16	4.82	4.38	010	
69020		A	Drainage external auditory canal, abscess	1.48	2.25	0.71	0.11	3.84	2.30	010	
69090		N	Ear piercing	0.34	0.27	0.27	0.04	0.64	0.64	XXX	■
69100		A	Biopsy external ear	0.81	1.44	0.41	0.04	2.29	1.26	000	
69105		A	Biopsy external auditory canal	0.85	1.51	1.02	0.06	2.42	1.93	000	
69110		A	Excision external ear; partial, simple repair	3.44	3.48	2.85	0.24	7.16	6.53	090	
69120		A	complete amputation	4.05	4.68	4.68	0.31	9.04	9.04	090	
69140		A	Excision exostosis(es), external auditory canal	7.97	8.24	8.24	0.56	16.77	16.77	090	
69145		A	Excision soft tissue lesion, external auditory canal	2.62	3.41	2.54	0.18	6.21	5.34	090	
69150		A	Radical excision external auditory canal lesion; without neck dissection	13.43	11.38	11.38	1.07	25.88	25.88	090	
69155		A	with neck dissection	20.80	16.26	16.26	1.51	38.57	38.57	090	
69200		A	Removal foreign body from external auditory canal; without general anesthesia	0.77	1.45	0.77	0.05	2.27	1.59	000	
69205		A	with general anesthesia	1.20	1.58	1.58	0.09	2.87	2.87	010	
69210		A	Removal impacted cerumen (separate procedure), one or both ears	0.61	0.59	0.25	0.04	1.24	0.90	000	

Surgery

■ RVU not developed by CMS. Gap-filled RVUs developed by Ingenix/CHEG.

Code	M	S	Description	Work Value	Non-Fac PE	Fac PE	Mal-practice	Non-Fac Total	Fac Total	Global	Gap
69220		A	Debridement, mastoidectomy cavity, simple (eg, routine cleaning)	0.83	1.53	0.44	0.06	2.42	1.33	000	
69222		A	Debridement, mastoidectomy cavity, complex (eg, with anesthesia or more than routine cleaning)	1.40	2.24	1.71	0.10	3.74	3.21	010	
69300		R	Otoplasty, protruding ear, with or without size reduction	6.36	4.38	4.38	0.43	11.17	11.17	YYY	
69310		A	Reconstruction of external auditory canal (meatoplasty) (eg, for stenosis due to injury, infection) (separate procedure)	10.79	9.86	9.86	0.77	21.42	21.42	090	
69320		A	Reconstruction external auditory canal for congenital atresia, single stage	16.96	13.77	13.77	1.17	31.90	31.90	090	
69399		C	Unlisted procedure, external ear	0.00	0.00	0.00	0.00	0.00	0.00	YYY	
69400		A	Eustachian tube inflation, transnasal; with catheterization	0.83	1.51	0.49	0.06	2.40	1.38	000	
69401		A	without catheterization	0.63	1.41	0.34	0.04	2.08	1.01	000	
69405		A	Eustachian tube catheterization, transtympanic	2.63	3.09	1.50	0.18	5.90	4.31	010	
69410		A	Focal application of phase control substance, middle ear (baffle technique)	0.33	1.39	0.17	0.02	1.74	0.52	000	
69420		A	Myringotomy including aspiration and/or eustachian tube inflation	1.33	2.35	0.75	0.10	3.78	2.18	010	
69421		A	Myringotomy including aspiration and/or eustachian tube inflation requiring general anesthesia	1.73	2.58	1.92	0.13	4.44	3.78	010	
69424		A	Ventilating tube removal when originally inserted by another physician	0.85	1.68	0.94	0.06	2.59	1.85	000	
69433		A	Tympanostomy (requiring insertion of ventilating tube), local or topical anesthesia	1.52	2.32	0.88	0.11	3.95	2.51	010	
69436		A	Tympanostomy (requiring insertion of ventilating tube), general anesthesia	1.96	2.05	2.05	0.14	4.15	4.15	010	
69440		A	Middle ear exploration through postauricular or ear canal incision	7.57	7.41	7.41	0.53	15.51	15.51	090	
69450		A	Tympanolysis, transcanal	5.57	6.18	6.18	0.39	12.14	12.14	090	
69501		A	Transmastoid antrotomy (simple mastoidectomy)	9.07	8.22	8.22	0.65	17.94	17.94	090	
69502		A	Mastoidectomy; complete	12.38	10.80	10.80	0.86	24.04	24.04	090	
69505		A	modified radical	12.99	10.94	10.94	0.92	24.85	24.85	090	
69511		A	radical	13.52	11.45	11.45	0.96	25.93	25.93	090	
69530		A	Petrous apicectomy including radical mastoidectomy	19.19	15.06	15.06	1.32	35.57	35.57	090	

■ RVU not developed by CMS. Gap-filled RVUs developed by Ingenix/CHEG.

Code	M	S	Description	Work Value	Non-Fac PE	Fac PE	Mal-prac-tice	Non-Fac Total	Fac Total	Global	Gap
69535		A	Resection temporal bone, external approach	36.14	25.13	25.13	2.59	63.86	63.86	090	
69540		A	Excision aural polyp	1.20	2.27	1.61	0.09	3.56	2.90	010	
69550		A	Excision aural glomus tumor; transcanal	10.99	9.97	9.97	0.80	21.76	21.76	090	
69552		A	transmastoid	19.46	14.81	14.81	1.36	35.63	35.63	090	
69554		A	extended (extratemporal)	33.16	21.79	21.79	2.32	57.27	57.27	090	
69601		A	Revision mastoidectomy; resulting in complete mastoidectomy	13.24	11.97	11.97	0.92	26.13	26.13	090	
69602		A	resulting in modified radical mastoidectomy	13.58	11.55	11.55	0.94	26.07	26.07	090	
69603		A	resulting in radical mastoidectomy	14.02	11.80	11.80	1.00	26.82	26.82	090	
69604		A	resulting in tympanoplasty	14.02	11.76	11.76	0.98	26.76	26.76	090	
69605		A	with apicectomy	18.49	14.37	14.37	1.29	34.15	34.15	090	
69610		A	Tympanic membrane repair, with or without site preparation or perforation for closure, with or without patch	4.43	4.27	3.47	0.31	9.01	8.21	010	
69620		A	Myringoplasty (surgery confined to drumhead and donor area)	5.89	6.90	3.40	0.40	13.19	9.69	090	
69631		A	Tympanoplasty without mastoidectomy (including canalplasty, atticotomy and/or middle ear surgery), initial or revision; without ossicular chain reconstruction	9.86	9.38	9.38	0.69	19.93	19.93	090	
69632		A	with ossicular chain reconstruction (eg, postfenestration)	12.75	11.73	11.73	0.89	25.37	25.37	090	
69633		A	with ossicular chain reconstruction and synthetic prosthesis (eg, partial ossicular replacement prosthesis, (PORP), total ossicular replacement prosthesis (TORP))	12.10	11.36	11.36	0.84	24.30	24.30	090	
69635		A	Tympanoplasty with antrotomy or mastoidotomy (including canalplasty, atticotomy, middle ear surgery, and/or tympanic membrane repair); without ossicular chain reconstruction	13.33	11.41	11.41	0.87	25.61	25.61	090	
69636		A	with ossicular chain reconstruction	15.22	13.23	13.23	1.07	29.52	29.52	090	
69637		A	with ossicular chain reconstruction and synthetic prosthesis (eg, partial ossicular replacement prosthesis, (PORP), total ossicular replacement prosthesis (TORP))	15.11	13.16	13.16	1.06	29.33	29.33	090	
69641		A	Tympanoplasty with mastoidectomy (including canalplasty, middle ear surgery, tympanic membrane repair); without ossicular chain reconstruction	12.71	11.06	11.06	0.89	24.66	24.66	090	
69642		A	with ossicular chain reconstruction	16.84	14.16	14.16	1.18	32.18	32.18	090	

Surgery

■ RVU not developed by CMS. Gap-filled RVUs developed by Ingenix/CHEG.

Code	M	S	Description	Work Value	Non-Fac PE	Fac PE	Mal-practice	Non-Fac Total	Fac Total	Global	Gap
69643		A	with intact or reconstructed wall, without ossicular chain reconstruction	15.32	13.24	13.24	1.08	29.64	29.64	090	
69644		A	with intact or reconstructed canal wall, with ossicular chain reconstruction	16.97	14.22	14.22	1.19	32.38	32.38	090	
69645		A	radical or complete, without ossicular chain reconstruction	16.38	13.77	13.77	1.16	31.31	31.31	090	
69646		A	radical or complete, with ossicular chain reconstruction	17.99	14.83	14.83	1.26	34.08	34.08	090	
69650		A	Stapes mobilization	9.66	8.53	8.53	0.68	18.87	18.87	090	
69660		A	Stapedectomy or stapedotomy with reestablishment of ossicular continuity, with or without use of foreign material;	11.90	9.86	9.86	0.84	22.60	22.60	090	
69661		A	with footplate drill out	15.74	12.63	12.63	1.10	29.47	29.47	090	
69662		A	Revision of stapedectomy or stapedotomy	15.44	12.56	12.56	1.08	29.08	29.08	090	
69666		A	Repair oval window fistula	9.75	8.65	8.65	0.68	19.08	19.08	090	
69667		A	Repair round window fistula	9.76	8.58	8.58	0.72	19.06	19.06	090	
69670		A	Mastoid obliteration (separate procedure)	11.51	10.36	10.36	0.78	22.65	22.65	090	
69676		A	Tympanic neurectomy	9.52	9.14	9.14	0.69	19.35	19.35	090	
69700		A	Closure postauricular fistula, mastoid (separate procedure)	8.23	5.77	5.77	0.55	14.55	14.55	090	
69710		N	Implantation or replacement of electromagnetic bone conduction hearing device in temporal bone	0.00	0.00	0.00	0.00	0.00	0.00	XXX	
69711		A	Removal or repair of electromagnetic bone conduction hearing device in temporal bone	10.44	9.62	9.62	0.62	20.68	20.68	090	
69714		A	Implantation, osseointegrated implant, temporal bone, with percutaneous attachment to external speech processor/cochlear stimulator; without mastoidectomy	14.00	11.53	11.53	1.01	26.54	26.54	090	
69715		A	with mastoidectomy	18.25	14.05	14.05	1.32	33.62	33.62	090	
69717		A	Replacement (including removal of existing device), osseointegrated implant, temporal bone, with percutaneous attachment to external speech processor/cochlear stimulator; without mastoidectomy	14.98	11.46	11.46	1.08	27.52	27.52	090	
69718		A	with mastoidectomy	18.50	14.20	14.20	1.34	34.04	34.04	090	
69720		A	Decompression facial nerve, intratemporal; lateral to geniculate ganglion	14.38	12.85	12.85	1.03	28.26	28.26	090	
69725		A	including medial to geniculate ganglion	25.38	17.97	17.97	1.78	45.13	45.13	090	

■ RVU not developed by CMS. Gap-filled RVUs developed by Ingenix/CHEG.

Code	M	S	Description	Work Value	Non-Fac PE	Fac PE	Mal-practice	Non-Fac Total	Fac Total	Global	Gap
69740		A	Suture facial nerve, intratemporal, with or without graft or decompression; lateral to geniculate ganglion	15.96	10.90	10.90	1.13	27.99	27.99	090	
69745		A	including medial to geniculate ganglion	16.69	12.80	12.80	1.00	30.49	30.49	090	
69799		C	Unlisted procedure, middle ear	0.00	0.00	0.00	0.00	0.00	0.00	YYY	
69801		A	Labyrinthotomy, with or without cryosurgery including other nonexcisional destructive procedures or perfusion of vestibuloactive drugs (single or multiple perfusions); transcanal	8.56	7.96	7.96	0.60	17.12	17.12	090	
69802		A	with mastoidectomy	13.10	11.37	11.37	0.91	25.38	25.38	090	
69805		A	Endolymphatic sac operation; without shunt	13.82	10.91	10.91	0.97	25.70	25.70	090	
69806		A	with shunt	12.35	10.82	10.82	0.86	24.03	24.03	090	
69820		A	Fenestration semicircular canal	10.34	8.78	8.78	0.66	19.78	19.78	090	
69840		A	Revision fenestration operation	10.26	9.00	9.00	0.64	19.90	19.90	090	
69905		A	Labyrinthectomy; transcanal	11.10	9.94	9.94	0.77	21.81	21.81	090	
69910		A	with mastoidectomy	13.63	11.42	11.42	0.94	25.99	25.99	090	
69915		A	Vestibular nerve section, translabyrinthine approach	21.23	15.88	15.88	1.54	38.65	38.65	090	
69930		A	Cochlear device implantation, with or without mastoidectomy	16.81	12.94	12.94	1.19	30.94	30.94	090	
69949		C	Unlisted procedure, inner ear	0.00	0.00	0.00	0.00	0.00	0.00	YYY	
69950		A	Vestibular nerve section, transcranial approach	25.64	16.71	16.71	2.90	45.25	45.25	090	
69955		A	Total facial nerve decompression and/or repair (may include graft)	27.04	18.39	18.39	1.89	47.32	47.32	090	
69960		A	Decompression internal auditory canal	27.04	18.40	18.40	2.43	47.87	47.87	090	
69970		A	Removal of tumor, temporal bone	30.04	19.12	19.12	2.34	51.50	51.50	090	
69979		C	Unlisted procedure, temporal bone, middle fossa approach	0.00	0.00	0.00	0.00	0.00	0.00	YYY	
69990		R	Microsurgical techniques, requiring use of operating microscope (List separately in addition to code for primary procedure)	3.47	1.87	1.87	0.56	5.90	5.90	ZZZ	

■ RVU not developed by CMS. Gap-filled RVUs developed by Ingenix/CHEG.

Radiology

The Introduction provides complete descriptions for the status column (abbreviated as S). If a relative value is not available for a procedure, it is indicated with a "0.00" in the individual units column.

I. **General:** Listed values for radiology procedures apply only when these services are performed by or under the supervision of a physician.

A. **Total:** When no modifier is listed, the unit value represents the global value of the procedure. The five-digit code is used to represent a global service inclusive of the professional services and technical value of providing that service. The following sections, professional and technical, provide additional definitions for each component.

B. **Professional:** The unit value listed next to the modifier column (modifier -26) is used to designate professional services. Modifier -26 is added to the procedure code to indicate the use of this value. The professional component includes examination of the patient, when indicated; performance and/or supervision of the procedure; interpretation and written report of the examination; and consultation with referring physicians.

C. **Technical:** The unit value listed next to the modifier column (modifier -TC) is used to designate the technical value of providing the service. Modifier -TC may be used to designate this component. The technical component includes personnel, materials, space, equipment, and other allocated facility overhead normally included in providing the service. **Note:** Modifier -TC is not CPT compatible and may not be accepted by all payers. Check with the specific payer prior to use of this modifier. -TC is accepted by Medicare.

II. **Supervision and Interpretation Only:** A code designated as "supervision and interpretation only" is used to indicate the radiological component of a service that has both a radiological and procedural component (e.g., injection, insertion of catheter, etc.). These two-component services may be performed by a single physician or two physicians, usually a radiologist and another physician (e.g., surgeon, cadiologist, urologist, etc.). When both components of the service are performed by a single physician, current CPT guidelines require the physician to report both the radiological supervision and interpretation component (70000 series code) and the procedural component (surgical or medicine code). When the procedure is performed by two physicians, each physician reports only the component provided, either the radiological supervision and interpretation component or the procedural component.

III. **Unlisted Services or Procedure:** A service or procedure that is not identified by a particular code should be listed under the appropriate "Unlisted Procedure." These procedures have "9" as the final digit. Values should be substantiated by report. *See "By Report."*

IV. **Unusual Procedural Services:** When a procedure of unusual nature is performed, modifier -22 should be added and value substantiated by report. *See "By Report."*

V. **By Report:** Value of a procedure should be established for any by report circumstance by identifying a similar service and justifying value difference. Procedures which require a report should include the following:

A. Accurate definition

B. Clinical history

C. Related procedure values

D. Reason for value adjustment

VI. Portable X-Ray: Use code Q0092 to indicate set-up of portable x-ray. Medicare will increase payment by 0.31.

VII. Separate or Multiple Procedures: Multiple procedures performed on the same date should be listed separately. Medicare allows 100 percent for each code between 70000–79999 billed on the same date. Codes falling in the 10000 - 69990 series are subject to the surgical guidelines, regardless of physician specialty.

VIII. Reduced Services: If a physician elects to reduce the value of a procedure, modifier -52 should be added to the procedure code. For example, modifier -52 and the appropriate code may be used to indicate a limited or follow-up CT scan.

IX. Services or Procedures Listed in Other Sections: Services or procedures provided by a radiologist may be listed in another section of the book (e.g., consultations listed in Evaluation and Management). The radiologist should use the procedure codes following the guidelines appropriate to that section.

X. Modifiers: A listing of CPT modifiers is provided in the Introduction.

XI. Global Values: This column indicates the number of days in the global period for which services directly related to the procedure are included. The majority of codes have a numerical designation (i.e., 0, 10, or 90).

A. MMM codes describe services furnished in uncomplicated maternity care. This includes antepartum, delivery, and postpartum care. The usual global surgical concept does not apply.

B. XXX codes indicate that the global surgery concept does not apply.

C. YYY codes indicate that the global period is to be set by the local carrier.

D. ZZZ codes indicate that the code is an add-on service and therefore is treated in the global period of the other procedure billed in conjunction with a ZZZ code. Do not bill these codes with modifier -51. They should not be reduced.

Radiology Values

Code	M	S	Description	Work Value	Non-Fac PE	Fac PE	Mal-practice	Non-Fac Total	Fac Total	Global	Gap
70010		A	Myelography, posterior fossa, radiological supervision and interpretation	1.19	4.53	4.53	0.24	5.96	5.96	XXX	
	26	A		1.19	0.42	0.42	0.06	1.67	1.67	XXX	
	TC	A		0.00	4.11	4.11	0.18	4.29	4.29	XXX	
70015		A	Cisternography, positive contrast, radiological supervision and interpretation	1.19	1.71	1.71	0.12	3.02	3.02	XXX	
	26	A		1.19	0.42	0.42	0.05	1.66	1.66	XXX	
	TC	A		0.00	1.29	1.29	0.07	1.36	1.36	XXX	
70030		A	Radiologic examination, eye, for detection of foreign body	0.17	0.45	0.45	0.03	0.65	0.65	XXX	
	26	A		0.17	0.06	0.06	0.01	0.24	0.24	XXX	
	TC	A		0.00	0.39	0.39	0.02	0.41	0.41	XXX	
70100		A	Radiologic examination, mandible; partial, less than four views	0.18	0.56	0.56	0.03	0.77	0.77	XXX	
	26	A		0.18	0.06	0.06	0.01	0.25	0.25	XXX	
	TC	A		0.00	0.50	0.50	0.02	0.52	0.52	XXX	
70110		A	complete, minimum of four views	0.25	0.68	0.68	0.04	0.97	0.97	XXX	
	26	A		0.25	0.09	0.09	0.01	0.35	0.35	XXX	
	TC	A		0.00	0.59	0.59	0.03	0.62	0.62	XXX	
70120		A	Radiologic examination, mastoids; less than three views per side	0.18	0.65	0.65	0.04	0.87	0.87	XXX	
	26	A		0.18	0.06	0.06	0.01	0.25	0.25	XXX	
	TC	A		0.00	0.59	0.59	0.03	0.62	0.62	XXX	
70130		A	complete, minimum of three views per side	0.34	0.86	0.86	0.05	1.25	1.25	XXX	
	26	A		0.34	0.12	0.12	0.01	0.47	0.47	XXX	
	TC	A		0.00	0.74	0.74	0.04	0.78	0.78	XXX	
70134		A	Radiologic examination, internal auditory meati, complete	0.34	0.82	0.82	0.05	1.21	1.21	XXX	
	26	A		0.34	0.12	0.12	0.01	0.47	0.47	XXX	
	TC	A		0.00	0.70	0.70	0.04	0.74	0.74	XXX	
70140		A	Radiologic examination, facial bones; less than three views	0.19	0.66	0.66	0.04	0.89	0.89	XXX	
	26	A		0.19	0.07	0.07	0.01	0.27	0.27	XXX	
	TC	A		0.00	0.59	0.59	0.03	0.62	0.62	XXX	
70150		A	complete, minimum of three views	0.26	0.83	0.83	0.05	1.14	1.14	XXX	
	26	A		0.26	0.09	0.09	0.01	0.36	0.36	XXX	
	TC	A		0.00	0.74	0.74	0.04	0.78	0.78	XXX	
70160		A	Radiologic examination, nasal bones, complete, minimum of three views	0.17	0.56	0.56	0.03	0.76	0.76	XXX	
	26	A		0.17	0.06	0.06	0.01	0.24	0.24	XXX	
	TC	A		0.00	0.50	0.50	0.02	0.52	0.52	XXX	
70170		A	Dacryocystography, nasolacrimal duct, radiological supervision and interpretation	0.30	1.01	1.01	0.06	1.37	1.37	XXX	
	26	A		0.30	0.11	0.11	0.01	0.42	0.42	XXX	
	TC	A		0.00	0.90	0.90	0.05	0.95	0.95	XXX	
70190		A	Radiologic examination; optic foramina	0.21	0.66	0.66	0.04	0.91	0.91	XXX	
	26	A		0.21	0.07	0.07	0.01	0.29	0.29	XXX	
	TC	A		0.00	0.59	0.59	0.03	0.62	0.62	XXX	
70200		A	orbits, complete, minimum of four views	0.28	0.84	0.84	0.05	1.17	1.17	XXX	
	26	A		0.28	0.10	0.10	0.01	0.39	0.39	XXX	
	TC	A		0.00	0.74	0.74	0.04	0.78	0.78	XXX	

Radiology

■ RVU not developed by CMS. Gap-filled RVUs developed by CHEG.

Code	M	S	Description	Work Value	Non-Fac PE	Fac PE	Mal-prac-tice	Non-Fac Total	Fac Total	Global	Gap
70210		A	Radiologic examination, sinuses, paranasal, less than three views	0.17	0.65	0.65	0.04	0.86	0.86	XXX	
	26	A		0.17	0.06	0.06	0.01	0.24	0.24	XXX	
	TC	A		0.00	0.59	0.59	0.03	0.62	0.62	XXX	
70220		A	Radiologic examination, sinuses, paranasal, complete, minimum of three views	0.25	0.83	0.83	0.05	1.13	1.13	XXX	
	26	A		0.25	0.09	0.09	0.01	0.35	0.35	XXX	
	TC	A		0.00	0.74	0.74	0.04	0.78	0.78	XXX	
70240		A	Radiologic examination, sella turcica	0.19	0.46	0.46	0.03	0.68	0.68	XXX	
	26	A		0.19	0.07	0.07	0.01	0.27	0.27	XXX	
	TC	A		0.00	0.39	0.39	0.02	0.41	0.41	XXX	
70250		A	Radiologic examination, skull; less than four views, with or without stereo	0.24	0.67	0.67	0.04	0.95	0.95	XXX	
	26	A		0.24	0.08	0.08	0.01	0.33	0.33	XXX	
	TC	A		0.00	0.59	0.59	0.03	0.62	0.62	XXX	
70260		A	complete, minimum of four views, with or without stereo	0.34	0.96	0.96	0.06	1.36	1.36	XXX	
	26	A		0.34	0.12	0.12	0.01	0.47	0.47	XXX	
	TC	A		0.00	0.84	0.84	0.05	0.89	0.89	XXX	
70300		A	Radiologic examination, teeth; single view	0.10	0.29	0.29	0.03	0.42	0.42	XXX	
	26	A		0.10	0.04	0.04	0.01	0.15	0.15	XXX	
	TC	A		0.00	0.25	0.25	0.02	0.27	0.27	XXX	
70310		A	partial examination, less than full mouth	0.16	0.46	0.46	0.03	0.65	0.65	XXX	
	26	A		0.16	0.07	0.07	0.01	0.24	0.24	XXX	
	TC	A		0.00	0.39	0.39	0.02	0.41	0.41	XXX	
70320		A	complete, full mouth	0.22	0.82	0.82	0.05	1.09	1.09	XXX	
	26	A		0.22	0.08	0.08	0.01	0.31	0.31	XXX	
	TC	A		0.00	0.74	0.74	0.04	0.78	0.78	XXX	
70328		A	Radiologic examination, temporomandibular joint, open and closed mouth; unilateral	0.18	0.53	0.53	0.03	0.74	0.74	XXX	
	26	A		0.18	0.06	0.06	0.01	0.25	0.25	XXX	
	TC	A		0.00	0.47	0.47	0.02	0.49	0.49	XXX	
70330		A	bilateral	0.24	0.88	0.88	0.05	1.17	1.17	XXX	
	26	A		0.24	0.08	0.08	0.01	0.33	0.33	XXX	
	TC	A		0.00	0.80	0.80	0.04	0.84	0.84	XXX	
70332		A	Temporomandibular joint arthrography, radiological supervision and interpretation	0.54	2.18	2.18	0.12	2.84	2.84	XXX	
	26	A		0.54	0.19	0.19	0.02	0.75	0.75	XXX	
	TC	A		0.00	1.99	1.99	0.10	2.09	2.09	XXX	
70336		A	Magnetic resonance (eg, proton) imaging, temporomandibular joint(s)	1.48	11.16	11.16	0.56	13.20	13.20	XXX	
	26	A		1.48	0.52	0.52	0.07	2.07	2.07	XXX	
	TC	A		0.00	10.64	10.64	0.49	11.13	11.13	XXX	
70350		A	Cephalogram, orthodontic	0.17	0.42	0.42	0.03	0.62	0.62	XXX	
	26	A		0.17	0.06	0.06	0.01	0.24	0.24	XXX	
	TC	A		0.00	0.36	0.36	0.02	0.38	0.38	XXX	
70355		A	Orthopantogram	0.20	0.61	0.61	0.04	0.85	0.85	XXX	
	26	A		0.20	0.07	0.07	0.01	0.28	0.28	XXX	
	TC	A		0.00	0.54	0.54	0.03	0.57	0.57	XXX	
70360		A	Radiologic examination; neck, soft tissue	0.17	0.45	0.45	0.03	0.65	0.65	XXX	
	26	A		0.17	0.06	0.06	0.01	0.24	0.24	XXX	
	TC	A		0.00	0.39	0.39	0.02	0.41	0.41	XXX	

■ RVU not developed by CMS. Gap-filled RVUs developed by CHEG.

Code	M	S	Description	Work Value	Non-Fac PE	Fac PE	Mal-practice	Non-Fac Total	Fac Total	Global	Gap
70370		A	pharynx or larynx, including fluoroscopy and/or magnification technique	0.32	1.35	1.35	0.07	1.74	1.74	XXX	
	26	A		0.32	0.11	0.11	0.01	0.44	0.44	XXX	
	TC	A		0.00	1.24	1.24	0.06	1.30	1.30	XXX	
70371		A	Complex dynamic pharyngeal and speech evaluation by cine or video recording	0.84	2.29	2.29	0.14	3.27	3.27	XXX	
	26	A		0.84	0.30	0.30	0.04	1.18	1.18	XXX	
	TC	A		0.00	1.99	1.99	0.10	2.09	2.09	XXX	
70373		A	Laryngography, contrast, radiological supervision and interpretation	0.44	1.84	1.84	0.11	2.39	2.39	XXX	
	26	A		0.44	0.15	0.15	0.02	0.61	0.61	XXX	
	TC	A		0.00	1.69	1.69	0.09	1.78	1.78	XXX	
70380		A	Radiologic examination, salivary gland for calculus	0.17	0.69	0.69	0.04	0.90	0.90	XXX	
	26	A		0.17	0.06	0.06	0.01	0.24	0.24	XXX	
	TC	A		0.00	0.63	0.63	0.03	0.66	0.66	XXX	
70390		A	Sialography, radiological supervision and interpretation	0.38	1.82	1.82	0.11	2.31	2.31	XXX	
	26	A		0.38	0.13	0.13	0.02	0.53	0.53	XXX	
	TC	A		0.00	1.69	1.69	0.09	1.78	1.78	XXX	
70450		A	Computerized axial tomography, head or brain; without contrast material	0.85	4.78	4.78	0.25	5.88	5.88	XXX	
	26	A		0.85	0.30	0.30	0.04	1.19	1.19	XXX	
	TC	A		0.00	4.48	4.48	0.21	4.69	4.69	XXX	
70460		A	with contrast material(s)	1.13	5.77	5.77	0.30	7.20	7.20	XXX	
	26	A		1.13	0.40	0.40	0.05	1.58	1.58	XXX	
	TC	A		0.00	5.37	5.37	0.25	5.62	5.62	XXX	
70470		A	without contrast material, followed by contrast material(s) and further sections	1.27	7.16	7.16	0.37	8.80	8.80	XXX	
	26	A		1.27	0.45	0.45	0.06	1.78	1.78	XXX	
	TC	A		0.00	6.71	6.71	0.31	7.02	7.02	XXX	
70480		A	Computerized axial tomography, orbit, sella, or posterior fossa or outer, middle, or inner ear; without contrast material	1.28	4.93	4.93	0.27	6.48	6.48	XXX	
	26	A		1.28	0.45	0.45	0.06	1.79	1.79	XXX	
	TC	A		0.00	4.48	4.48	0.21	4.69	4.69	XXX	
70481		A	with contrast material(s)	1.38	5.85	5.85	0.31	7.54	7.54	XXX	
	26	A		1.38	0.48	0.48	0.06	1.92	1.92	XXX	
	TC	A		0.00	5.37	5.37	0.25	5.62	5.62	XXX	
70482		A	without contrast material, followed by contrast material(s) and further sections	1.45	7.22	7.22	0.37	9.04	9.04	XXX	
	26	A		1.45	0.51	0.51	0.06	2.02	2.02	XXX	
	TC	A		0.00	6.71	6.71	0.31	7.02	7.02	XXX	
70486		A	Computerized axial tomography, maxillofacial area; without contrast material	1.14	4.88	4.88	0.26	6.28	6.28	XXX	
	26	A		1.14	0.40	0.40	0.05	1.59	1.59	XXX	
	TC	A		0.00	4.48	4.48	0.21	4.69	4.69	XXX	
70487		A	with contrast material(s)	1.30	5.83	5.83	0.31	7.44	7.44	XXX	
	26	A		1.30	0.46	0.46	0.06	1.82	1.82	XXX	
	TC	A		0.00	5.37	5.37	0.25	5.62	5.62	XXX	
70488		A	without contrast material, followed by contrast material(s) and further sections	1.42	7.21	7.21	0.37	9.00	9.00	XXX	
	26	A		1.42	0.50	0.50	0.06	1.98	1.98	XXX	
	TC	A		0.00	6.71	6.71	0.31	7.02	7.02	XXX	
70490		A	Computerized axial tomography, soft tissue neck; without contrast material	1.28	4.93	4.93	0.27	6.48	6.48	XXX	
	26	A		1.28	0.45	0.45	0.06	1.79	1.79	XXX	
	TC	A		0.00	4.48	4.48	0.21	4.69	4.69	XXX	

■ RVU not developed by CMS. Gap-filled RVUs developed by CHEG.

Code	M	S	Description	Work Value	Non-Fac PE	Fac PE	Mal-practice	Non-Fac Total	Fac Total	Global	Gap
70491		A	with contrast material(s)	1.38	5.85	5.85	0.31	7.54	7.54	XXX	
	26	A		1.38	0.48	0.48	0.06	1.92	1.92	XXX	
	TC	A		0.00	5.37	5.37	0.25	5.62	5.62	XXX	
70492		A	without contrast material followed by contrast material(s) and further sections	1.45	7.22	7.22	0.37	9.04	9.04	XXX	
	26	A		1.45	0.51	0.51	0.06	2.02	2.02	XXX	
	TC	A		0.00	6.71	6.71	0.31	7.02	7.02	XXX	
70496		A	Computed tomographic angiography, head, without contrast material(s), followed by contrast material(s) and further sections, including image post-processing	1.75	7.41	7.41	0.56	9.72	9.72	XXX	
	26	A		1.75	0.70	0.70	0.08	2.53	2.53	XXX	
	TC	A		0.00	6.71	6.71	0.48	7.19	7.19	XXX	
70498		A	Computed tomographic angiography, neck, without contrast material(s), followed by contrast material(s) and further sections, including image post-processing	1.75	7.41	7.41	0.56	9.72	9.72	XXX	
	26	A		1.75	0.70	0.70	0.08	2.53	2.53	XXX	
	TC	A		0.00	6.71	6.71	0.48	7.19	7.19	XXX	
70540		A	Magnetic resonance (eg, proton) imaging, orbit, face, and neck; without contrast material(s)	1.35	11.11	11.11	0.36	12.82	12.82	XXX	
	26	A		1.35	0.47	0.47	0.04	1.86	1.86	XXX	
	TC	A		0.00	10.64	10.64	0.32	10.96	10.96	XXX	
70542		A	with contrast material(s)	1.62	13.33	13.33	0.44	15.39	15.39	XXX	
	26	A		1.62	0.57	0.57	0.05	2.24	2.24	XXX	
	TC	A		0.00	12.76	12.76	0.39	13.15	13.15	XXX	
70543		A	without contrast material(s), followed by contrast material(s) and further sequences	2.15	24.39	24.39	0.77	27.31	27.31	XXX	
	26	A		2.15	0.75	0.75	0.07	2.97	2.97	XXX	
	TC	A		0.00	23.64	23.64	0.70	24.34	24.34	XXX	
70544		A	Magnetic resonance angiography, head; without contrast material(s)	1.20	11.06	11.06	0.54	12.80	12.80	XXX	
	26	A		1.20	0.42	0.42	0.05	1.67	1.67	XXX	
	TC	A		0.00	10.64	10.64	0.49	11.13	11.13	XXX	
70545		A	with contrast material(s)	1.20	11.06	11.06	0.54	12.80	12.80	XXX	
	26	A		1.20	0.42	0.42	0.05	1.67	1.67	XXX	
	TC	A		0.00	10.64	10.64	0.49	11.13	11.13	XXX	
70546		A	without contrast material(s), followed by contrast material(s) and further sequences	1.80	21.92	21.92	0.57	24.29	24.29	XXX	
	26	A		1.80	0.63	0.63	0.08	2.51	2.51	XXX	
	TC	A		0.00	21.29	21.29	0.49	21.78	21.78	XXX	
70547		A	Magnetic resonance angiography, neck; without contrast material(s)	1.20	11.06	11.06	0.54	12.80	12.80	XXX	
	26	A		1.20	0.42	0.42	0.05	1.67	1.67	XXX	
	TC	A		0.00	10.64	10.64	0.49	11.13	11.13	XXX	
70548		A	with contrast material(s)	1.20	11.06	11.06	0.54	12.80	12.80	XXX	
	26	A		1.20	0.42	0.42	0.05	1.67	1.67	XXX	
	TC	A		0.00	10.64	10.64	0.49	11.13	11.13	XXX	
70549		A	without contrast material(s), followed by contrast material(s) and further sequences	1.80	21.92	21.92	0.57	24.29	24.29	XXX	
	26	A		1.80	0.63	0.63	0.08	2.51	2.51	XXX	
	TC	A		0.00	21.29	21.29	0.49	21.78	21.78	XXX	
70551		A	Magnetic resonance (eg, proton) imaging, brain (including brain stem); without contrast material	1.48	11.16	11.16	0.56	13.20	13.20	XXX	
	26	A		1.48	0.52	0.52	0.07	2.07	2.07	XXX	
	TC	A		0.00	10.64	10.64	0.49	11.13	11.13	XXX	

■ RVU not developed by CMS. Gap-filled RVUs developed by CHEG.

Code	M	S	Description	Work Value	Non-Fac PE	Fac PE	Mal-practice	Non-Fac Total	Fac Total	Global	Gap
70552		A	with contrast material(s)	1.78	13.40	13.40	0.66	15.84	15.84	XXX	
	26	A		1.78	0.64	0.64	0.08	2.50	2.50	XXX	
	TC	A		0.00	12.76	12.76	0.58	13.34	13.34	XXX	
70553		A	without contrast material, followed by contrast material(s) and further sequences	2.36	24.47	24.47	1.19	28.02	28.02	XXX	
	26	A		2.36	0.83	0.83	0.10	3.29	3.29	XXX	
	TC	A		0.00	23.64	23.64	1.09	24.73	24.73	XXX	
71010		A	Radiologic examination, chest; single view, frontal	0.18	0.51	0.51	0.03	0.72	0.72	XXX	
	26	A		0.18	0.06	0.06	0.01	0.25	0.25	XXX	
	TC	A		0.00	0.45	0.45	0.02	0.47	0.47	XXX	
71015		A	stereo, frontal	0.21	0.57	0.57	0.03	0.81	0.81	XXX	
	26	A		0.21	0.07	0.07	0.01	0.29	0.29	XXX	
	TC	A		0.00	0.50	0.50	0.02	0.52	0.52	XXX	
71020		A	Radiologic examination, chest, two views, frontal and lateral;	0.22	0.67	0.67	0.04	0.93	0.93	XXX	
	26	A		0.22	0.08	0.08	0.01	0.31	0.31	XXX	
	TC	A		0.00	0.59	0.59	0.03	0.62	0.62	XXX	
71021		A	with apical lordotic procedure	0.27	0.79	0.79	0.05	1.11	1.11	XXX	
	26	A		0.27	0.09	0.09	0.01	0.37	0.37	XXX	
	TC	A		0.00	0.70	0.70	0.04	0.74	0.74	XXX	
71022		A	with oblique projections	0.31	0.81	0.81	0.06	1.18	1.18	XXX	
	26	A		0.31	0.11	0.11	0.02	0.44	0.44	XXX	
	TC	A		0.00	0.70	0.70	0.04	0.74	0.74	XXX	
71023		A	with fluoroscopy	0.38	0.88	0.88	0.06	1.32	1.32	XXX	
	26	A		0.38	0.14	0.14	0.02	0.54	0.54	XXX	
	TC	A		0.00	0.74	0.74	0.04	0.78	0.78	XXX	
71030		A	Radiologic examination, chest, complete, minimum of four views;	0.31	0.85	0.85	0.05	1.21	1.21	XXX	
	26	A		0.31	0.11	0.11	0.01	0.43	0.43	XXX	
	TC	A		0.00	0.74	0.74	0.04	0.78	0.78	XXX	
71034		A	with fluoroscopy	0.46	1.54	1.54	0.09	2.09	2.09	XXX	
	26	A		0.46	0.17	0.17	0.02	0.65	0.65	XXX	
	TC	A		0.00	1.37	1.37	0.07	1.44	1.44	XXX	
71035		A	Radiologic examination, chest, special views (eg, lateral decubitus, Bucky studies)	0.18	0.56	0.56	0.03	0.77	0.77	XXX	
	26	A		0.18	0.06	0.06	0.01	0.25	0.25	XXX	
	TC	A		0.00	0.50	0.50	0.02	0.52	0.52	XXX	
71040		A	Bronchography, unilateral, radiological supervision and interpretation	0.58	1.59	1.59	0.10	2.27	2.27	XXX	
	26	A		0.58	0.20	0.20	0.03	0.81	0.81	XXX	
	TC	A		0.00	1.39	1.39	0.07	1.46	1.46	XXX	
71060		A	Bronchography, bilateral, radiological supervision and interpretation	0.74	2.35	2.35	0.14	3.23	3.23	XXX	
	26	A		0.74	0.26	0.26	0.03	1.03	1.03	XXX	
	TC	A		0.00	2.09	2.09	0.11	2.20	2.20	XXX	
71090		A	Insertion pacemaker, fluoroscopy and radiography, radiological supervision and interpretation	0.54	1.82	1.82	0.11	2.47	2.47	XXX	
	26	A		0.54	0.22	0.22	0.02	0.78	0.78	XXX	
	TC	A		0.00	1.60	1.60	0.09	1.69	1.69	XXX	
71100		A	Radiologic examination, ribs, unilateral; two views	0.22	0.62	0.62	0.04	0.88	0.88	XXX	
	26	A		0.22	0.08	0.08	0.01	0.31	0.31	XXX	
	TC	A		0.00	0.54	0.54	0.03	0.57	0.57	XXX	

■ RVU not developed by CMS. Gap-filled RVUs developed by CHEG.

Code	M	S	Description	Work Value	Non-Fac PE	Fac PE	Mal-practice	Non-Fac Total	Fac Total	Global	Gap
71101		A	including posteroanterior chest, minimum of three views	0.27	0.72	0.72	0.04	1.03	1.03	XXX	
	26	A		0.27	0.09	0.09	0.01	0.37	0.37	XXX	
	TC	A		0.00	0.63	0.63	0.03	0.66	0.66	XXX	
71110		A	Radiologic examination, ribs, bilateral; three views	0.27	0.83	0.83	0.05	1.15	1.15	XXX	
	26	A		0.27	0.09	0.09	0.01	0.37	0.37	XXX	
	TC	A		0.00	0.74	0.74	0.04	0.78	0.78	XXX	
71111		A	including posteroanterior chest, minimum of four views	0.32	0.95	0.95	0.06	1.33	1.33	XXX	
	26	A		0.32	0.11	0.11	0.01	0.44	0.44	XXX	
	TC	A		0.00	0.84	0.84	0.05	0.89	0.89	XXX	
71120		A	Radiologic examination; sternum, minimum of two views	0.20	0.69	0.69	0.04	0.93	0.93	XXX	
	26	A		0.20	0.07	0.07	0.01	0.28	0.28	XXX	
	TC	A		0.00	0.62	0.62	0.03	0.65	0.65	XXX	
71130		A	sternoclavicular joint or joints, minimum of three views	0.22	0.75	0.75	0.04	1.01	1.01	XXX	
	26	A		0.22	0.08	0.08	0.01	0.31	0.31	XXX	
	TC	A		0.00	0.67	0.67	0.03	0.70	0.70	XXX	
71250		A	Computerized axial tomography, thorax; without contrast material	1.16	6.02	6.02	0.31	7.49	7.49	XXX	
	26	A		1.16	0.41	0.41	0.05	1.62	1.62	XXX	
	TC	A		0.00	5.61	5.61	0.26	5.87	5.87	XXX	
71260		A	with contrast material(s)	1.24	7.14	7.14	0.36	8.74	8.74	XXX	
	26	A		1.24	0.43	0.43	0.05	1.72	1.72	XXX	
	TC	A		0.00	6.71	6.71	0.31	7.02	7.02	XXX	
71270		A	without contrast material, followed by contrast material(s) and further sections	1.38	8.88	8.88	0.44	10.70	10.70	XXX	
	26	A		1.38	0.48	0.48	0.06	1.92	1.92	XXX	
	TC	A		0.00	8.40	8.40	0.38	8.78	8.78	XXX	
71275		A	Computed tomographic angiography, chest, without contrast material(s), followed by contrast material(s) and further sections, including image post-processing	1.92	9.17	9.17	0.38	11.47	11.47	XXX	
	26	A		1.92	0.77	0.77	0.06	2.75	2.75	XXX	
	TC	A		0.00	8.40	8.40	0.32	8.72	8.72	XXX	
71550		A	Magnetic resonance (eg, proton) imaging, chest (eg, for evaluation of hilar and mediastinal lymphadenopathy); without contrast material(s)	1.46	11.15	11.15	0.41	13.02	13.02	XXX	
	26	A		1.46	0.51	0.51	0.04	2.01	2.01	XXX	
	TC	A		0.00	10.64	10.64	0.37	11.01	11.01	XXX	
71551		A	with contrast material(s)	1.73	13.36	13.36	0.49	15.58	15.58	XXX	
	26	A		1.73	0.60	0.60	0.06	2.39	2.39	XXX	
	TC	A		0.00	12.76	12.76	0.43	13.19	13.19	XXX	
71552		A	without contrast material(s), followed by contrast material(s) and further sequences	2.26	24.43	24.43	0.64	27.33	27.33	XXX	
	26	A		2.26	0.79	0.79	0.08	3.13	3.13	XXX	
	TC	A		0.00	23.64	23.64	0.56	24.20	24.20	XXX	
71555		R	Magnetic resonance angiography, chest (excluding myocardium), with or without contrast material(s)	1.81	11.28	11.28	0.57	13.66	13.66	XXX	
	26	R		1.81	0.64	0.64	0.08	2.53	2.53	XXX	
	TC	R		0.00	10.64	10.64	0.49	11.13	11.13	XXX	
72010		A	Radiologic examination, spine, entire, survey study, anteroposterior and lateral	0.45	1.13	1.13	0.08	1.66	1.66	XXX	
	26	A		0.45	0.16	0.16	0.03	0.64	0.64	XXX	
	TC	A		0.00	0.97	0.97	0.05	1.02	1.02	XXX	

Radiology

■ RVU not developed by CMS. Gap-filled RVUs developed by CHEG.

Code	M	S	Description	Work Value	Non-Fac PE	Fac PE	Mal-practice	Non-Fac Total	Fac Total	Global	Gap
72020		A	Radiologic examination, spine, single view, specify level	0.15	0.44	0.44	0.03	0.62	0.62	XXX	
	26	A		0.15	0.05	0.05	0.01	0.21	0.21	XXX	
	TC	A		0.00	0.39	0.39	0.02	0.41	0.41	XXX	
72040		A	Radiologic examination, spine, cervical; two or three views	0.22	0.65	0.65	0.04	0.91	0.91	XXX	
	26	A		0.22	0.08	0.08	0.01	0.31	0.31	XXX	
	TC	A		0.00	0.57	0.57	0.03	0.60	0.60	XXX	
72050		A	minimum of four views	0.31	0.95	0.95	0.07	1.33	1.33	XXX	
	26	A		0.31	0.11	0.11	0.02	0.44	0.44	XXX	
	TC	A		0.00	0.84	0.84	0.05	0.89	0.89	XXX	
72052		A	complete, including oblique and flexion and/or extension studies	0.36	1.20	1.20	0.07	1.63	1.63	XXX	
	26	A		0.36	0.13	0.13	0.02	0.51	0.51	XXX	
	TC	A		0.00	1.07	1.07	0.05	1.12	1.12	XXX	
72069		A	Radiologic examination, spine, thoracolumbar, standing (scoliosis)	0.22	0.56	0.56	0.04	0.82	0.82	XXX	
	26	A		0.22	0.09	0.09	0.02	0.33	0.33	XXX	
	TC	A		0.00	0.47	0.47	0.02	0.49	0.49	XXX	
72070		A	Radiologic examination, spine; thoracic, two views	0.22	0.70	0.70	0.04	0.96	0.96	XXX	
	26	A		0.22	0.08	0.08	0.01	0.31	0.31	XXX	
	TC	A		0.00	0.62	0.62	0.03	0.65	0.65	XXX	
72072		A	thoracic, three views	0.22	0.78	0.78	0.05	1.05	1.05	XXX	
	26	A		0.22	0.08	0.08	0.01	0.31	0.31	XXX	
	TC	A		0.00	0.70	0.70	0.04	0.74	0.74	XXX	
72074		A	thoracic, minimum of four views	0.22	0.94	0.94	0.06	1.22	1.22	XXX	
	26	A		0.22	0.08	0.08	0.01	0.31	0.31	XXX	
	TC	A		0.00	0.86	0.86	0.05	0.91	0.91	XXX	
72080		A	thoracolumbar, two views	0.22	0.71	0.71	0.05	0.98	0.98	XXX	
	26	A		0.22	0.08	0.08	0.02	0.32	0.32	XXX	
	TC	A		0.00	0.63	0.63	0.03	0.66	0.66	XXX	
72090		A	scoliosis study, including supine and erect studies	0.28	0.73	0.73	0.05	1.06	1.06	XXX	
	26	A		0.28	0.10	0.10	0.02	0.40	0.40	XXX	
	TC	A		0.00	0.63	0.63	0.03	0.66	0.66	XXX	
72100		A	Radiologic examination, spine, lumbosacral; two or three views	0.22	0.71	0.71	0.05	0.98	0.98	XXX	
	26	A		0.22	0.08	0.08	0.02	0.32	0.32	XXX	
	TC	A		0.00	0.63	0.63	0.03	0.66	0.66	XXX	
72110		A	minimum of four views	0.31	0.97	0.97	0.07	1.35	1.35	XXX	
	26	A		0.31	0.11	0.11	0.02	0.44	0.44	XXX	
	TC	A		0.00	0.86	0.86	0.05	0.91	0.91	XXX	
72114		A	complete, including bending views	0.36	1.26	1.26	0.08	1.70	1.70	XXX	
	26	A		0.36	0.13	0.13	0.03	0.52	0.52	XXX	
	TC	A		0.00	1.13	1.13	0.05	1.18	1.18	XXX	
72120		A	Radiologic examination, spine, lumbosacral, bending views only, minimum of four views	0.22	0.92	0.92	0.07	1.21	1.21	XXX	
	26	A		0.22	0.08	0.08	0.02	0.32	0.32	XXX	
	TC	A		0.00	0.84	0.84	0.05	0.89	0.89	XXX	
72125		A	Computerized axial tomography, cervical spine; without contrast material	1.16	6.02	6.02	0.31	7.49	7.49	XXX	
	26	A		1.16	0.41	0.41	0.05	1.62	1.62	XXX	
	TC	A		0.00	5.61	5.61	0.26	5.87	5.87	XXX	

Radiology

■ RVU not developed by CMS. Gap-filled RVUs developed by CHEG.

Code	M	S	Description	Work Value	Non-Fac PE	Fac PE	Mal-practice	Non-Fac Total	Fac Total	Global	Gap
72126		A	with contrast material	1.22	7.14	7.14	0.36	8.72	8.72	XXX	
	26	A		1.22	0.43	0.43	0.05	1.70	1.70	XXX	
	TC	A		0.00	6.71	6.71	0.31	7.02	7.02	XXX	
72127		A	without contrast material, followed by contrast material(s) and further sections	1.27	8.85	8.85	0.44	10.56	10.56	XXX	
	26	A		1.27	0.45	0.45	0.06	1.78	1.78	XXX	
	TC	A		0.00	8.40	8.40	0.38	8.78	8.78	XXX	
72128		A	Computerized axial tomography, thoracic spine; without contrast material	1.16	6.02	6.02	0.31	7.49	7.49	XXX	
	26	A		1.16	0.41	0.41	0.05	1.62	1.62	XXX	
	TC	A		0.00	5.61	5.61	0.26	5.87	5.87	XXX	
72129		A	with contrast material	1.22	7.14	7.14	0.36	8.72	8.72	XXX	
	26	A		1.22	0.43	0.43	0.05	1.70	1.70	XXX	
	TC	A		0.00	6.71	6.71	0.31	7.02	7.02	XXX	
72130		A	without contrast material, followed by contrast material(s) and further sections	1.27	8.85	8.85	0.44	10.56	10.56	XXX	
	26	A		1.27	0.45	0.45	0.06	1.78	1.78	XXX	
	TC	A		0.00	8.40	8.40	0.38	8.78	8.78	XXX	
72131		A	Computerized axial tomography, lumbar spine; without contrast material	1.16	6.02	6.02	0.31	7.49	7.49	XXX	
	26	A		1.16	0.41	0.41	0.05	1.62	1.62	XXX	
	TC	A		0.00	5.61	5.61	0.26	5.87	5.87	XXX	
72132		A	with contrast material	1.22	7.14	7.14	0.37	8.73	8.73	XXX	
	26	A		1.22	0.43	0.43	0.06	1.71	1.71	XXX	
	TC	A		0.00	6.71	6.71	0.31	7.02	7.02	XXX	
72133		A	without contrast material, followed by contrast material(s) and further sections	1.27	8.85	8.85	0.44	10.56	10.56	XXX	
	26	A		1.27	0.45	0.45	0.06	1.78	1.78	XXX	
	TC	A		0.00	8.40	8.40	0.38	8.78	8.78	XXX	
72141		A	Magnetic resonance (eg, proton) imaging, spinal canal and contents, cervical; without contrast material	1.60	11.20	11.20	0.56	13.36	13.36	XXX	
	26	A		1.60	0.56	0.56	0.07	2.23	2.23	XXX	
	TC	A		0.00	10.64	10.64	0.49	11.13	11.13	XXX	
72142		A	with contrast material(s)	1.92	13.45	13.45	0.67	16.04	16.04	XXX	
	26	A		1.92	0.69	0.69	0.09	2.70	2.70	XXX	
	TC	A		0.00	12.76	12.76	0.58	13.34	13.34	XXX	
72146		A	Magnetic resonance (eg, proton) imaging, spinal canal and contents, thoracic; without contrast material	1.60	12.38	12.38	0.60	14.58	14.58	XXX	
	26	A		1.60	0.56	0.56	0.07	2.23	2.23	XXX	
	TC	A		0.00	11.82	11.82	0.53	12.35	12.35	XXX	
72147		A	with contrast material(s)	1.92	13.44	13.44	0.67	16.03	16.03	XXX	
	26	A		1.92	0.68	0.68	0.09	2.69	2.69	XXX	
	TC	A		0.00	12.76	12.76	0.58	13.34	13.34	XXX	
72148		A	Magnetic resonance (eg, proton) imaging, spinal canal and contents, lumbar; without contrast material	1.48	12.34	12.34	0.60	14.42	14.42	XXX	
	26	A		1.48	0.52	0.52	0.07	2.07	2.07	XXX	
	TC	A		0.00	11.82	11.82	0.53	12.35	12.35	XXX	
72149		A	with contrast material(s)	1.78	13.40	13.40	0.67	15.85	15.85	XXX	
	26	A		1.78	0.64	0.64	0.09	2.51	2.51	XXX	
	TC	A		0.00	12.76	12.76	0.58	13.34	13.34	XXX	

■ RVU not developed by CMS. Gap-filled RVUs developed by CHEG.

Code	M	S	Description	Work Value	Non-Fac PE	Fac PE	Mal-practice	Non-Fac Total	Fac Total	Global	Gap
72156		A	Magnetic resonance (eg, proton) imaging, spinal canal and contents, without contrast material, followed by contrast material(s) and further sequences; cervical	2.57	24.55	24.55	1.20	28.32	28.32	XXX	
	26	A		2.57	0.91	0.91	0.11	3.59	3.59	XXX	
	TC	A		0.00	23.64	23.64	1.09	24.73	24.73	XXX	
72157		A	thoracic	2.57	24.54	24.54	1.20	28.31	28.31	XXX	
	26	A		2.57	0.90	0.90	0.11	3.58	3.58	XXX	
	TC	A		0.00	23.64	23.64	1.09	24.73	24.73	XXX	
72158		A	lumbar	2.36	24.47	24.47	1.20	28.03	28.03	XXX	
	26	A		2.36	0.83	0.83	0.11	3.30	3.30	XXX	
	TC	A		0.00	23.64	23.64	1.09	24.73	24.73	XXX	
72159		N	Magnetic resonance angiography, spinal canal and contents, with or without contrast material(s)	1.80	12.54	12.54	0.61	14.95	14.95	XXX	
	26	N		1.80	0.72	0.72	0.08	2.60	2.60	XXX	
	TC	N		0.00	11.82	11.82	0.53	12.35	12.35	XXX	
72170		A	Radiologic examination, pelvis; one or two views	0.17	0.56	0.56	0.03	0.76	0.76	XXX	
	26	A		0.17	0.06	0.06	0.01	0.24	0.24	XXX	
	TC	A		0.00	0.50	0.50	0.02	0.52	0.52	XXX	
72190		A	complete, minimum of three views	0.21	0.70	0.70	0.04	0.95	0.95	XXX	
	26	A		0.21	0.07	0.07	0.01	0.29	0.29	XXX	
	TC	A		0.00	0.63	0.63	0.03	0.66	0.66	XXX	
72191		A	Computed tomographic angiography, pelvis, without contrast material(s), followed by contrast material(s) and further sections, including image post-processing	1.81	8.78	8.78	0.38	10.97	10.97	XXX	
	26	A		1.81	0.72	0.72	0.06	2.59	2.59	XXX	
	TC	A		0.00	8.06	8.06	0.32	8.38	8.38	XXX	
72192		A	Computerized axial tomography, pelvis; without contrast material	1.09	5.99	5.99	0.31	7.39	7.39	XXX	
	26	A		1.09	0.38	0.38	0.05	1.52	1.52	XXX	
	TC	A		0.00	5.61	5.61	0.26	5.87	5.87	XXX	
72193		A	with contrast material(s)	1.16	6.91	6.91	0.35	8.42	8.42	XXX	
	26	A		1.16	0.41	0.41	0.05	1.62	1.62	XXX	
	TC	A		0.00	6.50	6.50	0.30	6.80	6.80	XXX	
72194		A	without contrast material, followed by contrast material(s) and further sections	1.22	8.49	8.49	0.41	10.12	10.12	XXX	
	26	A		1.22	0.43	0.43	0.05	1.70	1.70	XXX	
	TC	A		0.00	8.06	8.06	0.36	8.42	8.42	XXX	
72195		A	Magnetic resonance (eg, proton) imaging, pelvis; without contrast material(s)	1.46	11.15	11.15	0.42	13.03	13.03	XXX	
	26	A		1.46	0.51	0.51	0.05	2.02	2.02	XXX	
	TC	A		0.00	10.64	10.64	0.37	11.01	11.01	XXX	
72196		A	with contrast material(s)	1.73	13.36	13.36	0.48	15.57	15.57	XXX	
	26	A		1.73	0.60	0.60	0.05	2.38	2.38	XXX	
	TC	A		0.00	12.76	12.76	0.43	13.19	13.19	XXX	
72197		A	without contrast material(s), followed by contrast material(s) and further sequences	2.26	24.43	24.43	0.84	27.53	27.53	XXX	
	26	A		2.26	0.79	0.79	0.08	3.13	3.13	XXX	
	TC	A		0.00	23.64	23.64	0.76	24.40	24.40	XXX	
72198		N	Magnetic resonance angiography, pelvis, with or without contrast material(s)	1.80	11.36	11.36	0.57	13.73	13.73	XXX	
	26	N		1.80	0.72	0.72	0.08	2.60	2.60	XXX	
	TC	N		0.00	10.64	10.64	0.49	11.13	11.13	XXX	

■ RVU not developed by CMS. Gap-filled RVUs developed by CHEG.

Code	M	S	Description	Work Value	Non-Fac PE	Fac PE	Mal-practice	Non-Fac Total	Fac Total	Global	Gap
72200		A	Radiologic examination, sacroiliac joints; less than three views	0.17	0.56	0.56	0.03	0.76	0.76	XXX	
	26	A		0.17	0.06	0.06	0.01	0.24	0.24	XXX	
	TC	A		0.00	0.50	0.50	0.02	0.52	0.52	XXX	
72202		A	three or more views	0.19	0.66	0.66	0.04	0.89	0.89	XXX	
	26	A		0.19	0.07	0.07	0.01	0.27	0.27	XXX	
	TC	A		0.00	0.59	0.59	0.03	0.62	0.62	XXX	
72220		A	Radiologic examination, sacrum and coccyx, minimum of two views	0.17	0.60	0.60	0.04	0.81	0.81	XXX	
	26	A		0.17	0.06	0.06	0.01	0.24	0.24	XXX	
	TC	A		0.00	0.54	0.54	0.03	0.57	0.57	XXX	
72240		A	Myelography, cervical, radiological supervision and interpretation	0.91	4.82	4.82	0.25	5.98	5.98	XXX	
	26	A		0.91	0.31	0.31	0.04	1.26	1.26	XXX	
	TC	A		0.00	4.51	4.51	0.21	4.72	4.72	XXX	
72255		A	Myelography, thoracic, radiological supervision and interpretation	0.91	4.41	4.41	0.22	5.54	5.54	XXX	
	26	A		0.91	0.30	0.30	0.04	1.25	1.25	XXX	
	TC	A		0.00	4.11	4.11	0.18	4.29	4.29	XXX	
72265		A	Myelography, lumbosacral, radiological supervision and interpretation	0.83	4.15	4.15	0.22	5.20	5.20	XXX	
	26	A		0.83	0.28	0.28	0.04	1.15	1.15	XXX	
	TC	A		0.00	3.87	3.87	0.18	4.05	4.05	XXX	
72270		A	Myelography, entire spinal canal, radiological supervision and interpretation	1.33	6.25	6.25	0.34	7.92	7.92	XXX	
	26	A		1.33	0.46	0.46	0.07	1.86	1.86	XXX	
	TC	A		0.00	5.79	5.79	0.27	6.06	6.06	XXX	
72275		A	Epidurography, radiological supervision and interpretation	0.76	2.20	2.20	0.21	3.17	3.17	XXX	
	26	A		0.76	0.21	0.21	0.03	1.00	1.00	XXX	
	TC	A		0.00	1.99	1.99	0.18	2.17	2.17	XXX	
72285		A	Diskography, cervical or thoracic, radiological supervision and interpretation	1.16	8.35	8.35	0.42	9.93	9.93	XXX	
	26	A		1.16	0.39	0.39	0.06	1.61	1.61	XXX	
	TC	A		0.00	7.96	7.96	0.36	8.32	8.32	XXX	
72295		A	Diskography, lumbar, radiological supervision and interpretation	0.83	7.76	7.76	0.37	8.96	8.96	XXX	
	26	A		0.83	0.29	0.29	0.04	1.16	1.16	XXX	
	TC	A		0.00	7.47	7.47	0.33	7.80	7.80	XXX	
73000		A	Radiologic examination; clavicle, complete	0.16	0.56	0.56	0.03	0.75	0.75	XXX	
	26	A		0.16	0.06	0.06	0.01	0.23	0.23	XXX	
	TC	A		0.00	0.50	0.50	0.02	0.52	0.52	XXX	
73010		A	scapula, complete	0.17	0.56	0.56	0.03	0.76	0.76	XXX	
	26	A		0.17	0.06	0.06	0.01	0.24	0.24	XXX	
	TC	A		0.00	0.50	0.50	0.02	0.52	0.52	XXX	
73020		A	Radiologic examination, shoulder; one view	0.15	0.50	0.50	0.03	0.68	0.68	XXX	
	26	A		0.15	0.05	0.05	0.01	0.21	0.21	XXX	
	TC	A		0.00	0.45	0.45	0.02	0.47	0.47	XXX	
73030		A	complete, minimum of two views	0.18	0.60	0.60	0.04	0.82	0.82	XXX	
	26	A		0.18	0.06	0.06	0.01	0.25	0.25	XXX	
	TC	A		0.00	0.54	0.54	0.03	0.57	0.57	XXX	
73040		A	Radiologic examination, shoulder, arthrography, radiological supervision and interpretation	0.54	2.18	2.18	0.13	2.85	2.85	XXX	
	26	A		0.54	0.19	0.19	0.03	0.76	0.76	XXX	
	TC	A		0.00	1.99	1.99	0.10	2.09	2.09	XXX	

■ RVU not developed by CMS. Gap-filled RVUs developed by CHEG.

Code	M	S	Description	Work Value	Non-Fac PE	Fac PE	Mal-practice	Non-Fac Total	Fac Total	Global	Gap
73050		A	Radiologic examination; acromioclavicular joints, bilateral, with or without weighted distraction	0.20	0.70	0.70	0.05	0.95	0.95	XXX	
	26	A		0.20	0.07	0.07	0.02	0.29	0.29	XXX	
	TC	A		0.00	0.63	0.63	0.03	0.66	0.66	XXX	
73060		A	humerus, minimum of two views	0.17	0.60	0.60	0.04	0.81	0.81	XXX	
	26	A		0.17	0.06	0.06	0.01	0.24	0.24	XXX	
	TC	A		0.00	0.54	0.54	0.03	0.57	0.57	XXX	
73070		A	Radiologic examination, elbow; two views	0.15	0.55	0.55	0.03	0.73	0.73	XXX	
	26	A		0.15	0.05	0.05	0.01	0.21	0.21	XXX	
	TC	A		0.00	0.50	0.50	0.02	0.52	0.52	XXX	
73080		A	complete, minimum of three views	0.17	0.60	0.60	0.04	0.81	0.81	XXX	
	26	A		0.17	0.06	0.06	0.01	0.24	0.24	XXX	
	TC	A		0.00	0.54	0.54	0.03	0.57	0.57	XXX	
73085		A	Radiologic examination, elbow, arthrography, radiological supervision and interpretation	0.54	2.19	2.19	0.13	2.86	2.86	XXX	
	26	A		0.54	0.20	0.20	0.03	0.77	0.77	XXX	
	TC	A		0.00	1.99	1.99	0.10	2.09	2.09	XXX	
73090		A	Radiologic examination; forearm, two views	0.16	0.56	0.56	0.03	0.75	0.75	XXX	
	26	A		0.16	0.06	0.06	0.01	0.23	0.23	XXX	
	TC	A		0.00	0.50	0.50	0.02	0.52	0.52	XXX	
73092		A	upper extremity, infant, minimum of two views	0.16	0.53	0.53	0.03	0.72	0.72	XXX	
	26	A		0.16	0.06	0.06	0.01	0.23	0.23	XXX	
	TC	A		0.00	0.47	0.47	0.02	0.49	0.49	XXX	
73100		A	Radiologic examination, wrist; two views	0.16	0.53	0.53	0.04	0.73	0.73	XXX	
	26	A		0.16	0.06	0.06	0.02	0.24	0.24	XXX	
	TC	A		0.00	0.47	0.47	0.02	0.49	0.49	XXX	
73110		A	complete, minimum of three views	0.17	0.57	0.57	0.03	0.77	0.77	XXX	
	26	A		0.17	0.06	0.06	0.01	0.24	0.24	XXX	
	TC	A		0.00	0.51	0.51	0.02	0.53	0.53	XXX	
73115		A	Radiologic examination, wrist, arthrography, radiological supervision and interpretation	0.54	1.70	1.70	0.11	2.35	2.35	XXX	
	26	A		0.54	0.20	0.20	0.03	0.77	0.77	XXX	
	TC	A		0.00	1.50	1.50	0.08	1.58	1.58	XXX	
73120		A	Radiologic examination, hand; two views	0.16	0.53	0.53	0.03	0.72	0.72	XXX	
	26	A		0.16	0.06	0.06	0.01	0.23	0.23	XXX	
	TC	A		0.00	0.47	0.47	0.02	0.49	0.49	XXX	
73130		A	minimum of three views	0.17	0.57	0.57	0.03	0.77	0.77	XXX	
	26	A		0.17	0.06	0.06	0.01	0.24	0.24	XXX	
	TC	A		0.00	0.51	0.51	0.02	0.53	0.53	XXX	
73140		A	Radiologic examination, finger(s), minimum of two views	0.13	0.44	0.44	0.03	0.60	0.60	XXX	
	26	A		0.13	0.05	0.05	0.01	0.19	0.19	XXX	
	TC	A		0.00	0.39	0.39	0.02	0.41	0.41	XXX	
73200		A	Computerized axial tomography, upper extremity; without contrast material	1.09	5.09	5.09	0.26	6.44	6.44	XXX	
	26	A		1.09	0.38	0.38	0.05	1.52	1.52	XXX	
	TC	A		0.00	4.71	4.71	0.21	4.92	4.92	XXX	
73201		A	with contrast material(s)	1.16	6.02	6.02	0.31	7.49	7.49	XXX	
	26	A		1.16	0.41	0.41	0.05	1.62	1.62	XXX	
	TC	A		0.00	5.61	5.61	0.26	5.87	5.87	XXX	

■ RVU not developed by CMS. Gap-filled RVUs developed by CHEG.

Radiology

Code	M	S	Description	Work Value	Non-Fac PE	Fac PE	Mal-practice	Non-Fac Total	Fac Total	Global	Gap
73202		A	without contrast material, followed by contrast material(s) and further sections	1.22	7.48	7.48	0.38	9.08	9.08	XXX	
	26	A		1.22	0.43	0.43	0.06	1.71	1.71	XXX	
	TC	A		0.00	7.05	7.05	0.32	7.37	7.37	XXX	
73206		A	Computed tomographic angiography, upper extremity, without contrast material(s), followed by contrast material(s) and further sections, including image post-processing	1.81	7.77	7.77	0.38	9.96	9.96	XXX	
	26	A		1.81	0.72	0.72	0.06	2.59	2.59	XXX	
	TC	A		0.00	7.05	7.05	0.32	7.37	7.37	XXX	
73218		A	Magnetic resonance (eg, proton) imaging, upper extremity, other than joint; without contrast material(s)	1.35	11.11	11.11	0.36	12.82	12.82	XXX	
	26	A		1.35	0.47	0.47	0.04	1.86	1.86	XXX	
	TC	A		0.00	10.64	10.64	0.32	10.96	10.96	XXX	
73219		A	with contrast material(s)	1.62	13.33	13.33	0.44	15.39	15.39	XXX	
	26	A		1.62	0.57	0.57	0.05	2.24	2.24	XXX	
	TC	A		0.00	12.76	12.76	0.39	13.15	13.15	XXX	
73220		A	without contrast material(s), followed by contrast material(s) and further sequences	2.15	24.39	24.39	0.78	27.32	27.32	XXX	
	26	A		2.15	0.75	0.75	0.08	2.98	2.98	XXX	
	TC	A		0.00	23.64	23.64	0.70	24.34	24.34	XXX	
73221		A	Magnetic resonance (eg, proton) imaging, any joint of upper extremity; without contrast material(s)	1.35	11.11	11.11	0.36	12.82	12.82	XXX	
	26	A		1.35	0.47	0.47	0.04	1.86	1.86	XXX	
	TC	A		0.00	10.64	10.64	0.32	10.96	10.96	XXX	
73222		A	with contrast material(s)	1.62	13.33	13.33	0.44	15.39	15.39	XXX	
	26	A		1.62	0.57	0.57	0.05	2.24	2.24	XXX	
	TC	A		0.00	12.76	12.76	0.39	13.15	13.15	XXX	
73223		A	without contrast material(s), followed by contrast material(s) and further sequences	2.15	24.39	24.39	0.77	27.31	27.31	XXX	
	26	A		2.15	0.75	0.75	0.07	2.97	2.97	XXX	
	TC	A		0.00	23.64	23.64	0.70	24.34	24.34	XXX	
73225		N	Magnetic resonance angiography, upper extremity, with or without contrast material(s)	1.73	11.33	11.33	0.57	13.63	13.63	XXX	
	26	N		1.73	0.69	0.69	0.08	2.50	2.50	XXX	
	TC	N		0.00	10.64	10.64	0.49	11.13	11.13	XXX	
73500		A	Radiologic examination, hip unilateral; one view	0.17	0.51	0.51	0.03	0.71	0.71	XXX	
	26	A		0.17	0.06	0.06	0.01	0.24	0.24	XXX	
	TC	A		0.00	0.45	0.45	0.02	0.47	0.47	XXX	
73510		A	complete, minimum of two views	0.21	0.61	0.61	0.05	0.87	0.87	XXX	
	26	A		0.21	0.07	0.07	0.02	0.30	0.30	XXX	
	TC	A		0.00	0.54	0.54	0.03	0.57	0.57	XXX	
73520		A	Radiologic examination, hips, bilateral, minimum of two views of each hip, including anteroposterior view of pelvis	0.26	0.72	0.72	0.05	1.03	1.03	XXX	
	26	A		0.26	0.09	0.09	0.02	0.37	0.37	XXX	
	TC	A		0.00	0.63	0.63	0.03	0.66	0.66	XXX	
73525		A	Radiologic examination, hip, arthrography, radiological supervision and interpretation	0.54	2.19	2.19	0.13	2.86	2.86	XXX	
	26	A		0.54	0.20	0.20	0.03	0.77	0.77	XXX	
	TC	A		0.00	1.99	1.99	0.10	2.09	2.09	XXX	
73530		A	Radiologic examination, hip, during operative procedure	0.29	0.60	0.60	0.03	0.92	0.92	XXX	
	26	A		0.29	0.10	0.10	0.01	0.40	0.40	XXX	
	TC	A		0.00	0.50	0.50	0.02	0.52	0.52	XXX	

Radiology

■ RVU not developed by CMS. Gap-filled RVUs developed by CHEG.

Code	M	S	Description	Work Value	Non-Fac PE	Fac PE	Mal-practice	Non-Fac Total	Fac Total	Global	Gap
73540		A	Radiologic examination, pelvis and hips, infant or child, minimum of two views	0.20	0.61	0.61	0.05	0.86	0.86	XXX	
	26	A		0.20	0.07	0.07	0.02	0.29	0.29	XXX	
	TC	A		0.00	0.54	0.54	0.03	0.57	0.57	XXX	
73542		A	Radiological examination, sacroiliac joint arthrography, radiological supervision and interpretation	0.59	2.16	2.16	0.13	2.88	2.88	XXX	
	26	A		0.59	0.17	0.17	0.03	0.79	0.79	XXX	
	TC	A		0.00	1.99	1.99	0.10	2.09	2.09	XXX	
73550		A	Radiologic examination, femur, two views	0.17	0.60	0.60	0.04	0.81	0.81	XXX	
	26	A		0.17	0.06	0.06	0.01	0.24	0.24	XXX	
	TC	A		0.00	0.54	0.54	0.03	0.57	0.57	XXX	
73560		A	Radiologic examination, knee; one or two views	0.17	0.56	0.56	0.04	0.77	0.77	XXX	
	26	A		0.17	0.06	0.06	0.02	0.25	0.25	XXX	
	TC	A		0.00	0.50	0.50	0.02	0.52	0.52	XXX	
73562		A	three views	0.18	0.60	0.60	0.05	0.83	0.83	XXX	
	26	A		0.18	0.06	0.06	0.02	0.26	0.26	XXX	
	TC	A		0.00	0.54	0.54	0.03	0.57	0.57	XXX	
73564		A	complete, four or more views	0.22	0.67	0.67	0.05	0.94	0.94	XXX	
	26	A		0.22	0.08	0.08	0.02	0.32	0.32	XXX	
	TC	A		0.00	0.59	0.59	0.03	0.62	0.62	XXX	
73565		A	both knees, standing, anteroposterior	0.17	0.54	0.54	0.04	0.75	0.75	XXX	
	26	A		0.17	0.07	0.07	0.02	0.26	0.26	XXX	
	TC	A		0.00	0.47	0.47	0.02	0.49	0.49	XXX	
73580		A	Radiologic examination, knee, arthrography, radiological supervision and interpretation	0.54	2.68	2.68	0.15	3.37	3.37	XXX	
	26	A		0.54	0.19	0.19	0.03	0.76	0.76	XXX	
	TC	A		0.00	2.49	2.49	0.12	2.61	2.61	XXX	
73590		A	Radiologic examination; tibia and fibula, two views	0.17	0.56	0.56	0.03	0.76	0.76	XXX	
	26	A		0.17	0.06	0.06	0.01	0.24	0.24	XXX	
	TC	A		0.00	0.50	0.50	0.02	0.52	0.52	XXX	
73592		A	lower extremity, infant, minimum of two views	0.16	0.53	0.53	0.03	0.72	0.72	XXX	
	26	A		0.16	0.06	0.06	0.01	0.23	0.23	XXX	
	TC	A		0.00	0.47	0.47	0.02	0.49	0.49	XXX	
73600		A	Radiologic examination, ankle; two views	0.16	0.53	0.53	0.03	0.72	0.72	XXX	
	26	A		0.16	0.06	0.06	0.01	0.23	0.23	XXX	
	TC	A		0.00	0.47	0.47	0.02	0.49	0.49	XXX	
73610		A	complete, minimum of three views	0.17	0.57	0.57	0.03	0.77	0.77	XXX	
	26	A		0.17	0.06	0.06	0.01	0.24	0.24	XXX	
	TC	A		0.00	0.51	0.51	0.02	0.53	0.53	XXX	
73615		A	Radiologic examination, ankle, arthrography, radiological supervision and interpretation	0.54	2.18	2.18	0.13	2.85	2.85	XXX	
	26	A		0.54	0.19	0.19	0.03	0.76	0.76	XXX	
	TC	A		0.00	1.99	1.99	0.10	2.09	2.09	XXX	
73620		A	Radiologic examination, foot; two views	0.16	0.53	0.53	0.03	0.72	0.72	XXX	
	26	A		0.16	0.06	0.06	0.01	0.23	0.23	XXX	
	TC	A		0.00	0.47	0.47	0.02	0.49	0.49	XXX	
73630		A	complete, minimum of three views	0.17	0.57	0.57	0.03	0.77	0.77	XXX	
	26	A		0.17	0.06	0.06	0.01	0.24	0.24	XXX	
	TC	A		0.00	0.51	0.51	0.02	0.53	0.53	XXX	

Radiology

■ RVU not developed by CMS. Gap-filled RVUs developed by CHEG.

Code	M	S	Description	Work Value	Non-Fac PE	Fac PE	Mal-practice	Non-Fac Total	Fac Total	Global	Gap
73650		A	Radiologic examination; calcaneus, minimum of two views	0.16	0.51	0.51	0.03	0.70	0.70	XXX	
	26	A		0.16	0.06	0.06	0.01	0.23	0.23	XXX	
	TC	A		0.00	0.45	0.45	0.02	0.47	0.47	XXX	
73660		A	toe(s), minimum of two views	0.13	0.44	0.44	0.03	0.60	0.60	XXX	
	26	A		0.13	0.05	0.05	0.01	0.19	0.19	XXX	
	TC	A		0.00	0.39	0.39	0.02	0.41	0.41	XXX	
73700		A	Computerized axial tomography, lower extremity; without contrast material	1.09	5.09	5.09	0.26	6.44	6.44	XXX	
	26	A		1.09	0.38	0.38	0.05	1.52	1.52	XXX	
	TC	A		0.00	4.71	4.71	0.21	4.92	4.92	XXX	
73701		A	with contrast material(s)	1.16	6.02	6.02	0.31	7.49	7.49	XXX	
	26	A		1.16	0.41	0.41	0.05	1.62	1.62	XXX	
	TC	A		0.00	5.61	5.61	0.26	5.87	5.87	XXX	
73702		A	without contrast material, followed by contrast material(s) and further sections	1.22	7.48	7.48	0.37	9.07	9.07	XXX	
	26	A		1.22	0.43	0.43	0.05	1.70	1.70	XXX	
	TC	A		0.00	7.05	7.05	0.32	7.37	7.37	XXX	
73706		A	Computed tomographic angiography, lower extremity, without contrast material(s), followed by contrast material(s) and further sections, including image post-processing	1.90	7.81	7.81	0.38	10.09	10.09	XXX	
	26	A		1.90	0.76	0.76	0.06	2.72	2.72	XXX	
	TC	A		0.00	7.05	7.05	0.32	7.37	7.37	XXX	
73718		A	Magnetic resonance (eg, proton) imaging, lower extremity other than joint; without contrast material(s)	1.35	11.11	11.11	0.36	12.82	12.82	XXX	
	26	A		1.35	0.47	0.47	0.04	1.86	1.86	XXX	
	TC	A		0.00	10.64	10.64	0.32	10.96	10.96	XXX	
73719		A	with contrast material(s)	1.62	13.32	13.32	0.44	15.38	15.38	XXX	
	26	A		1.62	0.56	0.56	0.05	2.23	2.23	XXX	
	TC	A		0.00	12.76	12.76	0.39	13.15	13.15	XXX	
73720		A	without contrast material(s), followed by contrast material(s) and further sequences	2.15	24.39	24.39	0.78	27.32	27.32	XXX	
	26	A		2.15	0.75	0.75	0.08	2.98	2.98	XXX	
	TC	A		0.00	23.64	23.64	0.70	24.34	24.34	XXX	
73721		A	Magnetic resonance (eg, proton) imaging, any joint of lower extremity; without contrast material	1.35	11.11	11.11	0.36	12.82	12.82	XXX	
	26	A		1.35	0.47	0.47	0.04	1.86	1.86	XXX	
	TC	A		0.00	10.64	10.64	0.32	10.96	10.96	XXX	
73722		A	with contrast material(s)	1.62	13.33	13.33	0.45	15.40	15.40	XXX	
	26	A		1.62	0.57	0.57	0.06	2.25	2.25	XXX	
	TC	A		0.00	12.76	12.76	0.39	13.15	13.15	XXX	
73723		A	without contrast material(s), followed by contrast material(s) and further sequences	2.15	24.39	24.39	0.77	27.31	27.31	XXX	
	26	A		2.15	0.75	0.75	0.07	2.97	2.97	XXX	
	TC	A		0.00	23.64	23.64	0.70	24.34	24.34	XXX	
73725		R	Magnetic resonance angiography, lower extremity, with or without contrast material(s)	1.82	11.28	11.28	0.57	13.67	13.67	XXX	
	26	R		1.82	0.64	0.64	0.08	2.54	2.54	XXX	
	TC	R		0.00	10.64	10.64	0.49	11.13	11.13	XXX	
74000		A	Radiologic examination, abdomen; single anteroposterior view	0.18	0.56	0.56	0.03	0.77	0.77	XXX	
	26	A		0.18	0.06	0.06	0.01	0.25	0.25	XXX	
	TC	A		0.00	0.50	0.50	0.02	0.52	0.52	XXX	

■ RVU not developed by CMS. Gap-filled RVUs developed by CHEG.

Code	M	S	Description	Work Value	Non-Fac PE	Fac PE	Mal-prac-tice	Non-Fac Total	Fac Total	Global	Gap
74010		A	anteroposterior and additional oblique and cone views	0.23	0.62	0.62	0.04	0.89	0.89	XXX	
	26	A		0.23	0.08	0.08	0.01	0.32	0.32	XXX	
	TC	A		0.00	0.54	0.54	0.03	0.57	0.57	XXX	
74020		A	complete, including decubitus and/or erect views	0.27	0.68	0.68	0.04	0.99	0.99	XXX	
	26	A		0.27	0.09	0.09	0.01	0.37	0.37	XXX	
	TC	A		0.00	0.59	0.59	0.03	0.62	0.62	XXX	
74022		A	complete acute abdomen series, including supine, erect, and/or decubitus views, upright PA chest	0.32	0.81	0.81	0.05	1.18	1.18	XXX	
	26	A		0.32	0.11	0.11	0.01	0.44	0.44	XXX	
	TC	A		0.00	0.70	0.70	0.04	0.74	0.74	XXX	
74150		A	Computerized axial tomography, abdomen; without contrast material	1.19	5.79	5.79	0.30	7.28	7.28	XXX	
	26	A		1.19	0.42	0.42	0.05	1.66	1.66	XXX	
	TC	A		0.00	5.37	5.37	0.25	5.62	5.62	XXX	
74160		A	with contrast material(s)	1.27	6.94	6.94	0.36	8.57	8.57	XXX	
	26	A		1.27	0.44	0.44	0.06	1.77	1.77	XXX	
	TC	A		0.00	6.50	6.50	0.30	6.80	6.80	XXX	
74170		A	without contrast material, followed by contrast material(s) and further sections	1.40	8.55	8.55	0.42	10.37	10.37	XXX	
	26	A		1.40	0.49	0.49	0.06	1.95	1.95	XXX	
	TC	A		0.00	8.06	8.06	0.36	8.42	8.42	XXX	
74175		A	Computed tomographic angiography, abdomen, without contrast material(s), followed by contrast material(s) and further sections, including image post-processing	1.90	8.82	8.82	0.38	11.10	11.10	XXX	
	26	A		1.90	0.76	0.76	0.06	2.72	2.72	XXX	
	TC	A		0.00	8.06	8.06	0.32	8.38	8.38	XXX	
74181		A	Magnetic resonance (eg, proton) imaging, abdomen; without contrast material(s)	1.46	11.15	11.15	0.41	13.02	13.02	XXX	
	26	A		1.46	0.51	0.51	0.04	2.01	2.01	XXX	
	TC	A		0.00	10.64	10.64	0.37	11.01	11.01	XXX	
74182		A	with contrast material(s)	1.73	13.36	13.36	0.49	15.58	15.58	XXX	
	26	A		1.73	0.60	0.60	0.06	2.39	2.39	XXX	
	TC	A		0.00	12.76	12.76	0.43	13.19	13.19	XXX	
74183		A	without contrast material(s), followed by with contrast material(s) and further sequences	2.26	24.43	24.43	0.84	27.53	27.53	XXX	
	26	A		2.26	0.79	0.79	0.08	3.13	3.13	XXX	
	TC	A		0.00	23.64	23.64	0.76	24.40	24.40	XXX	
74185		R	Magnetic resonance angiography, abdomen, with or without contrast material(s)	1.80	11.27	11.27	0.57	13.64	13.64	XXX	
	26	R		1.80	0.63	0.63	0.08	2.51	2.51	XXX	
	TC	R		0.00	10.64	10.64	0.49	11.13	11.13	XXX	
74190		A	Peritoneogram (eg, after injection of air or contrast), radiological supervision and interpretation	0.48	1.41	1.41	0.08	1.97	1.97	XXX	
	26	A		0.48	0.17	0.17	0.02	0.67	0.67	XXX	
	TC	A		0.00	1.24	1.24	0.06	1.30	1.30	XXX	
74210		A	Radiologic examination; pharynx and/or cervical esophagus	0.36	1.26	1.26	0.07	1.69	1.69	XXX	
	26	A		0.36	0.13	0.13	0.02	0.51	0.51	XXX	
	TC	A		0.00	1.13	1.13	0.05	1.18	1.18	XXX	
74220		A	esophagus	0.46	1.29	1.29	0.07	1.82	1.82	XXX	
	26	A		0.46	0.16	0.16	0.02	0.64	0.64	XXX	
	TC	A		0.00	1.13	1.13	0.05	1.18	1.18	XXX	

■ RVU not developed by CMS. Gap-filled RVUs developed by CHEG.

Code	M	S	Description	Work Value	Non-Fac PE	Fac PE	Mal-practice	Non-Fac Total	Fac Total	Global	Gap
74230		A	Swallowing function, with cineradiography/ videoradiography	0.53	1.43	1.43	0.08	2.04	2.04	XXX	
	26	A		0.53	0.19	0.19	0.02	0.74	0.74	XXX	
	TC	A		0.00	1.24	1.24	0.06	1.30	1.30	XXX	
74235		A	Removal of foreign body(s), esophageal, with use of balloon catheter, radiological supervision and interpretation	1.19	2.90	2.90	0.17	4.26	4.26	XXX	
	26	A		1.19	0.41	0.41	0.05	1.65	1.65	XXX	
	TC	A		0.00	2.49	2.49	0.12	2.61	2.61	XXX	
74240		A	Radiologic examination, gastrointestinal tract, upper; with or without delayed films, without KUB	0.69	1.63	1.63	0.10	2.42	2.42	XXX	
	26	A		0.69	0.24	0.24	0.03	0.96	0.96	XXX	
	TC	A		0.00	1.39	1.39	0.07	1.46	1.46	XXX	
74241		A	with or without delayed films, with KUB	0.69	1.65	1.65	0.10	2.44	2.44	XXX	
	26	A		0.69	0.24	0.24	0.03	0.96	0.96	XXX	
	TC	A		0.00	1.41	1.41	0.07	1.48	1.48	XXX	
74245		A	with small intestine, includes multiple serial films	0.91	2.58	2.58	0.15	3.64	3.64	XXX	
	26	A		0.91	0.32	0.32	0.04	1.27	1.27	XXX	
	TC	A		0.00	2.26	2.26	0.11	2.37	2.37	XXX	
74246		A	Radiological examination, gastrointestinal tract, upper, air contrast, with specific high density barium, effervescent agent, with or without glucagon; with or without delayed films, without KUB	0.69	1.80	1.80	0.11	2.60	2.60	XXX	
	26	A		0.69	0.24	0.24	0.03	0.96	0.96	XXX	
	TC	A		0.00	1.56	1.56	0.08	1.64	1.64	XXX	
74247		A	with or without delayed films, with KUB	0.69	1.84	1.84	0.12	2.65	2.65	XXX	
	26	A		0.69	0.24	0.24	0.03	0.96	0.96	XXX	
	TC	A		0.00	1.60	1.60	0.09	1.69	1.69	XXX	
74249		A	with small intestine follow-through	0.91	2.76	2.76	0.16	3.83	3.83	XXX	
	26	A		0.91	0.32	0.32	0.04	1.27	1.27	XXX	
	TC	A		0.00	2.44	2.44	0.12	2.56	2.56	XXX	
74250		A	Radiologic examination, small intestine, includes multiple serial films;	0.47	1.40	1.40	0.08	1.95	1.95	XXX	
	26	A		0.47	0.16	0.16	0.02	0.65	0.65	XXX	
	TC	A		0.00	1.24	1.24	0.06	1.30	1.30	XXX	
74251		A	via enteroclysis tube	0.69	1.48	1.48	0.09	2.26	2.26	XXX	
	26	A		0.69	0.24	0.24	0.03	0.96	0.96	XXX	
	TC	A		0.00	1.24	1.24	0.06	1.30	1.30	XXX	
74260		A	Duodenography, hypotonic	0.50	1.58	1.58	0.09	2.17	2.17	XXX	
	26	A		0.50	0.17	0.17	0.02	0.69	0.69	XXX	
	TC	A		0.00	1.41	1.41	0.07	1.48	1.48	XXX	
74270		A	Radiologic examination, colon; barium enema, with or without KUB	0.69	1.86	1.86	0.12	2.67	2.67	XXX	
	26	A		0.69	0.24	0.24	0.03	0.96	0.96	XXX	
	TC	A		0.00	1.62	1.62	0.09	1.71	1.71	XXX	
74280		A	air contrast with specific high density barium, with or without glucagon	0.99	2.47	2.47	0.15	3.61	3.61	XXX	
	26	A		0.99	0.35	0.35	0.04	1.38	1.38	XXX	
	TC	A		0.00	2.12	2.12	0.11	2.23	2.23	XXX	
74283		A	Therapeutic enema, contrast or air, for reduction of intussusception or other intraluminal obstruction (eg, meconium ileus)	2.02	3.14	3.14	0.21	5.37	5.37	XXX	
	26	A		2.02	0.71	0.71	0.09	2.82	2.82	XXX	
	TC	A		0.00	2.43	2.43	0.12	2.55	2.55	XXX	

■ RVU not developed by CMS. Gap-filled RVUs developed by CHEG.

Code	M	S	Description	Work Value	Non-Fac PE	Fac PE	Mal-practice	Non-Fac Total	Fac Total	Global	Gap
74290		A	Cholecystography, oral contrast;	0.32	0.81	0.81	0.05	1.18	1.18	XXX	
	26	A		0.32	0.11	0.11	0.01	0.44	0.44	XXX	
	TC	A		0.00	0.70	0.70	0.04	0.74	0.74	XXX	
74291		A	additional or repeat examination or multiple day examination	0.20	0.46	0.46	0.03	0.69	0.69	XXX	
	26	A		0.20	0.07	0.07	0.01	0.28	0.28	XXX	
	TC	A		0.00	0.39	0.39	0.02	0.41	0.41	XXX	
74300		C	Cholangiography and/or pancreatography; intraoperative, radiological supervision and interpretation	1.03	0.37	0.37	0.06	1.46	1.46	XXX	■
	26	A		0.36	0.13	0.13	0.02	0.51	0.51	XXX	
	TC	C		0.67	0.24	0.24	0.04	0.95	0.95	XXX	■
74301		C	additional set intraoperative, radiological supervision and interpretation (List separately in addition to code for primary procedure)	0.60	0.20	0.20	0.03	0.83	0.83	ZZZ	■
	26	A		0.21	0.07	0.07	0.01	0.29	0.29	ZZZ	
	TC	C		0.39	0.13	0.13	0.02	0.54	0.54	ZZZ	■
74305		A	through existing catheter, radiological supervision and interpretation	0.42	0.89	0.89	0.06	1.37	1.37	XXX	
	26	A		0.42	0.15	0.15	0.02	0.59	0.59	XXX	
	TC	A		0.00	0.74	0.74	0.04	0.78	0.78	XXX	
74320		A	Cholangiography, percutaneous, transhepatic, radiological supervision and interpretation	0.54	3.18	3.18	0.16	3.88	3.88	XXX	
	26	A		0.54	0.19	0.19	0.02	0.75	0.75	XXX	
	TC	A		0.00	2.99	2.99	0.14	3.13	3.13	XXX	
74327		A	Postoperative biliary duct calculus removal, percutaneous via T-tube tract, basket, or snare (eg, Burhenne technique), radiological supervision and interpretation	0.70	1.91	1.91	0.12	2.73	2.73	XXX	
	26	A		0.70	0.24	0.24	0.03	0.97	0.97	XXX	
	TC	A		0.00	1.67	1.67	0.09	1.76	1.76	XXX	
74328		A	Endoscopic catheterization of the biliary ductal system, radiological supervision and interpretation	0.70	3.24	3.24	0.17	4.11	4.11	XXX	
	26	A		0.70	0.25	0.25	0.03	0.98	0.98	XXX	
	TC	A		0.00	2.99	2.99	0.14	3.13	3.13	XXX	
74329		A	Endoscopic catheterization of the pancreatic ductal system, radiological supervision and interpretation	0.70	3.24	3.24	0.17	4.11	4.11	XXX	
	26	A		0.70	0.25	0.25	0.03	0.98	0.98	XXX	
	TC	A		0.00	2.99	2.99	0.14	3.13	3.13	XXX	
74330		A	Combined endoscopic catheterization of the biliary and pancreatic ductal systems, radiological supervision and interpretation	0.90	3.31	3.31	0.18	4.39	4.39	XXX	
	26	A		0.90	0.32	0.32	0.04	1.26	1.26	XXX	
	TC	A		0.00	2.99	2.99	0.14	3.13	3.13	XXX	
74340		A	Introduction of long gastrointestinal tube (eg, Miller-Abbott), including multiple fluoroscopies and films, radiological supervision and interpretation	0.54	2.68	2.68	0.14	3.36	3.36	XXX	
	26	A		0.54	0.19	0.19	0.02	0.75	0.75	XXX	
	TC	A		0.00	2.49	2.49	0.12	2.61	2.61	XXX	
74350		A	Percutaneous placement of gastrostomy tube, radiological supervision and interpretation	0.76	3.26	3.26	0.17	4.19	4.19	XXX	
	26	A		0.76	0.27	0.27	0.03	1.06	1.06	XXX	
	TC	A		0.00	2.99	2.99	0.14	3.13	3.13	XXX	
74355		A	Percutaneous placement of enteroclysis tube, radiological supervision and interpretation	0.76	2.75	2.75	0.15	3.66	3.66	XXX	
	26	A		0.76	0.26	0.26	0.03	1.05	1.05	XXX	
	TC	A		0.00	2.49	2.49	0.12	2.61	2.61	XXX	
74360		A	Intraluminal dilation of strictures and/or obstructions (eg, esophagus), radiological supervision and interpretation	0.54	3.18	3.18	0.16	3.88	3.88	XXX	
	26	A		0.54	0.19	0.19	0.02	0.75	0.75	XXX	
	TC	A		0.00	2.99	2.99	0.14	3.13	3.13	XXX	

■ RVU not developed by CMS. Gap-filled RVUs developed by CHEG.

Code	M	S	Description	Work Value	Non-Fac PE	Fac PE	Mal-practice	Non-Fac Total	Fac Total	Global	Gap
74363		A	Percutaneous transhepatic dilation of biliary duct stricture with or without placement of stent, radiological supervision and interpretation	0.88	6.10	6.10	0.31	7.29	7.29	XXX	
	26	A		0.88	0.31	0.31	0.04	1.23	1.23	XXX	
	TC	A		0.00	5.79	5.79	0.27	6.06	6.06	XXX	
74400		A	Urography (pyelography), intravenous, with or without KUB, with or without tomography;	0.49	1.77	1.77	0.11	2.37	2.37	XXX	
	26	A		0.49	0.17	0.17	0.02	0.68	0.68	XXX	
	TC	A		0.00	1.60	1.60	0.09	1.69	1.69	XXX	
74410		A	Urography, infusion, drip technique and/or bolus technique;	0.49	2.02	2.02	0.11	2.62	2.62	XXX	
	26	A		0.49	0.17	0.17	0.02	0.68	0.68	XXX	
	TC	A		0.00	1.85	1.85	0.09	1.94	1.94	XXX	
74415		A	with nephrotomography	0.49	2.18	2.18	0.12	2.79	2.79	XXX	
	26	A		0.49	0.17	0.17	0.02	0.68	0.68	XXX	
	TC	A		0.00	2.01	2.01	0.10	2.11	2.11	XXX	
74420		A	Urography, retrograde, with or without KUB	0.36	2.62	2.62	0.14	3.12	3.12	XXX	
	26	A		0.36	0.13	0.13	0.02	0.51	0.51	XXX	
	TC	A		0.00	2.49	2.49	0.12	2.61	2.61	XXX	
74425		A	Urography, antegrade, (pyelostogram, nephrostogram, loopogram), radiological supervision and interpretation	0.36	1.37	1.37	0.08	1.81	1.81	XXX	
	26	A		0.36	0.13	0.13	0.02	0.51	0.51	XXX	
	TC	A		0.00	1.24	1.24	0.06	1.30	1.30	XXX	
74430		A	Cystography, minimum of three views, radiological supervision and interpretation	0.32	1.11	1.11	0.07	1.50	1.50	XXX	
	26	A		0.32	0.11	0.11	0.02	0.45	0.45	XXX	
	TC	A		0.00	1.00	1.00	0.05	1.05	1.05	XXX	
74440		A	Vasography, vesiculography, or epididymography, radiological supervision and interpretation	0.38	1.20	1.20	0.07	1.65	1.65	XXX	
	26	A		0.38	0.13	0.13	0.02	0.53	0.53	XXX	
	TC	A		0.00	1.07	1.07	0.05	1.12	1.12	XXX	
74445		A	Corpora cavernosography, radiological supervision and interpretation	1.14	1.46	1.46	0.10	2.70	2.70	XXX	
	26	A		1.14	0.39	0.39	0.05	1.58	1.58	XXX	
	TC	A		0.00	1.07	1.07	0.05	1.12	1.12	XXX	
74450		A	Urethrocystography, retrograde, radiological supervision and interpretation	0.33	1.51	1.51	0.09	1.93	1.93	XXX	
	26	A		0.33	0.12	0.12	0.02	0.47	0.47	XXX	
	TC	A		0.00	1.39	1.39	0.07	1.46	1.46	XXX	
74455		A	Urethrocystography, voiding, radiological supervision and interpretation	0.33	1.61	1.61	0.10	2.04	2.04	XXX	
	26	A		0.33	0.11	0.11	0.02	0.46	0.46	XXX	
	TC	A		0.00	1.50	1.50	0.08	1.58	1.58	XXX	
74470		A	Radiologic examination, renal cyst study, translumbar, contrast visualization, radiological supervision and interpretation	0.54	1.37	1.37	0.08	1.99	1.99	XXX	
	26	A		0.54	0.19	0.19	0.02	0.75	0.75	XXX	
	TC	A		0.00	1.18	1.18	0.06	1.24	1.24	XXX	
74475		A	Introduction of intracatheter or catheter into renal pelvis for drainage and/or injection, percutaneous, radiological supervision and interpretation	0.54	4.06	4.06	0.20	4.80	4.80	XXX	
	26	A		0.54	0.19	0.19	0.02	0.75	0.75	XXX	
	TC	A		0.00	3.87	3.87	0.18	4.05	4.05	XXX	
74480		A	Introduction of ureteral catheter or stent into ureter through renal pelvis for drainage and/or injection, percutaneous, radiological supervision and interpretation	0.54	4.06	4.06	0.20	4.80	4.80	XXX	
	26	A		0.54	0.19	0.19	0.02	0.75	0.75	XXX	
	TC	A		0.00	3.87	3.87	0.18	4.05	4.05	XXX	

■ RVU not developed by CMS. Gap-filled RVUs developed by CHEG.

Code	M	S	Description	Work Value	Non-Fac PE	Fac PE	Mal-practice	Non-Fac Total	Fac Total	Global	Gap
74485		A	Dilation of nephrostomy, ureters, or urethra, radiological supervision and interpretation	0.54	3.18	3.18	0.17	3.89	3.89	XXX	
	26	A		0.54	0.19	0.19	0.03	0.76	0.76	XXX	
	TC	A		0.00	2.99	2.99	0.14	3.13	3.13	XXX	
74710		A	Pelvimetry, with or without placental localization	0.34	1.12	1.12	0.07	1.53	1.53	XXX	
	26	A		0.34	0.12	0.12	0.02	0.48	0.48	XXX	
	TC	A		0.00	1.00	1.00	0.05	1.05	1.05	XXX	
74740		A	Hysterosalpingography, radiological supervision and interpretation	0.38	1.37	1.37	0.08	1.83	1.83	XXX	
	26	A		0.38	0.13	0.13	0.02	0.53	0.53	XXX	
	TC	A		0.00	1.24	1.24	0.06	1.30	1.30	XXX	
74742		A	Transcervical catheterization of fallopian tube, radiological supervision and interpretation	0.61	3.23	3.23	0.16	4.00	4.00	XXX	
	26	A		0.61	0.24	0.24	0.02	0.87	0.87	XXX	
	TC	A		0.00	2.99	2.99	0.14	3.13	3.13	XXX	
74775		A	Perineogram (eg, vaginogram, for sex determination or extent of anomalies)	0.62	1.62	1.62	0.10	2.34	2.34	XXX	
	26	A		0.62	0.23	0.23	0.03	0.88	0.88	XXX	
	TC	A		0.00	1.39	1.39	0.07	1.46	1.46	XXX	
75552		A	Cardiac magnetic resonance imaging for morphology; without contrast material	1.60	11.20	11.20	0.56	13.36	13.36	XXX	
	26	A		1.60	0.56	0.56	0.07	2.23	2.23	XXX	
	TC	A		0.00	10.64	10.64	0.49	11.13	11.13	XXX	
75553		A	with contrast material	2.00	11.35	11.35	0.58	13.93	13.93	XXX	
	26	A		2.00	0.71	0.71	0.09	2.80	2.80	XXX	
	TC	A		0.00	10.64	10.64	0.49	11.13	11.13	XXX	
75554		A	Cardiac magnetic resonance imaging for funciton, with or without morphology; complete study	1.83	11.33	11.33	0.56	13.72	13.72	XXX	
	26	A		1.83	0.69	0.69	0.07	2.59	2.59	XXX	
	TC	A		0.00	10.64	10.64	0.49	11.13	11.13	XXX	
75555		A	limited study	1.74	11.32	11.32	0.56	13.62	13.62	XXX	
	26	A		1.74	0.68	0.68	0.07	2.49	2.49	XXX	
	TC	A		0.00	10.64	10.64	0.49	11.13	11.13	XXX	
75556		N	Cardiac magnetic resonance imaging for velocity flow mapping	0.00	0.00	0.00	0.00	0.00	0.00	XXX	
75600		A	Aortography, thoracic, without serialography, radiological supervision and interpretation	0.49	12.16	12.16	0.56	13.21	13.21	XXX	
	26	A		0.49	0.20	0.20	0.02	0.71	0.71	XXX	
	TC	A		0.00	11.96	11.96	0.54	12.50	12.50	XXX	
75605		A	Aortography, thoracic, by serialography, radiological supervision and interpretation	1.14	12.39	12.39	0.59	14.12	14.12	XXX	
	26	A		1.14	0.43	0.43	0.05	1.62	1.62	XXX	
	TC	A		0.00	11.96	11.96	0.54	12.50	12.50	XXX	
75625		A	Aortography, abdominal, by serialography, radiological supervision and interpretation	1.14	12.37	12.37	0.59	14.10	14.10	XXX	
	26	A		1.14	0.41	0.41	0.05	1.60	1.60	XXX	
	TC	A		0.00	11.96	11.96	0.54	12.50	12.50	XXX	
75630		A	Aortography, abdominal plus bilateral iliofemoral lower extremity, catheter, by serialography, radiological supervision and interpretation	1.79	13.14	13.14	0.65	15.58	15.58	XXX	
	26	A		1.79	0.67	0.67	0.08	2.54	2.54	XXX	
	TC	A		0.00	12.47	12.47	0.57	13.04	13.04	XXX	

Radiology

■ RVU not developed by CMS. Gap-filled RVUs developed by CHEG.

Code	M	S	Description	Work Value	Non-Fac PE	Fac PE	Mal-practice	Non-Fac Total	Fac Total	Global	Gap
75635		A	Computed tomographic angiography, abdominal aorta and bilateral iliofemoral lower extremity runoff, radiological supervision and interpretation, without contrast material(s), followed by contrast material(s) and further sections, including image post-processing	2.40	9.02	9.02	0.41	11.83	11.83	XXX	
	26	A		2.40	0.96	0.96	0.09	3.45	3.45	XXX	
	TC	A		0.00	8.06	8.06	0.32	8.38	8.38	XXX	
75650		A	Angiography, cervicocerebral, catheter, including vessel origin, radiological supervision and interpretation	1.49	12.49	12.49	0.61	14.59	14.59	XXX	
	26	A		1.49	0.53	0.53	0.07	2.09	2.09	XXX	
	TC	A		0.00	11.96	11.96	0.54	12.50	12.50	XXX	
75658		A	Angiography, brachial, retrograde, radiological supervision and interpretation	1.31	12.44	12.44	0.60	14.35	14.35	XXX	
	26	A		1.31	0.48	0.48	0.06	1.85	1.85	XXX	
	TC	A		0.00	11.96	11.96	0.54	12.50	12.50	XXX	
75660		A	Angiography, external carotid, unilateral, selective, radiological supervision and interpretation	1.31	12.44	12.44	0.60	14.35	14.35	XXX	
	26	A		1.31	0.48	0.48	0.06	1.85	1.85	XXX	
	TC	A		0.00	11.96	11.96	0.54	12.50	12.50	XXX	
75662		A	Angiography, external carotid, bilateral, selective, radiological supervision and interpretation	1.66	12.60	12.60	0.62	14.88	14.88	XXX	
	26	A		1.66	0.64	0.64	0.08	2.38	2.38	XXX	
	TC	A		0.00	11.96	11.96	0.54	12.50	12.50	XXX	
75665		A	Angiography, carotid, cerebral, unilateral, radiological supervision and interpretation	1.31	12.43	12.43	0.61	14.35	14.35	XXX	
	26	A		1.31	0.47	0.47	0.07	1.85	1.85	XXX	
	TC	A		0.00	11.96	11.96	0.54	12.50	12.50	XXX	
75671		A	Angiography, carotid, cerebral, bilateral, radiological supervision and interpretation	1.66	12.55	12.55	0.62	14.83	14.83	XXX	
	26	A		1.66	0.59	0.59	0.08	2.33	2.33	XXX	
	TC	A		0.00	11.96	11.96	0.54	12.50	12.50	XXX	
75676		A	Angiography, carotid, cervical, unilateral, radiological supervision and interpretation	1.31	12.43	12.43	0.61	14.35	14.35	XXX	
	26	A		1.31	0.47	0.47	0.07	1.85	1.85	XXX	
	TC	A		0.00	11.96	11.96	0.54	12.50	12.50	XXX	
75680		A	Angiography, carotid, cervical, bilateral, radiological supervision and interpretation	1.66	12.55	12.55	0.62	14.83	14.83	XXX	
	26	A		1.66	0.59	0.59	0.08	2.33	2.33	XXX	
	TC	A		0.00	11.96	11.96	0.54	12.50	12.50	XXX	
75685		A	Angiography, vertebral, cervical, and/or intracranial, radiological supervision and interpretation	1.31	12.43	12.43	0.60	14.34	14.34	XXX	
	26	A		1.31	0.47	0.47	0.06	1.84	1.84	XXX	
	TC	A		0.00	11.96	11.96	0.54	12.50	12.50	XXX	
75705		A	Angiography, spinal, selective, radiological supervision and interpretation	2.18	12.75	12.75	0.65	15.58	15.58	XXX	
	26	A		2.18	0.79	0.79	0.11	3.08	3.08	XXX	
	TC	A		0.00	11.96	11.96	0.54	12.50	12.50	XXX	
75710		A	Angiography, extremity, unilateral, radiological supervision and interpretation	1.14	12.38	12.38	0.60	14.12	14.12	XXX	
	26	A		1.14	0.42	0.42	0.06	1.62	1.62	XXX	
	TC	A		0.00	11.96	11.96	0.54	12.50	12.50	XXX	
75716		A	Angiography, extremity, bilateral, radiological supervision and interpretation	1.31	12.43	12.43	0.60	14.34	14.34	XXX	
	26	A		1.31	0.47	0.47	0.06	1.84	1.84	XXX	
	TC	A		0.00	11.96	11.96	0.54	12.50	12.50	XXX	
75722		A	Angiography, renal, unilateral, selective (including flush aortogram), radiological supervision and interpretation	1.14	12.39	12.39	0.59	14.12	14.12	XXX	
	26	A		1.14	0.43	0.43	0.05	1.62	1.62	XXX	
	TC	A		0.00	11.96	11.96	0.54	12.50	12.50	XXX	

■ RVU not developed by CMS. Gap-filled RVUs developed by CHEG.

Code	M	S	Description	Work Value	Non-Fac PE	Fac PE	Mal-prac-tice	Non-Fac Total	Fac Total	Global	Gap
75724		A	Angiography, renal, bilateral, selective (including flush aortogram), radiological supervision and interpretation	1.49	12.56	12.56	0.59	14.64	14.64	XXX	
	26	A		1.49	0.60	0.60	0.05	2.14	2.14	XXX	
	TC	A		0.00	11.96	11.96	0.54	12.50	12.50	XXX	
75726		A	Angiography, visceral, selective or supraselective, (with or without flush aortogram), radiological supervision and interpretation	1.14	12.36	12.36	0.59	14.09	14.09	XXX	
	26	A		1.14	0.40	0.40	0.05	1.59	1.59	XXX	
	TC	A		0.00	11.96	11.96	0.54	12.50	12.50	XXX	
75731		A	Angiography, adrenal, unilateral, selective, radiological supervision and interpretation	1.14	12.36	12.36	0.59	14.09	14.09	XXX	
	26	A		1.14	0.40	0.40	0.05	1.59	1.59	XXX	
	TC	A		0.00	11.96	11.96	0.54	12.50	12.50	XXX	
75733		A	Angiography, adrenal, bilateral, selective, radiological supervision and interpretation	1.31	12.43	12.43	0.60	14.34	14.34	XXX	
	26	A		1.31	0.47	0.47	0.06	1.84	1.84	XXX	
	TC	A		0.00	11.96	11.96	0.54	12.50	12.50	XXX	
75736		A	Angiography, pelvic, selective or supraselective, radiological supervision and interpretation	1.14	12.37	12.37	0.59	14.10	14.10	XXX	
	26	A		1.14	0.41	0.41	0.05	1.60	1.60	XXX	
	TC	A		0.00	11.96	11.96	0.54	12.50	12.50	XXX	
75741		A	Angiography, pulmonary, unilateral, selective, radiological supervision and interpretation	1.31	12.42	12.42	0.60	14.33	14.33	XXX	
	26	A		1.31	0.46	0.46	0.06	1.83	1.83	XXX	
	TC	A		0.00	11.96	11.96	0.54	12.50	12.50	XXX	
75743		A	Angiography, pulmonary, bilateral, selective, radiological supervision and interpretation	1.66	12.54	12.54	0.61	14.81	14.81	XXX	
	26	A		1.66	0.58	0.58	0.07	2.31	2.31	XXX	
	TC	A		0.00	11.96	11.96	0.54	12.50	12.50	XXX	
75746		A	Angiography, pulmonary, by nonselective catheter or venous injection, radiological supervision and interpretation	1.14	12.36	12.36	0.59	14.09	14.09	XXX	
	26	A		1.14	0.40	0.40	0.05	1.59	1.59	XXX	
	TC	A		0.00	11.96	11.96	0.54	12.50	12.50	XXX	
75756		A	Angiography, internal mammary, radiological supervision and interpretation	1.14	12.44	12.44	0.58	14.16	14.16	XXX	
	26	A		1.14	0.48	0.48	0.04	1.66	1.66	XXX	
	TC	A		0.00	11.96	11.96	0.54	12.50	12.50	XXX	
75774		A	Angiography, selective, each additional vessel studied after basic examination, radiological supervision and interpretation (List separately in addition to code for primary procedure)	0.36	12.09	12.09	0.56	13.01	13.01	ZZZ	
	26	A		0.36	0.13	0.13	0.02	0.51	0.51	ZZZ	
	TC	A		0.00	11.96	11.96	0.54	12.50	12.50	ZZZ	
75790		A	Angiography, arteriovenous shunt (eg, dialysis patient), radiological supervision and interpretation	1.84	1.93	1.93	0.16	3.93	3.93	XXX	
	26	A		1.84	0.64	0.64	0.09	2.57	2.57	XXX	
	TC	A		0.00	1.29	1.29	0.07	1.36	1.36	XXX	
75801		A	Lymphangiography, extremity only, unilateral, radiological supervision and interpretation	0.81	5.42	5.42	0.29	6.52	6.52	XXX	
	26	A		0.81	0.28	0.28	0.05	1.14	1.14	XXX	
	TC	A		0.00	5.14	5.14	0.24	5.38	5.38	XXX	
75803		A	Lymphangiography, extremity only, bilateral, radiological supervision and interpretation	1.17	5.55	5.55	0.29	7.01	7.01	XXX	
	26	A		1.17	0.41	0.41	0.05	1.63	1.63	XXX	
	TC	A		0.00	5.14	5.14	0.24	5.38	5.38	XXX	
75805		A	Lymphangiography, pelvic/abdominal, unilateral, radiological supervision and interpretation	0.81	6.08	6.08	0.31	7.20	7.20	XXX	
	26	A		0.81	0.29	0.29	0.04	1.14	1.14	XXX	
	TC	A		0.00	5.79	5.79	0.27	6.06	6.06	XXX	

■ RVU not developed by CMS. Gap-filled RVUs developed by CHEG.

Code	M	S	Description	Work Value	Non-Fac PE	Fac PE	Mal-prac-tice	Non-Fac Total	Fac Total	Global	Gap
75807		A	Lymphangiography, pelvic/abdominal, bilateral, radiological supervision and interpretation	1.17	6.20	6.20	0.32	7.69	7.69	XXX	
	26	A		1.17	0.41	0.41	0.05	1.63	1.63	XXX	
	TC	A		0.00	5.79	5.79	0.27	6.06	6.06	XXX	
75809		A	Shuntogram for investigation of previously placed indwelling nonvascular shunt (eg, LeVeen shunt, ventriculoperitoneal shunt, indwelling infusion pump), radiological supervision and interpretation	0.47	0.91	0.91	0.06	1.44	1.44	XXX	
	26	A		0.47	0.17	0.17	0.02	0.66	0.66	XXX	
	TC	A		0.00	0.74	0.74	0.04	0.78	0.78	XXX	
75810		A	Splenoportography, radiological supervision and interpretation	1.14	12.36	12.36	0.60	14.10	14.10	XXX	
	26	A		1.14	0.40	0.40	0.06	1.60	1.60	XXX	
	TC	A		0.00	11.96	11.96	0.54	12.50	12.50	XXX	
75820		A	Venography, extremity, unilateral, radiological supervision and interpretation	0.70	1.15	1.15	0.08	1.93	1.93	XXX	
	26	A		0.70	0.25	0.25	0.03	0.98	0.98	XXX	
	TC	A		0.00	0.90	0.90	0.05	0.95	0.95	XXX	
75822		A	Venography, extremity, bilateral, radiological supervision and interpretation	1.06	1.77	1.77	0.12	2.95	2.95	XXX	
	26	A		1.06	0.37	0.37	0.05	1.48	1.48	XXX	
	TC	A		0.00	1.40	1.40	0.07	1.47	1.47	XXX	
75825		A	Venography, caval, inferior, with serialography, radiological supervision and interpretation	1.14	12.36	12.36	0.60	14.10	14.10	XXX	
	26	A		1.14	0.40	0.40	0.06	1.60	1.60	XXX	
	TC	A		0.00	11.96	11.96	0.54	12.50	12.50	XXX	
75827		A	Venography, caval, superior, with serialography, radiological supervision and interpretation	1.14	12.36	12.36	0.59	14.09	14.09	XXX	
	26	A		1.14	0.40	0.40	0.05	1.59	1.59	XXX	
	TC	A		0.00	11.96	11.96	0.54	12.50	12.50	XXX	
75831		A	Venography, renal, unilateral, selective, radiological supervision and interpretation	1.14	12.36	12.36	0.59	14.09	14.09	XXX	
	26	A		1.14	0.40	0.40	0.05	1.59	1.59	XXX	
	TC	A		0.00	11.96	11.96	0.54	12.50	12.50	XXX	
75833		A	Venography, renal, bilateral, selective, radiological supervision and interpretation	1.49	12.49	12.49	0.61	14.59	14.59	XXX	
	26	A		1.49	0.53	0.53	0.07	2.09	2.09	XXX	
	TC	A		0.00	11.96	11.96	0.54	12.50	12.50	XXX	
75840		A	Venography, adrenal, unilateral, selective, radiological supervision and interpretation	1.14	12.38	12.38	0.61	14.13	14.13	XXX	
	26	A		1.14	0.42	0.42	0.07	1.63	1.63	XXX	
	TC	A		0.00	11.96	11.96	0.54	12.50	12.50	XXX	
75842		A	Venography, adrenal, bilateral, selective, radiological supervision and interpretation	1.49	12.48	12.48	0.61	14.58	14.58	XXX	
	26	A		1.49	0.52	0.52	0.07	2.08	2.08	XXX	
	TC	A		0.00	11.96	11.96	0.54	12.50	12.50	XXX	
75860		A	Venography, sinus or jugular, catheter, radiological supervision and interpretation	1.14	12.39	12.39	0.60	14.13	14.13	XXX	
	26	A		1.14	0.43	0.43	0.06	1.63	1.63	XXX	
	TC	A		0.00	11.96	11.96	0.54	12.50	12.50	XXX	
75870		A	Venography, superior sagittal sinus, radiological supervision and interpretation	1.14	12.38	12.38	0.60	14.12	14.12	XXX	
	26	A		1.14	0.42	0.42	0.06	1.62	1.62	XXX	
	TC	A		0.00	11.96	11.96	0.54	12.50	12.50	XXX	
75872		A	Venography, epidural, radiological supervision and interpretation	1.14	12.36	12.36	0.59	14.09	14.09	XXX	
	26	A		1.14	0.40	0.40	0.05	1.59	1.59	XXX	
	TC	A		0.00	11.96	11.96	0.54	12.50	12.50	XXX	

■ RVU not developed by CMS. Gap-filled RVUs developed by CHEG.

Code	M	S	Description	Work Value	Non-Fac PE	Fac PE	Mal-practice	Non-Fac Total	Fac Total	Global	Gap
75880		A	Venography, orbital, radiological supervision and interpretation	0.70	1.17	1.17	0.08	1.95	1.95	XXX	
	26	A		0.70	0.27	0.27	0.03	1.00	1.00	XXX	
	TC	A		0.00	0.90	0.90	0.05	0.95	0.95	XXX	
75885		A	Percutaneous transhepatic portography with hemodynamic evaluation, radiological supervision and interpretation	1.44	12.46	12.46	0.60	14.50	14.50	XXX	
	26	A		1.44	0.50	0.50	0.06	2.00	2.00	XXX	
	TC	A		0.00	11.96	11.96	0.54	12.50	12.50	XXX	
75887		A	Percutaneous transhepatic portography without hemodynamic evaluation, radiological supervision and interpretation	1.44	12.46	12.46	0.60	14.50	14.50	XXX	
	26	A		1.44	0.50	0.50	0.06	2.00	2.00	XXX	
	TC	A		0.00	11.96	11.96	0.54	12.50	12.50	XXX	
75889		A	Hepatic venography, wedged or free, with hemodynamic evaluation, radiological supervision and interpretation	1.14	12.36	12.36	0.59	14.09	14.09	XXX	
	26	A		1.14	0.40	0.40	0.05	1.59	1.59	XXX	
	TC	A		0.00	11.96	11.96	0.54	12.50	12.50	XXX	
75891		A	Hepatic venography, wedged or free, without hemodynamic evaluation, radiological supervision and interpretation	1.14	12.36	12.36	0.59	14.09	14.09	XXX	
	26	A		1.14	0.40	0.40	0.05	1.59	1.59	XXX	
	TC	A		0.00	11.96	11.96	0.54	12.50	12.50	XXX	
75893		A	Venous sampling through catheter, with or without angiography (eg, for parathyroid hormone, renin), radiological supervision and interpretation	0.54	12.15	12.15	0.56	13.25	13.25	XXX	
	26	A		0.54	0.19	0.19	0.02	0.75	0.75	XXX	
	TC	A		0.00	11.96	11.96	0.54	12.50	12.50	XXX	
75894		A	Transcatheter therapy, embolization, any method, radiological supervision and interpretation	1.31	23.38	23.38	1.12	25.81	25.81	XXX	
	26	A		1.31	0.46	0.46	0.07	1.84	1.84	XXX	
	TC	A		0.00	22.92	22.92	1.05	23.97	23.97	XXX	
75896		A	Transcatheter therapy, infusion, any method (eg, thrombolysis other than coronary), radiological supervision and interpretation	1.31	20.42	20.42	0.97	22.70	22.70	XXX	
	26	A		1.31	0.48	0.48	0.06	1.85	1.85	XXX	
	TC	A		0.00	19.94	19.94	0.91	20.85	20.85	XXX	
75898		A	Angiography through existing catheter for follow-up study for transcatheter therapy, embolization or infusion	1.65	1.60	1.60	0.12	3.37	3.37	XXX	
	26	A		1.65	0.60	0.60	0.07	2.32	2.32	XXX	
	TC	A		0.00	1.00	1.00	0.05	1.05	1.05	XXX	
75900		A	Exchange of a previously placed arterial catheter during thrombolytic therapy with contrast monitoring, radiological supervision and interpretation	0.49	20.09	20.09	0.94	21.52	21.52	XXX	
	26	A		0.49	0.17	0.17	0.02	0.68	0.68	XXX	
	TC	A		0.00	19.92	19.92	0.92	20.84	20.84	XXX	
75940		A	Percutaneous placement of IVC filter, radiological supervision and interpretation	0.54	12.15	12.15	0.57	13.26	13.26	XXX	
	26	A		0.54	0.19	0.19	0.03	0.76	0.76	XXX	
	TC	A		0.00	11.96	11.96	0.54	12.50	12.50	XXX	
75945		A	Intravascular ultrasound (non-coronary vessel), radiological supervision and interpretation; initial vessel	0.40	4.48	4.48	0.23	5.11	5.11	XXX	
	26	A		0.40	0.15	0.15	0.03	0.58	0.58	XXX	
	TC	A		0.00	4.33	4.33	0.20	4.53	4.53	XXX	
75946		A	each additional non-coronary vessel (List separately in addition to code for primary procedure)	0.40	2.32	2.32	0.14	2.86	2.86	ZZZ	
	26	A		0.40	0.14	0.14	0.03	0.57	0.57	ZZZ	
	TC	A		0.00	2.18	2.18	0.11	2.29	2.29	ZZZ	
75952		C	Endovascular repair of infrarenal abdominal aortic aneurysm or dissection, radiological supervision and interpretation	45.00	18.00	18.00	6.80	69.80	69.80	XXX	■
	26	A		4.50	1.80	1.80	0.68	6.98	6.98	XXX	
	TC	C		40.50	16.20	16.20	6.12	62.82	62.82	XXX	■

■ RVU not developed by CMS. Gap-filled RVUs developed by CHEG.

Code	M	S	Description	Work Value	Non-Fac PE	Fac PE	Mal-practice	Non-Fac Total	Fac Total	Global	Gap
75953		C	Placement of proximal or distal extension prosthesis for endovascular repair of infrarenal abdominal aortic aneurysm, radiological supervision and interpretation	13.60	5.40	5.40	6.80	25.80	25.80	XXX	■
	26	A		1.36	0.54	0.54	0.68	2.58	2.58	XXX	
	TC	C		12.24	4.86	4.86	6.12	23.22	23.22	XXX	■
75960		A	Transcatheter introduction of intravascular stent(s), (non-coronary vessel), percutaneous and/or open, radiological supervision and interpretation, each vessel	0.82	14.45	14.45	0.68	15.95	15.95	XXX	
	26	A		0.82	0.30	0.30	0.04	1.16	1.16	XXX	
	TC	A		0.00	14.15	14.15	0.64	14.79	14.79	XXX	
75961		A	Transcatheter retrieval, percutaneous, of intravascular foreign body (eg, fractured venous or arterial catheter), radiological supervision and interpretation	4.25	11.46	11.46	0.64	16.35	16.35	XXX	
	26	A		4.25	1.49	1.49	0.18	5.92	5.92	XXX	
	TC	A		0.00	9.97	9.97	0.46	10.43	10.43	XXX	
75962		A	Transluminal balloon angioplasty, peripheral artery, radiological supervision and interpretation	0.54	15.15	15.15	0.72	16.41	16.41	XXX	
	26	A		0.54	0.20	0.20	0.03	0.77	0.77	XXX	
	TC	A		0.00	14.95	14.95	0.69	15.64	15.64	XXX	
75964		A	Transluminal balloon angioplasty, each additional peripheral artery, radiological supervision and interpretation (List separately in addition to code for primary procedure)	0.36	8.10	8.10	0.38	8.84	8.84	ZZZ	
	26	A		0.36	0.13	0.13	0.02	0.51	0.51	ZZZ	
	TC	A		0.00	7.97	7.97	0.36	8.33	8.33	ZZZ	
75966		A	Transluminal balloon angioplasty, renal or other visceral artery, radiological supervision and interpretation	1.31	15.45	15.45	0.75	17.51	17.51	XXX	
	26	A		1.31	0.50	0.50	0.06	1.87	1.87	XXX	
	TC	A		0.00	14.95	14.95	0.69	15.64	15.64	XXX	
75968		A	Transluminal balloon angioplasty, each additional visceral artery, radiological supervision and interpretation (List separately in addition to code for primary procedure)	0.36	8.11	8.11	0.37	8.84	8.84	ZZZ	
	26	A		0.36	0.14	0.14	0.01	0.51	0.51	ZZZ	
	TC	A		0.00	7.97	7.97	0.36	8.33	8.33	ZZZ	
75970		A	Transcatheter biopsy, radiological supervision and interpretation	0.83	11.26	11.26	0.54	12.63	12.63	XXX	
	26	A		0.83	0.30	0.30	0.04	1.17	1.17	XXX	
	TC	A		0.00	10.96	10.96	0.50	11.46	11.46	XXX	
75978		A	Transluminal balloon angioplasty, venous (eg, subclavian stenosis), radiological supervision and interpretation	0.54	15.14	15.14	0.71	16.39	16.39	XXX	
	26	A		0.54	0.19	0.19	0.02	0.75	0.75	XXX	
	TC	A		0.00	14.95	14.95	0.69	15.64	15.64	XXX	
75980		A	Percutaneous transhepatic biliary drainage with contrast monitoring, radiological supervision and interpretation	1.44	5.64	5.64	0.30	7.38	7.38	XXX	
	26	A		1.44	0.50	0.50	0.06	2.00	2.00	XXX	
	TC	A		0.00	5.14	5.14	0.24	5.38	5.38	XXX	
75982		A	Percutaneous placement of drainage catheter for combined internal and external biliary drainage or of a drainage stent for internal biliary drainage in patients with an inoperable mechanical biliary obstruction, radiological supervision and interpretation	1.44	6.29	6.29	0.33	8.06	8.06	XXX	
	26	A		1.44	0.50	0.50	0.06	2.00	2.00	XXX	
	TC	A		0.00	5.79	5.79	0.27	6.06	6.06	XXX	
75984		A	Change of percutaneous tube or drainage catheter with contrast monitoring (eg, gastrointestinal system, genitourinary system, abscess), radiological supervision and interpretation	0.72	2.10	2.10	0.12	2.94	2.94	XXX	
	26	A		0.72	0.25	0.25	0.03	1.00	1.00	XXX	
	TC	A		0.00	1.85	1.85	0.09	1.94	1.94	XXX	

■ RVU not developed by CMS. Gap-filled RVUs developed by CHEG.

Code	M	S	Description	Work Value	Non-Fac PE	Fac PE	Mal-practice	Non-Fac Total	Fac Total	Global	Gap
75989		A	Radiological guidance for percutaneous drainage of abscess, or specimen collection (ie, fluoroscopy, ultrasound, or computed axial tomography), with placement of indwelling catheter, radiological supervision and interpretation	1.19	3.41	3.41	0.19	4.79	4.79	XXX	
	26	A		1.19	0.42	0.42	0.05	1.66	1.66	XXX	
	TC	A		0.00	2.99	2.99	0.14	3.13	3.13	XXX	
75992		A	Transluminal atherectomy, peripheral artery, radiological supervision and interpretation	0.54	15.15	15.15	0.71	16.40	16.40	XXX	
	26	A		0.54	0.20	0.20	0.02	0.76	0.76	XXX	
	TC	A		0.00	14.95	14.95	0.69	15.64	15.64	XXX	
75993		A	Transluminal atherectomy, each additional peripheral artery, radiological supervision and interpretation (List separately in addition to code for primary procedure)	0.36	8.11	8.11	0.37	8.84	8.84	ZZZ	
	26	A		0.36	0.14	0.14	0.01	0.51	0.51	ZZZ	
	TC	A		0.00	7.97	7.97	0.36	8.33	8.33	ZZZ	
75994		A	Transluminal atherectomy, renal, radiological supervision and interpretation	1.31	15.45	15.45	0.75	17.51	17.51	XXX	
	26	A		1.31	0.50	0.50	0.06	1.87	1.87	XXX	
	TC	A		0.00	14.95	14.95	0.69	15.64	15.64	XXX	
75995		A	Transluminal atherectomy, visceral, radiological supervision and interpretation	1.31	15.42	15.42	0.75	17.48	17.48	XXX	
	26	A		1.31	0.47	0.47	0.06	1.84	1.84	XXX	
	TC	A		0.00	14.95	14.95	0.69	15.64	15.64	XXX	
75996		A	Transluminal atherectomy, each additional visceral artery, radiological supervision and interpretation (List separately in addition to code for primary procedure)	0.36	8.09	8.09	0.37	8.82	8.82	ZZZ	
	26	A		0.36	0.12	0.12	0.01	0.49	0.49	ZZZ	
	TC	A		0.00	7.97	7.97	0.36	8.33	8.33	ZZZ	
76000		A	Fluoroscopy (separate procedure), up to one hour physician time, other than 71023 or 71034 (eg, cardiac fluoroscopy)	0.17	1.31	1.31	0.07	1.55	1.55	XXX	
	26	A		0.17	0.07	0.07	0.01	0.25	0.25	XXX	
	TC	A		0.00	1.24	1.24	0.06	1.30	1.30	XXX	
76001		A	Fluoroscopy, physician time more than one hour, assisting a non-radiologic physician (eg, nephrostolithotomy, ERCP, bronchoscopy, transbronchial biopsy)	0.67	2.73	2.73	0.15	3.55	3.55	XXX	
	26	A		0.67	0.24	0.24	0.03	0.94	0.94	XXX	
	TC	A		0.00	2.49	2.49	0.12	2.61	2.61	XXX	
76003		A	Fluoroscopic guidance for needle placement (eg, biopsy, aspiration, injection, localization device)	0.54	1.43	1.43	0.09	2.06	2.06	XXX	
	26	A		0.54	0.19	0.19	0.03	0.76	0.76	XXX	
	TC	A		0.00	1.24	1.24	0.06	1.30	1.30	XXX	
76005		A	Fluoroscopic guidance and localization of needle or catheter tip for spine or paraspinous diagnostic or therapeutic injection procedures (epidural, transforaminal epidural, subarachnoid, paravertebral facet joint, paravertebral facet joint nerve or sacroiliac joint), including neurolytic agent destruction	0.60	1.41	1.41	0.09	2.10	2.10	XXX	
	26	A		0.60	0.17	0.17	0.03	0.80	0.80	XXX	
	TC	A		0.00	1.24	1.24	0.06	1.30	1.30	XXX	
76006		A	Radiologic examination, stress view(s), any joint, stress applied by a physician (includes comparison views)	0.41	0.20	0.20	0.04	0.65	0.65	XXX	
	26			0.25	0.12	0.12	0.02	0.39	0.39	XXX	■
	TC			0.16	0.08	0.08	0.02	0.26	0.26	XXX	■
76010		A	Radiologic examination from nose to rectum for foreign body, single view, child	0.18	0.56	0.56	0.03	0.77	0.77	XXX	
	26	A		0.18	0.06	0.06	0.01	0.25	0.25	XXX	
	TC	A		0.00	0.50	0.50	0.02	0.52	0.52	XXX	

Radiology

■ RVU not developed by CMS. Gap-filled RVUs developed by CHEG.

Code	M	S	Description	Work Value	Non-Fac PE	Fac PE	Mal-prac-tice	Non-Fac Total	Fac Total	Global	Gap
76012		C	Radiological supervision and interpretation, percutaneous vertebroplasty, per vertebral body; under fluoroscopic guidance	3.74	1.49	1.49	0.66	5.89	5.89	XXX	■
	26	A		1.31	0.52	0.52	0.23	2.06	2.06	XXX	
	TC	C		2.43	0.97	0.97	0.43	3.83	3.83	XXX	■
76013		C	under CT guidance	6.90	2.75	2.75	2.40	12.05	12.05	XXX	■
	26	A		1.38	0.55	0.55	0.48	2.41	2.41	XXX	
	TC	C		5.52	2.20	2.20	1.92	9.64	9.64	XXX	■
76020		A	Bone age studies	0.19	0.57	0.57	0.03	0.79	0.79	XXX	
	26	A		0.19	0.07	0.07	0.01	0.27	0.27	XXX	
	TC	A		0.00	0.50	0.50	0.02	0.52	0.52	XXX	
76040		A	Bone length studies (orthoroentgenogram, scanogram)	0.27	0.84	0.84	0.07	1.18	1.18	XXX	
	26	A		0.27	0.10	0.10	0.03	0.40	0.40	XXX	
	TC	A		0.00	0.74	0.74	0.04	0.78	0.78	XXX	
76061		A	Radiologic examination, osseous survey; limited (eg, for metastases)	0.45	1.11	1.11	0.07	1.63	1.63	XXX	
	26	A		0.45	0.16	0.16	0.02	0.63	0.63	XXX	
	TC	A		0.00	0.95	0.95	0.05	1.00	1.00	XXX	
76062		A	complete (axial and appendicular skeleton)	0.54	1.56	1.56	0.09	2.19	2.19	XXX	
	26	A		0.54	0.19	0.19	0.02	0.75	0.75	XXX	
	TC	A		0.00	1.37	1.37	0.07	1.44	1.44	XXX	
76065		A	Radiologic examination, osseous survey, infant	0.70	0.95	0.95	0.05	1.70	1.70	XXX	
	26	A		0.70	0.25	0.25	0.01	0.96	0.96	XXX	
	TC	A		0.00	0.70	0.70	0.04	0.74	0.74	XXX	
76066		A	Joint survey, single view, one or more joints (specify)	0.31	1.17	1.17	0.07	1.55	1.55	XXX	
	26	A		0.31	0.11	0.11	0.02	0.44	0.44	XXX	
	TC	A		0.00	1.06	1.06	0.05	1.11	1.11	XXX	
76070		I	Computerized axial tomography bone density study, one or more sites	0.25	2.90	2.90	0.14	3.29	3.29	XXX	
	26	I		0.25	0.10	0.10	0.01	0.36	0.36	XXX	
	TC	I		0.00	2.80	2.80	0.13	2.93	2.93	XXX	
76075		A	Dual energy x-ray absorptiometry (DEXA), bone density study, one or more sites; axial skeleton (eg, hips, pelvis, spine)	0.30	3.05	3.05	0.15	3.50	3.50	XXX	
	26	A		0.30	0.11	0.11	0.01	0.42	0.42	XXX	
	TC	A		0.00	2.94	2.94	0.14	3.08	3.08	XXX	
76076		A	appendicular skeleton (peripheral) (eg, radius, wrist, heel)	0.22	0.80	0.80	0.05	1.07	1.07	XXX	
	26	A		0.22	0.08	0.08	0.01	0.31	0.31	XXX	
	TC	A		0.00	0.72	0.72	0.04	0.76	0.76	XXX	
76078		A	Radiographic absorptiometry (eg, photodensitometry, radiogrammetry), one or more sites	0.20	0.80	0.80	0.05	1.05	1.05	XXX	
	26	A		0.20	0.08	0.08	0.01	0.29	0.29	XXX	
	TC	A		0.00	0.72	0.72	0.04	0.76	0.76	XXX	
76080		A	Radiologic examination, abscess, fistula or sinus tract study, radiological supervision and interpretation	0.54	1.19	1.19	0.07	1.80	1.80	XXX	
	26	A		0.54	0.19	0.19	0.02	0.75	0.75	XXX	
	TC	A		0.00	1.00	1.00	0.05	1.05	1.05	XXX	
76085		A	Digitization of film radiographic images with computer analysis for lesion detection and further physician review for interpretation, screening mammography (List separately in addition to code for primary procedure)	0.06	0.31	0.31	0.02	0.39	0.39	ZZZ	
	26	A		0.06	0.02	0.02	0.01	0.09	0.09	ZZZ	
	TC	A		0.00	0.29	0.29	0.01	0.30	0.30	XXX	

■ RVU not developed by CMS. Gap-filled RVUs developed by CHEG.

Code	M	S	Description	Work Value	Non-Fac PE	Fac PE	Mal-practice	Non-Fac Total	Fac Total	Global	Gap
76086		A	Mammary ductogram or galactogram, single duct, radiological supervision and interpretation	0.36	2.62	2.62	0.14	3.12	3.12	XXX	
	26	A		0.36	0.13	0.13	0.02	0.51	0.51	XXX	
	TC	A		0.00	2.49	2.49	0.12	2.61	2.61	XXX	
76088		A	Mammary ductogram or galactogram, multiple ducts, radiological supervision and interpretation	0.45	3.64	3.64	0.18	4.27	4.27	XXX	
	26	A		0.45	0.16	0.16	0.02	0.63	0.63	XXX	
	TC	A		0.00	3.48	3.48	0.16	3.64	3.64	XXX	
76090		A	Mammography; unilateral	0.70	1.25	1.25	0.08	2.03	2.03	XXX	
	26	A		0.70	0.25	0.25	0.03	0.98	0.98	XXX	
	TC	A		0.00	1.00	1.00	0.05	1.05	1.05	XXX	
76091		A	bilateral	0.87	1.54	1.54	0.09	2.50	2.50	XXX	
	26	A		0.87	0.30	0.30	0.03	1.20	1.20	XXX	
	TC	A		0.00	1.24	1.24	0.06	1.30	1.30	XXX	
76092		A	Screening mammography, bilateral (two view film study of each breast)	0.70	1.44	1.44	0.09	2.23	2.23	XXX	
	26	A		0.70	0.25	0.25	0.03	0.98	0.98	XXX	
	TC	A		0.00	1.19	1.19	0.06	1.25	1.25	XXX	
76093		A	Magnetic resonance imaging, breast, without and/or with contrast material(s); unilateral	1.63	17.31	17.31	0.83	19.77	19.77	XXX	
	26	A		1.63	0.57	0.57	0.07	2.27	2.27	XXX	
	TC	A		0.00	16.74	16.74	0.76	17.50	17.50	XXX	
76094		A	bilateral	1.63	23.28	23.28	1.10	26.01	26.01	XXX	
	26	A		1.63	0.57	0.57	0.07	2.27	2.27	XXX	
	TC	A		0.00	22.71	22.71	1.03	23.74	23.74	XXX	
76095		A	Stereotactic localization guidance for breast biopsy or needle placement (eg, for wire localization or for injection), each lesion, radiological supervision and interpretation	1.59	7.36	7.36	0.40	9.35	9.35	XXX	
	26	A		1.59	0.56	0.56	0.09	2.24	2.24	XXX	
	TC	A		0.00	6.80	6.80	0.31	7.11	7.11	XXX	
76096		A	Mammographic guidance for needle placement, breast (eg, for wire localization or for injection), each lesion, radiological supervision and interpretation	0.56	1.44	1.44	0.09	2.09	2.09	XXX	
	26	A		0.56	0.20	0.20	0.03	0.79	0.79	XXX	
	TC	A		0.00	1.24	1.24	0.06	1.30	1.30	XXX	
76098		A	Radiological examination, surgical specimen	0.16	0.45	0.45	0.03	0.64	0.64	XXX	
	26	A		0.16	0.06	0.06	0.01	0.23	0.23	XXX	
	TC	A		0.00	0.39	0.39	0.02	0.41	0.41	XXX	
76100		A	Radiologic examination, single plane body section (eg, tomography), other than with urography	0.58	1.38	1.38	0.09	2.05	2.05	XXX	
	26	A		0.58	0.20	0.20	0.03	0.81	0.81	XXX	
	TC	A		0.00	1.18	1.18	0.06	1.24	1.24	XXX	
76101		A	Radiologic examination, complex motion (ie, hypercycloidal) body section (eg, mastoid polytomography), other than with urography; unilateral	0.58	1.55	1.55	0.10	2.23	2.23	XXX	
	26	A		0.58	0.20	0.20	0.03	0.81	0.81	XXX	
	TC	A		0.00	1.35	1.35	0.07	1.42	1.42	XXX	
76102		A	bilateral	0.58	1.84	1.84	0.12	2.54	2.54	XXX	
	26	A		0.58	0.20	0.20	0.03	0.81	0.81	XXX	
	TC	A		0.00	1.64	1.64	0.09	1.73	1.73	XXX	
76120		A	Cineradiography/videoradiography, except where specifically included	0.38	1.14	1.14	0.07	1.59	1.59	XXX	
	26	A		0.38	0.14	0.14	0.02	0.54	0.54	XXX	
	TC	A		0.00	1.00	1.00	0.05	1.05	1.05	XXX	

Radiology

■ RVU not developed by CMS. Gap-filled RVUs developed by CHEG.

Code	M	S	Description	Work Value	Non-Fac PE	Fac PE	Mal-practice	Non-Fac Total	Fac Total	Global	Gap
76125		A	Cineradiography/videoradiography to complement routine examination (List separately in addition to code for primary procedure)	0.27	0.84	0.84	0.05	1.16	1.16	ZZZ	
	26	A		0.27	0.10	0.10	0.01	0.38	0.38	ZZZ	
	TC	A		0.00	0.74	0.74	0.04	0.78	0.78	ZZZ	
76140		I	Consultation on x-ray examination made elsewhere, written report	0.00	0.00	0.00	0.00	0.00	0.00	XXX	
76150		A	Xeroradiography	0.00	0.39	0.39	0.02	0.41	0.41	XXX	
	26			0.00	0.00	0.00	0.00	0.00	0.00	XXX	■
	TC			0.00	0.39	0.39	0.02	0.41	0.41	XXX	■
76350		C	Subtraction in conjunction with contrast studies	0.15	0.82	0.82	0.04	1.01	1.01	XXX	■
	26			0.03	0.16	0.16	0.01	0.20	0.20	XXX	■
	TC			0.12	0.66	0.66	0.03	0.81	0.81	XXX	■
76355		A	Computerized axial tomographic guidance for stereotactic localization	1.21	8.28	8.28	0.41	9.90	9.90	XXX	
	26	A		1.21	0.44	0.44	0.06	1.71	1.71	XXX	
	TC	A		0.00	7.84	7.84	0.35	8.19	8.19	XXX	
76360		A	Computerized axial tomographic guidance for needle biopsy, radiological supervision and interpretation	1.16	8.24	8.24	0.40	9.80	9.80	XXX	
	26	A		1.16	0.40	0.40	0.05	1.61	1.61	XXX	
	TC	A		0.00	7.84	7.84	0.35	8.19	8.19	XXX	
76362		A	Computerized axial tomographic guidance for, and monitoring of, tissue ablation	4.00	9.24	9.24	1.38	14.62	14.62	XXX	
	26	A		4.00	1.40	1.40	0.17	5.57	5.57	XXX	
	TC	A		0.00	7.84	7.84	1.21	9.05	9.05	XXX	
76370		A	Computerized axial tomographic guidance for placement of radiation therapy fields	0.85	3.10	3.10	0.17	4.12	4.12	XXX	
	26	A		0.85	0.30	0.30	0.04	1.19	1.19	XXX	
	TC	A		0.00	2.80	2.80	0.13	2.93	2.93	XXX	
76375		A	Coronal, sagittal, multiplanar, oblique, 3-dimensional and/or holographic reconstruction of computerized axial tomography, magnetic resonance imaging, or other tomographic modality	0.16	3.42	3.42	0.16	3.74	3.74	XXX	
	26	A		0.16	0.06	0.06	0.01	0.23	0.23	XXX	
	TC	A		0.00	3.36	3.36	0.15	3.51	3.51	XXX	
76380		A	Computerized axial tomography, limited or localized follow-up study	0.98	3.66	3.66	0.19	4.83	4.83	XXX	
	26	A		0.98	0.34	0.34	0.04	1.36	1.36	XXX	
	TC	A		0.00	3.32	3.32	0.15	3.47	3.47	XXX	
76390		A	Magnetic resonance spectroscopy	1.40	11.14	11.14	0.55	13.09	13.09	XXX	
	26	A		1.40	0.50	0.50	0.06	1.96	1.96	XXX	
	TC	A		0.00	10.64	10.64	0.49	11.13	11.13	XXX	
76393		A	Magnetic resonance guidance for needle placement (eg, for biopsy, needle aspiration, injection, or placement of localization device) radiological supervision and interpretation	1.50	11.16	11.16	0.53	13.19	13.19	XXX	
	26	A		1.50	0.52	0.52	0.07	2.09	2.09	XXX	
	TC	A		0.00	10.64	10.64	0.46	11.10	11.10	XXX	
76394		A	Magnetic resonance guidance for, and monitoring of, tissue ablation	4.25	12.13	12.13	1.43	17.81	17.81	XXX	
	26	A		4.25	1.49	1.49	0.14	5.88	5.88	XXX	
	TC	A		0.00	10.64	10.64	1.29	11.93	11.93	XXX	
76400		A	Magnetic resonance (eg, proton) imaging, bone marrow blood supply	1.60	11.20	11.20	0.56	13.36	13.36	XXX	
	26	A		1.60	0.56	0.56	0.07	2.23	2.23	XXX	
	TC	A		0.00	10.64	10.64	0.49	11.13	11.13	XXX	

■ RVU not developed by CMS. Gap-filled RVUs developed by CHEG.

Code	M	S	Description	Work Value	Non-Fac PE	Fac PE	Mal-prac-tice	Non-Fac Total	Fac Total	Global	Gap
76490		A	Ultrasound guidance for, and monitoring of, tissue ablation	2.00	2.13	2.13	0.36	4.49	4.49	XXX	
	26	A		2.00	0.69	0.69	0.12	2.81	2.81	XXX	
	TC	A		0.00	1.44	1.44	0.24	1.68	1.68	XXX	
76499		C	Unlisted diagnostic radiologic procedure	0.00	0.00	0.00	0.00	0.00	0.00	XXX	
	26	C		0.00	0.00	0.00	0.00	0.00	0.00	XXX	
	TC	C		0.00	0.00	0.00	0.00	0.00	0.00	XXX	
76506		A	Echoencephalography, B-scan and/or real time with image documentation (gray scale) (for determination of ventricular size, delineation of cerebral contents and detection of fluid masses or other intracranial abnormalities), including A-mode encephalography as secondary component where indicated	0.63	1.61	1.61	0.10	2.34	2.34	XXX	
	26	A		0.63	0.26	0.26	0.03	0.92	0.92	XXX	
	TC	A		0.00	1.35	1.35	0.07	1.42	1.42	XXX	
76511		A	Ophthalmic ultrasound, echography, diagnostic; A-scan only, with amplitude quantification	0.94	2.37	2.37	0.08	3.39	3.39	XXX	
	26	A		0.94	0.45	0.45	0.02	1.41	1.41	XXX	
	TC	A		0.00	1.92	1.92	0.06	1.98	1.98	XXX	
76512		A	contact B-scan (with or without simultaneous A-scan)	0.66	2.49	2.49	0.09	3.24	3.24	XXX	
	26	A		0.66	0.31	0.31	0.01	0.98	0.98	XXX	
	TC	A		0.00	2.18	2.18	0.08	2.26	2.26	XXX	
76513		A	anterior segment ultrasound, immersion (water bath) B-scan or high resolution biomicroscopy	0.66	2.90	2.90	0.09	3.65	3.65	XXX	
	26	A		0.66	0.32	0.32	0.01	0.99	0.99	XXX	
	TC	A		0.00	2.58	2.58	0.08	2.66	2.66	XXX	
76516		A	Ophthalmic biometry by ultrasound echography, A-scan;	0.54	2.04	2.04	0.07	2.65	2.65	XXX	
	26	A		0.54	0.26	0.26	0.01	0.81	0.81	XXX	
	TC	A		0.00	1.78	1.78	0.06	1.84	1.84	XXX	
76519		A	with intraocular lens power calculation	0.54	1.91	1.91	0.07	2.52	2.52	XXX	
	26	A		0.54	0.26	0.26	0.01	0.81	0.81	XXX	
	TC	A		0.00	1.65	1.65	0.06	1.71	1.71	XXX	
76529		A	Ophthalmic ultrasonic foreign body localization	0.57	2.70	2.70	0.08	3.35	3.35	XXX	
	26	A		0.57	0.27	0.27	0.01	0.85	0.85	XXX	
	TC	A		0.00	2.43	2.43	0.07	2.50	2.50	XXX	
76536		A	Ultrasound, soft tissues of head and neck (eg, thyroid, parathyroid, parotid), B-scan and/or real time with image documentation	0.56	1.55	1.55	0.09	2.20	2.20	XXX	
	26	A		0.56	0.20	0.20	0.02	0.78	0.78	XXX	
	TC	A		0.00	1.35	1.35	0.07	1.42	1.42	XXX	
76604		A	Ultrasound, chest, B-scan (includes mediastinum) and/or real time with image documentation	0.55	1.43	1.43	0.08	2.06	2.06	XXX	
	26	A		0.55	0.19	0.19	0.02	0.76	0.76	XXX	
	TC	A		0.00	1.24	1.24	0.06	1.30	1.30	XXX	
76645		A	Ultrasound, breast(s) (unilateral or bilateral), B-scan and/or real time with image documentation	0.54	1.19	1.19	0.08	1.81	1.81	XXX	
	26	A		0.54	0.19	0.19	0.03	0.76	0.76	XXX	
	TC	A		0.00	1.00	1.00	0.05	1.05	1.05	XXX	
76700		A	Ultrasound, abdominal, B-scan and/or real time with image documentation; complete	0.81	2.15	2.15	0.13	3.09	3.09	XXX	
	26	A		0.81	0.28	0.28	0.04	1.13	1.13	XXX	
	TC	A		0.00	1.87	1.87	0.09	1.96	1.96	XXX	
76705		A	limited (eg, single organ, quadrant, follow-up)	0.59	1.56	1.56	0.10	2.25	2.25	XXX	
	26	A		0.59	0.21	0.21	0.03	0.83	0.83	XXX	
	TC	A		0.00	1.35	1.35	0.07	1.42	1.42	XXX	

Radiology

■ RVU not developed by CMS. Gap-filled RVUs developed by CHEG.

Code	M	S	Description	Work Value	Non-Fac PE	Fac PE	Mal-practice	Non-Fac Total	Fac Total	Global	Gap
76770		A	Ultrasound, retroperitoneal (eg, renal, aorta, nodes), B-scan and/or real time with image documentation; complete	0.74	2.13	2.13	0.12	2.99	2.99	XXX	
	26	A		0.74	0.26	0.26	0.03	1.03	1.03	XXX	
	TC	A		0.00	1.87	1.87	0.09	1.96	1.96	XXX	
76775		A	limited	0.58	1.55	1.55	0.10	2.23	2.23	XXX	
	26	A		0.58	0.20	0.20	0.03	0.81	0.81	XXX	
	TC	A		0.00	1.35	1.35	0.07	1.42	1.42	XXX	
76778		A	Ultrasound, transplanted kidney, B-scan and/or real time with image documentation, with or without duplex Doppler study	0.74	2.13	2.13	0.12	2.99	2.99	XXX	
	26	A		0.74	0.26	0.26	0.03	1.03	1.03	XXX	
	TC	A		0.00	1.87	1.87	0.09	1.96	1.96	XXX	
76800		A	Ultrasound, spinal canal and contents	1.13	1.73	1.73	0.11	2.97	2.97	XXX	
	26	A		1.13	0.38	0.38	0.04	1.55	1.55	XXX	
	TC	A		0.00	1.35	1.35	0.07	1.42	1.42	XXX	
76805		A	Ultrasound, pregnant uterus, B-scan and/or real time with image documentation; complete (complete fetal and maternal evaluation)	0.99	2.35	2.35	0.14	3.48	3.48	XXX	
	26	A		0.99	0.36	0.36	0.04	1.39	1.39	XXX	
	TC	A		0.00	1.99	1.99	0.10	2.09	2.09	XXX	
76810		A	complete (complete fetal and maternal evaluation), multiple gestation, after the first trimester	1.97	4.74	4.74	0.25	6.96	6.96	XXX	
	26	A		1.97	0.75	0.75	0.07	2.79	2.79	XXX	
	TC	A		0.00	3.99	3.99	0.18	4.17	4.17	XXX	
76815		A	limited (fetal size, heart beat, placental location, fetal position, or emergency in the delivery room)	0.65	1.60	1.60	0.09	2.34	2.34	XXX	
	26	A		0.65	0.25	0.25	0.02	0.92	0.92	XXX	
	TC	A		0.00	1.35	1.35	0.07	1.42	1.42	XXX	
76816		A	follow-up or repeat	0.57	1.28	1.28	0.07	1.92	1.92	XXX	
	26	A		0.57	0.22	0.22	0.02	0.81	0.81	XXX	
	TC	A		0.00	1.06	1.06	0.05	1.11	1.11	XXX	
76818		A	Fetal biophysical profile; with non-stress testing	1.05	1.94	1.94	0.12	3.11	3.11	XXX	
	26	A		1.05	0.41	0.41	0.04	1.50	1.50	XXX	
	TC	A		0.00	1.53	1.53	0.08	1.61	1.61	XXX	
76819		A	without non-stress testing	0.77	1.83	1.83	0.10	2.70	2.70	XXX	
	26	A		0.77	0.30	0.30	0.02	1.09	1.09	XXX	
	TC	A		0.00	1.53	1.53	0.08	1.61	1.61	XXX	
76825		A	Echocardiography, fetal, cardiovascular system, real time with image documentation (2D) with or without M-mode recording;	1.67	2.50	2.50	0.15	4.32	4.32	XXX	
	26	A		1.67	0.63	0.63	0.06	2.36	2.36	XXX	
	TC	A		0.00	1.87	1.87	0.09	1.96	1.96	XXX	
76826		A	follow-up or repeat study	0.83	0.97	0.97	0.07	1.87	1.87	XXX	
	26	A		0.83	0.30	0.30	0.03	1.16	1.16	XXX	
	TC	A		0.00	0.67	0.67	0.04	0.71	0.71	XXX	
76827		A	Doppler echocardiography, fetal, cardiovascular system, pulsed wave and/or continuous wave with spectral display; complete	0.58	1.85	1.85	0.12	2.55	2.55	XXX	
	26	A		0.58	0.22	0.22	0.02	0.82	0.82	XXX	
	TC	A		0.00	1.63	1.63	0.10	1.73	1.73	XXX	
76828		A	follow-up or repeat study	0.56	1.29	1.29	0.09	1.94	1.94	XXX	
	26	A		0.56	0.23	0.23	0.02	0.81	0.81	XXX	
	TC	A		0.00	1.06	1.06	0.07	1.13	1.13	XXX	
76830		A	Ultrasound, transvaginal	0.69	1.68	1.68	0.11	2.48	2.48	XXX	
	26	A		0.69	0.24	0.24	0.03	0.96	0.96	XXX	
	TC	A		0.00	1.44	1.44	0.08	1.52	1.52	XXX	

■ RVU not developed by CMS. Gap-filled RVUs developed by CHEG.

Code	M	S	Description	Work Value	Non-Fac PE	Fac PE	Mal-practice	Non-Fac Total	Fac Total	Global	Gap
76831		A	Hysterosonography, with or without color flow Doppler	0.72	1.71	1.71	0.10	2.53	2.53	XXX	
	26	A		0.72	0.27	0.27	0.02	1.01	1.01	XXX	
	TC	A		0.00	1.44	1.44	0.08	1.52	1.52	XXX	
76856		A	Ultrasound, pelvic (nonobstetric), B-scan and/or real time with image documentation; complete	0.69	1.68	1.68	0.11	2.48	2.48	XXX	
	26	A		0.69	0.24	0.24	0.03	0.96	0.96	XXX	
	TC	A		0.00	1.44	1.44	0.08	1.52	1.52	XXX	
76857		A	limited or follow-up (eg, for follicles)	0.38	1.13	1.13	0.07	1.58	1.58	XXX	
	26	A		0.38	0.13	0.13	0.02	0.53	0.53	XXX	
	TC	A		0.00	1.00	1.00	0.05	1.05	1.05	XXX	
76870		A	Ultrasound, scrotum and contents	0.64	1.66	1.66	0.11	2.41	2.41	XXX	
	26	A		0.64	0.22	0.22	0.03	0.89	0.89	XXX	
	TC	A		0.00	1.44	1.44	0.08	1.52	1.52	XXX	
76872		A	Echography, transrectal;	0.69	1.68	1.68	0.12	2.49	2.49	XXX	
	26	A		0.69	0.24	0.24	0.04	0.97	0.97	XXX	
	TC	A		0.00	1.44	1.44	0.08	1.52	1.52	XXX	
76873		A	prostate volume study for brachytherapy treatment planning (separate procedure)	1.55	2.53	2.53	0.21	4.29	4.29	XXX	
	26	A		1.55	0.54	0.54	0.08	2.17	2.17	XXX	
	TC	A		0.00	1.99	1.99	0.13	2.12	2.12	XXX	
76880		A	Ultrasound, extremity, non-vascular, B-scan and/or real time with image documentation	0.59	1.56	1.56	0.10	2.25	2.25	XXX	
	26	A		0.59	0.21	0.21	0.03	0.83	0.83	XXX	
	TC	A		0.00	1.35	1.35	0.07	1.42	1.42	XXX	
76885		A	Ultrasound, infant hips, real time with imaging documentation; dynamic (requiring physician manipulation)	0.74	1.70	1.70	0.11	2.55	2.55	XXX	
	26	A		0.74	0.26	0.26	0.03	1.03	1.03	XXX	
	TC	A		0.00	1.44	1.44	0.08	1.52	1.52	XXX	
76886		A	limited, static (not requiring physician manipulation)	0.62	1.57	1.57	0.10	2.29	2.29	XXX	
	26	A		0.62	0.22	0.22	0.03	0.87	0.87	XXX	
	TC	A		0.00	1.35	1.35	0.07	1.42	1.42	XXX	
76930		A	Ultrasonic guidance for pericardiocentesis, imaging supervision and interpretation	0.67	1.71	1.71	0.10	2.48	2.48	XXX	
	26	A		0.67	0.27	0.27	0.02	0.96	0.96	XXX	
	TC	A		0.00	1.44	1.44	0.08	1.52	1.52	XXX	
76932		A	Ultrasonic guidance for endomyocardial biopsy, imaging supervision and interpretation	0.67	1.71	1.71	0.10	2.48	2.48	XXX	
	26	A		0.67	0.27	0.27	0.02	0.96	0.96	XXX	
	TC	A		0.00	1.44	1.44	0.08	1.52	1.52	XXX	
76936		A	Ultrasound guided compression repair of arterial pseudo-aneurysm or arteriovenous fistulae (includes diagnostic ultrasound evaluation, compression of lesion and imaging)	1.99	6.68	6.68	0.39	9.06	9.06	XXX	
	26	A		1.99	0.70	0.70	0.11	2.80	2.80	XXX	
	TC	A		0.00	5.98	5.98	0.28	6.26	6.26	XXX	
76941		A	Ultrasonic guidance for intrauterine fetal transfusion or cordocentesis, imaging supervision and interpretation	1.34	1.98	1.98	0.13	3.45	3.45	XXX	
	26	A		1.34	0.53	0.53	0.06	1.93	1.93	XXX	
	TC	A		0.00	1.45	1.45	0.07	1.52	1.52	XXX	
76942		A	Ultrasonic guidance for needle placement (eg, biopsy, aspiration, injection, localization device), imaging supervision and interpretation	0.67	1.67	1.67	0.12	2.46	2.46	XXX	
	26	A		0.67	0.23	0.23	0.04	0.94	0.94	XXX	
	TC	A		0.00	1.44	1.44	0.08	1.52	1.52	XXX	

Radiology

■ RVU not developed by CMS. Gap-filled RVUs developed by CHEG.

Code	M	S	Description	Work Value	Non-Fac PE	Fac PE	Mal-practice	Non-Fac Total	Fac Total	Global	Gap
76945		A	Ultrasonic guidance for chorionic villus sampling, imaging supervision and interpretation	0.67	1.69	1.69	0.10	2.46	2.46	XXX	
	26	A		0.67	0.24	0.24	0.03	0.94	0.94	XXX	
	TC	A		0.00	1.45	1.45	0.07	1.52	1.52	XXX	
76946		A	Ultrasonic guidance for amniocentesis, imaging supervision and interpretation	0.38	1.59	1.59	0.09	2.06	2.06	XXX	
	26	A		0.38	0.15	0.15	0.01	0.54	0.54	XXX	
	TC	A		0.00	1.44	1.44	0.08	1.52	1.52	XXX	
76948		A	Ultrasonic guidance for aspiration of ova, imaging supervision and interpretation	0.38	1.57	1.57	0.10	2.05	2.05	XXX	
	26	A		0.38	0.13	0.13	0.02	0.53	0.53	XXX	
	TC	A		0.00	1.44	1.44	0.08	1.52	1.52	XXX	
76950		A	Ultrasonic guidance for placement of radiation therapy fields	0.58	1.45	1.45	0.09	2.12	2.12	XXX	
	26	A		0.58	0.21	0.21	0.03	0.82	0.82	XXX	
	TC	A		0.00	1.24	1.24	0.06	1.30	1.30	XXX	
76965		A	Ultrasonic guidance for interstitial radioelement application	1.34	5.75	5.75	0.31	7.40	7.40	XXX	
	26	A		1.34	0.46	0.46	0.07	1.87	1.87	XXX	
	TC	A		0.00	5.29	5.29	0.24	5.53	5.53	XXX	
76970		A	Ultrasound study follow-up (specify)	0.40	1.14	1.14	0.07	1.61	1.61	XXX	
	26	A		0.40	0.14	0.14	0.02	0.56	0.56	XXX	
	TC	A		0.00	1.00	1.00	0.05	1.05	1.05	XXX	
76975		A	Gastrointestinal endoscopic ultrasound, supervision and interpretation	0.81	1.73	1.73	0.11	2.65	2.65	XXX	
	26	A		0.81	0.29	0.29	0.03	1.13	1.13	XXX	
	TC	A		0.00	1.44	1.44	0.08	1.52	1.52	XXX	
76977		A	Ultrasound bone density measurement and interpretation, peripheral site(s), any method	0.05	0.80	0.80	0.05	0.90	0.90	XXX	
	26	A		0.05	0.02	0.02	0.01	0.08	0.08	XXX	
	TC	A		0.00	0.78	0.78	0.04	0.82	0.82	XXX	
76986		A	Ultrasonic guidance, intraoperative	1.20	2.91	2.91	0.19	4.30	4.30	XXX	
	26	A		1.20	0.42	0.42	0.07	1.69	1.69	XXX	
	TC	A		0.00	2.49	2.49	0.12	2.61	2.61	XXX	
76999		C	Unlisted ultrasound procedure	0.00	0.00	0.00	0.00	0.00	0.00	XXX	
	26	C		0.00	0.00	0.00	0.00	0.00	0.00	XXX	
	TC	C		0.00	0.00	0.00	0.00	0.00	0.00	XXX	
77261		A	Therapeutic radiology treatment planning; simple	1.39	0.56	0.56	0.06	2.01	2.01	XXX	
77262		A	intermediate	2.11	0.82	0.82	0.09	3.02	3.02	XXX	
77263		A	complex	3.14	1.23	1.23	0.13	4.50	4.50	XXX	
77280		A	Therapeutic radiology simulation-aided field setting; simple	0.70	3.55	3.55	0.18	4.43	4.43	XXX	
	26	A		0.70	0.25	0.25	0.03	0.98	0.98	XXX	
	TC	A		0.00	3.30	3.30	0.15	3.45	3.45	XXX	
77285		A	intermediate	1.05	5.67	5.67	0.29	7.01	7.01	XXX	
	26	A		1.05	0.38	0.38	0.04	1.47	1.47	XXX	
	TC	A		0.00	5.29	5.29	0.25	5.54	5.54	XXX	
77290		A	complex	1.56	6.74	6.74	0.35	8.65	8.65	XXX	
	26	A		1.56	0.56	0.56	0.06	2.18	2.18	XXX	
	TC	A		0.00	6.18	6.18	0.29	6.47	6.47	XXX	

■ RVU not developed by CMS. Gap-filled RVUs developed by CHEG.

Code	M	S	Description	Work Value	Non-Fac PE	Fac PE	Mal-practice	Non-Fac Total	Fac Total	Global	Gap
77295		A	three-dimensional	4.57	28.18	28.18	1.41	34.16	34.16	XXX	
	26	A		4.57	1.65	1.65	0.18	6.40	6.40	XXX	
	TC	A		0.00	26.53	26.53	1.23	27.76	27.76	XXX	
77299		C	Unlisted procedure, therapeutic radiology clinical treatment planning	0.00	0.00	0.00	0.00	0.00	0.00	XXX	
	26	C		0.00	0.00	0.00	0.00	0.00	0.00	XXX	
	TC	C		0.00	0.00	0.00	0.00	0.00	0.00	XXX	
77300		A	Basic radiation dosimetry calculation, central axis depth dose calculation, TDF, NSD, gap calculation, off axis factor, tissue inhomogeneity factors, calculation of non-ionizing radiation surface and depth dose, as required during course of treatment, only when prescribed by the treating physician	0.62	1.50	1.50	0.09	2.21	2.21	XXX	
	26	A		0.62	0.22	0.22	0.03	0.87	0.87	XXX	
	TC	A		0.00	1.28	1.28	0.06	1.34	1.34	XXX	
77301		A	Intensity modulated radiotherapy plan, including dose-volume histograms for target and critical structure partial tolerance specifications	8.00	29.72	29.72	1.41	39.13	39.13	XXX	
	26	A		8.00	3.19	3.19	0.18	11.37	11.37	XXX	
	TC	A		0.00	26.53	26.53	1.23	27.76	27.76	XXX	
77305		A	Teletherapy, isodose plan (whether hand or computer calculated); simple (one or two parallel opposed unmodified ports directed to a single area of interest)	0.70	2.01	2.01	0.12	2.83	2.83	XXX	
	26	A		0.70	0.25	0.25	0.03	0.98	0.98	XXX	
	TC	A		0.00	1.76	1.76	0.09	1.85	1.85	XXX	
77310		A	intermediate (three or more treatment ports directed to a single area of interest)	1.05	2.59	2.59	0.15	3.79	3.79	XXX	
	26	A		1.05	0.38	0.38	0.04	1.47	1.47	XXX	
	TC	A		0.00	2.21	2.21	0.11	2.32	2.32	XXX	
77315		A	complex (mantle or inverted Y, tangential ports, the use of wedges, compensators, complex blocking, rotational beam, or special beam considerations)	1.56	3.09	3.09	0.18	4.83	4.83	XXX	
	26	A		1.56	0.56	0.56	0.06	2.18	2.18	XXX	
	TC	A		0.00	2.53	2.53	0.12	2.65	2.65	XXX	
77321		A	Special teletherapy port plan, particles, hemibody, total body	0.95	4.18	4.18	0.21	5.34	5.34	XXX	
	26	A		0.95	0.34	0.34	0.04	1.33	1.33	XXX	
	TC	A		0.00	3.84	3.84	0.17	4.01	4.01	XXX	
77326		A	Brachytherapy isodose calculation; simple (calculation made from single plane, one to four sources/ribbon application, remote afterloading brachytherapy, 1 to 8 sources)	0.93	2.58	2.58	0.15	3.66	3.66	XXX	
	26	A		0.93	0.34	0.34	0.04	1.31	1.31	XXX	
	TC	A		0.00	2.24	2.24	0.11	2.35	2.35	XXX	
77327		A	intermediate (multiplane dosage calculations, application involving five to ten sources/ribbons, remote afterloading brachytherapy, 9 to 12 sources)	1.39	3.80	3.80	0.21	5.40	5.40	XXX	
	26	A		1.39	0.50	0.50	0.06	1.95	1.95	XXX	
	TC	A		0.00	3.30	3.30	0.15	3.45	3.45	XXX	
77328		A	complex (multiplane isodose plan, volume implant calculations, over 10 sources/ ribbons used, special spatial reconstruction, remote afterloading brachytherapy, over 12 sources)	2.09	5.46	5.46	0.30	7.85	7.85	XXX	
	26	A		2.09	0.75	0.75	0.09	2.93	2.93	XXX	
	TC	A		0.00	4.71	4.71	0.21	4.92	4.92	XXX	
77331		A	Special dosimetry (eg, TLD, microdosimetry) (specify), only when prescribed by the treating physician	0.87	0.79	0.79	0.06	1.72	1.72	XXX	
	26	A		0.87	0.31	0.31	0.04	1.22	1.22	XXX	
	TC	A		0.00	0.48	0.48	0.02	0.50	0.50	XXX	

Radiology

■ RVU not developed by CMS. Gap-filled RVUs developed by CHEG.

Code	M	S	Description	Work Value	Non-Fac PE	Fac PE	Mal-practice	Non-Fac Total	Fac Total	Global	Gap
77332		A	Treatment devices, design and construction; simple (simple block, simple bolus)	0.54	1.47	1.47	0.08	2.09	2.09	XXX	
	26	A		0.54	0.19	0.19	0.02	0.75	0.75	XXX	
	TC	A		0.00	1.28	1.28	0.06	1.34	1.34	XXX	
77333		A	intermediate (multiple blocks, stents, bite blocks, special bolus)	0.84	2.10	2.10	0.13	3.07	3.07	XXX	
	26	A		0.84	0.30	0.30	0.04	1.18	1.18	XXX	
	TC	A		0.00	1.80	1.80	0.09	1.89	1.89	XXX	
77334		A	complex (irregular blocks, special shields, compensators, wedges, molds or casts)	1.24	3.54	3.54	0.19	4.97	4.97	XXX	
	26	A		1.24	0.45	0.45	0.05	1.74	1.74	XXX	
	TC	A		0.00	3.09	3.09	0.14	3.23	3.23	XXX	
77336		A	Continuing medical physics consultation, including assessment of treatment parameters, quality assurance of dose delivery, and review of patient treatment documentation in support of the radiation oncologist, reported per week of therapy	0.00	2.83	2.83	0.13	2.96	2.96	XXX	
	26			0.00	0.00	0.00	0.00	0.00	0.00	XXX	■
	TC			0.00	2.83	2.83	0.13	2.96	2.96	XXX	■
77370		A	Special medical radiation physics consultation	0.00	3.31	3.31	0.15	3.46	3.46	XXX	
	26			0.00	0.00	0.00	0.00	0.00	0.00	XXX	■
	TC			0.00	3.31	3.31	0.15	3.46	3.46	XXX	■
77399		C	Unlisted procedure, medical radiation physics, dosimetry and treatment devices, and special services	0.00	0.00	0.00	0.00	0.00	0.00	XXX	
	26	C		0.00	0.00	0.00	0.00	0.00	0.00	XXX	
	TC	C		0.00	0.00	0.00	0.00	0.00	0.00	XXX	
77401		A	Radiation treatment delivery, superficial and/or ortho voltage	0.00	1.68	1.68	0.09	1.77	1.77	XXX	
	26			0.00	0.00	0.00	0.00	0.00	0.00	XXX	■
	TC			0.00	1.68	1.68	0.09	1.77	1.77	XXX	■
77402		A	Radiation treatment delivery, single treatment area, single port or parallel opposed ports, simple blocks or no blocks; up to 5 MeV	0.00	1.68	1.68	0.09	1.77	1.77	XXX	
	26			0.00	0.00	0.00	0.00	0.00	0.00	XXX	■
	TC			0.00	1.68	1.68	0.09	1.77	1.77	XXX	■
77403		A	6-10 MeV	0.00	1.68	1.68	0.09	1.77	1.77	XXX	
	26			0.00	0.00	0.00	0.00	0.00	0.00	XXX	■
	TC			0.00	1.68	1.68	0.09	1.77	1.77	XXX	■
77404		A	11-19 MeV	0.00	1.68	1.68	0.09	1.77	1.77	XXX	
	26			0.00	0.00	0.00	0.00	0.00	0.00	XXX	■
	TC			0.00	1.68	1.68	0.09	1.77	1.77	XXX	■
77406		A	20 MeV or greater	0.00	1.68	1.68	0.09	1.77	1.77	XXX	
	26			0.00	0.00	0.00	0.00	0.00	0.00	XXX	■
	TC			0.00	1.68	1.68	0.09	1.77	1.77	XXX	■
77407		A	Radiation treatment delivery, two separate treatment areas, three or more ports on a single treatment area, use of multiple blocks; up to 5 MeV	0.00	1.98	1.98	0.10	2.08	2.08	XXX	
	26			0.00	0.00	0.00	0.00	0.00	0.00	XXX	■
	TC			0.00	1.98	1.98	0.10	2.08	2.08	XXX	■
77408		A	6-10 MeV	0.00	1.98	1.98	0.10	2.08	2.08	XXX	
	26			0.00	0.00	0.00	0.00	0.00	0.00	XXX	■
	TC			0.00	1.98	1.98	0.10	2.08	2.08	XXX	■
77409		A	11-19 MeV	0.00	1.98	1.98	0.10	2.08	2.08	XXX	
	26			0.00	0.00	0.00	0.00	0.00	0.00	XXX	■
	TC			0.00	1.98	1.98	0.10	2.08	2.08	XXX	■

■ RVU not developed by CMS. Gap-filled RVUs developed by CHEG.

Code	M	S	Description	Work Value	Non-Fac PE	Fac PE	Mal-practice	Non-Fac Total	Fac Total	Global	Gap
77411		A	20 MeV or greater	0.00	1.98	1.98	0.10	2.08	2.08	XXX	
	26			0.00	0.00	0.00	0.00	0.00	0.00	XXX	■
	TC			0.00	1.98	1.98	0.10	2.08	2.08	XXX	■
77412		A	Radiation treatment delivery, three or more separate treatment areas, custom blocking, tangential ports, wedges, rotational beam, compensators, special particle beam (eg, electron or neutrons); up to 5 MeV	0.00	2.21	2.21	0.11	2.32	2.32	XXX	
	26			0.00	0.00	0.00	0.00	0.00	0.00	XXX	■
	TC			0.00	2.21	2.21	0.11	2.32	2.32	XXX	■
77413		A	6-10 MeV	0.00	2.21	2.21	0.11	2.32	2.32	XXX	
	26			0.00	0.00	0.00	0.00	0.00	0.00	XXX	■
	TC			0.00	2.21	2.21	0.11	2.32	2.32	XXX	■
77414		A	11-19 MeV	0.00	2.21	2.21	0.11	2.32	2.32	XXX	
	26			0.00	0.00	0.00	0.00	0.00	0.00	XXX	■
	TC			0.00	2.21	2.21	0.11	2.32	2.32	XXX	■
77416		A	20 MeV or greater	0.00	2.21	2.21	0.11	2.32	2.32	XXX	
	26			0.00	0.00	0.00	0.00	0.00	0.00	XXX	■
	TC			0.00	2.21	2.21	0.11	2.32	2.32	XXX	■
77417		A	Therapeutic radiology port film(s)	0.00	0.56	0.56	0.03	0.59	0.59	XXX	
	26			0.00	0.00	0.00	0.00	0.00	0.00	XXX	■
	TC			0.00	0.56	0.56	0.03	0.59	0.59	XXX	■
77418		A	Intensity modulated treatment delivery, single or multiple fields/arcs, via narrow spatially and temporally modulated beams (eg, binary, dynamic MLC), per treatment session	0.00	16.07	16.07	0.11	16.18	16.18	XXX	
	26			0.00	0.00	0.00	0.00	0.00	0.00	XXX	■
	TC			0.00	16.07	16.07	0.11	16.18	16.18	XXX	■
77427		A	Radiation treatment management, five treatments	3.31	1.19	1.19	0.14	4.64	4.64	XXX	
77431		A	Radiation therapy management with complete course of therapy consisting of one or two fractions only	1.81	0.73	0.73	0.07	2.61	2.61	XXX	
77432		A	Stereotactic radiation treatment management of cerebral lesion(s) (complete course of treatment consisting of one session)	7.93	3.25	3.25	0.33	11.51	11.51	XXX	
77470		A	Special treatment procedure (eg, total body irradiation, hemibody radiation, per oral, endocavitary or intraoperative cone irradiation)	2.09	11.34	11.34	0.58	14.01	14.01	XXX	
	26	A		2.09	0.75	0.75	0.09	2.93	2.93	XXX	
	TC	A		0.00	10.59	10.59	0.49	11.08	11.08	XXX	
77499		C	Unlisted procedure, therapeutic radiology treatment management	0.00	0.00	0.00	0.00	0.00	0.00	XXX	
	26	C		0.00	0.00	0.00	0.00	0.00	0.00	XXX	
	TC	C		0.00	0.00	0.00	0.00	0.00	0.00	XXX	
77520		C	Proton treatment delivery; simple, without compensation	0.00	0.00	0.00	0.00	0.00	0.00	XXX	
77522		C	simple, with compensation	0.00	0.00	0.00	0.00	0.00	0.00	XXX	
77523		C	intermediate	0.00	0.00	0.00	0.00	0.00	0.00	XXX	
77525		C	complex	0.00	0.00	0.00	0.00	0.00	0.00	XXX	

Radiology

■ RVU not developed by CMS. Gap-filled RVUs developed by CHEG.

Code	M	S	Description	Work Value	Non-Fac PE	Fac PE	Mal-practice	Non-Fac Total	Fac Total	Global	Gap
77600		R	Hyperthermia, externally generated; superficial (ie, heating to a depth of 4 cm or less)	1.56	3.44	3.44	0.21	5.21	5.21	XXX	
	26	R		1.56	0.55	0.55	0.08	2.19	2.19	XXX	
	TC	R		0.00	2.89	2.89	0.13	3.02	3.02	XXX	
77605		R	deep (ie, heating to depths greater than 4 cm)	2.09	4.62	4.62	0.31	7.02	7.02	XXX	
	26	R		2.09	0.76	0.76	0.13	2.98	2.98	XXX	
	TC	R		0.00	3.86	3.86	0.18	4.04	4.04	XXX	
77610		R	Hyperthermia generated by interstitial probe(s); 5 or fewer interstitial applicators	1.56	3.44	3.44	0.20	5.20	5.20	XXX	
	26	R		1.56	0.55	0.55	0.07	2.18	2.18	XXX	
	TC	R		0.00	2.89	2.89	0.13	3.02	3.02	XXX	
77615		R	more than 5 interstitial applicators	2.09	4.60	4.60	0.27	6.96	6.96	XXX	
	26	R		2.09	0.74	0.74	0.09	2.92	2.92	XXX	
	TC	R		0.00	3.86	3.86	0.18	4.04	4.04	XXX	
77620		R	Hyperthermia generated by intracavitary probe(s)	1.56	3.47	3.47	0.19	5.22	5.22	XXX	
	26	R		1.56	0.58	0.58	0.06	2.20	2.20	XXX	
	TC	R		0.00	2.89	2.89	0.13	3.02	3.02	XXX	
77750		A	Infusion or instillation of radioelement solution	4.91	3.04	3.04	0.23	8.18	8.18	090	
	26	A		4.91	1.77	1.77	0.17	6.85	6.85	090	
	TC	A		0.00	1.27	1.27	0.06	1.33	1.33	090	
77761		A	Intracavitary radiation source application; simple	3.81	3.51	3.51	0.28	7.60	7.60	090	
	26	A		3.81	1.13	1.13	0.16	5.10	5.10	090	
	TC	A		0.00	2.38	2.38	0.12	2.50	2.50	090	
77762		A	intermediate	5.72	5.42	5.42	0.38	11.52	11.52	090	
	26	A		5.72	1.99	1.99	0.22	7.93	7.93	090	
	TC	A		0.00	3.43	3.43	0.16	3.59	3.59	090	
77763		A	complex	8.57	7.38	7.38	0.53	16.48	16.48	090	
	26	A		8.57	3.12	3.12	0.34	12.03	12.03	090	
	TC	A		0.00	4.26	4.26	0.19	4.45	4.45	090	
77776		A	Interstitial radiation source application; simple	4.66	3.72	3.72	0.35	8.73	8.73	090	
	26	A		4.66	1.65	1.65	0.24	6.55	6.55	090	
	TC	A		0.00	2.07	2.07	0.11	2.18	2.18	090	
77777		A	intermediate	7.48	6.37	6.37	0.50	14.35	14.35	090	
	26	A		7.48	2.35	2.35	0.32	10.15	10.15	090	
	TC	A		0.00	4.02	4.02	0.18	4.20	4.20	090	
77778		A	complex	11.19	8.90	8.90	0.69	20.78	20.78	090	
	26	A		11.19	4.02	4.02	0.47	15.68	15.68	090	
	TC	A		0.00	4.88	4.88	0.22	5.10	5.10	090	
77781		A	Remote afterloading high intensity brachytherapy; 1-4 source positions or catheters	1.66	19.88	19.88	0.95	22.49	22.49	090	
	26	A		1.66	0.60	0.60	0.07	2.33	2.33	090	
	TC	A		0.00	19.28	19.28	0.88	20.16	20.16	090	
77782		A	5-8 source positions or catheters	2.49	20.18	20.18	0.98	23.65	23.65	090	
	26	A		2.49	0.90	0.90	0.10	3.49	3.49	090	
	TC	A		0.00	19.28	19.28	0.88	20.16	20.16	090	
77783		A	9-12 source positions or catheters	3.73	20.62	20.62	1.03	25.38	25.38	090	
	26	A		3.73	1.34	1.34	0.15	5.22	5.22	090	
	TC	A		0.00	19.28	19.28	0.88	20.16	20.16	090	

■ RVU not developed by CMS. Gap-filled RVUs developed by CHEG.

Code	M	S	Description	Work Value	Non-Fac PE	Fac PE	Mal-prac-tice	Non-Fac Total	Fac Total	Global	Gap
77784		A	over 12 source positions or catheters	5.61	21.30	21.30	1.10	28.01	28.01	090	
	26	A		5.61	2.02	2.02	0.22	7.85	7.85	090	
	TC	A		0.00	19.28	19.28	0.88	20.16	20.16	090	
77789		A	Surface application of radiation source	1.12	0.84	0.84	0.05	2.01	2.01	090	
	26	A		1.12	0.41	0.41	0.03	1.56	1.56	090	
	TC	A		0.00	0.43	0.43	0.02	0.45	0.45	090	
77790		A	Supervision, handling, loading of radiation source	1.05	0.86	0.86	0.06	1.97	1.97	XXX	
	26	A		1.05	0.38	0.38	0.04	1.47	1.47	XXX	
	TC	A		0.00	0.48	0.48	0.02	0.50	0.50	XXX	
77799		C	Unlisted procedure, clinical brachytherapy	0.00	0.00	0.00	0.00	0.00	0.00	XXX	
	26	C		0.00	0.00	0.00	0.00	0.00	0.00	XXX	
	TC	C		0.00	0.00	0.00	0.00	0.00	0.00	XXX	
78000		A	Thyroid uptake; single determination	0.19	0.99	0.99	0.06	1.24	1.24	XXX	
	26	A		0.19	0.07	0.07	0.01	0.27	0.27	XXX	
	TC	A		0.00	0.92	0.92	0.05	0.97	0.97	XXX	
78001		A	multiple determinations	0.26	1.33	1.33	0.07	1.66	1.66	XXX	
	26	A		0.26	0.09	0.09	0.01	0.36	0.36	XXX	
	TC	A		0.00	1.24	1.24	0.06	1.30	1.30	XXX	
78003		A	stimulation, suppression or discharge (not including initial uptake studies)	0.33	1.04	1.04	0.06	1.43	1.43	XXX	
	26	A		0.33	0.12	0.12	0.01	0.46	0.46	XXX	
	TC	A		0.00	0.92	0.92	0.05	0.97	0.97	XXX	
78006		A	Thyroid imaging, with uptake; single determination	0.49	2.44	2.44	0.13	3.06	3.06	XXX	
	26	A		0.49	0.18	0.18	0.02	0.69	0.69	XXX	
	TC	A		0.00	2.26	2.26	0.11	2.37	2.37	XXX	
78007		A	multiple determinations	0.50	2.62	2.62	0.14	3.26	3.26	XXX	
	26	A		0.50	0.18	0.18	0.02	0.70	0.70	XXX	
	TC	A		0.00	2.44	2.44	0.12	2.56	2.56	XXX	
78010		A	Thyroid imaging; only	0.39	1.87	1.87	0.11	2.37	2.37	XXX	
	26	A		0.39	0.14	0.14	0.02	0.55	0.55	XXX	
	TC	A		0.00	1.73	1.73	0.09	1.82	1.82	XXX	
78011		A	with vascular flow	0.45	2.45	2.45	0.13	3.03	3.03	XXX	
	26	A		0.45	0.16	0.16	0.02	0.63	0.63	XXX	
	TC	A		0.00	2.29	2.29	0.11	2.40	2.40	XXX	
78015		A	Thyroid carcinoma metastases imaging; limited area (eg, neck and chest only)	0.67	2.68	2.68	0.15	3.50	3.50	XXX	
	26	A		0.67	0.24	0.24	0.03	0.94	0.94	XXX	
	TC	A		0.00	2.44	2.44	0.12	2.56	2.56	XXX	
78016		A	with additional studies (eg, urinary recovery)	0.82	3.62	3.62	0.18	4.62	4.62	XXX	
	26	A		0.82	0.31	0.31	0.03	1.16	1.16	XXX	
	TC	A		0.00	3.31	3.31	0.15	3.46	3.46	XXX	
78018		A	whole body	0.86	5.47	5.47	0.27	6.60	6.60	XXX	
	26	A		0.86	0.32	0.32	0.03	1.21	1.21	XXX	
	TC	A		0.00	5.15	5.15	0.24	5.39	5.39	XXX	
78020		A	Thyroid carcinoma metastases uptake (List separately in addition to code for primary procedure)	0.60	1.47	1.47	0.14	2.21	2.21	ZZZ	
	26	A		0.60	0.23	0.23	0.02	0.85	0.85	ZZZ	
	TC	A		0.00	1.24	1.24	0.12	1.36	1.36	ZZZ	

■ RVU not developed by CMS. Gap-filled RVUs developed by CHEG.

Code	M	S	Description	Work Value	Non-Fac PE	Fac PE	Mal-prac-tice	Non-Fac Total	Fac Total	Global	Gap
78070		A	Parathyroid imaging	0.82	2.03	2.03	0.12	2.97	2.97	XXX	
	26	A		0.82	0.30	0.30	0.03	1.15	1.15	XXX	
	TC	A		0.00	1.73	1.73	0.09	1.82	1.82	XXX	
78075		A	Adrenal imaging, cortex and/or medulla	0.74	5.44	5.44	0.27	6.45	6.45	XXX	
	26	A		0.74	0.29	0.29	0.03	1.06	1.06	XXX	
	TC	A		0.00	5.15	5.15	0.24	5.39	5.39	XXX	
78099		C	Unlisted endocrine procedure, diagnostic nuclear medicine	0.00	0.00	0.00	0.00	0.00	0.00	XXX	
	26	C		0.00	0.00	0.00	0.00	0.00	0.00	XXX	
	TC	C		0.00	0.00	0.00	0.00	0.00	0.00	XXX	
78102		A	Bone marrow imaging; limited area	0.55	2.15	2.15	0.12	2.82	2.82	XXX	
	26	A		0.55	0.21	0.21	0.02	0.78	0.78	XXX	
	TC	A		0.00	1.94	1.94	0.10	2.04	2.04	XXX	
78103		A	multiple areas	0.75	3.28	3.28	0.17	4.20	4.20	XXX	
	26	A		0.75	0.27	0.27	0.03	1.05	1.05	XXX	
	TC	A		0.00	3.01	3.01	0.14	3.15	3.15	XXX	
78104		A	whole body	0.80	4.16	4.16	0.21	5.17	5.17	XXX	
	26	A		0.80	0.29	0.29	0.03	1.12	1.12	XXX	
	TC	A		0.00	3.87	3.87	0.18	4.05	4.05	XXX	
78110		A	Plasma volume, radiopharmaceutical volume-dilution technique (separate procedure); single sampling	0.19	0.97	0.97	0.06	1.22	1.22	XXX	
	26	A		0.19	0.07	0.07	0.01	0.27	0.27	XXX	
	TC	A		0.00	0.90	0.90	0.05	0.95	0.95	XXX	
78111		A	multiple samplings	0.22	2.52	2.52	0.13	2.87	2.87	XXX	
	26	A		0.22	0.08	0.08	0.01	0.31	0.31	XXX	
	TC	A		0.00	2.44	2.44	0.12	2.56	2.56	XXX	
78120		A	Red cell volume determination (separate procedure); single sampling	0.23	1.73	1.73	0.10	2.06	2.06	XXX	
	26	A		0.23	0.09	0.09	0.01	0.33	0.33	XXX	
	TC	A		0.00	1.64	1.64	0.09	1.73	1.73	XXX	
78121		A	multiple samplings	0.32	2.88	2.88	0.13	3.33	3.33	XXX	
	26	A		0.32	0.12	0.12	0.01	0.45	0.45	XXX	
	TC	A		0.00	2.76	2.76	0.12	2.88	2.88	XXX	
78122		A	Whole blood volume determination, including separate measurement of plasma volume and red cell volume (radiopharmaceutical volume-dilution technique)	0.45	4.54	4.54	0.22	5.21	5.21	XXX	
	26	A		0.45	0.17	0.17	0.02	0.64	0.64	XXX	
	TC	A		0.00	4.37	4.37	0.20	4.57	4.57	XXX	
78130		A	Red cell survival study;	0.61	2.93	2.93	0.15	3.69	3.69	XXX	
	26	A		0.61	0.22	0.22	0.03	0.86	0.86	XXX	
	TC	A		0.00	2.71	2.71	0.12	2.83	2.83	XXX	
78135		A	differential organ/tissue kinetics, (eg, splenic and/or hepatic sequestration)	0.64	4.86	4.86	0.24	5.74	5.74	XXX	
	26	A		0.64	0.23	0.23	0.03	0.90	0.90	XXX	
	TC	A		0.00	4.63	4.63	0.21	4.84	4.84	XXX	
78140		A	Labeled red cell sequestration, differential organ/tissue, (eg, splenic and/or hepatic)	0.61	3.95	3.95	0.20	4.76	4.76	XXX	
	26	A		0.61	0.21	0.21	0.03	0.85	0.85	XXX	
	TC	A		0.00	3.74	3.74	0.17	3.91	3.91	XXX	

Radiology

■ RVU not developed by CMS. Gap-filled RVUs developed by CHEG.

Code	M	S	Description	Work Value	Non-Fac PE	Fac PE	Mal-practice	Non-Fac Total	Fac Total	Global	Gap
78160		A	Plasma radioiron disappearance (turnover) rate	0.33	3.60	3.60	0.19	4.12	4.12	XXX	
	26	A		0.33	0.12	0.12	0.03	0.48	0.48	XXX	
	TC	A		0.00	3.48	3.48	0.16	3.64	3.64	XXX	
78162		A	Radioiron oral absorption	0.45	3.22	3.22	0.15	3.82	3.82	XXX	
	26	A		0.45	0.18	0.18	0.01	0.64	0.64	XXX	
	TC	A		0.00	3.04	3.04	0.14	3.18	3.18	XXX	
78170		A	Radioiron red cell utilization	0.41	5.19	5.19	0.27	5.87	5.87	XXX	
	26	A		0.41	0.15	0.15	0.04	0.60	0.60	XXX	
	TC	A		0.00	5.04	5.04	0.23	5.27	5.27	XXX	
78172		C	Chelatable iron for estimation of total body iron	2.12	0.80	0.80	0.08	3.00	3.00	XXX	■
	26	A		0.53	0.20	0.20	0.02	0.75	0.75	XXX	
	TC	C		1.59	0.60	0.60	0.06	2.25	2.25	XXX	■
78185		A	Spleen imaging only, with or without vascular flow	0.40	2.39	2.39	0.13	2.92	2.92	XXX	
	26	A		0.40	0.15	0.15	0.02	0.57	0.57	XXX	
	TC	A		0.00	2.24	2.24	0.11	2.35	2.35	XXX	
78190		A	Kinetics, study of platelet survival, with or without differential organ/tissue localization	1.09	5.83	5.83	0.31	7.23	7.23	XXX	
	26	A		1.09	0.40	0.40	0.06	1.55	1.55	XXX	
	TC	A		0.00	5.43	5.43	0.25	5.68	5.68	XXX	
78191		A	Platelet survival study	0.61	7.19	7.19	0.34	8.14	8.14	XXX	
	26	A		0.61	0.22	0.22	0.03	0.86	0.86	XXX	
	TC	A		0.00	6.97	6.97	0.31	7.28	7.28	XXX	
78195		A	Lymphatics and lymph nodes imaging	1.20	4.31	4.31	0.23	5.74	5.74	XXX	
	26	A		1.20	0.44	0.44	0.05	1.69	1.69	XXX	
	TC	A		0.00	3.87	3.87	0.18	4.05	4.05	XXX	
78199		C	Unlisted hematopoietic, reticuloendothelial and lymphatic procedure, diagnostic nuclear medicine	0.00	0.00	0.00	0.00	0.00	0.00	XXX	
	26	C		0.00	0.00	0.00	0.00	0.00	0.00	XXX	
	TC	C		0.00	0.00	0.00	0.00	0.00	0.00	XXX	
78201		A	Liver imaging; static only	0.44	2.40	2.40	0.13	2.97	2.97	XXX	
	26	A		0.44	0.16	0.16	0.02	0.62	0.62	XXX	
	TC	A		0.00	2.24	2.24	0.11	2.35	2.35	XXX	
78202		A	with vascular flow	0.51	2.93	2.93	0.14	3.58	3.58	XXX	
	26	A		0.51	0.19	0.19	0.02	0.72	0.72	XXX	
	TC	A		0.00	2.74	2.74	0.12	2.86	2.86	XXX	
78205		A	Liver imaging (SPECT)	0.71	5.87	5.87	0.29	6.87	6.87	XXX	
	26	A		0.71	0.26	0.26	0.03	1.00	1.00	XXX	
	TC	A		0.00	5.61	5.61	0.26	5.87	5.87	XXX	
78206		A	with vascular flow	0.96	5.96	5.96	0.13	7.05	7.05	XXX	
	26	A		0.96	0.35	0.35	0.04	1.35	1.35	XXX	
	TC	A		0.00	5.61	5.61	0.09	5.70	5.70	XXX	
78215		A	Liver and spleen imaging; static only	0.49	2.97	2.97	0.14	3.60	3.60	XXX	
	26	A		0.49	0.18	0.18	0.02	0.69	0.69	XXX	
	TC	A		0.00	2.79	2.79	0.12	2.91	2.91	XXX	
78216		A	with vascular flow	0.57	3.52	3.52	0.17	4.26	4.26	XXX	
	26	A		0.57	0.21	0.21	0.02	0.80	0.80	XXX	
	TC	A		0.00	3.31	3.31	0.15	3.46	3.46	XXX	

Radiology

■ RVU not developed by CMS. Gap-filled RVUs developed by CHEG.

Code	M	S	Description	Work Value	Non-Fac PE	Fac PE	Mal-practice	Non-Fac Total	Fac Total	Global	Gap
78220		A	Liver function study with hepatobiliary agents, with serial images	0.49	3.72	3.72	0.18	4.39	4.39	XXX	
	26	A		0.49	0.18	0.18	0.02	0.69	0.69	XXX	
	TC	A		0.00	3.54	3.54	0.16	3.70	3.70	XXX	
78223		A	Hepatobiliary ductal system imaging, including gallbladder, with or without pharmacologic intervention, with or without quantitative measurement of gallbladder function	0.84	3.78	3.78	0.20	4.82	4.82	XXX	
	26	A		0.84	0.30	0.30	0.04	1.18	1.18	XXX	
	TC	A		0.00	3.48	3.48	0.16	3.64	3.64	XXX	
78230		A	Salivary gland imaging;	0.45	2.23	2.23	0.13	2.81	2.81	XXX	
	26	A		0.45	0.16	0.16	0.02	0.63	0.63	XXX	
	TC	A		0.00	2.07	2.07	0.11	2.18	2.18	XXX	
78231		A	with serial images	0.52	3.21	3.21	0.16	3.89	3.89	XXX	
	26	A		0.52	0.20	0.20	0.02	0.74	0.74	XXX	
	TC	A		0.00	3.01	3.01	0.14	3.15	3.15	XXX	
78232		A	Salivary gland function study	0.47	3.54	3.54	0.16	4.17	4.17	XXX	
	26	A		0.47	0.18	0.18	0.01	0.66	0.66	XXX	
	TC	A		0.00	3.36	3.36	0.15	3.51	3.51	XXX	
78258		A	Esophageal motility	0.74	3.01	3.01	0.15	3.90	3.90	XXX	
	26	A		0.74	0.27	0.27	0.03	1.04	1.04	XXX	
	TC	A		0.00	2.74	2.74	0.12	2.86	2.86	XXX	
78261		A	Gastric mucosa imaging	0.69	4.15	4.15	0.21	5.05	5.05	XXX	
	26	A		0.69	0.26	0.26	0.03	0.98	0.98	XXX	
	TC	A		0.00	3.89	3.89	0.18	4.07	4.07	XXX	
78262		A	Gastroesophageal reflux study	0.68	4.29	4.29	0.21	5.18	5.18	XXX	
	26	A		0.68	0.25	0.25	0.03	0.96	0.96	XXX	
	TC	A		0.00	4.04	4.04	0.18	4.22	4.22	XXX	
78264		A	Gastric emptying study	0.78	4.20	4.20	0.21	5.19	5.19	XXX	
	26	A		0.78	0.28	0.28	0.03	1.09	1.09	XXX	
	TC	A		0.00	3.92	3.92	0.18	4.10	4.10	XXX	
78267		X	Urea breath test, C-14; acquisition for analysis	0.00	0.00	0.00	0.00	0.00	0.00	XXX	
78268		X	analysis	0.00	0.00	0.00	0.00	0.00	0.00	XXX	
78270		A	Vitamin B-12 absorption study (eg, Schilling test); without intrinsic factor	0.20	1.54	1.54	0.09	1.83	1.83	XXX	
	26	A		0.20	0.07	0.07	0.01	0.28	0.28	XXX	
	TC	A		0.00	1.47	1.47	0.08	1.55	1.55	XXX	
78271		A	with intrinsic factor	0.20	1.63	1.63	0.09	1.92	1.92	XXX	
	26	A		0.20	0.07	0.07	0.01	0.28	0.28	XXX	
	TC	A		0.00	1.56	1.56	0.08	1.64	1.64	XXX	
78272		A	Vitamin B-12 absorption studies combined, with and without intrinsic factor	0.27	2.30	2.30	0.12	2.69	2.69	XXX	
	26	A		0.27	0.10	0.10	0.01	0.38	0.38	XXX	
	TC	A		0.00	2.20	2.20	0.11	2.31	2.31	XXX	
78278		A	Acute gastrointestinal blood loss imaging	0.99	4.98	4.98	0.25	6.22	6.22	XXX	
	26	A		0.99	0.35	0.35	0.04	1.38	1.38	XXX	
	TC	A		0.00	4.63	4.63	0.21	4.84	4.84	XXX	

■ RVU not developed by CMS. Gap-filled RVUs developed by CHEG.

Code	M	S	Description	Work Value	Non-Fac PE	Fac PE	Mal-practice	Non-Fac Total	Fac Total	Global	Gap
78282		C	Gastrointestinal protein loss	1.52	0.52	0.52	0.08	2.12	2.12	XXX	■
	26	A		0.38	0.13	0.13	0.02	0.53	0.53	XXX	
	TC	C		1.14	0.39	0.39	0.06	1.59	1.59	XXX	■
78290		A	Intestine imaging (eg, ectopic gastric mucosa, Meckels localization, volvulus)	0.68	3.13	3.13	0.16	3.97	3.97	XXX	
	26	A		0.68	0.24	0.24	0.03	0.95	0.95	XXX	
	TC	A		0.00	2.89	2.89	0.13	3.02	3.02	XXX	
78291		A	Peritoneal-venous shunt patency test (eg, for LeVeen, Denver shunt)	0.88	3.23	3.23	0.17	4.28	4.28	XXX	
	26	A		0.88	0.32	0.32	0.04	1.24	1.24	XXX	
	TC	A		0.00	2.91	2.91	0.13	3.04	3.04	XXX	
78299		C	Unlisted gastrointestinal procedure, diagnostic nuclear medicine	0.00	0.00	0.00	0.00	0.00	0.00	XXX	
	26	C		0.00	0.00	0.00	0.00	0.00	0.00	XXX	
	TC	C		0.00	0.00	0.00	0.00	0.00	0.00	XXX	
78300		A	Bone and/or joint imaging; limited area	0.62	2.58	2.58	0.15	3.35	3.35	XXX	
	26	A		0.62	0.22	0.22	0.03	0.87	0.87	XXX	
	TC	A		0.00	2.36	2.36	0.12	2.48	2.48	XXX	
78305		A	multiple areas	0.83	3.78	3.78	0.19	4.80	4.80	XXX	
	26	A		0.83	0.30	0.30	0.03	1.16	1.16	XXX	
	TC	A		0.00	3.48	3.48	0.16	3.64	3.64	XXX	
78306		A	whole body	0.86	4.37	4.37	0.22	5.45	5.45	XXX	
	26	A		0.86	0.31	0.31	0.04	1.21	1.21	XXX	
	TC	A		0.00	4.06	4.06	0.18	4.24	4.24	XXX	
78315		A	three phase study	1.02	4.91	4.91	0.25	6.18	6.18	XXX	
	26	A		1.02	0.37	0.37	0.04	1.43	1.43	XXX	
	TC	A		0.00	4.54	4.54	0.21	4.75	4.75	XXX	
78320		A	tomographic (SPECT)	1.04	6.00	6.00	0.30	7.34	7.34	XXX	
	26	A		1.04	0.39	0.39	0.04	1.47	1.47	XXX	
	TC	A		0.00	5.61	5.61	0.26	5.87	5.87	XXX	
78350		A	Bone density (bone mineral content) study, one or more sites; single photon asorptiometry	0.22	0.80	0.80	0.05	1.07	1.07	XXX	
	26	A		0.22	0.08	0.08	0.01	0.31	0.31	XXX	
	TC	A		0.00	0.72	0.72	0.04	0.76	0.76	XXX	
78351		N	dual photon absorptiometry, one or more sites	0.30	1.64	0.12	0.01	1.95	0.43	XXX	
	26			0.09	0.49	0.04	0.00	0.59	0.13	XXX	■
	TC			0.21	1.15	0.08	0.01	1.37	0.30	XXX	■
78399		C	Unlisted musculoskeletal procedure, diagnostic nuclear medicine	0.00	0.00	0.00	0.00	0.00	0.00	XXX	
	26	C		0.00	0.00	0.00	0.00	0.00	0.00	XXX	
	TC	C		0.00	0.00	0.00	0.00	0.00	0.00	XXX	
78414		C	Determination of central c-v hemodynamics (non-imaging) (eg, ejection fraction with probe technique) with or without pharmacologic intervention or exercise, single or multiple determinations	1.50	0.53	0.53	0.07	2.10	2.10	XXX	■
	26	A		0.45	0.16	0.16	0.02	0.63	0.63	XXX	
	TC	C		1.05	0.37	0.37	0.05	1.47	1.47	XXX	■
78428		A	Cardiac shunt detection	0.78	2.46	2.46	0.14	3.38	3.38	XXX	
	26	A		0.78	0.32	0.32	0.03	1.13	1.13	XXX	
	TC	A		0.00	2.14	2.14	0.11	2.25	2.25	XXX	

■ RVU not developed by CMS. Gap-filled RVUs developed by CHEG.

Code	M	S	Description	Work Value	Non-Fac PE	Fac PE	Mal-practice	Non-Fac Total	Fac Total	Global	Gap
78445		A	Non-cardiac vascular flow imaging (ie, angiography, venography)	0.49	1.94	1.94	0.11	2.54	2.54	XXX	
	26	A		0.49	0.18	0.18	0.02	0.69	0.69	XXX	
	TC	A		0.00	1.76	1.76	0.09	1.85	1.85	XXX	
78455		A	Venous thrombosis study (eg, radioactive fibrinogen)	0.73	4.04	4.04	0.20	4.97	4.97	XXX	
	26	A		0.73	0.26	0.26	0.03	1.02	1.02	XXX	
	TC	A		0.00	3.78	3.78	0.17	3.95	3.95	XXX	
78456		A	Acute venous thrombosis imaging, peptide	1.00	4.15	4.15	0.28	5.43	5.43	XXX	
	26	A		1.00	0.37	0.37	0.04	1.41	1.41	XXX	
	TC	A		0.00	3.78	3.78	0.24	4.02	4.02	XXX	
78457		A	Venous thrombosis imaging, venogram; unilateral	0.77	2.81	2.81	0.15	3.73	3.73	XXX	
	26	A		0.77	0.28	0.28	0.03	1.08	1.08	XXX	
	TC	A		0.00	2.53	2.53	0.12	2.65	2.65	XXX	
78458		A	bilateral	0.90	4.17	4.17	0.20	5.27	5.27	XXX	
	26	A		0.90	0.35	0.35	0.03	1.28	1.28	XXX	
	TC	A		0.00	3.82	3.82	0.17	3.99	3.99	XXX	
78459		I	Myocardial imaging, positron emission tomography (PET), metabolic evaluation	0.00	0.00	0.00	0.00	0.00	0.00	XXX	
	26	I		1.88	0.75	0.75	0.08	2.71	2.71	XXX	
	TC	I		0.00	0.00	0.00	0.00	0.00	0.00	XXX	
78460		A	Myocardial perfusion imaging; (planar) single study, at rest or stress (exercise and/or pharmacologic), with or without quantification	0.86	2.55	2.55	0.14	3.55	3.55	XXX	
	26	A		0.86	0.31	0.31	0.03	1.20	1.20	XXX	
	TC	A		0.00	2.24	2.24	0.11	2.35	2.35	XXX	
78461		A	multiple studies, (planar) at rest and/or stress (exercise and/or pharmacologic), and redistribution and/or rest injection, with or without quantification	1.23	4.94	4.94	0.26	6.43	6.43	XXX	
	26	A		1.23	0.46	0.46	0.05	1.74	1.74	XXX	
	TC	A		0.00	4.48	4.48	0.21	4.69	4.69	XXX	
78464		A	tomographic (SPECT), single study at rest or stress (exercise and/or pharmacologic), with or without quantification	1.09	7.12	7.12	0.35	8.56	8.56	XXX	
	26	A		1.09	0.41	0.41	0.04	1.54	1.54	XXX	
	TC	A		0.00	6.71	6.71	0.31	7.02	7.02	XXX	
78465		A	tomographic (SPECT), multiple studies, at rest and/or stress (exercise and/or pharmacologic) and redistribution and/or rest injection, with or without quantification	1.46	11.76	11.76	0.56	13.78	13.78	XXX	
	26	A		1.46	0.56	0.56	0.05	2.07	2.07	XXX	
	TC	A		0.00	11.20	11.20	0.51	11.71	11.71	XXX	
78466		A	Myocardial imaging, infarct avid, planar; qualitative or quantitative	0.69	2.75	2.75	0.15	3.59	3.59	XXX	
	26	A		0.69	0.26	0.26	0.03	0.98	0.98	XXX	
	TC	A		0.00	2.49	2.49	0.12	2.61	2.61	XXX	
78468		A	with ejection fraction by first pass technique	0.80	3.78	3.78	0.19	4.77	4.77	XXX	
	26	A		0.80	0.30	0.30	0.03	1.13	1.13	XXX	
	TC	A		0.00	3.48	3.48	0.16	3.64	3.64	XXX	
78469		A	tomographic SPECT with or without quantification	0.92	5.31	5.31	0.26	6.49	6.49	XXX	
	26	A		0.92	0.35	0.35	0.03	1.30	1.30	XXX	
	TC	A		0.00	4.96	4.96	0.23	5.19	5.19	XXX	
78472		A	Cardiac blood pool imaging, gated equilibrium; planar, single study at rest or stress (exercise and/or pharmacologic), wall motion study plus ejection fraction, with or without additional quantitative processing	0.98	5.60	5.60	0.29	6.87	6.87	XXX	
	26	A		0.98	0.37	0.37	0.04	1.39	1.39	XXX	
	TC	A		0.00	5.23	5.23	0.25	5.48	5.48	XXX	

■ RVU not developed by CMS. Gap-filled RVUs developed by CHEG.

Code	M	S	Description	Work Value	Non-Fac PE	Fac PE	Mal-practice	Non-Fac Total	Fac Total	Global	Gap
78473		A	multiple studies, wall motion study plus ejection fraction, at rest and stress (exercise and/or pharmacologic), with or without additional quantification	1.47	8.40	8.40	0.40	10.27	10.27	XXX	
	26	A		1.47	0.56	0.56	0.05	2.08	2.08	XXX	
	TC	A		0.00	7.84	7.84	0.35	8.19	8.19	XXX	
78478		A	Myocardial perfusion study with wall motion, qualitative or quantitative study (List separately in addition to code for primary procedure)	0.62	1.72	1.72	0.10	2.44	2.44	ZZZ	
	26	A		0.62	0.24	0.24	0.02	0.88	0.88	ZZZ	
	TC	A		0.00	1.48	1.48	0.08	1.56	1.56	ZZZ	
78480		A	Myocardial perfusion study with ejection fraction (List separately in addition to code for primary procedure)	0.62	1.72	1.72	0.10	2.44	2.44	ZZZ	
	26	A		0.62	0.24	0.24	0.02	0.88	0.88	ZZZ	
	TC	A		0.00	1.48	1.48	0.08	1.56	1.56	ZZZ	
78481		A	Cardiac blood pool imaging, (planar), first pass technique; single study, at rest or with stress (exercise and/or pharmacologic), wall motion study plus ejection fraction, with or without quantification	0.98	5.35	5.35	0.26	6.59	6.59	XXX	
	26	A		0.98	0.39	0.39	0.03	1.40	1.40	XXX	
	TC	A		0.00	4.96	4.96	0.23	5.19	5.19	XXX	
78483		A	multiple studies, at rest and with stress (exercise and/or pharmacologic), wall motion study plus ejection fraction, with or without quantification	1.47	8.05	8.05	0.39	9.91	9.91	XXX	
	26	A		1.47	0.58	0.58	0.05	2.10	2.10	XXX	
	TC	A		0.00	7.47	7.47	0.34	7.81	7.81	XXX	
78491		I	Myocardial imaging, positron emission tomography (PET), perfusion; single study at rest or stress	0.00	0.00	0.00	0.00	0.00	0.00	XXX	
	26	I		1.50	0.60	0.60	0.05	2.15	2.15	XXX	
	TC	I		0.00	0.00	0.00	0.00	0.00	0.00	XXX	
78492		I	multiple studies at rest and/or stress	0.00	0.00	0.00	0.00	0.00	0.00	XXX	
	26	I		1.87	0.75	0.75	0.06	2.68	2.68	XXX	
	TC	I		0.00	0.00	0.00	0.00	0.00	0.00	XXX	
78494		A	Cardiac blood pool imaging, gated equilibrium, SPECT, at rest, wall motion study plus ejection fraction, with or without quantitative processing	1.19	7.15	7.15	0.29	8.63	8.63	XXX	
	26	A		1.19	0.44	0.44	0.04	1.67	1.67	XXX	
	TC	A		0.00	6.71	6.71	0.25	6.96	6.96	XXX	
78496		A	Cardiac blood pool imaging, gated equilibrium, single study, at rest, with right ventricular ejection fraction by first pass technique (List separately in addition to code for primary procedure)	0.50	6.91	6.91	0.27	7.68	7.68	ZZZ	
	26	A		0.50	0.20	0.20	0.02	0.72	0.72	ZZZ	
	TC	A		0.00	6.71	6.71	0.25	6.96	6.96	ZZZ	
78499		C	Unlisted cardiovascular procedure, diagnostic nuclear medicine	0.00	0.00	0.00	0.00	0.00	0.00	XXX	
	26	C		0.00	0.00	0.00	0.00	0.00	0.00	XXX	
	TC	C		0.00	0.00	0.00	0.00	0.00	0.00	XXX	
78580		A	Pulmonary perfusion imaging, particulate	0.74	3.53	3.53	0.18	4.45	4.45	XXX	
	26	A		0.74	0.27	0.27	0.03	1.04	1.04	XXX	
	TC	A		0.00	3.26	3.26	0.15	3.41	3.41	XXX	
78584		A	Pulmonary perfusion imaging, particulate, with ventilation; single breath	0.99	3.39	3.39	0.18	4.56	4.56	XXX	
	26	A		0.99	0.35	0.35	0.04	1.38	1.38	XXX	
	TC	A		0.00	3.04	3.04	0.14	3.18	3.18	XXX	
78585		A	rebreathing and washout, with or without single breath	1.09	5.74	5.74	0.30	7.13	7.13	XXX	
	26	A		1.09	0.39	0.39	0.05	1.53	1.53	XXX	
	TC	A		0.00	5.35	5.35	0.25	5.60	5.60	XXX	

■ RVU not developed by CMS. Gap-filled RVUs developed by CHEG.

Code	M	S	Description	Work Value	Non-Fac PE	Fac PE	Mal-practice	Non-Fac Total	Fac Total	Global	Gap
78586		A	Pulmonary ventilation imaging, aerosol; single projection	0.40	2.60	2.60	0.14	3.14	3.14	XXX	
	26	A		0.40	0.14	0.14	0.02	0.56	0.56	XXX	
	TC	A		0.00	2.46	2.46	0.12	2.58	2.58	XXX	
78587		A	multiple projections (eg, anterior, posterior, lateral views)	0.49	2.84	2.84	0.14	3.47	3.47	XXX	
	26	A		0.49	0.18	0.18	0.02	0.69	0.69	XXX	
	TC	A		0.00	2.66	2.66	0.12	2.78	2.78	XXX	
78588		A	Pulmonary perfusion imaging, particulate, with ventilation imaging, aerosol, one or multiple projections	1.09	3.43	3.43	0.20	4.72	4.72	XXX	
	26	A		1.09	0.39	0.39	0.05	1.53	1.53	XXX	
	TC	A		0.00	3.04	3.04	0.15	3.19	3.19	XXX	
78591		A	Pulmonary ventilation imaging, gaseous, single breath, single projection	0.40	2.86	2.86	0.14	3.40	3.40	XXX	
	26	A		0.40	0.15	0.15	0.02	0.57	0.57	XXX	
	TC	A		0.00	2.71	2.71	0.12	2.83	2.83	XXX	
78593		A	Pulmonary ventilation imaging, gaseous, with rebreathing and washout with or without single breath; single projection	0.49	3.46	3.46	0.17	4.12	4.12	XXX	
	26	A		0.49	0.18	0.18	0.02	0.69	0.69	XXX	
	TC	A		0.00	3.28	3.28	0.15	3.43	3.43	XXX	
78594		A	multiple projections (eg, anterior, posterior, lateral views)	0.53	4.92	4.92	0.23	5.68	5.68	XXX	
	26	A		0.53	0.19	0.19	0.02	0.74	0.74	XXX	
	TC	A		0.00	4.73	4.73	0.21	4.94	4.94	XXX	
78596		A	Pulmonary quantitative differential function (ventilation/perfusion) study	1.27	7.17	7.17	0.36	8.80	8.80	XXX	
	26	A		1.27	0.46	0.46	0.05	1.78	1.78	XXX	
	TC	A		0.00	6.71	6.71	0.31	7.02	7.02	XXX	
78599		C	Unlisted respiratory procedure, diagnostic nuclear medicine	0.00	0.00	0.00	0.00	0.00	0.00	XXX	
	26	C		0.00	0.00	0.00	0.00	0.00	0.00	XXX	
	TC	C		0.00	0.00	0.00	0.00	0.00	0.00	XXX	
78600		A	Brain imaging, limited procedure; static	0.44	2.90	2.90	0.14	3.48	3.48	XXX	
	26	A		0.44	0.16	0.16	0.02	0.62	0.62	XXX	
	TC	A		0.00	2.74	2.74	0.12	2.86	2.86	XXX	
78601		A	with vascular flow	0.51	3.41	3.41	0.17	4.09	4.09	XXX	
	26	A		0.51	0.18	0.18	0.02	0.71	0.71	XXX	
	TC	A		0.00	3.23	3.23	0.15	3.38	3.38	XXX	
78605		A	Brain imaging, complete study; static	0.53	3.42	3.42	0.17	4.12	4.12	XXX	
	26	A		0.53	0.19	0.19	0.02	0.74	0.74	XXX	
	TC	A		0.00	3.23	3.23	0.15	3.38	3.38	XXX	
78606		A	with vascular flow	0.64	3.90	3.90	0.20	4.74	4.74	XXX	
	26	A		0.64	0.23	0.23	0.03	0.90	0.90	XXX	
	TC	A		0.00	3.67	3.67	0.17	3.84	3.84	XXX	
78607		A	tomographic (SPECT)	1.23	6.70	6.70	0.34	8.27	8.27	XXX	
	26	A		1.23	0.47	0.47	0.05	1.75	1.75	XXX	
	TC	A		0.00	6.23	6.23	0.29	6.52	6.52	XXX	
78608		N	Brain imaging, positron emission tomography (PET); metabolic evaluation	0.00	0.00	0.00	0.00	0.00	0.00	XXX	
78609		N	perfusion evaluation	0.00	0.00	0.00	0.00	0.00	0.00	XXX	

■ RVU not developed by CMS. Gap-filled RVUs developed by CHEG.

Code	M	S	Description	Work Value	Non-Fac PE	Fac PE	Mal-practice	Non-Fac Total	Fac Total	Global	Gap
78610		**A**	Brain imaging, vascular flow only	0.30	1.61	1.61	0.09	2.00	2.00	XXX	
	26	**A**		0.30	0.11	0.11	0.01	0.42	0.42	XXX	
	TC	**A**		0.00	1.50	1.50	0.08	1.58	1.58	XXX	
78615		**A**	Cerebral vascular flow	0.42	3.81	3.81	0.19	4.42	4.42	XXX	
	26	**A**		0.42	0.16	0.16	0.02	0.60	0.60	XXX	
	TC	**A**		0.00	3.65	3.65	0.17	3.82	3.82	XXX	
78630		**A**	Cerebrospinal fluid flow, imaging (not	0.68	5.02	5.02	0.25	5.95	5.95	XXX	
	26	**A**	including introduction of material);	0.68	0.24	0.24	0.03	0.95	0.95	XXX	
	TC	**A**	cisternography	0.00	4.78	4.78	0.22	5.00	5.00	XXX	
78635		**A**	ventriculography	0.61	2.67	2.67	0.14	3.42	3.42	XXX	
	26	**A**		0.61	0.25	0.25	0.02	0.88	0.88	XXX	
	TC	**A**		0.00	2.42	2.42	0.12	2.54	2.54	XXX	
78645		**A**	shunt evaluation	0.57	3.47	3.47	0.17	4.21	4.21	XXX	
	26	**A**		0.57	0.21	0.21	0.02	0.80	0.80	XXX	
	TC	**A**		0.00	3.26	3.26	0.15	3.41	3.41	XXX	
78647		**A**	tomographic (SPECT)	0.90	5.94	5.94	0.29	7.13	7.13	XXX	
	26	**A**		0.90	0.33	0.33	0.03	1.26	1.26	XXX	
	TC	**A**		0.00	5.61	5.61	0.26	5.87	5.87	XXX	
78650		**A**	Cerebrospinal fluid leakage detection and	0.61	4.63	4.63	0.22	5.46	5.46	XXX	
	26	**A**	localization	0.61	0.22	0.22	0.02	0.85	0.85	XXX	
	TC	**A**		0.00	4.41	4.41	0.20	4.61	4.61	XXX	
78660		**A**	Radiopharmaceutical dacryocystography	0.53	2.20	2.20	0.12	2.85	2.85	XXX	
	26	**A**		0.53	0.19	0.19	0.02	0.74	0.74	XXX	
	TC	**A**		0.00	2.01	2.01	0.10	2.11	2.11	XXX	
78699		**C**	Unlisted nervous system procedure, diagnostic	0.00	0.00	0.00	0.00	0.00	0.00	XXX	
	26	**C**	nuclear medicine	0.00	0.00	0.00	0.00	0.00	0.00	XXX	
	TC	**C**		0.00	0.00	0.00	0.00	0.00	0.00	XXX	
78700		**A**	Kidney imaging; static only	0.45	3.05	3.05	0.15	3.65	3.65	XXX	
	26	**A**		0.45	0.16	0.16	0.02	0.63	0.63	XXX	
	TC	**A**		0.00	2.89	2.89	0.13	3.02	3.02	XXX	
78701		**A**	with vascular flow	0.49	3.55	3.55	0.17	4.21	4.21	XXX	
	26	**A**		0.49	0.17	0.17	0.02	0.68	0.68	XXX	
	TC	**A**		0.00	3.38	3.38	0.15	3.53	3.53	XXX	
78704		**A**	with function study (ie, imaging	0.74	4.03	4.03	0.20	4.97	4.97	XXX	
	26	**A**	renogram)	0.74	0.27	0.27	0.03	1.04	1.04	XXX	
	TC	**A**		0.00	3.76	3.76	0.17	3.93	3.93	XXX	
78707		**A**	Kidney imaging with vascular flow and	0.96	4.59	4.59	0.23	5.78	5.78	XXX	
	26	**A**	function; single study without pharmacological	0.96	0.35	0.35	0.04	1.35	1.35	XXX	
	TC	**A**	intervention	0.00	4.24	4.24	0.19	4.43	4.43	XXX	
78708		**A**	single study, with pharmacological	1.21	4.68	4.68	0.24	6.13	6.13	XXX	
	26	**A**	intervention (eg, angiotensin converting	1.21	0.44	0.44	0.05	1.70	1.70	XXX	
	TC	**A**	enzyme inhibitor and/or diuretic	0.00	4.24	4.24	0.19	4.43	4.43	XXX	

Radiology

■ RVU not developed by CMS. Gap-filled RVUs developed by CHEG.

Code	M	S	Description	Work Value	Non-Fac PE	Fac PE	Mal-prac-tice	Non-Fac Total	Fac Total	Global	Gap
78709		A	multiple studies, with and without	1.41	4.75	4.75	0.25	6.41	6.41	XXX	
	26	A	pharmacological intervention (eg,	1.41	0.51	0.51	0.06	1.98	1.98	XXX	
	TC	A	angiotensin converting enzyme inhibitor and/or diuretic)	0.00	4.24	4.24	0.19	4.43	4.43	XXX	
78710		A	Kidney imaging, tomographic (SPECT)	0.66	5.84	5.84	0.29	6.79	6.79	XXX	
	26	A		0.66	0.23	0.23	0.03	0.92	0.92	XXX	
	TC	A		0.00	5.61	5.61	0.26	5.87	5.87	XXX	
78715		A	Kidney vascular flow only	0.30	1.61	1.61	0.09	2.00	2.00	XXX	
	26	A		0.30	0.11	0.11	0.01	0.42	0.42	XXX	
	TC	A		0.00	1.50	1.50	0.08	1.58	1.58	XXX	
78725		A	Kidney function study, non-imaging	0.38	1.83	1.83	0.10	2.31	2.31	XXX	
	26	A	radioisotopic study	0.38	0.14	0.14	0.01	0.53	0.53	XXX	
	TC	A		0.00	1.69	1.69	0.09	1.78	1.78	XXX	
78730		A	Urinary bladder residual study	0.36	1.52	1.52	0.09	1.97	1.97	XXX	
	26	A		0.36	0.13	0.13	0.02	0.51	0.51	XXX	
	TC	A		0.00	1.39	1.39	0.07	1.46	1.46	XXX	
78740		A	Ureteral reflux study (radiopharmaceutical	0.57	2.22	2.22	0.12	2.91	2.91	XXX	
	26	A	voiding cystogram)	0.57	0.21	0.21	0.02	0.80	0.80	XXX	
	TC	A		0.00	2.01	2.01	0.10	2.11	2.11	XXX	
78760		A	Testicular imaging;	0.66	2.77	2.77	0.15	3.58	3.58	XXX	
	26	A		0.66	0.23	0.23	0.03	0.92	0.92	XXX	
	TC	A		0.00	2.54	2.54	0.12	2.66	2.66	XXX	
78761		A	with vascular flow	0.71	3.30	3.30	0.17	4.18	4.18	XXX	
	26	A		0.71	0.26	0.26	0.03	1.00	1.00	XXX	
	TC	A		0.00	3.04	3.04	0.14	3.18	3.18	XXX	
78799		C	Unlisted genitourinary procedure, diagnostic	0.00	0.00	0.00	0.00	0.00	0.00	XXX	
	26	C	nuclear medicine	0.00	0.00	0.00	0.00	0.00	0.00	XXX	
	TC	C		0.00	0.00	0.00	0.00	0.00	0.00	XXX	
78800		A	Radiopharmaceutical localization of tumor;	0.66	3.46	3.46	0.18	4.30	4.30	XXX	
	26	A	limited area	0.66	0.23	0.23	0.03	0.92	0.92	XXX	
	TC	A		0.00	3.23	3.23	0.15	3.38	3.38	XXX	
78801		A	multiple areas	0.79	4.30	4.30	0.21	5.30	5.30	XXX	
	26	A		0.79	0.29	0.29	0.03	1.11	1.11	XXX	
	TC	A		0.00	4.01	4.01	0.18	4.19	4.19	XXX	
78802		A	whole body	0.86	5.57	5.57	0.28	6.71	6.71	XXX	
	26	A		0.86	0.32	0.32	0.03	1.21	1.21	XXX	
	TC	A		0.00	5.25	5.25	0.25	5.50	5.50	XXX	
78803		A	tomographic (SPECT)	1.09	6.64	6.64	0.33	8.06	8.06	XXX	
	26	A		1.09	0.41	0.41	0.04	1.54	1.54	XXX	
	TC	A		0.00	6.23	6.23	0.29	6.52	6.52	XXX	
78805		A	Radiopharmaceutical localization of	0.73	3.50	3.50	0.18	4.41	4.41	XXX	
	26	A	inflammatory process; limited area	0.73	0.27	0.27	0.03	1.03	1.03	XXX	
	TC	A		0.00	3.23	3.23	0.15	3.38	3.38	XXX	

■ RVU not developed by CMS. Gap-filled RVUs developed by CHEG.

Code	M	S	Description	Work Value	Non-Fac PE	Fac PE	Mal-practice	Non-Fac Total	Fac Total	Global	Gap
78806		A	whole body	0.86	6.43	6.43	0.32	7.61	7.61	XXX	
	26	A		0.86	0.32	0.32	0.03	1.21	1.21	XXX	
	TC	A		0.00	6.11	6.11	0.29	6.40	6.40	XXX	
78807		A	tomographic (SPECT)	1.09	6.66	6.66	0.33	8.08	8.08	XXX	
	26	A		1.09	0.43	0.43	0.04	1.56	1.56	XXX	
	TC	A		0.00	6.23	6.23	0.29	6.52	6.52	XXX	
78810		N	Tumor imaging, positron emission tomography (PET), metabolic evaluation	0.00	0.00	0.00	0.00	0.00	0.00	XXX	
	26	N		1.93	0.77	0.77	0.09	2.79	2.79	XXX	
	TC	N		0.00	0.00	0.00	0.00	0.00	0.00	XXX	
78890		B	Generation of automated data: interactive process involving nuclear physician and/or allied health professional personnel; simple manipulations and interpretation, not to exceed 30 minutes	0.05	1.26	1.26	0.06	1.37	1.37	XXX	
	26	B		0.05	0.02	0.02	0.01	0.08	0.08	XXX	
	TC	B		0.00	1.24	1.24	0.05	1.29	1.29	XXX	
78891		B	complex manipulations and interpretation, exceeding 30 minutes	0.10	2.53	2.53	0.12	2.75	2.75	XXX	
	26	B		0.10	0.04	0.04	0.01	0.15	0.15	XXX	
	TC	B		0.00	2.49	2.49	0.11	2.60	2.60	XXX	
78990		I	Provision of diagnostic radiopharmaceutical(s)	0.00	0.00	0.00	0.00	0.00	0.00	XXX	
78999		C	Unlisted miscellaneous procedure, diagnostic nuclear medicine	0.00	0.00	0.00	0.00	0.00	0.00	XXX	
	26	C		0.00	0.00	0.00	0.00	0.00	0.00	XXX	
	TC	C		0.00	0.00	0.00	0.00	0.00	0.00	XXX	
79000		A	Radiopharmaceutical therapy, hyperthyroidism; initial, including evaluation of patient	1.80	3.14	3.14	0.19	5.13	5.13	XXX	
	26	A		1.80	0.65	0.65	0.07	2.52	2.52	XXX	
	TC	A		0.00	2.49	2.49	0.12	2.61	2.61	XXX	
79001		A	subsequent, each therapy	1.05	1.63	1.63	0.10	2.78	2.78	XXX	
	26	A		1.05	0.39	0.39	0.04	1.48	1.48	XXX	
	TC	A		0.00	1.24	1.24	0.06	1.30	1.30	XXX	
79020		A	Radiopharmaceutical therapy, thyroid suppression (euthyroid cardiac disease), including evaluation of patient	1.81	3.13	3.13	0.19	5.13	5.13	XXX	
	26	A		1.81	0.64	0.64	0.07	2.52	2.52	XXX	
	TC	A		0.00	2.49	2.49	0.12	2.61	2.61	XXX	
79030		A	Radiopharmaceutical ablation of gland for thyroid carcinoma	2.10	3.26	3.26	0.20	5.56	5.56	XXX	
	26	A		2.10	0.77	0.77	0.08	2.95	2.95	XXX	
	TC	A		0.00	2.49	2.49	0.12	2.61	2.61	XXX	
79035		A	Radiopharmaceutical therapy for metastases of thyroid carcinoma	2.52	3.43	3.43	0.21	6.16	6.16	XXX	
	26	A		2.52	0.94	0.94	0.09	3.55	3.55	XXX	
	TC	A		0.00	2.49	2.49	0.12	2.61	2.61	XXX	
79100		A	Radiopharmaceutical therapy, polycythemia vera, chronic leukemia, each treatment	1.32	3.00	3.00	0.17	4.49	4.49	XXX	
	26	A		1.32	0.51	0.51	0.05	1.88	1.88	XXX	
	TC	A		0.00	2.49	2.49	0.12	2.61	2.61	XXX	
79200		A	Intracavitary radioactive colloid therapy	1.99	3.23	3.23	0.19	5.41	5.41	XXX	
	26	A		1.99	0.74	0.74	0.07	2.80	2.80	XXX	
	TC	A		0.00	2.49	2.49	0.12	2.61	2.61	XXX	
79300		C	Interstitial radioactive colloid therapy	2.67	1.13	1.13	0.12	3.92	3.92	XXX	■
	26	A		1.60	0.68	0.68	0.07	2.35	2.35	XXX	
	TC	C		1.07	0.45	0.45	0.05	1.57	1.57	XXX	■

■ RVU not developed by CMS. Gap-filled RVUs developed by CHEG.

Radiology

Code	M	S	Description	Work Value	Non-Fac PE	Fac PE	Mal-prac-tice	Non-Fac Total	Fac Total	Global	Gap
79400		A	Radiopharmaceutical therapy, nonthyroid, nonhematologic	1.96	3.22	3.22	0.20	5.38	5.38	XXX	
	26	A		1.96	0.73	0.73	0.08	2.77	2.77	XXX	
	TC	A		0.00	2.49	2.49	0.12	2.61	2.61	XXX	
79420		C	Intravascular radiopharmaceutical therapy, particulate	0.00	0.00	0.00	0.00	0.00	0.00	XXX	
	26	A		1.51	0.54	0.54	0.06	2.11	2.11	XXX	
	TC	C		0.00	0.00	0.00	0.00	0.00	0.00	XXX	
79440		A	Intra-articular radiopharmaceutical therapy	1.99	3.29	3.29	0.20	5.48	5.48	XXX	
	26	A		1.99	0.80	0.80	0.08	2.87	2.87	XXX	
	TC	A		0.00	2.49	2.49	0.12	2.61	2.61	XXX	
79900		C	Provision of therapeutic radiopharmaceutical(s)	0.00	0.00	0.00	0.00	0.00	0.00	XXX	
79999		C	Unlisted radiopharmaceutical therapeutic procedure	0.00	0.00	0.00	0.00	0.00	0.00	XXX	
	26	C		0.00	0.00	0.00	0.00	0.00	0.00	XXX	
	TC	C		0.00	0.00	0.00	0.00	0.00	0.00	XXX	

■ RVU not developed by CMS. Gap-filled RVUs developed by CHEG.

Pathology and Laboratory

The Introduction provides complete descriptions for the status column (abbreviated as S). If a relative value is not available for a procedure, it is indicated with a "0.00" in the individual units column.

I. **General:** Values in this section include recording of the specimen, performance of the test, and reporting of the result. They do not include specimen collection, transfer, or individual patient administrative services.

   A. **Total:** When no modifier is listed, the unit value represents the global value of the procedure. The five-digit code is used to represent a global service inclusive of the professional services and technical cost of providing that service.

   B. **Professional:** The unit value listed next to the modifier column (modifier -26) is used to designate professional services. Modifier -26 is added to the procedure code to indicate the use of this value. The professional component includes examination of the patient, when indicated; performance and/or supervision of the procedure or lab test; interpretation and/or written report concerning the examination or lab test; and consultation with referring physicians.

   C. **Technical:** The unit value listed next to the modifier column (modifier -TC) is used to designate the technical value of providing the service, Modifier -T may be used to designate this component. The technical component includes personnel, materials, space, equipment, and other allocated facility overhead normally included in providing the service. **Note:** Modifier -TC is not CPT compatible and may not be accepted by all payers. Check with the specific payer prior to use of this modifier. Medicare will accept -TC'.

II. **Unlisted Service or Procedure:** A service or procedure that is not identified by a particular code should be listed under the appropriate "Unlisted Procedure." These procedures have "9" as the final digit. Values should be substantiated by report. *See "By Report."*

III. **Unusual Procedural Services:** When a procedure of unusual nature is performed, modifier -22 should be added and value substantiated by report. *See "By Report."*

IV. **By Report:** Value of a procedure should be established for any "By Report" circumstance by identifying a similar service and justifying the difference. Procedures which require a report should include the following:

   A. Accurate definition

   B. Clinical history

   C. Related procedure values

   D. Reason for value adjustment

V. **Reference (Outside) Laboratory:** The laboratory tests and services listed in this section, when performed by other than the physician, require the applicable procedure number with the appropriate modifier (-90). *See Introduction for complete modifier description.*

VI. **Repeat Clinical Diagnostic Laboratory Test:** Tests repeated the same day for the same patient to obtain multiple results require use of modifier -91'. *See Introduction for complete modifier description.*

VII. **Collection and Handling:** Collection and handling of laboratory and pathology specimens may be reported separately. To report handling of specimens, see codes 99000 and 99001 in the Medicine section. Collection is reported using codes from the Surgery section. For routine venipuncture, see 36415. For venipuncture over age three years, requiring physician skill, see 36410. For venipuncture under age three years (femoral, jugular, sagittal sinus, scalp or other vein)

Pathology

see 36400-36406. For venipuncture by cutdown, see 36420-36425. For collection of specimen from implanted venous access device, see 36540. For routine arterial puncture, see 36600. For arterial catheterization, see 36620-36625. See Guidelines for reporting these services in the appropriate section (Medicine or Surgery) and use the appropriate conversion factor. Medicare requires the use of HCPCS Level II code G0001 for routine venipuncture and may not pay for handling charges (99000-99001).

VIII. Multiple Procedures: Multiple procedures performed on the same date should be listed using modifier -51'. Customarily each procedure is allowed 100 percent of the listed value.

IX. Reduced Services: If a physician elects to reduce the value of a procedure, modifier -52 should be added to the procedure code.

X. Consultation: Several consultation codes are listed for various types of pathology consults. (See 80500–80502, 88321–88392). Medicine codes may also be used, if appropriate.

XI. Services or Procedures Listed in Other Sections: Services or procedures provided by a pathologist may be listed in an alternate section of the book (i.e., consultations listed in Medicine). The pathologist should use these procedure codes following the guidelines appropriate to that section.

XII. Modifiers: A comprehensive listing of modifiers is provided in the Introduction.

XIII. Global Values: This column indicates the number of days in the global period for which services directly related to the procedure are included. The majority of codes have a numerical designation (i.e., 0, 10, or 90).

A. MMM codes describe services furnished in uncomplicated maternity care. This includes antepartum, delivery, and postpartum care. The usual global surgical concept does not apply.

B. XXX codes indicate that the global surgery concept does not apply.

C. YYY codes indicate that the global period is to be set by the local carrier.

D. ZZZ codes indicate that the code is an add-on service and therefore is treated in the global period of the other procedure billed in conjunction with a ZZZ code. Do not bill these codes with modifier -51'. They should not be reduced.

Pathology

XIV. Clinical Laboratory Improvements Amendments (CLIA): CMS has identified a number of simple laboratory procedures that can be performed in physicians offices after obtaining a Certificate of Waiver. Waived tests are subject to change at any time, so review all Medicare mailings for changes to the waived tests. Waived tests submitted to Medicare should be reported exactly as they appear on the Medicare list of waived procedures. Those identified with HCPCS Level II modifier -QW on the list, should be submitted with the -QW modifier appended to the code. If the code is not identified with a -QW on the list, do not append the modifier.

Pathology and Laboratory Values

Code	M	S	Description	Work Value	Non-Fac PE	Fac PE	Mal-prac-tice	Non-Fac Total	Fac Total	Global	Gap
80048		X	Basic metabolic panel This panel must include the following: Calcium (82310) Carbon dioxide (82374) Chloride (82435) Creatinine (82565) Glucose (82947) Potassium (84132) Sodium (84295) Urea Nitrogen (BUN) (84520)	0.00	0.31	0.31	0.00	0.31	0.31	XXX	■
	26			0.00	0.00	0.00	0.00	0.00	0.00	XXX	■
	TC			0.00	0.31	0.31	0.00	0.31	0.31	XXX	■
80050		N	General health panel This panel must include the following: Comprehensive metabolic panel (80053) Hemogram, automated, and manual differential WBC count (CBC) (85022) OR Hemogram and platelet count, automated, and automated complete differential WBC count (CBC) (85025) Thyroid stimulating hormone (TSH) (84443)	0.00	0.81	0.81	0.00	0.81	0.81	XXX	■
	26			0.00	0.00	0.00	0.00	0.00	0.00	XXX	■
	TC			0.00	0.81	0.81	0.00	0.81	0.81	XXX	■
80051		X	Electrolyte panel This panel must include the following: carbon dioxide (82374), chloride (82435), potassium (84132), sodium (84295)	0.00	0.25	0.25	0.00	0.25	0.25	XXX	■
	26			0.00	0.00	0.00	0.00	0.00	0.00	XXX	■
	TC			0.00	0.25	0.25	0.00	0.25	0.25	XXX	■
80053		X	Comprehensive metabolic panel This panel must include the following: Albumin (82040) Bilirubin, total (82247) Calcium (82310) Carbon dioxide (bicarbonate) (82374) Chloride (82435) Creatinine (82565) Glucose (82947) Phosphatase, alkaline (84075) Potassium (84132) Protein, total (84155) Sodium (84295) Transferase, alanine amino (ALT) (SGPT) (84460) Transferase, aspartate amino (AST) (SGOT) (84450) Urea Nitrogen (BUN) (84520)	0.00	0.42	0.42	0.00	0.42	0.42	XXX	■
	26			0.00	0.00	0.00	0.00	0.00	0.00	XXX	■
	TC			0.00	0.42	0.42	0.00	0.42	0.42	XXX	■
80055		I	Obstetric panel This panel must include the following: Hemogram, automated, and manual differential WBC count (CBC) (85022) OR Hemogram and platelet count, automated, and automated complete differential WBC count (CBC) (85025) Hepatitis B surface antigen (HBsAg) (87340) Antibody, rubella (86762) Syphilis test, qualitative (eg, VDRL, RPR, ART) (86592) Antibody screen, RBC, each serum technique (86850) Blood typing, ABO (86900) AND Blood typing, Rh (D) (86901)	0.00	0.92	0.92	0.00	0.92	0.92	XXX	■
	26			0.00	0.00	0.00	0.00	0.00	0.00	XXX	■
	TC			0.00	0.92	0.92	0.00	0.92	0.92	XXX	■
80061		X	Lipid panel This panel must include the following: Cholesterol, serum, total (82465) Lipoprotein, direct measurement, high density cholesterol (HDL cholesterol) (83718) Triglycerides (84478)	0.00	0.56	0.56	0.00	0.56	0.56	XXX	■
	26			0.00	0.00	0.00	0.00	0.00	0.00	XXX	■
	TC			0.00	0.56	0.56	0.00	0.56	0.56	XXX	■
80069		X	Renal function panel This panel must include the following: Albumin (82040) Calcium (82310) Carbon dioxide (bicarbonate) (82374) Chloride (82435) Creatinine (82565) Glucose (82947) Phosphorus inorganic (phosphate) (84100) Potassium (84132) Sodium (84295) Urea nitrogen (BUN) (84520)	0.00	0.34	0.34	0.00	0.34	0.34	XXX	■
	26			0.00	0.00	0.00	0.00	0.00	0.00	XXX	■
	TC			0.00	0.34	0.34	0.00	0.34	0.34	XXX	■

■ RVU not developed by CMS. Gap-filled RVUs developed by Ingenix/CHEG.

Code	M	S	Description	Work Value	Non-Fac PE	Fac PE	Mal-practice	Non-Fac Total	Fac Total	Global	Gap
80074		X	Acute hepatitis panel This panel must include the following: Hepatitis A antibody (HAAb), IgM antibody (86709) Hepatitis B core antibody (HbcAb), IgM antibody (86705) Hepatitis B surface antigen (HbsAg) (87340) Hepatitis C antibody (86803)	0.00	1.38	1.38	0.00	1.38	1.38	XXX	■
	26			0.00	0.00	0.00	0.00	0.00	0.00	XXX	■
	TC			0.00	1.38	1.38	0.00	1.38	1.38	XXX	■
80076		X	Hepatic function panel This panel must include the following: Albumin (82040) Bilirubin, total (82247) Bilirubin, direct (82248) Phosphatase, alkaline (84075) Protein, total (84155) Transferase, alanine amino (ALT) (SGPT) (84460) Transferase, aspartate amino (AST) (SGOT) (84450)	0.00	0.29	0.29	0.00	0.29	0.29	XXX	■
	26			0.00	0.00	0.00	0.00	0.00	0.00	XXX	■
	TC			0.00	0.29	0.29	0.00	0.29	0.29	XXX	■
80090		X	TORCH antibody panel This panel must include the following tests: Antibody, cytomegalovirus (CMV) (86644) Antibody, herpes simplex, non-specific type test (86694) Antibody, rubella (86762) Antibody, toxoplasma (86777)	0.00	1.10	1.10	0.00	1.10	1.10	XXX	■
	26			0.00	0.00	0.00	0.00	0.00	0.00	XXX	■
	TC			0.00	1.10	1.10	0.00	1.10	1.10	XXX	■
80100		X	Drug screen, qualitative; multiple drug classes chromatographic method, each procedure	0.00	0.64	0.64	0.00	0.64	0.64	XXX	■
	26			0.00	0.00	0.00	0.00	0.00	0.00	XXX	■
	TC			0.00	0.64	0.64	0.00	0.64	0.64	XXX	■
80101		X	single drug class method (eg, immunoassay, enzyme assay), each drug class	0.00	0.51	0.51	0.00	0.51	0.51	XXX	■
	26			0.00	0.00	0.00	0.00	0.00	0.00	XXX	■
	TC			0.00	0.51	0.51	0.00	0.51	0.51	XXX	■
80102		X	Drug confirmation, each procedure	0.00	0.73	0.73	0.00	0.73	0.73	XXX	■
	26			0.00	0.00	0.00	0.00	0.00	0.00	XXX	■
	TC			0.00	0.73	0.73	0.00	0.73	0.73	XXX	■
80103		X	Tissue preparation for drug analysis	0.00	0.37	0.37	0.00	0.37	0.37	XXX	■
	26			0.00	0.00	0.00	0.00	0.00	0.00	XXX	■
	TC			0.00	0.37	0.37	0.00	0.37	0.37	XXX	■
80150		X	Amikacin	0.00	0.66	0.66	0.00	0.66	0.66	XXX	■
	26			0.00	0.00	0.00	0.00	0.00	0.00	XXX	■
	TC			0.00	0.66	0.66	0.00	0.66	0.66	XXX	■
80152		X	Amitriptyline	0.00	0.73	0.73	0.00	0.73	0.73	XXX	■
	26			0.00	0.00	0.00	0.00	0.00	0.00	XXX	■
	TC			0.00	0.73	0.73	0.00	0.73	0.73	XXX	■
80154		X	Benzodiazepines	0.00	0.73	0.73	0.00	0.73	0.73	XXX	■
	26			0.00	0.00	0.00	0.00	0.00	0.00	XXX	■
	TC			0.00	0.73	0.73	0.00	0.73	0.73	XXX	■
80156		X	Carbamazepine; total	0.00	0.59	0.59	0.00	0.59	0.59	XXX	■
	26			0.00	0.00	0.00	0.00	0.00	0.00	XXX	■
	TC			0.00	0.59	0.59	0.00	0.59	0.59	XXX	■
80157		X	free	0.00	0.59	0.59	0.00	0.59	0.59	XXX	■
	26			0.00	0.00	0.00	0.00	0.00	0.00	XXX	■
	TC			0.00	0.59	0.59	0.00	0.59	0.59	XXX	■

Pathology

■ RVU not developed by CMS. Gap-filled RVUs developed by Ingenix/CHEG.

Code	M	S	Description	Work Value	Non-Fac PE	Fac PE	Mal-prac-tice	Non-Fac Total	Fac Total	Global	Gap
80158		X	Cyclosporine	0.00	0.88	0.88	0.00	0.88	0.88	XXX	■
	26			0.00	0.00	0.00	0.00	0.00	0.00	XXX	■
	TC			0.00	0.88	0.88	0.00	0.88	0.88	XXX	■
80160		X	Desipramine	0.00	0.73	0.73	0.00	0.73	0.73	XXX	■
	26			0.00	0.00	0.00	0.00	0.00	0.00	XXX	■
	TC			0.00	0.73	0.73	0.00	0.73	0.73	XXX	■
80162		X	Digoxin	0.00	0.56	0.56	0.00	0.56	0.56	XXX	■
	26			0.00	0.00	0.00	0.00	0.00	0.00	XXX	■
	TC			0.00	0.56	0.56	0.00	0.56	0.56	XXX	■
80164		X	Dipropylacetic acid (valproic acid)	0.00	0.59	0.59	0.00	0.59	0.59	XXX	■
	26			0.00	0.00	0.00	0.00	0.00	0.00	XXX	■
	TC			0.00	0.59	0.59	0.00	0.59	0.59	XXX	■
80166		X	Doxepin	0.00	0.73	0.73	0.00	0.73	0.73	XXX	■
	26			0.00	0.00	0.00	0.00	0.00	0.00	XXX	■
	TC			0.00	0.73	0.73	0.00	0.73	0.73	XXX	■
80168		X	Ethosuximide	0.00	0.66	0.66	0.00	0.66	0.66	XXX	■
	26			0.00	0.00	0.00	0.00	0.00	0.00	XXX	■
	TC			0.00	0.66	0.66	0.00	0.66	0.66	XXX	■
80170		X	Gentamicin	0.00	0.59	0.59	0.00	0.59	0.59	XXX	■
	26			0.00	0.00	0.00	0.00	0.00	0.00	XXX	■
	TC			0.00	0.59	0.59	0.00	0.59	0.59	XXX	■
80172		X	Gold	0.00	0.59	0.59	0.00	0.59	0.59	XXX	■
	26			0.00	0.00	0.00	0.00	0.00	0.00	XXX	■
	TC			0.00	0.59	0.59	0.00	0.59	0.59	XXX	■
80173		X	Haloperidol	0.00	0.73	0.73	0.00	0.73	0.73	XXX	■
	26			0.00	0.00	0.00	0.00	0.00	0.00	XXX	■
	TC			0.00	0.73	0.73	0.00	0.73	0.73	XXX	■
80174		X	Imipramine	0.00	0.73	0.73	0.00	0.73	0.73	XXX	■
	26			0.00	0.00	0.00	0.00	0.00	0.00	XXX	■
	TC			0.00	0.73	0.73	0.00	0.73	0.73	XXX	■
80176		X	Lidocaine	0.00	0.59	0.59	0.00	0.59	0.59	XXX	■
	26			0.00	0.00	0.00	0.00	0.00	0.00	XXX	■
	TC			0.00	0.59	0.59	0.00	0.59	0.59	XXX	■
80178		X	Lithium	0.00	0.34	0.34	0.00	0.34	0.34	XXX	■
	26			0.00	0.00	0.00	0.00	0.00	0.00	XXX	■
	TC			0.00	0.34	0.34	0.00	0.34	0.34	XXX	■
80182		X	Nortriptyline	0.00	0.73	0.73	0.00	0.73	0.73	XXX	■
	26			0.00	0.00	0.00	0.00	0.00	0.00	XXX	■
	TC			0.00	0.73	0.73	0.00	0.73	0.73	XXX	■
80184		X	Phenobarbital	0.00	0.59	0.59	0.00	0.59	0.59	XXX	■
	26			0.00	0.00	0.00	0.00	0.00	0.00	XXX	■
	TC			0.00	0.59	0.59	0.00	0.59	0.59	XXX	■
80185		X	Phenytoin; total	0.00	0.56	0.56	0.00	0.56	0.56	XXX	■
	26			0.00	0.00	0.00	0.00	0.00	0.00	XXX	■
	TC			0.00	0.56	0.56	0.00	0.56	0.56	XXX	■

Pathology

■ RVU not developed by CMS. Gap-filled RVUs developed by Ingenix/CHEG.

Code	M	S	Description	Work Value	Non-Fac PE	Fac PE	Mal-practice	Non-Fac Total	Fac Total	Global	Gap
80186		X	free	0.00	0.59	0.59	0.00	0.59	0.59	XXX	■
	26			0.00	0.00	0.00	0.00	0.00	0.00	XXX	■
	TC			0.00	0.59	0.59	0.00	0.59	0.59	XXX	■
80188		X	Primidone	0.00	0.59	0.59	0.00	0.59	0.59	XXX	■
	26			0.00	0.00	0.00	0.00	0.00	0.00	XXX	■
	TC			0.00	0.59	0.59	0.00	0.59	0.59	XXX	■
80190		X	Procainamide;	0.00	0.59	0.59	0.00	0.59	0.59	XXX	■
	26			0.00	0.00	0.00	0.00	0.00	0.00	XXX	■
	TC			0.00	0.59	0.59	0.00	0.59	0.59	XXX	■
80192		X	with metabolites (eg, n-acetyl procainamide)	0.00	0.81	0.81	0.00	0.81	0.81	XXX	■
	26			0.00	0.00	0.00	0.00	0.00	0.00	XXX	■
	TC			0.00	0.81	0.81	0.00	0.81	0.81	XXX	■
80194		X	Quinidine	0.00	0.59	0.59	0.00	0.59	0.59	XXX	■
	26			0.00	0.00	0.00	0.00	0.00	0.00	XXX	■
	TC			0.00	0.59	0.59	0.00	0.59	0.59	XXX	■
80196		X	Salicylate	0.00	0.35	0.35	0.00	0.35	0.35	XXX	■
	26			0.00	0.00	0.00	0.00	0.00	0.00	XXX	■
	TC			0.00	0.35	0.35	0.00	0.35	0.35	XXX	■
80197		X	Tacrolimus	0.00	0.88	0.88	0.00	0.88	0.88	XXX	■
	26			0.00	0.00	0.00	0.00	0.00	0.00	XXX	■
	TC			0.00	0.88	0.88	0.00	0.88	0.88	XXX	■
80198		X	Theophylline	0.00	0.56	0.56	0.00	0.56	0.56	XXX	■
	26			0.00	0.00	0.00	0.00	0.00	0.00	XXX	■
	TC			0.00	0.56	0.56	0.00	0.56	0.56	XXX	■
80200		X	Tobramycin	0.00	0.66	0.66	0.00	0.66	0.66	XXX	■
	26			0.00	0.00	0.00	0.00	0.00	0.00	XXX	■
	TC			0.00	0.66	0.66	0.00	0.66	0.66	XXX	■
80201		X	Topiramate	0.00	0.59	0.59	0.00	0.59	0.59	XXX	■
	26			0.00	0.00	0.00	0.00	0.00	0.00	XXX	■
	TC			0.00	0.59	0.59	0.00	0.59	0.59	XXX	■
80202		X	Vancomycin	0.00	0.59	0.59	0.00	0.59	0.59	XXX	■
	26			0.00	0.00	0.00	0.00	0.00	0.00	XXX	■
	TC			0.00	0.59	0.59	0.00	0.59	0.59	XXX	■
80299		X	Quantitation of drug, not elsewhere specified	0.00	0.73	0.73	0.00	0.73	0.73	XXX	■
	26			0.00	0.00	0.00	0.00	0.00	0.00	XXX	■
	TC			0.00	0.73	0.73	0.00	0.73	0.73	XXX	■
80400		X	ACTH stimulation panel; for adrenal insufficiency This panel must include the following: Cortisol (82533 x 2)	0.00	1.38	1.38	0.00	1.38	1.38	XXX	■
	26			0.00	0.00	0.00	0.00	0.00	0.00	XXX	■
	TC			0.00	1.38	1.38	0.00	1.38	1.38	XXX	■
80402		X	for 21 hydroxylase deficiency This panel must include the following: Cortisol (82533 x 2) 17 hydroxyprogesterone (83498 x 2)	0.00	2.53	2.53	0.00	2.53	2.53	XXX	■
	26			0.00	0.00	0.00	0.00	0.00	0.00	XXX	■
	TC			0.00	2.53	2.53	0.00	2.53	2.53	XXX	■

■ RVU not developed by CMS. Gap-filled RVUs developed by Ingenix/CHEG.

Code	M	S	Description	Work Value	Non-Fac PE	Fac PE	Mal-prac-tice	Non-Fac Total	Fac Total	Global	Gap
80406		X	for 3 beta-hydroxydehydrogenase deficiency This panel must include the following: Cortisol (82533 x 2) 17 hydroxypregnenolone (84143 x 2)	0.00	2.36	2.36	0.00	2.36	2.36	XXX	■
	26			0.00	0.00	0.00	0.00	0.00	0.00	XXX	■
	TC			0.00	2.36	2.36	0.00	2.36	2.36	XXX	■
80408		X	Aldosterone suppression evaluation panel (eg, saline infusion) This panel must include the following: Aldosterone (82088 x 2) Renin (84244 x 2)	0.00	3.16	3.16	0.00	3.16	3.16	XXX	■
	26			0.00	0.00	0.00	0.00	0.00	0.00	XXX	■
	TC			0.00	3.16	3.16	0.00	3.16	3.16	XXX	■
80410		X	Calcitonin stimulation panel (eg, calcium, pentagastrin) This panel must include the following: Calcitonin (82308 x 3)	0.00	2.83	2.83	0.00	2.83	2.83	XXX	■
	26			0.00	0.00	0.00	0.00	0.00	0.00	XXX	■
	TC			0.00	2.83	2.83	0.00	2.83	2.83	XXX	■
80412		X	Corticotropic releasing hormone (CRH) stimulation panel This panel must include the following: Cortisol (82533 x 6) Adrenocorticotropic hormone (ACTH) (82024 x 6)	0.00	7.03	7.03	0.00	7.03	7.03	XXX	■
	26			0.00	0.00	0.00	0.00	0.00	0.00	XXX	■
	TC			0.00	7.03	7.03	0.00	7.03	7.03	XXX	■
80414		X	Chorionic gonadotropin stimulation panel; testosterone response This panel must include the following: Testosterone (84403 x 2 on three pooled blood samples)	0.00	1.04	1.04	0.00	1.04	1.04	XXX	■
	26			0.00	0.00	0.00	0.00	0.00	0.00	XXX	■
	TC			0.00	1.04	1.04	0.00	1.04	1.04	XXX	■
80415		X	estradiol response This panel must include the following: Estradiol (82670 x 2 on three pooled blood samples)	0.00	1.04	1.04	0.00	1.04	1.04	XXX	■
	26			0.00	0.00	0.00	0.00	0.00	0.00	XXX	■
	TC			0.00	1.04	1.04	0.00	1.04	1.04	XXX	■
80416		X	Renal vein renin stimulation panel (eg, captopril) This panel must include the following: Renin (84244 x 6)	0.00	3.28	3.28	0.00	3.28	3.28	XXX	■
	26			0.00	0.00	0.00	0.00	0.00	0.00	XXX	■
	TC			0.00	3.28	3.28	0.00	3.28	3.28	XXX	■
80417		X	Peripheral vein renin stimulation panel (eg, captopril) This panel must include the following: Renin (84244 x 2)	0.00	1.41	1.41	0.00	1.41	1.41	XXX	■
	26			0.00	0.00	0.00	0.00	0.00	0.00	XXX	■
	TC			0.00	1.41	1.41	0.00	1.41	1.41	XXX	■
80418		X	Combined rapid anterior pituitary evaluation panel This panel must include the following: Adrenocorticotropic hormone (ACTH) (82024 x 4) Luteinizing hormone (LH) (83002 x 4) Follicle stimulating hormone (FSH) (83001 x 4) Prolactin (84146 x 4) Human growth hormone (HGH) (83003 x 4) Cortisol (82533 x 4) Thyroid stimulating hormone (TSH) (84443 x 4)	0.00	19.59	19.59	0.00	19.59	19.59	XXX	■
	26			0.00	0.00	0.00	0.00	0.00	0.00	XXX	■
	TC			0.00	19.59	19.59	0.00	19.59	19.59	XXX	■
80420		X	Dexamethasone suppression panel, 48 hour This panel must include the following: Free cortisol, urine (82530 x 2) Cortisol (82533 x 2) Volume measurement for timed collection (81050 x 2) (For single dose dexamethasone, use 82533)	0.00	2.49	2.49	0.00	2.49	2.49	XXX	■
	26			0.00	0.00	0.00	0.00	0.00	0.00	XXX	■
	TC			0.00	2.49	2.49	0.00	2.49	2.49	XXX	■
80422		X	Glucagon tolerance panel; for insulinoma This panel must include the following: Glucose (82947 x 3) Insulin (83525 x 3)	0.00	1.55	1.55	0.00	1.55	1.55	XXX	■
	26			0.00	0.00	0.00	0.00	0.00	0.00	XXX	■
	TC			0.00	1.55	1.55	0.00	1.55	1.55	XXX	■

Pathology

■ RVU not developed by CMS. Gap-filled RVUs developed by Ingenix/CHEG.

Code	M	S	Description	Work Value	Non-Fac PE	Fac PE	Mal-practice	Non-Fac Total	Fac Total	Global	Gap
80424		X	for pheochromocytoma This panel must include the following: Catecholamines, fractionated (82384 x 2)	0.00	1.51	1.51	0.00	1.51	1.51	XXX	■
	26			0.00	0.00	0.00	0.00	0.00	0.00	XXX	■
	TC			0.00	1.51	1.51	0.00	1.51	1.51	XXX	■
80426		X	Gonadotropin releasing hormone stimulation panel This panel must include the following: Follicle stimulating hormone (FSH) (83001 x 4) Luteinizing hormone (LH) (83002 x 4)	0.00	3.66	3.66	0.00	3.66	3.66	XXX	■
	26			0.00	0.00	0.00	0.00	0.00	0.00	XXX	■
	TC			0.00	3.66	3.66	0.00	3.66	3.66	XXX	■
80428		X	Growth hormone stimulation panel (eg, arginine infusion, l-dopa administration) This panel must include the following: Human growth hormone (HGH) (83003 x 4)	0.00	1.83	1.83	0.00	1.83	1.83	XXX	■
	26			0.00	0.00	0.00	0.00	0.00	0.00	XXX	■
	TC			0.00	1.83	1.83	0.00	1.83	1.83	XXX	■
80430		X	Growth hormone suppression panel (glucose administration) This panel must include the following: Glucose (82947 x 3) Human growth hormone (HGH) (83003 x 4)	0.00	2.23	2.23	0.00	2.23	2.23	XXX	■
	26			0.00	0.00	0.00	0.00	0.00	0.00	XXX	■
	TC			0.00	2.23	2.23	0.00	2.23	2.23	XXX	■
80432		X	Insulin-induced C-peptide suppression panel This panel must include the following: Insulin (83525) C-peptide (84681 x 5) Glucose (82947 x 5)	0.00	3.97	3.97	0.00	3.97	3.97	XXX	■
	26			0.00	0.00	0.00	0.00	0.00	0.00	XXX	■
	TC			0.00	3.97	3.97	0.00	3.97	3.97	XXX	■
80434		X	Insulin tolerance panel; for ACTH insufficiency This panel must include the following: Cortisol (82533 x 5) Glucose (82947 x 5)	0.00	2.64	2.64	0.00	2.64	2.64	XXX	■
	26			0.00	0.00	0.00	0.00	0.00	0.00	XXX	■
	TC			0.00	2.64	2.64	0.00	2.64	2.64	XXX	■
80435		X	for growth hormone deficiency This panel must include the following: Glucose (82947 x 5) Human growth hormone (HGH) (83003 x 5)	0.00	2.80	2.80	0.00	2.80	2.80	XXX	■
	26			0.00	0.00	0.00	0.00	0.00	0.00	XXX	■
	TC			0.00	2.80	2.80	0.00	2.80	2.80	XXX	■
80436		X	Metyrapone panel This panel must include the following: Cortisol (82533 x 2) 11 deoxycortisol (82634 x 2)	0.00	2.58	2.58	0.00	2.58	2.58	XXX	■
	26			0.00	0.00	0.00	0.00	0.00	0.00	XXX	■
	TC			0.00	2.58	2.58	0.00	2.58	2.58	XXX	■
80438		X	Thyrotropin releasing hormone (TRH) stimulation panel; one hour This panel must include the following: Thyroid stimulating hormone (TSH) (84443 x 3)	0.00	1.23	1.23	0.00	1.23	1.23	XXX	■
	26			0.00	0.00	0.00	0.00	0.00	0.00	XXX	■
	TC			0.00	1.23	1.23	0.00	1.23	1.23	XXX	■
80439		X	two hour This panel must include the following: Thyroid stimulating hormone (TSH) (84443 x 4)	0.00	1.54	1.54	0.00	1.54	1.54	XXX	■
	26			0.00	0.00	0.00	0.00	0.00	0.00	XXX	■
	TC			0.00	1.54	1.54	0.00	1.54	1.54	XXX	■
80440		X	for hyperprolactinemia This panel must include the following: Prolactin (84146 x 3)	0.00	1.47	1.47	0.00	1.47	1.47	XXX	■
	26			0.00	0.00	0.00	0.00	0.00	0.00	XXX	■
	TC			0.00	1.47	1.47	0.00	1.47	1.47	XXX	■
80500		A	Clinical pathology consultation; limited, without review of patient's history and medical records	0.37	0.21	0.17	0.01	0.59	0.55	XXX	
80502		A	comprehensive, for a complex diagnostic problem, with review of patient's history and medical records	1.33	0.63	0.61	0.05	2.01	1.99	XXX	

Pathology

■ RVU not developed by CMS. Gap-filled RVUs developed by Ingenix/CHEG.

Code	M	S	Description	Work Value	Non-Fac PE	Fac PE	Mal-practice	Non-Fac Total	Fac Total	Global	Gap
81000		X	Urinalysis, by dip stick or tablet reagent for bilirubin, glucose, hemoglobin, ketones, leukocytes, nitrite, pH, protein, specific gravity, urobilinogen, any number of these constituents; non-automated, with microscopy	0.00	0.17	0.17	0.00	0.17	0.17	XXX	■
	26			0.00	0.00	0.00	0.00	0.00	0.00	XXX	■
	TC			0.00	0.17	0.17	0.00	0.17	0.17	XXX	■
81001		X	automated, with microscopy	0.00	0.17	0.17	0.00	0.17	0.17	XXX	■
	26			0.00	0.00	0.00	0.00	0.00	0.00	XXX	■
	TC			0.00	0.17	0.17	0.00	0.17	0.17	XXX	■
81002		X	non-automated, without microscopy	0.00	0.13	0.13	0.00	0.13	0.13	XXX	■
	26			0.00	0.00	0.00	0.00	0.00	0.00	XXX	■
	TC			0.00	0.13	0.13	0.00	0.13	0.13	XXX	■
81003		X	automated, without microscopy	0.00	0.13	0.13	0.00	0.13	0.13	XXX	■
	26			0.00	0.00	0.00	0.00	0.00	0.00	XXX	■
	TC			0.00	0.13	0.13	0.00	0.13	0.13	XXX	■
81005		X	Urinalysis; qualitative or semiquantitative, except immunoassays	0.00	0.12	0.12	0.00	0.12	0.12	XXX	■
	26			0.00	0.00	0.00	0.00	0.00	0.00	XXX	■
	TC			0.00	0.12	0.12	0.00	0.12	0.12	XXX	■
81007		X	bacteriuria screen, except by culture or dipstick	0.00	0.18	0.18	0.00	0.18	0.18	XXX	■
	26			0.00	0.00	0.00	0.00	0.00	0.00	XXX	■
	TC			0.00	0.18	0.18	0.00	0.18	0.18	XXX	■
81015		X	microscopic only	0.00	0.13	0.13	0.00	0.13	0.13	XXX	■
	26			0.00	0.00	0.00	0.00	0.00	0.00	XXX	■
	TC			0.00	0.13	0.13	0.00	0.13	0.13	XXX	■
81020		X	two or three glass test	0.00	0.16	0.16	0.00	0.16	0.16	XXX	■
	26			0.00	0.00	0.00	0.00	0.00	0.00	XXX	■
	TC			0.00	0.16	0.16	0.00	0.16	0.16	XXX	■
81025		X	Urine pregnancy test, by visual color comparison methods	0.00	0.25	0.25	0.00	0.25	0.25	XXX	■
	26			0.00	0.00	0.00	0.00	0.00	0.00	XXX	■
	TC			0.00	0.25	0.25	0.00	0.25	0.25	XXX	■
81050		X	Volume measurement for timed collection, each	0.00	0.12	0.12	0.00	0.12	0.12	XXX	■
	26			0.00	0.00	0.00	0.00	0.00	0.00	XXX	■
	TC			0.00	0.12	0.12	0.00	0.12	0.12	XXX	■
81099		X	Unlisted urinalysis procedure	0.00	0.00	0.00	0.00	0.00	0.00	XXX	
82000		X	Acetaldehyde, blood	0.00	0.67	0.67	0.00	0.67	0.67	XXX	■
	26			0.00	0.00	0.00	0.00	0.00	0.00	XXX	■
	TC			0.00	0.67	0.67	0.00	0.67	0.67	XXX	■
82003		X	Acetaminophen	0.00	0.66	0.66	0.00	0.66	0.66	XXX	■
	26			0.00	0.00	0.00	0.00	0.00	0.00	XXX	■
	TC			0.00	0.66	0.66	0.00	0.66	0.66	XXX	■
82009		X	Acetone or other ketone bodies, serum; qualitative	0.00	0.15	0.15	0.00	0.15	0.15	XXX	■
	26			0.00	0.00	0.00	0.00	0.00	0.00	XXX	■
	TC			0.00	0.15	0.15	0.00	0.15	0.15	XXX	■
82010		X	quantitative	0.00	0.29	0.29	0.00	0.29	0.29	XXX	■
	26			0.00	0.00	0.00	0.00	0.00	0.00	XXX	■
	TC			0.00	0.29	0.29	0.00	0.29	0.29	XXX	■

■ RVU not developed by CMS. Gap-filled RVUs developed by Ingenix/CHEG.

Code	M	S	Description	Work Value	Non-Fac PE	Fac PE	Mal-prac-tice	Non-Fac Total	Fac Total	Global	Gap
82013		X	Acetylcholinesterase	0.00	0.59	0.59	0.00	0.59	0.59	XXX	■
	26			0.00	0.00	0.00	0.00	0.00	0.00	XXX	■
	TC			0.00	0.59	0.59	0.00	0.59	0.59	XXX	■
82016		X	Acylcarnitines; qualitative, each specimen	0.00	0.82	0.82	0.00	0.82	0.82	XXX	■
	26			0.00	0.00	0.00	0.00	0.00	0.00	XXX	■
	TC			0.00	0.82	0.82	0.00	0.82	0.82	XXX	■
82017		X	quantitative, each specimen	0.00	0.64	0.64	0.00	0.64	0.64	XXX	■
	26			0.00	0.00	0.00	0.00	0.00	0.00	XXX	■
	TC			0.00	0.64	0.64	0.00	0.64	0.64	XXX	■
82024		X	Adrenocorticotropic hormone (ACTH)	0.00	1.32	1.32	0.00	1.32	1.32	XXX	■
	26			0.00	0.00	0.00	0.00	0.00	0.00	XXX	■
	TC			0.00	1.32	1.32	0.00	1.32	1.32	XXX	■
82030		X	Adenosine, 5'-monophosphate, cyclic (cyclic AMP)	0.00	1.03	1.03	0.00	1.03	1.03	XXX	■
	26			0.00	0.00	0.00	0.00	0.00	0.00	XXX	■
	TC			0.00	1.03	1.03	0.00	1.03	1.03	XXX	■
82040		X	Albumin; serum	0.00	0.19	0.19	0.00	0.19	0.19	XXX	■
	26			0.00	0.00	0.00	0.00	0.00	0.00	XXX	■
	TC			0.00	0.19	0.19	0.00	0.19	0.19	XXX	■
82042		X	urine or other source, quantitative, each specimen	0.00	0.23	0.23	0.00	0.23	0.23	XXX	■
	26			0.00	0.00	0.00	0.00	0.00	0.00	XXX	■
	TC			0.00	0.23	0.23	0.00	0.23	0.23	XXX	■
82043		X	urine, microalbumin, quantitative	0.00	0.51	0.51	0.00	0.51	0.51	XXX	■
	26			0.00	0.00	0.00	0.00	0.00	0.00	XXX	■
	TC			0.00	0.51	0.51	0.00	0.51	0.51	XXX	■
82044		X	urine, microalbumin, semiquantitative (eg, reagent strip assay)	0.00	0.26	0.26	0.00	0.26	0.26	XXX	■
	26			0.00	0.00	0.00	0.00	0.00	0.00	XXX	■
	TC			0.00	0.26	0.26	0.00	0.26	0.26	XXX	■
82055		X	Alcohol (ethanol); any specimen except breath	0.00	0.44	0.44	0.00	0.44	0.44	XXX	■
	26			0.00	0.00	0.00	0.00	0.00	0.00	XXX	■
	TC			0.00	0.44	0.44	0.00	0.44	0.44	XXX	■
82075		X	breath	0.00	0.26	0.26	0.00	0.26	0.26	XXX	■
	26			0.00	0.00	0.00	0.00	0.00	0.00	XXX	■
	TC			0.00	0.26	0.26	0.00	0.26	0.26	XXX	■
82085		X	Aldolase	0.00	0.44	0.44	0.00	0.44	0.44	XXX	■
	26			0.00	0.00	0.00	0.00	0.00	0.00	XXX	■
	TC			0.00	0.44	0.44	0.00	0.44	0.44	XXX	■
82088		X	Aldosterone	0.00	1.17	1.17	0.00	1.17	1.17	XXX	■
	26			0.00	0.00	0.00	0.00	0.00	0.00	XXX	■
	TC			0.00	1.17	1.17	0.00	1.17	1.17	XXX	■
82101		X	Alkaloids, urine, quantitative	0.00	0.73	0.73	0.00	0.73	0.73	XXX	■
	26			0.00	0.00	0.00	0.00	0.00	0.00	XXX	■
	TC			0.00	0.73	0.73	0.00	0.73	0.73	XXX	■
82103		X	Alpha-1-antitrypsin; total	0.00	0.59	0.59	0.00	0.59	0.59	XXX	■
	26			0.00	0.00	0.00	0.00	0.00	0.00	XXX	■
	TC			0.00	0.59	0.59	0.00	0.59	0.59	XXX	■

■ RVU not developed by CMS. Gap-filled RVUs developed by Ingenix/CHEG.

Code	M	S	Description	Work Value	Non-Fac PE	Fac PE	Mal-practice	Non-Fac Total	Fac Total	Global	Gap
82104		X	phenotype	0.00	0.81	0.81	0.00	0.81	0.81	XXX	■
	26			0.00	0.00	0.00	0.00	0.00	0.00	XXX	■
	TC			0.00	0.81	0.81	0.00	0.81	0.81	XXX	■
82105		X	Alpha-fetoprotein; serum	0.00	0.69	0.69	0.00	0.69	0.69	XXX	■
	26			0.00	0.00	0.00	0.00	0.00	0.00	XXX	■
	TC			0.00	0.69	0.69	0.00	0.69	0.69	XXX	■
82106		X	amniotic fluid	0.00	0.69	0.69	0.00	0.69	0.69	XXX	■
	26			0.00	0.00	0.00	0.00	0.00	0.00	XXX	■
	TC			0.00	0.69	0.69	0.00	0.69	0.69	XXX	■
82108		X	Aluminum	0.00	0.88	0.88	0.00	0.88	0.88	XXX	■
	26			0.00	0.00	0.00	0.00	0.00	0.00	XXX	■
	TC			0.00	0.88	0.88	0.00	0.88	0.88	XXX	■
82120		X	Amines, vaginal fluid, qualitative	0.00	0.14	0.14	0.00	0.14	0.14	XXX	■
	26			0.00	0.00	0.00	0.00	0.00	0.00	XXX	■
	TC			0.00	0.14	0.14	0.00	0.14	0.14	XXX	■
82127		X	Amino acids; single, qualitative, each specimen	0.00	0.42	0.42	0.00	0.42	0.42	XXX	■
	26			0.00	0.00	0.00	0.00	0.00	0.00	XXX	■
	TC			0.00	0.42	0.42	0.00	0.42	0.42	XXX	■
82128		X	multiple, qualitative, each specimen	0.00	0.42	0.42	0.00	0.42	0.42	XXX	■
	26			0.00	0.00	0.00	0.00	0.00	0.00	XXX	■
	TC			0.00	0.42	0.42	0.00	0.42	0.42	XXX	■
82131		X	single, quantitative, each specimen	0.00	1.98	1.98	0.00	1.98	1.98	XXX	■
	26			0.00	0.00	0.00	0.00	0.00	0.00	XXX	■
	TC			0.00	1.98	1.98	0.00	1.98	1.98	XXX	■
82135		X	Aminolevulinic acid, delta (ALA)	0.00	0.64	0.64	0.00	0.64	0.64	XXX	■
	26			0.00	0.00	0.00	0.00	0.00	0.00	XXX	■
	TC			0.00	0.64	0.64	0.00	0.64	0.64	XXX	■
82136		X	Amino acids, 2 to 5 amino acids, quantitative, each specimen	0.00	1.98	1.98	0.00	1.98	1.98	XXX	■
	26			0.00	0.00	0.00	0.00	0.00	0.00	XXX	■
	TC			0.00	1.98	1.98	0.00	1.98	1.98	XXX	■
82139		X	Amino acids, 6 or more amino acids, quantitative, each specimen	0.00	1.98	1.98	0.00	1.98	1.98	XXX	■
	26			0.00	0.00	0.00	0.00	0.00	0.00	XXX	■
	TC			0.00	1.98	1.98	0.00	1.98	1.98	XXX	■
82140		X	Ammonia	0.00	0.51	0.51	0.00	0.51	0.51	XXX	■
	26			0.00	0.00	0.00	0.00	0.00	0.00	XXX	■
	TC			0.00	0.51	0.51	0.00	0.51	0.51	XXX	■
82143		X	Amniotic fluid scan (spectrophotometric)	0.00	0.54	0.54	0.00	0.54	0.54	XXX	■
	26			0.00	0.00	0.00	0.00	0.00	0.00	XXX	■
	TC			0.00	0.54	0.54	0.00	0.54	0.54	XXX	■
82145		X	Amphetamine or methamphetamine	0.00	0.73	0.73	0.00	0.73	0.73	XXX	■
	26			0.00	0.00	0.00	0.00	0.00	0.00	XXX	■
	TC			0.00	0.73	0.73	0.00	0.73	0.73	XXX	■
82150		X	Amylase	0.00	0.23	0.23	0.00	0.23	0.23	XXX	■
	26			0.00	0.00	0.00	0.00	0.00	0.00	XXX	■
	TC			0.00	0.23	0.23	0.00	0.23	0.23	XXX	■

■ RVU not developed by CMS. Gap-filled RVUs developed by Ingenix/CHEG.

Code	M	S	Description	Work Value	Non-Fac PE	Fac PE	Mal-practice	Non-Fac Total	Fac Total	Global	Gap
82154		X	Androstanediol glucuronide	0.00	0.95	0.95	0.00	0.95	0.95	XXX	■
	26			0.00	0.00	0.00	0.00	0.00	0.00	XXX	■
	TC			0.00	0.95	0.95	0.00	0.95	0.95	XXX	■
82157		X	Androstenedione	0.00	0.88	0.88	0.00	0.88	0.88	XXX	■
	26			0.00	0.00	0.00	0.00	0.00	0.00	XXX	■
	TC			0.00	0.88	0.88	0.00	0.88	0.88	XXX	■
82160		X	Androsterone	0.00	0.95	0.95	0.00	0.95	0.95	XXX	■
	26			0.00	0.00	0.00	0.00	0.00	0.00	XXX	■
	TC			0.00	0.95	0.95	0.00	0.95	0.95	XXX	■
82163		X	Angiotensin II	0.00	0.88	0.88	0.00	0.88	0.88	XXX	■
	26			0.00	0.00	0.00	0.00	0.00	0.00	XXX	■
	TC			0.00	0.88	0.88	0.00	0.88	0.88	XXX	■
82164		X	Angiotensin I - converting enzyme (ACE)	0.00	0.73	0.73	0.00	0.73	0.73	XXX	■
	26			0.00	0.00	0.00	0.00	0.00	0.00	XXX	■
	TC			0.00	0.73	0.73	0.00	0.73	0.73	XXX	■
82172		X	Apolipoprotein, each	0.00	0.48	0.48	0.00	0.48	0.48	XXX	■
	26			0.00	0.00	0.00	0.00	0.00	0.00	XXX	■
	TC			0.00	0.48	0.48	0.00	0.48	0.48	XXX	■
82175		X	Arsenic	0.00	0.81	0.81	0.00	0.81	0.81	XXX	■
	26			0.00	0.00	0.00	0.00	0.00	0.00	XXX	■
	TC			0.00	0.81	0.81	0.00	0.81	0.81	XXX	■
82180		X	Ascorbic acid (Vitamin C), blood	0.00	0.42	0.42	0.00	0.42	0.42	XXX	■
	26			0.00	0.00	0.00	0.00	0.00	0.00	XXX	■
	TC			0.00	0.42	0.42	0.00	0.42	0.42	XXX	■
82190		X	Atomic absorption spectroscopy, each analyte	0.00	0.88	0.88	0.00	0.88	0.88	XXX	■
	26			0.00	0.00	0.00	0.00	0.00	0.00	XXX	■
	TC			0.00	0.88	0.88	0.00	0.88	0.88	XXX	■
82205		X	Barbiturates, not elsewhere specified	0.00	0.59	0.59	0.00	0.59	0.59	XXX	■
	26			0.00	0.00	0.00	0.00	0.00	0.00	XXX	■
	TC			0.00	0.59	0.59	0.00	0.59	0.59	XXX	■
82232		X	Beta-2 microglobulin	0.00	0.81	0.81	0.00	0.81	0.81	XXX	■
	26			0.00	0.00	0.00	0.00	0.00	0.00	XXX	■
	TC			0.00	0.81	0.81	0.00	0.81	0.81	XXX	■
82239		X	Bile acids; total	0.00	0.47	0.47	0.00	0.47	0.47	XXX	■
	26			0.00	0.00	0.00	0.00	0.00	0.00	XXX	■
	TC			0.00	0.47	0.47	0.00	0.47	0.47	XXX	■
82240		X	cholylglycine	0.00	1.04	1.04	0.00	1.04	1.04	XXX	■
	26			0.00	0.00	0.00	0.00	0.00	0.00	XXX	■
	TC			0.00	1.04	1.04	0.00	1.04	1.04	XXX	■
82247		X	Bilirubin; total	0.00	0.19	0.19	0.00	0.19	0.19	XXX	■
	26			0.00	0.00	0.00	0.00	0.00	0.00	XXX	■
	TC			0.00	0.19	0.19	0.00	0.19	0.19	XXX	■
82248		X	direct	0.00	0.19	0.19	0.00	0.19	0.19	XXX	■
	26			0.00	0.00	0.00	0.00	0.00	0.00	XXX	■
	TC			0.00	0.19	0.19	0.00	0.19	0.19	XXX	■

■ RVU not developed by CMS. Gap-filled RVUs developed by Ingenix/CHEG.

Pathology

Code	M	S	Description	Work Value	Non-Fac PE	Fac PE	Mal-practice	Non-Fac Total	Fac Total	Global	Gap
82252		X	feces, qualitative	0.00	0.13	0.13	0.00	0.13	0.13	XXX	■
	26			0.00	0.00	0.00	0.00	0.00	0.00	XXX	■
	TC			0.00	0.13	0.13	0.00	0.13	0.13	XXX	■
82261		X	Biotinidase, each specimen	0.00	0.21	0.21	0.00	0.21	0.21	XXX	■
	26			0.00	0.00	0.00	0.00	0.00	0.00	XXX	■
	TC			0.00	0.21	0.21	0.00	0.21	0.21	XXX	■
82270		X	Blood, occult, by peroxidase activity (eg,	0.00	0.15	0.15	0.00	0.15	0.15	XXX	■
	26		guaiac), qualitative; feces, 1-3 simultaneous	0.00	0.00	0.00	0.00	0.00	0.00	XXX	■
	TC		determinations	0.00	0.15	0.15	0.00	0.15	0.15	XXX	■
82273		X	other sources	0.00	0.15	0.15	0.00	0.15	0.15	XXX	■
	26			0.00	0.00	0.00	0.00	0.00	0.00	XXX	■
	TC			0.00	0.15	0.15	0.00	0.15	0.15	XXX	■
82274		X	Blood, occult, by fecal hemoglobin	0.00	0.73	0.73	0.00	0.73	0.73	XXX	■
	26		determination by immunoassay, qualitative,	0.00	0.00	0.00	0.00	0.00	0.00	XXX	■
	TC		feces, 1-3 simultaneous determinations	0.00	0.73	0.73	0.00	0.73	0.73	XXX	■
82286		X	Bradykinin	0.00	1.17	1.17	0.00	1.17	1.17	XXX	■
	26			0.00	0.00	0.00	0.00	0.00	0.00	XXX	■
	TC			0.00	1.17	1.17	0.00	1.17	1.17	XXX	■
82300		X	Cadmium	0.00	0.81	0.81	0.00	0.81	0.81	XXX	■
	26			0.00	0.00	0.00	0.00	0.00	0.00	XXX	■
	TC			0.00	0.81	0.81	0.00	0.81	0.81	XXX	■
82306		X	Calcifediol (25-OH Vitamin D-3)	0.00	1.10	1.10	0.00	1.10	1.10	XXX	■
	26			0.00	0.00	0.00	0.00	0.00	0.00	XXX	■
	TC			0.00	1.10	1.10	0.00	1.10	1.10	XXX	■
82307		X	Calciferol (Vitamin D)	0.00	1.10	1.10	0.00	1.10	1.10	XXX	■
	26			0.00	0.00	0.00	0.00	0.00	0.00	XXX	■
	TC			0.00	1.10	1.10	0.00	1.10	1.10	XXX	■
82308		X	Calcitonin	0.00	1.13	1.13	0.00	1.13	1.13	XXX	■
	26			0.00	0.00	0.00	0.00	0.00	0.00	XXX	■
	TC			0.00	1.13	1.13	0.00	1.13	1.13	XXX	■
82310		X	Calcium; total	0.00	0.19	0.19	0.00	0.19	0.19	XXX	■
	26			0.00	0.00	0.00	0.00	0.00	0.00	XXX	■
	TC			0.00	0.19	0.19	0.00	0.19	0.19	XXX	■
82330		X	ionized	0.00	0.54	0.54	0.00	0.54	0.54	XXX	■
	26			0.00	0.00	0.00	0.00	0.00	0.00	XXX	■
	TC			0.00	0.54	0.54	0.00	0.54	0.54	XXX	■
82331		X	after calcium infusion test	0.00	0.23	0.23	0.00	0.23	0.23	XXX	■
	26			0.00	0.00	0.00	0.00	0.00	0.00	XXX	■
	TC			0.00	0.23	0.23	0.00	0.23	0.23	XXX	■
82340		X	urine quantitative, timed specimen	0.00	0.23	0.23	0.00	0.23	0.23	XXX	■
	26			0.00	0.00	0.00	0.00	0.00	0.00	XXX	■
	TC			0.00	0.23	0.23	0.00	0.23	0.23	XXX	■
82355		X	Calculus; qualitative analysis	0.00	0.51	0.51	0.00	0.51	0.51	XXX	■
	26			0.00	0.00	0.00	0.00	0.00	0.00	XXX	■
	TC			0.00	0.51	0.51	0.00	0.51	0.51	XXX	■

■ RVU not developed by CMS. Gap-filled RVUs developed by Ingenix/CHEG.

Code	M	S	Description	Work Value	Non-Fac PE	Fac PE	Mal-prac-tice	Non-Fac Total	Fac Total	Global	Gap
82360		X	quantitative analysis, chemical	0.00	0.56	0.56	0.00	0.56	0.56	XXX	■
	26			0.00	0.00	0.00	0.00	0.00	0.00	XXX	■
	TC			0.00	0.56	0.56	0.00	0.56	0.56	XXX	■
82365		X	infrared spectroscopy	0.00	0.56	0.56	0.00	0.56	0.56	XXX	■
	26			0.00	0.00	0.00	0.00	0.00	0.00	XXX	■
	TC			0.00	0.56	0.56	0.00	0.56	0.56	XXX	■
82370		X	x-ray diffraction	0.00	0.51	0.51	0.00	0.51	0.51	XXX	■
	26			0.00	0.00	0.00	0.00	0.00	0.00	XXX	■
	TC			0.00	0.51	0.51	0.00	0.51	0.51	XXX	■
82373		X	Carbohydrate deficient transferrin	0.00	0.51	0.51	0.00	0.51	0.51	XXX	■
	26			0.00	0.00	0.00	0.00	0.00	0.00	XXX	■
	TC			0.00	0.51	0.51	0.00	0.51	0.51	XXX	■
82374		X	Carbon dioxide (bicarbonate)	0.00	0.19	0.19	0.00	0.19	0.19	XXX	■
	26			0.00	0.00	0.00	0.00	0.00	0.00	XXX	■
	TC			0.00	0.19	0.19	0.00	0.19	0.19	XXX	■
82375		X	Carbon monoxide, (carboxyhemoglobin); quantitative	0.00	0.50	0.50	0.00	0.50	0.50	XXX	■
	26			0.00	0.00	0.00	0.00	0.00	0.00	XXX	■
	TC			0.00	0.50	0.50	0.00	0.50	0.50	XXX	■
82376		X	qualitative	0.00	0.18	0.18	0.00	0.18	0.18	XXX	■
	26			0.00	0.00	0.00	0.00	0.00	0.00	XXX	■
	TC			0.00	0.18	0.18	0.00	0.18	0.18	XXX	■
82378		X	Carcinoembryonic antigen (CEA)	0.00	0.76	0.76	0.00	0.76	0.76	XXX	■
	26			0.00	0.00	0.00	0.00	0.00	0.00	XXX	■
	TC			0.00	0.76	0.76	0.00	0.76	0.76	XXX	■
82379		X	Carnitine (total and free), quantitative, each specimen	0.00	0.76	0.76	0.00	0.76	0.76	XXX	■
	26			0.00	0.00	0.00	0.00	0.00	0.00	XXX	■
	TC			0.00	0.76	0.76	0.00	0.76	0.76	XXX	■
82380		X	Carotene	0.00	0.44	0.44	0.00	0.44	0.44	XXX	■
	26			0.00	0.00	0.00	0.00	0.00	0.00	XXX	■
	TC			0.00	0.44	0.44	0.00	0.44	0.44	XXX	■
82382		X	Catecholamines; total urine	0.00	0.76	0.76	0.00	0.76	0.76	XXX	■
	26			0.00	0.00	0.00	0.00	0.00	0.00	XXX	■
	TC			0.00	0.76	0.76	0.00	0.76	0.76	XXX	■
82383		X	blood	0.00	1.10	1.10	0.00	1.10	1.10	XXX	■
	26			0.00	0.00	0.00	0.00	0.00	0.00	XXX	■
	TC			0.00	1.10	1.10	0.00	1.10	1.10	XXX	■
82384		X	fractionated	0.00	1.10	1.10	0.00	1.10	1.10	XXX	■
	26			0.00	0.00	0.00	0.00	0.00	0.00	XXX	■
	TC			0.00	1.10	1.10	0.00	1.10	1.10	XXX	■
82387		X	Cathepsin-D	0.00	1.03	1.03	0.00	1.03	1.03	XXX	■
	26			0.00	0.00	0.00	0.00	0.00	0.00	XXX	■
	TC			0.00	1.03	1.03	0.00	1.03	1.03	XXX	■
82390		X	Ceruloplasmin	0.00	0.47	0.47	0.00	0.47	0.47	XXX	■
	26			0.00	0.00	0.00	0.00	0.00	0.00	XXX	■
	TC			0.00	0.47	0.47	0.00	0.47	0.47	XXX	■

■ RVU not developed by CMS. Gap-filled RVUs developed by Ingenix/CHEG.

Code	M	S	Description	Work Value	Non-Fac PE	Fac PE	Mal-practice	Non-Fac Total	Fac Total	Global	Gap
82397		X	Chemiluminescent assay	0.00	0.54	0.54	0.00	0.54	0.54	XXX	■
	26			0.00	0.00	0.00	0.00	0.00	0.00	XXX	■
	TC			0.00	0.54	0.54	0.00	0.54	0.54	XXX	■
82415		X	Chloramphenicol	0.00	0.73	0.73	0.00	0.73	0.73	XXX	■
	26			0.00	0.00	0.00	0.00	0.00	0.00	XXX	■
	TC			0.00	0.73	0.73	0.00	0.73	0.73	XXX	■
82435		X	Chloride; blood	0.00	0.19	0.19	0.00	0.19	0.19	XXX	■
	26			0.00	0.00	0.00	0.00	0.00	0.00	XXX	■
	TC			0.00	0.19	0.19	0.00	0.19	0.19	XXX	■
82436		X	urine	0.00	0.21	0.21	0.00	0.21	0.21	XXX	■
	26			0.00	0.00	0.00	0.00	0.00	0.00	XXX	■
	TC			0.00	0.21	0.21	0.00	0.21	0.21	XXX	■
82438		X	other source	0.00	0.21	0.21	0.00	0.21	0.21	XXX	■
	26			0.00	0.00	0.00	0.00	0.00	0.00	XXX	■
	TC			0.00	0.21	0.21	0.00	0.21	0.21	XXX	■
82441		X	Chlorinated hydrocarbons, screen	0.00	0.53	0.53	0.00	0.53	0.53	XXX	■
	26			0.00	0.00	0.00	0.00	0.00	0.00	XXX	■
	TC			0.00	0.53	0.53	0.00	0.53	0.53	XXX	■
82465		X	Cholesterol, serum or whole blood, total	0.00	0.19	0.19	0.00	0.19	0.19	XXX	■
	26			0.00	0.00	0.00	0.00	0.00	0.00	XXX	■
	TC			0.00	0.19	0.19	0.00	0.19	0.19	XXX	■
82480		X	Cholinesterase; serum	0.00	0.35	0.35	0.00	0.35	0.35	XXX	■
	26			0.00	0.00	0.00	0.00	0.00	0.00	XXX	■
	TC			0.00	0.35	0.35	0.00	0.35	0.35	XXX	■
82482		X	RBC	0.00	0.53	0.53	0.00	0.53	0.53	XXX	■
	26			0.00	0.00	0.00	0.00	0.00	0.00	XXX	■
	TC			0.00	0.53	0.53	0.00	0.53	0.53	XXX	■
82485		X	Chondroitin B sulfate, quantitative	0.00	0.88	0.88	0.00	0.88	0.88	XXX	■
	26			0.00	0.00	0.00	0.00	0.00	0.00	XXX	■
	TC			0.00	0.88	0.88	0.00	0.88	0.88	XXX	■
82486		X	Chromatography, qualitative; column (eg, gas liquid or HPLC), analyte not elsewhere specified	0.00	0.82	0.82	0.00	0.82	0.82	XXX	■
	26			0.00	0.00	0.00	0.00	0.00	0.00	XXX	■
	TC			0.00	0.82	0.82	0.00	0.82	0.82	XXX	■
82487		X	paper, 1-dimensional, analyte not elsewhere specified	0.00	0.64	0.64	0.00	0.64	0.64	XXX	■
	26			0.00	0.00	0.00	0.00	0.00	0.00	XXX	■
	TC			0.00	0.64	0.64	0.00	0.64	0.64	XXX	■
82488		X	paper, 2-dimensional, analyte not elsewhere specified	0.00	0.86	0.86	0.00	0.86	0.86	XXX	■
	26			0.00	0.00	0.00	0.00	0.00	0.00	XXX	■
	TC			0.00	0.86	0.86	0.00	0.86	0.86	XXX	■
82489		X	thin layer, analyte not elsewhere specified	0.00	0.64	0.64	0.00	0.64	0.64	XXX	■
	26			0.00	0.00	0.00	0.00	0.00	0.00	XXX	■
	TC			0.00	0.64	0.64	0.00	0.64	0.64	XXX	■
82491		X	Chromatography, quantitative, column (eg, gas liquid or HPLC); single analyte not elsewhere specified, single stationary and mobile phase	0.00	0.73	0.73	0.00	0.73	0.73	XXX	■
	26			0.00	0.00	0.00	0.00	0.00	0.00	XXX	■
	TC			0.00	0.73	0.73	0.00	0.73	0.73	XXX	■

■ RVU not developed by CMS. Gap-filled RVUs developed by Ingenix/CHEG.

Pathology

Code	M	S	Description	Work Value	Non-Fac PE	Fac PE	Mal-practice	Non-Fac Total	Fac Total	Global	Gap
82492		X	multiple analytes, single stationary and mobile phase	0.00	0.73	0.73	0.00	0.73	0.73	XXX	■
	26			0.00	0.00	0.00	0.00	0.00	0.00	XXX	■
	TC			0.00	0.73	0.73	0.00	0.73	0.73	XXX	■
82495		X	Chromium	0.00	0.88	0.88	0.00	0.88	0.88	XXX	■
	26			0.00	0.00	0.00	0.00	0.00	0.00	XXX	■
	TC			0.00	0.88	0.88	0.00	0.88	0.88	XXX	■
82507		X	Citrate	0.00	1.10	1.10	0.00	1.10	1.10	XXX	■
	26			0.00	0.00	0.00	0.00	0.00	0.00	XXX	■
	TC			0.00	1.10	1.10	0.00	1.10	1.10	XXX	■
82520		X	Cocaine or metabolite	0.00	0.73	0.73	0.00	0.73	0.73	XXX	■
	26			0.00	0.00	0.00	0.00	0.00	0.00	XXX	■
	TC			0.00	0.73	0.73	0.00	0.73	0.73	XXX	■
82523		X	Collagen cross links, any method	0.00	0.71	0.71	0.00	0.71	0.71	XXX	■
	26			0.00	0.00	0.00	0.00	0.00	0.00	XXX	■
	TC			0.00	0.71	0.71	0.00	0.71	0.71	XXX	■
82525		X	Copper	0.00	0.59	0.59	0.00	0.59	0.59	XXX	■
	26			0.00	0.00	0.00	0.00	0.00	0.00	XXX	■
	TC			0.00	0.59	0.59	0.00	0.59	0.59	XXX	■
82528		X	Corticosterone	0.00	0.88	0.88	0.00	0.88	0.88	XXX	■
	26			0.00	0.00	0.00	0.00	0.00	0.00	XXX	■
	TC			0.00	0.88	0.88	0.00	0.88	0.88	XXX	■
82530		X	Cortisol; free	0.00	0.81	0.81	0.00	0.81	0.81	XXX	■
	26			0.00	0.00	0.00	0.00	0.00	0.00	XXX	■
	TC			0.00	0.81	0.81	0.00	0.81	0.81	XXX	■
82533		X	total	0.00	0.69	0.69	0.00	0.69	0.69	XXX	■
	26			0.00	0.00	0.00	0.00	0.00	0.00	XXX	■
	TC			0.00	0.69	0.69	0.00	0.69	0.69	XXX	■
82540		X	Creatine	0.00	0.21	0.21	0.00	0.21	0.21	XXX	■
	26			0.00	0.00	0.00	0.00	0.00	0.00	XXX	■
	TC			0.00	0.21	0.21	0.00	0.21	0.21	XXX	■
82541		X	Column chromatography/mass spectrometry (eg, GC/MS, or HPLC/MS), analyte not elsewhere specified; qualitative, single stationary and mobile phase	0.00	0.59	0.59	0.00	0.59	0.59	XXX	■
	26			0.00	0.00	0.00	0.00	0.00	0.00	XXX	■
	TC			0.00	0.59	0.59	0.00	0.59	0.59	XXX	■
82542		X	quantitative, single stationary and mobile phase	0.00	0.59	0.59	0.00	0.59	0.59	XXX	■
	26			0.00	0.00	0.00	0.00	0.00	0.00	XXX	■
	TC			0.00	0.59	0.59	0.00	0.59	0.59	XXX	■
82543		X	stable isotope dilution, single analyte, quantitative, single stationary and mobile phase	0.00	0.59	0.59	0.00	0.59	0.59	XXX	■
	26			0.00	0.00	0.00	0.00	0.00	0.00	XXX	■
	TC			0.00	0.59	0.59	0.00	0.59	0.59	XXX	■
82544		X	stable isotope dilution, multiple analytes, quantitative, single stationary and mobile phase	0.00	0.59	0.59	0.00	0.59	0.59	XXX	■
	26			0.00	0.00	0.00	0.00	0.00	0.00	XXX	■
	TC			0.00	0.59	0.59	0.00	0.59	0.59	XXX	■

■ RVU not developed by CMS. Gap-filled RVUs developed by Ingenix/CHEG.

Code	M	S	Description	Work Value	Non-Fac PE	Fac PE	Mal-practice	Non-Fac Total	Fac Total	Global	Gap
82550		X	Creatine kinase (CK), (CPK); total	0.00	0.19	0.19	0.00	0.19	0.19	XXX	■
	26			0.00	0.00	0.00	0.00	0.00	0.00	XXX	■
	TC			0.00	0.19	0.19	0.00	0.19	0.19	XXX	■
82552		X	isoenzymes	0.00	0.59	0.59	0.00	0.59	0.59	XXX	■
	26			0.00	0.00	0.00	0.00	0.00	0.00	XXX	■
	TC			0.00	0.59	0.59	0.00	0.59	0.59	XXX	■
82553		X	MB fraction only	0.00	0.27	0.27	0.00	0.27	0.27	XXX	■
	26			0.00	0.00	0.00	0.00	0.00	0.00	XXX	■
	TC			0.00	0.27	0.27	0.00	0.27	0.27	XXX	■
82554		X	isoforms	0.00	0.51	0.51	0.00	0.51	0.51	XXX	■
	26			0.00	0.00	0.00	0.00	0.00	0.00	XXX	■
	TC			0.00	0.51	0.51	0.00	0.51	0.51	XXX	■
82565		X	Creatinine; blood	0.00	0.19	0.19	0.00	0.19	0.19	XXX	■
	26			0.00	0.00	0.00	0.00	0.00	0.00	XXX	■
	TC			0.00	0.19	0.19	0.00	0.19	0.19	XXX	■
82570		X	other source	0.00	0.23	0.23	0.00	0.23	0.23	XXX	■
	26			0.00	0.00	0.00	0.00	0.00	0.00	XXX	■
	TC			0.00	0.23	0.23	0.00	0.23	0.23	XXX	■
82575		X	clearance	0.00	0.42	0.42	0.00	0.42	0.42	XXX	■
	26			0.00	0.00	0.00	0.00	0.00	0.00	XXX	■
	TC			0.00	0.42	0.42	0.00	0.42	0.42	XXX	■
82585		X	Cryofibrinogen	0.00	0.29	0.29	0.00	0.29	0.29	XXX	■
	26			0.00	0.00	0.00	0.00	0.00	0.00	XXX	■
	TC			0.00	0.29	0.29	0.00	0.29	0.29	XXX	■
82595		X	Cryoglobulin, qualitative or semi-quantitative (eg, cryocrit)	0.00	0.29	0.29	0.00	0.29	0.29	XXX	■
	26			0.00	0.00	0.00	0.00	0.00	0.00	XXX	■
	TC			0.00	0.29	0.29	0.00	0.29	0.29	XXX	■
82600		X	Cyanide	0.00	0.59	0.59	0.00	0.59	0.59	XXX	■
	26			0.00	0.00	0.00	0.00	0.00	0.00	XXX	■
	TC			0.00	0.59	0.59	0.00	0.59	0.59	XXX	■
82607		X	Cyanocobalamin (Vitamin B-12);	0.00	0.59	0.59	0.00	0.59	0.59	XXX	■
	26			0.00	0.00	0.00	0.00	0.00	0.00	XXX	■
	TC			0.00	0.59	0.59	0.00	0.59	0.59	XXX	■
82608		X	unsaturated binding capacity	0.00	0.67	0.67	0.00	0.67	0.67	XXX	■
	26			0.00	0.00	0.00	0.00	0.00	0.00	XXX	■
	TC			0.00	0.67	0.67	0.00	0.67	0.67	XXX	■
82615		X	Cystine and homocystine, urine, qualitative	0.00	0.44	0.44	0.00	0.44	0.44	XXX	■
	26			0.00	0.00	0.00	0.00	0.00	0.00	XXX	■
	TC			0.00	0.44	0.44	0.00	0.44	0.44	XXX	■
82626		X	Dehydroepiandrosterone (DHEA)	0.00	1.02	1.02	0.00	1.02	1.02	XXX	■
	26			0.00	0.00	0.00	0.00	0.00	0.00	XXX	■
	TC			0.00	1.02	1.02	0.00	1.02	1.02	XXX	■
82627		X	Dehydroepiandrosterone-sulfate (DHEA-S)	0.00	0.88	0.88	0.00	0.88	0.88	XXX	■
	26			0.00	0.00	0.00	0.00	0.00	0.00	XXX	■
	TC			0.00	0.88	0.88	0.00	0.88	0.88	XXX	■

■ RVU not developed by CMS. Gap-filled RVUs developed by Ingenix/CHEG.

Code	M	S	Description	Work Value	Non-Fac PE	Fac PE	Mal-practice	Non-Fac Total	Fac Total	Global	Gap
82633		X	Desoxycorticosterone, 11-	0.00	1.17	1.17	0.00	1.17	1.17	XXX	■
	26			0.00	0.00	0.00	0.00	0.00	0.00	XXX	■
	TC			0.00	1.17	1.17	0.00	1.17	1.17	XXX	■
82634		X	Deoxycortisol, 11-	0.00	1.03	1.03	0.00	1.03	1.03	XXX	■
	26			0.00	0.00	0.00	0.00	0.00	0.00	XXX	■
	TC			0.00	1.03	1.03	0.00	1.03	1.03	XXX	■
82638		X	Dibucaine number	0.00	0.41	0.41	0.00	0.41	0.41	XXX	■
	26			0.00	0.00	0.00	0.00	0.00	0.00	XXX	■
	TC			0.00	0.41	0.41	0.00	0.41	0.41	XXX	■
82646		X	Dihydrocodeinone	0.00	0.73	0.73	0.00	0.73	0.73	XXX	■
	26			0.00	0.00	0.00	0.00	0.00	0.00	XXX	■
	TC			0.00	0.73	0.73	0.00	0.73	0.73	XXX	■
82649		X	Dihydromorphinone	0.00	0.73	0.73	0.00	0.73	0.73	XXX	■
	26			0.00	0.00	0.00	0.00	0.00	0.00	XXX	■
	TC			0.00	0.73	0.73	0.00	0.73	0.73	XXX	■
82651		X	Dihydrotestosterone (DHT)	0.00	0.88	0.88	0.00	0.88	0.88	XXX	■
	26			0.00	0.00	0.00	0.00	0.00	0.00	XXX	■
	TC			0.00	0.88	0.88	0.00	0.88	0.88	XXX	■
82652		X	Dihydroxyvitamin D, 1,25-	0.00	1.17	1.17	0.00	1.17	1.17	XXX	■
	26			0.00	0.00	0.00	0.00	0.00	0.00	XXX	■
	TC			0.00	1.17	1.17	0.00	1.17	1.17	XXX	■
82654		X	Dimethadione	0.00	0.73	0.73	0.00	0.73	0.73	XXX	■
	26			0.00	0.00	0.00	0.00	0.00	0.00	XXX	■
	TC			0.00	0.73	0.73	0.00	0.73	0.73	XXX	■
82657		X	Enzyme activity in blood cells, cultured cells, or tissue, not elsewhere specified; nonradioactive substrate, each specimen	0.00	0.69	0.69	0.00	0.69	0.69	XXX	■
	26			0.00	0.00	0.00	0.00	0.00	0.00	XXX	■
	TC			0.00	0.69	0.69	0.00	0.69	0.69	XXX	■
82658		X	radioactive substrate, each specimen	0.00	0.62	0.62	0.00	0.62	0.62	XXX	■
	26			0.00	0.00	0.00	0.00	0.00	0.00	XXX	■
	TC			0.00	0.62	0.62	0.00	0.62	0.62	XXX	■
82664		X	Electrophoretic technique, not elsewhere specified	0.00	0.67	0.67	0.00	0.67	0.67	XXX	■
	26			0.00	0.00	0.00	0.00	0.00	0.00	XXX	■
	TC			0.00	0.67	0.67	0.00	0.67	0.67	XXX	■
82666		X	Epiandrosterone	0.00	0.88	0.88	0.00	0.88	0.88	XXX	■
	26			0.00	0.00	0.00	0.00	0.00	0.00	XXX	■
	TC			0.00	0.88	0.88	0.00	0.88	0.88	XXX	■
82668		X	Erythropoietin	0.00	0.95	0.95	0.00	0.95	0.95	XXX	■
	26			0.00	0.00	0.00	0.00	0.00	0.00	XXX	■
	TC			0.00	0.95	0.95	0.00	0.95	0.95	XXX	■
82670		X	Estradiol	0.00	0.69	0.69	0.00	0.69	0.69	XXX	■
	26			0.00	0.00	0.00	0.00	0.00	0.00	XXX	■
	TC			0.00	0.69	0.69	0.00	0.69	0.69	XXX	■
82671		X	Estrogens; fractionated	0.00	1.23	1.23	0.00	1.23	1.23	XXX	■
	26			0.00	0.00	0.00	0.00	0.00	0.00	XXX	■
	TC			0.00	1.23	1.23	0.00	1.23	1.23	XXX	■

■ RVU not developed by CMS. Gap-filled RVUs developed by Ingenix/CHEG.

Code	M	S	Description	Work Value	Non-Fac PE	Fac PE	Mal-practice	Non-Fac Total	Fac Total	Global	Gap
82672		X	total	0.00	0.88	0.88	0.00	0.88	0.88	XXX	■
	26			0.00	0.00	0.00	0.00	0.00	0.00	XXX	■
	TC			0.00	0.88	0.88	0.00	0.88	0.88	XXX	■
82677		X	Estriol	0.00	0.63	0.63	0.00	0.63	0.63	XXX	■
	26			0.00	0.00	0.00	0.00	0.00	0.00	XXX	■
	TC			0.00	0.63	0.63	0.00	0.63	0.63	XXX	■
82679		X	Estrone	0.00	0.95	0.95	0.00	0.95	0.95	XXX	■
	26			0.00	0.00	0.00	0.00	0.00	0.00	XXX	■
	TC			0.00	0.95	0.95	0.00	0.95	0.95	XXX	■
82690		X	Ethchlorvynol	0.00	0.48	0.48	0.00	0.48	0.48	XXX	■
	26			0.00	0.00	0.00	0.00	0.00	0.00	XXX	■
	TC			0.00	0.48	0.48	0.00	0.48	0.48	XXX	■
82693		X	Ethylene glycol	0.00	0.73	0.73	0.00	0.73	0.73	XXX	■
	26			0.00	0.00	0.00	0.00	0.00	0.00	XXX	■
	TC			0.00	0.73	0.73	0.00	0.73	0.73	XXX	■
82696		X	Etiocholanolone	0.00	1.03	1.03	0.00	1.03	1.03	XXX	■
	26			0.00	0.00	0.00	0.00	0.00	0.00	XXX	■
	TC			0.00	1.03	1.03	0.00	1.03	1.03	XXX	■
82705		X	Fat or lipids, feces; qualitative	0.00	0.22	0.22	0.00	0.22	0.22	XXX	■
	26			0.00	0.00	0.00	0.00	0.00	0.00	XXX	■
	TC			0.00	0.22	0.22	0.00	0.22	0.22	XXX	■
82710		X	quantitative	0.00	0.82	0.82	0.00	0.82	0.82	XXX	■
	26			0.00	0.00	0.00	0.00	0.00	0.00	XXX	■
	TC			0.00	0.82	0.82	0.00	0.82	0.82	XXX	■
82715		X	Fat differential, feces, quantitative	0.00	0.35	0.35	0.00	0.35	0.35	XXX	■
	26			0.00	0.00	0.00	0.00	0.00	0.00	XXX	■
	TC			0.00	0.35	0.35	0.00	0.35	0.35	XXX	■
82725		X	Fatty acids, nonesterified	0.00	0.35	0.35	0.00	0.35	0.35	XXX	■
	26			0.00	0.00	0.00	0.00	0.00	0.00	XXX	■
	TC			0.00	0.35	0.35	0.00	0.35	0.35	XXX	■
82726		X	Very long chain fatty acids	0.00	0.69	0.69	0.00	0.69	0.69	XXX	■
	26			0.00	0.00	0.00	0.00	0.00	0.00	XXX	■
	TC			0.00	0.69	0.69	0.00	0.69	0.69	XXX	■
82728		X	Ferritin	0.00	0.54	0.54	0.00	0.54	0.54	XXX	■
	26			0.00	0.00	0.00	0.00	0.00	0.00	XXX	■
	TC			0.00	0.54	0.54	0.00	0.54	0.54	XXX	■
82731		X	Fetal fibronectin, cervicovaginal secretions,	0.00	0.54	0.54	0.00	0.54	0.54	XXX	■
	26		semi-quantitative	0.00	0.00	0.00	0.00	0.00	0.00	XXX	■
	TC			0.00	0.54	0.54	0.00	0.54	0.54	XXX	■
82735		X	Fluoride	0.00	0.63	0.63	0.00	0.63	0.63	XXX	■
	26			0.00	0.00	0.00	0.00	0.00	0.00	XXX	■
	TC			0.00	0.63	0.63	0.00	0.63	0.63	XXX	■
82742		X	Flurazepam	0.00	0.73	0.73	0.00	0.73	0.73	XXX	■
	26			0.00	0.00	0.00	0.00	0.00	0.00	XXX	■
	TC			0.00	0.73	0.73	0.00	0.73	0.73	XXX	■

■ RVU not developed by CMS. Gap-filled RVUs developed by Ingenix/CHEG.

Code	M	S	Description	Work Value	Non-Fac PE	Fac PE	Mal-practice	Non-Fac Total	Fac Total	Global	Gap
82746		X	Folic acid; serum	0.00	0.60	0.60	0.00	0.60	0.60	XXX	■
	26			0.00	0.00	0.00	0.00	0.00	0.00	XXX	■
	TC			0.00	0.60	0.60	0.00	0.60	0.60	XXX	■
82747		X	RBC	0.00	0.72	0.72	0.00	0.72	0.72	XXX	■
	26			0.00	0.00	0.00	0.00	0.00	0.00	XXX	■
	TC			0.00	0.72	0.72	0.00	0.72	0.72	XXX	■
82757		X	Fructose, semen	0.00	0.38	0.38	0.00	0.38	0.38	XXX	■
	26			0.00	0.00	0.00	0.00	0.00	0.00	XXX	■
	TC			0.00	0.38	0.38	0.00	0.38	0.38	XXX	■
82759		X	Galactokinase, RBC	0.00	0.47	0.47	0.00	0.47	0.47	XXX	■
	26			0.00	0.00	0.00	0.00	0.00	0.00	XXX	■
	TC			0.00	0.47	0.47	0.00	0.47	0.47	XXX	■
82760		X	Galactose	0.00	0.48	0.48	0.00	0.48	0.48	XXX	■
	26			0.00	0.00	0.00	0.00	0.00	0.00	XXX	■
	TC			0.00	0.48	0.48	0.00	0.48	0.48	XXX	■
82775		X	Galactose-1-phosphate uridyl transferase; quantitative	0.00	0.62	0.62	0.00	0.62	0.62	XXX	■
	26			0.00	0.00	0.00	0.00	0.00	0.00	XXX	■
	TC			0.00	0.62	0.62	0.00	0.62	0.62	XXX	■
82776		X	screen	0.00	0.20	0.20	0.00	0.20	0.20	XXX	■
	26			0.00	0.00	0.00	0.00	0.00	0.00	XXX	■
	TC			0.00	0.20	0.20	0.00	0.20	0.20	XXX	■
82784		X	Gammaglobulin; IgA, IgD, IgG, IgM, each	0.00	0.50	0.50	0.00	0.50	0.50	XXX	■
	26			0.00	0.00	0.00	0.00	0.00	0.00	XXX	■
	TC			0.00	0.50	0.50	0.00	0.50	0.50	XXX	■
82785		X	IgE	0.00	0.63	0.63	0.00	0.63	0.63	XXX	■
	26			0.00	0.00	0.00	0.00	0.00	0.00	XXX	■
	TC			0.00	0.63	0.63	0.00	0.63	0.63	XXX	■
82787		X	immunoglobulin subclasses, (IgG1, 2, 3, or 4), each	0.00	1.57	1.57	0.00	1.57	1.57	XXX	■
	26			0.00	0.00	0.00	0.00	0.00	0.00	XXX	■
	TC			0.00	1.57	1.57	0.00	1.57	1.57	XXX	■
82800		X	Gases, blood, pH only	0.00	0.38	0.38	0.00	0.38	0.38	XXX	■
	26			0.00	0.00	0.00	0.00	0.00	0.00	XXX	■
	TC			0.00	0.38	0.38	0.00	0.38	0.38	XXX	■
82803		X	Gases, blood, any combination of pH, pCO2, pO2, CO2, HCO3 (including calculated O2 saturation);	0.00	0.75	0.75	0.00	0.75	0.75	XXX	■
	26			0.00	0.00	0.00	0.00	0.00	0.00	XXX	■
	TC			0.00	0.75	0.75	0.00	0.75	0.75	XXX	■
82805		X	with O2 saturation, by direct measurement, except pulse oximetry	0.00	0.81	0.81	0.00	0.81	0.81	XXX	■
	26			0.00	0.00	0.00	0.00	0.00	0.00	XXX	■
	TC			0.00	0.81	0.81	0.00	0.81	0.81	XXX	■
82810		X	Gases, blood, O2 saturation only, by direct measurement, except pulse oximetry	0.00	0.41	0.41	0.00	0.41	0.41	XXX	■
	26			0.00	0.00	0.00	0.00	0.00	0.00	XXX	■
	TC			0.00	0.41	0.41	0.00	0.41	0.41	XXX	■
82820		X	Hemoglobin-oxygen affinity (pO2 for 50% hemoglobin saturation with oxygen)	0.00	0.51	0.51	0.00	0.51	0.51	XXX	■
	26			0.00	0.00	0.00	0.00	0.00	0.00	XXX	■
	TC			0.00	0.51	0.51	0.00	0.51	0.51	XXX	■

■ RVU not developed by CMS. Gap-filled RVUs developed by Ingenix/CHEG.

Pathology

Code	M	S	Description	Work Value	Non-Fac PE	Fac PE	Mal-practice	Non-Fac Total	Fac Total	Global	Gap
82926		**X**	Gastric acid, free and total, each specimen	0.00	0.23	0.23	0.00	0.23	0.23	XXX	■
	26			0.00	0.00	0.00	0.00	0.00	0.00	XXX	■
	TC			0.00	0.23	0.23	0.00	0.23	0.23	XXX	■
82928		**X**	Gastric acid, free or total; each specimen	0.00	0.22	0.22	0.00	0.22	0.22	XXX	■
	26			0.00	0.00	0.00	0.00	0.00	0.00	XXX	■
	TC			0.00	0.22	0.22	0.00	0.22	0.22	XXX	■
82938		**X**	Gastrin after secretin stimulation	0.00	0.72	0.72	0.00	0.72	0.72	XXX	■
	26			0.00	0.00	0.00	0.00	0.00	0.00	XXX	■
	TC			0.00	0.72	0.72	0.00	0.72	0.72	XXX	■
82941		**X**	Gastrin	0.00	0.72	0.72	0.00	0.72	0.72	XXX	■
	26			0.00	0.00	0.00	0.00	0.00	0.00	XXX	■
	TC			0.00	0.72	0.72	0.00	0.72	0.72	XXX	■
82943		**X**	Glucagon	0.00	0.86	0.86	0.00	0.86	0.86	XXX	■
	26			0.00	0.00	0.00	0.00	0.00	0.00	XXX	■
	TC			0.00	0.86	0.86	0.00	0.86	0.86	XXX	■
82945		**X**	Glucose, body fluid, other than blood	0.00	0.63	0.63	0.00	0.63	0.63	XXX	■
	26			0.00	0.00	0.00	0.00	0.00	0.00	XXX	■
	TC			0.00	0.63	0.63	0.00	0.63	0.63	XXX	■
82946		**X**	Glucagon tolerance test	0.00	0.48	0.48	0.00	0.48	0.48	XXX	■
	26			0.00	0.00	0.00	0.00	0.00	0.00	XXX	■
	TC			0.00	0.48	0.48	0.00	0.48	0.48	XXX	■
82947		**X**	Glucose; quantitative, blood (except reagent	0.00	0.19	0.19	0.00	0.19	0.19	XXX	■
	26		strip)	0.00	0.00	0.00	0.00	0.00	0.00	XXX	■
	TC			0.00	0.19	0.19	0.00	0.19	0.19	XXX	■
82948		**X**	blood, reagent strip	0.00	0.15	0.15	0.00	0.15	0.15	XXX	■
	26			0.00	0.00	0.00	0.00	0.00	0.00	XXX	■
	TC			0.00	0.15	0.15	0.00	0.15	0.15	XXX	■
82950		**X**	post glucose dose (includes glucose)	0.00	0.25	0.25	0.00	0.25	0.25	XXX	■
	26			0.00	0.00	0.00	0.00	0.00	0.00	XXX	■
	TC			0.00	0.25	0.25	0.00	0.25	0.25	XXX	■
82951		**X**	tolerance test (GTT), three specimens	0.00	0.54	0.54	0.00	0.54	0.54	XXX	■
	26		(includes glucose)	0.00	0.00	0.00	0.00	0.00	0.00	XXX	■
	TC			0.00	0.54	0.54	0.00	0.54	0.54	XXX	■
82952		**X**	tolerance test, each additional beyond	0.00	0.15	0.15	0.00	0.15	0.15	XXX	■
	26		three specimens	0.00	0.00	0.00	0.00	0.00	0.00	XXX	■
	TC			0.00	0.15	0.15	0.00	0.15	0.15	XXX	■
82953		**X**	tolbutamide tolerance test	0.00	0.63	0.63	0.00	0.63	0.63	XXX	■
	26			0.00	0.00	0.00	0.00	0.00	0.00	XXX	■
	TC			0.00	0.63	0.63	0.00	0.63	0.63	XXX	■
82955		**X**	Glucose-6-phosphate dehydrogenase (G6PD);	0.00	0.56	0.56	0.00	0.56	0.56	XXX	■
	26		quantitative	0.00	0.00	0.00	0.00	0.00	0.00	XXX	■
	TC			0.00	0.56	0.56	0.00	0.56	0.56	XXX	■
82960		**X**	screen	0.00	0.29	0.29	0.00	0.29	0.29	XXX	■
	26			0.00	0.00	0.00	0.00	0.00	0.00	XXX	■
	TC			0.00	0.29	0.29	0.00	0.29	0.29	XXX	■

■ RVU not developed by CMS. Gap-filled RVUs developed by Ingenix/CHEG.

Code	M	S	Description	Work Value	Non-Fac PE	Fac PE	Mal-prac-tice	Non-Fac Total	Fac Total	Global	Gap
82962		X	Glucose, blood by glucose monitoring device(s) cleared by the FDA specifically for home use	0.00	0.15	0.15	0.00	0.15	0.15	XXX	■
	26			0.00	0.00	0.00	0.00	0.00	0.00	XXX	■
	TC			0.00	0.15	0.15	0.00	0.15	0.15	XXX	■
82963		X	Glucosidase, beta	0.00	0.73	0.73	0.00	0.73	0.73	XXX	■
	26			0.00	0.00	0.00	0.00	0.00	0.00	XXX	■
	TC			0.00	0.73	0.73	0.00	0.73	0.73	XXX	■
82965		X	Glutamate dehydrogenase	0.00	0.21	0.21	0.00	0.21	0.21	XXX	■
	26			0.00	0.00	0.00	0.00	0.00	0.00	XXX	■
	TC			0.00	0.21	0.21	0.00	0.21	0.21	XXX	■
82975		X	Glutamine (glutamic acid amide)	0.00	0.50	0.50	0.00	0.50	0.50	XXX	■
	26			0.00	0.00	0.00	0.00	0.00	0.00	XXX	■
	TC			0.00	0.50	0.50	0.00	0.50	0.50	XXX	■
82977		X	Glutamyltransferase, gamma (GGT)	0.00	0.19	0.19	0.00	0.19	0.19	XXX	■
	26			0.00	0.00	0.00	0.00	0.00	0.00	XXX	■
	TC			0.00	0.19	0.19	0.00	0.19	0.19	XXX	■
82978		X	Glutathione	0.00	0.51	0.51	0.00	0.51	0.51	XXX	■
	26			0.00	0.00	0.00	0.00	0.00	0.00	XXX	■
	TC			0.00	0.51	0.51	0.00	0.51	0.51	XXX	■
82979		X	Glutathione reductase, RBC	0.00	0.37	0.37	0.00	0.37	0.37	XXX	■
	26			0.00	0.00	0.00	0.00	0.00	0.00	XXX	■
	TC			0.00	0.37	0.37	0.00	0.37	0.37	XXX	■
82980		X	Glutethimide	0.00	0.73	0.73	0.00	0.73	0.73	XXX	■
	26			0.00	0.00	0.00	0.00	0.00	0.00	XXX	■
	TC			0.00	0.73	0.73	0.00	0.73	0.73	XXX	■
82985		X	Glycated protein	0.00	0.31	0.31	0.00	0.31	0.31	XXX	■
	26			0.00	0.00	0.00	0.00	0.00	0.00	XXX	■
	TC			0.00	0.31	0.31	0.00	0.31	0.31	XXX	■
83001		X	Gonadotropin; follicle stimulating hormone (FSH)	0.00	0.73	0.73	0.00	0.73	0.73	XXX	■
	26			0.00	0.00	0.00	0.00	0.00	0.00	XXX	■
	TC			0.00	0.73	0.73	0.00	0.73	0.73	XXX	■
83002		X	luteinizing hormone (LH)	0.00	0.73	0.73	0.00	0.73	0.73	XXX	■
	26			0.00	0.00	0.00	0.00	0.00	0.00	XXX	■
	TC			0.00	0.73	0.73	0.00	0.73	0.73	XXX	■
83003		X	Growth hormone, human (HGH) (somatotropin)	0.00	0.73	0.73	0.00	0.73	0.73	XXX	■
	26			0.00	0.00	0.00	0.00	0.00	0.00	XXX	■
	TC			0.00	0.73	0.73	0.00	0.73	0.73	XXX	■
83008		X	Guanosine monophosphate (GMP), cyclic	0.00	0.88	0.88	0.00	0.88	0.88	XXX	■
	26			0.00	0.00	0.00	0.00	0.00	0.00	XXX	■
	TC			0.00	0.88	0.88	0.00	0.88	0.88	XXX	■
83010		X	Haptoglobin; quantitative	0.00	0.54	0.54	0.00	0.54	0.54	XXX	■
	26			0.00	0.00	0.00	0.00	0.00	0.00	XXX	■
	TC			0.00	0.54	0.54	0.00	0.54	0.54	XXX	■
83012		X	phenotypes	0.00	0.59	0.59	0.00	0.59	0.59	XXX	■
	26			0.00	0.00	0.00	0.00	0.00	0.00	XXX	■
	TC			0.00	0.59	0.59	0.00	0.59	0.59	XXX	■

■ RVU not developed by CMS. Gap-filled RVUs developed by Ingenix/CHEG.

Code	M	S	Description	Work Value	Non-Fac PE	Fac PE	Mal-practice	Non-Fac Total	Fac Total	Global	Gap
83013		X	Helicobacter pylori; analysis for urease activity,	0.00	2.57	2.57	0.00	2.57	2.57	XXX	■
	26		non-radioactive isotope	0.00	0.00	0.00	0.00	0.00	0.00	XXX	■
	TC			0.00	2.57	2.57	0.00	2.57	2.57	XXX	■
83014		X	drug administration and sample collection	0.00	0.30	0.30	0.00	0.30	0.30	XXX	■
	26			0.00	0.00	0.00	0.00	0.00	0.00	XXX	■
	TC			0.00	0.30	0.30	0.00	0.30	0.30	XXX	■
83015		X	Heavy metal (arsenic, barium, beryllium,	0.00	0.97	0.97	0.00	0.97	0.97	XXX	■
	26		bismuth, antimony, mercury); screen	0.00	0.00	0.00	0.00	0.00	0.00	XXX	■
	TC			0.00	0.97	0.97	0.00	0.97	0.97	XXX	■
83018		X	quantitative, each	0.00	1.03	1.03	0.00	1.03	1.03	XXX	■
	26			0.00	0.00	0.00	0.00	0.00	0.00	XXX	■
	TC			0.00	1.03	1.03	0.00	1.03	1.03	XXX	■
83020		X	Hemoglobin fractionation and quantitation;	0.37	0.66	0.66	0.01	1.04	1.04	XXX	■
	26	A	electrophoresis (eg, A2, S, C, and/or F)	0.37	0.17	0.17	0.01	0.55	0.55	XXX	
	TC			0.00	0.49	0.49	0.00	0.49	0.49	XXX	■
83021		X	chromatography (eg, A2, S, C, and/or F)	0.00	0.73	0.73	0.00	0.73	0.73	XXX	■
	26			0.00	0.00	0.00	0.00	0.00	0.00	XXX	■
	TC			0.00	0.73	0.73	0.00	0.73	0.73	XXX	■
83026		X	Hemoglobin; by copper sulfate method, non-	0.00	0.13	0.13	0.00	0.13	0.13	XXX	■
	26		automated	0.00	0.00	0.00	0.00	0.00	0.00	XXX	■
	TC			0.00	0.13	0.13	0.00	0.13	0.13	XXX	■
83030		X	F(fetal), chemical	0.00	0.38	0.38	0.00	0.38	0.38	XXX	■
	26			0.00	0.00	0.00	0.00	0.00	0.00	XXX	■
	TC			0.00	0.38	0.38	0.00	0.38	0.38	XXX	■
83033		X	F (fetal), qualitative	0.00	0.22	0.22	0.00	0.22	0.22	XXX	■
	26			0.00	0.00	0.00	0.00	0.00	0.00	XXX	■
	TC			0.00	0.22	0.22	0.00	0.22	0.22	XXX	■
83036		X	glycated	0.00	0.42	0.42	0.00	0.42	0.42	XXX	■
	26			0.00	0.00	0.00	0.00	0.00	0.00	XXX	■
	TC			0.00	0.42	0.42	0.00	0.42	0.42	XXX	■
83045		X	methemoglobin, qualitative	0.00	0.15	0.15	0.00	0.15	0.15	XXX	■
	26			0.00	0.00	0.00	0.00	0.00	0.00	XXX	■
	TC			0.00	0.15	0.15	0.00	0.15	0.15	XXX	■
83050		X	methemoglobin, quantitative	0.00	0.18	0.18	0.00	0.18	0.18	XXX	■
	26			0.00	0.00	0.00	0.00	0.00	0.00	XXX	■
	TC			0.00	0.18	0.18	0.00	0.18	0.18	XXX	■
83051		X	plasma	0.00	0.19	0.19	0.00	0.19	0.19	XXX	■
	26			0.00	0.00	0.00	0.00	0.00	0.00	XXX	■
	TC			0.00	0.19	0.19	0.00	0.19	0.19	XXX	■
83055		X	sulfhemoglobin, qualitative	0.00	0.24	0.24	0.00	0.24	0.24	XXX	■
	26			0.00	0.00	0.00	0.00	0.00	0.00	XXX	■
	TC			0.00	0.24	0.24	0.00	0.24	0.24	XXX	■
83060		X	sulfhemoglobin, quantitative	0.00	0.34	0.34	0.00	0.34	0.34	XXX	■
	26			0.00	0.00	0.00	0.00	0.00	0.00	XXX	■
	TC			0.00	0.34	0.34	0.00	0.34	0.34	XXX	■

■ RVU not developed by CMS. Gap-filled RVUs developed by Ingenix/CHEG.

Code	M	S	Description	Work Value	Non-Fac PE	Fac PE	Mal-practice	Non-Fac Total	Fac Total	Global	Gap
83065		X	thermolabile	0.00	0.12	0.12	0.00	0.12	0.12	XXX	■
	26			0.00	0.00	0.00	0.00	0.00	0.00	XXX	■
	TC			0.00	0.12	0.12	0.00	0.12	0.12	XXX	■
83068		X	unstable, screen	0.00	0.16	0.16	0.00	0.16	0.16	XXX	■
	26			0.00	0.00	0.00	0.00	0.00	0.00	XXX	■
	TC			0.00	0.16	0.16	0.00	0.16	0.16	XXX	■
83069		X	urine	0.00	0.12	0.12	0.00	0.12	0.12	XXX	■
	26			0.00	0.00	0.00	0.00	0.00	0.00	XXX	■
	TC			0.00	0.12	0.12	0.00	0.12	0.12	XXX	■
83070		X	Hemosiderin; qualitative	0.00	0.18	0.18	0.00	0.18	0.18	XXX	■
	26			0.00	0.00	0.00	0.00	0.00	0.00	XXX	■
	TC			0.00	0.18	0.18	0.00	0.18	0.18	XXX	■
83071		X	quantitative	0.00	0.18	0.18	0.00	0.18	0.18	XXX	■
	26			0.00	0.00	0.00	0.00	0.00	0.00	XXX	■
	TC			0.00	0.18	0.18	0.00	0.18	0.18	XXX	■
83080		X	b-Hexosaminidase, each assay	0.00	0.45	0.45	0.00	0.45	0.45	XXX	■
	26			0.00	0.00	0.00	0.00	0.00	0.00	XXX	■
	TC			0.00	0.45	0.45	0.00	0.45	0.45	XXX	■
83088		X	Histamine	0.00	1.13	1.13	0.00	1.13	1.13	XXX	■
	26			0.00	0.00	0.00	0.00	0.00	0.00	XXX	■
	TC			0.00	1.13	1.13	0.00	1.13	1.13	XXX	■
83090		X	Homocystine	0.00	0.42	0.42	0.00	0.42	0.42	XXX	■
	26			0.00	0.00	0.00	0.00	0.00	0.00	XXX	■
	TC			0.00	0.42	0.42	0.00	0.42	0.42	XXX	■
83150		X	Homovanillic acid (HVA)	0.00	0.73	0.73	0.00	0.73	0.73	XXX	■
	26			0.00	0.00	0.00	0.00	0.00	0.00	XXX	■
	TC			0.00	0.73	0.73	0.00	0.73	0.73	XXX	■
83491		X	Hydroxycorticosteroids, 17- (17-OHCS)	0.00	0.86	0.86	0.00	0.86	0.86	XXX	■
	26			0.00	0.00	0.00	0.00	0.00	0.00	XXX	■
	TC			0.00	0.86	0.86	0.00	0.86	0.86	XXX	■
83497		X	Hydroxyindolacetic acid, 5-(HIAA)	0.00	0.69	0.69	0.00	0.69	0.69	XXX	■
	26			0.00	0.00	0.00	0.00	0.00	0.00	XXX	■
	TC			0.00	0.69	0.69	0.00	0.69	0.69	XXX	■
83498		X	Hydroxyprogesterone, 17-d	0.00	1.00	1.00	0.00	1.00	1.00	XXX	■
	26			0.00	0.00	0.00	0.00	0.00	0.00	XXX	■
	TC			0.00	1.00	1.00	0.00	1.00	1.00	XXX	■
83499		X	Hydroxyprogesterone, 20-	0.00	0.78	0.78	0.00	0.78	0.78	XXX	■
	26			0.00	0.00	0.00	0.00	0.00	0.00	XXX	■
	TC			0.00	0.78	0.78	0.00	0.78	0.78	XXX	■
83500		X	Hydroxyproline; free	0.00	0.73	0.73	0.00	0.73	0.73	XXX	■
	26			0.00	0.00	0.00	0.00	0.00	0.00	XXX	■
	TC			0.00	0.73	0.73	0.00	0.73	0.73	XXX	■
83505		X	total	0.00	0.95	0.95	0.00	0.95	0.95	XXX	■
	26			0.00	0.00	0.00	0.00	0.00	0.00	XXX	■
	TC			0.00	0.95	0.95	0.00	0.95	0.95	XXX	■

■ RVU not developed by CMS. Gap-filled RVUs developed by Ingenix/CHEG.

Code	M	S	Description	Work Value	Non-Fac PE	Fac PE	Mal-practice	Non-Fac Total	Fac Total	Global	Gap
83516		X	Immunoassay for analyte other than infectious agent antibody or infectious agent antigen, qualitative or semiquantitative; multiple step method	0.00	0.47	0.47	0.00	0.47	0.47	XXX	■
	26			0.00	0.00	0.00	0.00	0.00	0.00	XXX	■
	TC			0.00	0.47	0.47	0.00	0.47	0.47	XXX	■
83518		X	single step method (eg, reagent strip)	0.00	0.29	0.29	0.00	0.29	0.29	XXX	■
	26			0.00	0.00	0.00	0.00	0.00	0.00	XXX	■
	TC			0.00	0.29	0.29	0.00	0.29	0.29	XXX	■
83519		X	Immunoassay, analyte, quantitative; by radiopharmaceutical technique (eg, RIA)	0.00	0.62	0.62	0.00	0.62	0.62	XXX	■
	26			0.00	0.00	0.00	0.00	0.00	0.00	XXX	■
	TC			0.00	0.62	0.62	0.00	0.62	0.62	XXX	■
83520		X	not otherwise specified	0.00	0.53	0.53	0.00	0.53	0.53	XXX	■
	26			0.00	0.00	0.00	0.00	0.00	0.00	XXX	■
	TC			0.00	0.53	0.53	0.00	0.53	0.53	XXX	■
83525		X	Insulin; total	0.00	0.57	0.57	0.00	0.57	0.57	XXX	■
	26			0.00	0.00	0.00	0.00	0.00	0.00	XXX	■
	TC			0.00	0.57	0.57	0.00	0.57	0.57	XXX	■
83527		X	free	0.00	0.64	0.64	0.00	0.64	0.64	XXX	■
	26			0.00	0.00	0.00	0.00	0.00	0.00	XXX	■
	TC			0.00	0.64	0.64	0.00	0.64	0.64	XXX	■
83528		X	Intrinsic factor	0.00	0.76	0.76	0.00	0.76	0.76	XXX	■
	26			0.00	0.00	0.00	0.00	0.00	0.00	XXX	■
	TC			0.00	0.76	0.76	0.00	0.76	0.76	XXX	■
83540		X	Iron	0.00	0.19	0.19	0.00	0.19	0.19	XXX	■
	26			0.00	0.00	0.00	0.00	0.00	0.00	XXX	■
	TC			0.00	0.19	0.19	0.00	0.19	0.19	XXX	■
83550		X	Iron binding capacity	0.00	0.26	0.26	0.00	0.26	0.26	XXX	■
	26			0.00	0.00	0.00	0.00	0.00	0.00	XXX	■
	TC			0.00	0.26	0.26	0.00	0.26	0.26	XXX	■
83570		X	Isocitric dehydrogenase (IDH)	0.00	0.35	0.35	0.00	0.35	0.35	XXX	■
	26			0.00	0.00	0.00	0.00	0.00	0.00	XXX	■
	TC			0.00	0.35	0.35	0.00	0.35	0.35	XXX	■
83582		X	Ketogenic steroids, fractionation	0.00	0.60	0.60	0.00	0.60	0.60	XXX	■
	26			0.00	0.00	0.00	0.00	0.00	0.00	XXX	■
	TC			0.00	0.60	0.60	0.00	0.60	0.60	XXX	■
83586		X	Ketosteroids, 17- (17-KS); total	0.00	0.59	0.59	0.00	0.59	0.59	XXX	■
	26			0.00	0.00	0.00	0.00	0.00	0.00	XXX	■
	TC			0.00	0.59	0.59	0.00	0.59	0.59	XXX	■
83593		X	fractionation	0.00	1.29	1.29	0.00	1.29	1.29	XXX	■
	26			0.00	0.00	0.00	0.00	0.00	0.00	XXX	■
	TC			0.00	1.29	1.29	0.00	1.29	1.29	XXX	■
83605		X	Lactate (lactic acid)	0.00	0.47	0.47	0.00	0.47	0.47	XXX	■
	26			0.00	0.00	0.00	0.00	0.00	0.00	XXX	■
	TC			0.00	0.47	0.47	0.00	0.47	0.47	XXX	■

Pathology

■ RVU not developed by CMS. Gap-filled RVUs developed by Ingenix/CHEG.

Code	M	S	Description	Work Value	Non-Fac PE	Fac PE	Mal-practice	Non-Fac Total	Fac Total	Global	Gap
83615		X	Lactate dehydrogenase (LD), (LDH);	0.00	0.19	0.19	0.00	0.19	0.19	XXX	■
	26			0.00	0.00	0.00	0.00	0.00	0.00	XXX	■
	TC			0.00	0.19	0.19	0.00	0.19	0.19	XXX	■
83625		X	isoenzymes, separation and quantitation	0.00	0.59	0.59	0.00	0.59	0.59	XXX	■
	26			0.00	0.00	0.00	0.00	0.00	0.00	XXX	■
	TC			0.00	0.59	0.59	0.00	0.59	0.59	XXX	■
83632		X	Lactogen, human placental (HPL) human chorionic somatomammotropin	0.00	0.94	0.94	0.00	0.94	0.94	XXX	■
	26			0.00	0.00	0.00	0.00	0.00	0.00	XXX	■
	TC			0.00	0.94	0.94	0.00	0.94	0.94	XXX	■
83633		X	Lactose, urine; qualitative	0.00	0.18	0.18	0.00	0.18	0.18	XXX	■
	26			0.00	0.00	0.00	0.00	0.00	0.00	XXX	■
	TC			0.00	0.18	0.18	0.00	0.18	0.18	XXX	■
83634		X	quantitative	0.00	0.32	0.32	0.00	0.32	0.32	XXX	■
	26			0.00	0.00	0.00	0.00	0.00	0.00	XXX	■
	TC			0.00	0.32	0.32	0.00	0.32	0.32	XXX	■
83655		X	Lead	0.00	0.37	0.37	0.00	0.37	0.37	XXX	■
	26			0.00	0.00	0.00	0.00	0.00	0.00	XXX	■
	TC			0.00	0.37	0.37	0.00	0.37	0.37	XXX	■
83661		X	Fetal lung maturity assessment; lecithin sphingomyelin (L/S) ratio	0.00	1.26	1.26	0.00	1.26	1.26	XXX	■
	26			0.00	0.00	0.00	0.00	0.00	0.00	XXX	■
	TC			0.00	1.26	1.26	0.00	1.26	1.26	XXX	■
83662		X	foam stability test	0.00	0.37	0.37	0.00	0.37	0.37	XXX	■
	26			0.00	0.00	0.00	0.00	0.00	0.00	XXX	■
	TC			0.00	0.37	0.37	0.00	0.37	0.37	XXX	■
83663		X	fluorescence polarization	0.00	0.37	0.37	0.00	0.37	0.37	XXX	■
	26			0.00	0.00	0.00	0.00	0.00	0.00	XXX	■
	TC			0.00	0.37	0.37	0.00	0.37	0.37	XXX	■
83664		X	lamellar body density	0.00	0.37	0.37	0.00	0.37	0.37	XXX	■
	26			0.00	0.00	0.00	0.00	0.00	0.00	XXX	■
	TC			0.00	0.37	0.37	0.00	0.37	0.37	XXX	■
83670		X	Leucine aminopeptidase (LAP)	0.00	0.53	0.53	0.00	0.53	0.53	XXX	■
	26			0.00	0.00	0.00	0.00	0.00	0.00	XXX	■
	TC			0.00	0.53	0.53	0.00	0.53	0.53	XXX	■
83690		X	Lipase	0.00	0.34	0.34	0.00	0.34	0.34	XXX	■
	26			0.00	0.00	0.00	0.00	0.00	0.00	XXX	■
	TC			0.00	0.34	0.34	0.00	0.34	0.34	XXX	■
83715		X	Lipoprotein, blood; electrophoretic separation and quantitation	0.00	0.45	0.45	0.00	0.45	0.45	XXX	■
	26			0.00	0.00	0.00	0.00	0.00	0.00	XXX	■
	TC			0.00	0.45	0.45	0.00	0.45	0.45	XXX	■
83716		X	high resolution fractionation and quantitation of lipoprotein cholesterols (eg, electrophoresis, nuclear magnetic resonance, ultracentrifugation)	0.00	0.95	0.95	0.00	0.95	0.95	XXX	■
	26			0.00	0.00	0.00	0.00	0.00	0.00	XXX	■
	TC			0.00	0.95	0.95	0.00	0.95	0.95	XXX	■

■ RVU not developed by CMS. Gap-filled RVUs developed by Ingenix/CHEG.

Code	M	S	Description	Work Value	Non-Fac PE	Fac PE	Mal-prac-tice	Non-Fac Total	Fac Total	Global	Gap
83718		X	Lipoprotein, direct measurement; high density cholesterol (HDL cholesterol)	0.00	0.28	0.28	0.00	0.28	0.28	XXX	■
	26			0.00	0.00	0.00	0.00	0.00	0.00	XXX	■
	TC			0.00	0.28	0.28	0.00	0.28	0.28	XXX	■
83719		X	direct measurement VLDL cholesterol	0.00	0.31	0.31	0.00	0.31	0.31	XXX	■
	26			0.00	0.00	0.00	0.00	0.00	0.00	XXX	■
	TC			0.00	0.31	0.31	0.00	0.31	0.31	XXX	■
83721		X	direct measurement LDL cholesterol	0.00	0.29	0.29	0.00	0.29	0.29	XXX	■
	26			0.00	0.00	0.00	0.00	0.00	0.00	XXX	■
	TC			0.00	0.29	0.29	0.00	0.29	0.29	XXX	■
83727		X	Luteinizing releasing factor (LRH)	0.00	0.81	0.81	0.00	0.81	0.81	XXX	■
	26			0.00	0.00	0.00	0.00	0.00	0.00	XXX	■
	TC			0.00	0.81	0.81	0.00	0.81	0.81	XXX	■
83735		X	Magnesium	0.00	0.21	0.21	0.00	0.21	0.21	XXX	■
	26			0.00	0.00	0.00	0.00	0.00	0.00	XXX	■
	TC			0.00	0.21	0.21	0.00	0.21	0.21	XXX	■
83775		X	Malate dehydrogenase	0.00	0.34	0.34	0.00	0.34	0.34	XXX	■
	26			0.00	0.00	0.00	0.00	0.00	0.00	XXX	■
	TC			0.00	0.34	0.34	0.00	0.34	0.34	XXX	■
83785		X	Manganese	0.00	0.88	0.88	0.00	0.88	0.88	XXX	■
	26			0.00	0.00	0.00	0.00	0.00	0.00	XXX	■
	TC			0.00	0.88	0.88	0.00	0.88	0.88	XXX	■
83788		X	Mass spectrometry and tandem mass spectrometry (MS, MS/MS), analyte not elsewhere specified; qualitative, each specimen	0.00	0.69	0.69	0.00	0.69	0.69	XXX	■
	26			0.00	0.00	0.00	0.00	0.00	0.00	XXX	■
	TC			0.00	0.69	0.69	0.00	0.69	0.69	XXX	■
83789		X	quantitative, each specimen	0.00	0.69	0.69	0.00	0.69	0.69	XXX	■
	26			0.00	0.00	0.00	0.00	0.00	0.00	XXX	■
	TC			0.00	0.69	0.69	0.00	0.69	0.69	XXX	■
83805		X	Meprobamate	0.00	0.73	0.73	0.00	0.73	0.73	XXX	■
	26			0.00	0.00	0.00	0.00	0.00	0.00	XXX	■
	TC			0.00	0.73	0.73	0.00	0.73	0.73	XXX	■
83825		X	Mercury, quantitative	0.00	0.76	0.76	0.00	0.76	0.76	XXX	■
	26			0.00	0.00	0.00	0.00	0.00	0.00	XXX	■
	TC			0.00	0.76	0.76	0.00	0.76	0.76	XXX	■
83835		X	Metanephrines	0.00	0.76	0.76	0.00	0.76	0.76	XXX	■
	26			0.00	0.00	0.00	0.00	0.00	0.00	XXX	■
	TC			0.00	0.76	0.76	0.00	0.76	0.76	XXX	■
83840		X	Methadone	0.00	0.73	0.73	0.00	0.73	0.73	XXX	■
	26			0.00	0.00	0.00	0.00	0.00	0.00	XXX	■
	TC			0.00	0.73	0.73	0.00	0.73	0.73	XXX	■
83857		X	Methemalbumin	0.00	0.44	0.44	0.00	0.44	0.44	XXX	■
	26			0.00	0.00	0.00	0.00	0.00	0.00	XXX	■
	TC			0.00	0.44	0.44	0.00	0.44	0.44	XXX	■
83858		X	Methsuximide	0.00	0.73	0.73	0.00	0.73	0.73	XXX	■
	26			0.00	0.00	0.00	0.00	0.00	0.00	XXX	■
	TC			0.00	0.73	0.73	0.00	0.73	0.73	XXX	■

■ RVU not developed by CMS. Gap-filled RVUs developed by Ingenix/CHEG.

Code	M	S	Description	Work Value	Non-Fac PE	Fac PE	Mal-practice	Non-Fac Total	Fac Total	Global	Gap
83864		X	Mucopolysaccharides, acid; quantitative	0.00	0.44	0.44	0.00	0.44	0.44	XXX	■
	26			0.00	0.00	0.00	0.00	0.00	0.00	XXX	■
	TC			0.00	0.44	0.44	0.00	0.44	0.44	XXX	■
83866		X	screen	0.00	0.28	0.28	0.00	0.28	0.28	XXX	■
	26			0.00	0.00	0.00	0.00	0.00	0.00	XXX	■
	TC			0.00	0.28	0.28	0.00	0.28	0.28	XXX	■
83872		X	Mucin, synovial fluid (Ropes test)	0.00	0.19	0.19	0.00	0.19	0.19	XXX	■
	26			0.00	0.00	0.00	0.00	0.00	0.00	XXX	■
	TC			0.00	0.19	0.19	0.00	0.19	0.19	XXX	■
83873		X	Myelin basic protein, cerebrospinal fluid	0.00	0.81	0.81	0.00	0.81	0.81	XXX	■
	26			0.00	0.00	0.00	0.00	0.00	0.00	XXX	■
	TC			0.00	0.81	0.81	0.00	0.81	0.81	XXX	■
83874		X	Myoglobin	0.00	0.66	0.66	0.00	0.66	0.66	XXX	■
	26			0.00	0.00	0.00	0.00	0.00	0.00	XXX	■
	TC			0.00	0.66	0.66	0.00	0.66	0.66	XXX	■
83883		X	Nephelometry, each analyte not elsewhere specified	0.00	0.54	0.54	0.00	0.54	0.54	XXX	■
	26			0.00	0.00	0.00	0.00	0.00	0.00	XXX	■
	TC			0.00	0.54	0.54	0.00	0.54	0.54	XXX	■
83885		X	Nickel	0.00	0.78	0.78	0.00	0.78	0.78	XXX	■
	26			0.00	0.00	0.00	0.00	0.00	0.00	XXX	■
	TC			0.00	0.78	0.78	0.00	0.78	0.78	XXX	■
83887		X	Nicotine	0.00	0.73	0.73	0.00	0.73	0.73	XXX	■
	26			0.00	0.00	0.00	0.00	0.00	0.00	XXX	■
	TC			0.00	0.73	0.73	0.00	0.73	0.73	XXX	■
83890		X	Molecular diagnostics; molecular isolation or extraction	0.00	0.37	0.37	0.00	0.37	0.37	XXX	■
	26			0.00	0.00	0.00	0.00	0.00	0.00	XXX	■
	TC			0.00	0.37	0.37	0.00	0.37	0.37	XXX	■
83891		X	isolation or extraction of highly purified nucleic acid	0.00	0.37	0.37	0.00	0.37	0.37	XXX	■
	26			0.00	0.00	0.00	0.00	0.00	0.00	XXX	■
	TC			0.00	0.37	0.37	0.00	0.37	0.37	XXX	■
83892		X	enzymatic digestion	0.00	0.29	0.29	0.00	0.29	0.29	XXX	■
	26			0.00	0.00	0.00	0.00	0.00	0.00	XXX	■
	TC			0.00	0.29	0.29	0.00	0.29	0.29	XXX	■
83893		X	dot/slot blot production	0.00	0.51	0.51	0.00	0.51	0.51	XXX	■
	26			0.00	0.00	0.00	0.00	0.00	0.00	XXX	■
	TC			0.00	0.51	0.51	0.00	0.51	0.51	XXX	■
83894		X	separation by gel electrophoresis (eg, agarose, polyacrylamide)	0.00	0.51	0.51	0.00	0.51	0.51	XXX	■
	26			0.00	0.00	0.00	0.00	0.00	0.00	XXX	■
	TC			0.00	0.51	0.51	0.00	0.51	0.51	XXX	■
83896		X	nucleic acid probe, each	0.00	0.51	0.51	0.00	0.51	0.51	XXX	■
	26			0.00	0.00	0.00	0.00	0.00	0.00	XXX	■
	TC			0.00	0.51	0.51	0.00	0.51	0.51	XXX	■
83897		X	nucleic acid transfer (eg, Southern, Northern)	0.00	0.15	0.15	0.00	0.15	0.15	XXX	■
	26			0.00	0.00	0.00	0.00	0.00	0.00	XXX	■
	TC			0.00	0.15	0.15	0.00	0.15	0.15	XXX	■

■ RVU not developed by CMS. Gap-filled RVUs developed by Ingenix/CHEG.

Pathology

Code	M	S	Description	Work Value	Non-Fac PE	Fac PE	Mal-prac-tice	Non-Fac Total	Fac Total	Global	Gap
83898		**X**	amplification of patient nucleic acid (eg, PCR, LCR), single primer pair, each primer pair	0.00	1.08	1.08	0.00	1.08	1.08	XXX	■
	26			0.00	0.00	0.00	0.00	0.00	0.00	XXX	■
	TC			0.00	1.08	1.08	0.00	1.08	1.08	XXX	■
83901		**X**	amplification of patient nucleic acid, multiplex, each multiplex reaction	0.00	1.08	1.08	0.00	1.08	1.08	XXX	■
	26			0.00	0.00	0.00	0.00	0.00	0.00	XXX	■
	TC			0.00	1.08	1.08	0.00	1.08	1.08	XXX	■
83902		**X**	reverse transcription	0.00	0.54	0.54	0.00	0.54	0.54	XXX	■
	26			0.00	0.00	0.00	0.00	0.00	0.00	XXX	■
	TC			0.00	0.54	0.54	0.00	0.54	0.54	XXX	■
83903		**X**	mutation scanning, by physical properties (eg, single strand conformational polymorphisms (SSCP), heteroduplex, denaturing gradient gel electrophoresis (DGGE), RNA'ase A), single segment, each	0.00	0.64	0.64	0.00	0.64	0.64	XXX	■
	26			0.00	0.00	0.00	0.00	0.00	0.00	XXX	■
	TC			0.00	0.64	0.64	0.00	0.64	0.64	XXX	■
83904		**X**	mutation identification by sequencing, single segment, each segment	0.00	0.64	0.64	0.00	0.64	0.64	XXX	■
	26			0.00	0.00	0.00	0.00	0.00	0.00	XXX	■
	TC			0.00	0.64	0.64	0.00	0.64	0.64	XXX	■
83905		**X**	mutation identification by allele specific transcription, single segment, each segment	0.00	0.64	0.64	0.00	0.64	0.64	XXX	■
	26			0.00	0.00	0.00	0.00	0.00	0.00	XXX	■
	TC			0.00	0.64	0.64	0.00	0.64	0.64	XXX	■
83906		**X**	mutation identification by allele specific translation, single segment, each segment	0.00	0.64	0.64	0.00	0.64	0.64	XXX	■
	26			0.00	0.00	0.00	0.00	0.00	0.00	XXX	■
	TC			0.00	0.64	0.64	0.00	0.64	0.64	XXX	■
83912		**X**	interpretation and report	0.37	0.32	0.32	0.01	0.70	0.70	XXX	■
	26	**A**		0.37	0.17	0.17	0.01	0.55	0.55	XXX	
	TC			0.00	0.15	0.15	0.00	0.15	0.15	XXX	■
83915		**X**	Nucleotidase 5-	0.00	0.41	0.41	0.00	0.41	0.41	XXX	■
	26			0.00	0.00	0.00	0.00	0.00	0.00	XXX	■
	TC			0.00	0.41	0.41	0.00	0.41	0.41	XXX	■
83916		**X**	Oligoclonal immune (oligoclonal bands)	0.00	0.70	0.70	0.00	0.70	0.70	XXX	■
	26			0.00	0.00	0.00	0.00	0.00	0.00	XXX	■
	TC			0.00	0.70	0.70	0.00	0.70	0.70	XXX	■
83918		**X**	Organic acids; total, quantitative, each specimen	0.00	1.10	1.10	0.00	1.10	1.10	XXX	■
	26			0.00	0.00	0.00	0.00	0.00	0.00	XXX	■
	TC			0.00	1.10	1.10	0.00	1.10	1.10	XXX	■
83919		**X**	qualitative, each specimen	0.00	0.73	0.73	0.00	0.73	0.73	XXX	■
	26			0.00	0.00	0.00	0.00	0.00	0.00	XXX	■
	TC			0.00	0.73	0.73	0.00	0.73	0.73	XXX	■
83921		**X**	Organic acid, single, quantitative	0.00	0.73	0.73	0.00	0.73	0.73	XXX	■
	26			0.00	0.00	0.00	0.00	0.00	0.00	XXX	■
	TC			0.00	0.73	0.73	0.00	0.73	0.73	XXX	■
83925		**X**	Opiates, (eg, morphine, meperidine)	0.00	0.73	0.73	0.00	0.73	0.73	XXX	■
	26			0.00	0.00	0.00	0.00	0.00	0.00	XXX	■
	TC			0.00	0.73	0.73	0.00	0.73	0.73	XXX	■

■ RVU not developed by CMS. Gap-filled RVUs developed by Ingenix/CHEG.

Code	M	S	Description	Work Value	Non-Fac PE	Fac PE	Mal-practice	Non-Fac Total	Fac Total	Global	Gap
83930		X	Osmolality; blood	0.00	0.22	0.22	0.00	0.22	0.22	XXX	■
	26			0.00	0.00	0.00	0.00	0.00	0.00	XXX	■
	TC			0.00	0.22	0.22	0.00	0.22	0.22	XXX	■
83935		X	urine	0.00	0.32	0.32	0.00	0.32	0.32	XXX	■
	26			0.00	0.00	0.00	0.00	0.00	0.00	XXX	■
	TC			0.00	0.32	0.32	0.00	0.32	0.32	XXX	■
83937		X	Osteocalcin (bone gla protein)	0.00	1.05	1.05	0.00	1.05	1.05	XXX	■
	26			0.00	0.00	0.00	0.00	0.00	0.00	XXX	■
	TC			0.00	1.05	1.05	0.00	1.05	1.05	XXX	■
83945		X	Oxalate	0.00	0.53	0.53	0.00	0.53	0.53	XXX	■
	26			0.00	0.00	0.00	0.00	0.00	0.00	XXX	■
	TC			0.00	0.53	0.53	0.00	0.53	0.53	XXX	■
83950		X	Oncoprotein, HER-2/neu	0.00	0.76	0.76	0.00	0.76	0.76	XXX	■
	26			0.00	0.00	0.00	0.00	0.00	0.00	XXX	■
	TC			0.00	0.76	0.76	0.00	0.76	0.76	XXX	■
83970		X	Parathormone (parathyroid hormone)	0.00	1.17	1.17	0.00	1.17	1.17	XXX	■
	26			0.00	0.00	0.00	0.00	0.00	0.00	XXX	■
	TC			0.00	1.17	1.17	0.00	1.17	1.17	XXX	■
83986		X	pH, body fluid, except blood	0.00	0.16	0.16	0.00	0.16	0.16	XXX	■
	26			0.00	0.00	0.00	0.00	0.00	0.00	XXX	■
	TC			0.00	0.16	0.16	0.00	0.16	0.16	XXX	■
83992		X	Phencyclidine (PCP)	0.00	0.73	0.73	0.00	0.73	0.73	XXX	■
	26			0.00	0.00	0.00	0.00	0.00	0.00	XXX	■
	TC			0.00	0.73	0.73	0.00	0.73	0.73	XXX	■
84022		X	Phenothiazine	0.00	0.60	0.60	0.00	0.60	0.60	XXX	■
	26			0.00	0.00	0.00	0.00	0.00	0.00	XXX	■
	TC			0.00	0.60	0.60	0.00	0.60	0.60	XXX	■
84030		X	Phenylalanine (PKU), blood	0.00	0.21	0.21	0.00	0.21	0.21	XXX	■
	26			0.00	0.00	0.00	0.00	0.00	0.00	XXX	■
	TC			0.00	0.21	0.21	0.00	0.21	0.21	XXX	■
84035		X	Phenylketones, qualitative	0.00	0.15	0.15	0.00	0.15	0.15	XXX	■
	26			0.00	0.00	0.00	0.00	0.00	0.00	XXX	■
	TC			0.00	0.15	0.15	0.00	0.15	0.15	XXX	■
84060		X	Phosphatase, acid; total	0.00	0.37	0.37	0.00	0.37	0.37	XXX	■
	26			0.00	0.00	0.00	0.00	0.00	0.00	XXX	■
	TC			0.00	0.37	0.37	0.00	0.37	0.37	XXX	■
84061		X	forensic examination	0.00	0.41	0.41	0.00	0.41	0.41	XXX	■
	26			0.00	0.00	0.00	0.00	0.00	0.00	XXX	■
	TC			0.00	0.41	0.41	0.00	0.41	0.41	XXX	■
84066		X	prostatic	0.00	0.48	0.48	0.00	0.48	0.48	XXX	■
	26			0.00	0.00	0.00	0.00	0.00	0.00	XXX	■
	TC			0.00	0.48	0.48	0.00	0.48	0.48	XXX	■
84075		X	Phosphatase, alkaline;	0.00	0.19	0.19	0.00	0.19	0.19	XXX	■
	26			0.00	0.00	0.00	0.00	0.00	0.00	XXX	■
	TC			0.00	0.19	0.19	0.00	0.19	0.19	XXX	■

■ RVU not developed by CMS. Gap-filled RVUs developed by Ingenix/CHEG.

Pathology

Code	M	S	Description	Work Value	Non-Fac PE	Fac PE	Mal-practice	Non-Fac Total	Fac Total	Global	Gap
84078		X	heat stable (total not included)	0.00	0.36	0.36	0.00	0.36	0.36	XXX	■
	26			0.00	0.00	0.00	0.00	0.00	0.00	XXX	■
	TC			0.00	0.36	0.36	0.00	0.36	0.36	XXX	■
84080		X	isoenzymes	0.00	0.63	0.63	0.00	0.63	0.63	XXX	■
	26			0.00	0.00	0.00	0.00	0.00	0.00	XXX	■
	TC			0.00	0.63	0.63	0.00	0.63	0.63	XXX	■
84081		X	Phosphatidylglycerol	0.00	0.88	0.88	0.00	0.88	0.88	XXX	■
	26			0.00	0.00	0.00	0.00	0.00	0.00	XXX	■
	TC			0.00	0.88	0.88	0.00	0.88	0.88	XXX	■
84085		X	Phosphogluconate, 6-, dehydrogenase, RBC	0.00	0.38	0.38	0.00	0.38	0.38	XXX	■
	26			0.00	0.00	0.00	0.00	0.00	0.00	XXX	■
	TC			0.00	0.38	0.38	0.00	0.38	0.38	XXX	■
84087		X	Phosphohexose isomerase	0.00	0.41	0.41	0.00	0.41	0.41	XXX	■
	26			0.00	0.00	0.00	0.00	0.00	0.00	XXX	■
	TC			0.00	0.41	0.41	0.00	0.41	0.41	XXX	■
84100		X	Phosphorus inorganic (phosphate);	0.00	0.19	0.19	0.00	0.19	0.19	XXX	■
	26			0.00	0.00	0.00	0.00	0.00	0.00	XXX	■
	TC			0.00	0.19	0.19	0.00	0.19	0.19	XXX	■
84105		X	urine	0.00	0.23	0.23	0.00	0.23	0.23	XXX	■
	26			0.00	0.00	0.00	0.00	0.00	0.00	XXX	■
	TC			0.00	0.23	0.23	0.00	0.23	0.23	XXX	■
84106		X	Porphobilinogen, urine; qualitative	0.00	0.28	0.28	0.00	0.28	0.28	XXX	■
	26			0.00	0.00	0.00	0.00	0.00	0.00	XXX	■
	TC			0.00	0.28	0.28	0.00	0.28	0.28	XXX	■
84110		X	quantitative	0.00	0.37	0.37	0.00	0.37	0.37	XXX	■
	26			0.00	0.00	0.00	0.00	0.00	0.00	XXX	■
	TC			0.00	0.37	0.37	0.00	0.37	0.37	XXX	■
84119		X	Porphyrins, urine; qualitative	0.00	0.38	0.38	0.00	0.38	0.38	XXX	■
	26			0.00	0.00	0.00	0.00	0.00	0.00	XXX	■
	TC			0.00	0.38	0.38	0.00	0.38	0.38	XXX	■
84120		X	quantitation and fractionation	0.00	0.69	0.69	0.00	0.69	0.69	XXX	■
	26			0.00	0.00	0.00	0.00	0.00	0.00	XXX	■
	TC			0.00	0.69	0.69	0.00	0.69	0.69	XXX	■
84126		X	Porphyrins, feces; quantitative	0.00	0.66	0.66	0.00	0.66	0.66	XXX	■
	26			0.00	0.00	0.00	0.00	0.00	0.00	XXX	■
	TC			0.00	0.66	0.66	0.00	0.66	0.66	XXX	■
84127		X	qualitative	0.00	0.19	0.19	0.00	0.19	0.19	XXX	■
	26			0.00	0.00	0.00	0.00	0.00	0.00	XXX	■
	TC			0.00	0.19	0.19	0.00	0.19	0.19	XXX	■
84132		X	Potassium; serum	0.00	0.19	0.19	0.00	0.19	0.19	XXX	■
	26			0.00	0.00	0.00	0.00	0.00	0.00	XXX	■
	TC			0.00	0.19	0.19	0.00	0.19	0.19	XXX	■
84133		X	urine	0.00	0.21	0.21	0.00	0.21	0.21	XXX	■
	26			0.00	0.00	0.00	0.00	0.00	0.00	XXX	■
	TC			0.00	0.21	0.21	0.00	0.21	0.21	XXX	■

■ RVU not developed by CMS. Gap-filled RVUs developed by Ingenix/CHEG.

Code	M	S	Description	Work Value	Non-Fac PE	Fac PE	Mal-practice	Non-Fac Total	Fac Total	Global	Gap
84134		X	Prealbumin	0.00	0.44	0.44	0.00	0.44	0.44	XXX	■
	26			0.00	0.00	0.00	0.00	0.00	0.00	XXX	■
	TC			0.00	0.44	0.44	0.00	0.44	0.44	XXX	■
84135		X	Pregnanediol	0.00	0.73	0.73	0.00	0.73	0.73	XXX	■
	26			0.00	0.00	0.00	0.00	0.00	0.00	XXX	■
	TC			0.00	0.73	0.73	0.00	0.73	0.73	XXX	■
84138		X	Pregnanetriol	0.00	0.73	0.73	0.00	0.73	0.73	XXX	■
	26			0.00	0.00	0.00	0.00	0.00	0.00	XXX	■
	TC			0.00	0.73	0.73	0.00	0.73	0.73	XXX	■
84140		X	Pregnenolone	0.00	0.88	0.88	0.00	0.88	0.88	XXX	■
	26			0.00	0.00	0.00	0.00	0.00	0.00	XXX	■
	TC			0.00	0.88	0.88	0.00	0.88	0.88	XXX	■
84143		X	17-hydroxypregnenolone	0.00	0.88	0.88	0.00	0.88	0.88	XXX	■
	26			0.00	0.00	0.00	0.00	0.00	0.00	XXX	■
	TC			0.00	0.88	0.88	0.00	0.88	0.88	XXX	■
84144		X	Progesterone	0.00	0.73	0.73	0.00	0.73	0.73	XXX	■
	26			0.00	0.00	0.00	0.00	0.00	0.00	XXX	■
	TC			0.00	0.73	0.73	0.00	0.73	0.73	XXX	■
84146		X	Prolactin	0.00	0.73	0.73	0.00	0.73	0.73	XXX	■
	26			0.00	0.00	0.00	0.00	0.00	0.00	XXX	■
	TC			0.00	0.73	0.73	0.00	0.73	0.73	XXX	■
84150		X	Prostaglandin, each	0.00	0.81	0.81	0.00	0.81	0.81	XXX	■
	26			0.00	0.00	0.00	0.00	0.00	0.00	XXX	■
	TC			0.00	0.81	0.81	0.00	0.81	0.81	XXX	■
84152		X	Prostate specific antigen (PSA); complexed (direct measurement)	0.00	0.73	0.73	0.00	0.73	0.73	XXX	■
	26			0.00	0.00	0.00	0.00	0.00	0.00	XXX	■
	TC			0.00	0.73	0.73	0.00	0.73	0.73	XXX	■
84153		X	Prostate specific antigen (PSA); total	0.00	0.73	0.73	0.00	0.73	0.73	XXX	■
	26			0.00	0.00	0.00	0.00	0.00	0.00	XXX	■
	TC			0.00	0.73	0.73	0.00	0.73	0.73	XXX	■
84154		X	free	0.00	0.73	0.73	0.00	0.73	0.73	XXX	■
	26			0.00	0.00	0.00	0.00	0.00	0.00	XXX	■
	TC			0.00	0.73	0.73	0.00	0.73	0.73	XXX	■
84155		X	Protein; total, except refractometry	0.00	0.19	0.19	0.00	0.19	0.19	XXX	■
	26			0.00	0.00	0.00	0.00	0.00	0.00	XXX	■
	TC			0.00	0.19	0.19	0.00	0.19	0.19	XXX	■
84160		X	refractometric	0.00	0.15	0.15	0.00	0.15	0.15	XXX	■
	26			0.00	0.00	0.00	0.00	0.00	0.00	XXX	■
	TC			0.00	0.15	0.15	0.00	0.15	0.15	XXX	■
84165		X	electrophoretic fractionation and quantitation	0.37	0.58	0.58	0.01	0.96	0.96	XXX	■
	26	A		0.37	0.17	0.17	0.01	0.55	0.55	XXX	
	TC			0.00	0.41	0.41	0.00	0.41	0.41	XXX	■
84181		X	Western Blot, with interpretation and report, blood or other body fluid	0.37	0.80	0.80	0.01	1.18	1.18	XXX	■
	26	A		0.37	0.15	0.15	0.01	0.53	0.53	XXX	
	TC			0.00	0.65	0.65	0.00	0.65	0.65	XXX	■

■ RVU not developed by CMS. Gap-filled RVUs developed by Ingenix/CHEG.

Pathology

Code	M	S	Description	Work Value	Non-Fac PE	Fac PE	Mal-prac-tice	Non-Fac Total	Fac Total	Global	Gap
84182		X	Western Blot, with interpretation and report, blood or other body fluid, immunological probe for band identification, each	0.37	0.84	0.84	0.01	1.22	1.22	XXX	■
	26	A		0.37	0.15	0.15	0.01	0.53	0.53	XXX	
	TC			0.00	0.69	0.69	0.00	0.69	0.69	XXX	■
84202		X	Protoporphyrin, RBC; quantitative	0.00	0.47	0.47	0.00	0.47	0.47	XXX	■
	26			0.00	0.00	0.00	0.00	0.00	0.00	XXX	■
	TC			0.00	0.47	0.47	0.00	0.47	0.47	XXX	■
84203		X	screen	0.00	0.26	0.26	0.00	0.26	0.26	XXX	■
	26			0.00	0.00	0.00	0.00	0.00	0.00	XXX	■
	TC			0.00	0.26	0.26	0.00	0.26	0.26	XXX	■
84206		X	Proinsulin	0.00	1.10	1.10	0.00	1.10	1.10	XXX	■
	26			0.00	0.00	0.00	0.00	0.00	0.00	XXX	■
	TC			0.00	1.10	1.10	0.00	1.10	1.10	XXX	■
84207		X	Pyridoxal phosphate (Vitamin B-6)	0.00	1.10	1.10	0.00	1.10	1.10	XXX	■
	26			0.00	0.00	0.00	0.00	0.00	0.00	XXX	■
	TC			0.00	1.10	1.10	0.00	1.10	1.10	XXX	■
84210		X	Pyruvate	0.00	0.53	0.53	0.00	0.53	0.53	XXX	■
	26			0.00	0.00	0.00	0.00	0.00	0.00	XXX	■
	TC			0.00	0.53	0.53	0.00	0.53	0.53	XXX	■
84220		X	Pyruvate kinase	0.00	0.44	0.44	0.00	0.44	0.44	XXX	■
	26			0.00	0.00	0.00	0.00	0.00	0.00	XXX	■
	TC			0.00	0.44	0.44	0.00	0.44	0.44	XXX	■
84228		X	Quinine	0.00	0.59	0.59	0.00	0.59	0.59	XXX	■
	26			0.00	0.00	0.00	0.00	0.00	0.00	XXX	■
	TC			0.00	0.59	0.59	0.00	0.59	0.59	XXX	■
84233		X	Receptor assay; estrogen	0.00	1.04	1.04	0.00	1.04	1.04	XXX	■
	26			0.00	0.00	0.00	0.00	0.00	0.00	XXX	■
	TC			0.00	1.04	1.04	0.00	1.04	1.04	XXX	■
84234		X	progesterone	0.00	1.04	1.04	0.00	1.04	1.04	XXX	■
	26			0.00	0.00	0.00	0.00	0.00	0.00	XXX	■
	TC			0.00	1.04	1.04	0.00	1.04	1.04	XXX	■
84235		X	endocrine, other than estrogen or progesterone (specify hormone)	0.00	1.04	1.04	0.00	1.04	1.04	XXX	■
	26			0.00	0.00	0.00	0.00	0.00	0.00	XXX	■
	TC			0.00	1.04	1.04	0.00	1.04	1.04	XXX	■
84238		X	non-endocrine (eg, acetylcholine) (specify receptor)	0.00	1.47	1.47	0.00	1.47	1.47	XXX	■
	26			0.00	0.00	0.00	0.00	0.00	0.00	XXX	■
	TC			0.00	1.47	1.47	0.00	1.47	1.47	XXX	■
84244		X	Renin	0.00	0.94	0.94	0.00	0.94	0.94	XXX	■
	26			0.00	0.00	0.00	0.00	0.00	0.00	XXX	■
	TC			0.00	0.94	0.94	0.00	0.94	0.94	XXX	■
84252		X	Riboflavin (Vitamin B-2)	0.00	0.62	0.62	0.00	0.62	0.62	XXX	■
	26			0.00	0.00	0.00	0.00	0.00	0.00	XXX	■
	TC			0.00	0.62	0.62	0.00	0.62	0.62	XXX	■

■ RVU not developed by CMS. Gap-filled RVUs developed by Ingenix/CHEG.

Code	M	S	Description	Work Value	Non-Fac PE	Fac PE	Mal-practice	Non-Fac Total	Fac Total	Global	Gap
84255		X	Selenium	0.00	0.73	0.73	0.00	0.73	0.73	XXX	■
	26			0.00	0.00	0.00	0.00	0.00	0.00	XXX	■
	TC			0.00	0.73	0.73	0.00	0.73	0.73	XXX	■
84260		X	Serotonin	0.00	1.35	1.35	0.00	1.35	1.35	XXX	■
	26			0.00	0.00	0.00	0.00	0.00	0.00	XXX	■
	TC			0.00	1.35	1.35	0.00	1.35	1.35	XXX	■
84270		X	Sex hormone binding globulin (SHBG)	0.00	0.78	0.78	0.00	0.78	0.78	XXX	■
	26			0.00	0.00	0.00	0.00	0.00	0.00	XXX	■
	TC			0.00	0.78	0.78	0.00	0.78	0.78	XXX	■
84275		X	Sialic acid	0.00	0.47	0.47	0.00	0.47	0.47	XXX	■
	26			0.00	0.00	0.00	0.00	0.00	0.00	XXX	■
	TC			0.00	0.47	0.47	0.00	0.47	0.47	XXX	■
84285		X	Silica	0.00	1.00	1.00	0.00	1.00	1.00	XXX	■
	26			0.00	0.00	0.00	0.00	0.00	0.00	XXX	■
	TC			0.00	1.00	1.00	0.00	1.00	1.00	XXX	■
84295		X	Sodium; serum	0.00	0.19	0.19	0.00	0.19	0.19	XXX	■
	26			0.00	0.00	0.00	0.00	0.00	0.00	XXX	■
	TC			0.00	0.19	0.19	0.00	0.19	0.19	XXX	■
84300		X	urine	0.00	0.21	0.21	0.00	0.21	0.21	XXX	■
	26			0.00	0.00	0.00	0.00	0.00	0.00	XXX	■
	TC			0.00	0.21	0.21	0.00	0.21	0.21	XXX	■
84305		X	Somatomedin	0.00	1.10	1.10	0.00	1.10	1.10	XXX	■
	26			0.00	0.00	0.00	0.00	0.00	0.00	XXX	■
	TC			0.00	1.10	1.10	0.00	1.10	1.10	XXX	■
84307		X	Somatostatin	0.00	0.81	0.81	0.00	0.81	0.81	XXX	■
	26			0.00	0.00	0.00	0.00	0.00	0.00	XXX	■
	TC			0.00	0.81	0.81	0.00	0.81	0.81	XXX	■
84311		X	Spectrophotometry, analyte not elsewhere specified	0.00	0.32	0.32	0.00	0.32	0.32	XXX	■
	26			0.00	0.00	0.00	0.00	0.00	0.00	XXX	■
	TC			0.00	0.32	0.32	0.00	0.32	0.32	XXX	■
84315		X	Specific gravity (except urine)	0.00	0.10	0.10	0.00	0.10	0.10	XXX	■
	26			0.00	0.00	0.00	0.00	0.00	0.00	XXX	■
	TC			0.00	0.10	0.10	0.00	0.10	0.10	XXX	■
84375		X	Sugars, chromatographic, TLC or paper chromatography	0.00	0.59	0.59	0.00	0.59	0.59	XXX	■
	26			0.00	0.00	0.00	0.00	0.00	0.00	XXX	■
	TC			0.00	0.59	0.59	0.00	0.59	0.59	XXX	■
84376		X	Sugars (mono-, di-, and oligosaccharides); single qualitative, each specimen	0.00	0.21	0.21	0.00	0.21	0.21	XXX	■
	26			0.00	0.00	0.00	0.00	0.00	0.00	XXX	■
	TC			0.00	0.21	0.21	0.00	0.21	0.21	XXX	■
84377		X	multiple qualitative, each specimen	0.00	0.21	0.21	0.00	0.21	0.21	XXX	■
	26			0.00	0.00	0.00	0.00	0.00	0.00	XXX	■
	TC			0.00	0.21	0.21	0.00	0.21	0.21	XXX	■
84378		X	single quantitative, each specimen	0.00	0.44	0.44	0.00	0.44	0.44	XXX	■
	26			0.00	0.00	0.00	0.00	0.00	0.00	XXX	■
	TC			0.00	0.44	0.44	0.00	0.44	0.44	XXX	■

■ RVU not developed by CMS. Gap-filled RVUs developed by Ingenix/CHEG.

Pathology

Code	M	S	Description	Work Value	Non-Fac PE	Fac PE	Mal-practice	Non-Fac Total	Fac Total	Global	Gap
84379		X	multiple quantitative, each specimen	0.00	0.44	0.44	0.00	0.44	0.44	XXX	■
	26			0.00	0.00	0.00	0.00	0.00	0.00	XXX	■
	TC			0.00	0.44	0.44	0.00	0.44	0.44	XXX	■
84392		X	Sulfate, urine	0.00	0.18	0.18	0.00	0.18	0.18	XXX	■
	26			0.00	0.00	0.00	0.00	0.00	0.00	XXX	■
	TC			0.00	0.18	0.18	0.00	0.18	0.18	XXX	■
84402		X	Testosterone; free	0.00	0.84	0.84	0.00	0.84	0.84	XXX	■
	26			0.00	0.00	0.00	0.00	0.00	0.00	XXX	■
	TC			0.00	0.84	0.84	0.00	0.84	0.84	XXX	■
84403		X	total	0.00	0.69	0.69	0.00	0.69	0.69	XXX	■
	26			0.00	0.00	0.00	0.00	0.00	0.00	XXX	■
	TC			0.00	0.69	0.69	0.00	0.69	0.69	XXX	■
84425		X	Thiamine (Vitamin B-1)	0.00	0.81	0.81	0.00	0.81	0.81	XXX	■
	26			0.00	0.00	0.00	0.00	0.00	0.00	XXX	■
	TC			0.00	0.81	0.81	0.00	0.81	0.81	XXX	■
84430		X	Thiocyanate	0.00	0.51	0.51	0.00	0.51	0.51	XXX	■
	26			0.00	0.00	0.00	0.00	0.00	0.00	XXX	■
	TC			0.00	0.51	0.51	0.00	0.51	0.51	XXX	■
84432		X	Thyroglobulin	0.00	0.73	0.73	0.00	0.73	0.73	XXX	■
	26			0.00	0.00	0.00	0.00	0.00	0.00	XXX	■
	TC			0.00	0.73	0.73	0.00	0.73	0.73	XXX	■
84436		X	Thyroxine; total	0.00	0.26	0.26	0.00	0.26	0.26	XXX	■
	26			0.00	0.00	0.00	0.00	0.00	0.00	XXX	■
	TC			0.00	0.26	0.26	0.00	0.26	0.26	XXX	■
84437		X	requiring elution (eg, neonatal)	0.00	0.29	0.29	0.00	0.29	0.29	XXX	■
	26			0.00	0.00	0.00	0.00	0.00	0.00	XXX	■
	TC			0.00	0.29	0.29	0.00	0.29	0.29	XXX	■
84439		X	free	0.00	0.44	0.44	0.00	0.44	0.44	XXX	■
	26			0.00	0.00	0.00	0.00	0.00	0.00	XXX	■
	TC			0.00	0.44	0.44	0.00	0.44	0.44	XXX	■
84442		X	Thyroxine binding globulin (TBG)	0.00	0.51	0.51	0.00	0.51	0.51	XXX	■
	26			0.00	0.00	0.00	0.00	0.00	0.00	XXX	■
	TC			0.00	0.51	0.51	0.00	0.51	0.51	XXX	■
84443		X	Thyroid stimulating hormone (TSH)	0.00	0.62	0.62	0.00	0.62	0.62	XXX	■
	26			0.00	0.00	0.00	0.00	0.00	0.00	XXX	■
	TC			0.00	0.62	0.62	0.00	0.62	0.62	XXX	■
84445		X	Thyroid stimulating immune globulins (TSI)	0.00	1.90	1.90	0.00	1.90	1.90	XXX	■
	26			0.00	0.00	0.00	0.00	0.00	0.00	XXX	■
	TC			0.00	1.90	1.90	0.00	1.90	1.90	XXX	■
84446		X	Tocopherol alpha (Vitamin E)	0.00	0.59	0.59	0.00	0.59	0.59	XXX	■
	26			0.00	0.00	0.00	0.00	0.00	0.00	XXX	■
	TC			0.00	0.59	0.59	0.00	0.59	0.59	XXX	■
84449		X	Transcortin (cortisol binding globulin)	0.00	0.70	0.70	0.00	0.70	0.70	XXX	■
	26			0.00	0.00	0.00	0.00	0.00	0.00	XXX	■
	TC			0.00	0.70	0.70	0.00	0.70	0.70	XXX	■

■ RVU not developed by CMS. Gap-filled RVUs developed by Ingenix/CHEG.

Code	M	S	Description	Work Value	Non-Fac PE	Fac PE	Mal-practice	Non-Fac Total	Fac Total	Global	Gap
84450		X	Transferase; aspartate amino (AST) (SGOT)	0.00	0.19	0.19	0.00	0.19	0.19	XXX	■
	26			0.00	0.00	0.00	0.00	0.00	0.00	XXX	■
	TC			0.00	0.19	0.19	0.00	0.19	0.19	XXX	■
84460		X	alanine amino (ALT) (SGPT)	0.00	0.19	0.19	0.00	0.19	0.19	XXX	■
	26			0.00	0.00	0.00	0.00	0.00	0.00	XXX	■
	TC			0.00	0.19	0.19	0.00	0.19	0.19	XXX	■
84466		X	Transferrin	0.00	0.51	0.51	0.00	0.51	0.51	XXX	■
	26			0.00	0.00	0.00	0.00	0.00	0.00	XXX	■
	TC			0.00	0.51	0.51	0.00	0.51	0.51	XXX	■
84478		X	Triglycerides	0.00	0.19	0.19	0.00	0.19	0.19	XXX	■
	26			0.00	0.00	0.00	0.00	0.00	0.00	XXX	■
	TC			0.00	0.19	0.19	0.00	0.19	0.19	XXX	■
84479		X	Thyroid hormone (T3 or T4) uptake or thyroid hormone binding ratio (THBR)	0.00	0.26	0.26	0.00	0.26	0.26	XXX	■
	26			0.00	0.00	0.00	0.00	0.00	0.00	XXX	■
	TC			0.00	0.26	0.26	0.00	0.26	0.26	XXX	■
84480		X	Triiodothyronine T3; total (TT-3)	0.00	0.59	0.59	0.00	0.59	0.59	XXX	■
	26			0.00	0.00	0.00	0.00	0.00	0.00	XXX	■
	TC			0.00	0.59	0.59	0.00	0.59	0.59	XXX	■
84481		X	free	0.00	0.78	0.78	0.00	0.78	0.78	XXX	■
	26			0.00	0.00	0.00	0.00	0.00	0.00	XXX	■
	TC			0.00	0.78	0.78	0.00	0.78	0.78	XXX	■
84482		X	reverse	0.00	0.66	0.66	0.00	0.66	0.66	XXX	■
	26			0.00	0.00	0.00	0.00	0.00	0.00	XXX	■
	TC			0.00	0.66	0.66	0.00	0.66	0.66	XXX	■
84484		X	Troponin, quantitative	0.00	0.38	0.38	0.00	0.38	0.38	XXX	■
	26			0.00	0.00	0.00	0.00	0.00	0.00	XXX	■
	TC			0.00	0.38	0.38	0.00	0.38	0.38	XXX	■
84485		X	Trypsin; duodenal fluid	0.00	0.29	0.29	0.00	0.29	0.29	XXX	■
	26			0.00	0.00	0.00	0.00	0.00	0.00	XXX	■
	TC			0.00	0.29	0.29	0.00	0.29	0.29	XXX	■
84488		X	feces, qualitative	0.00	0.19	0.19	0.00	0.19	0.19	XXX	■
	26			0.00	0.00	0.00	0.00	0.00	0.00	XXX	■
	TC			0.00	0.19	0.19	0.00	0.19	0.19	XXX	■
84490		X	feces, quantitative, 24-hour collection	0.00	0.22	0.22	0.00	0.22	0.22	XXX	■
	26			0.00	0.00	0.00	0.00	0.00	0.00	XXX	■
	TC			0.00	0.22	0.22	0.00	0.22	0.22	XXX	■
84510		X	Tyrosine	0.00	0.38	0.38	0.00	0.38	0.38	XXX	■
	26			0.00	0.00	0.00	0.00	0.00	0.00	XXX	■
	TC			0.00	0.38	0.38	0.00	0.38	0.38	XXX	■
84512		X	Troponin, qualitative	0.00	0.29	0.29	0.00	0.29	0.29	XXX	■
	26			0.00	0.00	0.00	0.00	0.00	0.00	XXX	■
	TC			0.00	0.29	0.29	0.00	0.29	0.29	XXX	■
84520		X	Urea nitrogen; quantitative	0.00	0.19	0.19	0.00	0.19	0.19	XXX	■
	26			0.00	0.00	0.00	0.00	0.00	0.00	XXX	■
	TC			0.00	0.19	0.19	0.00	0.19	0.19	XXX	■

■ RVU not developed by CMS. Gap-filled RVUs developed by Ingenix/CHEG.

Pathology

Code	M	S	Description	Work Value	Non-Fac PE	Fac PE	Mal-practice	Non-Fac Total	Fac Total	Global	Gap
84525		X	semiquantitative (eg, reagent strip test)	0.00	0.15	0.15	0.00	0.15	0.15	XXX	■
	26			0.00	0.00	0.00	0.00	0.00	0.00	XXX	■
	TC			0.00	0.15	0.15	0.00	0.15	0.15	XXX	■
84540		X	Urea nitrogen, urine	0.00	0.23	0.23	0.00	0.23	0.23	XXX	■
	26			0.00	0.00	0.00	0.00	0.00	0.00	XXX	■
	TC			0.00	0.23	0.23	0.00	0.23	0.23	XXX	■
84545		X	Urea nitrogen, clearance	0.00	0.29	0.29	0.00	0.29	0.29	XXX	■
	26			0.00	0.00	0.00	0.00	0.00	0.00	XXX	■
	TC			0.00	0.29	0.29	0.00	0.29	0.29	XXX	■
84550		X	Uric acid; blood	0.00	0.19	0.19	0.00	0.19	0.19	XXX	■
	26			0.00	0.00	0.00	0.00	0.00	0.00	XXX	■
	TC			0.00	0.19	0.19	0.00	0.19	0.19	XXX	■
84560		X	other source	0.00	0.23	0.23	0.00	0.23	0.23	XXX	■
	26			0.00	0.00	0.00	0.00	0.00	0.00	XXX	■
	TC			0.00	0.23	0.23	0.00	0.23	0.23	XXX	■
84577		X	Urobilinogen, feces, quantitative	0.00	0.29	0.29	0.00	0.29	0.29	XXX	■
	26			0.00	0.00	0.00	0.00	0.00	0.00	XXX	■
	TC			0.00	0.29	0.29	0.00	0.29	0.29	XXX	■
84578		X	Urobilinogen, urine; qualitative	0.00	0.13	0.13	0.00	0.13	0.13	XXX	■
	26			0.00	0.00	0.00	0.00	0.00	0.00	XXX	■
	TC			0.00	0.13	0.13	0.00	0.13	0.13	XXX	■
84580		X	quantitative, timed specimen	0.00	0.28	0.28	0.00	0.28	0.28	XXX	■
	26			0.00	0.00	0.00	0.00	0.00	0.00	XXX	■
	TC			0.00	0.28	0.28	0.00	0.28	0.28	XXX	■
84583		X	semiquantitative	0.00	0.13	0.13	0.00	0.13	0.13	XXX	■
	26			0.00	0.00	0.00	0.00	0.00	0.00	XXX	■
	TC			0.00	0.13	0.13	0.00	0.13	0.13	XXX	■
84585		X	Vanillylmandelic acid (VMA), urine	0.00	0.73	0.73	0.00	0.73	0.73	XXX	■
	26			0.00	0.00	0.00	0.00	0.00	0.00	XXX	■
	TC			0.00	0.73	0.73	0.00	0.73	0.73	XXX	■
84586		X	Vasoactive intestinal peptide (VIP)	0.00	1.13	1.13	0.00	1.13	1.13	XXX	■
	26			0.00	0.00	0.00	0.00	0.00	0.00	XXX	■
	TC			0.00	1.13	1.13	0.00	1.13	1.13	XXX	■
84588		X	Vasopressin (antidiuretic hormone, ADH)	0.00	1.20	1.20	0.00	1.20	1.20	XXX	■
	26			0.00	0.00	0.00	0.00	0.00	0.00	XXX	■
	TC			0.00	1.20	1.20	0.00	1.20	1.20	XXX	■
84590		X	Vitamin A	0.00	0.69	0.69	0.00	0.69	0.69	XXX	■
	26			0.00	0.00	0.00	0.00	0.00	0.00	XXX	■
	TC			0.00	0.69	0.69	0.00	0.69	0.69	XXX	■
84591		X	Vitamin, not otherwise specified	0.00	0.67	0.67	0.00	0.67	0.67	XXX	■
	26			0.00	0.00	0.00	0.00	0.00	0.00	XXX	■
	TC			0.00	0.67	0.67	0.00	0.67	0.67	XXX	■
84597		X	Vitamin K	0.00	0.67	0.67	0.00	0.67	0.67	XXX	■
	26			0.00	0.00	0.00	0.00	0.00	0.00	XXX	■
	TC			0.00	0.67	0.67	0.00	0.67	0.67	XXX	■

■ RVU not developed by CMS. Gap-filled RVUs developed by Ingenix/CHEG.

Code	M	S	Description	Work Value	Non-Fac PE	Fac PE	Mal-practice	Non-Fac Total	Fac Total	Global	Gap
84600		X	Volatiles (eg, acetic anhydride, carbon tetrachloride, dichloroethane, dichloromethane, diethylether, isopropyl alcohol, methanol)	0.00	0.51	0.51	0.00	0.51	0.51	XXX	■
	26			0.00	0.00	0.00	0.00	0.00	0.00	XXX	■
	TC			0.00	0.51	0.51	0.00	0.51	0.51	XXX	■
84620		X	Xylose absorption test, blood and/or urine	0.00	0.64	0.64	0.00	0.64	0.64	XXX	■
	26			0.00	0.00	0.00	0.00	0.00	0.00	XXX	■
	TC			0.00	0.64	0.64	0.00	0.64	0.64	XXX	■
84630		X	Zinc	0.00	0.59	0.59	0.00	0.59	0.59	XXX	■
	26			0.00	0.00	0.00	0.00	0.00	0.00	XXX	■
	TC			0.00	0.59	0.59	0.00	0.59	0.59	XXX	■
84681		X	C-peptide	0.00	0.88	0.88	0.00	0.88	0.88	XXX	■
	26			0.00	0.00	0.00	0.00	0.00	0.00	XXX	■
	TC			0.00	0.88	0.88	0.00	0.88	0.88	XXX	■
84702		X	Gonadotropin, chorionic (hCG); quantitative	0.00	0.59	0.59	0.00	0.59	0.59	XXX	■
	26			0.00	0.00	0.00	0.00	0.00	0.00	XXX	■
	TC			0.00	0.59	0.59	0.00	0.59	0.59	XXX	■
84703		X	qualitative	0.00	0.34	0.34	0.00	0.34	0.34	XXX	■
	26			0.00	0.00	0.00	0.00	0.00	0.00	XXX	■
	TC			0.00	0.34	0.34	0.00	0.34	0.34	XXX	■
84830		X	Ovulation tests, by visual color comparison methods for human luteinizing hormone	0.00	0.37	0.37	0.00	0.37	0.37	XXX	■
	26			0.00	0.00	0.00	0.00	0.00	0.00	XXX	■
	TC			0.00	0.37	0.37	0.00	0.37	0.37	XXX	■
84999		X	Unlisted chemistry procedure	0.00	0.00	0.00	0.00	0.00	0.00	XXX	
85002		X	Bleeding time	0.00	0.63	0.63	0.00	0.63	0.63	XXX	■
	26			0.00	0.00	0.00	0.00	0.00	0.00	XXX	■
	TC			0.00	0.63	0.63	0.00	0.63	0.63	XXX	■
85007		X	Blood count; manual differential WBC count (includes RBC morphology and platelet estimation)	0.00	0.36	0.36	0.00	0.36	0.36	XXX	■
	26			0.00	0.00	0.00	0.00	0.00	0.00	XXX	■
	TC			0.00	0.36	0.36	0.00	0.36	0.36	XXX	■
85008		X	manual blood smear examination without differential parameters	0.00	0.24	0.24	0.00	0.24	0.24	XXX	■
	26			0.00	0.00	0.00	0.00	0.00	0.00	XXX	■
	TC			0.00	0.24	0.24	0.00	0.24	0.24	XXX	■
85009		X	differential WBC count, buffy coat	0.00	0.36	0.36	0.00	0.36	0.36	XXX	■
	26			0.00	0.00	0.00	0.00	0.00	0.00	XXX	■
	TC			0.00	0.36	0.36	0.00	0.36	0.36	XXX	■
85013		X	spun microhematocrit	0.00	0.27	0.27	0.00	0.27	0.27	XXX	■
	26			0.00	0.00	0.00	0.00	0.00	0.00	XXX	■
	TC			0.00	0.27	0.27	0.00	0.27	0.27	XXX	■
85014		X	other than spun hematocrit	0.00	0.27	0.27	0.00	0.27	0.27	XXX	■
	26			0.00	0.00	0.00	0.00	0.00	0.00	XXX	■
	TC			0.00	0.27	0.27	0.00	0.27	0.27	XXX	■
85018		X	hemoglobin	0.00	0.27	0.27	0.00	0.27	0.27	XXX	■
	26			0.00	0.00	0.00	0.00	0.00	0.00	XXX	■
	TC			0.00	0.27	0.27	0.00	0.27	0.27	XXX	■

Pathology

■ RVU not developed by CMS. Gap-filled RVUs developed by Ingenix/CHEG.

Code	M	S	Description	Work Value	Non-Fac PE	Fac PE	Mal-prac-tice	Non-Fac Total	Fac Total	Global	Gap
85021		X	hemogram, automated (RBC, WBC, Hgb, Hct and indices only)	0.00	0.45	0.45	0.00	0.45	0.45	XXX	■
	26			0.00	0.00	0.00	0.00	0.00	0.00	XXX	■
	TC			0.00	0.45	0.45	0.00	0.45	0.45	XXX	■
85022		X	hemogram, automated, and manual differential WBC count (CBC)	0.00	0.53	0.53	0.00	0.53	0.53	XXX	■
	26			0.00	0.00	0.00	0.00	0.00	0.00	XXX	■
	TC			0.00	0.53	0.53	0.00	0.53	0.53	XXX	■
85023		X	hemogram and platelet count, automated, and manual differential WBC count (CBC)	0.00	0.67	0.67	0.00	0.67	0.67	XXX	■
	26			0.00	0.00	0.00	0.00	0.00	0.00	XXX	■
	TC			0.00	0.67	0.67	0.00	0.67	0.67	XXX	■
85024		X	hemogram and platelet count, automated, and automated partial differential WBC count (CBC)	0.00	0.54	0.54	0.00	0.54	0.54	XXX	■
	26			0.00	0.00	0.00	0.00	0.00	0.00	XXX	■
	TC			0.00	0.54	0.54	0.00	0.54	0.54	XXX	■
85025		X	hemogram and platelet count, automated, and automated complete differential WBC count (CBC)	0.00	0.56	0.56	0.00	0.56	0.56	XXX	■
	26			0.00	0.00	0.00	0.00	0.00	0.00	XXX	■
	TC			0.00	0.56	0.56	0.00	0.56	0.56	XXX	■
85027		X	hemogram and platelet count, automated	0.00	0.53	0.53	0.00	0.53	0.53	XXX	■
	26			0.00	0.00	0.00	0.00	0.00	0.00	XXX	■
	TC			0.00	0.53	0.53	0.00	0.53	0.53	XXX	■
85031		X	Blood count; hemogram, manual, complete CBC (RBC, WBC, Hgb, Hct, differential and indices)	0.00	0.56	0.56	0.00	0.56	0.56	XXX	■
	26			0.00	0.00	0.00	0.00	0.00	0.00	XXX	■
	TC			0.00	0.56	0.56	0.00	0.56	0.56	XXX	■
85041		X	red blood cell (RBC) only	0.00	0.26	0.26	0.00	0.26	0.26	XXX	■
	26			0.00	0.00	0.00	0.00	0.00	0.00	XXX	■
	TC			0.00	0.26	0.26	0.00	0.26	0.26	XXX	■
85044		X	reticulocyte count, manual	0.00	0.45	0.45	0.00	0.45	0.45	XXX	■
	26			0.00	0.00	0.00	0.00	0.00	0.00	XXX	■
	TC			0.00	0.45	0.45	0.00	0.45	0.45	XXX	■
85045		X	reticulocyte count, flow cytometry	0.00	0.42	0.42	0.00	0.42	0.42	XXX	■
	26			0.00	0.00	0.00	0.00	0.00	0.00	XXX	■
	TC			0.00	0.42	0.42	0.00	0.42	0.42	XXX	■
85046		X	reticulocytes, hemoglobin concentration	0.00	0.21	0.21	0.00	0.21	0.21	XXX	■
	26			0.00	0.00	0.00	0.00	0.00	0.00	XXX	■
	TC			0.00	0.21	0.21	0.00	0.21	0.21	XXX	■
85048		X	white blood cell (WBC)	0.00	0.30	0.30	0.00	0.30	0.30	XXX	■
	26			0.00	0.00	0.00	0.00	0.00	0.00	XXX	■
	TC			0.00	0.30	0.30	0.00	0.30	0.30	XXX	■
85060		A	Blood smear, peripheral, interpretation by physician with written report	0.45	0.19	0.19	0.02	0.66	0.66	XXX	
85097		A	Bone marrow, smear interpretation	0.94	1.75	0.43	0.03	2.72	1.40	XXX	
85130		X	Chromogenic substrate assay	0.00	0.91	0.91	0.00	0.91	0.91	XXX	■
	26			0.00	0.00	0.00	0.00	0.00	0.00	XXX	■
	TC			0.00	0.91	0.91	0.00	0.91	0.91	XXX	■

Pathology

■ RVU not developed by CMS. Gap-filled RVUs developed by Ingenix/CHEG.

Code	M	S	Description	Work Value	Non-Fac PE	Fac PE	Mal-practice	Non-Fac Total	Fac Total	Global	Gap
85170		X	Clot retraction	0.00	0.32	0.32	0.00	0.32	0.32	XXX	■
	26			0.00	0.00	0.00	0.00	0.00	0.00	XXX	■
	TC			0.00	0.32	0.32	0.00	0.32	0.32	XXX	■
85175		X	Clot lysis time, whole blood dilution	0.00	0.60	0.60	0.00	0.60	0.60	XXX	■
	26			0.00	0.00	0.00	0.00	0.00	0.00	XXX	■
	TC			0.00	0.60	0.60	0.00	0.60	0.60	XXX	■
85210		X	Clotting; factor II, prothrombin, specific	0.00	0.91	0.91	0.00	0.91	0.91	XXX	■
	26			0.00	0.00	0.00	0.00	0.00	0.00	XXX	■
	TC			0.00	0.91	0.91	0.00	0.91	0.91	XXX	■
85220		X	factor V (AcG or proaccelerin), labile factor	0.00	1.81	1.81	0.00	1.81	1.81	XXX	■
	26			0.00	0.00	0.00	0.00	0.00	0.00	XXX	■
	TC			0.00	1.81	1.81	0.00	1.81	1.81	XXX	■
85230		X	factor VII (proconvertin, stable factor)	0.00	1.81	1.81	0.00	1.81	1.81	XXX	■
	26			0.00	0.00	0.00	0.00	0.00	0.00	XXX	■
	TC			0.00	1.81	1.81	0.00	1.81	1.81	XXX	■
85240		X	factor VIII (AHG), one stage	0.00	1.96	1.96	0.00	1.96	1.96	XXX	■
	26			0.00	0.00	0.00	0.00	0.00	0.00	XXX	■
	TC			0.00	1.96	1.96	0.00	1.96	1.96	XXX	■
85244		X	factor VIII related antigen	0.00	2.42	2.42	0.00	2.42	2.42	XXX	■
	26			0.00	0.00	0.00	0.00	0.00	0.00	XXX	■
	TC			0.00	2.42	2.42	0.00	2.42	2.42	XXX	■
85245		X	factor VIII, VW factor, ristocetin cofactor	0.00	1.51	1.51	0.00	1.51	1.51	XXX	■
	26			0.00	0.00	0.00	0.00	0.00	0.00	XXX	■
	TC			0.00	1.51	1.51	0.00	1.51	1.51	XXX	■
85246		X	factor VIII, VW factor antigen	0.00	2.42	2.42	0.00	2.42	2.42	XXX	■
	26			0.00	0.00	0.00	0.00	0.00	0.00	XXX	■
	TC			0.00	2.42	2.42	0.00	2.42	2.42	XXX	■
85247		X	factor VIII, von Willebrand factor, multimetric analysis	0.00	2.42	2.42	0.00	2.42	2.42	XXX	■
	26			0.00	0.00	0.00	0.00	0.00	0.00	XXX	■
	TC			0.00	2.42	2.42	0.00	2.42	2.42	XXX	■
85250		X	factor IX (PTC or Christmas)	0.00	1.96	1.96	0.00	1.96	1.96	XXX	■
	26			0.00	0.00	0.00	0.00	0.00	0.00	XXX	■
	TC			0.00	1.96	1.96	0.00	1.96	1.96	XXX	■
85260		X	factor X (Stuart-Prower)	0.00	1.81	1.81	0.00	1.81	1.81	XXX	■
	26			0.00	0.00	0.00	0.00	0.00	0.00	XXX	■
	TC			0.00	1.81	1.81	0.00	1.81	1.81	XXX	■
85270		X	factor XI (PTA)	0.00	1.96	1.96	0.00	1.96	1.96	XXX	■
	26			0.00	0.00	0.00	0.00	0.00	0.00	XXX	■
	TC			0.00	1.96	1.96	0.00	1.96	1.96	XXX	■
85280		X	factor XII (Hageman)	0.00	1.96	1.96	0.00	1.96	1.96	XXX	■
	26			0.00	0.00	0.00	0.00	0.00	0.00	XXX	■
	TC			0.00	1.96	1.96	0.00	1.96	1.96	XXX	■
85290		X	factor XIII (fibrin stabilizing)	0.00	1.81	1.81	0.00	1.81	1.81	XXX	■
	26			0.00	0.00	0.00	0.00	0.00	0.00	XXX	■
	TC			0.00	1.81	1.81	0.00	1.81	1.81	XXX	■

■ RVU not developed by CMS. Gap-filled RVUs developed by Ingenix/CHEG.

Pathology

Code	M	S	Description	Work Value	Non-Fac PE	Fac PE	Mal-practice	Non-Fac Total	Fac Total	Global	Gap
85291		X	factor XIII (fibrin stabilizing), screen	0.00	0.88	0.88	0.00	0.88	0.88	XXX	■
	26		solubility	0.00	0.00	0.00	0.00	0.00	0.00	XXX	■
	TC			0.00	0.88	0.88	0.00	0.88	0.88	XXX	■
85292		X	prekallikrein assay (Fletcher factor assay)	0.00	1.81	1.81	0.00	1.81	1.81	XXX	■
	26			0.00	0.00	0.00	0.00	0.00	0.00	XXX	■
	TC			0.00	1.81	1.81	0.00	1.81	1.81	XXX	■
85293		X	high molecular weight kininogen assay	0.00	1.81	1.81	0.00	1.81	1.81	XXX	■
	26		(Fitzgerald factor assay)	0.00	0.00	0.00	0.00	0.00	0.00	XXX	■
	TC			0.00	1.81	1.81	0.00	1.81	1.81	XXX	■
85300		X	Clotting inhibitors or anticoagulants;	0.00	1.60	1.60	0.00	1.60	1.60	XXX	■
	26		antithrombin III, activity	0.00	0.00	0.00	0.00	0.00	0.00	XXX	■
	TC			0.00	1.60	1.60	0.00	1.60	1.60	XXX	■
85301		X	antithrombin III, antigen assay	0.00	1.51	1.51	0.00	1.51	1.51	XXX	■
	26			0.00	0.00	0.00	0.00	0.00	0.00	XXX	■
	TC			0.00	1.51	1.51	0.00	1.51	1.51	XXX	■
85302		X	protein C, antigen	0.00	1.66	1.66	0.00	1.66	1.66	XXX	■
	26			0.00	0.00	0.00	0.00	0.00	0.00	XXX	■
	TC			0.00	1.66	1.66	0.00	1.66	1.66	XXX	■
85303		X	protein C, activity	0.00	1.81	1.81	0.00	1.81	1.81	XXX	■
	26			0.00	0.00	0.00	0.00	0.00	0.00	XXX	■
	TC			0.00	1.81	1.81	0.00	1.81	1.81	XXX	■
85305		X	protein S, total	0.00	1.96	1.96	0.00	1.96	1.96	XXX	■
	26			0.00	0.00	0.00	0.00	0.00	0.00	XXX	■
	TC			0.00	1.96	1.96	0.00	1.96	1.96	XXX	■
85306		X	protein S, free	0.00	1.96	1.96	0.00	1.96	1.96	XXX	■
	26			0.00	0.00	0.00	0.00	0.00	0.00	XXX	■
	TC			0.00	1.96	1.96	0.00	1.96	1.96	XXX	■
85307		X	Activated Protein C (APC) resistance assay	0.00	1.66	1.66	0.00	1.66	1.66	XXX	■
	26			0.00	0.00	0.00	0.00	0.00	0.00	XXX	■
	TC			0.00	1.66	1.66	0.00	1.66	1.66	XXX	■
85335		X	Factor inhibitor test	0.00	0.82	0.82	0.00	0.82	0.82	XXX	■
	26			0.00	0.00	0.00	0.00	0.00	0.00	XXX	■
	TC			0.00	0.82	0.82	0.00	0.82	0.82	XXX	■
85337		X	Thrombomodulin	0.00	1.51	1.51	0.00	1.51	1.51	XXX	■
	26			0.00	0.00	0.00	0.00	0.00	0.00	XXX	■
	TC			0.00	1.51	1.51	0.00	1.51	1.51	XXX	■
85345		X	Coagulation time; Lee and White	0.00	0.30	0.30	0.00	0.30	0.30	XXX	■
	26			0.00	0.00	0.00	0.00	0.00	0.00	XXX	■
	TC			0.00	0.30	0.30	0.00	0.30	0.30	XXX	■
85347		X	activated	0.00	0.30	0.30	0.00	0.30	0.30	XXX	■
	26			0.00	0.00	0.00	0.00	0.00	0.00	XXX	■
	TC			0.00	0.30	0.30	0.00	0.30	0.30	XXX	■
85348		X	other methods	0.00	0.48	0.48	0.00	0.48	0.48	XXX	■
	26			0.00	0.00	0.00	0.00	0.00	0.00	XXX	■
	TC			0.00	0.48	0.48	0.00	0.48	0.48	XXX	■

■ RVU not developed by CMS. Gap-filled RVUs developed by Ingenix/CHEG.

Code	M	S	Description	Work Value	Non-Fac PE	Fac PE	Mal-practice	Non-Fac Total	Fac Total	Global	Gap
85360		X	Euglobulin lysis	0.00	0.97	0.97	0.00	0.97	0.97	XXX	■
	26			0.00	0.00	0.00	0.00	0.00	0.00	XXX	■
	TC			0.00	0.97	0.97	0.00	0.97	0.97	XXX	■
85362		X	Fibrin(ogen) degradation (split) products (FDP)(FSP); agglutination slide, semiquantitative	0.00	0.67	0.67	0.00	0.67	0.67	XXX	■
	26			0.00	0.00	0.00	0.00	0.00	0.00	XXX	■
	TC			0.00	0.67	0.67	0.00	0.67	0.67	XXX	■
85366		X	paracoagulation	0.00	0.97	0.97	0.00	0.97	0.97	XXX	■
	26			0.00	0.00	0.00	0.00	0.00	0.00	XXX	■
	TC			0.00	0.97	0.97	0.00	0.97	0.97	XXX	■
85370		X	quantitative	0.00	0.97	0.97	0.00	0.97	0.97	XXX	■
	26			0.00	0.00	0.00	0.00	0.00	0.00	XXX	■
	TC			0.00	0.97	0.97	0.00	0.97	0.97	XXX	■
85378		X	Fibrin degradation products, D-dimer; semiquantitative	0.00	0.79	0.79	0.00	0.79	0.79	XXX	■
	26			0.00	0.00	0.00	0.00	0.00	0.00	XXX	■
	TC			0.00	0.79	0.79	0.00	0.79	0.79	XXX	■
85379		X	quantitative	0.00	0.91	0.91	0.00	0.91	0.91	XXX	■
	26			0.00	0.00	0.00	0.00	0.00	0.00	XXX	■
	TC			0.00	0.91	0.91	0.00	0.91	0.91	XXX	■
85384		X	Fibrinogen; activity	0.00	0.60	0.60	0.00	0.60	0.60	XXX	■
	26			0.00	0.00	0.00	0.00	0.00	0.00	XXX	■
	TC			0.00	0.60	0.60	0.00	0.60	0.60	XXX	■
85385		X	antigen	0.00	0.76	0.76	0.00	0.76	0.76	XXX	■
	26			0.00	0.00	0.00	0.00	0.00	0.00	XXX	■
	TC			0.00	0.76	0.76	0.00	0.76	0.76	XXX	■
85390		X	Fibrinolysins or coagulopathy screen, interpretation and report	0.37	0.12	0.12	0.01	0.50	0.50	XXX	■
	26	A		0.37	0.12	0.12	0.01	0.50	0.50	XXX	
	TC			0.00	0.00	0.00	0.00	0.00	0.00	XXX	■
85400		X	Fibrinolytic factors and inhibitors; plasmin	0.00	1.45	1.45	0.00	1.45	1.45	XXX	■
	26			0.00	0.00	0.00	0.00	0.00	0.00	XXX	■
	TC			0.00	1.45	1.45	0.00	1.45	1.45	XXX	■
85410		X	alpha-2 antiplasmin	0.00	1.45	1.45	0.00	1.45	1.45	XXX	■
	26			0.00	0.00	0.00	0.00	0.00	0.00	XXX	■
	TC			0.00	1.45	1.45	0.00	1.45	1.45	XXX	■
85415		X	plasminogen activator	0.00	1.12	1.12	0.00	1.12	1.12	XXX	■
	26			0.00	0.00	0.00	0.00	0.00	0.00	XXX	■
	TC			0.00	1.12	1.12	0.00	1.12	1.12	XXX	■
85420		X	plasminogen, except antigenic assay	0.00	1.45	1.45	0.00	1.45	1.45	XXX	■
	26			0.00	0.00	0.00	0.00	0.00	0.00	XXX	■
	TC			0.00	1.45	1.45	0.00	1.45	1.45	XXX	■
85421		X	plasminogen, antigenic assay	0.00	1.81	1.81	0.00	1.81	1.81	XXX	■
	26			0.00	0.00	0.00	0.00	0.00	0.00	XXX	■
	TC			0.00	1.81	1.81	0.00	1.81	1.81	XXX	■
85441		X	Heinz bodies; direct	0.00	0.27	0.27	0.00	0.27	0.27	XXX	■
	26			0.00	0.00	0.00	0.00	0.00	0.00	XXX	■
	TC			0.00	0.27	0.27	0.00	0.27	0.27	XXX	■

■ RVU not developed by CMS. Gap-filled RVUs developed by Ingenix/CHEG.

Code	M	S	Description	Work Value	Non-Fac PE	Fac PE	Mal-practice	Non-Fac Total	Fac Total	Global	Gap
85445		X	induced, acetyl phenylhydrazine	0.00	0.42	0.42	0.00	0.42	0.42	XXX	■
	26			0.00	0.00	0.00	0.00	0.00	0.00	XXX	■
	TC			0.00	0.42	0.42	0.00	0.42	0.42	XXX	■
85460		X	Hemoglobin or RBCs, fetal, for fetomaternal hemorrhage; differential lysis (Kleihauer-Betke)	0.00	0.82	0.82	0.00	0.82	0.82	XXX	■
	26			0.00	0.00	0.00	0.00	0.00	0.00	XXX	■
	TC			0.00	0.82	0.82	0.00	0.82	0.82	XXX	■
85461		X	rosette	0.00	0.82	0.82	0.00	0.82	0.82	XXX	■
	26			0.00	0.00	0.00	0.00	0.00	0.00	XXX	■
	TC			0.00	0.82	0.82	0.00	0.82	0.82	XXX	■
85475		X	Hemolysin, acid	0.00	1.03	1.03	0.00	1.03	1.03	XXX	■
	26			0.00	0.00	0.00	0.00	0.00	0.00	XXX	■
	TC			0.00	1.03	1.03	0.00	1.03	1.03	XXX	■
85520		X	Heparin assay	0.00	1.21	1.21	0.00	1.21	1.21	XXX	■
	26			0.00	0.00	0.00	0.00	0.00	0.00	XXX	■
	TC			0.00	1.21	1.21	0.00	1.21	1.21	XXX	■
85525		X	Heparin neutralization	0.00	1.21	1.21	0.00	1.21	1.21	XXX	■
	26			0.00	0.00	0.00	0.00	0.00	0.00	XXX	■
	TC			0.00	1.21	1.21	0.00	1.21	1.21	XXX	■
85530		X	Heparin-protamine tolerance test	0.00	1.21	1.21	0.00	1.21	1.21	XXX	■
	26			0.00	0.00	0.00	0.00	0.00	0.00	XXX	■
	TC			0.00	1.21	1.21	0.00	1.21	1.21	XXX	■
85536		X	Iron stain, peripheral blood	0.00	0.51	0.51	0.00	0.51	0.51	XXX	■
	26			0.00	0.00	0.00	0.00	0.00	0.00	XXX	■
	TC			0.00	0.51	0.51	0.00	0.51	0.51	XXX	■
85540		X	Leukocyte alkaline phosphatase with count	0.00	0.76	0.76	0.00	0.76	0.76	XXX	■
	26			0.00	0.00	0.00	0.00	0.00	0.00	XXX	■
	TC			0.00	0.76	0.76	0.00	0.76	0.76	XXX	■
85547		X	Mechanical fragility, RBC	0.00	0.70	0.70	0.00	0.70	0.70	XXX	■
	26			0.00	0.00	0.00	0.00	0.00	0.00	XXX	■
	TC			0.00	0.70	0.70	0.00	0.70	0.70	XXX	■
85549		X	Muramidase	0.00	1.54	1.54	0.00	1.54	1.54	XXX	■
	26			0.00	0.00	0.00	0.00	0.00	0.00	XXX	■
	TC			0.00	1.54	1.54	0.00	1.54	1.54	XXX	■
85555		X	Osmotic fragility, RBC; unincubated	0.00	0.76	0.76	0.00	0.76	0.76	XXX	■
	26			0.00	0.00	0.00	0.00	0.00	0.00	XXX	■
	TC			0.00	0.76	0.76	0.00	0.76	0.76	XXX	■
85557		X	incubated	0.00	1.51	1.51	0.00	1.51	1.51	XXX	■
	26			0.00	0.00	0.00	0.00	0.00	0.00	XXX	■
	TC			0.00	1.51	1.51	0.00	1.51	1.51	XXX	■
85576		X	Platelet; aggregation (in vitro), each agent	0.37	0.98	0.98	0.01	1.36	1.36	XXX	■
	26	A		0.37	0.16	0.16	0.01	0.54	0.54	XXX	
	TC			0.00	0.82	0.82	0.00	0.82	0.82	XXX	■
85585		X	estimation on smear, only	0.00	0.24	0.24	0.00	0.24	0.24	XXX	■
	26			0.00	0.00	0.00	0.00	0.00	0.00	XXX	■
	TC			0.00	0.24	0.24	0.00	0.24	0.24	XXX	■

■ RVU not developed by CMS. Gap-filled RVUs developed by Ingenix/CHEG.

Pathology

Code	M	S	Description	Work Value	Non-Fac PE	Fac PE	Mal-practice	Non-Fac Total	Fac Total	Global	Gap
85590		X	manual count	0.00	0.36	0.36	0.00	0.36	0.36	XXX	■
	26			0.00	0.00	0.00	0.00	0.00	0.00	XXX	■
	TC			0.00	0.36	0.36	0.00	0.36	0.36	XXX	■
85595		X	automated count	0.00	0.36	0.36	0.00	0.36	0.36	XXX	■
	26			0.00	0.00	0.00	0.00	0.00	0.00	XXX	■
	TC			0.00	0.36	0.36	0.00	0.36	0.36	XXX	■
85597		X	Platelet neutralization	0.00	1.06	1.06	0.00	1.06	1.06	XXX	■
	26			0.00	0.00	0.00	0.00	0.00	0.00	XXX	■
	TC			0.00	1.06	1.06	0.00	1.06	1.06	XXX	■
85610		X	Prothrombin time;	0.00	0.42	0.42	0.00	0.42	0.42	XXX	■
	26			0.00	0.00	0.00	0.00	0.00	0.00	XXX	■
	TC			0.00	0.42	0.42	0.00	0.42	0.42	XXX	■
85611		X	substitution, plasma fractions, each	0.00	0.45	0.45	0.00	0.45	0.45	XXX	■
	26			0.00	0.00	0.00	0.00	0.00	0.00	XXX	■
	TC			0.00	0.45	0.45	0.00	0.45	0.45	XXX	■
85612		X	Russell viper venom time (includes venom); undiluted	0.00	0.85	0.85	0.00	0.85	0.85	XXX	■
	26			0.00	0.00	0.00	0.00	0.00	0.00	XXX	■
	TC			0.00	0.85	0.85	0.00	0.85	0.85	XXX	■
85613		X	diluted	0.00	1.00	1.00	0.00	1.00	1.00	XXX	■
	26			0.00	0.00	0.00	0.00	0.00	0.00	XXX	■
	TC			0.00	1.00	1.00	0.00	1.00	1.00	XXX	■
85635		X	Reptilase test	0.00	0.60	0.60	0.00	0.60	0.60	XXX	■
	26			0.00	0.00	0.00	0.00	0.00	0.00	XXX	■
	TC			0.00	0.60	0.60	0.00	0.60	0.60	XXX	■
85651		X	Sedimentation rate, erythrocyte; non-automated	0.00	0.38	0.38	0.00	0.38	0.38	XXX	■
	26			0.00	0.00	0.00	0.00	0.00	0.00	XXX	■
	TC			0.00	0.38	0.38	0.00	0.38	0.38	XXX	■
85652		X	automated	0.00	0.38	0.38	0.00	0.38	0.38	XXX	■
	26			0.00	0.00	0.00	0.00	0.00	0.00	XXX	■
	TC			0.00	0.38	0.38	0.00	0.38	0.38	XXX	■
85660		X	Sickling of RBC, reduction	0.00	0.42	0.42	0.00	0.42	0.42	XXX	■
	26			0.00	0.00	0.00	0.00	0.00	0.00	XXX	■
	TC			0.00	0.42	0.42	0.00	0.42	0.42	XXX	■
85670		X	Thrombin time; plasma	0.00	0.57	0.57	0.00	0.57	0.57	XXX	■
	26			0.00	0.00	0.00	0.00	0.00	0.00	XXX	■
	TC			0.00	0.57	0.57	0.00	0.57	0.57	XXX	■
85675		X	titer	0.00	0.63	0.63	0.00	0.63	0.63	XXX	■
	26			0.00	0.00	0.00	0.00	0.00	0.00	XXX	■
	TC			0.00	0.63	0.63	0.00	0.63	0.63	XXX	■
85705		X	Thromboplastin inhibition; tissue	0.00	1.15	1.15	0.00	1.15	1.15	XXX	■
	26			0.00	0.00	0.00	0.00	0.00	0.00	XXX	■
	TC			0.00	1.15	1.15	0.00	1.15	1.15	XXX	■
85730		X	Thromboplastin time, partial (PTT); plasma or whole blood	0.00	0.51	0.51	0.00	0.51	0.51	XXX	■
	26			0.00	0.00	0.00	0.00	0.00	0.00	XXX	■
	TC			0.00	0.51	0.51	0.00	0.51	0.51	XXX	■

■ RVU not developed by CMS. Gap-filled RVUs developed by Ingenix/CHEG.

Code	M	S	Description	Work Value	Non-Fac PE	Fac PE	Mal-practice	Non-Fac Total	Fac Total	Global	Gap
85732		X	substitution, plasma fractions, each	0.00	0.60	0.60	0.00	0.60	0.60	XXX	■
	26			0.00	0.00	0.00	0.00	0.00	0.00	XXX	■
	TC			0.00	0.60	0.60	0.00	0.60	0.60	XXX	■
85810		X	Viscosity	0.00	0.70	0.70	0.00	0.70	0.70	XXX	■
	26			0.00	0.00	0.00	0.00	0.00	0.00	XXX	■
	TC			0.00	0.70	0.70	0.00	0.70	0.70	XXX	■
85999		X	Unlisted hematology and coagulation procedure	0.00	0.00	0.00	0.00	0.00	0.00	XXX	
86000		X	Agglutinins, febrile (eg, Brucella, Francisella, Murine typhus, Q fever, Rocky Mountain spotted fever, scrub typhus), each antigen	0.00	0.38	0.38	0.00	0.38	0.38	XXX	■
	26			0.00	0.00	0.00	0.00	0.00	0.00	XXX	■
	TC			0.00	0.38	0.38	0.00	0.38	0.38	XXX	■
86001		X	Allergen specific IgG quantitative or semiquantitative, each allergen	0.00	0.18	0.18	0.00	0.18	0.18	XXX	■
	26			0.00	0.00	0.00	0.00	0.00	0.00	XXX	■
	TC			0.00	0.18	0.18	0.00	0.18	0.18	XXX	■
86003		X	Allergen specific IgE; quantitative or semiquantitative, each allergen	0.00	0.18	0.18	0.00	0.18	0.18	XXX	■
	26			0.00	0.00	0.00	0.00	0.00	0.00	XXX	■
	TC			0.00	0.18	0.18	0.00	0.18	0.18	XXX	■
86005		X	qualitative, multiallergen screen (dipstick, paddle or disk)	0.00	0.82	0.82	0.00	0.82	0.82	XXX	■
	26			0.00	0.00	0.00	0.00	0.00	0.00	XXX	■
	TC			0.00	0.82	0.82	0.00	0.82	0.82	XXX	■
86021		X	Antibody identification; leukocyte antibodies	0.00	0.98	0.98	0.00	0.98	0.98	XXX	■
	26			0.00	0.00	0.00	0.00	0.00	0.00	XXX	■
	TC			0.00	0.98	0.98	0.00	0.98	0.98	XXX	■
86022		X	platelet antibodies	0.00	1.49	1.49	0.00	1.49	1.49	XXX	■
	26			0.00	0.00	0.00	0.00	0.00	0.00	XXX	■
	TC			0.00	1.49	1.49	0.00	1.49	1.49	XXX	■
86023		X	platelet associated immunoglobulin assay	0.00	0.82	0.82	0.00	0.82	0.82	XXX	■
	26			0.00	0.00	0.00	0.00	0.00	0.00	XXX	■
	TC			0.00	0.82	0.82	0.00	0.82	0.82	XXX	■
86038		X	Antinuclear antibodies (ANA);	0.00	0.57	0.57	0.00	0.57	0.57	XXX	■
	26			0.00	0.00	0.00	0.00	0.00	0.00	XXX	■
	TC			0.00	0.57	0.57	0.00	0.57	0.57	XXX	■
86039		X	titer	0.00	0.57	0.57	0.00	0.57	0.57	XXX	■
	26			0.00	0.00	0.00	0.00	0.00	0.00	XXX	■
	TC			0.00	0.57	0.57	0.00	0.57	0.57	XXX	■
86060		X	Antistreptolysin 0; titer	0.00	0.39	0.39	0.00	0.39	0.39	XXX	■
	26			0.00	0.00	0.00	0.00	0.00	0.00	XXX	■
	TC			0.00	0.39	0.39	0.00	0.39	0.39	XXX	■
86063		X	screen	0.00	0.29	0.29	0.00	0.29	0.29	XXX	■
	26			0.00	0.00	0.00	0.00	0.00	0.00	XXX	■
	TC			0.00	0.29	0.29	0.00	0.29	0.29	XXX	■
86077		A	Blood bank physician services; difficult cross match and/or evaluation of irregular antibody(s), interpretation and written report	0.94	0.48	0.43	0.03	1.45	1.40	XXX	

■ RVU not developed by CMS. Gap-filled RVUs developed by Ingenix/CHEG.

Code	M	S	Description	Work Value	Non-Fac PE	Fac PE	Mal-practice	Non-Fac Total	Fac Total	Global	Gap
86078		A	investigation of transfusion reaction including suspicion of transmissible disease, interpretation and written report	0.94	0.51	0.43	0.03	1.48	1.40	XXX	
86079		A	authorization for deviation from standard blood banking procedures (eg, use of outdated blood, transfusion of Rh incompatible units), with written report	0.94	0.50	0.44	0.03	1.47	1.41	XXX	
86140		X	C-reactive protein;	0.00	0.31	0.31	0.00	0.31	0.31	XXX	■
	26			0.00	0.00	0.00	0.00	0.00	0.00	XXX	■
	TC			0.00	0.31	0.31	0.00	0.31	0.31	XXX	■
86141		X	high sensitivity (hsCRP)	0.00	0.39	0.39	0.00	0.39	0.39	XXX	■
	26			0.00	0.00	0.00	0.00	0.00	0.00	XXX	■
	TC			0.00	0.39	0.39	0.00	0.39	0.39	XXX	■
86146		X	Beta 2 Glycoprotein I antibody, each	0.00	1.14	1.14	0.00	1.14	1.14	XXX	■
	26			0.00	0.00	0.00	0.00	0.00	0.00	XXX	■
	TC			0.00	1.14	1.14	0.00	1.14	1.14	XXX	■
86147		X	Cardiolipin (phospholipid) antibody, each Ig class	0.00	1.14	1.14	0.00	1.14	1.14	XXX	■
	26			0.00	0.00	0.00	0.00	0.00	0.00	XXX	■
	TC			0.00	1.14	1.14	0.00	1.14	1.14	XXX	■
86148		X	Anti-phosphatidylserine (phospholipid) antibody	0.00	0.61	0.61	0.00	0.61	0.61	XXX	■
	26			0.00	0.00	0.00	0.00	0.00	0.00	XXX	■
	TC			0.00	0.61	0.61	0.00	0.61	0.61	XXX	■
86155		X	Chemotaxis assay, specify method	0.00	0.44	0.44	0.00	0.44	0.44	XXX	■
	26			0.00	0.00	0.00	0.00	0.00	0.00	XXX	■
	TC			0.00	0.44	0.44	0.00	0.44	0.44	XXX	■
86156		X	Cold agglutinin; screen	0.00	0.29	0.29	0.00	0.29	0.29	XXX	■
	26			0.00	0.00	0.00	0.00	0.00	0.00	XXX	■
	TC			0.00	0.29	0.29	0.00	0.29	0.29	XXX	■
86157		X	titer	0.00	0.38	0.38	0.00	0.38	0.38	XXX	■
	26			0.00	0.00	0.00	0.00	0.00	0.00	XXX	■
	TC			0.00	0.38	0.38	0.00	0.38	0.38	XXX	■
86160		X	Complement; antigen, each component	0.00	0.72	0.72	0.00	0.72	0.72	XXX	■
	26			0.00	0.00	0.00	0.00	0.00	0.00	XXX	■
	TC			0.00	0.72	0.72	0.00	0.72	0.72	XXX	■
86161		X	functional activity, each component	0.00	0.72	0.72	0.00	0.72	0.72	XXX	■
	26			0.00	0.00	0.00	0.00	0.00	0.00	XXX	■
	TC			0.00	0.72	0.72	0.00	0.72	0.72	XXX	■
86162		X	total hemolytic (CH50)	0.00	1.01	1.01	0.00	1.01	1.01	XXX	■
	26			0.00	0.00	0.00	0.00	0.00	0.00	XXX	■
	TC			0.00	1.01	1.01	0.00	1.01	1.01	XXX	■
86171		X	Complement fixation tests, each antigen	0.00	0.47	0.47	0.00	0.47	0.47	XXX	■
	26			0.00	0.00	0.00	0.00	0.00	0.00	XXX	■
	TC			0.00	0.47	0.47	0.00	0.47	0.47	XXX	■

Pathology

■ RVU not developed by CMS. Gap-filled RVUs developed by Ingenix/CHEG.

Code	M	S	Description	Work Value	Non-Fac PE	Fac PE	Mal-practice	Non-Fac Total	Fac Total	Global	Gap
86185		X	Counterimmunoelectrophoresis, each antigen	0.00	0.46	0.46	0.00	0.46	0.46	XXX	■
	26			0.00	0.00	0.00	0.00	0.00	0.00	XXX	■
	TC			0.00	0.46	0.46	0.00	0.46	0.46	XXX	■
86215		X	Deoxyribonuclease, antibody	0.00	0.64	0.64	0.00	0.64	0.64	XXX	■
	26			0.00	0.00	0.00	0.00	0.00	0.00	XXX	■
	TC			0.00	0.64	0.64	0.00	0.64	0.64	XXX	■
86225		X	Deoxyribonucleic acid (DNA) antibody; native or double stranded	0.00	0.70	0.70	0.00	0.70	0.70	XXX	■
	26			0.00	0.00	0.00	0.00	0.00	0.00	XXX	■
	TC			0.00	0.70	0.70	0.00	0.70	0.70	XXX	■
86226		X	single stranded	0.00	0.70	0.70	0.00	0.70	0.70	XXX	■
	26			0.00	0.00	0.00	0.00	0.00	0.00	XXX	■
	TC			0.00	0.70	0.70	0.00	0.70	0.70	XXX	■
86235		X	Extractable nuclear antigen, antibody to, any method (eg, nRNP, SS-A, SS-B, Sm, RNP, Sc170, J01), each antibody	0.00	0.62	0.62	0.00	0.62	0.62	XXX	■
	26			0.00	0.00	0.00	0.00	0.00	0.00	XXX	■
	TC			0.00	0.62	0.62	0.00	0.62	0.62	XXX	■
86243		X	Fc receptor	0.00	0.77	0.77	0.00	0.77	0.77	XXX	■
	26			0.00	0.00	0.00	0.00	0.00	0.00	XXX	■
	TC			0.00	0.77	0.77	0.00	0.77	0.77	XXX	■
86255		X	Fluorescent noninfectious agent antibody; screen, each antibody	0.37	0.63	0.63	0.01	1.01	1.01	XXX	■
	26	A		0.37	0.17	0.17	0.01	0.55	0.55	XXX	
	TC			0.00	0.46	0.46	0.00	0.46	0.46	XXX	■
86256		X	titer, each antibody	0.37	0.63	0.63	0.01	1.01	1.01	XXX	■
	26	A		0.37	0.17	0.17	0.01	0.55	0.55	XXX	
	TC			0.00	0.46	0.46	0.00	0.46	0.46	XXX	■
86277		X	Growth hormone, human (HGH), antibody	0.00	0.57	0.57	0.00	0.57	0.57	XXX	■
	26			0.00	0.00	0.00	0.00	0.00	0.00	XXX	■
	TC			0.00	0.57	0.57	0.00	0.57	0.57	XXX	■
86280		X	Hemagglutination inhibition test (HAI)	0.00	0.47	0.47	0.00	0.47	0.47	XXX	■
	26			0.00	0.00	0.00	0.00	0.00	0.00	XXX	■
	TC			0.00	0.47	0.47	0.00	0.47	0.47	XXX	■
86294		X	Immunoassay for tumor antigen, qualitative or semiquantitative (eg, bladder tumor antigen)	0.00	0.85	0.85	0.00	0.85	0.85	XXX	■
	26			0.00	0.00	0.00	0.00	0.00	0.00	XXX	■
	TC			0.00	0.85	0.85	0.00	0.85	0.85	XXX	■
86300		X	Immunoassay for tumor antigen, quantitative; CA 15-3 (27.29)	0.00	0.85	0.85	0.00	0.85	0.85	XXX	■
	26			0.00	0.00	0.00	0.00	0.00	0.00	XXX	■
	TC			0.00	0.85	0.85	0.00	0.85	0.85	XXX	■
86301		X	CA 19-9	0.00	0.85	0.85	0.00	0.85	0.85	XXX	■
	26			0.00	0.00	0.00	0.00	0.00	0.00	XXX	■
	TC			0.00	0.85	0.85	0.00	0.85	0.85	XXX	■
86304		X	CA 125	0.00	0.85	0.85	0.00	0.85	0.85	XXX	■
	26			0.00	0.00	0.00	0.00	0.00	0.00	XXX	■
	TC			0.00	0.85	0.85	0.00	0.85	0.85	XXX	■
86308		X	Heterophile antibodies; screening	0.00	0.28	0.28	0.00	0.28	0.28	XXX	■
	26			0.00	0.00	0.00	0.00	0.00	0.00	XXX	■
	TC			0.00	0.28	0.28	0.00	0.28	0.28	XXX	■

■ RVU not developed by CMS. Gap-filled RVUs developed by Ingenix/CHEG.

Code	M	S	Description	Work Value	Non-Fac PE	Fac PE	Mal-practice	Non-Fac Total	Fac Total	Global	Gap
86309		X	titer	0.00	0.36	0.36	0.00	0.36	0.36	XXX	■
	26			0.00	0.00	0.00	0.00	0.00	0.00	XXX	■
	TC			0.00	0.36	0.36	0.00	0.36	0.36	XXX	■
86310		X	titers after absorption with beef cells and guinea pig kidney	0.00	0.41	0.41	0.00	0.41	0.41	XXX	■
	26			0.00	0.00	0.00	0.00	0.00	0.00	XXX	■
	TC			0.00	0.41	0.41	0.00	0.41	0.41	XXX	■
86316		X	Immunoassay for tumor antigen; other antigen, quantitative (eg, CA 50, 72-4, 549), each	0.00	0.85	0.85	0.00	0.85	0.85	XXX	■
	26			0.00	0.00	0.00	0.00	0.00	0.00	XXX	■
	TC			0.00	0.85	0.85	0.00	0.85	0.85	XXX	■
86317		X	Immunoassay for infectious agent antibody, quantitative, not otherwise specified	0.00	0.39	0.39	0.00	0.39	0.39	XXX	■
	26			0.00	0.00	0.00	0.00	0.00	0.00	XXX	■
	TC			0.00	0.39	0.39	0.00	0.39	0.39	XXX	■
86318		X	Immunoassay for infectious agent antibody, qualitative or semiquantitative, single step method (eg, reagent strip)	0.00	0.39	0.39	0.00	0.39	0.39	XXX	■
	26			0.00	0.00	0.00	0.00	0.00	0.00	XXX	■
	TC			0.00	0.39	0.39	0.00	0.39	0.39	XXX	■
86320		X	Immunoelectrophoresis; serum	0.37	1.03	1.03	0.01	1.41	1.41	XXX	■
	26	A		0.37	0.17	0.17	0.01	0.55	0.55	XXX	
	TC			0.00	0.86	0.86	0.00	0.86	0.86	XXX	■
86325		X	other fluids (eg, urine, cerebrospinal fluid) with concentration	0.37	1.02	1.02	0.01	1.40	1.40	XXX	■
	26	A		0.37	0.17	0.17	0.01	0.55	0.55	XXX	
	TC			0.00	0.85	0.85	0.00	0.85	0.85	XXX	■
86327		X	crossed (2-dimensional assay)	0.42	1.07	1.07	0.01	1.50	1.50	XXX	■
	26	A		0.42	0.20	0.20	0.01	0.63	0.63	XXX	
	TC			0.00	0.87	0.87	0.00	0.87	0.87	XXX	■
86329		X	Immunodiffusion; not elsewhere specified	0.00	0.78	0.78	0.00	0.78	0.78	XXX	■
	26			0.00	0.00	0.00	0.00	0.00	0.00	XXX	■
	TC			0.00	0.78	0.78	0.00	0.78	0.78	XXX	■
86331		X	gel diffusion, qualitative (Ouchterlony), each antigen or antibody	0.00	0.73	0.73	0.00	0.73	0.73	XXX	■
	26			0.00	0.00	0.00	0.00	0.00	0.00	XXX	■
	TC			0.00	0.73	0.73	0.00	0.73	0.73	XXX	■
86332		X	Immune complex assay	0.00	0.93	0.93	0.00	0.93	0.93	XXX	■
	26			0.00	0.00	0.00	0.00	0.00	0.00	XXX	■
	TC			0.00	0.93	0.93	0.00	0.93	0.93	XXX	■
86334		X	Immunofixation electrophoresis	0.37	1.02	1.02	0.01	1.40	1.40	XXX	■
	26	A		0.37	0.17	0.17	0.01	0.55	0.55	XXX	
	TC			0.00	0.85	0.85	0.00	0.85	0.85	XXX	■
86336		X	Inhibin A	0.00	0.82	0.82	0.00	0.82	0.82	XXX	■
	26			0.00	0.00	0.00	0.00	0.00	0.00	XXX	■
	TC			0.00	0.82	0.82	0.00	0.82	0.82	XXX	■
86337		X	Insulin antibodies	0.00	1.03	1.03	0.00	1.03	1.03	XXX	■
	26			0.00	0.00	0.00	0.00	0.00	0.00	XXX	■
	TC			0.00	1.03	1.03	0.00	1.03	1.03	XXX	■
86340		X	Intrinsic factor antibodies	0.00	0.72	0.72	0.00	0.72	0.72	XXX	■
	26			0.00	0.00	0.00	0.00	0.00	0.00	XXX	■
	TC			0.00	0.72	0.72	0.00	0.72	0.72	XXX	■

■ RVU not developed by CMS. Gap-filled RVUs developed by Ingenix/CHEG.

Code	M	S	Description	Work Value	Non-Fac PE	Fac PE	Mal-practice	Non-Fac Total	Fac Total	Global	Gap
86341		X	Islet cell antibody	0.00	0.57	0.57	0.00	0.57	0.57	XXX	■
	26			0.00	0.00	0.00	0.00	0.00	0.00	XXX	■
	TC			0.00	0.57	0.57	0.00	0.57	0.57	XXX	■
86343		X	Leukocyte histamine release test (LHR)	0.00	0.70	0.70	0.00	0.70	0.70	XXX	■
	26			0.00	0.00	0.00	0.00	0.00	0.00	XXX	■
	TC			0.00	0.70	0.70	0.00	0.70	0.70	XXX	■
86344		X	Leukocyte phagocytosis	0.00	0.41	0.41	0.00	0.41	0.41	XXX	■
	26			0.00	0.00	0.00	0.00	0.00	0.00	XXX	■
	TC			0.00	0.41	0.41	0.00	0.41	0.41	XXX	■
86353		X	Lymphocyte transformation, mitogen (phytomitogen) or antigen induced blastogenesis	0.00	2.28	2.28	0.00	2.28	2.28	XXX	■
	26			0.00	0.00	0.00	0.00	0.00	0.00	XXX	■
	TC			0.00	2.28	2.28	0.00	2.28	2.28	XXX	■
86359		X	T cells; total count	0.00	1.08	1.08	0.00	1.08	1.08	XXX	■
	26			0.00	0.00	0.00	0.00	0.00	0.00	XXX	■
	TC			0.00	1.08	1.08	0.00	1.08	1.08	XXX	■
86360		X	absolute CD4 and CD8 count, including ratio	0.00	1.63	1.63	0.00	1.63	1.63	XXX	■
	26			0.00	0.00	0.00	0.00	0.00	0.00	XXX	■
	TC			0.00	1.63	1.63	0.00	1.63	1.63	XXX	■
86361		X	absolute CD4 count	0.00	1.35	1.35	0.00	1.35	1.35	XXX	■
	26			0.00	0.00	0.00	0.00	0.00	0.00	XXX	■
	TC			0.00	1.35	1.35	0.00	1.35	1.35	XXX	■
86376		X	Microsomal antibodies (eg, thyroid or liver-kidney), each	0.00	0.69	0.69	0.00	0.69	0.69	XXX	■
	26			0.00	0.00	0.00	0.00	0.00	0.00	XXX	■
	TC			0.00	0.69	0.69	0.00	0.69	0.69	XXX	■
86378		X	Migration inhibitory factor test (MIF)	0.00	0.73	0.73	0.00	0.73	0.73	XXX	■
	26			0.00	0.00	0.00	0.00	0.00	0.00	XXX	■
	TC			0.00	0.73	0.73	0.00	0.73	0.73	XXX	■
86382		X	Neutralization test, viral	0.00	0.75	0.75	0.00	0.75	0.75	XXX	■
	26			0.00	0.00	0.00	0.00	0.00	0.00	XXX	■
	TC			0.00	0.75	0.75	0.00	0.75	0.75	XXX	■
86384		X	Nitroblue tetrazolium dye test (NTD)	0.00	0.57	0.57	0.00	0.57	0.57	XXX	■
	26			0.00	0.00	0.00	0.00	0.00	0.00	XXX	■
	TC			0.00	0.57	0.57	0.00	0.57	0.57	XXX	■
86403		X	Particle agglutination; screen, each antibody	0.00	0.26	0.26	0.00	0.26	0.26	XXX	■
	26			0.00	0.00	0.00	0.00	0.00	0.00	XXX	■
	TC			0.00	0.26	0.26	0.00	0.26	0.26	XXX	■
86406		X	titer, each antibody	0.00	0.30	0.30	0.00	0.30	0.30	XXX	■
	26			0.00	0.00	0.00	0.00	0.00	0.00	XXX	■
	TC			0.00	0.30	0.30	0.00	0.30	0.30	XXX	■
86430		X	Rheumatoid factor; qualitative	0.00	0.31	0.31	0.00	0.31	0.31	XXX	■
	26			0.00	0.00	0.00	0.00	0.00	0.00	XXX	■
	TC			0.00	0.31	0.31	0.00	0.31	0.31	XXX	■
86431		X	quantitative	0.00	0.36	0.36	0.00	0.36	0.36	XXX	■
	26			0.00	0.00	0.00	0.00	0.00	0.00	XXX	■
	TC			0.00	0.36	0.36	0.00	0.36	0.36	XXX	■

■ RVU not developed by CMS. Gap-filled RVUs developed by Ingenix/CHEG.

Code	M	S	Description	Work Value	Non-Fac PE	Fac PE	Mal-practice	Non-Fac Total	Fac Total	Global	Gap
86485		C	Skin test; candida	0.00	0.24	0.24	0.00	0.24	0.24	XXX	■
	26			0.00	0.00	0.00	0.00	0.00	0.00	XXX	■
	TC			0.00	0.24	0.24	0.00	0.24	0.24	XXX	■
86490		A	coccidioidomycosis	0.00	0.28	0.28	0.02	0.30	0.30	XXX	
	26			0.00	0.00	0.00	0.00	0.00	0.00	XXX	■
	TC			0.00	0.28	0.28	0.02	0.30	0.30	XXX	■
86510		A	histoplasmosis	0.00	0.30	0.30	0.02	0.32	0.32	XXX	
	26			0.00	0.00	0.00	0.00	0.00	0.00	XXX	■
	TC			0.00	0.30	0.30	0.02	0.32	0.32	XXX	■
86580		A	tuberculosis, intradermal	0.00	0.24	0.24	0.02	0.26	0.26	XXX	
	26			0.00	0.00	0.00	0.00	0.00	0.00	XXX	■
	TC			0.00	0.24	0.24	0.02	0.26	0.26	XXX	■
86585		A	tuberculosis, tine test	0.00	0.19	0.19	0.01	0.20	0.20	XXX	
	26			0.00	0.00	0.00	0.00	0.00	0.00	XXX	■
	TC			0.00	0.19	0.19	0.01	0.20	0.20	XXX	■
86586		C	unlisted antigen, each	0.00	0.24	0.24	0.00	0.24	0.24	XXX	■
	26			0.00	0.00	0.00	0.00	0.00	0.00	XXX	■
	TC			0.00	0.24	0.24	0.00	0.24	0.24	XXX	■
86590		X	Streptokinase, antibody	0.00	0.29	0.29	0.00	0.29	0.29	XXX	■
	26			0.00	0.00	0.00	0.00	0.00	0.00	XXX	■
	TC			0.00	0.29	0.29	0.00	0.29	0.29	XXX	■
86592		X	Syphilis test; qualitative (eg, VDRL, RPR, ART)	0.00	0.21	0.21	0.00	0.21	0.21	XXX	■
	26			0.00	0.00	0.00	0.00	0.00	0.00	XXX	■
	TC			0.00	0.21	0.21	0.00	0.21	0.21	XXX	■
86593		X	quantitative	0.00	0.23	0.23	0.00	0.23	0.23	XXX	■
	26			0.00	0.00	0.00	0.00	0.00	0.00	XXX	■
	TC			0.00	0.23	0.23	0.00	0.23	0.23	XXX	■
86602		X	Antibody; actinomyces	0.00	0.65	0.65	0.00	0.65	0.65	XXX	■
	26			0.00	0.00	0.00	0.00	0.00	0.00	XXX	■
	TC			0.00	0.65	0.65	0.00	0.65	0.65	XXX	■
86603		X	adenovirus	0.00	0.65	0.65	0.00	0.65	0.65	XXX	■
	26			0.00	0.00	0.00	0.00	0.00	0.00	XXX	■
	TC			0.00	0.65	0.65	0.00	0.65	0.65	XXX	■
86606		X	Aspergillus	0.00	0.72	0.72	0.00	0.72	0.72	XXX	■
	26			0.00	0.00	0.00	0.00	0.00	0.00	XXX	■
	TC			0.00	0.72	0.72	0.00	0.72	0.72	XXX	■
86609		X	bacterium, not elsewhere specified	0.00	0.90	0.90	0.00	0.90	0.90	XXX	■
	26			0.00	0.00	0.00	0.00	0.00	0.00	XXX	■
	TC			0.00	0.90	0.90	0.00	0.90	0.90	XXX	■
86611		X	Bartonella	0.00	0.73	0.73	0.00	0.73	0.73	XXX	■
	26			0.00	0.00	0.00	0.00	0.00	0.00	XXX	■
	TC			0.00	0.73	0.73	0.00	0.73	0.73	XXX	■
86612		X	Blastomyces	0.00	0.72	0.72	0.00	0.72	0.72	XXX	■
	26			0.00	0.00	0.00	0.00	0.00	0.00	XXX	■
	TC			0.00	0.72	0.72	0.00	0.72	0.72	XXX	■

■ RVU not developed by CMS. Gap-filled RVUs developed by Ingenix/CHEG.

Code	M	S	Description	Work Value	Non-Fac PE	Fac PE	Mal-practice	Non-Fac Total	Fac Total	Global	Gap
86615		X	Bordetella	0.00	0.82	0.82	0.00	0.82	0.82	XXX	■
	26			0.00	0.00	0.00	0.00	0.00	0.00	XXX	■
	TC			0.00	0.82	0.82	0.00	0.82	0.82	XXX	■
86617		X	Borrelia burgdorferi (Lyme disease) confirmatory test (eg, Western blot or immunoblot)	0.00	0.86	0.86	0.00	0.86	0.86	XXX	■
	26			0.00	0.00	0.00	0.00	0.00	0.00	XXX	■
	TC			0.00	0.86	0.86	0.00	0.86	0.86	XXX	■
86618		X	Borrelia burgdorferi (Lyme disease)	0.00	0.82	0.82	0.00	0.82	0.82	XXX	■
	26			0.00	0.00	0.00	0.00	0.00	0.00	XXX	■
	TC			0.00	0.82	0.82	0.00	0.82	0.82	XXX	■
86619		X	Borrelia (relapsing fever)	0.00	0.65	0.65	0.00	0.65	0.65	XXX	■
	26			0.00	0.00	0.00	0.00	0.00	0.00	XXX	■
	TC			0.00	0.65	0.65	0.00	0.65	0.65	XXX	■
86622		X	Brucella	0.00	0.49	0.49	0.00	0.49	0.49	XXX	■
	26			0.00	0.00	0.00	0.00	0.00	0.00	XXX	■
	TC			0.00	0.49	0.49	0.00	0.49	0.49	XXX	■
86625		X	Campylobacter	0.00	0.82	0.82	0.00	0.82	0.82	XXX	■
	26			0.00	0.00	0.00	0.00	0.00	0.00	XXX	■
	TC			0.00	0.82	0.82	0.00	0.82	0.82	XXX	■
86628		X	Candida	0.00	0.78	0.78	0.00	0.78	0.78	XXX	■
	26			0.00	0.00	0.00	0.00	0.00	0.00	XXX	■
	TC			0.00	0.78	0.78	0.00	0.78	0.78	XXX	■
86631		X	Chlamydia	0.00	0.57	0.57	0.00	0.57	0.57	XXX	■
	26			0.00	0.00	0.00	0.00	0.00	0.00	XXX	■
	TC			0.00	0.57	0.57	0.00	0.57	0.57	XXX	■
86632		X	Chlamydia, IgM	0.00	0.64	0.64	0.00	0.64	0.64	XXX	■
	26			0.00	0.00	0.00	0.00	0.00	0.00	XXX	■
	TC			0.00	0.64	0.64	0.00	0.64	0.64	XXX	■
86635		X	Coccidioides	0.00	0.78	0.78	0.00	0.78	0.78	XXX	■
	26			0.00	0.00	0.00	0.00	0.00	0.00	XXX	■
	TC			0.00	0.78	0.78	0.00	0.78	0.78	XXX	■
86638		X	Coxiella Brunetii (Q fever)	0.00	0.65	0.65	0.00	0.65	0.65	XXX	■
	26			0.00	0.00	0.00	0.00	0.00	0.00	XXX	■
	TC			0.00	0.65	0.65	0.00	0.65	0.65	XXX	■
86641		X	Cryptococcus	0.00	0.49	0.49	0.00	0.49	0.49	XXX	■
	26			0.00	0.00	0.00	0.00	0.00	0.00	XXX	■
	TC			0.00	0.49	0.49	0.00	0.49	0.49	XXX	■
86644		X	cytomegalovirus (CMV)	0.00	0.75	0.75	0.00	0.75	0.75	XXX	■
	26			0.00	0.00	0.00	0.00	0.00	0.00	XXX	■
	TC			0.00	0.75	0.75	0.00	0.75	0.75	XXX	■
86645		X	cytomegalovirus (CMV), IgM	0.00	0.83	0.83	0.00	0.83	0.83	XXX	■
	26			0.00	0.00	0.00	0.00	0.00	0.00	XXX	■
	TC			0.00	0.83	0.83	0.00	0.83	0.83	XXX	■
86648		X	Diphtheria	0.00	0.72	0.72	0.00	0.72	0.72	XXX	■
	26			0.00	0.00	0.00	0.00	0.00	0.00	XXX	■
	TC			0.00	0.72	0.72	0.00	0.72	0.72	XXX	■

■ RVU not developed by CMS. Gap-filled RVUs developed by Ingenix/CHEG.

Pathology

Code	M	S	Description	Work Value	Non-Fac PE	Fac PE	Mal-practice	Non-Fac Total	Fac Total	Global	Gap
86651		**X**	encephalitis, California (La Crosse)	0.00	0.65	0.65	0.00	0.65	0.65	XXX	■
	26			0.00	0.00	0.00	0.00	0.00	0.00	XXX	■
	TC			0.00	0.65	0.65	0.00	0.65	0.65	XXX	■
86652		**X**	encephalitis, Eastern equine	0.00	0.65	0.65	0.00	0.65	0.65	XXX	■
	26			0.00	0.00	0.00	0.00	0.00	0.00	XXX	■
	TC			0.00	0.65	0.65	0.00	0.65	0.65	XXX	■
86653		**X**	encephalitis, St. Louis	0.00	0.65	0.65	0.00	0.65	0.65	XXX	■
	26			0.00	0.00	0.00	0.00	0.00	0.00	XXX	■
	TC			0.00	0.65	0.65	0.00	0.65	0.65	XXX	■
86654		**X**	encephalitis, Western equine	0.00	0.65	0.65	0.00	0.65	0.65	XXX	■
	26			0.00	0.00	0.00	0.00	0.00	0.00	XXX	■
	TC			0.00	0.65	0.65	0.00	0.65	0.65	XXX	■
86658		**X**	enterovirus (eg, coxsackie, echo, polio)	0.00	0.65	0.65	0.00	0.65	0.65	XXX	■
	26			0.00	0.00	0.00	0.00	0.00	0.00	XXX	■
	TC			0.00	0.65	0.65	0.00	0.65	0.65	XXX	■
86663		**X**	Epstein-Barr (EB) virus, early antigen (EA)	0.00	0.78	0.78	0.00	0.78	0.78	XXX	■
	26			0.00	0.00	0.00	0.00	0.00	0.00	XXX	■
	TC			0.00	0.78	0.78	0.00	0.78	0.78	XXX	■
86664		**X**	Epstein-Barr (EB) virus, nuclear antigen (EBNA)	0.00	0.78	0.78	0.00	0.78	0.78	XXX	■
	26			0.00	0.00	0.00	0.00	0.00	0.00	XXX	■
	TC			0.00	0.78	0.78	0.00	0.78	0.78	XXX	■
86665		**X**	Epstein-Barr (EB) virus, viral capsid (VCA)	0.00	0.85	0.85	0.00	0.85	0.85	XXX	■
	26			0.00	0.00	0.00	0.00	0.00	0.00	XXX	■
	TC			0.00	0.85	0.85	0.00	0.85	0.85	XXX	■
86666		**X**	Ehrlichia	0.00	0.73	0.73	0.00	0.73	0.73	XXX	■
	26			0.00	0.00	0.00	0.00	0.00	0.00	XXX	■
	TC			0.00	0.73	0.73	0.00	0.73	0.73	XXX	■
86668		**X**	Francisella Tularensis	0.00	0.49	0.49	0.00	0.49	0.49	XXX	■
	26			0.00	0.00	0.00	0.00	0.00	0.00	XXX	■
	TC			0.00	0.49	0.49	0.00	0.49	0.49	XXX	■
86671		**X**	fungus, not elsewhere specified	0.00	0.90	0.90	0.00	0.90	0.90	XXX	■
	26			0.00	0.00	0.00	0.00	0.00	0.00	XXX	■
	TC			0.00	0.90	0.90	0.00	0.90	0.90	XXX	■
86674		**X**	Giardia Lamblia	0.00	0.65	0.65	0.00	0.65	0.65	XXX	■
	26			0.00	0.00	0.00	0.00	0.00	0.00	XXX	■
	TC			0.00	0.65	0.65	0.00	0.65	0.65	XXX	■
86677		**X**	Helicobacter Pylori	0.00	0.88	0.88	0.00	0.88	0.88	XXX	■
	26			0.00	0.00	0.00	0.00	0.00	0.00	XXX	■
	TC			0.00	0.88	0.88	0.00	0.88	0.88	XXX	■
86682		**X**	helminth, not elsewhere specified	0.00	0.90	0.90	0.00	0.90	0.90	XXX	■
	26			0.00	0.00	0.00	0.00	0.00	0.00	XXX	■
	TC			0.00	0.90	0.90	0.00	0.90	0.90	XXX	■
86684		**X**	Hemophilus influenza	0.00	0.82	0.82	0.00	0.82	0.82	XXX	■
	26			0.00	0.00	0.00	0.00	0.00	0.00	XXX	■
	TC			0.00	0.82	0.82	0.00	0.82	0.82	XXX	■

■ RVU not developed by CMS. Gap-filled RVUs developed by Ingenix/CHEG.

Code	M	S	Description	Work Value	Non-Fac PE	Fac PE	Mal-practice	Non-Fac Total	Fac Total	Global	Gap
86687		X	HTLV I	0.00	0.65	0.65	0.00	0.65	0.65	XXX	■
	26			0.00	0.00	0.00	0.00	0.00	0.00	XXX	■
	TC			0.00	0.65	0.65	0.00	0.65	0.65	XXX	■
86688		X	HTLV-II	0.00	0.62	0.62	0.00	0.62	0.62	XXX	■
	26			0.00	0.00	0.00	0.00	0.00	0.00	XXX	■
	TC			0.00	0.62	0.62	0.00	0.62	0.62	XXX	■
86689		X	HTLV or HIV antibody, confirmatory test (eg, Western Blot)	0.00	0.86	0.86	0.00	0.86	0.86	XXX	■
	26			0.00	0.00	0.00	0.00	0.00	0.00	XXX	■
	TC			0.00	0.86	0.86	0.00	0.86	0.86	XXX	■
86692		X	hepatitis, delta agent	0.00	0.82	0.82	0.00	0.82	0.82	XXX	■
	26			0.00	0.00	0.00	0.00	0.00	0.00	XXX	■
	TC			0.00	0.82	0.82	0.00	0.82	0.82	XXX	■
86694		X	herpes simplex, non-specific type test	0.00	0.72	0.72	0.00	0.72	0.72	XXX	■
	26			0.00	0.00	0.00	0.00	0.00	0.00	XXX	■
	TC			0.00	0.72	0.72	0.00	0.72	0.72	XXX	■
86695		X	herpes simplex, type I	0.00	0.72	0.72	0.00	0.72	0.72	XXX	■
	26			0.00	0.00	0.00	0.00	0.00	0.00	XXX	■
	TC			0.00	0.72	0.72	0.00	0.72	0.72	XXX	■
86696		X	herpes simplex, type 2	0.00	0.72	0.72	0.00	0.72	0.72	XXX	■
	26			0.00	0.00	0.00	0.00	0.00	0.00	XXX	■
	TC			0.00	0.72	0.72	0.00	0.72	0.72	XXX	■
86698		X	histoplasma	0.00	0.65	0.65	0.00	0.65	0.65	XXX	■
	26			0.00	0.00	0.00	0.00	0.00	0.00	XXX	■
	TC			0.00	0.65	0.65	0.00	0.65	0.65	XXX	■
86701		X	HIV-1	0.00	0.55	0.55	0.00	0.55	0.55	XXX	■
	26			0.00	0.00	0.00	0.00	0.00	0.00	XXX	■
	TC			0.00	0.55	0.55	0.00	0.55	0.55	XXX	■
86702		X	HIV-2	0.00	0.82	0.82	0.00	0.82	0.82	XXX	■
	26			0.00	0.00	0.00	0.00	0.00	0.00	XXX	■
	TC			0.00	0.82	0.82	0.00	0.82	0.82	XXX	■
86703		X	HIV-1 and HIV-2, single assay	0.00	0.55	0.55	0.00	0.55	0.55	XXX	■
	26			0.00	0.00	0.00	0.00	0.00	0.00	XXX	■
	TC			0.00	0.55	0.55	0.00	0.55	0.55	XXX	■
86704		X	Hepatitis B core antibody (HBcAb); total	0.00	0.57	0.57	0.00	0.57	0.57	XXX	■
	26			0.00	0.00	0.00	0.00	0.00	0.00	XXX	■
	TC			0.00	0.57	0.57	0.00	0.57	0.57	XXX	■
86705		X	IgM antibody	0.00	0.62	0.62	0.00	0.62	0.62	XXX	■
	26			0.00	0.00	0.00	0.00	0.00	0.00	XXX	■
	TC			0.00	0.62	0.62	0.00	0.62	0.62	XXX	■
86706		X	Hepatitis B surface antibody (HBsAb)	0.00	0.51	0.51	0.00	0.51	0.51	XXX	■
	26			0.00	0.00	0.00	0.00	0.00	0.00	XXX	■
	TC			0.00	0.51	0.51	0.00	0.51	0.51	XXX	■
86707		X	Hepatitis Be antibody (HBeAb)	0.00	0.55	0.55	0.00	0.55	0.55	XXX	■
	26			0.00	0.00	0.00	0.00	0.00	0.00	XXX	■
	TC			0.00	0.55	0.55	0.00	0.55	0.55	XXX	■

■ RVU not developed by CMS. Gap-filled RVUs developed by Ingenix/CHEG.

Code	M	S	Description	Work Value	Non-Fac PE	Fac PE	Mal-practice	Non-Fac Total	Fac Total	Global	Gap
86708		X	Hepatitis A antibody (HAAb); total	0.00	0.60	0.60	0.00	0.60	0.60	XXX	■
	26			0.00	0.00	0.00	0.00	0.00	0.00	XXX	■
	TC			0.00	0.60	0.60	0.00	0.60	0.60	XXX	■
86709		X	IgM antibody	0.00	0.57	0.57	0.00	0.57	0.57	XXX	■
	26			0.00	0.00	0.00	0.00	0.00	0.00	XXX	■
	TC			0.00	0.57	0.57	0.00	0.57	0.57	XXX	■
86710		X	Antibody; influenza virus	0.00	0.54	0.54	0.00	0.54	0.54	XXX	■
	26			0.00	0.00	0.00	0.00	0.00	0.00	XXX	■
	TC			0.00	0.54	0.54	0.00	0.54	0.54	XXX	■
86713		X	Legionella	0.00	0.78	0.78	0.00	0.78	0.78	XXX	■
	26			0.00	0.00	0.00	0.00	0.00	0.00	XXX	■
	TC			0.00	0.78	0.78	0.00	0.78	0.78	XXX	■
86717		X	Leishmania	0.00	0.65	0.65	0.00	0.65	0.65	XXX	■
	26			0.00	0.00	0.00	0.00	0.00	0.00	XXX	■
	TC			0.00	0.65	0.65	0.00	0.65	0.65	XXX	■
86720		X	Leptospira	0.00	0.65	0.65	0.00	0.65	0.65	XXX	■
	26			0.00	0.00	0.00	0.00	0.00	0.00	XXX	■
	TC			0.00	0.65	0.65	0.00	0.65	0.65	XXX	■
86723		X	Listeria monocytogenes	0.00	0.65	0.65	0.00	0.65	0.65	XXX	■
	26			0.00	0.00	0.00	0.00	0.00	0.00	XXX	■
	TC			0.00	0.65	0.65	0.00	0.65	0.65	XXX	■
86727		X	lymphocytic choriomeningitis	0.00	0.65	0.65	0.00	0.65	0.65	XXX	■
	26			0.00	0.00	0.00	0.00	0.00	0.00	XXX	■
	TC			0.00	0.65	0.65	0.00	0.65	0.65	XXX	■
86729		X	Lymphogranuloma Venereum	0.00	0.65	0.65	0.00	0.65	0.65	XXX	■
	26			0.00	0.00	0.00	0.00	0.00	0.00	XXX	■
	TC			0.00	0.65	0.65	0.00	0.65	0.65	XXX	■
86732		X	mucormycosis	0.00	0.65	0.65	0.00	0.65	0.65	XXX	■
	26			0.00	0.00	0.00	0.00	0.00	0.00	XXX	■
	TC			0.00	0.65	0.65	0.00	0.65	0.65	XXX	■
86735		X	mumps	0.00	0.65	0.65	0.00	0.65	0.65	XXX	■
	26			0.00	0.00	0.00	0.00	0.00	0.00	XXX	■
	TC			0.00	0.65	0.65	0.00	0.65	0.65	XXX	■
86738		X	Mycoplasma	0.00	0.65	0.65	0.00	0.65	0.65	XXX	■
	26			0.00	0.00	0.00	0.00	0.00	0.00	XXX	■
	TC			0.00	0.65	0.65	0.00	0.65	0.65	XXX	■
86741		X	Neisseria meningitidis	0.00	0.65	0.65	0.00	0.65	0.65	XXX	■
	26			0.00	0.00	0.00	0.00	0.00	0.00	XXX	■
	TC			0.00	0.65	0.65	0.00	0.65	0.65	XXX	■
86744		X	Nocardia	0.00	0.65	0.65	0.00	0.65	0.65	XXX	■
	26			0.00	0.00	0.00	0.00	0.00	0.00	XXX	■
	TC			0.00	0.65	0.65	0.00	0.65	0.65	XXX	■
86747		X	parvovirus	0.00	0.82	0.82	0.00	0.82	0.82	XXX	■
	26			0.00	0.00	0.00	0.00	0.00	0.00	XXX	■
	TC			0.00	0.82	0.82	0.00	0.82	0.82	XXX	■

Pathology

■ RVU not developed by CMS. Gap-filled RVUs developed by Ingenix/CHEG.

Code	M	S	Description	Work Value	Non-Fac PE	Fac PE	Mal-practice	Non-Fac Total	Fac Total	Global	Gap
86750		X	Plasmodium (malaria)	0.00	0.65	0.65	0.00	0.65	0.65	XXX	■
	26			0.00	0.00	0.00	0.00	0.00	0.00	XXX	■
	TC			0.00	0.65	0.65	0.00	0.65	0.65	XXX	■
86753		X	protozoa, not elsewhere specified	0.00	0.90	0.90	0.00	0.90	0.90	XXX	■
	26			0.00	0.00	0.00	0.00	0.00	0.00	XXX	■
	TC			0.00	0.90	0.90	0.00	0.90	0.90	XXX	■
86756		X	respiratory syncytial virus	0.00	0.65	0.65	0.00	0.65	0.65	XXX	■
	26			0.00	0.00	0.00	0.00	0.00	0.00	XXX	■
	TC			0.00	0.65	0.65	0.00	0.65	0.65	XXX	■
86757		X	Rickettsia	0.00	0.65	0.65	0.00	0.65	0.65	XXX	■
	26			0.00	0.00	0.00	0.00	0.00	0.00	XXX	■
	TC			0.00	0.65	0.65	0.00	0.65	0.65	XXX	■
86759		X	rotavirus	0.00	0.65	0.65	0.00	0.65	0.65	XXX	■
	26			0.00	0.00	0.00	0.00	0.00	0.00	XXX	■
	TC			0.00	0.65	0.65	0.00	0.65	0.65	XXX	■
86762		X	rubella	0.00	0.38	0.38	0.00	0.38	0.38	XXX	■
	26			0.00	0.00	0.00	0.00	0.00	0.00	XXX	■
	TC			0.00	0.38	0.38	0.00	0.38	0.38	XXX	■
86765		X	rubeola	0.00	0.82	0.82	0.00	0.82	0.82	XXX	■
	26			0.00	0.00	0.00	0.00	0.00	0.00	XXX	■
	TC			0.00	0.82	0.82	0.00	0.82	0.82	XXX	■
86768		X	Salmonella	0.00	0.65	0.65	0.00	0.65	0.65	XXX	■
	26			0.00	0.00	0.00	0.00	0.00	0.00	XXX	■
	TC			0.00	0.65	0.65	0.00	0.65	0.65	XXX	■
86771		X	Shigella	0.00	0.65	0.65	0.00	0.65	0.65	XXX	■
	26			0.00	0.00	0.00	0.00	0.00	0.00	XXX	■
	TC			0.00	0.65	0.65	0.00	0.65	0.65	XXX	■
86774		X	tetanus	0.00	0.82	0.82	0.00	0.82	0.82	XXX	■
	26			0.00	0.00	0.00	0.00	0.00	0.00	XXX	■
	TC			0.00	0.82	0.82	0.00	0.82	0.82	XXX	■
86777		X	Toxoplasma	0.00	0.62	0.62	0.00	0.62	0.62	XXX	■
	26			0.00	0.00	0.00	0.00	0.00	0.00	XXX	■
	TC			0.00	0.62	0.62	0.00	0.62	0.62	XXX	■
86778		X	Toxoplasma, IgM	0.00	0.77	0.77	0.00	0.77	0.77	XXX	■
	26			0.00	0.00	0.00	0.00	0.00	0.00	XXX	■
	TC			0.00	0.77	0.77	0.00	0.77	0.77	XXX	■
86781		X	Treponema Pallidum, confirmatory test (eg, FTA-abs)	0.00	0.55	0.55	0.00	0.55	0.55	XXX	■
	26			0.00	0.00	0.00	0.00	0.00	0.00	XXX	■
	TC			0.00	0.55	0.55	0.00	0.55	0.55	XXX	■
86784		X	trichinella	0.00	0.65	0.65	0.00	0.65	0.65	XXX	■
	26			0.00	0.00	0.00	0.00	0.00	0.00	XXX	■
	TC			0.00	0.65	0.65	0.00	0.65	0.65	XXX	■
86787		X	varicella-zoster	0.00	0.72	0.72	0.00	0.72	0.72	XXX	■
	26			0.00	0.00	0.00	0.00	0.00	0.00	XXX	■
	TC			0.00	0.72	0.72	0.00	0.72	0.72	XXX	■

■ RVU not developed by CMS. Gap-filled RVUs developed by Ingenix/CHEG.

Pathology

Code	M	S	Description	Work Value	Non-Fac PE	Fac PE	Mal-practice	Non-Fac Total	Fac Total	Global	Gap
86790		X	virus, not elsewhere specified	0.00	0.90	0.90	0.00	0.90	0.90	XXX	■
	26			0.00	0.00	0.00	0.00	0.00	0.00	XXX	■
	TC			0.00	0.90	0.90	0.00	0.90	0.90	XXX	■
86793		X	Yersinia	0.00	0.65	0.65	0.00	0.65	0.65	XXX	■
	26			0.00	0.00	0.00	0.00	0.00	0.00	XXX	■
	TC			0.00	0.65	0.65	0.00	0.65	0.65	XXX	■
86800		X	Thyroglobulin antibody	0.00	0.70	0.70	0.00	0.70	0.70	XXX	■
	26			0.00	0.00	0.00	0.00	0.00	0.00	XXX	■
	TC			0.00	0.70	0.70	0.00	0.70	0.70	XXX	■
86803		X	Hepatitis C antibody;	0.00	0.80	0.80	0.00	0.80	0.80	XXX	■
	26			0.00	0.00	0.00	0.00	0.00	0.00	XXX	■
	TC			0.00	0.80	0.80	0.00	0.80	0.80	XXX	■
86804		X	confirmatory test (eg, immunoblot)	0.00	1.14	1.14	0.00	1.14	1.14	XXX	■
	26			0.00	0.00	0.00	0.00	0.00	0.00	XXX	■
	TC			0.00	1.14	1.14	0.00	1.14	1.14	XXX	■
86805		X	Lymphocytotoxicity assay, visual crossmatch; with titration	0.00	2.42	2.42	0.00	2.42	2.42	XXX	■
	26			0.00	0.00	0.00	0.00	0.00	0.00	XXX	■
	TC			0.00	2.42	2.42	0.00	2.42	2.42	XXX	■
86806		X	without titration	0.00	0.80	0.80	0.00	0.80	0.80	XXX	■
	26			0.00	0.00	0.00	0.00	0.00	0.00	XXX	■
	TC			0.00	0.80	0.80	0.00	0.80	0.80	XXX	■
86807		X	Serum screening for cytotoxic percent reactive antibody (PRA); standard method	0.00	0.80	0.80	0.00	0.80	0.80	XXX	■
	26			0.00	0.00	0.00	0.00	0.00	0.00	XXX	■
	TC			0.00	0.80	0.80	0.00	0.80	0.80	XXX	■
86808		X	quick method	0.00	0.90	0.90	0.00	0.90	0.90	XXX	■
	26			0.00	0.00	0.00	0.00	0.00	0.00	XXX	■
	TC			0.00	0.90	0.90	0.00	0.90	0.90	XXX	■
86812		X	HLA typing; A, B, or C (eg, A10, B7, B27), single antigen	0.00	1.14	1.14	0.00	1.14	1.14	XXX	■
	26			0.00	0.00	0.00	0.00	0.00	0.00	XXX	■
	TC			0.00	1.14	1.14	0.00	1.14	1.14	XXX	■
86813		X	A, B, or C, multiple antigens	0.00	1.63	1.63	0.00	1.63	1.63	XXX	■
	26			0.00	0.00	0.00	0.00	0.00	0.00	XXX	■
	TC			0.00	1.63	1.63	0.00	1.63	1.63	XXX	■
86816		X	DR/DQ, single antigen	0.00	1.55	1.55	0.00	1.55	1.55	XXX	■
	26			0.00	0.00	0.00	0.00	0.00	0.00	XXX	■
	TC			0.00	1.55	1.55	0.00	1.55	1.55	XXX	■
86817		X	DR/DQ, multiple antigens	0.00	4.46	4.46	0.00	4.46	4.46	XXX	■
	26			0.00	0.00	0.00	0.00	0.00	0.00	XXX	■
	TC			0.00	4.46	4.46	0.00	4.46	4.46	XXX	■
86821		X	lymphocyte culture, mixed (MLC)	0.00	3.48	3.48	0.00	3.48	3.48	XXX	■
	26			0.00	0.00	0.00	0.00	0.00	0.00	XXX	■
	TC			0.00	3.48	3.48	0.00	3.48	3.48	XXX	■
86822		X	lymphocyte culture, primed (PLC)	0.00	1.14	1.14	0.00	1.14	1.14	XXX	■
	26			0.00	0.00	0.00	0.00	0.00	0.00	XXX	■
	TC			0.00	1.14	1.14	0.00	1.14	1.14	XXX	■

■ RVU not developed by CMS. Gap-filled RVUs developed by Ingenix/CHEG.

Code	M	S	Description	Work Value	Non-Fac PE	Fac PE	Mal-practice	Non-Fac Total	Fac Total	Global	Gap
86849		X	Unlisted immunology procedure	0.00	0.00	0.00	0.00	0.00	0.00	XXX	
86850		X	Antibody screen, RBC, each serum technique	0.00	0.33	0.33	0.00	0.33	0.33	XXX	■
	26			0.00	0.00	0.00	0.00	0.00	0.00	XXX	■
	TC			0.00	0.33	0.33	0.00	0.33	0.33	XXX	■
86860		X	Antibody elution (RBC), each elution	0.00	0.33	0.33	0.00	0.33	0.33	XXX	■
	26			0.00	0.00	0.00	0.00	0.00	0.00	XXX	■
	TC			0.00	0.33	0.33	0.00	0.33	0.33	XXX	■
86870		X	Antibody identification, RBC antibodies, each panel for each serum technique	0.00	0.57	0.57	0.00	0.57	0.57	XXX	■
	26			0.00	0.00	0.00	0.00	0.00	0.00	XXX	■
	TC			0.00	0.57	0.57	0.00	0.57	0.57	XXX	■
86880		X	Antihuman globulin test (Coombs test); direct, each antiserum	0.00	0.18	0.18	0.00	0.18	0.18	XXX	■
	26			0.00	0.00	0.00	0.00	0.00	0.00	XXX	■
	TC			0.00	0.18	0.18	0.00	0.18	0.18	XXX	■
86885		X	indirect, qualitative, each antiserum	0.00	0.23	0.23	0.00	0.23	0.23	XXX	■
	26			0.00	0.00	0.00	0.00	0.00	0.00	XXX	■
	TC			0.00	0.23	0.23	0.00	0.23	0.23	XXX	■
86886		X	indirect, titer, each antiserum	0.00	0.29	0.29	0.00	0.29	0.29	XXX	■
	26			0.00	0.00	0.00	0.00	0.00	0.00	XXX	■
	TC			0.00	0.29	0.29	0.00	0.29	0.29	XXX	■
86890		X	Autologous blood or component, collection processing and storage; predeposited	0.00	1.31	1.31	0.00	1.31	1.31	XXX	■
	26			0.00	0.00	0.00	0.00	0.00	0.00	XXX	■
	TC			0.00	1.31	1.31	0.00	1.31	1.31	XXX	■
86891		X	intra- or postoperative salvage	0.00	2.04	2.04	0.00	2.04	2.04	XXX	■
	26			0.00	0.00	0.00	0.00	0.00	0.00	XXX	■
	TC			0.00	2.04	2.04	0.00	2.04	2.04	XXX	■
86900		X	Blood typing; ABO	0.00	0.18	0.18	0.00	0.18	0.18	XXX	■
	26			0.00	0.00	0.00	0.00	0.00	0.00	XXX	■
	TC			0.00	0.18	0.18	0.00	0.18	0.18	XXX	■
86901		X	Rh (D)	0.00	0.16	0.16	0.00	0.16	0.16	XXX	■
	26			0.00	0.00	0.00	0.00	0.00	0.00	XXX	■
	TC			0.00	0.16	0.16	0.00	0.16	0.16	XXX	■
86903		X	antigen screening for compatible blood unit using reagent serum, per unit screened	0.00	0.26	0.26	0.00	0.26	0.26	XXX	■
	26			0.00	0.00	0.00	0.00	0.00	0.00	XXX	■
	TC			0.00	0.26	0.26	0.00	0.26	0.26	XXX	■
86904		X	antigen screening for compatible unit using patient serum, per unit screened	0.00	0.24	0.24	0.00	0.24	0.24	XXX	■
	26			0.00	0.00	0.00	0.00	0.00	0.00	XXX	■
	TC			0.00	0.24	0.24	0.00	0.24	0.24	XXX	■
86905		X	RBC antigens, other than ABO or Rh (D), each	0.00	0.20	0.20	0.00	0.20	0.20	XXX	■
	26			0.00	0.00	0.00	0.00	0.00	0.00	XXX	■
	TC			0.00	0.20	0.20	0.00	0.20	0.20	XXX	■
86906		X	Rh phenotyping, complete	0.00	0.28	0.28	0.00	0.28	0.28	XXX	■
	26			0.00	0.00	0.00	0.00	0.00	0.00	XXX	■
	TC			0.00	0.28	0.28	0.00	0.28	0.28	XXX	■

Pathology

■ RVU not developed by CMS. Gap-filled RVUs developed by Ingenix/CHEG.

Code	M	S	Description	Work Value	Non-Fac PE	Fac PE	Mal-prac-tice	Non-Fac Total	Fac Total	Global	Gap
86910		N	Blood typing, for paternity testing, per individual; ABO, Rh and MN	0.00	0.36	0.36	0.00	0.36	0.36	XXX	■
	26			0.00	0.00	0.00	0.00	0.00	0.00	XXX	■
	TC			0.00	0.36	0.36	0.00	0.36	0.36	XXX	■
86911		N	each additional antigen system	0.00	0.28	0.28	0.00	0.28	0.28	XXX	■
	26			0.00	0.00	0.00	0.00	0.00	0.00	XXX	■
	TC			0.00	0.28	0.28	0.00	0.28	0.28	XXX	■
86915		X	Bone marrow or peripheral stem cell harvest, modification or treatment to eliminate cell type(s) (eg, T-cells, metastatic carcinoma)	0.00	1.71	1.71	0.00	1.71	1.71	XXX	■
	26			0.00	0.00	0.00	0.00	0.00	0.00	XXX	■
	TC			0.00	1.71	1.71	0.00	1.71	1.71	XXX	■
86920		X	Compatibility test each unit; immediate spin technique	0.00	0.36	0.36	0.00	0.36	0.36	XXX	■
	26			0.00	0.00	0.00	0.00	0.00	0.00	XXX	■
	TC			0.00	0.36	0.36	0.00	0.36	0.36	XXX	■
86921		X	incubation technique	0.00	0.33	0.33	0.00	0.33	0.33	XXX	■
	26			0.00	0.00	0.00	0.00	0.00	0.00	XXX	■
	TC			0.00	0.33	0.33	0.00	0.33	0.33	XXX	■
86922		X	antiglobulin technique	0.00	0.20	0.20	0.00	0.20	0.20	XXX	■
	26			0.00	0.00	0.00	0.00	0.00	0.00	XXX	■
	TC			0.00	0.20	0.20	0.00	0.20	0.20	XXX	■
86927		X	Fresh frozen plasma, thawing, each unit	0.00	0.18	0.18	0.00	0.18	0.18	XXX	■
	26			0.00	0.00	0.00	0.00	0.00	0.00	XXX	■
	TC			0.00	0.18	0.18	0.00	0.18	0.18	XXX	■
86930		X	Frozen blood, preparation for freezing, each unit;	0.00	1.63	1.63	0.00	1.63	1.63	XXX	■
	26			0.00	0.00	0.00	0.00	0.00	0.00	XXX	■
	TC			0.00	1.63	1.63	0.00	1.63	1.63	XXX	■
86931		X	with thawing	0.00	1.80	1.80	0.00	1.80	1.80	XXX	■
	26			0.00	0.00	0.00	0.00	0.00	0.00	XXX	■
	TC			0.00	1.80	1.80	0.00	1.80	1.80	XXX	■
86932		X	with freezing and thawing	0.00	1.96	1.96	0.00	1.96	1.96	XXX	■
	26			0.00	0.00	0.00	0.00	0.00	0.00	XXX	■
	TC			0.00	1.96	1.96	0.00	1.96	1.96	XXX	■
86940		X	Hemolysins and agglutinins; auto, screen, each	0.00	0.34	0.34	0.00	0.34	0.34	XXX	■
	26			0.00	0.00	0.00	0.00	0.00	0.00	XXX	■
	TC			0.00	0.34	0.34	0.00	0.34	0.34	XXX	■
86941		X	incubated	0.00	0.36	0.36	0.00	0.36	0.36	XXX	■
	26			0.00	0.00	0.00	0.00	0.00	0.00	XXX	■
	TC			0.00	0.36	0.36	0.00	0.36	0.36	XXX	■
86945		X	Irradiation of blood product, each unit	0.00	0.49	0.49	0.00	0.49	0.49	XXX	■
	26			0.00	0.00	0.00	0.00	0.00	0.00	XXX	■
	TC			0.00	0.49	0.49	0.00	0.49	0.49	XXX	■
86950		X	Leukocyte transfusion	0.00	0.90	0.90	0.00	0.90	0.90	XXX	■
	26			0.00	0.00	0.00	0.00	0.00	0.00	XXX	■
	TC			0.00	0.90	0.90	0.00	0.90	0.90	XXX	■
86965		X	Pooling of platelets or other blood products	0.00	0.23	0.23	0.00	0.23	0.23	XXX	■
	26			0.00	0.00	0.00	0.00	0.00	0.00	XXX	■
	TC			0.00	0.23	0.23	0.00	0.23	0.23	XXX	■

■ RVU not developed by CMS. Gap-filled RVUs developed by Ingenix/CHEG.

Code	M	S	Description	Work Value	Non-Fac PE	Fac PE	Mal-practice	Non-Fac Total	Fac Total	Global	Gap
86970		X	Pretreatment of RBC's for use in RBC antibody detection, identification, and/or compatibility testing; incubation with chemical agents or drugs, each	0.00	0.26	0.26	0.00	0.26	0.26	XXX	■
	26			0.00	0.00	0.00	0.00	0.00	0.00	XXX	■
	TC			0.00	0.26	0.26	0.00	0.26	0.26	XXX	■
86971		X	incubation with enzymes, each	0.00	0.26	0.26	0.00	0.26	0.26	XXX	■
	26			0.00	0.00	0.00	0.00	0.00	0.00	XXX	■
	TC			0.00	0.26	0.26	0.00	0.26	0.26	XXX	■
86972		X	by density gradient separation	0.00	0.24	0.24	0.00	0.24	0.24	XXX	■
	26			0.00	0.00	0.00	0.00	0.00	0.00	XXX	■
	TC			0.00	0.24	0.24	0.00	0.24	0.24	XXX	■
86975		X	Pretreatment of serum for use in RBC antibody identification; incubation with drugs, each	0.00	0.16	0.16	0.00	0.16	0.16	XXX	■
	26			0.00	0.00	0.00	0.00	0.00	0.00	XXX	■
	TC			0.00	0.16	0.16	0.00	0.16	0.16	XXX	■
86976		X	by dilution	0.00	0.13	0.13	0.00	0.13	0.13	XXX	■
	26			0.00	0.00	0.00	0.00	0.00	0.00	XXX	■
	TC			0.00	0.13	0.13	0.00	0.13	0.13	XXX	■
86977		X	incubation with inhibitors, each	0.00	0.16	0.16	0.00	0.16	0.16	XXX	■
	26			0.00	0.00	0.00	0.00	0.00	0.00	XXX	■
	TC			0.00	0.16	0.16	0.00	0.16	0.16	XXX	■
86978		X	by differential red cell absorption using patient RBC's or RBC's of known phenotype, each absorption	0.00	0.36	0.36	0.00	0.36	0.36	XXX	■
	26			0.00	0.00	0.00	0.00	0.00	0.00	XXX	■
	TC			0.00	0.36	0.36	0.00	0.36	0.36	XXX	■
86985		X	Splitting of blood or blood products, each unit	0.00	0.34	0.34	0.00	0.34	0.34	XXX	■
	26			0.00	0.00	0.00	0.00	0.00	0.00	XXX	■
	TC			0.00	0.34	0.34	0.00	0.34	0.34	XXX	■
86999		X	Unlisted transfusion medicine procedure	0.00	0.00	0.00	0.00	0.00	0.00	XXX	
87001		X	Animal inoculation, small animal; with observation	0.00	0.56	0.56	0.00	0.56	0.56	XXX	■
	26			0.00	0.00	0.00	0.00	0.00	0.00	XXX	■
	TC			0.00	0.56	0.56	0.00	0.56	0.56	XXX	■
87003		X	with observation and dissection	0.00	0.83	0.83	0.00	0.83	0.83	XXX	■
	26			0.00	0.00	0.00	0.00	0.00	0.00	XXX	■
	TC			0.00	0.83	0.83	0.00	0.83	0.83	XXX	■
87015		X	Concentration (any type), for infectious agents	0.00	0.44	0.44	0.00	0.44	0.44	XXX	■
	26			0.00	0.00	0.00	0.00	0.00	0.00	XXX	■
	TC			0.00	0.44	0.44	0.00	0.44	0.44	XXX	■
87040		X	Culture, bacterial; blood, with isolation and presumptive identification of isolates (includes anaerobic culture, if appropriate)	0.00	0.58	0.58	0.00	0.58	0.58	XXX	■
	26			0.00	0.00	0.00	0.00	0.00	0.00	XXX	■
	TC			0.00	0.58	0.58	0.00	0.58	0.58	XXX	■
87045		X	feces, with isolation and preliminary examination (eg, KIA, LIA), Salmonella and Shigella species	0.00	0.58	0.58	0.00	0.58	0.58	XXX	■
	26			0.00	0.00	0.00	0.00	0.00	0.00	XXX	■
	TC			0.00	0.58	0.58	0.00	0.58	0.58	XXX	■
87046		X	stool, additional pathogens, isolation and preliminary examination (eg, Campylobacter, Yersinia, Vibro, E. coli O157), each plate	0.00	0.58	0.58	0.00	0.58	0.58	XXX	■
	26			0.00	0.00	0.00	0.00	0.00	0.00	XXX	■
	TC			0.00	0.58	0.58	0.00	0.58	0.58	XXX	■

■ RVU not developed by CMS. Gap-filled RVUs developed by Ingenix/CHEG.

Pathology

Code	M	S	Description	Work Value	Non-Fac PE	Fac PE	Mal-practice	Non-Fac Total	Fac Total	Global	Gap
87070		X	any other source except urine, blood or stool, with isolation and presumptive identification of isolates	0.00	0.56	0.56	0.00	0.56	0.56	XXX	■
	26			0.00	0.00	0.00	0.00	0.00	0.00	XXX	■
	TC			0.00	0.56	0.56	0.00	0.56	0.56	XXX	■
87071		X	quantitative, aerobic with isolation and presumptive identification of isolates, any source except urine, blood or stool	0.00	0.58	0.58	0.00	0.58	0.58	XXX	■
	26			0.00	0.00	0.00	0.00	0.00	0.00	XXX	■
	TC			0.00	0.58	0.58	0.00	0.58	0.58	XXX	■
87073		X	quantitative, anaerobic with isolation and presumptive identification of isolates, any source except urine, blood or stool	0.00	0.64	0.64	0.00	0.64	0.64	XXX	■
	26			0.00	0.00	0.00	0.00	0.00	0.00	XXX	■
	TC			0.00	0.64	0.64	0.00	0.64	0.64	XXX	■
87075		X	any source, anaerobic with isolation and presumptive identification of isolates	0.00	0.64	0.64	0.00	0.64	0.64	XXX	■
	26			0.00	0.00	0.00	0.00	0.00	0.00	XXX	■
	TC			0.00	0.64	0.64	0.00	0.64	0.64	XXX	■
87076		X	anaerobic isolate, additional methods required for definitive identification, each isolate	0.00	0.64	0.64	0.00	0.64	0.64	XXX	■
	26			0.00	0.00	0.00	0.00	0.00	0.00	XXX	■
	TC			0.00	0.64	0.64	0.00	0.64	0.64	XXX	■
87077		X	aerobic isolate, additional methods required for definitive identification, each isolate	0.00	0.64	0.64	0.00	0.64	0.64	XXX	■
	26			0.00	0.00	0.00	0.00	0.00	0.00	XXX	■
	TC			0.00	0.64	0.64	0.00	0.64	0.64	XXX	■
87081		X	Culture, presumptive, pathogenic organisms, screening only;	0.00	0.33	0.33	0.00	0.33	0.33	XXX	■
	26			0.00	0.00	0.00	0.00	0.00	0.00	XXX	■
	TC			0.00	0.33	0.33	0.00	0.33	0.33	XXX	■
87084		X	with colony estimation from density chart	0.00	0.42	0.42	0.00	0.42	0.42	XXX	■
	26			0.00	0.00	0.00	0.00	0.00	0.00	XXX	■
	TC			0.00	0.42	0.42	0.00	0.42	0.42	XXX	■
87086		X	Culture, bacterial; quantitative colony count, urine	0.00	0.52	0.52	0.00	0.52	0.52	XXX	■
	26			0.00	0.00	0.00	0.00	0.00	0.00	XXX	■
	TC			0.00	0.52	0.52	0.00	0.52	0.52	XXX	■
87088		X	with isolation and presumptive identification of isolates, urine	0.00	0.50	0.50	0.00	0.50	0.50	XXX	■
	26			0.00	0.00	0.00	0.00	0.00	0.00	XXX	■
	TC			0.00	0.50	0.50	0.00	0.50	0.50	XXX	■
87101		X	Culture, fungi (mold or yeast) isolation, with presumptive identification of isolates; skin, hair, or nail	0.00	0.44	0.44	0.00	0.44	0.44	XXX	■
	26			0.00	0.00	0.00	0.00	0.00	0.00	XXX	■
	TC			0.00	0.44	0.44	0.00	0.44	0.44	XXX	■
87102		X	other source (except blood)	0.00	0.54	0.54	0.00	0.54	0.54	XXX	■
	26			0.00	0.00	0.00	0.00	0.00	0.00	XXX	■
	TC			0.00	0.54	0.54	0.00	0.54	0.54	XXX	■
87103		X	blood	0.00	0.62	0.62	0.00	0.62	0.62	XXX	■
	26			0.00	0.00	0.00	0.00	0.00	0.00	XXX	■
	TC			0.00	0.62	0.62	0.00	0.62	0.62	XXX	■
87106		X	Culture, fungi, definitive identification, each organism; yeast	0.00	0.56	0.56	0.00	0.56	0.56	XXX	■
	26			0.00	0.00	0.00	0.00	0.00	0.00	XXX	■
	TC			0.00	0.56	0.56	0.00	0.56	0.56	XXX	■
87107		X	mold	0.00	0.56	0.56	0.00	0.56	0.56	XXX	■
	26			0.00	0.00	0.00	0.00	0.00	0.00	XXX	■
	TC			0.00	0.56	0.56	0.00	0.56	0.56	XXX	■

■ RVU not developed by CMS. Gap-filled RVUs developed by Ingenix/CHEG.

Code	M	S	Description	Work Value	Non-Fac PE	Fac PE	Mal-practice	Non-Fac Total	Fac Total	Global	Gap
87109		X	Culture, mycoplasma, any source	0.00	1.19	1.19	0.00	1.19	1.19	XXX	■
	26			0.00	0.00	0.00	0.00	0.00	0.00	XXX	■
	TC			0.00	1.19	1.19	0.00	1.19	1.19	XXX	■
87110		X	Culture, chlamydia, any source	0.00	0.83	0.83	0.00	0.83	0.83	XXX	■
	26			0.00	0.00	0.00	0.00	0.00	0.00	XXX	■
	TC			0.00	0.83	0.83	0.00	0.83	0.83	XXX	■
87116		X	Culture, tubercle or other acid-fast bacilli (eg, TB, AFB, mycobacteria) any source, with isolation and presumptive identification of isolates	0.00	0.66	0.66	0.00	0.66	0.66	XXX	■
	26			0.00	0.00	0.00	0.00	0.00	0.00	XXX	■
	TC			0.00	0.66	0.66	0.00	0.66	0.66	XXX	■
87118		X	Culture, mycobacterial, definitive identification, each isolate	0.00	0.54	0.54	0.00	0.54	0.54	XXX	■
	26			0.00	0.00	0.00	0.00	0.00	0.00	XXX	■
	TC			0.00	0.54	0.54	0.00	0.54	0.54	XXX	■
87140		X	Culture, typing; immunofluorescent method, each antiserum	0.00	0.33	0.33	0.00	0.33	0.33	XXX	■
	26			0.00	0.00	0.00	0.00	0.00	0.00	XXX	■
	TC			0.00	0.33	0.33	0.00	0.33	0.33	XXX	■
87143		X	gas liquid chromatography (GLC) or high pressure liquid chromatography (HPLC) method	0.00	0.79	0.79	0.00	0.79	0.79	XXX	■
	26			0.00	0.00	0.00	0.00	0.00	0.00	XXX	■
	TC			0.00	0.79	0.79	0.00	0.79	0.79	XXX	■
87147		X	immunologic method, other than immunofluorescence (eg, agglutination grouping), per antiserum	0.00	0.29	0.29	0.00	0.29	0.29	XXX	■
	26			0.00	0.00	0.00	0.00	0.00	0.00	XXX	■
	TC			0.00	0.29	0.29	0.00	0.29	0.29	XXX	■
87149		X	identification by nucleic acid probe	0.00	0.83	0.83	0.00	0.83	0.83	XXX	■
	26			0.00	0.00	0.00	0.00	0.00	0.00	XXX	■
	TC			0.00	0.83	0.83	0.00	0.83	0.83	XXX	■
87152		X	identification by pulse field gel typing	0.00	0.20	0.20	0.00	0.20	0.20	XXX	■
	26			0.00	0.00	0.00	0.00	0.00	0.00	XXX	■
	TC			0.00	0.20	0.20	0.00	0.20	0.20	XXX	■
87158		X	other methods	0.00	0.28	0.28	0.00	0.28	0.28	XXX	■
	26			0.00	0.00	0.00	0.00	0.00	0.00	XXX	■
	TC			0.00	0.28	0.28	0.00	0.28	0.28	XXX	■
87164		X	Dark field examination, any source (eg, penile, vaginal, oral, skin); includes specimen collection	0.37	0.53	0.52	0.01	0.91	0.90	XXX	■
	26	A		0.37	0.12	0.11	0.01	0.50	0.49	XXX	
	TC			0.00	0.41	0.41	0.00	0.41	0.41	XXX	■
87166		X	without collection	0.00	0.52	0.52	0.00	0.52	0.52	XXX	■
	26			0.00	0.00	0.00	0.00	0.00	0.00	XXX	■
	TC			0.00	0.52	0.52	0.00	0.52	0.52	XXX	■
87168		X	Macroscopic examination; arthropod	0.00	0.17	0.17	0.00	0.17	0.17	XXX	■
	26			0.00	0.00	0.00	0.00	0.00	0.00	XXX	■
	TC			0.00	0.17	0.17	0.00	0.17	0.17	XXX	■
87169		X	parasite	0.00	0.17	0.17	0.00	0.17	0.17	XXX	■
	26			0.00	0.00	0.00	0.00	0.00	0.00	XXX	■
	TC			0.00	0.17	0.17	0.00	0.17	0.17	XXX	■

Pathology

■ RVU not developed by CMS. Gap-filled RVUs developed by Ingenix/CHEG.

Code	M	S	Description	Work Value	Non-Fac PE	Fac PE	Mal-practice	Non-Fac Total	Fac Total	Global	Gap
87172		X	Pinworm exam (eg, cellophane tape prep)	0.00	0.17	0.17	0.00	0.17	0.17	XXX	■
	26			0.00	0.00	0.00	0.00	0.00	0.00	XXX	■
	TC			0.00	0.17	0.17	0.00	0.17	0.17	XXX	■
87176		X	Homogenization, tissue, for culture	0.00	0.37	0.37	0.00	0.37	0.37	XXX	■
	26			0.00	0.00	0.00	0.00	0.00	0.00	XXX	■
	TC			0.00	0.37	0.37	0.00	0.37	0.37	XXX	■
87177		X	Ova and parasites, direct smears, concentration and identification	0.00	0.62	0.62	0.00	0.62	0.62	XXX	■
	26			0.00	0.00	0.00	0.00	0.00	0.00	XXX	■
	TC			0.00	0.62	0.62	0.00	0.62	0.62	XXX	■
87181		X	Susceptibility studies, antimicrobial agent; agar dilution method, per agent (eg, antibiotic gradient strip)	0.00	0.35	0.35	0.00	0.35	0.35	XXX	■
	26			0.00	0.00	0.00	0.00	0.00	0.00	XXX	■
	TC			0.00	0.35	0.35	0.00	0.35	0.35	XXX	■
87184		X	disk method, per plate (12 or fewer agents)	0.00	0.42	0.42	0.00	0.42	0.42	XXX	■
	26			0.00	0.00	0.00	0.00	0.00	0.00	XXX	■
	TC			0.00	0.42	0.42	0.00	0.42	0.42	XXX	■
87185		X	enzyme detection (eg, beta lactamase), per enzyme	0.00	0.42	0.42	0.00	0.42	0.42	XXX	■
	26			0.00	0.00	0.00	0.00	0.00	0.00	XXX	■
	TC			0.00	0.42	0.42	0.00	0.42	0.42	XXX	■
87186		X	microdilution or agar dilution (minimum inhibitory concentration (MIC) or breakpoint), each multi-antimicrobial, per plate	0.00	0.48	0.48	0.00	0.48	0.48	XXX	■
	26			0.00	0.00	0.00	0.00	0.00	0.00	XXX	■
	TC			0.00	0.48	0.48	0.00	0.48	0.48	XXX	■
87187		X	microdilution or agar dilution, minimum lethal concentration (MLC), each plate (List separately in addition to code for primary procedure)	0.00	0.48	0.48	0.00	0.48	0.48	XXX	■
	26			0.00	0.00	0.00	0.00	0.00	0.00	XXX	■
	TC			0.00	0.48	0.48	0.00	0.48	0.48	XXX	■
87188		X	macrobroth dilution method, each agent	0.00	0.48	0.48	0.00	0.48	0.48	XXX	■
	26			0.00	0.00	0.00	0.00	0.00	0.00	XXX	■
	TC			0.00	0.48	0.48	0.00	0.48	0.48	XXX	■
87190		X	mycobacteria, proportion method, each agent	0.00	0.31	0.31	0.00	0.31	0.31	XXX	■
	26			0.00	0.00	0.00	0.00	0.00	0.00	XXX	■
	TC			0.00	0.31	0.31	0.00	0.31	0.31	XXX	■
87197		X	Serum bactericidal titer (Schlicter test)	0.00	0.66	0.66	0.00	0.66	0.66	XXX	■
	26			0.00	0.00	0.00	0.00	0.00	0.00	XXX	■
	TC			0.00	0.66	0.66	0.00	0.66	0.66	XXX	■
87198		X	Cytomegalovirus, direct fluorescent antibody (DFA)	0.00	0.83	0.83	0.00	0.83	0.83	XXX	■
	26			0.00	0.00	0.00	0.00	0.00	0.00	XXX	■
	TC			0.00	0.83	0.83	0.00	0.83	0.83	XXX	■
87199		X	Enterovirus, direct fluorescent antibody (DFA)	0.00	0.83	0.83	0.00	0.83	0.83	XXX	■
	26			0.00	0.00	0.00	0.00	0.00	0.00	XXX	■
	TC			0.00	0.83	0.83	0.00	0.83	0.83	XXX	■
87205		X	Smear, primary source with interpretation; Gram or Giemsa stain for bacteria, fungi, or cell types	0.00	0.27	0.27	0.00	0.27	0.27	XXX	■
	26			0.00	0.00	0.00	0.00	0.00	0.00	XXX	■
	TC			0.00	0.27	0.27	0.00	0.27	0.27	XXX	■

Pathology

■ RVU not developed by CMS. Gap-filled RVUs developed by Ingenix/CHEG.

Code	M	S	Description	Work Value	Non-Fac PE	Fac PE	Mal-practice	Non-Fac Total	Fac Total	Global	Gap
87206		X	fluorescent and/or acid fast stain for bacteria, fungi, parasites, viruses or cell types	0.00	0.48	0.48	0.00	0.48	0.48	XXX	■
	26			0.00	0.00	0.00	0.00	0.00	0.00	XXX	■
	TC			0.00	0.48	0.48	0.00	0.48	0.48	XXX	■
87207		X	special stain for inclusion bodies or intracellular parasites (eg, malaria, coccidia, microsporidia, cytomegalovirus, herpes viruses)	0.37	0.41	0.40	0.01	0.79	0.78	XXX	■
	26	A		0.37	0.18	0.17	0.01	0.56	0.55	XXX	
	TC			0.00	0.23	0.23	0.00	0.23	0.23	XXX	■
87210		X	wet mount for infectious agents (eg, saline, India ink, KOH preps)	0.00	0.25	0.25	0.00	0.25	0.25	XXX	■
	26			0.00	0.00	0.00	0.00	0.00	0.00	XXX	■
	TC			0.00	0.25	0.25	0.00	0.25	0.25	XXX	■
87220		X	Tissue examination by KOH slide of samples from skin, hair, or nails for fungi or ectoparasite ova or mites (eg, scabies)	0.00	0.31	0.31	0.00	0.31	0.31	XXX	■
	26			0.00	0.00	0.00	0.00	0.00	0.00	XXX	■
	TC			0.00	0.31	0.31	0.00	0.31	0.31	XXX	■
87230		X	Toxin or antitoxin assay, tissue culture (eg, Clostridium difficile toxin)	0.00	0.94	0.94	0.00	0.94	0.94	XXX	■
	26			0.00	0.00	0.00	0.00	0.00	0.00	XXX	■
	TC			0.00	0.94	0.94	0.00	0.94	0.94	XXX	■
87250		X	Virus isolation; inoculation of embryonated eggs, or small animal, includes observation and dissection	0.00	1.12	1.12	0.00	1.12	1.12	XXX	■
	26			0.00	0.00	0.00	0.00	0.00	0.00	XXX	■
	TC			0.00	1.12	1.12	0.00	1.12	1.12	XXX	■
87252		X	tissue culture inoculation, observation, and presumptive identification by cytopathic effect	0.00	1.04	1.04	0.00	1.04	1.04	XXX	■
	26			0.00	0.00	0.00	0.00	0.00	0.00	XXX	■
	TC			0.00	1.04	1.04	0.00	1.04	1.04	XXX	■
87253		X	tissue culture, additional studies or definitive identification (eg, hemabsorption, neutralization, immunofluorescence stain), each isolate	0.00	1.04	1.04	0.00	1.04	1.04	XXX	■
	26			0.00	0.00	0.00	0.00	0.00	0.00	XXX	■
	TC			0.00	1.04	1.04	0.00	1.04	1.04	XXX	■
87254		X	shell vial, includes identification with immunofluorescence stain, each virus	0.00	1.04	1.04	0.00	1.04	1.04	XXX	■
	26			0.00	0.00	0.00	0.00	0.00	0.00	XXX	■
	TC			0.00	1.04	1.04	0.00	1.04	1.04	XXX	■
87260		X	Infectious agent antigen detection by immunofluorescent technique; adenovirus	0.00	0.83	0.83	0.00	0.83	0.83	XXX	■
	26			0.00	0.00	0.00	0.00	0.00	0.00	XXX	■
	TC			0.00	0.83	0.83	0.00	0.83	0.83	XXX	■
87265		X	Bordetella pertussis/parapertussis	0.00	0.83	0.83	0.00	0.83	0.83	XXX	■
	26			0.00	0.00	0.00	0.00	0.00	0.00	XXX	■
	TC			0.00	0.83	0.83	0.00	0.83	0.83	XXX	■
87270		X	Chlamydia trachomatis	0.00	0.83	0.83	0.00	0.83	0.83	XXX	■
	26			0.00	0.00	0.00	0.00	0.00	0.00	XXX	■
	TC			0.00	0.83	0.83	0.00	0.83	0.83	XXX	■
87272		X	cryptosporidium/giardia	0.00	0.83	0.83	0.00	0.83	0.83	XXX	■
	26			0.00	0.00	0.00	0.00	0.00	0.00	XXX	■
	TC			0.00	0.83	0.83	0.00	0.83	0.83	XXX	■
87273		X	Herpes simplex virus type 2	0.00	0.83	0.83	0.00	0.83	0.83	XXX	■
	26			0.00	0.00	0.00	0.00	0.00	0.00	XXX	■
	TC			0.00	0.83	0.83	0.00	0.83	0.83	XXX	■

Pathology

■ RVU not developed by CMS. Gap-filled RVUs developed by Ingenix/CHEG.

Code	M	S	Description	Work Value	Non-Fac PE	Fac PE	Mal-practice	Non-Fac Total	Fac Total	Global	Gap
87274		X	Herpes simplex virus type 1	0.00	0.83	0.83	0.00	0.83	0.83	XXX	■
	26			0.00	0.00	0.00	0.00	0.00	0.00	XXX	■
	TC			0.00	0.83	0.83	0.00	0.83	0.83	XXX	■
87275		X	Influenza B virus	0.00	0.83	0.83	0.00	0.83	0.83	XXX	■
	26			0.00	0.00	0.00	0.00	0.00	0.00	XXX	■
	TC			0.00	0.83	0.83	0.00	0.83	0.83	XXX	■
87276		X	Influenza A virus	0.00	0.83	0.83	0.00	0.83	0.83	XXX	■
	26			0.00	0.00	0.00	0.00	0.00	0.00	XXX	■
	TC			0.00	0.83	0.83	0.00	0.83	0.83	XXX	■
87277		X	Legionella micdadei	0.00	0.83	0.83	0.00	0.83	0.83	XXX	■
	26			0.00	0.00	0.00	0.00	0.00	0.00	XXX	■
	TC			0.00	0.83	0.83	0.00	0.83	0.83	XXX	■
87278		X	Legionella pneumophila	0.00	0.83	0.83	0.00	0.83	0.83	XXX	■
	26			0.00	0.00	0.00	0.00	0.00	0.00	XXX	■
	TC			0.00	0.83	0.83	0.00	0.83	0.83	XXX	■
87279		X	Parainfluenza virus, each type	0.00	0.83	0.83	0.00	0.83	0.83	XXX	■
	26			0.00	0.00	0.00	0.00	0.00	0.00	XXX	■
	TC			0.00	0.83	0.83	0.00	0.83	0.83	XXX	■
87280		X	respiratory syncytial virus	0.00	0.83	0.83	0.00	0.83	0.83	XXX	■
	26			0.00	0.00	0.00	0.00	0.00	0.00	XXX	■
	TC			0.00	0.83	0.83	0.00	0.83	0.83	XXX	■
87281		X	Pneumocystis carinii	0.00	0.83	0.83	0.00	0.83	0.83	XXX	■
	26			0.00	0.00	0.00	0.00	0.00	0.00	XXX	■
	TC			0.00	0.83	0.83	0.00	0.83	0.83	XXX	■
87283		X	Rubeola	0.00	0.83	0.83	0.00	0.83	0.83	XXX	■
	26			0.00	0.00	0.00	0.00	0.00	0.00	XXX	■
	TC			0.00	0.83	0.83	0.00	0.83	0.83	XXX	■
87285		X	Treponema pallidum	0.00	0.83	0.83	0.00	0.83	0.83	XXX	■
	26			0.00	0.00	0.00	0.00	0.00	0.00	XXX	■
	TC			0.00	0.83	0.83	0.00	0.83	0.83	XXX	■
87290		X	Varicella zoster virus	0.00	0.83	0.83	0.00	0.83	0.83	XXX	■
	26			0.00	0.00	0.00	0.00	0.00	0.00	XXX	■
	TC			0.00	0.83	0.83	0.00	0.83	0.83	XXX	■
87299		X	not otherwise specified, each organism	0.00	0.83	0.83	0.00	0.83	0.83	XXX	■
	26			0.00	0.00	0.00	0.00	0.00	0.00	XXX	■
	TC			0.00	0.83	0.83	0.00	0.83	0.83	XXX	■
87300		X	Infectious agent antigen detection by immunofluorescent technique, polyvalent for multiple organisms, each polyvalent antiserum	0.00	0.23	0.23	0.00	0.23	0.23	XXX	■
	26			0.00	0.00	0.00	0.00	0.00	0.00	XXX	■
	TC			0.00	0.23	0.23	0.00	0.23	0.23	XXX	■
87301		X	Infectious agent antigen detection by enzyme immunoassay technique, qualitative or semiquantitative, multiple step method; adenovirus enteric types 40/41	0.00	0.46	0.46	0.00	0.46	0.46	XXX	■
	26			0.00	0.00	0.00	0.00	0.00	0.00	XXX	■
	TC			0.00	0.46	0.46	0.00	0.46	0.46	XXX	■

■ RVU not developed by CMS. Gap-filled RVUs developed by Ingenix/CHEG.

Code	M	S	Description	Work Value	Non-Fac PE	Fac PE	Mal-prac-tice	Non-Fac Total	Fac Total	Global	Gap
87320		X	Chlamydia trachomatis	0.00	0.46	0.46	0.00	0.46	0.46	XXX	■
	26			0.00	0.00	0.00	0.00	0.00	0.00	XXX	■
	TC			0.00	0.46	0.46	0.00	0.46	0.46	XXX	■
87324		X	Clostridium difficile toxin(s)	0.00	0.46	0.46	0.00	0.46	0.46	XXX	■
	26			0.00	0.00	0.00	0.00	0.00	0.00	XXX	■
	TC			0.00	0.46	0.46	0.00	0.46	0.46	XXX	■
87327		X	Cryptococcus neoformans	0.00	0.46	0.46	0.00	0.46	0.46	XXX	■
	26			0.00	0.00	0.00	0.00	0.00	0.00	XXX	■
	TC			0.00	0.46	0.46	0.00	0.46	0.46	XXX	■
87328		X	cryptosporidum/giardia	0.00	0.46	0.46	0.00	0.46	0.46	XXX	■
	26			0.00	0.00	0.00	0.00	0.00	0.00	XXX	■
	TC			0.00	0.46	0.46	0.00	0.46	0.46	XXX	■
87332		X	cytomegalovirus	0.00	0.46	0.46	0.00	0.46	0.46	XXX	■
	26			0.00	0.00	0.00	0.00	0.00	0.00	XXX	■
	TC			0.00	0.46	0.46	0.00	0.46	0.46	XXX	■
87335		X	Escherichia coli 0157	0.00	0.46	0.46	0.00	0.46	0.46	XXX	■
	26			0.00	0.00	0.00	0.00	0.00	0.00	XXX	■
	TC			0.00	0.46	0.46	0.00	0.46	0.46	XXX	■
87336		X	Entamoeba histolytica dispar group	0.00	0.46	0.46	0.00	0.46	0.46	XXX	■
	26			0.00	0.00	0.00	0.00	0.00	0.00	XXX	■
	TC			0.00	0.46	0.46	0.00	0.46	0.46	XXX	■
87337		X	Entamoeba histolytica group	0.00	0.46	0.46	0.00	0.46	0.46	XXX	■
	26			0.00	0.00	0.00	0.00	0.00	0.00	XXX	■
	TC			0.00	0.46	0.46	0.00	0.46	0.46	XXX	■
87338		X	Infectious agent antigen detection by enzyme immunoassay technique, qualitative or semiquantitative, multiple step method; Helicobacter pylori, stool	0.00	0.55	0.55	0.00	0.55	0.55	XXX	■
	26			0.00	0.00	0.00	0.00	0.00	0.00	XXX	■
	TC			0.00	0.55	0.55	0.00	0.55	0.55	XXX	■
87339		X	Helicobacter pylori	0.00	0.46	0.46	0.00	0.46	0.46	XXX	■
	26			0.00	0.00	0.00	0.00	0.00	0.00	XXX	■
	TC			0.00	0.46	0.46	0.00	0.46	0.46	XXX	■
87340		X	hepatitis B surface antigen (HBsAg)	0.00	0.60	0.60	0.00	0.60	0.60	XXX	■
	26			0.00	0.00	0.00	0.00	0.00	0.00	XXX	■
	TC			0.00	0.60	0.60	0.00	0.60	0.60	XXX	■
87341		X	hepatitis B surface antigen (HBsAg) neutralization	0.00	0.46	0.46	0.00	0.46	0.46	XXX	■
	26			0.00	0.00	0.00	0.00	0.00	0.00	XXX	■
	TC			0.00	0.46	0.46	0.00	0.46	0.46	XXX	■
87350		X	hepatitis Be antigen (HBeAg)	0.00	0.71	0.71	0.00	0.71	0.71	XXX	■
	26			0.00	0.00	0.00	0.00	0.00	0.00	XXX	■
	TC			0.00	0.71	0.71	0.00	0.71	0.71	XXX	■
87380		X	hepatitis, delta agent	0.00	0.79	0.79	0.00	0.79	0.79	XXX	■
	26			0.00	0.00	0.00	0.00	0.00	0.00	XXX	■
	TC			0.00	0.79	0.79	0.00	0.79	0.79	XXX	■

Pathology

■ RVU not developed by CMS. Gap-filled RVUs developed by Ingenix/CHEG.

Code	M	S	Description	Work Value	Non-Fac PE	Fac PE	Mal-practice	Non-Fac Total	Fac Total	Global	Gap
87385		X	Histoplasma capsulatum	0.00	0.46	0.46	0.00	0.46	0.46	XXX	■
	26			0.00	0.00	0.00	0.00	0.00	0.00	XXX	■
	TC			0.00	0.46	0.46	0.00	0.46	0.46	XXX	■
87390		X	HIV-1	0.00	0.98	0.98	0.00	0.98	0.98	XXX	■
	26			0.00	0.00	0.00	0.00	0.00	0.00	XXX	■
	TC			0.00	0.98	0.98	0.00	0.98	0.98	XXX	■
87391		X	HIV-2	0.00	0.98	0.98	0.00	0.98	0.98	XXX	■
	26			0.00	0.00	0.00	0.00	0.00	0.00	XXX	■
	TC			0.00	0.98	0.98	0.00	0.98	0.98	XXX	■
87400		X	Influenza, A or B, each	0.00	0.46	0.46	0.00	0.46	0.46	XXX	■
	26			0.00	0.00	0.00	0.00	0.00	0.00	XXX	■
	TC			0.00	0.46	0.46	0.00	0.46	0.46	XXX	■
87420		X	respiratory syncytial virus	0.00	0.46	0.46	0.00	0.46	0.46	XXX	■
	26			0.00	0.00	0.00	0.00	0.00	0.00	XXX	■
	TC			0.00	0.46	0.46	0.00	0.46	0.46	XXX	■
87425		X	rotavirus	0.00	0.46	0.46	0.00	0.46	0.46	XXX	■
	26			0.00	0.00	0.00	0.00	0.00	0.00	XXX	■
	TC			0.00	0.46	0.46	0.00	0.46	0.46	XXX	■
87427		X	Shiga-like toxin	0.00	0.46	0.46	0.00	0.46	0.46	XXX	■
	26			0.00	0.00	0.00	0.00	0.00	0.00	XXX	■
	TC			0.00	0.46	0.46	0.00	0.46	0.46	XXX	■
87430		X	Streptococcus, group A	0.00	0.46	0.46	0.00	0.46	0.46	XXX	■
	26			0.00	0.00	0.00	0.00	0.00	0.00	XXX	■
	TC			0.00	0.46	0.46	0.00	0.46	0.46	XXX	■
87449		X	Infectious agent antigen detection by enzyme immunoassay technique qualitative or semiquantitative; multiple step method, not otherwise specified, each organism	0.00	0.46	0.46	0.00	0.46	0.46	XXX	■
	26			0.00	0.00	0.00	0.00	0.00	0.00	XXX	■
	TC			0.00	0.46	0.46	0.00	0.46	0.46	XXX	■
87450		X	single step method, not otherwise specified, each organism	0.00	0.46	0.46	0.00	0.46	0.46	XXX	■
	26			0.00	0.00	0.00	0.00	0.00	0.00	XXX	■
	TC			0.00	0.46	0.46	0.00	0.46	0.46	XXX	■
87451		X	multiple step method, polyvalent for multiple organisms, each polyvalent antiserum	0.00	0.37	0.37	0.00	0.37	0.37	XXX	■
	26			0.00	0.00	0.00	0.00	0.00	0.00	XXX	■
	TC			0.00	0.37	0.37	0.00	0.37	0.37	XXX	■
87470		X	Infectious agent detection by nucleic acid (DNA or RNA); Bartonella henselae and Bartonella quintana, direct probe technique	0.00	0.83	0.83	0.00	0.83	0.83	XXX	■
	26			0.00	0.00	0.00	0.00	0.00	0.00	XXX	■
	TC			0.00	0.83	0.83	0.00	0.83	0.83	XXX	■
87471		X	Bartonella henselae and Bartonella quintana, amplified probe technique	0.00	1.66	1.66	0.00	1.66	1.66	XXX	■
	26			0.00	0.00	0.00	0.00	0.00	0.00	XXX	■
	TC			0.00	1.66	1.66	0.00	1.66	1.66	XXX	■
87472		X	Bartonella henselae and Bartonella quintana, quantification	0.00	1.67	1.67	0.00	1.67	1.67	XXX	■
	26			0.00	0.00	0.00	0.00	0.00	0.00	XXX	■
	TC			0.00	1.67	1.67	0.00	1.67	1.67	XXX	■

■ RVU not developed by CMS. Gap-filled RVUs developed by Ingenix/CHEG.

Code	M	S	Description	Work Value	Non-Fac PE	Fac PE	Mal-practice	Non-Fac Total	Fac Total	Global	Gap
87475		X	Borrelia burgdorferi, direct probe technique	0.00	0.83	0.83	0.00	0.83	0.83	XXX	■
	26			0.00	0.00	0.00	0.00	0.00	0.00	XXX	■
	TC			0.00	0.83	0.83	0.00	0.83	0.83	XXX	■
87476		X	Borrelia burgdorferi, amplified probe technique	0.00	1.66	1.66	0.00	1.66	1.66	XXX	■
	26			0.00	0.00	0.00	0.00	0.00	0.00	XXX	■
	TC			0.00	1.66	1.66	0.00	1.66	1.66	XXX	■
87477		X	Borrelia burgdorferi, quantification	0.00	1.67	1.67	0.00	1.67	1.67	XXX	■
	26			0.00	0.00	0.00	0.00	0.00	0.00	XXX	■
	TC			0.00	1.67	1.67	0.00	1.67	1.67	XXX	■
87480		X	Candida species, direct probe technique	0.00	0.83	0.83	0.00	0.83	0.83	XXX	■
	26			0.00	0.00	0.00	0.00	0.00	0.00	XXX	■
	TC			0.00	0.83	0.83	0.00	0.83	0.83	XXX	■
87481		X	Candida species, amplified probe technique	0.00	1.66	1.66	0.00	1.66	1.66	XXX	■
	26			0.00	0.00	0.00	0.00	0.00	0.00	XXX	■
	TC			0.00	1.66	1.66	0.00	1.66	1.66	XXX	■
87482		X	Candida species, quantification	0.00	1.67	1.67	0.00	1.67	1.67	XXX	■
	26			0.00	0.00	0.00	0.00	0.00	0.00	XXX	■
	TC			0.00	1.67	1.67	0.00	1.67	1.67	XXX	■
87485		X	Chlamydia pneumoniae, direct probe technique	0.00	0.83	0.83	0.00	0.83	0.83	XXX	■
	26			0.00	0.00	0.00	0.00	0.00	0.00	XXX	■
	TC			0.00	0.83	0.83	0.00	0.83	0.83	XXX	■
87486		X	Chlamydia pneumoniae, amplified probe technique	0.00	1.66	1.66	0.00	1.66	1.66	XXX	■
	26			0.00	0.00	0.00	0.00	0.00	0.00	XXX	■
	TC			0.00	1.66	1.66	0.00	1.66	1.66	XXX	■
87487		X	Chlamydia pneumoniae, quantification	0.00	1.67	1.67	0.00	1.67	1.67	XXX	■
	26			0.00	0.00	0.00	0.00	0.00	0.00	XXX	■
	TC			0.00	1.67	1.67	0.00	1.67	1.67	XXX	■
87490		X	Chlamydia trachomatis, direct probe technique	0.00	0.83	0.83	0.00	0.83	0.83	XXX	■
	26			0.00	0.00	0.00	0.00	0.00	0.00	XXX	■
	TC			0.00	0.83	0.83	0.00	0.83	0.83	XXX	■
87491		X	Chlamydia trachomatis, amplified probe technique	0.00	1.66	1.66	0.00	1.66	1.66	XXX	■
	26			0.00	0.00	0.00	0.00	0.00	0.00	XXX	■
	TC			0.00	1.66	1.66	0.00	1.66	1.66	XXX	■
87492		X	Chlamydia trachomatis, quantification	0.00	1.67	1.67	0.00	1.67	1.67	XXX	■
	26			0.00	0.00	0.00	0.00	0.00	0.00	XXX	■
	TC			0.00	1.67	1.67	0.00	1.67	1.67	XXX	■
87495		X	cytomegalovirus, direct probe technique	0.00	0.83	0.83	0.00	0.83	0.83	XXX	■
	26			0.00	0.00	0.00	0.00	0.00	0.00	XXX	■
	TC			0.00	0.83	0.83	0.00	0.83	0.83	XXX	■
87496		X	cytomegalovirus, amplified probe technique	0.00	1.66	1.66	0.00	1.66	1.66	XXX	■
	26			0.00	0.00	0.00	0.00	0.00	0.00	XXX	■
	TC			0.00	1.66	1.66	0.00	1.66	1.66	XXX	■
87497		X	cytomegalovirus, quantification	0.00	1.67	1.67	0.00	1.67	1.67	XXX	■
	26			0.00	0.00	0.00	0.00	0.00	0.00	XXX	■
	TC			0.00	1.67	1.67	0.00	1.67	1.67	XXX	■

■ RVU not developed by CMS. Gap-filled RVUs developed by Ingenix/CHEG.

Code	M	S	Description	Work Value	Non-Fac PE	Fac PE	Mal-practice	Non-Fac Total	Fac Total	Global	Gap
87510		X	Gardnerella vaginalis, direct probe technique	0.00	0.83	0.83	0.00	0.83	0.83	XXX	■
	26			0.00	0.00	0.00	0.00	0.00	0.00	XXX	■
	TC			0.00	0.83	0.83	0.00	0.83	0.83	XXX	■
87511		X	Gardnerella vaginalis, amplified probe technique	0.00	1.66	1.66	0.00	1.66	1.66	XXX	■
	26			0.00	0.00	0.00	0.00	0.00	0.00	XXX	■
	TC			0.00	1.66	1.66	0.00	1.66	1.66	XXX	■
87512		X	Gardnerella vaginalis, quantification	0.00	1.67	1.67	0.00	1.67	1.67	XXX	■
	26			0.00	0.00	0.00	0.00	0.00	0.00	XXX	■
	TC			0.00	1.67	1.67	0.00	1.67	1.67	XXX	■
87515		X	hepatitis B virus, direct probe technique	0.00	0.83	0.83	0.00	0.83	0.83	XXX	■
	26			0.00	0.00	0.00	0.00	0.00	0.00	XXX	■
	TC			0.00	0.83	0.83	0.00	0.83	0.83	XXX	■
87516		X	hepatitis B virus, amplified probe technique	0.00	1.66	1.66	0.00	1.66	1.66	XXX	■
	26			0.00	0.00	0.00	0.00	0.00	0.00	XXX	■
	TC			0.00	1.66	1.66	0.00	1.66	1.66	XXX	■
87517		X	hepatitis B virus, quantification	0.00	1.67	1.67	0.00	1.67	1.67	XXX	■
	26			0.00	0.00	0.00	0.00	0.00	0.00	XXX	■
	TC			0.00	1.67	1.67	0.00	1.67	1.67	XXX	■
87520		X	hepatitis C, direct probe technique	0.00	0.83	0.83	0.00	0.83	0.83	XXX	■
	26			0.00	0.00	0.00	0.00	0.00	0.00	XXX	■
	TC			0.00	0.83	0.83	0.00	0.83	0.83	XXX	■
87521		X	hepatitis C, amplified probe technique	0.00	1.66	1.66	0.00	1.66	1.66	XXX	■
	26			0.00	0.00	0.00	0.00	0.00	0.00	XXX	■
	TC			0.00	1.66	1.66	0.00	1.66	1.66	XXX	■
87522		X	hepatitis C, quantification	0.00	1.67	1.67	0.00	1.67	1.67	XXX	■
	26			0.00	0.00	0.00	0.00	0.00	0.00	XXX	■
	TC			0.00	1.67	1.67	0.00	1.67	1.67	XXX	■
87525		X	hepatitis G, direct probe technique	0.00	0.83	0.83	0.00	0.83	0.83	XXX	■
	26			0.00	0.00	0.00	0.00	0.00	0.00	XXX	■
	TC			0.00	0.83	0.83	0.00	0.83	0.83	XXX	■
87526		X	hepatitis G, amplified probe technique	0.00	1.66	1.66	0.00	1.66	1.66	XXX	■
	26			0.00	0.00	0.00	0.00	0.00	0.00	XXX	■
	TC			0.00	1.66	1.66	0.00	1.66	1.66	XXX	■
87527		X	hepatitis G, quantification	0.00	1.67	1.67	0.00	1.67	1.67	XXX	■
	26			0.00	0.00	0.00	0.00	0.00	0.00	XXX	■
	TC			0.00	1.67	1.67	0.00	1.67	1.67	XXX	■
87528		X	Herpes simplex virus, direct probe technique	0.00	0.83	0.83	0.00	0.83	0.83	XXX	■
	26			0.00	0.00	0.00	0.00	0.00	0.00	XXX	■
	TC			0.00	0.83	0.83	0.00	0.83	0.83	XXX	■
87529		X	Herpes simplex virus, amplified probe technique	0.00	1.66	1.66	0.00	1.66	1.66	XXX	■
	26			0.00	0.00	0.00	0.00	0.00	0.00	XXX	■
	TC			0.00	1.66	1.66	0.00	1.66	1.66	XXX	■
87530		X	Herpes simplex virus, quantification	0.00	1.67	1.67	0.00	1.67	1.67	XXX	■
	26			0.00	0.00	0.00	0.00	0.00	0.00	XXX	■
	TC			0.00	1.67	1.67	0.00	1.67	1.67	XXX	■

■ RVU not developed by CMS. Gap-filled RVUs developed by Ingenix/CHEG.

Pathology

Code	M	S	Description	Work Value	Non-Fac PE	Fac PE	Mal-prac-tice	Non-Fac Total	Fac Total	Global	Gap
87531		X	Herpes virus-6, direct probe technique	0.00	0.83	0.83	0.00	0.83	0.83	XXX	■
	26			0.00	0.00	0.00	0.00	0.00	0.00	XXX	■
	TC			0.00	0.83	0.83	0.00	0.83	0.83	XXX	■
87532		X	Herpes virus-6, amplified probe technique	0.00	1.66	1.66	0.00	1.66	1.66	XXX	■
	26			0.00	0.00	0.00	0.00	0.00	0.00	XXX	■
	TC			0.00	1.66	1.66	0.00	1.66	1.66	XXX	■
87533		X	Herpes virus-6, quantification	0.00	1.67	1.67	0.00	1.67	1.67	XXX	■
	26			0.00	0.00	0.00	0.00	0.00	0.00	XXX	■
	TC			0.00	1.67	1.67	0.00	1.67	1.67	XXX	■
87534		X	HIV-1, direct probe technique	0.00	0.83	0.83	0.00	0.83	0.83	XXX	■
	26			0.00	0.00	0.00	0.00	0.00	0.00	XXX	■
	TC			0.00	0.83	0.83	0.00	0.83	0.83	XXX	■
87535		X	HIV-1, amplified probe technique	0.00	1.66	1.66	0.00	1.66	1.66	XXX	■
	26			0.00	0.00	0.00	0.00	0.00	0.00	XXX	■
	TC			0.00	1.66	1.66	0.00	1.66	1.66	XXX	■
87536		X	HIV-1, quantification	0.00	1.67	1.67	0.00	1.67	1.67	XXX	■
	26			0.00	0.00	0.00	0.00	0.00	0.00	XXX	■
	TC			0.00	1.67	1.67	0.00	1.67	1.67	XXX	■
87537		X	HIV-2, direct probe technique	0.00	0.83	0.83	0.00	0.83	0.83	XXX	■
	26			0.00	0.00	0.00	0.00	0.00	0.00	XXX	■
	TC			0.00	0.83	0.83	0.00	0.83	0.83	XXX	■
87538		X	HIV-2, amplified probe technique	0.00	1.66	1.66	0.00	1.66	1.66	XXX	■
	26			0.00	0.00	0.00	0.00	0.00	0.00	XXX	■
	TC			0.00	1.66	1.66	0.00	1.66	1.66	XXX	■
87539		X	HIV-2, quantification	0.00	1.67	1.67	0.00	1.67	1.67	XXX	■
	26			0.00	0.00	0.00	0.00	0.00	0.00	XXX	■
	TC			0.00	1.67	1.67	0.00	1.67	1.67	XXX	■
87540		X	Legionella pneumophila, direct probe technique	0.00	0.83	0.83	0.00	0.83	0.83	XXX	■
	26			0.00	0.00	0.00	0.00	0.00	0.00	XXX	■
	TC			0.00	0.83	0.83	0.00	0.83	0.83	XXX	■
87541		X	Legionella pneumophila, amplified probe technique	0.00	1.66	1.66	0.00	1.66	1.66	XXX	■
	26			0.00	0.00	0.00	0.00	0.00	0.00	XXX	■
	TC			0.00	1.66	1.66	0.00	1.66	1.66	XXX	■
87542		X	Legionella pneumophila, quantification	0.00	1.67	1.67	0.00	1.67	1.67	XXX	■
	26			0.00	0.00	0.00	0.00	0.00	0.00	XXX	■
	TC			0.00	1.67	1.67	0.00	1.67	1.67	XXX	■
87550		X	Mycobacteria species, direct probe technique	0.00	0.83	0.83	0.00	0.83	0.83	XXX	■
	26			0.00	0.00	0.00	0.00	0.00	0.00	XXX	■
	TC			0.00	0.83	0.83	0.00	0.83	0.83	XXX	■
87551		X	Mycobacteria species, amplified probe technique	0.00	1.66	1.66	0.00	1.66	1.66	XXX	■
	26			0.00	0.00	0.00	0.00	0.00	0.00	XXX	■
	TC			0.00	1.66	1.66	0.00	1.66	1.66	XXX	■
87552		X	Mycobacteria species, quantification	0.00	1.67	1.67	0.00	1.67	1.67	XXX	■
	26			0.00	0.00	0.00	0.00	0.00	0.00	XXX	■
	TC			0.00	1.67	1.67	0.00	1.67	1.67	XXX	■

■ RVU not developed by CMS. Gap-filled RVUs developed by Ingenix/CHEG.

Pathology

Code	M	S	Description	Work Value	Non-Fac PE	Fac PE	Mal-practice	Non-Fac Total	Fac Total	Global	Gap
87555		X	Mycobacteria tuberculosis, direct probe technique	0.00	0.83	0.83	0.00	0.83	0.83	XXX	■
	26			0.00	0.00	0.00	0.00	0.00	0.00	XXX	■
	TC			0.00	0.83	0.83	0.00	0.83	0.83	XXX	■
87556		X	Mycobacteria tuberculosis, amplified probe technique	0.00	1.66	1.66	0.00	1.66	1.66	XXX	■
	26			0.00	0.00	0.00	0.00	0.00	0.00	XXX	■
	TC			0.00	1.66	1.66	0.00	1.66	1.66	XXX	■
87557		X	Mycobacteria tuberculosis, quantification	0.00	1.67	1.67	0.00	1.67	1.67	XXX	■
	26			0.00	0.00	0.00	0.00	0.00	0.00	XXX	■
	TC			0.00	1.67	1.67	0.00	1.67	1.67	XXX	■
87560		X	Mycobacteria avium-intracellulare, direct probe technique	0.00	0.83	0.83	0.00	0.83	0.83	XXX	■
	26			0.00	0.00	0.00	0.00	0.00	0.00	XXX	■
	TC			0.00	0.83	0.83	0.00	0.83	0.83	XXX	■
87561		X	Mycobacteria avium-intracellulare, amplified probe technique	0.00	1.66	1.66	0.00	1.66	1.66	XXX	■
	26			0.00	0.00	0.00	0.00	0.00	0.00	XXX	■
	TC			0.00	1.66	1.66	0.00	1.66	1.66	XXX	■
87562		X	Mycobacteria avium-intracellulare, quantification	0.00	1.67	1.67	0.00	1.67	1.67	XXX	■
	26			0.00	0.00	0.00	0.00	0.00	0.00	XXX	■
	TC			0.00	1.67	1.67	0.00	1.67	1.67	XXX	■
87580		X	Mycoplasma pneumoniae, direct probe technique	0.00	0.83	0.83	0.00	0.83	0.83	XXX	■
	26			0.00	0.00	0.00	0.00	0.00	0.00	XXX	■
	TC			0.00	0.83	0.83	0.00	0.83	0.83	XXX	■
87581		X	Mycoplasma pneumoniae, amplified probe technique	0.00	1.66	1.66	0.00	1.66	1.66	XXX	■
	26			0.00	0.00	0.00	0.00	0.00	0.00	XXX	■
	TC			0.00	1.66	1.66	0.00	1.66	1.66	XXX	■
87582		X	Mycoplasma pneumoniae, quantification	0.00	1.67	1.67	0.00	1.67	1.67	XXX	■
	26			0.00	0.00	0.00	0.00	0.00	0.00	XXX	■
	TC			0.00	1.67	1.67	0.00	1.67	1.67	XXX	■
87590		X	Neisseria gonorrhoeae, direct probe technique	0.00	0.83	0.83	0.00	0.83	0.83	XXX	■
	26			0.00	0.00	0.00	0.00	0.00	0.00	XXX	■
	TC			0.00	0.83	0.83	0.00	0.83	0.83	XXX	■
87591		X	Neisseria gonorrhoeae, amplified probe technique	0.00	1.66	1.66	0.00	1.66	1.66	XXX	■
	26			0.00	0.00	0.00	0.00	0.00	0.00	XXX	■
	TC			0.00	1.66	1.66	0.00	1.66	1.66	XXX	■
87592		X	Neisseria gonorrhoeae, quantification	0.00	1.67	1.67	0.00	1.67	1.67	XXX	■
	26			0.00	0.00	0.00	0.00	0.00	0.00	XXX	■
	TC			0.00	1.67	1.67	0.00	1.67	1.67	XXX	■
87620		X	papillomavirus, human, direct probe technique	0.00	0.83	0.83	0.00	0.83	0.83	XXX	■
	26			0.00	0.00	0.00	0.00	0.00	0.00	XXX	■
	TC			0.00	0.83	0.83	0.00	0.83	0.83	XXX	■
87621		X	papillomavirus, human, amplified probe technique	0.00	1.66	1.66	0.00	1.66	1.66	XXX	■
	26			0.00	0.00	0.00	0.00	0.00	0.00	XXX	■
	TC			0.00	1.66	1.66	0.00	1.66	1.66	XXX	■
87622		X	papillomavirus, human, quantification	0.00	1.67	1.67	0.00	1.67	1.67	XXX	■
	26			0.00	0.00	0.00	0.00	0.00	0.00	XXX	■
	TC			0.00	1.67	1.67	0.00	1.67	1.67	XXX	■

■ RVU not developed by CMS. Gap-filled RVUs developed by Ingenix/CHEG.

Code	M	S	Description	Work Value	Non-Fac PE	Fac PE	Mal-prac-tice	Non-Fac Total	Fac Total	Global	Gap
87650		X	Streptococcus, group A, direct probe technique	0.00	0.83	0.83	0.00	0.83	0.83	XXX	■
	26			0.00	0.00	0.00	0.00	0.00	0.00	XXX	■
	TC			0.00	0.83	0.83	0.00	0.83	0.83	XXX	■
87651		X	Streptococcus, group A, amplified probe technique	0.00	1.66	1.66	0.00	1.66	1.66	XXX	■
	26			0.00	0.00	0.00	0.00	0.00	0.00	XXX	■
	TC			0.00	1.66	1.66	0.00	1.66	1.66	XXX	■
87652		X	Streptococcus, group A, quantification	0.00	1.67	1.67	0.00	1.67	1.67	XXX	■
	26			0.00	0.00	0.00	0.00	0.00	0.00	XXX	■
	TC			0.00	1.67	1.67	0.00	1.67	1.67	XXX	■
87797		X	Infectious agent detection by nucleic acid (DNA or RNA), not otherwise specified; direct probe technique, each organism	0.00	0.83	0.83	0.00	0.83	0.83	XXX	■
	26			0.00	0.00	0.00	0.00	0.00	0.00	XXX	■
	TC			0.00	0.83	0.83	0.00	0.83	0.83	XXX	■
87798		X	amplified probe technique, each organism	0.00	1.66	1.66	0.00	1.66	1.66	XXX	■
	26			0.00	0.00	0.00	0.00	0.00	0.00	XXX	■
	TC			0.00	1.66	1.66	0.00	1.66	1.66	XXX	■
87799		X	quantification, each organism	0.00	1.67	1.67	0.00	1.67	1.67	XXX	■
	26			0.00	0.00	0.00	0.00	0.00	0.00	XXX	■
	TC			0.00	1.67	1.67	0.00	1.67	1.67	XXX	■
87800		X	Infectious agent detection by nucleic acid (DNA or RNA), multiple organisms; direct probe(s) technique	0.00	0.77	0.77	0.00	0.77	0.77	XXX	■
	26			0.00	0.00	0.00	0.00	0.00	0.00	XXX	■
	TC			0.00	0.77	0.77	0.00	0.77	0.77	XXX	■
87801		X	amplified probe(s) technique	0.00	1.34	1.34	0.00	1.34	1.34	XXX	■
	26			0.00	0.00	0.00	0.00	0.00	0.00	XXX	■
	TC			0.00	1.34	1.34	0.00	1.34	1.34	XXX	■
87802		X	Infectious agent antigen detection by immunoassay with direct optical observation; Streptococcus, group B	0.00	0.73	0.73	0.00	0.73	0.73	XXX	■
	26			0.00	0.00	0.00	0.00	0.00	0.00	XXX	■
	TC			0.00	0.73	0.73	0.00	0.73	0.73	XXX	■
87803		X	Clostridium difficile toxin A	0.00	0.73	0.73	0.00	0.73	0.73	XXX	■
	26			0.00	0.00	0.00	0.00	0.00	0.00	XXX	■
	TC			0.00	0.73	0.73	0.00	0.73	0.73	XXX	■
87804		X	Influenza	0.00	0.73	0.73	0.00	0.73	0.73	XXX	■
	26			0.00	0.00	0.00	0.00	0.00	0.00	XXX	■
	TC			0.00	0.73	0.73	0.00	0.73	0.73	XXX	■
87810		X	Infectious agent detection by immunoassay with direct optical observation; Chlamydia trachomatis	0.00	0.73	0.73	0.00	0.73	0.73	XXX	■
	26			0.00	0.00	0.00	0.00	0.00	0.00	XXX	■
	TC			0.00	0.73	0.73	0.00	0.73	0.73	XXX	■
87850		X	Neisseria gonorrhoeae	0.00	0.73	0.73	0.00	0.73	0.73	XXX	■
	26			0.00	0.00	0.00	0.00	0.00	0.00	XXX	■
	TC			0.00	0.73	0.73	0.00	0.73	0.73	XXX	■
87880		X	Streptococcus, group A	0.00	0.73	0.73	0.00	0.73	0.73	XXX	■
	26			0.00	0.00	0.00	0.00	0.00	0.00	XXX	■
	TC			0.00	0.73	0.73	0.00	0.73	0.73	XXX	■
87899		X	not otherwise specified	0.00	0.73	0.73	0.00	0.73	0.73	XXX	■
	26			0.00	0.00	0.00	0.00	0.00	0.00	XXX	■
	TC			0.00	0.73	0.73	0.00	0.73	0.73	XXX	■

Pathology

■ RVU not developed by CMS. Gap-filled RVUs developed by Ingenix/CHEG.

Code	M	S	Description	Work Value	Non-Fac PE	Fac PE	Mal-practice	Non-Fac Total	Fac Total	Global	Gap
87901		X	Infectious agent genotype analysis by nucleic acid (DNA or RNA), HIV 1, reverse transcriptase and protease	0.00	9.83	9.83	0.00	9.83	9.83	XXX	■
	26			0.00	0.00	0.00	0.00	0.00	0.00	XXX	■
	TC			0.00	9.83	9.83	0.00	9.83	9.83	XXX	■
87902		X	Hepatitis C virus	0.00	9.83	9.83	0.00	9.83	9.83	XXX	■
	26			0.00	0.00	0.00	0.00	0.00	0.00	XXX	■
	TC			0.00	9.83	9.83	0.00	9.83	9.83	XXX	■
87903		X	Infectious agent phenotype analysis by nucleic acid (DNA or RNA) with drug resistance tissue culture analysis, HIV 1; first through 10 drugs tested	0.00	18.65	18.65	0.00	18.65	18.65	XXX	■
	26			0.00	0.00	0.00	0.00	0.00	0.00	XXX	■
	TC			0.00	18.65	18.65	0.00	18.65	18.65	XXX	■
87904		X	Infectious agent phenotype analysis by nucleic acid (DNA or RNA) with drug resistance tissue culture analysis, HIV 1; each additional 1 through 5 drugs tested (List separately in addition to code for primary procedure)	0.00	1.00	1.00	0.00	1.00	1.00	XXX	■
	26			0.00	0.00	0.00	0.00	0.00	0.00	XXX	■
	TC			0.00	1.00	1.00	0.00	1.00	1.00	XXX	■
87999		X	Unlisted microbiology procedure	0.00	0.00	0.00	0.00	0.00	0.00	XXX	
88000		N	Necropsy (autopsy), gross examination only; without CNS	0.00	6.27	6.27	0.00	6.27	6.27	XXX	■
88005		N	with brain	0.00	6.97	6.97	0.00	6.97	6.97	XXX	■
88007		N	with brain and spinal cord	0.00	7.67	7.67	0.00	7.67	7.67	XXX	■
88012		N	infant with brain	0.00	5.78	5.78	0.00	5.78	5.78	XXX	■
88014		N	stillborn or newborn with brain	0.00	5.78	5.78	0.00	5.78	5.78	XXX	■
88016		N	macerated stillborn	0.00	7.02	7.02	0.00	7.02	7.02	XXX	■
88020		N	Necropsy (autopsy), gross and microscopic; without CNS	0.00	9.01	9.01	0.00	9.01	9.01	XXX	■
88025		N	with brain	0.00	9.71	9.71	0.00	9.71	9.71	XXX	■
88027		N	with brain and spinal cord	0.00	10.41	10.41	0.00	10.41	10.41	XXX	■
88028		N	infant with brain	0.00	5.78	5.78	0.00	5.78	5.78	XXX	■
88029		N	stillborn or newborn with brain	0.00	5.78	5.78	0.00	5.78	5.78	XXX	■
88036		N	Necropsy (autopsy), limited, gross and/or microscopic; regional	0.00	3.74	3.74	0.00	3.74	3.74	XXX	■
88037		N	single organ	0.00	2.74	2.74	0.00	2.74	2.74	XXX	■
88040		N	Necropsy (autopsy); forensic examination	0.00	14.94	14.94	0.00	14.94	14.94	XXX	■
88045		N	coroner's call	0.00	1.25	1.25	0.00	1.25	1.25	XXX	■
88099		N	Unlisted necropsy (autopsy) procedure	0.00	0.00	0.00	0.00	0.00	0.00	XXX	
88104		A	Cytopathology, fluids, washings or brushings, except cervical or vaginal; smears with interpretation	0.56	0.72	0.72	0.04	1.32	1.32	XXX	
	26	A		0.56	0.26	0.26	0.02	0.84	0.84	XXX	
	TC	A		0.00	0.46	0.46	0.02	0.48	0.48	XXX	

Pathology

■ RVU not developed by CMS. Gap-filled RVUs developed by Ingenix/CHEG.

Code	M	S	Description	Work Value	Non-Fac PE	Fac PE	Mal-practice	Non-Fac Total	Fac Total	Global	Gap
88106		A	filter method only with interpretation	0.56	0.72	0.72	0.04	1.32	1.32	XXX	
	26	A		0.56	0.26	0.26	0.02	0.84	0.84	XXX	
	TC	A		0.00	0.46	0.46	0.02	0.48	0.48	XXX	
88107		A	smears and filter preparation with interpretation	0.76	1.01	1.01	0.05	1.82	1.82	XXX	
	26	A		0.76	0.35	0.35	0.03	1.14	1.14	XXX	
	TC	A		0.00	0.66	0.66	0.02	0.68	0.68	XXX	
88108		A	Cytopathology, concentration technique, smears and interpretation (eg, Saccomanno technique)	0.56	0.94	0.94	0.04	1.54	1.54	XXX	
	26	A		0.56	0.26	0.26	0.02	0.84	0.84	XXX	
	TC	A		0.00	0.68	0.68	0.02	0.70	0.70	XXX	
88125		A	Cytopathology, forensic (eg, sperm)	0.26	0.30	0.30	0.02	0.58	0.58	XXX	
	26	A		0.26	0.12	0.12	0.01	0.39	0.39	XXX	
	TC	A		0.00	0.18	0.18	0.01	0.19	0.19	XXX	
88130		X	Sex chromatin identification; Barr bodies	0.00	0.62	0.62	0.00	0.62	0.62	XXX	■
	26			0.00	0.06	0.06	0.00	0.06	0.06	XXX	■
	TC			0.00	0.56	0.56	0.00	0.56	0.56	XXX	■
88140		X	peripheral blood smear, polymorphonuclear drumsticks	0.00	0.50	0.50	0.00	0.50	0.50	XXX	■
	26			0.00	0.00	0.00	0.00	0.00	0.00	XXX	■
	TC			0.00	0.50	0.50	0.00	0.50	0.50	XXX	■
88141		A	Cytopathology, cervical or vaginal (any reporting system); requiring interpretation by physician (List separately in addition to code for technical service)	0.42	0.19	0.19	0.01	0.62	0.62	XXX	
88142		X	Cytopathology, cervical or vaginal (any reporting system), collected in preservative fluid, automated thin layer preparation; manual screening under physician supervision	0.00	0.42	0.42	0.00	0.42	0.42	XXX	■
	26			0.00	0.00	0.00	0.00	0.00	0.00	XXX	■
	TC			0.00	0.42	0.42	0.00	0.42	0.42	XXX	■
88143		X	with manual screening and rescreening under physician supervision	0.00	0.47	0.47	0.00	0.47	0.47	XXX	■
	26			0.00	0.00	0.00	0.00	0.00	0.00	XXX	■
	TC			0.00	0.47	0.47	0.00	0.47	0.47	XXX	■
88144		X	with manual screening and computer-assisted rescreening under physician supervision	0.00	0.44	0.44	0.00	0.44	0.44	XXX	■
	26			0.00	0.00	0.00	0.00	0.00	0.00	XXX	■
	TC			0.00	0.44	0.44	0.00	0.44	0.44	XXX	■
88145		X	with manual screening and computer-assisted rescreening using cell selection and review under physician supervision	0.00	0.49	0.49	0.00	0.49	0.49	XXX	■
	26			0.00	0.00	0.00	0.00	0.00	0.00	XXX	■
	TC			0.00	0.49	0.49	0.00	0.49	0.49	XXX	■
88147		X	Cytopathology smears, cervical or vaginal; screening by automated system under physician supervision	0.00	0.44	0.44	0.00	0.44	0.44	XXX	■
	26			0.00	0.00	0.00	0.00	0.00	0.00	XXX	■
	TC			0.00	0.44	0.44	0.00	0.44	0.44	XXX	■
88148		X	screening by automated system with manual rescreening under physician supervision	0.00	0.47	0.47	0.00	0.47	0.47	XXX	■
	26			0.00	0.00	0.00	0.00	0.00	0.00	XXX	■
	TC			0.00	0.47	0.47	0.00	0.47	0.47	XXX	■
88150		X	Cytopathology, slides, cervical or vaginal; manual screening under physician supervision	0.00	0.42	0.42	0.00	0.42	0.42	XXX	■
	26			0.00	0.00	0.00	0.00	0.00	0.00	XXX	■
	TC			0.00	0.42	0.42	0.00	0.42	0.42	XXX	■

Pathology

■ RVU not developed by CMS. Gap-filled RVUs developed by Ingenix/CHEG.

Code	M	S	Description	Work Value	Non-Fac PE	Fac PE	Mal-practice	Non-Fac Total	Fac Total	Global	Gap
88152		X	with manual screening and computer-assisted rescreening under physician supervision	0.00	0.44	0.44	0.00	0.44	0.44	XXX	■
	26			0.00	0.00	0.00	0.00	0.00	0.00	XXX	■
	TC			0.00	0.44	0.44	0.00	0.44	0.44	XXX	■
88153		X	with manual screening and rescreening under physician supervision	0.00	0.47	0.47	0.00	0.47	0.47	XXX	■
	26			0.00	0.00	0.00	0.00	0.00	0.00	XXX	■
	TC			0.00	0.47	0.47	0.00	0.47	0.47	XXX	■
88154		X	with manual screening and computer-assisted rescreening using cell selection and review under physician supervision	0.00	0.49	0.49	0.00	0.49	0.49	XXX	■
	26			0.00	0.00	0.00	0.00	0.00	0.00	XXX	■
	TC			0.00	0.49	0.49	0.00	0.49	0.49	XXX	■
88155		X	Cytopathology, slides, cervical or vaginal, definitive hormonal evaluation (eg, maturation index, karyopyknotic index, estrogenic index) (List separately in addition to code(s) for other technical and interpretation services)	0.00	0.47	0.47	0.00	0.47	0.47	XXX	■
	26			0.00	0.00	0.00	0.00	0.00	0.00	XXX	■
	TC			0.00	0.47	0.47	0.00	0.47	0.47	XXX	■
88160		A	Cytopathology, smears, any other source; screening and interpretation	0.50	1.01	1.01	0.04	1.55	1.55	XXX	
	26	A		0.50	0.23	0.23	0.02	0.75	0.75	XXX	
	TC	A		0.00	0.78	0.78	0.02	0.80	0.80	XXX	
88161		A	preparation, screening and interpretation	0.50	1.22	1.22	0.04	1.76	1.76	XXX	
	26	A		0.50	0.23	0.23	0.02	0.75	0.75	XXX	
	TC	A		0.00	0.99	0.99	0.02	1.01	1.01	XXX	
88162		A	extended study involving over 5 slides and/or multiple stains	0.76	0.73	0.73	0.05	1.54	1.54	XXX	
	26	A		0.76	0.35	0.35	0.03	1.14	1.14	XXX	
	TC	A		0.00	0.38	0.38	0.02	0.40	0.40	XXX	
88164		X	Cytopathology, slides, cervical or vaginal (the Bethesda System); manual screening under physician supervision	0.00	0.42	0.42	0.00	0.42	0.42	XXX	■
	26			0.00	0.00	0.00	0.00	0.00	0.00	XXX	■
	TC			0.00	0.42	0.42	0.00	0.42	0.42	XXX	■
88165		X	with manual screening and rescreening under physician supervision	0.00	0.47	0.47	0.00	0.47	0.47	XXX	■
	26			0.00	0.00	0.00	0.00	0.00	0.00	XXX	■
	TC			0.00	0.47	0.47	0.00	0.47	0.47	XXX	■
88166		X	with manual screening and computer-assisted rescreening under physician supervision	0.00	0.44	0.44	0.00	0.44	0.44	XXX	■
	26			0.00	0.00	0.00	0.00	0.00	0.00	XXX	■
	TC			0.00	0.44	0.44	0.00	0.44	0.44	XXX	■
88167		X	with manual screening and computer-assisted rescreening using cell selection and review under physician supervision	0.00	0.49	0.49	0.00	0.49	0.49	XXX	■
	26			0.00	0.00	0.00	0.00	0.00	0.00	XXX	■
	TC			0.00	0.49	0.49	0.00	0.49	0.49	XXX	■
88172		A	Cytopathology, evaluation of fine needle aspirate; immediate cytohistologic study to determine adequacy of specimen(s)	0.60	0.68	0.68	0.04	1.32	1.32	XXX	
	26	A		0.60	0.28	0.28	0.02	0.90	0.90	XXX	
	TC	A		0.00	0.40	0.40	0.02	0.42	0.42	XXX	
88173		A	interpretation and report	1.39	1.80	1.80	0.07	3.26	3.26	XXX	
	26	A		1.39	0.64	0.64	0.05	2.08	2.08	XXX	
	TC	A		0.00	1.16	1.16	0.02	1.18	1.18	XXX	
88180		A	Flow cytometry; each cell surface, cytoplasmic or nuclear marker	0.36	0.60	0.60	0.03	0.99	0.99	XXX	
	26	A		0.36	0.17	0.17	0.01	0.54	0.54	XXX	
	TC	A		0.00	0.43	0.43	0.02	0.45	0.45	XXX	

Pathology

■ RVU not developed by CMS. Gap-filled RVUs developed by Ingenix/CHEG.

Code	M	S	Description	Work Value	Non-Fac PE	Fac PE	Mal-practice	Non-Fac Total	Fac Total	Global	Gap
88182		A	cell cycle or DNA analysis	0.77	1.81	1.81	0.06	2.64	2.64	XXX	
	26	A		0.77	0.36	0.36	0.03	1.16	1.16	XXX	
	TC	A		0.00	1.45	1.45	0.03	1.48	1.48	XXX	
88199		C	Unlisted cytopathology procedure	0.00	0.00	0.00	0.00	0.00	0.00	XXX	
	26	C		0.00	0.00	0.00	0.00	0.00	0.00	XXX	
	TC	C		0.00	0.00	0.00	0.00	0.00	0.00	XXX	
88230		X	Tissue culture for non-neoplastic disorders; lymphocyte	0.00	2.08	2.08	0.00	2.08	2.08	XXX	■
	26			0.00	0.00	0.00	0.00	0.00	0.00	XXX	■
	TC			0.00	2.08	2.08	0.00	2.08	2.08	XXX	■
88233		X	skin or other solid tissue biopsy	0.00	0.79	0.79	0.00	0.79	0.79	XXX	■
	26			0.00	0.00	0.00	0.00	0.00	0.00	XXX	■
	TC			0.00	0.79	0.79	0.00	0.79	0.79	XXX	■
88235		X	amniotic fluid or chorionic villus cells	0.00	4.43	4.43	0.00	4.43	4.43	XXX	■
	26			0.00	0.00	0.00	0.00	0.00	0.00	XXX	■
	TC			0.00	4.43	4.43	0.00	4.43	4.43	XXX	■
88237		X	Tissue culture for neoplastic disorders; bone marrow, blood cells	0.00	3.41	3.41	0.00	3.41	3.41	XXX	■
	26			0.00	0.00	0.00	0.00	0.00	0.00	XXX	■
	TC			0.00	3.41	3.41	0.00	3.41	3.41	XXX	■
88239		X	solid tumor	0.00	1.35	1.35	0.00	1.35	1.35	XXX	■
	26			0.00	0.00	0.00	0.00	0.00	0.00	XXX	■
	TC			0.00	1.35	1.35	0.00	1.35	1.35	XXX	■
88240		X	Cryopreservation, freezing and storage of cells, each cell line	0.00	1.93	1.93	0.00	1.93	1.93	XXX	■
	26			0.00	0.00	0.00	0.00	0.00	0.00	XXX	■
	TC			0.00	1.93	1.93	0.00	1.93	1.93	XXX	■
88241		X	Thawing and expansion of frozen cells, each aliquot	0.00	2.12	2.12	0.00	2.12	2.12	XXX	■
	26			0.00	0.00	0.00	0.00	0.00	0.00	XXX	■
	TC			0.00	2.12	2.12	0.00	2.12	2.12	XXX	■
88245		X	Chromosome analysis for breakage syndromes; baseline Sister Chromatid Exchange (SCE), 20-25 cells	0.00	2.60	2.60	0.00	2.60	2.60	XXX	■
	26			0.00	0.00	0.00	0.00	0.00	0.00	XXX	■
	TC			0.00	2.60	2.60	0.00	2.60	2.60	XXX	■
88248		X	baseline breakage, score 50-100 cells, count 20 cells, 2 karyotypes (eg, for ataxia telangiectasia, Fanconi anemia, fragile X)	0.00	5.20	5.20	0.00	5.20	5.20	XXX	■
	26			0.00	0.00	0.00	0.00	0.00	0.00	XXX	■
	TC			0.00	5.20	5.20	0.00	5.20	5.20	XXX	■
88249		X	score 100 cells, clastogen stress (eg, diepoxybutane, mitomycin C, ionizing radiation, UV radiation)	0.00	5.78	5.78	0.00	5.78	5.78	XXX	■
	26			0.00	0.00	0.00	0.00	0.00	0.00	XXX	■
	TC			0.00	5.78	5.78	0.00	5.78	5.78	XXX	■
88261		X	Chromosome analysis; count 5 cells, 1 karyotype, with banding	0.00	4.52	4.52	0.00	4.52	4.52	XXX	■
	26			0.00	0.00	0.00	0.00	0.00	0.00	XXX	■
	TC			0.00	4.52	4.52	0.00	4.52	4.52	XXX	■
88262		X	count 15-20 cells, 2 karyotypes, with banding	0.00	6.06	6.06	0.00	6.06	6.06	XXX	■
	26			0.00	0.00	0.00	0.00	0.00	0.00	XXX	■
	TC			0.00	6.06	6.06	0.00	6.06	6.06	XXX	■
88263		X	count 45 cells for mosaicism, 2 karyotypes, with banding	0.00	6.24	6.24	0.00	6.24	6.24	XXX	■
	26			0.00	0.00	0.00	0.00	0.00	0.00	XXX	■
	TC			0.00	6.24	6.24	0.00	6.24	6.24	XXX	■

■ RVU not developed by CMS. Gap-filled RVUs developed by Ingenix/CHEG.

Code	M	S	Description	Work Value	Non-Fac PE	Fac PE	Mal-practice	Non-Fac Total	Fac Total	Global	Gap
88264		X	analyze 20-25 cells	0.00	4.76	4.76	0.00	4.76	4.76	XXX	■
	26			0.00	0.00	0.00	0.00	0.00	0.00	XXX	■
	TC			0.00	4.76	4.76	0.00	4.76	4.76	XXX	■
88267		X	Chromosome analysis, amniotic fluid or chorionic villus, count 15 cells, 1 karyotype, with banding	0.00	6.83	6.83	0.00	6.83	6.83	XXX	■
	26			0.00	0.00	0.00	0.00	0.00	0.00	XXX	■
	TC			0.00	6.83	6.83	0.00	6.83	6.83	XXX	■
88269		X	Chromosome analysis, in situ for amniotic fluid cells, count cells from 6-12 colonies, 1 karyotype, with banding	0.00	6.01	6.01	0.00	6.01	6.01	XXX	■
	26			0.00	0.00	0.00	0.00	0.00	0.00	XXX	■
	TC			0.00	6.01	6.01	0.00	6.01	6.01	XXX	■
88271		X	Molecular cytogenetics; DNA probe, each (eg, FISH)	0.00	0.82	0.82	0.00	0.82	0.82	XXX	■
	26			0.00	0.00	0.00	0.00	0.00	0.00	XXX	■
	TC			0.00	0.82	0.82	0.00	0.82	0.82	XXX	■
88272		X	chromosomal in situ hybridization, analyze 3-5 cells (eg, for derivatives and markers)	0.00	1.02	1.02	0.00	1.02	1.02	XXX	■
	26			0.00	0.00	0.00	0.00	0.00	0.00	XXX	■
	TC			0.00	1.02	1.02	0.00	1.02	1.02	XXX	■
88273		X	chromosomal in situ hybridization, analyze 10-30 cells (eg, for microdeletions)	0.00	1.23	1.23	0.00	1.23	1.23	XXX	■
	26			0.00	0.00	0.00	0.00	0.00	0.00	XXX	■
	TC			0.00	1.23	1.23	0.00	1.23	1.23	XXX	■
88274		X	interphase in situ hybridization, analyze 25-99 cells	0.00	1.33	1.33	0.00	1.33	1.33	XXX	■
	26			0.00	0.00	0.00	0.00	0.00	0.00	XXX	■
	TC			0.00	1.33	1.33	0.00	1.33	1.33	XXX	■
88275		X	interphase in situ hybridization, analyze 100-300 cells	0.00	1.53	1.53	0.00	1.53	1.53	XXX	■
	26			0.00	0.00	0.00	0.00	0.00	0.00	XXX	■
	TC			0.00	1.53	1.53	0.00	1.53	1.53	XXX	■
88280		X	Chromosome analysis; additional karyotypes, each study	0.00	1.98	1.98	0.00	1.98	1.98	XXX	■
	26			0.00	0.00	0.00	0.00	0.00	0.00	XXX	■
	TC			0.00	1.98	1.98	0.00	1.98	1.98	XXX	■
88283		X	additional specialized banding technique (eg, NOR, C-banding)	0.00	1.56	1.56	0.00	1.56	1.56	XXX	■
	26			0.00	0.00	0.00	0.00	0.00	0.00	XXX	■
	TC			0.00	1.56	1.56	0.00	1.56	1.56	XXX	■
88285		X	additional cells counted, each study	0.00	1.81	1.81	0.00	1.81	1.81	XXX	■
	26			0.00	0.00	0.00	0.00	0.00	0.00	XXX	■
	TC			0.00	1.81	1.81	0.00	1.81	1.81	XXX	■
88289		X	additional high resolution study	0.00	1.29	1.29	0.00	1.29	1.29	XXX	■
	26			0.00	0.00	0.00	0.00	0.00	0.00	XXX	■
	TC			0.00	1.29	1.29	0.00	1.29	1.29	XXX	■
88291		A	Cytogenetics and molecular cytogenetics, interpretation and report	0.52	0.23	0.23	0.02	0.77	0.77	XXX	
88299		C	Unlisted cytogenetic study	0.00	0.00	0.00	0.00	0.00	0.00	XXX	
88300		A	Level I - Surgical pathology, gross examination only	0.08	0.34	0.34	0.02	0.44	0.44	XXX	
	26	A		0.08	0.04	0.04	0.01	0.13	0.13	XXX	
	TC	A		0.00	0.30	0.30	0.01	0.31	0.31	XXX	

Pathology

■ RVU not developed by CMS. Gap-filled RVUs developed by Ingenix/CHEG.

Code	M	S	Description	Work Value	Non-Fac PE	Fac PE	Mal-prac-tice	Non-Fac Total	Fac Total	Global	Gap
88302		A	Level II - Surgical pathology, gross and microscopic examination: Appendix, Incidental; Fallopian Tube, Sterilization; Fingers/Toes, Amputation,Traumatic; Foreskin, Newborn, Hernia Sac, Any Location; Hydrocele Sac; Nerve; Skin, Plastic Repair; Sympathetic Ganglion; Testis, Castration; Vaginal Mucosa, Incidental; Vas Deferens, Sterilization	0.13	0.73	0.73	0.03	0.89	0.89	XXX	
	26	A		0.13	0.06	0.06	0.01	0.20	0.20	XXX	
	TC	A		0.00	0.67	0.67	0.02	0.69	0.69	XXX	
88304		A	Level III - Surgical pathology, gross and microscopic examination Abortion, Induced Abscess Aneurysm - Arterial/Ventricular Anus, Tag Appendix, Other than Incidental Artery, Atheromatous Plaque Bartholin's Gland Cyst Bone Fragment(s), Other than Pathologic Fracture Bursa/Synovial Cyst Carpal Tunnel Tissue Cartilage, Shavings Cholesteatoma Colon, Colostomy Stoma Conjunctiva - Biopsy/ Pterygium Cornea Diverticulum - Esophagus/ Small Intestine Dupuytren's Contracture Tissue Femoral Head, Other than Fracture Fissure/ Fistula Foreskin, Other than Newborn Gallbladder Ganglion Cyst Hematoma Hemorrhoids Hydatid of Morgagni Intervertebral Disc Joint, Loose Body Meniscus Mucocele, Salivary Neuroma - Morton's/ Traumatic Pilonidal Cyst/Sinus Polyps, Inflammatory - Nasal/Sinusoidal Skin - Cyst/ Tag/Debridement Soft Tissue, Debridement Soft Tissue, Lipoma Spermatocele Tendon/Tendon Sheath Testicular Appendage Thrombus or Embolus Tonsil and/or Adenoids Varicocele Vas Deferens, Other than Sterilization Vein, Varicosity	0.22	0.95	0.95	0.03	1.20	1.20	XXX	
	26	A		0.22	0.10	0.10	0.01	0.33	0.33	XXX	
	TC	A		0.00	0.85	0.85	0.02	0.87	0.87	XXX	

■ RVU not developed by CMS. Gap-filled RVUs developed by Ingenix/CHEG.

Code	M	S	Description	Work Value	Non-Fac PE	Fac PE	Mal-practice	Non-Fac Total	Fac Total	Global	Gap
88305		A	Level IV - Surgical pathology, gross and microscopic examination Abortion - Spontaneous/Missed Artery, Biopsy Bone Marrow, Biopsy Bone Exostosis Brain/Meninges, Other than for Tumor Resection Breast, Biopsy, Not Requiring Microscopic Evaluation of Surgical Margins Breast, Reduction Mammoplasty Bronchus, Biopsy Cell Block, Any Source Cervix, Biopsy Colon, Biopsy Duodenum, Biopsy Endocervix, Curettings/ Biopsy Endometrium, Curettings/Biopsy Esophagus, Biopsy Extremity, Amputation, Traumatic Fallopian Tube, Biopsy Fallopian Tube, Ectopic Pregnancy Femoral Head, Fracture Fingers/Toes, Amputation, Non-traumatic Gingiva/Oral Mucosa, Biopsy Heart Valve Joint, Resection Kidney, Biopsy Larynx, Biopsy Leiomyoma(s), Uterine Myomectomy - without Uterus Lip, Biopsy/Wedge Resection Lung, Transbronchial Biopsy Lymph Node, Biopsy Muscle, Biopsy Nasal Mucosa, Biopsy Nasopharynx/Oropharynx, Biopsy Nerve, Biopsy Odontogenic/Dental Cyst Omentum, Biopsy Ovary with or without Tube, Non-neoplastic Ovary, Biopsy/Wedge Resection Parathyroid Gland Peritoneum, Biopsy Pituitary Tumor Placenta, Other than Third Trimester Pleura/Pericardium - Biopsy/Tissue Polyp, Cervical/Endometrial Polyp, Colorectal Polyp, Stomach/Small Intestine Prostate, Needle Biopsy Prostate, TUR Salivary Gland, Biopsy Sinus, Paranasal Biopsy Skin, Other than Cyst/ Tag/Debridement/Plastic Repair Small Intestine, Biopsy Soft Tissue, Other than Tumor/Mass/ Lipoma/Debridement Spleen Stomach, Biopsy Synovium Testis, Other than Tumor/Biopsy/ Castration Thyroglossal Duct/Brachial Cleft Cyst Tongue, Biopsy Tonsil, Biopsy Trachea, Biopsy Ureter, Biopsy Urethra, Biopsy Urinary Bladder, Biopsy Uterus, with or without Tubes and Ovaries, for Prolapse Vagina, Biopsy Vulva/ Labia, Biopsy	0.75	1.78	1.78	0.05	2.58	2.58	XXX	
	26	A		0.75	0.35	0.35	0.02	1.12	1.12	XXX	
	TC	A		0.00	1.43	1.43	0.03	1.46	1.46	XXX	

Pathology

■ RVU not developed by CMS. Gap-filled RVUs developed by Ingenix/CHEG.

Code	M	S	Description	Work Value	Non-Fac PE	Fac PE	Mal-practice	Non-Fac Total	Fac Total	Global	Gap
88307		A	Level V - Surgical pathology, gross and microscopic examination: Adrenal, Resection; Bone - Biopsy/Curettings; Bone Fragment(s), Pathologic Fracture; Brain, Biopsy; Brain/ Meninges, Tumor Resection; Breast, Excision of Lesion, Requiring Microscopic Evaluation of Surgical Margins; Breast, Mastectomy - Partial/ Simple; Cervix, Conization; Colon, Segmental Resection, Other than for Tumor; Extremity, Amputation, Non-Traumatic; Eye, Enucleation; Kidney, Partial/Total Nephrectomy; Larynx, Partial/Total Resection; Liver, Biopsy - Needle/ Wedge; Liver, Partial Resection; Lung, Wedge Biopsy; Lymph Nodes, Regional Resection; Mediastinum, Mass; Myocardium, Biopsy; Odontogenic Tumor; Ovary with or without Tube, Neoplastic; Pancreas, Biopsy; Placenta, Third Trimester; Prostate, Except Radical Resection; Salivary Gland; Sentinel Lymph Node; Small Intestine; Resection, Other than for Tumor; Soft Tissue Mass (except Lipoma) - Biopsy/Simple Excision; Stomach - Subtotal/ Total Resection, Other than for Tumor; Testis, Biopsy; Thymus, Tumor; Thyroid, Total/Lobe; Ureter, Resection; Urinary Bladder, TUR; Uterus, with or without Tubes and Ovaries, Other than Neoplastic/Prolapse	1.59	2.71	2.71	0.11	4.41	4.41	XXX	
	26	A		1.59	0.74	0.74	0.06	2.39	2.39	XXX	
	TC	A		0.00	1.97	1.97	0.05	2.02	2.02	XXX	
88309		A	Level VI - Surgical pathology, gross and microscopic examination: Bone Resection; Breast, Mastectomy - with Regional Lymph Nodes; Colon, Segmental Resection for Tumor; Colon, Total Resection; Esophagus, Partial/Total Resection; Extremity, Disarticulation; Fetus, with Dissection; Larynx, Partial/Total Resection - with Regional Lymph Nodes; Lung - Total/ Lobe/Segment Resection; Pancreas, Total/ Subtotal Resection; Prostate, Radical Resection; Small Intestine, Resection for Tumor; Soft Tissue Tumor, Extensive Resection; Stomach - Subtotal/Total Resection for Tumor; Testis, Tumor; Tongue/Tonsil - Resection for Tumor; Urinary Bladder, Partial/Total Resection; Uterus, with or without Tubes & Ovaries, Neoplastic; Vulva, Total/Subtotal Resection	2.28	3.40	3.40	0.13	5.81	5.81	XXX	
	26	A		2.28	1.05	1.05	0.08	3.41	3.41	XXX	
	TC	A		0.00	2.35	2.35	0.05	2.40	2.40	XXX	
88311		A	Decalcification procedure (List separately in addition to code for surgical pathology examination)	0.24	0.21	0.21	0.02	0.47	0.47	XXX	
	26	A		0.24	0.11	0.11	0.01	0.36	0.36	XXX	
	TC	A		0.00	0.10	0.10	0.01	0.11	0.11	XXX	
88312		A	Special stains (List separately in addition to code for surgical pathology examination); Group I for microorganisms (eg, Gridley, acid fast, methenamine silver), each	0.54	1.69	1.69	0.03	2.26	2.26	XXX	
	26	A		0.54	0.25	0.25	0.02	0.81	0.81	XXX	
	TC	A		0.00	1.44	1.44	0.01	1.45	1.45	XXX	
88313		A	Group II, all other, (eg, iron, trichrome), except immunocytochemistry and immunoperoxidase stains, each	0.24	1.47	1.47	0.02	1.73	1.73	XXX	
	26	A		0.24	0.11	0.11	0.01	0.36	0.36	XXX	
	TC	A		0.00	1.36	1.36	0.01	1.37	1.37	XXX	

Pathology

■ RVU not developed by CMS. Gap-filled RVUs developed by Ingenix/CHEG.

Code	M	S	Description	Work Value	Non-Fac PE	Fac PE	Mal-practice	Non-Fac Total	Fac Total	Global	Gap
88314		A	histochemical staining with frozen section(s)	0.45	0.86	0.86	0.04	1.35	1.35	XXX	
	26	A		0.45	0.20	0.20	0.02	0.67	0.67	XXX	
	TC	A		0.00	0.66	0.66	0.02	0.68	0.68	XXX	
88318		A	Determinative histochemistry to identify chemical components (eg, copper, zinc)	0.42	0.59	0.59	0.02	1.03	1.03	XXX	
	26	A		0.42	0.20	0.20	0.01	0.63	0.63	XXX	
	TC	A		0.00	0.39	0.39	0.01	0.40	0.40	XXX	
88319		A	Determinative histochemistry or cytochemistry to identify enzyme constituents, each	0.53	2.45	2.45	0.04	3.02	3.02	XXX	
	26	A		0.53	0.24	0.24	0.02	0.79	0.79	XXX	
	TC	A		0.00	2.21	2.21	0.02	2.23	2.23	XXX	
88321		A	Consultation and report on referred slides prepared elsewhere	1.30	0.62	0.60	0.04	1.96	1.94	XXX	
88323		A	Consultation and report on referred material requiring preparation of slides	1.35	1.37	1.37	0.07	2.79	2.79	XXX	
	26	A		1.35	0.63	0.63	0.05	2.03	2.03	XXX	
	TC	A		0.00	0.74	0.74	0.02	0.76	0.76	XXX	
88325		A	Consultation, comprehensive, with review of records and specimens, with report on referred material	2.22	0.98	0.98	0.08	3.28	3.28	XXX	
88329		A	Pathology consultation during surgery;	0.67	0.39	0.31	0.02	1.08	1.00	XXX	
88331		A	first tissue block, with frozen section(s), single specimen	1.19	0.87	0.87	0.07	2.13	2.13	XXX	
	26	A		1.19	0.55	0.55	0.04	1.78	1.78	XXX	
	TC	A		0.00	0.32	0.32	0.03	0.35	0.35	XXX	
88332		A	each additional tissue block with frozen section(s)	0.59	0.47	0.47	0.04	1.10	1.10	XXX	
	26	A		0.59	0.27	0.27	0.02	0.88	0.88	XXX	
	TC	A		0.00	0.20	0.20	0.02	0.22	0.22	XXX	
88342		A	Immunocytochemistry (including tissue immunoperoxidase), each antibody	0.85	1.43	1.43	0.05	2.33	2.33	XXX	
	26	A		0.85	0.39	0.39	0.03	1.27	1.27	XXX	
	TC	A		0.00	1.04	1.04	0.02	1.06	1.06	XXX	
88346		A	Immunofluorescent study, each antibody; direct method	0.86	1.20	1.20	0.05	2.11	2.11	XXX	
	26	A		0.86	0.39	0.39	0.03	1.28	1.28	XXX	
	TC	A		0.00	0.81	0.81	0.02	0.83	0.83	XXX	
88347		A	indirect method	0.86	1.90	1.90	0.05	2.81	2.81	XXX	
	26	A		0.86	0.38	0.38	0.03	1.27	1.27	XXX	
	TC	A		0.00	1.52	1.52	0.02	1.54	1.54	XXX	
88348		A	Electron microscopy; diagnostic	1.51	6.96	6.96	0.11	8.58	8.58	XXX	
	26	A		1.51	0.69	0.69	0.05	2.25	2.25	XXX	
	TC	A		0.00	6.27	6.27	0.06	6.33	6.33	XXX	
88349		A	scanning	0.76	8.51	8.51	0.08	9.35	9.35	XXX	
	26	A		0.76	0.35	0.35	0.03	1.14	1.14	XXX	
	TC	A		0.00	8.16	8.16	0.05	8.21	8.21	XXX	
88355		A	Morphometric analysis; skeletal muscle	1.85	2.41	2.41	0.12	4.38	4.38	XXX	
	26	A		1.85	0.86	0.86	0.07	2.78	2.78	XXX	
	TC	A		0.00	1.55	1.55	0.05	1.60	1.60	XXX	

Pathology

■ RVU not developed by CMS. Gap-filled RVUs developed by Ingenix/CHEG.

Code	M	S	Description	Work Value	Non-Fac PE	Fac PE	Mal-prac-tice	Non-Fac Total	Fac Total	Global	Gap
88356		A	nerve	3.02	4.96	4.96	0.16	8.14	8.14	XXX	
	26	A		3.02	1.37	1.37	0.10	4.49	4.49	XXX	
	TC	A		0.00	3.59	3.59	0.06	3.65	3.65	XXX	
88358		A	tumor	2.82	1.76	1.76	0.16	4.74	4.74	XXX	
	26	A		2.82	1.30	1.30	0.10	4.22	4.22	XXX	
	TC	A		0.00	0.46	0.46	0.06	0.52	0.52	XXX	
88362		A	Nerve teasing preparations	2.17	3.36	3.36	0.12	5.65	5.65	XXX	
	26	A		2.17	0.99	0.99	0.07	3.23	3.23	XXX	
	TC	A		0.00	2.37	2.37	0.05	2.42	2.42	XXX	
88365		A	Tissue in situ hybridization, interpretation and report	0.93	2.03	2.03	0.05	3.01	3.01	XXX	
	26	A		0.93	0.43	0.43	0.03	1.39	1.39	XXX	
	TC	A		0.00	1.60	1.60	0.02	1.62	1.62	XXX	
88371		X	Protein analysis of tissue by Western Blot, with interpretation and report;	0.37	1.00	0.99	0.01	1.38	1.37	XXX	■
	26	A		0.37	0.15	0.14	0.01	0.53	0.52	XXX	
	TC			0.00	0.85	0.85	0.00	0.85	0.85	XXX	■
88372		X	immunological probe for band identification, each	0.37	1.04	1.04	0.01	1.42	1.42	XXX	■
	26	A		0.37	0.17	0.17	0.01	0.55	0.55	XXX	
	TC			0.00	0.87	0.87	0.00	0.87	0.87	XXX	■
88380		C	Microdissection (eg, mechanical, laser capture)	0.00	0.00	0.00	0.00	0.00	0.00	XXX	
	26	C		0.00	0.00	0.00	0.00	0.00	0.00	XXX	
	TC	C		0.00	0.00	0.00	0.00	0.00	0.00	XXX	
88399		C	Unlisted surgical pathology procedure	0.00	0.00	0.00	0.00	0.00	0.00	XXX	
	26	C		0.00	0.00	0.00	0.00	0.00	0.00	XXX	
	TC	C		0.00	0.00	0.00	0.00	0.00	0.00	XXX	
88400		X	Bilirubin, total, transcutaneous	0.00	0.10	0.10	0.00	0.10	0.10	XXX	■
	26			0.00	0.00	0.00	0.00	0.00	0.00	XXX	■
	TC			0.00	0.10	0.10	0.00	0.10	0.10	XXX	■
89050		X	Cell count, miscellaneous body fluids (eg, cerebrospinal fluid, joint fluid), except blood;	0.00	0.73	0.73	0.00	0.73	0.73	XXX	■
	26			0.00	0.00	0.00	0.00	0.00	0.00	XXX	■
	TC			0.00	0.73	0.73	0.00	0.73	0.73	XXX	■
89051		X	with differential count	0.00	0.87	0.87	0.00	0.87	0.87	XXX	■
	26			0.00	0.00	0.00	0.00	0.00	0.00	XXX	■
	TC			0.00	0.87	0.87	0.00	0.87	0.87	XXX	■
89060		X	Crystal identification by light microscopy with or without polarizing lens analysis, any body fluid (except urine)	0.37	0.45	0.44	0.01	0.83	0.82	XXX	■
	26	A		0.37	0.18	0.17	0.01	0.56	0.55	XXX	
	TC			0.00	0.27	0.27	0.00	0.27	0.27	XXX	■
89100		A	Duodenal intubation and aspiration; single specimen (eg, simple bile study or afferent loop culture) plus appropriate test procedure	0.60	2.29	0.23	0.02	2.91	0.85	XXX	
89105		A	collection of multiple fractional specimens with pancreatic or gallbladder stimulation, single or double lumen tube	0.50	2.25	0.18	0.02	2.77	0.70	XXX	
89125		X	Fat stain, feces, urine, or respiratory secretions	0.00	0.68	0.68	0.00	0.68	0.68	XXX	■
	26			0.00	0.00	0.00	0.00	0.00	0.00	XXX	■
	TC			0.00	0.68	0.68	0.00	0.68	0.68	XXX	■

■ RVU not developed by CMS. Gap-filled RVUs developed by Ingenix/CHEG.

Code	M	S	Description	Work Value	Non-Fac PE	Fac PE	Mal-prac-tice	Non-Fac Total	Fac Total	Global	Gap
89130		A	Gastric intubation and aspiration, diagnostic, each specimen, for chemical analyses or cytopathology;	0.45	2.21	0.13	0.02	2.68	0.60	XXX	
89132		A	after stimulation	0.19	1.15	0.05	0.01	1.35	0.25	XXX	
89135		A	Gastric intubation, aspiration, and fractional collections (eg, gastric secretory study); one hour	0.79	2.53	0.25	0.03	3.35	1.07	XXX	
89136		A	two hours	0.21	2.05	0.08	0.01	2.27	0.30	XXX	
89140		A	two hours including gastric stimulation (eg, histalog, pentagastrin)	0.94	2.36	0.19	0.03	3.33	1.16	XXX	
89141		A	three hours, including gastric stimulation	0.85	3.14	0.40	0.03	4.02	1.28	XXX	
89160		X	Meat fibers, feces	0.00	0.41	0.41	0.00	0.41	0.41	XXX	■
	26			0.00	0.00	0.00	0.00	0.00	0.00	XXX	■
	TC			0.00	0.41	0.41	0.00	0.41	0.41	XXX	■
89190		X	Nasal smear for eosinophils	0.00	0.64	0.64	0.00	0.64	0.64	XXX	■
	26			0.00	0.00	0.00	0.00	0.00	0.00	XXX	■
	TC			0.00	0.64	0.64	0.00	0.64	0.64	XXX	■
89250		X	Culture and fertilization of oocyte(s);	0.00	30.64	30.64	0.00	30.64	30.64	XXX	■
	26			0.00	0.00	0.00	0.00	0.00	0.00	XXX	■
	TC			0.00	30.64	30.64	0.00	30.64	30.64	XXX	■
89251		X	with co-culture of embryos	0.00	0.00	0.00	0.00	0.00	0.00	XXX	
89252		X	Assisted oocyte fertilization, microtechnique (any method)	0.00	0.00	0.00	0.00	0.00	0.00	XXX	
89253		X	Assisted embryo hatching, microtechniques (any method)	0.00	0.00	0.00	0.00	0.00	0.00	XXX	
89254		X	Oocyte identification from follicular fluid	0.00	0.00	0.00	0.00	0.00	0.00	XXX	
89255		X	Preparation of embryo for transfer (any method)	0.00	0.00	0.00	0.00	0.00	0.00	XXX	
89256		X	Preparation of cryopreserved embryos for transfer (includes thaw)	0.00	0.00	0.00	0.00	0.00	0.00	XXX	
89257		X	Sperm identification from aspiration (other than seminal fluid)	0.00	0.00	0.00	0.00	0.00	0.00	XXX	
89258		X	Cryopreservation; embryo	0.00	0.00	0.00	0.00	0.00	0.00	XXX	
89259		X	sperm	0.00	0.00	0.00	0.00	0.00	0.00	XXX	
89260		X	Sperm isolation; simple prep (eg, sperm wash and swim-up) for insemination or diagnosis with semen analysis	0.00	0.00	0.00	0.00	0.00	0.00	XXX	
89261		X	complex prep (eg, Percoll gradient, albumin gradient) for insemination or diagnosis with semen analysis	0.00	0.00	0.00	0.00	0.00	0.00	XXX	

Pathology

■ RVU not developed by CMS. Gap-filled RVUs developed by Ingenix/CHEG.

Code	M	S	Description	Work Value	Non-Fac PE	Fac PE	Mal-practice	Non-Fac Total	Fac Total	Global	Gap
89264		X	Sperm identification from testis tissue, fresh or cryopreserved	0.00	0.00	0.00	0.00	0.00	0.00	XXX	
89300		X	Semen analysis; presence and/or motility of sperm including Huhner test (post coital)	0.00	1.59	1.59	0.00	1.59	1.59	XXX	■
	26			0.00	0.00	0.00	0.00	0.00	0.00	XXX	■
	TC			0.00	1.59	1.59	0.00	1.59	1.59	XXX	■
89310		X	motility and count	0.00	1.50	1.50	0.00	1.50	1.50	XXX	■
	26			0.00	0.00	0.00	0.00	0.00	0.00	XXX	■
	TC			0.00	1.50	1.50	0.00	1.50	1.50	XXX	■
89320		X	complete (volume, count, motility and differential)	0.00	2.28	2.28	0.00	2.28	2.28	XXX	■
	26			0.00	0.00	0.00	0.00	0.00	0.00	XXX	■
	TC			0.00	2.28	2.28	0.00	2.28	2.28	XXX	■
89321		X	Semen analysis, presence and/or motility of sperm	0.00	1.37	1.37	0.00	1.37	1.37	XXX	■
	26			0.00	0.00	0.00	0.00	0.00	0.00	XXX	■
	TC			0.00	1.37	1.37	0.00	1.37	1.37	XXX	■
89325		X	Sperm antibodies	0.00	3.87	3.87	0.00	3.87	3.87	XXX	■
	26			0.00	0.00	0.00	0.00	0.00	0.00	XXX	■
	TC			0.00	3.87	3.87	0.00	3.87	3.87	XXX	■
89329		X	Sperm evaluation; hamster penetration test	0.00	10.24	10.24	0.00	10.24	10.24	XXX	■
	26			0.00	0.00	0.00	0.00	0.00	0.00	XXX	■
	TC			0.00	10.24	10.24	0.00	10.24	10.24	XXX	■
89330		X	cervical mucus penetration test, with or without spinnbarkeit test	0.00	2.60	2.60	0.00	2.60	2.60	XXX	■
	26			0.00	0.00	0.00	0.00	0.00	0.00	XXX	■
	TC			0.00	2.60	2.60	0.00	2.60	2.60	XXX	■
89350		A	Sputum, obtaining specimen, aerosol induced technique (separate procedure)	0.00	0.39	0.39	0.02	0.41	0.41	XXX	
	26			0.00	0.00	0.00	0.00	0.00	0.00	XXX	■
	TC			0.00	0.39	0.39	0.02	0.41	0.41	XXX	■
89355		X	Starch granules, feces	0.00	0.46	0.46	0.00	0.46	0.46	XXX	■
	26			0.00	0.00	0.00	0.00	0.00	0.00	XXX	■
	TC			0.00	0.46	0.46	0.00	0.46	0.46	XXX	■
89360		A	Sweat collection by iontophoresis	0.00	0.43	0.43	0.02	0.45	0.45	XXX	
	26			0.00	0.00	0.00	0.00	0.00	0.00	XXX	■
	TC			0.00	0.43	0.43	0.02	0.45	0.45	XXX	■
89365		X	Water load test	0.00	1.09	1.09	0.00	1.09	1.09	XXX	■
	26			0.00	0.00	0.00	0.00	0.00	0.00	XXX	■
	TC			0.00	1.09	1.09	0.00	1.09	1.09	XXX	■
89399		C	Unlisted miscellaneous pathology test	0.00	0.00	0.00	0.00	0.00	0.00	XXX	
	26	C		0.00	0.00	0.00	0.00	0.00	0.00	XXX	
	TC	C		0.00	0.00	0.00	0.00	0.00	0.00	XXX	

■ RVU not developed by CMS. Gap-filled RVUs developed by Ingenix/CHEG.

Medicine

The Introduction provides complete descriptions for the status column (abbreviated as S). If a relative value is not available for a procedure, it is indicated with a "0.00" in the individual units column.

I. **Separate Procedures:** Procedures identified as "separate procedures" are frequently included in the global value of other procedures. Listing of a "separate procedure" code and full value is appropriate if the procedure is not included in the global value of another. Listing of "separate procedure" codes is not appropriate when the procedure is included in the global value of another.

II. **Unusual Procedural Services:** A service may necessitate skills and time of the physician over and above listed services and values. If substantiated "By Report" (BR), additional values may be warranted. Use modifier -22 to indicate these procedures.

III. **Unlisted Service Or Procedure:** When a service or procedure provided is not adequately identified, use of the unlisted procedure code for the related anatomical area is appropriate. Most codes of this type have "9" for the last digit. Value should be substantiated "By Report" (BR).

IV. **By Report:** Value of a procedure should be established for any "By Report" circumstance by identifying a similar service and justifying value difference. When a report is required, the report should include the following:

A. Accurate procedure definition or description

B. Justification for procedural variance, when appropriate

C. Similar procedure and value

D. Justification for value difference

V. **Reduced Services:** Under some circumstances, the value for a procedure may be reduced. Use modifier -52 to identify reduced value services.

VI. **Multiple Modifiers:** If circumstances require the use of more than one modifier with any one procedure code, modifier -99 should be added to the procedure code. Other modifiers are then attached to the procedure code and listed separately with appropriate values for each.

VII. **Materials Supplied By Physician:** CPT code 99070 or the specific HCPCS Level II code may be used to identify materials provided by the physician (e.g., sterile trays, drugs) over and above those usually indicated with the office visit. Medicare no longer provides separate payment for a sterile supply tray when the service is provided in the physician's office as these supplies are now included in the value of the non-facility practice expense component.

VIII. **Professional Component:** The unit value listed next to the modifier column (modifier -26) is used to designate professional services. Modifier -26 is added to the procedure code to indicate the use of this value. The professional component includes examination of the patient, when indicated; performance and/or supervision of the procedure or lab test; interpretation and/or written report concerning the examination or lab test; and consultation with referring physicians.

IX. **Global Values:** This column indicates the number of days in the global period for which services directly related to the procedure are included. The majority of codes have a numerical designation (i.e., 0, 10, or 90).

A. MMM codes describe services furnished in uncomplicated maternity care. This includes antepartum, delivery and postpartum care. The usual global surgical concept does not apply.

B. XXX codes indicate that the global surgery concept does not apply.

C. YYY codes indicate that the global period is to be set by the local carrier.

D. ZZZ codes indicate that the code is an add-on service and therefore is treated in the global period of the other procedure billed in conjunction with a ZZZ code. Do not bill these codes with modifier -51. They should not be reduced.

Medicine Values

Code	M	S	Description	Work Value	Non-Fac PE	Fac PE	Mal-practice	Non-Fac Total	Fac Total	Global	Gap
90281		I	Immune globulin (IG), human, for intramuscular use	0.00	0.00	0.00	0.00	0.00	0.00	XXX	
90283		I	Immune globulin (IGIV), human, for intravenous use	0.00	0.00	0.00	0.00	0.00	0.00	XXX	
90287		I	Botulinum antitoxin, equine, any route	0.00	0.00	0.00	0.00	0.00	0.00	XXX	
90288		I	Botulism immune globulin, human, for intravenous use	0.00	0.00	0.00	0.00	0.00	0.00	XXX	
90291		I	Cytomegalovirus immune globulin (CMV-IGIV), human, for intravenous use	0.00	0.00	0.00	0.00	0.00	0.00	XXX	
90296		E	Diphtheria antitoxin, equine, any route	0.00	0.00	0.00	0.00	0.00	0.00	XXX	
90371		E	Hepatitis B immune globulin (HBIG), human, for intramuscular use	0.00	0.00	0.00	0.00	0.00	0.00	XXX	
90375		E	Rabies immune globulin (RIG), human, for intramuscular use and/or subcutaneous use	0.00	4.41	4.41	0.00	4.41	4.41	XXX	■
90376		E	Rabies immune globulin, heat-treated (RIG-HT), human, for intramuscular and/or subcutaneous use	0.00	4.14	4.14	0.00	4.14	4.14	XXX	■
90378		X	Respiratory syncytial virus immune globulin (RSV-IgIM), for intramuscular use, 50 mg, each	0.00	0.00	0.00	0.00	0.00	0.00	XXX	
90379		I	Respiratory syncytial virus immune globulin (RSV-IGIV), human, for intravenous use	0.00	0.00	0.00	0.00	0.00	0.00	XXX	
90384		I	Rho(D) immune globulin (RhIG), human, full-dose, for intramuscular use	0.00	0.00	0.00	0.00	0.00	0.00	XXX	
90385		E	Rho(D) immune globulin (RhIG), human, mini-dose, for intramuscular use	0.00	0.00	0.00	0.00	0.00	0.00	XXX	
90386		I	Rho(D) immune globulin (RhIGIV), human, for intravenous use	0.00	0.00	0.00	0.00	0.00	0.00	XXX	
90389		I	Tetanus immune globulin (TIG), human, for intramuscular use	0.00	2.98	2.98	0.00	2.98	2.98	XXX	■
90393		E	Vaccinia immune globulin, human, for intramuscular use	0.00	0.00	0.00	0.00	0.00	0.00	XXX	
90396		E	Varicella-zoster immune globulin, human, for intramuscular use	0.00	0.00	0.00	0.00	0.00	0.00	XXX	
90399		I	Unlisted immune globulin	0.00	0.00	0.00	0.00	0.00	0.00	XXX	
90471		A	Immunization administration (includes percutaneous, intradermal, subcutaneous, intramuscular and jet injections); one vaccine (single or combination vaccine/toxoid)	0.00	0.10	0.10	0.01	0.11	0.11	XXX	

■ RVU not developed by CMS. Gap-filled RVUs developed by Ingenix/CHEG.

Code	M	S	Description	Work Value	Non-Fac PE	Fac PE	Mal-practice	Non-Fac Total	Fac Total	Global	Gap
90472		A	each additional vaccine (single or combination vaccine/toxoid) (List separately in addition to code for primary procedure)	0.00	0.10	0.10	0.01	0.11	0.11	ZZZ	
90473		N	Immunization administration by intranasal or oral route; one vaccine (single or combination vaccine/toxoid)	0.00	0.11	0.11	0.00	0.11	0.11	XXX	■
90474		N	each additional vaccine (single or combination vaccine/toxoid) (List separately in addition to code for primary procedure)	0.00	0.11	0.11	0.00	0.11	0.11	ZZZ	■
90476		E	Adenovirus vaccine, type 4, live, for oral use	0.00	0.00	0.00	0.00	0.00	0.00	XXX	
90477		E	Adenovirus vaccine, type 7, live, for oral use	0.00	0.00	0.00	0.00	0.00	0.00	XXX	
90581		E	Anthrax vaccine, for subcutaneous use	0.00	3.67	3.67	0.00	3.67	3.67	XXX	■
90585		E	Bacillus Calmette-Guerin vaccine (BCG) for tuberculosis, live, for percutaneous use	0.00	4.65	4.65	0.00	4.65	4.65	XXX	■
90586		E	Bacillus Calmette-Guerin vaccine (BCG) for bladder cancer, live, for intravesical use	0.00	4.84	4.84	0.00	4.84	4.84	XXX	■
90632		E	Hepatitis A vaccine, adult dosage, for intramuscular use	0.00	1.54	1.54	0.00	1.54	1.54	XXX	■
90633		E	Hepatitis A vaccine, pediatric/adolescent dosage-2 dose schedule, for intramuscular use	0.00	0.85	0.85	0.00	0.85	0.85	XXX	■
90634		E	Hepatitis A vaccine, pediatric/adolescent dosage-3 dose schedule, for intramuscular use	0.00	0.85	0.85	0.00	0.85	0.85	XXX	■
90636		E	Hepatitis A and hepatitis B vaccine (HepA-HepB), adult dosage, for intramuscular use	0.00	0.00	0.00	0.00	0.00	0.00	XXX	
90645		E	Hemophilus influenza b vaccine (Hib), HbOC conjugate (4 dose schedule), for intramuscular use	0.00	0.75	0.75	0.00	0.75	0.75	XXX	■
90646		E	Hemophilus influenza b vaccine (Hib), PRP-D conjugate, for booster use only, intramuscular use	0.00	0.00	0.00	0.00	0.00	0.00	XXX	
90647		E	Hemophilus influenza b vaccine (Hib), PRP-OMP conjugate (3 dose schedule), for intramuscular use	0.00	0.67	0.67	0.00	0.67	0.67	XXX	■
90648		E	Hemophilus influenza b vaccine (Hib),PRP-T conjugate (4 dose schedule), for intramuscular use	0.00	0.69	0.69	0.00	0.69	0.69	XXX	■
90657		X	Influenza virus vaccine, split virus, 6-35 months dosage, for intramuscular or jet injection use	0.00	0.18	0.18	0.00	0.18	0.18	XXX	■
90658		X	Influenza virus vaccine, split virus, 3 years and above dosage, for intramuscular or jet injection use	0.00	0.18	0.18	0.00	0.18	0.18	XXX	■

■ RVU not developed by CMS. Gap-filled RVUs developed by Ingenix/CHEG.

Code	M	S	Description	Work Value	Non-Fac PE	Fac PE	Mal-practice	Non-Fac Total	Fac Total	Global	Gap
90659		X	Influenza virus vaccine, whole virus, for intramuscular or jet injection use	0.00	0.00	0.00	0.00	0.00	0.00	XXX	
90660		X	Influenza virus vaccine, live, for intranasal use	0.00	0.06	0.06	0.00	0.06	0.06	XXX	■
90665		E	Lyme disease vaccine, adult dosage, for intramuscular use	0.00	1.72	1.72	0.00	1.72	1.72	XXX	■
90669		N	Pneumococcal conjugate vaccine, polyvalent, for children under five years, for intramuscular use	0.00	2.02	2.02	0.00	2.02	2.02	XXX	■
90675		E	Rabies vaccine, for intramuscular use	0.00	3.69	3.69	0.00	3.69	3.69	XXX	■
90676		E	Rabies vaccine, for intradermal use	0.00	0.00	0.00	0.00	0.00	0.00	XXX	
90680		E	Rotavirus vaccine, tetravalent, live, for oral use	0.00	0.00	0.00	0.00	0.00	0.00	XXX	
90690		E	Typhoid vaccine, live, oral	0.00	0.87	0.87	0.00	0.87	0.87	XXX	■
90691		E	Typhoid vaccine, Vi capsular polysaccharide (ViCPs), for intramuscular use	0.00	1.22	1.22	0.00	1.22	1.22	XXX	■
90692		E	Typhoid vaccine, heat- and phenol-inactivated (H-P), for subcutaneous or intradermal use	0.00	0.00	0.00	0.00	0.00	0.00	XXX	
90693		E	Typhoid vaccine, acetone-killed, dried (AKD), for subcutaneous or jet injection use (U.S. military)	0.00	0.00	0.00	0.00	0.00	0.00	XXX	
90700		E	Diphtheria, tetanus toxoids, and acellular pertussis vaccine (DTaP), for intramuscular use	0.00	0.60	0.60	0.00	0.60	0.60	XXX	■
90701		E	Diphtheria, tetanus toxoids, and whole cell pertussis vaccine (DTP), for intramuscular use	0.00	0.00	0.00	0.00	0.00	0.00	XXX	
90702		E	Diphtheria and tetanus toxoids (DT) adsorbed for use in individuals younger than seven years, for intramuscular use	0.00	0.20	0.20	0.00	0.20	0.20	XXX	■
90703		E	Tetanus toxoid adsorbed, for intramuscular or jet injection use	0.00	0.08	0.08	0.00	0.08	0.08	XXX	■
90704		E	Mumps virus vaccine, live, for subcutaneous or jet injection use	0.00	0.50	0.50	0.00	0.50	0.50	XXX	■
90705		E	Measles virus vaccine, live, for subcutaneous or jet injection use	0.00	0.41	0.41	0.00	0.41	0.41	XXX	■
90706		E	Rubella virus vaccine, live, for subcutaneous or jet injection use	0.00	0.44	0.44	0.00	0.44	0.44	XXX	■
90707		E	Measles, mumps and rubella virus vaccine (MMR), live, for subcutaneous or jet injection use	0.00	1.09	1.09	0.00	1.09	1.09	XXX	■
90708		E	Measles and rubella virus vaccine, live, for subcutaneous or jet injection use	0.00	0.00	0.00	0.00	0.00	0.00	XXX	
90709		E	Rubella and mumps virus vaccine, live, for subcutaneous use	0.00	0.00	0.00	0.00	0.00	0.00	XXX	

■ RVU not developed by CMS. Gap-filled RVUs developed by Ingenix/CHEG.

Code	M	S	Description	Work Value	Non-Fac PE	Fac PE	Mal-practice	Non-Fac Total	Fac Total	Global	Gap
90710		E	Measles, mumps, rubella, and varicella vaccine (MMRV), live, for subcutaneous use	0.00	0.00	0.00	0.00	0.00	0.00	XXX	
90712		E	Poliovirus vaccine, (any type(s)) (OPV), live, for oral use	0.00	0.58	0.58	0.00	0.58	0.58	XXX	■
90713		E	Poliovirus vaccine, inactivated, (IPV), for subcutaneous use	0.00	0.72	0.72	0.00	0.72	0.72	XXX	■
90716		E	Varicella virus vaccine, live, for subcutaneous use	0.00	1.70	1.70	0.00	1.70	1.70	XXX	■
90717		E	Yellow fever vaccine, live, for subcutaneous use	0.00	1.82	1.82	0.00	1.82	1.82	XXX	■
90718		E	Tetanus and diphtheria toxoids (Td) adsorbed for use in individuals seven years or older, for intramuscular or jet injection	0.00	0.15	0.15	0.00	0.15	0.15	XXX	■
90719		E	Diphtheria toxoid, for intramuscular use	0.00	0.00	0.00	0.00	0.00	0.00	XXX	
90720		E	Diphtheria, tetanus toxoids, and whole cell pertussis vaccine and Hemophilus influenza B vaccine (DTP-Hib), for intramuscular use	0.00	1.06	1.06	0.00	1.06	1.06	XXX	■
90721		E	Diphtheria, tetanus toxoids, and acellular pertussis vaccine and Hemophilus influenza B vaccine (DtaP-Hib), for intramuscular use	0.00	1.17	1.17	0.00	1.17	1.17	XXX	■
90723		X	Diphtheria, tetanus toxoids, acellular pertussis vaccine, Hepatitis B, and poliovirus vaccine, inactivated (DtaP-HepB-IPV), for intramuscular use	0.00	0.00	0.00	0.00	0.00	0.00	XXX	
90725		E	Cholera vaccine for injectable use	0.00	0.00	0.00	0.00	0.00	0.00	XXX	
90727		E	Plague vaccine, for intramuscular or jet injection use	0.00	0.20	0.20	0.00	0.20	0.20	XXX	■
90732		X	Pneumococcal polysaccharide vaccine, 23-valent, adult or immunosuppressed patient dosage, for use in individuals 2 years or older, for subcutaneous or intramuscular use	0.00	0.49	0.49	0.00	0.49	0.49	XXX	■
90733		E	Meningococcal polysaccharide vaccine (any group(s)), for subcutaneous or jet injection use	0.00	1.94	1.94	0.00	1.94	1.94	XXX	■
90735		E	Japanese encephalitis virus vaccine, for subcutaneous use	0.00	2.34	2.34	0.00	2.34	2.34	XXX	■
90740		X	Hepatitis B vaccine, dialysis or immunosuppressed patient dosage (3 dose schedule), for intramuscular use	0.00	5.22	5.22	0.00	5.22	5.22	XXX	■
90743		X	Hepatitis B vaccine, adolescent (2 dose schedule), for intramuscular use	0.00	0.75	0.75	0.00	0.75	0.75	XXX	■
90744		X	Hepatitis B vaccine, pediatric/adolescent dosage (3 dose schedule), for intramuscular use	0.00	0.75	0.75	0.00	0.75	0.75	XXX	■
90746		X	Hepatitis B vaccine, adult dosage, for intramuscular use	0.00	1.52	1.52	0.00	1.52	1.52	XXX	■

Medicine

■ RVU not developed by CMS. Gap-filled RVUs developed by Ingenix/CHEG.

Code	M	S	Description	Work Value	Non-Fac PE	Fac PE	Mal-prac-tice	Non-Fac Total	Fac Total	Global	Gap
90747		X	Hepatitis B vaccine, dialysis or immunosuppressed patient dosage (4 dose schedule), for intramuscular use	0.00	5.22	5.22	0.00	5.22	5.22	XXX	■
90748		E	Hepatitis B and Hemophilus influenza b vaccine (HepB-Hib), for intramuscular use	0.00	1.39	1.39	0.00	1.39	1.39	XXX	■
90749		E	Unlisted vaccine/toxoid	0.00	0.00	0.00	0.00	0.00	0.00	XXX	
90780		A	Intravenous infusion for therapy/diagnosis, administered by physician or under direct supervision of physician; up to one hour	0.00	1.06	1.06	0.06	1.12	1.12	XXX	
90781		A	each additional hour, up to eight (8) hours (List separately in addition to code for primary procedure)	0.00	0.53	0.53	0.03	0.56	0.56	ZZZ	
90782		T	Therapeutic, prophylactic or diagnostic injection (specify material injected); subcutaneous or intramuscular	0.00	0.10	0.10	0.01	0.11	0.11	XXX	
90783		T	intra-arterial	0.00	0.39	0.39	0.02	0.41	0.41	XXX	
90784		T	intravenous	0.00	0.45	0.45	0.03	0.48	0.48	XXX	
90788		T	Intramuscular injection of antibiotic (specify)	0.00	0.11	0.11	0.01	0.12	0.12	XXX	
90799		C	Unlisted therapeutic, prophylactic or diagnostic injection	0.00	0.00	0.00	0.00	0.00	0.00	XXX	
90801		A	Psychiatric diagnostic interview examination	2.80	1.14	0.93	0.06	4.00	3.79	XXX	
90802		A	Interactive psychiatric diagnostic interview examination using play equipment, physical devices, language interpreter, or other mechanisms of communication	3.01	1.17	0.99	0.07	4.25	4.07	XXX	
90804		A	Individual psychotherapy, insight oriented, behavior modifying and/or supportive, in an office or outpatient facility, approximately 20 to 30 minutes face-to-face with the patient;	1.21	0.53	0.4	0.03	1.77	1.64	XXX	
90805		A	with medical evaluation and management services	1.37	0.59	0.44	0.03	1.99	1.84	XXX	
90806		A	Individual psychotherapy, insight oriented, behavior modifying and/or supportive, in an office or outpatient facility, approximately 45 to 50 minutes face-to-face with the patient;	1.86	0.75	0.62	0.04	2.65	2.52	XXX	
90807		A	with medical evaluation and management services	2.02	0.79	0.66	0.05	2.86	2.73	XXX	
90808		A	Individual psychotherapy, insight oriented, behavior modifying and/or supportive, in an office or outpatient facility, approximately 75 to 80 minutes face-to-face with the patient;	2.79	1.06	0.93	0.07	3.92	3.79	XXX	
90809		A	with medical evaluation and management services	2.95	1.11	0.97	0.07	4.13	3.99	XXX	

Medicine

■ RVU not developed by CMS. Gap-filled RVUs developed by Ingenix/CHEG.

Code	M	S	Description	Work Value	Non-Fac PE	Fac PE	Mal-practice	Non-Fac Total	Fac Total	Global	Gap
90810		A	Individual psychotherapy, interactive, using play equipment, physical devices, language interpreter, or other mechanisms of nonverbal communication, in an office or outpatient facility, approximately 20 to 30 minutes face-to-face with the patient;	1.32	0.56	0.44	0.03	1.91	1.79	XXX	
90811		A	with medical evaluation and management services	1.48	0.63	0.48	0.03	2.14	1.99	XXX	
90812		A	Individual psychotherapy, interactive, using play equipment, physical devices, language interpreter, or other mechanisms of nonverbal communication, in an office or outpatient facility, approximately 45 to 50 minutes face-to-face with the patient;	1.97	0.80	0.69	0.05	2.82	2.71	XXX	
90813		A	with medical evaluation and management services	2.13	0.87	0.71	0.05	3.05	2.89	XXX	
90814		A	Individual psychotherapy, interactive, using play equipment, physical devices, language interpreter, or other mechanisms of nonverbal communication, in an office or outpatient facility, approximately 75 to 80 minutes face-to-face with the patient;	2.90	1.15	1.01	0.07	4.12	3.98	XXX	
90815		A	with medical evaluation and management services	3.06	1.15	1.02	0.07	4.28	4.15	XXX	
90816		A	Individual psychotherapy, insight oriented, behavior modifying and/or supportive, in an inpatient hospital, partial hospital or residential care setting, approximately 20 to 30 minutes face-to-face with the patient;	1.25	0.57	0.43	0.03	1.85	1.71	XXX	
90817		A	with medical evaluation and management services	1.41	0.62	0.45	0.03	2.06	1.89	XXX	
90818		A	Individual psychotherapy, insight oriented, behavior modifying and/or supportive, in an inpatient hospital, partial hospital or residential care setting, approximately 45 to 50 minutes face-to-face with the patient;	1.89	0.80	0.65	0.04	2.73	2.58	XXX	
90819		A	with medical evaluation and management services	2.05	0.83	0.66	0.05	2.93	2.76	XXX	
90821		A	Individual psychotherapy, insight oriented, behavior modifying and/or supportive, in an inpatient hospital, partial hospital or residential care setting, approximately 75 to 80 minutes face-to-face with the patient;	2.83	1.11	0.97	0.06	4.00	3.86	XXX	
90822		A	with medical evaluation and management services	2.99	1.30	0.97	0.07	4.36	4.03	XXX	

■ RVU not developed by CMS. Gap-filled RVUs developed by Ingenix/CHEG.

Code	M	S	Description	Work Value	Non-Fac PE	Fac PE	Mal-practice	Non-Fac Total	Fac Total	Global	Gap
90823		A	Individual psychotherapy, interactive, using play equipment, physical devices, language interpreter, or other mechanisms of nonverbal communication, in an inpatient hospital, partial hospital or residential care setting, approximately 20 to 30 minutes face-to-face with the patient;	1.36	0.65	0.45	0.03	2.04	1.84	XXX	
90824		A	with medical evaluation and management services	1.52	0.70	0.50	0.03	2.25	2.05	XXX	
90826		A	Individual psychotherapy, interactive, using play equipment, physical devices, language interpreter, or other mechanisms of nonverbal communication, in an inpatient hospital, partial hospital or residential care setting, approximately 45 to 50 minutes face-to-face with the patient;	2.01	0.89	0.68	0.04	2.94	2.73	XXX	
90827		A	with medical evaluation and management services	2.16	0.91	0.70	0.05	3.12	2.91	XXX	
90828		A	Individual psychotherapy, interactive, using play equipment, physical devices, language interpreter, or other mechanisms of nonverbal communication, in an inpatient hospital, partial hospital or residential care setting, approximately 75 to 80 minutes face-to-face with the patient;	2.94	1.90	1.02	0.07	4.91	4.03	XXX	
90829		A	with medical evaluation and management services	3.10	1.23	1.02	0.07	4.40	4.19	XXX	
90845		A	Psychoanalysis	1.79	0.71	0.57	0.04	2.54	2.40	XXX	
90846		R	Family psychotherapy (without the patient present)	1.83	0.73	0.62	0.04	2.60	2.49	XXX	
90847		R	Family psychotherapy (conjoint psychotherapy) (with patient present)	2.21	0.86	0.75	0.05	3.12	3.01	XXX	
90849		R	Multiple-family group psychotherapy	0.59	0.31	0.20	0.01	0.91	0.80	XXX	
90853		A	Group psychotherapy (other than of a multiple-family group)	0.59	0.35	0.20	0.01	0.95	0.80	XXX	
90857		A	Interactive group psychotherapy	0.63	0.37	0.21	0.02	1.02	0.86	XXX	
90862		A	Pharmacologic management, including prescription, use, and review of medication with no more than minimal medical psychotherapy	0.95	0.44	0.31	0.02	1.41	1.28	XXX	
90865		A	Narcosynthesis for psychiatric diagnostic and therapeutic purposes (eg, sodium amobarbital (Amytal) interview)	2.84	1.70	0.94	0.07	4.61	3.85	XXX	
90870		A	Electroconvulsive therapy (includes necessary monitoring); single seizure	1.88	0.74	0.74	0.04	2.66	2.66	000	
90871		A	multiple seizures, per day	2.72	1.04	1.04	0.06	3.82	3.82	000	

■ RVU not developed by CMS. Gap-filled RVUs developed by Ingenix/CHEG.

Medicine

Code	M	S	Description	Work Value	Non-Fac PE	Fac PE	Mal-practice	Non-Fac Total	Fac Total	Global	Gap
90875		N	Individual psychophysiological therapy incorporating biofeedback training by any modality (face-to-face with the patient), with psychotherapy (eg, insight oriented, behavior modifying or supportive psychotherapy); approximately 20-30 minutes	1.20	0.90	0.48	0.03	2.13	1.71	XXX	
90876		N	approximately 45-50 minutes	1.90	1.18	0.76	0.04	3.12	2.70	XXX	
90880		A	Hypnotherapy	2.19	0.91	0.71	0.05	3.15	2.95	XXX	
90882		N	Environmental intervention for medical management purposes on a psychiatric patient's behalf with agencies, employers, or institutions	0.66	1.51	1.51	0.09	2.26	2.26	XXX	■
90885		B	Psychiatric evaluation of hospital records, other psychiatric reports, psychometric and/or projective tests, and other accumulated data for medical diagnostic purposes	0.97	0.39	0.39	0.02	1.38	1.38	XXX	
90887		B	Interpretation or explanation of results of psychiatric, other medical examinations and procedures, or other accumulated data to family or other responsible persons, or advising them how to assist patient	1.48	0.83	0.59	0.03	2.34	2.10	XXX	
90889		B	Preparation of report of patient's psychiatric status, history, treatment, or progress (other than for legal or consultative purposes) for other physicians, agencies, or insurance carriers	0.57	1.31	1.31	0.08	1.95	1.95	XXX	■
90899		C	Unlisted psychiatric service or procedure	0.00	0.00	0.00	0.00	0.00	0.00	XXX	
90901		A	Biofeedback training by any modality	0.41	0.82	0.17	0.02	1.25	0.60	000	
90911		A	Biofeedback training, perineal muscles, anorectal or urethral sphincter, including EMG and/or manometry	0.89	0.87	0.39	0.04	1.80	1.32	000	
90918		A	End stage renal disease (ESRD) related services per full month; for patients under 2 years of age to include monitoring for the adequacy of nutrition, assessment of growth and development, and counseling of parents	11.18	5.53	5.53	0.3	17.01	17.01	XXX	
90919		A	for patients between two and eleven years of age to include monitoring for the adequacy of nutrition, assessment of growth and development, and counseling of parents	8.54	4.53	4.53	0.24	13.31	13.31	XXX	
90920		A	for patients between twelve and nineteen years of age to include monitoring for the adequacy of nutrition, assessment of growth and development, and counseling of parents	7.27	4.02	4.02	0.19	11.48	11.48	XXX	
90921		A	for patients twenty years of age and over	4.47	2.96	2.96	0.12	7.55	7.55	XXX	

■ RVU not developed by CMS. Gap-filled RVUs developed by Ingenix/CHEG.

Code	M	S	Description	Work Value	Non-Fac PE	Fac PE	Mal-practice	Non-Fac Total	Fac Total	Global	Gap
90922		A	End stage renal disease (ESRD) related services (less than full month), per day; for patients under two years of age	0.37	0.17	0.17	0.01	0.55	0.55	XXX	
90923		A	for patients between two and eleven years of age	0.28	0.15	0.15	0.01	0.44	0.44	XXX	
90924		A	for patients between twelve and nineteen years of age	0.24	0.13	0.13	0.01	0.38	0.38	XXX	
90925		A	for patients twenty years of age and over	0.15	0.10	0.10	0.01	0.26	0.26	XXX	
90935		A	Hemodialysis procedure with single physician evaluation	1.22	0.86	0.86	0.03	2.11	2.11	000	
90937		A	Hemodialysis procedure requiring repeated evaluation(s) with or without substantial revision of dialysis prescription	2.11	1.20	1.20	0.06	3.37	3.37	000	
90939		X	Hemodialysis access flow study to determine blood flow in grafts and arteriovenous fistulae by an indicator dilution method, hook-up; transcutaneous measurement and disconnection	0.64	1.47	1.47	0.09	2.20	2.20	XXX	■
	26			0.26	0.59	0.59	0.04	0.88	0.88	XXX	■
	TC			0.38	0.88	0.88	0.05	1.32	1.32	XXX	■
90940		X	Hemodialysis access flow study to determine blood flow in grafts and arteriovenous fistulae by an indicator dilution method, hook-up; measurement and disconnection	0.64	1.47	1.47	0.09	2.20	2.20	XXX	■
	26			0.26	0.59	0.59	0.04	0.88	0.88	XXX	■
	TC			0.38	0.88	0.88	0.05	1.32	1.32	XXX	■
90945		A	Dialysis procedure other than hemodialysis (eg, peritoneal dialysis, hemofiltration, or other continuous renal replacement therapies), with single physician evaluation	1.28	0.89	0.89	0.04	2.21	2.21	000	
90947		A	Dialysis procedure other than hemodialysis (eg, peritoneal dialysis, hemofiltration, or other continuous renal replacement therapies) requiring repeated physician evaluations, with or without substantial revision of dialysis prescription	2.16	1.24	1.24	0.06	3.46	3.46	000	
90989		X	Dialysis training, patient, including helper where applicable, any mode, completed course	4.17	9.63	9.63	0.58	14.38	14.38	XXX	■
90993		X	Dialysis training, patient, including helper where applicable, any mode, course not completed, per training session	0.70	1.62	1.62	0.10	2.42	2.42	XXX	■
90997		A	Hemoperfusion (eg, with activated charcoal or resin)	1.84	1.10	1.10	0.05	2.99	2.99	000	
90999		C	Unlisted dialysis procedure, inpatient or outpatient	0.00	0.00	0.00	0.00	0.00	0.00	XXX	
91000		A	Esophageal intubation and collection of washings for cytology, including preparation of specimens (separate procedure)	0.73	0.32	0.32	0.04	1.09	1.09	000	
	26	A		0.73	0.25	0.25	0.03	1.01	1.01	000	
	TC	A		0.00	0.07	0.07	0.01	0.08	0.08	000	

Medicine

■ RVU not developed by CMS. Gap-filled RVUs developed by Ingenix/CHEG.

Code	M	S	Description	Work Value	Non-Fac PE	Fac PE	Mal-prac-tice	Non-Fac Total	Fac Total	Global	Gap
91010		A	Esophageal motility (manometric study of the esophagus and/or gastroesophageal junction) study;	1.25	2.60	2.60	0.10	3.95	3.95	000	
	26	A		1.25	0.46	0.46	0.05	1.76	1.76	000	
	TC	A		0.00	2.14	2.14	0.05	2.19	2.19	000	
91011		A	with mecholyl or similar stimulant	1.50	2.71	2.71	0.10	4.31	4.31	000	
	26	A		1.50	0.55	0.55	0.05	2.10	2.10	000	
	TC	A		0.00	2.16	2.16	0.05	2.21	2.21	000	
91012		A	with acid perfusion studies	1.46	2.35	2.35	0.12	3.93	3.93	000	
	26	A		1.46	0.54	0.54	0.06	2.06	2.06	000	
	TC	A		0.00	1.81	1.81	0.06	1.87	1.87	000	
91020		A	Gastric motility (manometric) studies	1.44	2.96	2.96	0.11	4.51	4.51	000	
	26	A		1.44	0.51	0.51	0.06	2.01	2.01	000	
	TC	A		0.00	2.45	2.45	0.05	2.50	2.50	000	
91030		A	Esophagus, acid perfusion (Bernstein) test for esophagitis	0.91	2.27	2.27	0.05	3.23	3.23	000	
	26	A		0.91	0.34	0.34	0.03	1.28	1.28	000	
	TC	A		0.00	1.93	1.93	0.02	1.95	1.95	000	
91032		A	Esophagus, acid reflux test, with intraluminal pH electrode for detection of gastroesophageal reflux;	1.21	2.26	2.26	0.1	3.57	3.57	000	
	26	A		1.21	0.44	0.44	0.05	1.70	1.70	000	
	TC	A		0.00	1.82	1.82	0.05	1.87	1.87	000	
91033		A	prolonged recording	1.30	2.64	2.64	0.14	4.08	4.08	000	
	26	A		1.30	0.48	0.48	0.05	1.83	1.83	000	
	TC	A		0.00	2.16	2.16	0.09	2.25	2.25	000	
91052		A	Gastric analysis test with injection of stimulant of gastric secretion (eg, histamine, insulin, pentagastrin, calcium and secretin)	0.79	2.19	2.19	0.05	3.03	3.03	000	
	26	A		0.79	0.29	0.29	0.03	1.11	1.11	000	
	TC	A		0.00	1.90	1.90	0.02	1.92	1.92	000	
91055		A	Gastric intubation, washings, and preparing slides for cytology (separate procedure)	0.94	2.22	2.22	0.06	3.22	3.22	000	
	26	A		0.94	0.28	0.28	0.04	1.26	1.26	000	
	TC	A		0.00	1.94	1.94	0.02	1.96	1.96	000	
91060		A	Gastric saline load test	0.45	0.28	0.28	0.04	0.77	0.77	000	
	26	A		0.45	0.15	0.15	0.02	0.62	0.62	000	
	TC	A		0.00	0.13	0.13	0.02	0.15	0.15	000	
91065		A	Breath hydrogen test (eg, for detection of lactase deficiency)	0.20	4.55	4.55	0.03	4.78	4.78	000	
	26	A		0.20	0.07	0.07	0.01	0.28	0.28	000	
	TC	A		0.00	4.48	4.48	0.02	4.50	4.50	000	
91100		A	Intestinal bleeding tube, passage, positioning and monitoring	1.08	0.48	0.48	0.06	1.62	1.62	000	
91105		A	Gastric intubation, and aspiration or lavage for treatment (eg, for ingested poisons)	0.37	0.21	0.21	0.02	0.60	0.60	000	
91122		A	Anorectal manometry	1.77	2.77	2.77	0.17	4.71	4.71	000	
	26	A		1.77	0.63	0.63	0.10	2.50	2.50	000	
	TC	A		0.00	2.14	2.14	0.07	2.21	2.21	000	
91123		B	Pulsed irrigation of fecal impaction	0.00	0.00	0.00	0.00	0.00	0.00	XXX	
91132		C	Electrogastrography, diagnostic, transcutaneous;	0.80	0.32	0.32	0.05	1.17	1.17	XXX	■
	26	A		0.52	0.21	0.21	0.03	0.76	0.76	XXX	
	TC	C		0.28	0.11	0.11	0.02	0.41	0.41	XXX	■

■ RVU not developed by CMS. Gap-filled RVUs developed by Ingenix/CHEG.

Code	M	S	Description	Work Value	Non-Fac PE	Fac PE	Mal-practice	Non-Fac Total	Fac Total	Global	Gap
91133		C	with provocative testing	1.02	0.40	0.40	0.05	1.46	1.46	XXX	■
	26	A		0.66	0.26	0.26	0.03	0.95	0.95	XXX	
	TC	C		0.36	0.14	0.14	0.02	0.51	0.51	XXX	■
91299		C	Unlisted diagnostic gastroenterology procedure	0.00	0.00	0.00	0.00	0.00	0.00	XXX	
	26	C		0.00	0.00	0.00	0.00	0.00	0.00	XXX	
	TC	C		0.00	0.00	0.00	0.00	0.00	0.00	XXX	
92002		A	Ophthalmological services: medical examination and evaluation with initiation of diagnostic and treatment program; intermediate, new patient	0.88	0.96	0.38	0.02	1.86	1.28	XXX	
92004		A	comprehensive, new patient, one or more visits	1.67	1.71	0.73	0.03	3.41	2.43	XXX	
92012		A	Ophthalmological services: medical examination and evaluation, with initiation or continuation of diagnostic and treatment program; intermediate, established patient	0.67	1.01	0.31	0.01	1.69	0.99	XXX	
92014		A	comprehensive, established patient, one or more visits	1.10	1.40	0.50	0.02	2.52	1.62	XXX	
92015		N	Determination of refractive state	0.38	1.51	0.15	0.01	1.90	0.54	XXX	
92018		A	Ophthalmological examination and evaluation, under general anesthesia, with or without manipulation of globe for passive range of motion or other manipulation to facilitate diagnostic examination; complete	2.50	1.14	1.14	0.03	3.67	3.67	XXX	
92019		A	limited	1.31	0.61	0.61	0.03	1.95	1.95	XXX	
92020		A	Gonioscopy (separate procedure)	0.37	0.95	0.17	0.01	1.33	0.55	XXX	
92060		A	Sensorimotor examination with multiple measurements of ocular deviation (eg, restrictive or paretic muscle with diplopia) with interpretation and report (separate procedure)	0.69	0.74	0.74	0.02	1.45	1.45	XXX	
	26	A		0.69	0.31	0.31	0.01	1.01	1.01	XXX	
	TC	A		0.00	0.43	0.43	0.01	0.44	0.44	XXX	
92065		A	Orthoptic and/or pleoptic training, with continuing medical direction and evaluation	0.37	1.19	1.19	0.02	1.58	1.58	XXX	
	26	A		0.37	0.15	0.15	0.01	0.53	0.53	XXX	
	TC	A		0.00	1.04	1.04	0.01	1.05	1.05	XXX	
92070		A	Fitting of contact lens for treatment of disease, including supply of lens	0.70	1.12	0.34	0.01	1.83	1.05	XXX	
92081		A	Visual field examination, unilateral or bilateral, with interpretation and report; limited examination (eg, tangent screen, Autoplot, arc perimeter, or single stimulus level automated test, such as Octopus 3 or 7 equivalent)	0.36	1.84	1.84	0.02	2.22	2.22	XXX	
	26	A		0.36	0.16	0.16	0.01	0.53	0.53	XXX	
	TC	A		0.00	1.68	1.68	0.01	1.69	1.69	XXX	
92082		A	intermediate examination (eg, at least 2 isopters on Goldmann perimeter, or semiquantitative, automated suprathreshold screening program, Humphrey suprathreshold automatic diagnostic test, Octopus program 33)	0.44	0.85	0.85	0.02	1.31	1.31	XXX	
	26	A		0.44	0.20	0.20	0.01	0.65	0.65	XXX	
	TC	A		0.00	0.65	0.65	0.01	0.66	0.66	XXX	

■ RVU not developed by CMS. Gap-filled RVUs developed by Ingenix/CHEG.

Code	M	S	Description	Work Value	Non-Fac PE	Fac PE	Mal-practice	Non-Fac Total	Fac Total	Global	Gap
92083		A	extended examination (eg, Goldmann visual fields with at least 3 isopters plotted and static determination within the central 30 degrees, or quantitative, automated threshold perimetry, Octopus programs G-1, 32 or 42, Humphrey visual field analyzer full threshold programs 30-2, 24-2, or 30/60-2)	0.50	1.51	1.51	0.02	2.03	2.03	XXX	
	26	A		0.50	0.23	0.23	0.01	0.74	0.74	XXX	
	TC	A		0.00	1.28	1.28	0.01	1.29	1.29	XXX	
92100		A	Serial tonometry (separate procedure) with multiple measurements of intraocular pressure over an extended time period with interpretation and report, same day (eg, diurnal curve or medical treatment of acute elevation of intraocular pressure)	0.92	0.75	0.40	0.02	1.69	1.34	XXX	
92120		A	Tonography with interpretation and report, recording indentation tonometer method or perilimbal suction method	0.81	0.81	0.31	0.02	1.64	1.14	XXX	
92130		A	Tonography with water provocation	0.81	0.92	0.32	0.02	1.75	1.15	XXX	
92135		A	Scanning computerized ophthalmic diagnostic imaging (eg, scanning laser) with interpretation and report, unilateral	0.35	1.48	1.48	0.02	1.85	1.85	XXX	
	26	A		0.35	0.17	0.17	0.01	0.53	0.53	XXX	
	TC	A		0.00	1.31	1.31	0.01	1.32	1.32	XXX	
92136		A	Ophthalmic biometry by partial coherence interferometry with intraocular lens power calculation	0.54	1.52	1.52	0.07	2.13	2.13	XXX	
	26	A		0.54	0.22	0.22	0.01	0.77	0.77	XXX	
	TC	A		0.00	1.30	1.30	0.06	1.36	1.36	XXX	
92140		A	Provocative tests for glaucoma, with interpretation and report, without tonography	0.50	1.01	0.22	0.01	1.52	0.73	XXX	
92225		A	Ophthalmoscopy, extended, with retinal drawing (eg, for retinal detachment, melanoma), with interpretation and report; initial	0.38	0.23	0.17	0.01	0.62	0.56	XXX	
92226		A	subsequent	0.33	0.22	0.15	0.01	0.56	0.49	XXX	
92230		A	Fluorescein angioscopy with interpretation and report	0.60	1.73	0.21	0.02	2.35	0.83	XXX	
92235		A	Fluorescein angiography (includes multiframe imaging) with interpretation and report	0.81	2.62	2.62	0.07	3.50	3.50	XXX	
	26	A		0.81	0.39	0.39	0.02	1.22	1.22	XXX	
	TC	A		0.00	2.23	2.23	0.05	2.28	2.28	XXX	
92240		A	Indocyanine-green angiography (includes multiframe imaging) with interpretation and report)	1.10	5.24	5.24	0.07	6.41	6.41	XXX	
	26	A		1.10	0.53	0.53	0.02	1.65	1.65	XXX	
	TC	A		0.00	4.71	4.71	0.05	4.76	4.76	XXX	
92250		A	Fundus photography with interpretation and report	0.44	1.37	1.37	0.02	1.83	1.83	XXX	
	26	A		0.44	0.20	0.20	0.01	0.65	0.65	XXX	
	TC	A		0.00	1.17	1.17	0.01	1.18	1.18	XXX	
92260		A	Ophthalmodynamometry	0.20	0.24	0.10	0.01	0.45	0.31	XXX	
92265		A	Needle oculoelectromyography, one or more extraocular muscles, one or both eyes, with interpretation and report	0.81	1.23	1.23	0.04	2.08	2.08	XXX	
	26	A		0.81	0.38	0.38	0.02	1.21	1.21	XXX	
	TC	A		0.00	0.85	0.85	0.02	0.87	0.87	XXX	

■ RVU not developed by CMS. Gap-filled RVUs developed by Ingenix/CHEG.

Code	M	S	Description	Work Value	Non-Fac PE	Fac PE	Mal-prac-tice	Non-Fac Total	Fac Total	Global	Gap
92270		A	Electro-oculography with interpretation and report	0.81	1.15	1.15	0.05	2.01	2.01	XXX	
	26	A		0.81	0.37	0.37	0.03	1.21	1.21	XXX	
	TC	A		0.00	0.78	0.78	0.02	0.80	0.80	XXX	
92275		A	Electroretinography with interpretation and report	1.01	1.25	1.25	0.04	2.30	2.30	XXX	
	26	A		1.01	0.46	0.46	0.02	1.49	1.49	XXX	
	TC	A		0.00	0.79	0.79	0.02	0.81	0.81	XXX	
92283		A	Color vision examination, extended, eg, anomaloscope or equivalent	0.17	0.74	0.74	0.02	0.93	0.93	XXX	
	26	A		0.17	0.07	0.07	0.01	0.25	0.25	XXX	
	TC	A		0.00	0.67	0.67	0.01	0.68	0.68	XXX	
92284		A	Dark adaptation examination, with interpretation and report	0.24	1.75	1.75	0.02	2.01	2.01	XXX	
	26	A		0.24	0.09	0.09	0.01	0.34	0.34	XXX	
	TC	A		0.00	1.66	1.66	0.01	1.67	1.67	XXX	
92285		A	External ocular photography with interpretation and report for documentation of medical progress (eg, close-up photography, slit lamp photography, goniophotography, stereo-photography)	0.20	0.80	0.80	0.02	1.02	1.02	XXX	
	26	A		0.20	0.09	0.09	0.01	0.30	0.30	XXX	
	TC	A		0.00	0.71	0.71	0.01	0.72	0.72	XXX	
92286		A	Special anterior segment photography with interpretation and report; with specular endothelial microscopy and cell count	0.66	3.00	3.00	0.03	3.69	3.69	XXX	
	26	A		0.66	0.32	0.32	0.01	0.99	0.99	XXX	
	TC	A		0.00	2.68	2.68	0.02	2.70	2.70	XXX	
92287		A	with fluorescein angiography	0.81	3.16	0.31	0.02	3.99	1.14	XXX	
	26			0.24	0.95	0.09	0.01	1.20	0.34	XXX	■
	TC			0.57	2.21	0.22	0.01	2.79	0.80	XXX	■
92310		N	Prescription of optical and physical characteristics of and fitting of contact lens, with medical supervision of adaptation; corneal lens, both eyes, except for aphakia	1.17	1.10	0.47	0.03	2.30	1.67	XXX	
92311		A	corneal lens for aphakia, one eye	1.08	1.17	0.31	0.03	2.28	1.42	XXX	
92312		A	corneal lens for aphakia, both eyes	1.26	1.17	0.45	0.03	2.46	1.74	XXX	
92313		A	corneoscleral lens	0.92	1.21	0.33	0.02	2.15	1.27	XXX	
92314		N	Prescription of optical and physical characteristics of contact lens, with medical supervision of adaptation and direction of fitting by independent technician; corneal lens, both eyes, except for aphakia	0.69	0.91	0.28	0.01	1.61	0.98	XXX	
92315		A	corneal lens for aphakia, one eye	0.45	0.95	0.17	0.01	1.41	0.63	XXX	
92316		A	corneal lens for aphakia, both eyes	0.68	1.03	0.30	0.01	1.72	0.99	XXX	
92317		A	corneoscleral lens	0.45	0.97	0.18	0.01	1.43	0.64	XXX	
92325		A	Modification of contact lens (separate procedure), with medical supervision of adaptation	0.00	0.38	0.38	0.01	0.39	0.39	XXX	
92326		A	Replacement of contact lens	0.00	1.55	1.55	0.05	1.60	1.60	XXX	

Medicine

■ RVU not developed by CMS. Gap-filled RVUs developed by Ingenix/CHEG.

Code	M	S	Description	Work Value	Non-Fac PE	Fac PE	Mal-practice	Non-Fac Total	Fac Total	Global	Gap
92330		A	Prescription, fitting, and supply of ocular prosthesis (artificial eye), with medical supervision of adaptation	1.08	1.01	0.38	0.04	2.13	1.50	XXX	
92335		A	Prescription of ocular prosthesis (artificial eye) and direction of fitting and supply by independent technician, with medical supervision of adaptation	0.45	0.99	0.17	0.01	1.45	0.63	XXX	
92340		N	Fitting of spectacles, except for aphakia; monofocal	0.37	0.68	0.15	0.01	1.06	0.53	XXX	
92341		N	bifocal	0.47	0.72	0.19	0.01	1.20	0.67	XXX	
92342		N	multifocal, other than bifocal	0.53	0.74	0.21	0.01	1.28	0.75	XXX	
92352		B	Fitting of spectacle prosthesis for aphakia; monofocal	0.37	0.68	0.15	0.01	1.06	0.53	XXX	
92353		B	multifocal	0.50	0.73	0.20	0.02	1.25	0.72	XXX	
92354		B	Fitting of spectacle mounted low vision aid; single element system	0.00	8.41	8.41	0.08	8.49	8.49	XXX	
92355		B	telescopic or other compound lens system	0.00	4.11	4.11	0.01	4.12	4.12	XXX	
92358		B	Prosthesis service for aphakia, temporary (disposable or loan, including materials)	0.00	0.92	0.92	0.04	0.96	0.96	XXX	
92370		N	Repair and refitting spectacles; except for aphakia	0.32	0.54	0.13	0.02	0.88	0.47	XXX	
92371		B	spectacle prosthesis for aphakia	0.00	0.59	0.59	0.02	0.61	0.61	XXX	
92390		N	Supply of spectacles, except prosthesis for aphakia and low vision aids	0.00	0.00	0.00	0.00	0.00	0.00	XXX	
92391		N	Supply of contact lenses, except prosthesis for aphakia	0.00	0.00	0.00	0.00	0.00	0.00	XXX	
92392		I	Supply of low vision aids (A low vision aid is any lens or device used to aid or improve visual function in a person whose vision cannot be normalized by conventional spectacle correction. Includes reading additions up to 4D.)	0.00	3.84	3.84	0.02	3.86	3.86	XXX	
92393		I	Supply of ocular prosthesis (artificial eye)	0.00	11.92	11.92	0.47	12.39	12.39	XXX	
92395		I	Supply of permanent prosthesis for aphakia; spectacles	0.00	1.30	1.30	0.08	1.38	1.38	XXX	
92396		I	contact lenses	0.00	2.19	2.19	0.06	2.25	2.25	XXX	
92499		C	Unlisted ophthalmological service or procedure	0.00	0.00	0.00	0.00	0.00	0.00	XXX	
	26	C		0.00	0.00	0.00	0.00	0.00	0.00	XXX	
	TC	C		0.00	0.00	0.00	0.00	0.00	0.00	XXX	
92502		A	Otolaryngologic examination under general anesthesia	1.51	1.28	1.28	0.06	2.85	2.85	000	

■ RVU not developed by CMS. Gap-filled RVUs developed by Ingenix/CHEG.

Code	M	S	Description	Work Value	Non-Fac PE	Fac PE	Mal-practice	Non-Fac Total	Fac Total	Global	Gap
92504		A	Binocular microscopy (separate diagnostic procedure)	0.18	1.10	0.09	0.01	1.29	0.28	XXX	
92506		A	Evaluation of speech, language, voice, communication, auditory processing, and/or aural rehabilitation status	0.86	1.72	0.43	0.04	2.62	1.33	XXX	
92507		A	Treatment of speech, language, voice, communication, and/or auditory processing disorder (includes aural rehabilitation); individual	0.52	1.54	0.28	0.02	2.08	0.82	XXX	
92508		A	group, two or more individuals	0.26	1.77	0.15	0.01	2.04	0.42	XXX	
92510		A	Aural rehabilitation following cochlear implant (includes evaluation of aural rehabilitation status and hearing, therapeutic services) with or without speech processor programming	1.50	2.11	0.83	0.06	3.67	2.39	XXX	
92511		A	Nasopharyngoscopy with endoscope (separate procedure)	0.84	1.36	0.42	0.03	2.23	1.29	000	
92512		A	Nasal function studies (eg, rhinomanometry)	0.55	1.13	0.17	0.02	1.70	0.74	XXX	
92516		A	Facial nerve function studies (eg, electroneuronography)	0.43	0.94	0.24	0.02	1.39	0.69	XXX	
92520		A	Laryngeal function studies	0.76	0.52	0.43	0.03	1.31	1.22	XXX	
92525		I	Evaluation of swallowing and oral function for feeding	1.50	1.69	0.60	0.07	3.26	2.17	XXX	
92526		A	Treatment of swallowing dysfunction and/or oral function for feeding	0.55	1.55	0.27	0.02	2.12	0.84	XXX	
92531		B	Spontaneous nystagmus, including gaze	0.24	0.55	0.55	0.03	0.82	0.82	XXX	■
92532		B	Positional nystagmus test	0.28	0.64	0.64	0.04	0.96	0.96	XXX	■
92533		B	Caloric vestibular test, each irrigation (binaural, bithermal stimulation constitutes four tests)	0.44	1.02	1.02	0.06	1.52	1.52	XXX	■
92534		B	Optokinetic nystagmus test	0.19	0.45	0.45	0.03	0.67	0.67	XXX	■
92541		A	Spontaneous nystagmus test, including gaze and fixation nystagmus, with recording	0.40	1.45	1.45	0.04	1.89	1.89	XXX	
	26	A		0.40	0.20	0.20	0.02	0.62	0.62	XXX	
	TC	A		0.00	1.25	1.25	0.02	1.27	1.27	XXX	
92542		A	Positional nystagmus test, minimum of 4 positions, with recording	0.33	1.39	1.39	0.03	1.75	1.75	XXX	
	26	A		0.33	0.17	0.17	0.01	0.51	0.51	XXX	
	TC	A		0.00	1.22	1.22	0.02	1.24	1.24	XXX	
92543		A	Caloric vestibular test, each irrigation (binaural, bithermal stimulation constitutes four tests), with recording	0.10	0.39	0.39	0.02	0.51	0.51	XXX	
	26	A		0.10	0.05	0.05	0.01	0.16	0.16	XXX	
	TC	A		0.00	0.34	0.34	0.01	0.35	0.35	XXX	
92544		A	Optokinetic nystagmus test, bidirectional, foveal or peripheral stimulation, with recording	0.26	1.35	1.35	0.03	1.64	1.64	XXX	
	26	A		0.26	0.13	0.13	0.01	0.40	0.40	XXX	
	TC	A		0.00	1.22	1.22	0.02	1.24	1.24	XXX	

■ RVU not developed by CMS. Gap-filled RVUs developed by Ingenix/CHEG.

Code	M	S	Description	Work Value	Non-Fac PE	Fac PE	Mal-prac-tice	Non-Fac Total	Fac Total	Global	Gap
92545		A	Oscillating tracking test, with recording	0.23	1.32	1.32	0.03	1.58	1.58	XXX	
	26	A		0.23	0.12	0.12	0.01	0.36	0.36	XXX	
	TC	A		0.00	1.20	1.20	0.02	1.22	1.22	XXX	
92546		A	Sinusoidal vertical axis rotational testing	0.29	2.22	2.22	0.03	2.54	2.54	XXX	
	26	A		0.29	0.14	0.14	0.01	0.44	0.44	XXX	
	TC	A		0.00	2.08	2.08	0.02	2.10	2.10	XXX	
92547		A	Use of vertical electrodes (List separately in addition to code for primary procedure)	0.00	1.21	1.21	0.05	1.26	1.26	ZZZ	
	26			0.00	0.97	0.97	0.04	1.01	1.01	ZZZ	■
	TC			0.00	0.24	0.24	0.01	0.25	0.25	ZZZ	■
92548		A	Computerized dynamic posturography	0.50	2.09	2.09	0.13	2.72	2.72	XXX	
	26	A		0.50	0.28	0.28	0.02	0.80	0.80	XXX	
	TC	A		0.00	1.81	1.81	0.11	1.92	1.92	XXX	
92551		N	Screening test, pure tone, air only	0.08	0.19	0.19	0.01	0.28	0.28	XXX	■
92552		A	Pure tone audiometry (threshold); air only	0.00	0.42	0.42	0.03	0.45	0.45	XXX	
92553		A	air and bone	0.00	0.62	0.62	0.05	0.67	0.67	XXX	
92555		A	Speech audiometry threshold;	0.00	0.36	0.36	0.03	0.39	0.39	XXX	
92556		A	with speech recognition	0.00	0.54	0.54	0.05	0.59	0.59	XXX	
92557		A	Comprehensive audiometry threshold evaluation and speech recognition (92553 and 92556 combined)	0.00	1.13	1.13	0.10	1.23	1.23	XXX	
92559		N	Audiometric testing of groups	0.26	0.60	0.60	0.04	0.90	0.90	XXX	■
92560		N	Bekesy audiometry; screening	0.16	0.36	0.36	0.02	0.54	0.54	XXX	■
92561		A	diagnostic	0.00	0.68	0.68	0.05	0.73	0.73	XXX	
92562		A	Loudness balance test, alternate binaural or monaural	0.00	0.39	0.39	0.03	0.42	0.42	XXX	
92563		A	Tone decay test	0.00	0.36	0.36	0.03	0.39	0.39	XXX	
92564		A	Short increment sensitivity index (SISI)	0.00	0.45	0.45	0.04	0.49	0.49	XXX	
92565		A	Stenger test, pure tone	0.00	0.38	0.38	0.03	0.41	0.41	XXX	
92567		A	Tympanometry (impedance testing)	0.00	0.50	0.50	0.05	0.55	0.55	XXX	
92568		A	Acoustic reflex testing	0.00	0.36	0.36	0.03	0.39	0.39	XXX	
92569		A	Acoustic reflex decay test	0.00	0.39	0.39	0.03	0.42	0.42	XXX	
92571		A	Filtered speech test	0.00	0.37	0.37	0.03	0.40	0.40	XXX	
92572		A	Staggered spondaic word test	0.00	0.08	0.08	0.01	0.09	0.09	XXX	
92573		A	Lombard test	0.00	0.33	0.33	0.03	0.36	0.36	XXX	
92575		A	Sensorineural acuity level test	0.00	0.28	0.28	0.02	0.30	0.30	XXX	
92576		A	Synthetic sentence identification test	0.00	0.42	0.42	0.04	0.46	0.46	XXX	

■ RVU not developed by CMS. Gap-filled RVUs developed by Ingenix/CHEG.

Code	M	S	Description	Work Value	Non-Fac PE	Fac PE	Mal-practice	Non-Fac Total	Fac Total	Global	Gap
92577		A	Stenger test, speech	0.00	0.68	0.68	0.06	0.74	0.74	XXX	
92579		A	Visual reinforcement audiometry (VRA)	0.00	0.69	0.69	0.05	0.74	0.74	XXX	
92582		A	Conditioning play audiometry	0.00	0.69	0.69	0.05	0.74	0.74	XXX	
92583		A	Select picture audiometry	0.00	0.84	0.84	0.07	0.91	0.91	XXX	
92584		A	Electrocochleography	0.00	2.35	2.35	0.17	2.52	2.52	XXX	
92585		A	Auditory evoked potentials for evoked response audiometry and/or testing of the central nervous system; comprehensive	0.50	1.98	1.98	0.14	2.62	2.62	XXX	
	26	A		0.50	0.23	0.23	0.02	0.75	0.75	XXX	
	TC	A		0.00	1.75	1.75	0.12	1.87	1.87	XXX	
92586		A	limited	0.00	1.75	1.75	0.12	1.87	1.87	XXX	
92587		A	Evoked otoacoustic emissions; limited (single stimulus level, either transient or distortion products)	0.13	1.31	1.31	0.10	1.54	1.54	XXX	
	26	A		0.13	0.07	0.07	0.01	0.21	0.21	XXX	
	TC	A		0.00	1.24	1.24	0.09	1.33	1.33	XXX	
92588		A	comprehensive or diagnostic evaluation (comparison of transient and/or distortion product otoacoustic emissions at multiple levels and frequencies)	0.36	1.58	1.58	0.12	2.06	2.06	XXX	
	26	A		0.36	0.18	0.18	0.01	0.55	0.55	XXX	
	TC	A		0.00	1.40	1.40	0.11	1.51	1.51	XXX	
92589		A	Central auditory function test(s) (specify)	0.00	0.51	0.51	0.05	0.56	0.56	XXX	
92590		N	Hearing aid examination and selection; monaural	0.31	0.72	0.72	0.04	1.07	1.07	XXX	■
92591		N	binaural	0.47	1.08	1.08	0.06	1.61	1.61	XXX	■
92592		N	Hearing aid check; monaural	0.14	0.31	0.31	0.02	0.47	0.47	XXX	■
92593		N	binaural	0.21	0.48	0.48	0.03	0.71	0.71	XXX	■
92594		N	Electroacoustic evaluation for hearing aid; monaural	0.15	0.34	0.34	0.02	0.51	0.51	XXX	■
92595		N	binaural	0.22	0.52	0.52	0.03	0.77	0.77	XXX	■
92596		A	Ear protector attenuation measurements	0.00	0.56	0.56	0.05	0.61	0.61	XXX	
92597		G	Evaluation for use and/or fitting of voice prosthetic or augmentative/alternative communication device to supplement oral speech **Note:** This code was omitted from the November 1, 2001, *Federal Register.* The values published here are from the August 2, 2001, *Federal Register/Proposed Rules.*	1.35	0.53	1.60	0.05	1.93	3.00	XXX	
92598		G	Modification of voice prosthetic or augmentative/alternative communication device to supplement oral speech **Note:** This code was omitted from the November 1, 2001, *Federal Register.* The values published here are from the August 2, 2001, *Federal Register/Proposed Rules.*	0.99	0.39	0.80	0.04	1.42	1.83	XXX	

■ RVU not developed by CMS. Gap-filled RVUs developed by Ingenix/CHEG.

Code	M	S	Description	Work Value	Non-Fac PE	Fac PE	Mal-practice	Non-Fac Total	Fac Total	Global	Gap
92599		C	Unlisted otorhinolaryngological service or procedure	0.00	0.00	0.00	0.00	0.00	0.00	XXX	
	26	C		0.00	0.00	0.00	0.00	0.00	0.00	XXX	
	TC	C		0.00	0.00	0.00	0.00	0.00	0.00	XXX	
92950		A	Cardiopulmonary resuscitation (eg, in cardiac arrest)	3.80	1.59	1.18	0.21	5.60	5.19	000	
92953		A	Temporary transcutaneous pacing	0.23	0.23	0.23	0.01	0.47	0.47	000	
92960		A	Cardioversion, elective, electrical conversion of arrhythmia; external	2.25	2.23	0.91	0.08	4.56	3.24	000	
92961		A	internal (separate procedure)	4.60	1.85	1.85	0.17	6.62	6.62	000	
	26			2.53	1.02	1.02	0.09	3.64	3.64	000	■
	TC			2.07	0.83	0.83	0.08	2.98	2.98	000	■
92970		A	Cardioassist-method of circulatory assist; internal	3.52	1.27	1.27	0.17	4.96	4.96	000	
92971		A	external	1.77	0.86	0.86	0.06	2.69	2.69	000	
92973		A	Percutaneous transluminal coronary thrombectomy (List separately in addition to code for primary procedure)	3.28	1.37	1.37	0.17	4.82	4.82	ZZZ	
92974		A	Transcatheter placement of radiation delivery device for subsequent coronary intravascular brachytherapy (List separately in addition to code for primary procedure)	3.00	1.26	1.26	1.18	5.44	5.44	ZZZ	
92975		A	Thrombolysis, coronary; by intracoronary infusion, including selective coronary angiography	7.25	3.01	3.01	0.22	10.48	10.48	000	
92977		A	by intravenous infusion	0.00	7.65	7.65	0.38	8.03	8.03	XXX	
92978		A	Intravascular ultrasound (coronary vessel or graft) during diagnostic evaluation and/or therapeutic intervention including imaging supervision, interpretation and report; initial vessel (List separately in addition to code for primary procedure)	1.80	5.09	5.09	0.26	7.15	7.15	ZZZ	
	26	A		1.80	0.76	0.76	0.06	2.62	2.62	ZZZ	
	TC	A		0.00	4.33	4.33	0.20	4.53	4.53	ZZZ	
92979		A	each additional vessel (List separately in addition to code for primary procedure)	1.44	2.76	2.76	0.15	4.35	4.35	ZZZ	
	26	A		1.44	0.58	0.58	0.04	2.06	2.06	ZZZ	
	TC	A		0.00	2.18	2.18	0.11	2.29	2.29	ZZZ	
92980		A	Transcatheter placement of an intracoronary stent(s), percutaneous, with or without other therapeutic intervention, any method; single vessel	14.84	6.22	6.22	0.78	21.84	21.84	000	
92981		A	each additional vessel (List separately in addition to code for primary procedure)	4.17	1.75	1.75	0.21	6.13	6.13	ZZZ	
92982		A	Percutaneous transluminal coronary balloon angioplasty; single vessel	10.98	4.59	4.59	0.57	16.14	16.14	000	
92984		A	each additional vessel (List separately in addition to code for primary procedure)	2.97	1.24	1.24	0.16	4.37	4.37	ZZZ	

■ RVU not developed by CMS. Gap-filled RVUs developed by Ingenix/CHEG.

Medicine

Code	M	S	Description	Work Value	Non-Fac PE	Fac PE	Mal-practice	Non-Fac Total	Fac Total	Global	Gap
92986		A	Percutaneous balloon valvuloplasty; aortic valve	21.8	10.43	10.43	1.14	33.37	33.37	090	
92987		A	mitral valve	22.7	10.85	10.85	1.18	34.73	34.73	090	
92990		A	pulmonary valve	17.34	8.41	8.41	0.90	26.65	26.65	090	
92992		C	Atrial septectomy or septostomy; transvenous method, balloon, (eg, Rashkind type) (includes cardiac catheterization)	8.74	20.19	20.19	1.21	30.13	30.13	090	■
92993		C	blade method (Park septostomy) (includes cardiac catheterization)	6.12	14.14	14.14	0.84	21.11	21.11	090	■
92995		A	Percutaneous transluminal coronary atherectomy, by mechanical or other method, with or without balloon angioplasty; single vessel	12.09	5.06	5.06	0.63	17.78	17.78	000	
92996		A	each additional vessel (List separately in addition to code for primary procedure)	3.26	1.37	1.37	0.17	4.80	4.80	ZZZ	
92997		A	Percutaneous transluminal pulmonary artery balloon angioplasty; single vessel	12.00	4.55	4.55	0.63	17.18	17.18	000	
92998		A	each additional vessel (List separately in addition to code for primary procedure)	6.00	2.06	2.06	0.31	8.37	8.37	ZZZ	
93000		A	Electrocardiogram, routine ECG with at least 12 leads; with interpretation and report	0.17	0.50	0.50	0.03	0.70	0.70	XXX	
93005		A	tracing only, without interpretation and report	0.00	0.43	0.43	0.02	0.45	0.45	XXX	
	26			0.00	0.00	0.00	0.00	0.00	0.00	XXX	■
	TC			0.00	0.43	0.43	0.02	0.45	0.45	XXX	■
93010		A	interpretation and report only	0.17	0.07	0.07	0.01	0.25	0.25	XXX	
93012		A	Telephonic transmission of post-symptom electrocardiogram rhythm strip(s), per 30 day period of time; tracing only	0.00	2.24	2.24	0.15	2.39	2.39	XXX	
	26			0.00	0.00	0.00	0.00	0.00	0.00	XXX	■
	TC			0.00	2.24	2.24	0.15	2.39	2.39	XXX	■
93014		A	physician review with interpretation and report only	0.52	0.19	0.19	0.02	0.73	0.73	XXX	
93015		A	Cardiovascular stress test using maximal or submaximal treadmill or bicycle exercise, continous electrocardiographic monitoring, and/or pharmacological stress; with physician supervision, with interpretation and report	0.75	1.90	1.90	0.11	2.76	2.76	XXX	
93016		A	physician supervision only, without interpretation and report	0.45	0.18	0.18	0.01	0.64	0.64	XXX	
93017		A	tracing only, without interpretation and report	0.00	1.60	1.60	0.09	1.69	1.69	XXX	
	26			0.00	0.00	0.00	0.00	0.00	0.00	XXX	■
	TC			0.00	1.60	1.60	0.09	1.69	1.69	XXX	■
93018		A	interpretation and report only	0.30	0.12	0.12	0.01	0.43	0.43	XXX	

Medicine

■ RVU not developed by CMS. Gap-filled RVUs developed by Ingenix/CHEG.

Code	M	S	Description	Work Value	Non-Fac PE	Fac PE	Mal-practice	Non-Fac Total	Fac Total	Global	Gap
93024		A	Ergonovine provocation test	1.17	1.55	1.55	0.11	2.83	2.83	XXX	
	26	A		1.17	0.48	0.48	0.04	1.69	1.69	XXX	
	TC	A		0.00	1.07	1.07	0.07	1.14	1.14	XXX	
93025		A	Microvolt T-wave alternans for assessment of ventricular arrhythmias	0.75	6.42	6.42	0.11	7.28	7.28	XXX	
93040		A	Rhythm ECG, one to three leads; with interpretation and report	0.16	0.19	0.19	0.02	0.37	0.37	XXX	
93041		A	tracing only without interpretation and report	0.00	0.14	0.14	0.01	0.15	0.15	XXX	
	26			0.00	0.00	0.00	0.00	0.00	0.00	XXX	■
	TC			0.00	0.14	0.14	0.01	0.15	0.15	XXX	■
93042		A	interpretation and report only	0.16	0.05	0.05	0.01	0.22	0.22	XXX	
93224		A	Electrocardiographic monitoring for 24 hours by continuous original ECG waveform recording and storage, with visual superimposition scanning; includes recording, scanning analysis with report, physician review and interpretation	0.52	3.47	3.47	0.21	4.20	4.20	XXX	
93225		A	recording (includes hook-up, recording, and disconnection)	0.00	1.18	1.18	0.07	1.25	1.25	XXX	
	26			0.00	0.00	0.00	0.00	0.00	0.00	XXX	■
	TC			0.00	1.18	1.18	0.07	1.25	1.25	XXX	■
93226		A	scanning analysis with report	0.00	2.08	2.08	0.12	2.20	2.20	XXX	
	26			0.00	0.00	0.00	0.00	0.00	0.00	XXX	■
	TC			0.00	2.08	2.08	0.12	2.20	2.20	XXX	■
93227		A	physician review and interpretation	0.52	0.21	0.21	0.02	0.75	0.75	XXX	
93230		A	Electrocardiographic monitoring for 24 hours by continuous original ECG waveform recording and storage without superimposition scanning utilizing a device capable of producing a full miniaturized printout; includes recording, microprocessor-based analysis with report, physician review and interpretation	0.52	3.72	3.72	0.22	4.46	4.46	XXX	
93231		A	recording (includes hook-up, recording, and disconnection)	0.00	1.44	1.44	0.09	1.53	1.53	XXX	
	26			0.00	0.00	0.00	0.00	0.00	0.00	XXX	■
	TC			0.00	1.44	1.44	0.09	1.53	1.53	XXX	■
93232		A	microprocessor-based analysis with report	0.00	2.07	2.07	0.11	2.18	2.18	XXX	
	26			0.00	0.00	0.00	0.00	0.00	0.00	XXX	■
	TC			0.00	2.07	2.07	0.11	2.18	2.18	XXX	■
93233		A	physician review and interpretation	0.52	0.21	0.21	0.02	0.75	0.75	XXX	
93235		A	Electrocardiographic monitoring for 24 hours by continuous computerized monitoring and non-continuous recording, and real-time data analysis utilizing a device capable of producing intermittent full-sized waveform tracings, possibly patient activated; includes monitoring and real time data analysis with report, physician review and interpretation	0.45	2.66	2.66	0.13	3.24	3.24	XXX	

■ RVU not developed by CMS. Gap-filled RVUs developed by Ingenix/CHEG.

Code	M	S	Description	Work Value	Non-Fac PE	Fac PE	Mal-prac-tice	Non-Fac Total	Fac Total	Global	Gap
93236		A	monitoring and real-time data analysis with report	0.00	2.49	2.49	0.12	2.61	2.61	XXX	
	26			0.00	0.00	0.00	0.00	0.00	0.00	XXX	■
	TC			0.00	2.49	2.49	0.12	2.61	2.61	XXX	■
93237		A	physician review and interpretation	0.45	0.17	0.17	0.01	0.63	0.63	XXX	
93268		A	Patient demand single or multiple event recording with presymptom memory loop, per 30 day period of time; includes transmission, physician review and interpretation	0.52	3.62	3.62	0.24	4.38	4.38	XXX	
93270		A	recording (includes hook-up, recording and disconnection)	0.00	1.18	1.18	0.07	1.25	1.25	XXX	
	26			0.00	0.00	0.00	0.00	0.00	0.00	XXX	■
	TC			0.00	1.18	1.18	0.07	1.25	1.25	XXX	■
93271		A	monitoring, receipt of transmissions, and analysis	0.00	2.24	2.24	0.15	2.39	2.39	XXX	
	26			0.00	0.00	0.00	0.00	0.00	0.00	XXX	■
	TC			0.00	2.24	2.24	0.15	2.39	2.39	XXX	■
93272		A	physician review and interpretation only	0.52	0.20	0.20	0.02	0.74	0.74	XXX	
93278		A	Signal-averaged electrocardiography (SAECG), with or without ECG	0.25	1.19	1.19	0.10	1.54	1.54	XXX	
	26	A		0.25	0.10	0.10	0.01	0.36	0.36	XXX	
	TC	A		0.00	1.09	1.09	0.09	1.18	1.18	XXX	
93303		A	Transthoracic echocardiography for congenital cardiac anomalies; complete	1.30	4.16	4.16	0.23	5.69	5.69	XXX	
	26	A		1.30	0.50	0.50	0.04	1.84	1.84	XXX	
	TC	A		0.00	3.66	3.66	0.19	3.85	3.85	XXX	
93304		A	follow-up or limited study	0.75	2.15	2.15	0.13	3.03	3.03	XXX	
	26	A		0.75	0.30	0.30	0.02	1.07	1.07	XXX	
	TC	A		0.00	1.85	1.85	0.11	1.96	1.96	XXX	
93307		A	Echocardiography, transthoracic, real-time with image documentation (2D) with or without M-mode recording; complete	0.92	4.04	4.04	0.22	5.18	5.18	XXX	
	26	A		0.92	0.38	0.38	0.03	1.33	1.33	XXX	
	TC	A		0.00	3.66	3.66	0.19	3.85	3.85	XXX	
93308		A	follow-up or limited study	0.53	2.07	2.07	0.13	2.73	2.73	XXX	
	26	A		0.53	0.22	0.22	0.02	0.77	0.77	XXX	
	TC	A		0.00	1.85	1.85	0.11	1.96	1.96	XXX	
93312		A	Echocardiography, transesophageal, real time with image documentation (2D) (with or without M-mode recording); including probe placement, image acquisition, interpretation and report	2.20	4.45	4.45	0.32	6.97	6.97	XXX	
	26	A		2.20	0.86	0.86	0.08	3.14	3.14	XXX	
	TC	A		0.00	3.59	3.59	0.24	3.83	3.83	XXX	
93313		A	placement of transesophageal probe only	0.95	5.29	0.22	0.05	6.29	1.22	XXX	
93314		A	image acquisition, interpretation and report only	1.25	4.10	4.10	0.28	5.63	5.63	XXX	
	26	A		1.25	0.51	0.51	0.04	1.80	1.80	XXX	
	TC	A		0.00	3.59	3.59	0.24	3.83	3.83	XXX	
93315		A	Transesophageal echocardiography for congential cardiac anomalies; including probe placement, image acquisisiton, interpretation and report	2.78	4.70	4.70	0.34	7.82	7.82	XXX	
	26	A		2.78	1.11	1.11	0.1	3.99	3.99	XXX	
	TC	A		0.00	3.59	3.59	0.24	3.83	3.83	XXX	
93316		A	placement of transesophageal probe only	0.95	6.39	0.25	0.05	7.39	1.25	XXX	

■ RVU not developed by CMS. Gap-filled RVUs developed by Ingenix/CHEG.

Medicine

Code	M	S	Description	Work Value	Non-Fac PE	Fac PE	Mal-practice	Non-Fac Total	Fac Total	Global	Gap
93317		A	image acquisition, interpretation and report only	1.83	4.31	4.31	0.30	6.44	6.44	XXX	
	26	A		1.83	0.72	0.72	0.06	2.61	2.61	XXX	
	TC	A		0.00	3.59	3.59	0.24	3.83	3.83	XXX	
93318		C	Echocardiography, transesophageal (TEE) for monitoring purposes, including probe placement, real time 2-dimensional image acquisition and interpretation leading to ongoing (continuous) assessment of (dynamically changing) cardiac pumping function and to therapeutic measures on an immediate time basis	4.89	1.96	1.96	0.13	6.98	6.98	XXX	■
	26	A		2.20	0.88	0.88	0.06	3.14	3.14	XXX	
	TC	C		2.69	1.08	1.08	0.07	3.84	3.84	XXX	■
93320		A	Doppler echocardiography, pulsed wave and/or continuous wave with spectral display (List separately in addition to codes for echocardiographic imaging); complete	0.38	1.79	1.79	0.11	2.28	2.28	ZZZ	
	26	A		0.38	0.16	0.16	0.01	0.55	0.55	ZZZ	
	TC	A		0.00	1.63	1.63	0.10	1.73	1.73	ZZZ	
93321		A	follow-up or limited study (List separately in addition to codes for echocardiographic imaging)	0.15	1.12	1.12	0.08	1.35	1.35	ZZZ	
	26	A		0.15	0.06	0.06	0.01	0.22	0.22	ZZZ	
	TC	A		0.00	1.06	1.06	0.07	1.13	1.13	ZZZ	
93325		A	Doppler echocardiography color flow velocity mapping (List separately in addition to codes for echocardiography)	0.07	2.78	2.78	0.18	3.03	3.03	ZZZ	
	26	A		0.07	0.03	0.03	0.01	0.11	0.11	ZZZ	
	TC	A		0.00	2.75	2.75	0.17	2.92	2.92	ZZZ	
93350		A	Echocardiography, transthoracic, real-time with image documentation (2D, with or without M-mode recording) during rest and cardiovascular stress test using treadmill, bicycle exercise and/or pharmacologically induced stress, with interpretation and report	1.48	2.28	2.28	0.13	3.89	3.89	XXX	
	26	A		1.48	0.61	0.61	0.02	2.11	2.11	XXX	
	TC	A		0.00	1.67	1.67	0.11	1.78	1.78	XXX	
93501		A	Right heart catheterization	3.02	17.23	17.23	1.03	21.28	21.28	000	
	26	A		3.02	1.24	1.24	0.16	4.42	4.42	000	
	TC	A		0.00	15.99	15.99	0.87	16.86	16.86	000	
93503		A	Insertion and placement of flow directed catheter (eg, Swan-Ganz) for monitoring purposes	2.91	0.71	0.71	0.16	3.78	3.78	000	
93505		A	Endomyocardial biopsy	4.38	3.67	3.67	0.36	8.41	8.41	000	
	26	A		4.38	1.80	1.80	0.23	6.41	6.41	000	
	TC	A		0.00	1.87	1.87	0.13	2.00	2.00	000	
93508		A	Catheter placement in coronary artery(s), arterial coronary conduit(s), and/or venous coronary bypass graft(s) for coronary angiography without concomitant left heart catheterization	4.10	13.64	13.64	0.75	18.49	18.49	000	
	26	A		4.10	1.71	1.71	0.21	6.02	6.02	000	
	TC	A		0.00	11.93	11.93	0.54	12.47	12.47	000	
93510		A	Left heart catheterization, retrograde, from the brachial artery, axillary artery or femoral artery; percutaneous	4.33	36.77	36.77	2.13	43.23	43.23	000	
	26	A		4.33	1.82	1.82	0.22	6.37	6.37	000	
	TC	A		0.00	34.95	34.95	1.91	36.86	36.86	000	
93511		A	by cutdown	5.03	36.12	36.12	2.11	43.26	43.26	000	
	26	A		5.03	2.10	2.10	0.26	7.39	7.39	000	
	TC	A		0.00	34.02	34.02	1.85	35.87	35.87	000	

■ RVU not developed by CMS. Gap-filled RVUs developed by Ingenix/CHEG.

Code	M	S	Description	Work Value	Non-Fac PE	Fac PE	Mal-prac-tice	Non-Fac Total	Fac Total	Global	Gap
93514		A	Left heart catheterization by left ventricular puncture	7.05	36.79	36.79	2.22	46.06	46.06	000	
	26	A		7.05	2.77	2.77	0.37	10.19	10.19	000	
	TC	A		0.00	34.02	34.02	1.85	35.87	35.87	000	
93524		A	Combined transseptal and retrograde left heart catheterization	6.95	47.32	47.32	2.79	57.06	57.06	000	
	26	A		6.95	2.86	2.86	0.36	10.17	10.17	000	
	TC	A		0.00	44.46	44.46	2.43	46.89	46.89	000	
93526		A	Combined right heart catheterization and retrograde left heart catheterization	5.99	48.18	48.18	2.81	56.98	56.98	000	
	26	A		5.99	2.50	2.50	0.31	8.80	8.80	000	
	TC	A		0.00	45.68	45.68	2.50	48.18	48.18	000	
93527		A	Combined right heart catheterization and transseptal left heart catheterization through intact septum (with or without retrograde left heart catheterization)	7.28	47.49	47.49	2.81	57.58	57.58	000	
	26	A		7.28	3.03	3.03	0.38	10.69	10.69	000	
	TC	A		0.00	44.46	44.46	2.43	46.89	46.89	000	
93528		A	Combined right heart catheterization with left ventricular puncture (with or without retrograde left heart catheterization)	9.00	48.27	48.27	2.90	60.17	60.17	000	
	26	A		9.00	3.81	3.81	0.47	13.28	13.28	000	
	TC	A		0.00	44.46	44.46	2.43	46.89	46.89	000	
93529		A	Combined right heart catheterization and left heart catheterization through existing septal opening (with or without retrograde left heart catheterization)	4.80	46.46	46.46	2.68	53.94	53.94	000	
	26	A		4.80	2.00	2.00	0.25	7.05	7.05	000	
	TC	A		0.00	44.46	44.46	2.43	46.89	46.89	000	
93530		A	Right heart catheterization, for congenital cardiac anomalies	4.23	17.59	17.59	1.11	22.93	22.93	000	
	26	A		4.23	1.60	1.60	0.24	6.07	6.07	000	
	TC	A		0.00	15.99	15.99	0.87	16.86	16.86	000	
93531		A	Combined right heart catheterization and retrograde left heart catheterization, for congenital cardiac anomalies	8.35	48.92	48.92	2.96	60.23	60.23	000	
	26	A		8.35	3.24	3.24	0.46	12.05	12.05	000	
	TC	A		0.00	45.68	45.68	2.50	48.18	48.18	000	
93532		A	Combined right heart catheterization and transseptal left heart catheterization through intact septum with or without retrograde left heart catheterization, for congenital cardiac anomalies	10.00	48.58	48.58	2.95	61.53	61.53	000	
	26	A		10.00	4.12	4.12	0.52	14.64	14.64	000	
	TC	A		0.00	44.46	44.46	2.43	46.89	46.89	000	
93533		A	Combined right heart catheterization and transseptal left heart catheterization through existing septal opening, with or without retrograde left heart catheterization, for congenital cardiac anomalies	6.70	47.01	47.01	2.86	56.57	56.57	000	
	26	A		6.70	2.55	2.55	0.43	9.68	9.68	000	
	TC	A		0.00	44.46	44.46	2.43	46.89	46.89	000	
93539		A	Injection procedure during cardiac catheterization; for selective opacification of arterial conduits (eg, internal mammary), whether native or used for bypass	0.40	0.84	0.17	0.01	1.25	0.58	000	
93540		A	for selective opacification of aortocoronary venous bypass grafts, one or more coronary arteries	0.43	0.86	0.18	0.01	1.30	0.62	000	
93541		A	for pulmonary angiography	0.29	0.12	0.12	0.01	0.42	0.42	000	
93542		A	for selective right ventricular or right atrial angiography	0.29	0.12	0.12	0.01	0.42	0.42	000	

■ RVU not developed by CMS. Gap-filled RVUs developed by Ingenix/CHEG.

Code	M	S	Description	Work Value	Non-Fac PE	Fac PE	Mal-practice	Non-Fac Total	Fac Total	Global	Gap
93543		A	for selective left ventricular or left atrial angiography	0.29	0.55	0.12	0.01	0.85	0.42	000	
93544		A	for aortography	0.25	0.53	0.10	0.01	0.79	0.36	000	
93545		A	for selective coronary angiography (injection of radiopaque material may be by hand)	0.40	0.85	0.17	0.01	1.26	0.58	000	
93555		A	Imaging supervision, interpretation and report for injection procedure(s) during cardiac catheterization; ventricular and/or atrial angiography	0.81	6.27	6.27	0.31	7.39	7.39	XXX	
	26	A		0.81	0.34	0.34	0.03	1.18	1.18	XXX	
	TC	A		0.00	5.93	5.93	0.28	6.21	6.21	XXX	
93556		A	pulmonary angiography, aortography, and/or selective coronary angiography including venous bypass grafts and arterial conduits (whether native or used in bypass)	0.83	9.71	9.71	0.45	10.99	10.99	XXX	
	26	A		0.83	0.35	0.35	0.03	1.21	1.21	XXX	
	TC	A		0.00	9.36	9.36	0.42	9.78	9.78	XXX	
93561		A	Indicator dilution studies such as dye or thermal dilution, including arterial and/or venous catheterization; with cardiac output measurement (separate procedure)	0.50	0.67	0.67	0.07	1.24	1.24	000	
	26	A		0.50	0.16	0.16	0.02	0.68	0.68	000	
	TC	A		0.00	0.51	0.51	0.05	0.56	0.56	000	
93562		A	subsequent measurement of cardiac output	0.16	0.34	0.34	0.04	0.54	0.54	000	
	26	A		0.16	0.05	0.05	0.01	0.22	0.22	000	
	TC	A		0.00	0.29	0.29	0.03	0.32	0.32	000	
93571		A	Intravascular doppler velocity and/or pressure derived coronary flow reserve measurement (coronary vessel or graft) during coronary angiography including pharmacologically induced stress; initial vessel (List separately in addition to code for primary procedure)	1.80	5.06	5.06	0.31	7.17	7.17	ZZZ	
	26	A		1.80	0.73	0.73	0.11	2.64	2.64	ZZZ	
	TC	A		0.00	4.33	4.33	0.20	4.53	4.53	ZZZ	
93572		A	each additional vessel (List separately in addition to code for primary procedure)	1.44	2.70	2.70	0.28	4.42	4.42	ZZZ	
	26	A		1.44	0.52	0.52	0.17	2.13	2.13	ZZZ	
	TC	A		0.00	2.18	2.18	0.11	2.29	2.29	ZZZ	
93600		A	Bundle of His recording	2.12	2.74	2.74	0.22	5.08	5.08	000	
	26	A		2.12	0.89	0.89	0.11	3.12	3.12	000	
	TC	A		0.00	1.85	1.85	0.11	1.96	1.96	000	
93602		A	Intra-atrial recording	2.12	1.94	1.94	0.18	4.24	4.24	000	
	26	A		2.12	0.88	0.88	0.12	3.12	3.12	000	
	TC	A		0.00	1.06	1.06	0.06	1.12	1.12	000	
93603		A	Right ventricular recording	2.12	2.46	2.46	0.20	4.78	4.78	000	
	26	A		2.12	0.86	0.86	0.11	3.09	3.09	000	
	TC	A		0.00	1.60	1.60	0.09	1.69	1.69	000	
93609		A	Intraventricular and/or intra-atrial mapping of tachycardia site(s) with catheter manipulation to record from multiple sites to identify origin of tachycardia (List separately in addition to code for primary procedure)	4.81	4.59	4.59	0.66	10.06	10.06	ZZZ	
	26	A		4.81	2.01	2.01	0.52	7.34	7.34	ZZZ	
	TC	A		0.00	2.58	2.58	0.14	2.72	2.72	ZZZ	

Medicine

■ RVU not developed by CMS. Gap-filled RVUs developed by Ingenix/CHEG.

Code	M	S	Description	Work Value	Non-Fac PE	Fac PE	Mal-prac-tice	Non-Fac Total	Fac Total	Global	Gap
93610		A	Intra-atrial pacing	3.02	2.52	2.52	0.25	5.79	5.79	000	
	26	A		3.02	1.23	1.23	0.17	4.42	4.42	000	
	TC	A		0.00	1.29	1.29	0.08	1.37	1.37	000	
93612		A	Intraventricular pacing	3.02	2.76	2.76	0.26	6.04	6.04	000	
	26	A		3.02	1.23	1.23	0.17	4.42	4.42	000	
	TC	A		0.00	1.53	1.53	0.09	1.62	1.62	000	
93613		C	Intracardiac electrophysiologic 3-dimensional mapping (List separately in addition to code for primary procedure)	0.00	0.00	0.00	0.00	0.00	0.00	XXX	
	26	A		7.00	2.79	2.79	0.52	10.31	10.31	XXX	
	TC	C		0.00	0.00	0.00	0.00	0.00	0.00	XXX	
93615		A	Esophageal recording of atrial electrogram with or without ventricular electrogram(s);	0.99	0.66	0.66	0.05	1.70	1.70	000	
	26	A		0.99	0.36	0.36	0.03	1.38	1.38	000	
	TC	A		0.00	0.30	0.30	0.02	0.32	0.32	000	
93616		A	with pacing	1.49	0.80	0.80	0.08	2.37	2.37	000	
	26	A		1.49	0.50	0.50	0.06	2.05	2.05	000	
	TC	A		0.00	0.30	0.30	0.02	0.32	0.32	000	
93618		A	Induction of arrhythmia by electrical pacing	4.26	5.54	5.54	0.42	10.22	10.22	000	
	26	A		4.26	1.78	1.78	0.22	6.26	6.26	000	
	TC	A		0.00	3.76	3.76	0.20	3.96	3.96	000	
93619		A	Comprehensive electrophysiologic evaluation with right atrial pacing and recording, right ventricular pacing and recording, His bundle recording, including insertion and repositioning of multiple electrode catheters, without induction or attempted induction of arrhythmia	7.32	10.32	10.32	0.77	18.41	18.41	000	
	26	A		7.32	3.00	3.00	0.38	10.70	10.70	000	
	TC	A		0.00	7.32	7.32	0.39	7.71	7.71	000	
93620		A	Comprehensive electrophysiologic evaluation with right atrial pacing and recording, right ventricular pacing and recording, His bundle recording, including insertion and repositioning of multiple electrode catheters with induction or attempted induction of arrhythmia;	11.59	13.33	13.33	1.04	25.96	25.96	000	
	26	A		11.59	4.82	4.82	0.60	17.01	17.01	000	
	TC	A		0.00	8.51	8.51	0.44	8.95	8.95	000	
93621		C	with left atrial pacing and recording from coronary sinus or left atrium (List separately in addition to code for primary procedure)	3.82	1.60	1.60	0.27	5.69	5.69	ZZZ	■
	26	A		2.10	0.88	0.88	0.15	3.13	3.13	ZZZ	
	TC	C		1.72	0.72	0.72	0.12	2.56	2.56	ZZZ	■
93622		C	with left ventricular pacing and recording (List separately in addition to code for primary procedure)	5.64	2.36	2.36	1.22	9.22	9.22	ZZZ	■
	26	A		3.10	1.30	1.30	0.67	5.07	5.07	ZZZ	
	TC	C		2.54	1.06	1.06	0.55	4.15	4.15	ZZZ	■
93623		C	Programmed stimulation and pacing after intravenous drug infusion (List separately in addition to code for primary procedure)	5.18	2.16	2.16	0.27	7.62	7.62	ZZZ	■
	26	A		2.85	1.19	1.19	0.15	4.19	4.19	ZZZ	
	TC	C		2.33	0.97	0.97	0.12	3.43	3.43	ZZZ	■
93624		A	Electrophysiologic follow-up study with pacing and recording to test effectiveness of therapy, including induction or attempted induction of arrhythmia	4.81	3.87	3.87	0.36	9.04	9.04	000	
	26	A		4.81	1.99	1.99	0.25	7.05	7.05	000	
	TC	A		0.00	1.88	1.88	0.11	1.99	1.99	000	

Medicine

■ RVU not developed by CMS. Gap-filled RVUs developed by Ingenix/CHEG.

Code	M	S	Description	Work Value	Non-Fac PE	Fac PE	Mal-practice	Non-Fac Total	Fac Total	Global	Gap
93631		A	Intra-operative epicardial and endocardial pacing and mapping to localize the site of tachycardia or zone of slow conduction for surgical correction	7.60	8.65	8.65	1.17	17.42	17.42	000	
	26	A		7.60	2.81	2.81	0.66	11.07	11.07	000	
	TC	A		0.00	5.84	5.84	0.51	6.35	6.35	000	
93640		A	Electrophysiologic evaluation of single or dual chamber pacing cardioverter-defibrillator leads including defibrillation threshold evaluation (induction of arrhythmia, evaluation of sensing and pacing for arrhythmia termination) at time of initial implantation or replacement;	3.52	8.27	8.27	0.53	12.32	12.32	000	
	26	A		3.52	1.46	1.46	0.18	5.16	5.16	000	
	TC	A		0.00	6.81	6.81	0.35	7.16	7.16	000	
93641		A	with testing of single or dual chamber pacing cardioverter-defibrillator pulse generator	5.93	9.28	9.28	0.66	15.87	15.87	000	
	26	A		5.93	2.47	2.47	0.31	8.71	8.71	000	
	TC	A		0.00	6.81	6.81	0.35	7.16	7.16	000	
93642		A	Electrophysiologic evaluation of single or dual chamber pacing cardioverter-defibrillator (includes defibrillation threshold evaluation, induction of arrhythmia, evaluation of sensing and pacing for arrhythmia termination, and programming or reprogramming of sensing or therapeutic parameters)	4.89	8.85	8.85	0.51	14.25	14.25	000	
	26	A		4.89	2.04	2.04	0.16	7.09	7.09	000	
	TC	A		0.00	6.81	6.81	0.35	7.16	7.16	000	
93650		A	Intracardiac catheter ablation of atrioventricular node function, atrioventricular conduction for creation of complete heart block, with or without temporary pacemaker placement	10.51	4.32	4.32	0.55	15.38	15.38	000	
	26			5.78	2.38	2.38	0.30	8.46	8.46	000	■
	TC			4.73	1.94	1.94	0.25	6.92	6.92	000	■
93651		A	Intracardiac catheter ablation of arrhythmogenic focus; for treatment of supraventricular tachycardia by ablation of fast or slow atrioventricular pathways, accessory atrioventricular connections or other atrial foci, singly or in combination	16.25	6.78	6.78	0.85	23.88	23.88	000	
	26			8.94	3.73	3.73	0.47	13.13	13.13	000	■
	TC			7.31	3.05	3.05	0.38	10.75	10.75	000	■
93652		A	for treatment of ventricular tachycardia	17.68	7.36	7.36	0.92	25.96	25.96	000	
	26			9.72	4.05	4.05	0.51	14.28	14.28	000	■
	TC			7.96	3.31	3.31	0.41	11.68	11.68	000	■
93660		A	Evaluation of cardiovascular function with tilt table evaluation, with continuous ECG monitoring and intermittent blood pressure monitoring, with or without pharmacological intervention	1.89	2.39	2.39	0.08	4.36	4.36	000	
	26	A		1.89	0.79	0.79	0.06	2.74	2.74	000	
	TC	A		0.00	1.60	1.60	0.02	1.62	1.62	000	
93662		C	Intracardiac echocardiography during therapeutic/diagnostic intervention, including imaging supervision and interpretation (List separately in addition to code for primary procedure)	5.09	2.04	2.04	0.75	7.87	7.87	ZZZ	■
	26	A		2.80	1.12	1.12	0.41	4.33	4.33	ZZZ	
	TC	C		2.29	0.92	0.92	0.34	3.54	3.54	XXX	■
93668		N	Peripheral arterial disease (PAD) rehabilitation, per session	0.40	0.92	0.92	0.05	1.37	1.37	XXX	■
	26			0.00	0.00	0.00	0.00	0.00	0.00	XXX	■
	TC			0.40	0.92	0.92	0.05	1.37	1.37	XXX	■
93701		A	Bioimpedance, thoracic, electrical	0.17	0.78	0.78	0.02	0.97	0.97	XXX	
	26	A		0.17	0.07	0.07	0.01	0.25	0.25	XXX	
	TC	A		0.00	0.71	0.71	0.01	0.72	0.72	XXX	

■ RVU not developed by CMS. Gap-filled RVUs developed by Ingenix/CHEG.

Code	M	S	Description	Work Value	Non-Fac PE	Fac PE	Mal-practice	Non-Fac Total	Fac Total	Global	Gap
93720		A	Plethysmography, total body; with interpretation and report	0.17	0.73	0.73	0.06	0.96	0.96	XXX	
	26			0.07	0.29	0.29	0.02	0.38	0.38	XXX	■
	TC			0.10	0.44	0.44	0.04	0.58	0.58	XXX	■
93721		A	tracing only, without interpretation and report	0.00	0.67	0.67	0.05	0.72	0.72	XXX	
	26			0.00	0.00	0.00	0.00	0.00	0.00	XXX	■
	TC			0.00	0.67	0.67	0.05	0.72	0.72	XXX	■
93722		A	interpretation and report only	0.17	0.06	0.06	0.01	0.24	0.24	XXX	
93724		A	Electronic analysis of antitachycardia pacemaker system (includes electrocardiographic recording, programming of device, induction and termination of tachycardia via implanted pacemaker, and interpretation of recordings)	4.89	5.80	5.80	0.38	11.07	11.07	000	
	26	A		4.89	2.04	2.04	0.18	7.11	7.11	000	
	TC	A		0.00	3.76	3.76	0.20	3.96	3.96	000	
93727		A	Electronic analysis of implantable loop recorder (ILR) system (includes retrieval of recorded and stored ECG data, physician review and interpretation of retrieved ECG data and reprogramming)	0.52	0.21	0.21	0.05	0.78	0.78	XXX	
	26			0.36	0.15	0.15	0.04	0.55	0.55	XXX	■
	TC			0.16	0.06	0.06	0.02	0.23	0.23	XXX	■
93731		A	Electronic analysis of dual-chamber pacemaker system (includes evaluation of programmable parameters at rest and during activity where applicable, using electrocardiographic recording and interpretation of recordings at rest and during exercise, analysis of event markers and device response); without reprogramming	0.45	0.66	0.66	0.05	1.16	1.16	XXX	
	26	A		0.45	0.19	0.19	0.02	0.66	0.66	XXX	
	TC	A		0.00	0.47	0.47	0.03	0.50	0.50	XXX	
93732		A	with reprogramming	0.92	0.87	0.87	0.06	1.85	1.85	XXX	
	26	A		0.92	0.38	0.38	0.03	1.33	1.33	XXX	
	TC	A		0.00	0.49	0.49	0.03	0.52	0.52	XXX	
93733		A	Electronic analysis of dual chamber internal pacemaker system (may include rate, pulse amplitude and duration, configuration of wave form, and/or testing of sensory function of pacemaker), telephonic analysis	0.17	0.76	0.76	0.06	0.99	0.99	XXX	
	26	A		0.17	0.07	0.07	0.01	0.25	0.25	XXX	
	TC	A		0.00	0.69	0.69	0.05	0.74	0.74	XXX	
93734		A	Electronic analysis of single chamber pacemaker system (includes evaluation of programmable parameters at rest and during activity where applicable, using electrocardiographic recording and interpretation of recordings at rest and during exercise, analysis of event markers and device response); without reprogramming	0.38	0.49	0.49	0.03	0.90	0.90	XXX	
	26	A		0.38	0.16	0.16	0.01	0.55	0.55	XXX	
	TC	A		0.00	0.33	0.33	0.02	0.35	0.35	XXX	
93735		A	with reprogramming	0.74	0.72	0.72	0.06	1.52	1.52	XXX	
	26	A		0.74	0.30	0.30	0.03	1.07	1.07	XXX	
	TC	A		0.00	0.42	0.42	0.03	0.45	0.45	XXX	
93736		A	Electronic analysis of single chamber internal pacemaker system (may include rate, pulse amplitude and duration, configuration of wave form, and/or testing of sensory function of pacemaker), telephonic analysis	0.15	0.66	0.66	0.06	0.87	0.87	XXX	
	26	A		0.15	0.06	0.06	0.01	0.22	0.22	XXX	
	TC	A		0.00	0.60	0.60	0.05	0.65	0.65	XXX	

■ RVU not developed by CMS. Gap-filled RVUs developed by Ingenix/CHEG.

Code	M	S	Description	Work Value	Non-Fac PE	Fac PE	Mal-practice	Non-Fac Total	Fac Total	Global	Gap
93740		B	Temperature gradient studies	0.16	0.21	0.21	0.02	0.39	0.39	XXX	
	26	B		0.16	0.06	0.06	0.01	0.23	0.23	XXX	
	TC	B		0.00	0.15	0.15	0.01	0.16	0.16	XXX	
93741		A	Electronic analysis of pacing cardioverter-defibrillator (includes interrogation, evaluation of pulse generator status, evaluation of programmable parameters at rest and during activity where applicable, using electrocardiographic recording and interpretation of recordings at rest and during exercise, analysis of event markers and device response); single chamber, without reprogramming	0.80	0.96	0.96	0.05	1.81	1.81	XXX	
	26	A		0.80	0.33	0.33	0.02	1.15	1.15	XXX	
	TC	A		0.00	0.63	0.63	0.03	0.66	0.66	XXX	
93742		A	single chamber, with reprogramming	0.91	1.01	1.01	0.05	1.97	1.97	XXX	
	26	A		0.91	0.38	0.38	0.02	1.31	1.31	XXX	
	TC	A		0.00	0.63	0.63	0.03	0.66	0.66	XXX	
93743		A	dual chamber, without reprogramming	1.03	1.13	1.13	0.06	2.22	2.22	XXX	
	26	A		1.03	0.43	0.43	0.03	1.49	1.49	XXX	
	TC	A		0.00	0.70	0.70	0.03	0.73	0.73	XXX	
93744		A	dual chamber, with reprogramming	1.18	1.12	1.12	0.06	2.36	2.36	XXX	
	26	A		1.18	0.49	0.49	0.03	1.70	1.70	XXX	
	TC	A		0.00	0.63	0.63	0.03	0.66	0.66	XXX	
93760		N	Thermogram; cephalic	0.47	1.09	1.09	0.07	1.63	1.63	XXX	■
	26			0.09	0.22	0.22	0.01	0.33	0.33	XXX	■
	TC			0.38	0.87	0.87	0.06	1.30	1.30	XXX	■
93762		N	peripheral	0.70	1.61	1.61	0.10	2.40	2.40	XXX	■
	26			0.14	0.32	0.32	0.02	0.48	0.48	XXX	■
	TC			0.56	1.29	1.29	0.08	1.92	1.92	XXX	■
93770		B	Determination of venous pressure	0.16	0.09	0.09	0.02	0.27	0.27	XXX	
	26	B		0.16	0.06	0.06	0.01	0.23	0.23	XXX	
	TC	B		0.00	0.03	0.03	0.01	0.04	0.04	XXX	
93784		N	Ambulatory blood pressure monitoring, utilizing a system such as magnetic tape and/or computer disk, for 24 hours or longer; including recording, scanning analysis, interpretation and report	0.86	2.00	2.00	0.12	2.98	2.98	XXX	■
93786		N	recording only	0.13	0.30	0.30	0.02	0.45	0.45	XXX	■
	26			0.00	0.00	0.00	0.00	0.00	0.00	XXX	■
	TC			0.13	0.30	0.30	0.02	0.45	0.45	XXX	■
93788		N	scanning analysis with report	0.39	0.90	0.90	0.05	1.34	1.34	XXX	■
	26			0.00	0.00	0.00	0.00	0.00	0.00	XXX	■
	TC			0.39	0.90	0.90	0.05	1.34	1.34	XXX	■
93790		N	physician review with interpretation and report	0.35	0.80	0.80	0.05	1.19	1.19	XXX	■
93797		A	Physician services for outpatient cardiac rehabilitation; without continuous ECG monitoring (per session)	0.18	0.33	0.07	0.01	0.52	0.26	000	

■ RVU not developed by CMS. Gap-filled RVUs developed by Ingenix/CHEG.

Code	M	S	Description	Work Value	Non-Fac PE	Fac PE	Mal-practice	Non-Fac Total	Fac Total	Global	Gap
93798		A	with continuous ECG monitoring (per session)	0.28	0.44	0.11	0.01	0.73	0.40	000	
93799		C	Unlisted cardiovascular service or procedure	0.00	0.00	0.00	0.00	0.00	0.00	XXX	
	26	C		0.00	0.00	0.00	0.00	0.00	0.00	XXX	
	TC	C		0.00	0.00	0.00	0.00	0.00	0.00	XXX	
93875		A	Noninvasive physiologic studies of extracranial arteries, complete bilateral study (eg, periorbital flow direction with arterial compression, ocular pneumoplethysmography, Doppler ultrasound spectral analysis)	0.22	1.13	1.13	0.10	1.45	1.45	XXX	
	26	A		0.22	0.08	0.08	0.01	0.31	0.31	XXX	
	TC	A		0.00	1.05	1.05	0.09	1.14	1.14	XXX	
93880		A	Duplex scan of extracranial arteries; complete bilateral study	0.60	3.76	3.76	0.33	4.69	4.69	XXX	
	26	A		0.60	0.22	0.22	0.04	0.86	0.86	XXX	
	TC	A		0.00	3.54	3.54	0.29	3.83	3.83	XXX	
93882		A	unilateral or limited study	0.40	2.50	2.50	0.22	3.12	3.12	XXX	
	26	A		0.40	0.15	0.15	0.04	0.59	0.59	XXX	
	TC	A		0.00	2.35	2.35	0.18	2.53	2.53	XXX	
93886		A	Transcranial Doppler study of the intracranial arteries; complete study	0.94	4.40	4.40	0.37	5.71	5.71	XXX	
	26	A		0.94	0.40	0.40	0.05	1.39	1.39	XXX	
	TC	A		0.00	4.00	4.00	0.32	4.32	4.32	XXX	
93888		A	limited study	0.62	2.91	2.91	0.26	3.79	3.79	XXX	
	26	A		0.62	0.24	0.24	0.04	0.90	0.90	XXX	
	TC	A		0.00	2.67	2.67	0.22	2.89	2.89	XXX	
93922		A	Noninvasive physiologic studies of upper or lower extremity arteries, single level, bilateral (eg, ankle/brachial indices, Doppler waveform analysis, volume plethysmography, transcutaneous oxygen tension measurement)	0.25	1.18	1.18	0.13	1.56	1.56	XXX	
	26	A		0.25	0.09	0.09	0.02	0.36	0.36	XXX	
	TC	A		0.00	1.09	1.09	0.11	1.20	1.20	XXX	
93923		A	Non-invasive physiologic studies of upper or lower extremity arteries, multiple levels or with provocative functional maneuvers, complete bilateral study (eg, segmental blood pressure measurements, segmental Doppler waveform analysis, segmental volume plethysmography, segmental transcutaneous oxygen tension measurements, measurements with postural provocative tests, measurements with reactive hyperemia)	0.45	2.24	2.24	0.22	2.91	2.91	XXX	
	26	A		0.45	0.16	0.16	0.04	0.65	0.65	XXX	
	TC	A		0.00	2.08	2.08	0.18	2.26	2.26	XXX	
93924		A	Non-invasive physiologic studies of lower extremity arteries, at rest and following treadmill stress testing, complete bilateral study	0.50	2.43	2.43	0.26	3.19	3.19	XXX	
	26	A		0.50	0.18	0.18	0.05	0.73	0.73	XXX	
	TC	A		0.00	2.25	2.25	0.21	2.46	2.46	XXX	
93925		A	Duplex scan of lower extremity arteries or arterial bypass grafts; complete bilateral study	0.58	3.76	3.76	0.33	4.67	4.67	XXX	
	26	A		0.58	0.21	0.21	0.04	0.83	0.83	XXX	
	TC	A		0.00	3.55	3.55	0.29	3.84	3.84	XXX	
93926		A	unilateral or limited study	0.39	2.51	2.51	0.22	3.12	3.12	XXX	
	26	A		0.39	0.14	0.14	0.03	0.56	0.56	XXX	
	TC	A		0.00	2.37	2.37	0.19	2.56	2.56	XXX	

Medicine

■ RVU not developed by CMS. Gap-filled RVUs developed by Ingenix/CHEG.

Code	M	S	Description	Work Value	Non-Fac PE	Fac PE	Mal-practice	Non-Fac Total	Fac Total	Global	Gap
93930		A	Duplex scan of upper extremity arteries or arterial bypass grafts; complete bilateral study	0.46	3.93	3.93	0.34	4.73	4.73	XXX	
	26	A		0.46	0.16	0.16	0.03	0.65	0.65	XXX	
	TC	A		0.00	3.77	3.77	0.31	4.08	4.08	XXX	
93931		A	unilateral or limited study	0.31	2.62	2.62	0.22	3.15	3.15	XXX	
	26	A		0.31	0.11	0.11	0.02	0.44	0.44	XXX	
	TC	A		0.00	2.51	2.51	0.20	2.71	2.71	XXX	
93965		A	Non-invasive physiologic studies of extremity veins, complete bilateral study (eg, Doppler waveform analysis with responses to compression and other maneuvers, phleborheography, impedance plethysmography)	0.35	1.17	1.17	0.12	1.64	1.64	XXX	
	26	A		0.35	0.13	0.13	0.02	0.50	0.50	XXX	
	TC	A		0.00	1.04	1.04	0.10	1.14	1.14	XXX	
93970		A	Duplex scan of extremity veins including responses to compression and other maneuvers; complete bilateral study	0.68	4.16	4.16	0.38	5.22	5.22	XXX	
	26	A		0.68	0.24	0.24	0.05	0.97	0.97	XXX	
	TC	A		0.00	3.92	3.92	0.33	4.25	4.25	XXX	
93971		A	unilateral or limited study	0.45	2.77	2.77	0.25	3.47	3.47	XXX	
	26	A		0.45	0.16	0.16	0.03	0.64	0.64	XXX	
	TC	A		0.00	2.61	2.61	0.22	2.83	2.83	XXX	
93975		A	Duplex scan of arterial inflow and venous outflow of abdominal, pelvic, scrotal contents and/or retroperitoneal organs; complete study	1.80	5.10	5.10	0.47	7.37	7.37	XXX	
	26	A		1.80	0.64	0.64	0.11	2.55	2.55	XXX	
	TC	A		0.00	4.46	4.46	0.36	4.82	4.82	XXX	
93976		A	limited study	1.21	3.41	3.41	0.31	4.93	4.93	XXX	
	26	A		1.21	0.43	0.43	0.06	1.70	1.70	XXX	
	TC	A		0.00	2.98	2.98	0.25	3.23	3.23	XXX	
93978		A	Duplex scan of aorta, inferior vena cava, iliac vasculature, or bypass grafts; complete study	0.65	3.88	3.88	0.36	4.89	4.89	XXX	
	26	A		0.65	0.23	0.23	0.05	0.93	0.93	XXX	
	TC	A		0.00	3.65	3.65	0.31	3.96	3.96	XXX	
93979		A	unilateral or limited study	0.44	2.59	2.59	0.24	3.27	3.27	XXX	
	26	A		0.44	0.16	0.16	0.04	0.64	0.64	XXX	
	TC	A		0.00	2.43	2.43	0.20	2.63	2.63	XXX	
93980		A	Duplex scan of arterial inflow and venous outflow of penile vessels; complete study	1.25	3.75	3.75	0.35	5.35	5.35	XXX	
	26	A		1.25	0.44	0.44	0.07	1.76	1.76	XXX	
	TC	A		0.00	3.31	3.31	0.28	3.59	3.59	XXX	
93981		A	follow-up or limited study	0.44	3.21	3.21	0.28	3.93	3.93	XXX	
	26	A		0.44	0.15	0.15	0.02	0.61	0.61	XXX	
	TC	A		0.00	3.06	3.06	0.26	3.32	3.32	XXX	
93990		A	Duplex scan of hemodialysis access (including arterial inflow, body of access and venous outflow)	0.25	2.46	2.46	0.21	2.92	2.92	XXX	
	26	A		0.25	0.09	0.09	0.02	0.36	0.36	XXX	
	TC	A		0.00	2.37	2.37	0.19	2.56	2.56	XXX	
94010		A	Spirometry, including graphic record, total and timed vital capacity, expiratory flow rate measurement(s), with or without maximal voluntary ventilation	0.17	0.82	0.82	0.03	1.02	1.02	XXX	
	26	A		0.17	0.06	0.06	0.01	0.24	0.24	XXX	
	TC	A		0.00	0.76	0.76	0.02	0.78	0.78	XXX	

Medicine

■ RVU not developed by CMS. Gap-filled RVUs developed by Ingenix/CHEG.

Code	M	S	Description	Work Value	Non-Fac PE	Fac PE	Mal-prac-tice	Non-Fac Total	Fac Total	Global	Gap
94014		A	Patient-initiated spirometric recording per 30-day period of time; includes reinforced education, transmission of spirometric tracing, data capture, analysis of transmitted data, periodic recalibration and physician review and interpretation	0.52	0.46	0.46	0.03	1.01	1.01	XXX	
	26			0.21	0.18	0.18	0.01	0.40	0.40	XXX	■
	TC			0.31	0.28	0.28	0.02	0.61	0.61	XXX	■
94015		A	recording (includes hook-up, reinforced education, data transmission, data capture, trend analysis, and periodic recalibration)	0.00	0.29	0.29	0.01	0.30	0.30	XXX	
	26			0.00	0.00	0.00	0.00	0.00	0.00	XXX	■
	TC			0.00	0.29	0.29	0.01	0.30	0.30	XXX	■
94016		A	physician review and interpretation only	0.52	0.17	0.17	0.02	0.71	0.71	XXX	
94060		A	Bronchospasm evaluation: spirometry as in 94010, before and after bronchodilator (aerosol or parenteral)	0.31	1.36	1.36	0.06	1.73	1.73	XXX	
	26	A		0.31	0.10	0.10	0.01	0.42	0.42	XXX	
	TC	A		0.00	1.26	1.26	0.05	1.31	1.31	XXX	
94070		A	Prolonged postexposure evaluation of bronchospasm with multiple spirometric determinations after antigen, cold air, methacholine or other chemical agent, with subsequent spirometrics	0.60	3.38	3.38	0.10	4.08	4.08	XXX	
	26	A		0.60	0.19	0.19	0.02	0.81	0.81	XXX	
	TC	A		0.00	3.19	3.19	0.08	3.27	3.27	XXX	
94150		B	Vital capacity, total (separate procedure)	0.07	0.63	0.63	0.02	0.72	0.72	XXX	
	26	B		0.07	0.03	0.03	0.01	0.11	0.11	XXX	
	TC	B		0.00	0.60	0.60	0.01	0.61	0.61	XXX	
94200		A	Maximum breathing capacity, maximal voluntary ventilation	0.11	0.33	0.33	0.03	0.47	0.47	XXX	
	26	A		0.11	0.04	0.04	0.01	0.16	0.16	XXX	
	TC	A		0.00	0.29	0.29	0.02	0.31	0.31	XXX	
94240		A	Functional residual capacity or residual volume: helium method, nitrogen open circuit method, or other method	0.26	1.26	1.26	0.05	1.57	1.57	XXX	
	26	A		0.26	0.08	0.08	0.01	0.35	0.35	XXX	
	TC	A		0.00	1.18	1.18	0.04	1.22	1.22	XXX	
94250		A	Expired gas collection, quantitative, single procedure (separate procedure)	0.11	0.61	0.61	0.02	0.74	0.74	XXX	
	26	A		0.11	0.04	0.04	0.01	0.16	0.16	XXX	
	TC	A		0.00	0.57	0.57	0.01	0.58	0.58	XXX	
94260		A	Thoracic gas volume	0.13	0.38	0.38	0.04	0.55	0.55	XXX	
	26	A		0.13	0.04	0.04	0.01	0.18	0.18	XXX	
	TC	A		0.00	0.34	0.34	0.03	0.37	0.37	XXX	
94350		A	Determination of maldistribution of inspired gas: multiple breath nitrogen washout curve including alveolar nitrogen or helium equilibration time	0.26	1.01	1.01	0.04	1.31	1.31	XXX	
	26	A		0.26	0.08	0.08	0.01	0.35	0.35	XXX	
	TC	A		0.00	0.93	0.93	0.03	0.96	0.96	XXX	
94360		A	Determination of resistance to airflow, oscillatory or plethysmographic methods	0.26	0.50	0.50	0.06	0.82	0.82	XXX	
	26	A		0.26	0.08	0.08	0.01	0.35	0.35	XXX	
	TC	A		0.00	0.42	0.42	0.05	0.47	0.47	XXX	
94370		A	Determination of airway closing volume, single breath tests	0.26	2.03	2.03	0.03	2.32	2.32	XXX	
	26	A		0.26	0.08	0.08	0.01	0.35	0.35	XXX	
	TC	A		0.00	1.95	1.95	0.02	1.97	1.97	XXX	
94375		A	Respiratory flow volume loop	0.31	0.46	0.46	0.03	0.80	0.80	XXX	
	26	A		0.31	0.10	0.10	0.01	0.42	0.42	XXX	
	TC	A		0.00	0.36	0.36	0.02	0.38	0.38	XXX	

■ RVU not developed by CMS. Gap-filled RVUs developed by Ingenix/CHEG.

Code	M	S	Description	Work Value	Non-Fac PE	Fac PE	Mal-prac-tice	Non-Fac Total	Fac Total	Global	Gap
94400		A	Breathing response to CO2 (CO2 response curve)	0.40	0.70	0.70	0.06	1.16	1.16	XXX	
	26	A		0.40	0.13	0.13	0.01	0.54	0.54	XXX	
	TC	A		0.00	0.57	0.57	0.05	0.62	0.62	XXX	
94450		A	Breathing response to hypoxia (hypoxia response curve)	0.40	0.85	0.85	0.04	1.29	1.29	XXX	
	26	A		0.40	0.12	0.12	0.02	0.54	0.54	XXX	
	TC	A		0.00	0.73	0.73	0.02	0.75	0.75	XXX	
94620		A	Pulmonary stress testing; simple (eg, prolonged exercise test for bronchospasm with pre- and post-spirometry)	0.64	1.66	1.66	0.10	2.40	2.40	XXX	
	26	A		0.64	0.21	0.21	0.02	0.87	0.87	XXX	
	TC	A		0.00	1.45	1.45	0.08	1.53	1.53	XXX	
94621		A	complex (including measurements of CO2 production, O2 uptake, and electrocardiographic recordings)	1.42	1.25	1.25	0.13	2.80	2.80	XXX	
	26	A		1.42	0.47	0.47	0.05	1.94	1.94	XXX	
	TC	A		0.00	0.78	0.78	0.08	0.86	0.86	XXX	
94640		A	Nonpressurized inhalation treatment for acute airway obstruction	0.00	0.74	0.74	0.02	0.76	0.76	XXX	
94642		C	Aerosol inhalation of pentamidine for pneumocystis carinii pneumonia treatment or prophylaxis	0.47	1.09	1.09	0.07	1.63	1.63	XXX	■
94650		A	Intermittent positive pressure breathing (IPPB) treatment, air or oxygen, with or without nebulized medication; initial demonstration and/or evaluation	0.00	0.67	0.67	0.02	0.69	0.69	XXX	
94651		A	subsequent	0.00	0.62	0.62	0.02	0.64	0.64	XXX	
94652		A	newborn infants	0.00	0.77	0.77	0.06	0.83	0.83	XXX	
94656		A	Ventilation assist and management, initiation of pressure or volume preset ventilators for assisted or controlled breathing; first day	1.22	0.33	0.33	0.06	1.61	1.61	XXX	
94657		A	subsequent days	0.83	0.26	0.26	0.03	1.12	1.12	XXX	
94660		A	Continuous positive airway pressure ventilation (CPAP), initiation and management	0.76	0.67	0.24	0.03	1.46	1.03	XXX	
94662		A	Continuous negative pressure ventilation (CNP), initiation and management	0.76	0.24	0.24	0.02	1.02	1.02	XXX	
94664		A	Aerosol or vapor inhalations for sputum mobilization, bronchodilation, or sputum induction for diagnostic purposes; initial demonstration and/or evaluation	0.00	0.53	0.53	0.03	0.56	0.56	XXX	
94665		A	subsequent	0.00	0.53	0.53	0.04	0.57	0.57	XXX	
94667		A	Manipulation chest wall, such as cupping, percussing, and vibration to facilitate lung function; initial demonstration and/or evaluation	0.00	1.01	1.01	0.04	1.05	1.05	XXX	
94668		A	subsequent	0.00	0.75	0.75	0.02	0.77	0.77	XXX	
94680		A	Oxygen uptake, expired gas analysis; rest and exercise, direct, simple	0.26	1.17	1.17	0.06	1.49	1.49	XXX	
	26	A		0.26	0.09	0.09	0.01	0.36	0.36	XXX	
	TC	A		0.00	1.08	1.08	0.05	1.13	1.13	XXX	

■ RVU not developed by CMS. Gap-filled RVUs developed by Ingenix/CHEG.

Code	M	S	Description	Work Value	Non-Fac PE	Fac PE	Mal-practice	Non-Fac Total	Fac Total	Global	Gap
94681		A	including CO2 output, percentage oxygen extracted	0.20	1.32	1.32	0.11	1.63	1.63	XXX	
	26	A		0.20	0.07	0.07	0.01	0.28	0.28	XXX	
	TC	A		0.00	1.25	1.25	0.10	1.35	1.35	XXX	
94690		A	rest, indirect (separate procedure)	0.07	1.59	1.59	0.04	1.70	1.70	XXX	
	26	A		0.07	0.02	0.02	0.01	0.10	0.10	XXX	
	TC	A		0.00	1.57	1.57	0.03	1.60	1.60	XXX	
94720		A	Carbon monoxide diffusing capacity (eg, single breath, steady state)	0.26	1.32	1.32	0.06	1.64	1.64	XXX	
	26	A		0.26	0.08	0.08	0.01	0.35	0.35	XXX	
	TC	A		0.00	1.24	1.24	0.05	1.29	1.29	XXX	
94725		A	Membrane diffusion capacity	0.26	0.71	0.71	0.11	1.08	1.08	XXX	
	26	A		0.26	0.08	0.08	0.01	0.35	0.35	XXX	
	TC	A		0.00	0.63	0.63	0.10	0.73	0.73	XXX	
94750		A	Pulmonary compliance study (eg, plethysmography, volume and pressure measurements)	0.23	1.06	1.06	0.04	1.33	1.33	XXX	
	26	A		0.23	0.07	0.07	0.01	0.31	0.31	XXX	
	TC	A		0.00	0.99	0.99	0.03	1.02	1.02	XXX	
94760		T	Noninvasive ear or pulse oximetry for oxygen saturation; single determination	0.00	0.10	0.10	0.02	0.12	0.12	XXX	
	26			0.00	0.00	0.00	0.00	0.00	0.00	XXX	■
	TC			0.00	0.10	0.10	0.02	0.12	0.12	XXX	■
94761		T	multiple determinations (eg, during exercise)	0.00	0.14	0.14	0.05	0.19	0.19	XXX	
	26			0.00	0.00	0.00	0.00	0.00	0.00	XXX	■
	TC			0.00	0.14	0.14	0.05	0.19	0.19	XXX	■
94762		A	by continuous overnight monitoring (separate procedure)	0.00	0.74	0.74	0.08	0.82	0.82	XXX	
	26			0.00	0.00	0.00	0.00	0.00	0.00	XXX	■
	TC			0.00	0.74	0.74	0.08	0.82	0.82	XXX	■
94770		A	Carbon dioxide, expired gas determination by infrared analyzer	0.15	0.91	0.91	0.07	1.13	1.13	XXX	
	26	A		0.15	0.04	0.04	0.01	0.20	0.20	XXX	
	TC	A		0.00	0.87	0.87	0.06	0.93	0.93	XXX	
94772		C	Circadian respiratory pattern recording (pediatric pneumogram), 12 to 24 hour continuous recording, infant	0.00	0.00	0.00	0.00	0.00	0.00	XXX	
	26	C		0.00	0.00	0.00	0.00	0.00	0.00	XXX	
	TC	C		0.00	0.00	0.00	0.00	0.00	0.00	XXX	
94799		C	Unlisted pulmonary service or procedure	0.00	0.00	0.00	0.00	0.00	0.00	XXX	
	26	C		0.00	0.00	0.00	0.00	0.00	0.00	XXX	
	TC	C		0.00	0.00	0.00	0.00	0.00	0.00	XXX	
95004		A	Percutaneous tests (scratch, puncture, prick) with allergenic extracts, immediate type reaction, specify number of tests	0.00	0.09	0.09	0.01	0.10	0.10	XXX	
95010		A	Percutaneous tests (scratch, puncture, prick) sequential and incremental, with drugs, biologicals or venoms, immediate type reaction, specify number of tests	0.15	0.45	0.07	0.01	0.61	0.23	XXX	
95015		A	Intracutaneous (intradermal) tests, sequential and incremental, with drugs, biologicals, or venoms, immediate type reaction, specify number of tests	0.15	0.39	0.06	0.01	0.55	0.22	XXX	

Medicine

■ RVU not developed by CMS. Gap-filled RVUs developed by Ingenix/CHEG.

Code	M	S	Description	Work Value	Non-Fac PE	Fac PE	Mal-practice	Non-Fac Total	Fac Total	Global	Gap
95024		A	Intracutaneous (intradermal) tests with allergenic extracts, immediate type reaction, specify number of tests	0.00	0.14	0.14	0.01	0.15	0.15	XXX	
95027		A	Skin end point titration	0.00	0.14	0.14	0.01	0.15	0.15	XXX	
95028		A	Intracutaneous (intradermal) tests with allergenic extracts, delayed type reaction, including reading, specify number of tests	0.00	0.22	0.22	0.01	0.23	0.23	XXX	
95044		A	Patch or application test(s) (specify number of tests)	0.00	0.19	0.19	0.01	0.20	0.20	XXX	
95052		A	Photo patch test(s) (specify number of tests)	0.00	0.24	0.24	0.01	0.25	0.25	XXX	
95056		A	Photo tests	0.00	0.17	0.17	0.01	0.18	0.18	XXX	
95060		A	Ophthalmic mucous membrane tests	0.00	0.33	0.33	0.02	0.35	0.35	XXX	
95065		A	Direct nasal mucous membrane test	0.00	0.19	0.19	0.01	0.20	0.20	XXX	
95070		A	Inhalation bronchial challenge testing (not including necessary pulmonary function tests); with histamine, methacholine, or similar compounds	0.00	2.17	2.17	0.02	2.19	2.19	XXX	
95071		A	with antigens or gases, specify	0.00	2.77	2.77	0.02	2.79	2.79	XXX	
95075		A	Ingestion challenge test (sequential and incremental ingestion of test items, eg, food, drug or other substance such as metabisulfite)	0.95	0.80	0.43	0.03	1.78	1.41	XXX	
95078		A	Provocative testing (eg, Rinkel test)	0.00	0.24	0.24	0.02	0.26	0.26	XXX	
95115		A	Professional services for allergen immunotherapy not including provision of allergenic extracts; single injection	0.00	0.37	0.37	0.02	0.39	0.39	000	
95117		A	two or more injections	0.00	0.48	0.48	0.02	0.50	0.50	000	
95120		I	Professional services for allergen immunotherapy in prescribing physician's office or institution, including provision of allergenic extract; single injection	0.14	0.33	0.33	0.02	0.49	0.49	XXX	■
95125		I	two or more injections	0.17	0.40	0.40	0.02	0.60	0.60	XXX	■
95130		I	single stinging insect venom	0.25	0.57	0.57	0.03	0.85	0.85	XXX	■
95131		I	two stinging insect venoms	0.31	0.72	0.72	0.04	1.07	1.07	XXX	■
95132		I	three stinging insect venoms	0.37	0.86	0.86	0.05	1.29	1.29	XXX	■
95133		I	four stinging insect venoms	0.45	1.05	1.05	0.06	1.56	1.56	XXX	■
95134		I	five stinging insect venoms	0.54	1.25	1.25	0.07	1.87	1.87	XXX	■
95144		A	Professional services for the supervision of preparation and provision of antigens for allergen immunotherapy; single dose vial(s) (specify number of vials)	0.06	0.25	0.03	0.01	0.32	0.10	000	

■ RVU not developed by CMS. Gap-filled RVUs developed by Ingenix/CHEG.

Code	M	S	Description	Work Value	Non-Fac PE	Fac PE	Mal-practice	Non-Fac Total	Fac Total	Global	Gap
95145		A	Professional services for the supervision of preparation and provision of antigens for allergen immunotherapy (specify number of doses); single stinging insect venom	0.06	0.47	0.03	0.01	0.54	0.10	000	
95146		A	two single stinging insect venoms	0.06	0.62	0.03	0.01	0.69	0.10	000	
95147		A	three single stinging insect venoms	0.06	0.91	0.03	0.01	0.98	0.10	000	
95148		A	four single stinging insect venoms	0.06	0.81	0.03	0.01	0.88	0.10	000	
95149		A	five single stinging insect venoms	0.06	1.04	0.03	0.01	1.11	0.10	000	
95165		A	Professional services for the supervision of preparation and provision of antigens for allergen immunotherapy; single or multiple antigens (specify number of doses)	0.06	0.21	0.02	0.01	0.28	0.09	000	
95170		A	whole body extract of biting insect or other arthropod (specify number of doses)	0.06	0.26	0.02	0.01	0.33	0.09	000	
95180		A	Rapid desensitization procedure, each hour (eg, insulin, penicillin, equine serum)	2.01	1.66	0.85	0.04	3.71	2.90	000	
95199		C	Unlisted allergy/clinical immunologic service or procedure	0.00	0.00	0.00	0.00	0.00	0.00	000	
95250		A	Glucose monitoring for up to 72 hours by continuous recording and storage of glucose values from interstitial tissue fluid via a subcutaneous sensor (includes hook-up, calibration, patient initiation and training, recording, disconnection, downloading with printout of data)	0.00	1.44	1.44	0.01	1.45	1.45	XXX	
	26			0.00	0.00	0.00	0.00	0.00	0.00	XXX	■
	TC			0.00	1.44	1.44	0.01	1.45	1.45	XXX	■
95805		A	Multiple sleep latency or maintenance of wakefulness testing, recording, analysis and interpretation of physiological measurements of sleep during multiple trials to assess sleepiness	1.88	5.89	5.89	0.34	8.11	8.11	XXX	
	26	A		1.88	0.70	0.70	0.06	2.64	2.64	XXX	
	TC	A		0.00	5.19	5.19	0.28	5.47	5.47	XXX	
95806		A	Sleep study, simultaneous recording of ventilation, respiratory effort, ECG or heart rate, and oxygen saturation, unattended by a technologist	1.66	4.31	4.31	0.32	6.29	6.29	XXX	
	26	A		1.66	0.57	0.57	0.06	2.29	2.29	XXX	
	TC	A		0.00	3.74	3.74	0.26	4.00	4.00	XXX	
95807		A	Sleep study, simultaneous recording of ventilation, respiratory effort, ECG or heart rate, and oxygen saturation, attended by a technologist	1.66	10.70	10.70	0.40	12.76	12.76	XXX	
	26	A		1.66	0.56	0.56	0.05	2.27	2.27	XXX	
	TC	A		0.00	10.14	10.14	0.35	10.49	10.49	XXX	
95808		A	Polysomnography; sleep staging with 1-3 additional parameters of sleep, attended by a technologist	2.65	9.54	9.54	0.44	12.63	12.63	XXX	
	26	A		2.65	0.99	0.99	0.09	3.73	3.73	XXX	
	TC	A		0.00	8.55	8.55	0.35	8.90	8.90	XXX	
95810		A	sleep staging with 4 or more additional parameters of sleep, attended by a technologist	3.53	16.92	16.92	0.47	20.92	20.92	XXX	
	26	A		3.53	1.26	1.26	0.12	4.91	4.91	XXX	
	TC	A		0.00	15.66	15.66	0.35	16.01	16.01	XXX	

Medicine

■ RVU not developed by CMS. Gap-filled RVUs developed by Ingenix/CHEG.

Code	M	S	Description	Work Value	Non-Fac PE	Fac PE	Mal-practice	Non-Fac Total	Fac Total	Global	Gap
95811		A	sleep staging with 4 or more additional parameters of sleep, with initiation of continuous positive airway pressure therapy or bilevel ventilation, attended by a technologist	3.80	17.19	17.19	0.49	21.48	21.48	XXX	
	26	A		3.80	1.34	1.34	0.13	5.27	5.27	XXX	
	TC	A		0.00	15.85	15.85	0.36	16.21	16.21	XXX	
95812		A	Electroencephalogram (EEG) extended monitoring; up to one hour	1.08	3.96	3.96	0.13	5.17	5.17	XXX	
	26	A		1.08	0.48	0.48	0.04	1.60	1.60	XXX	
	TC	A		0.00	3.48	3.48	0.09	3.57	3.57	XXX	
95813		A	greater than one hour	1.73	5.53	5.53	0.15	7.41	7.41	XXX	
	26	A		1.73	0.73	0.73	0.06	2.52	2.52	XXX	
	TC	A		0.00	4.80	4.80	0.09	4.89	4.89	XXX	
95816		A	Electroencephalogram (EEG) including recording awake and drowsy (including hyperventilation and/or photic stimulation when appropriate)	1.08	3.42	3.42	0.12	4.62	4.62	XXX	
	26	A		1.08	0.49	0.49	0.04	1.61	1.61	XXX	
	TC	A		0.00	2.93	2.93	0.08	3.01	3.01	XXX	
95819		A	Electroencephalogram (EEG) including recording awake and asleep (including hyperventilation and/or photic stimulation when appropriate)	1.08	4.34	4.34	0.12	5.54	5.54	XXX	
	26	A		1.08	0.49	0.49	0.04	1.61	1.61	XXX	
	TC	A		0.00	3.85	3.85	0.08	3.93	3.93	XXX	
95822		A	Electroencephalogram (EEG); sleep only	1.08	1.78	1.78	0.15	3.01	3.01	XXX	
	26	A		1.08	0.49	0.49	0.04	1.61	1.61	XXX	
	TC	A		0.00	1.29	1.29	0.11	1.40	1.40	XXX	
95824		C	cerebral death evaluation only	1.85	0.75	0.75	0.13	2.73	2.73	XXX	■
	26	A		0.74	0.30	0.30	0.05	1.09	1.09	ZZZ	
	TC	C		1.11	0.45	0.45	0.08	1.64	1.64	XXX	■
95827		A	all night sleep only	1.08	2.64	2.64	0.15	3.87	3.87	XXX	
	26	A		1.08	0.46	0.46	0.03	1.57	1.57	XXX	
	TC	A		0.00	2.18	2.18	0.12	2.30	2.30	XXX	
95829		A	Electrocorticogram at surgery (separate procedure)	6.21	31.39	31.39	0.33	37.93	37.93	XXX	
	26	A		6.21	2.90	2.90	0.31	9.42	9.42	XXX	
	TC	A		0.00	28.49	28.49	0.02	28.51	28.51	XXX	
95830		A	Insertion by physician of sphenoidal electrodes for electroencephalographic (EEG) recording	1.70	3.76	0.78	0.07	5.53	2.55	XXX	
95831		A	Muscle testing, manual (separate procedure) with report; extremity (excluding hand) or trunk	0.28	0.52	0.12	0.01	0.81	0.41	XXX	
95832		A	hand, with or without comparison with normal side	0.29	0.48	0.11	0.01	0.78	0.41	XXX	
95833		A	total evaluation of body, excluding hands	0.47	0.54	0.24	0.01	1.02	0.72	XXX	
95834		A	total evaluation of body, including hands	0.60	0.59	0.28	0.02	1.21	0.90	XXX	
95851		A	Range of motion measurements and report (separate procedure); each extremity (excluding hand) or each trunk section (spine)	0.16	0.55	0.08	0.01	0.72	0.25	XXX	
95852		A	hand, with or without comparison with normal side	0.11	0.49	0.05	0.01	0.61	0.17	XXX	

■ RVU not developed by CMS. Gap-filled RVUs developed by Ingenix/CHEG.

Code	M	S	Description	Work Value	Non-Fac PE	Fac PE	Mal-practice	Non-Fac Total	Fac Total	Global	Gap
95857		A	Tensilon test for myasthenia gravis;	0.53	0.66	0.24	0.02	1.21	0.79	XXX	
95858		A	with electromyographic recording	1.56	1.10	1.10	0.07	2.73	2.73	XXX	
	26	A		1.56	0.72	0.72	0.04	2.32	2.32	XXX	
	TC	A		0.00	0.38	0.38	0.03	0.41	0.41	XXX	
95860		A	Needle electromyography, one extremity with or without related paraspinal areas	0.96	1.18	1.18	0.05	2.19	2.19	XXX	
	26	A		0.96	0.45	0.45	0.03	1.44	1.44	XXX	
	TC	A		0.00	0.73	0.73	0.02	0.75	0.75	XXX	
95861		A	Needle electromyography, two extremities with or without related paraspinal areas	1.54	1.42	1.42	0.10	3.06	3.06	XXX	
	26	A		1.54	0.72	0.72	0.05	2.31	2.31	XXX	
	TC	A		0.00	0.70	0.70	0.05	0.75	0.75	XXX	
95863		A	Needle electromyography, three extremities with or without related paraspinal areas	1.87	1.76	1.76	0.11	3.74	3.74	XXX	
	26	A		1.87	0.87	0.87	0.06	2.80	2.80	XXX	
	TC	A		0.00	0.89	0.89	0.05	0.94	0.94	XXX	
95864		A	Needle electromyography, four extremities with or without related paraspinal areas	1.99	2.62	2.62	0.16	4.77	4.77	XXX	
	26	A		1.99	0.93	0.93	0.06	2.98	2.98	XXX	
	TC	A		0.00	1.69	1.69	0.10	1.79	1.79	XXX	
95867		A	Needle electromyography, cranial nerve supplied muscles, unilateral	0.79	0.92	0.92	0.06	1.77	1.77	XXX	
	26	A		0.79	0.37	0.37	0.03	1.19	1.19	XXX	
	TC	A		0.00	0.55	0.55	0.03	0.58	0.58	XXX	
95868		A	Needle electromyography, cranial nerve supplied muscles, bilateral	1.18	1.23	1.23	0.08	2.49	2.49	XXX	
	26	A		1.18	0.57	0.57	0.04	1.79	1.79	XXX	
	TC	A		0.00	0.66	0.66	0.04	0.70	0.70	XXX	
95869		A	Needle electromyography; thoracic paraspinal muscles	0.37	0.37	0.37	0.03	0.77	0.77	XXX	
	26	A		0.37	0.17	0.17	0.01	0.55	0.55	XXX	
	TC	A		0.00	0.20	0.20	0.02	0.22	0.22	XXX	
95870		A	limited study of muscles in one extremity or non-limb (axial) muscles (unilateral or bilateral), other than thoracic paraspinal, cranial nerve supplied muscles, or sphincters	0.37	0.37	0.37	0.03	0.77	0.77	XXX	
	26	A		0.37	0.17	0.17	0.01	0.55	0.55	XXX	
	TC	A		0.00	0.20	0.20	0.02	0.22	0.22	XXX	
95872		A	Needle electromyography using single fiber electrode, with quantitative measurement of jitter, blocking and/or fiber density, any/all sites of each muscle studied	1.50	1.25	1.25	0.08	2.83	2.83	XXX	
	26	A		1.50	0.68	0.68	0.04	2.22	2.22	XXX	
	TC	A		0.00	0.57	0.57	0.04	0.61	0.61	XXX	
95875		A	Ischemic limb exercise test with serial specimen(s) acquisition for muscle metabolite(s)	1.10	1.38	1.38	0.09	2.57	2.57	XXX	
	26	A		1.10	0.49	0.49	0.04	1.63	1.63	XXX	
	TC	A		0.00	0.89	0.89	0.05	0.94	0.94	XXX	
95900		A	Nerve conduction, amplitude and latency/velocity study, each nerve; motor, without F-wave study	0.42	0.73	0.73	0.03	1.18	1.18	XXX	
	26	A		0.42	0.20	0.20	0.01	0.63	0.63	XXX	
	TC	A		0.00	0.53	0.53	0.02	0.55	0.55	XXX	
95903		A	motor, with F-wave study	0.60	0.51	0.51	0.04	1.15	1.15	XXX	
	26	A		0.60	0.27	0.27	0.02	0.89	0.89	XXX	
	TC	A		0.00	0.24	0.24	0.02	0.26	0.26	XXX	

Medicine

■ RVU not developed by CMS. Gap-filled RVUs developed by Ingenix/CHEG.

Code	M	S	Description	Work Value	Non-Fac PE	Fac PE	Mal-practice	Non-Fac Total	Fac Total	Global	Gap
95904		A	sensory	0.34	0.64	0.64	0.03	1.01	1.01	XXX	
	26	A		0.34	0.16	0.16	0.01	0.51	0.51	XXX	
	TC	A		0.00	0.48	0.48	0.02	0.50	0.50	XXX	
95920		A	Intraoperative neurophysiology testing, per hour (List separately in addition to code for primary procedure)	2.11	2.23	2.23	0.20	4.54	4.54	ZZZ	
	26	A		2.11	0.99	0.99	0.14	3.24	3.24	ZZZ	
	TC	A		0.00	1.24	1.24	0.06	1.30	1.30	ZZZ	
95921		A	Testing of autonomic nervous system function; cardiovagal innervation (parasympathetic function), including two or more of the following; heart rate response to deep breathing with recorded R-R interval, Valsalva ratio, and 30:15 ratio	0.90	0.70	0.70	0.05	1.65	1.65	XXX	
	26	A		0.90	0.34	0.34	0.03	1.27	1.27	XXX	
	TC	A		0.00	0.36	0.36	0.02	0.38	0.38	XXX	
95922		A	vasomotor adrenergic innervation (sympathetic adrenergic function), including beat-to-beat blood pressure and R-R interval changes during Valsalva maneuver and at least five minutes of passive tilt	0.96	0.79	0.79	0.05	1.80	1.80	XXX	
	26	A		0.96	0.43	0.43	0.03	1.42	1.42	XXX	
	TC	A		0.00	0.36	0.36	0.02	0.38	0.38	XXX	
95923		A	sudomotor, including one or more of the following: quantitative sudomotor axon reflex test (QSART), silastic sweat imprint, thermoregulatory sweat test, and changes in sympathetic skin potential	0.90	2.57	2.57	0.05	3.52	3.52	XXX	
	26	A		0.90	0.40	0.40	0.03	1.33	1.33	XXX	
	TC	A		0.00	2.17	2.17	0.02	2.19	2.19	XXX	
95925		A	Short-latency somatosensory evoked potential study, stimulation of any/all peripheral nerves or skin sites, recording from the central nervous system; in upper limbs	0.54	1.10	1.10	0.07	1.71	1.71	XXX	
	26	A		0.54	0.24	0.24	0.02	0.80	0.80	XXX	
	TC	A		0.00	0.86	0.86	0.05	0.91	0.91	XXX	
95926		A	in lower limbs	0.54	1.11	1.11	0.07	1.72	1.72	XXX	
	26	A		0.54	0.25	0.25	0.02	0.81	0.81	XXX	
	TC	A		0.00	0.86	0.86	0.05	0.91	0.91	XXX	
95927		A	in the trunk or head	0.54	1.13	1.13	0.08	1.75	1.75	XXX	
	26	A		0.54	0.27	0.27	0.03	0.84	0.84	XXX	
	TC	A		0.00	0.86	0.86	0.05	0.91	0.91	XXX	
95930		A	Visual evoked potential (VEP) testing central nervous system, checkerboard or flash	0.35	0.84	0.84	0.02	1.21	1.21	XXX	
	26	A		0.35	0.16	0.16	0.01	0.52	0.52	XXX	
	TC	A		0.00	0.68	0.68	0.01	0.69	0.69	XXX	
95933		A	Orbicularis oculi (blink) reflex, by electrodiagnostic testing	0.59	1.01	1.01	0.07	1.67	1.67	XXX	
	26	A		0.59	0.27	0.27	0.02	0.88	0.88	XXX	
	TC	A		0.00	0.74	0.74	0.05	0.79	0.79	XXX	
95934		A	H-reflex, amplitude and latency study; record gastrocnemius/soleus muscle	0.51	0.44	0.44	0.04	0.99	0.99	XXX	
	26	A		0.51	0.24	0.24	0.02	0.77	0.77	XXX	
	TC	A		0.00	0.20	0.20	0.02	0.22	0.22	XXX	
95936		A	record muscle other than gastrocnemius/soleus muscle	0.55	0.45	0.45	0.04	1.04	1.04	XXX	
	26	A		0.55	0.25	0.25	0.02	0.82	0.82	XXX	
	TC	A		0.00	0.20	0.20	0.02	0.22	0.22	XXX	
95937		A	Neuromuscular junction testing (repetitive stimulation, paired stimuli), each nerve, any one method	0.65	0.60	0.60	0.04	1.29	1.29	XXX	
	26	A		0.65	0.28	0.28	0.02	0.95	0.95	XXX	
	TC	A		0.00	0.32	0.32	0.02	0.34	0.34	XXX	

■ RVU not developed by CMS. Gap-filled RVUs developed by Ingenix/CHEG.

Code	M	S	Description	Work Value	Non-Fac PE	Fac PE	Mal-practice	Non-Fac Total	Fac Total	Global	Gap
95950		A	Monitoring for identification and lateralization of cerebral seizure focus, electroencephalographic (eg, 8 channel EEG) recording and interpretation, each 24 hours	1.51	4.93	4.93	0.44	6.88	6.88	XXX	
	26	A		1.51	0.70	0.70	0.08	2.29	2.29	XXX	
	TC	A		0.00	4.23	4.23	0.36	4.59	4.59	XXX	
95951		A	Monitoring for localization of cerebral seizure focus by cable or radio, 16 or more channel telemetry, combined electroencephalographic (EEG) and video recording and interpretation (eg, for presurgical localization), each 24 hours	6.00	16.38	16.38	0.58	22.96	22.96	XXX	
	26	A		6.00	2.72	2.72	0.20	8.92	8.92	XXX	
	TC	A		0.00	13.66	13.66	0.38	14.04	14.04	XXX	
95953		A	Monitoring for localization of cerebral seizure focus by computerized portable 16 or more channel EEG; electroencephalographic (EEG) recording and interpretation, each 24 hours	3.08	7.39	7.39	0.46	10.93	10.93	XXX	
	26	A		3.08	1.38	1.38	0.10	4.56	4.56	XXX	
	TC	A		0.00	6.01	6.01	0.36	6.37	6.37	XXX	
95954		A	Pharmacological or physical activation requiring physician attendance during EEG recording of activation phase (eg, thiopental activation test)	2.45	4.43	4.43	0.15	7.03	7.03	XXX	
	26	A		2.45	1.07	1.07	0.10	3.62	3.62	XXX	
	TC	A		0.00	3.36	3.36	0.05	3.41	3.41	XXX	
95955		A	Electroencephalogram (EEG) during nonintracranial surgery (eg, carotid surgery)	1.01	2.26	2.26	0.19	3.46	3.46	XXX	
	26	A		1.01	0.40	0.40	0.05	1.46	1.46	XXX	
	TC	A		0.00	1.86	1.86	0.14	2.00	2.00	XXX	
95956		A	Monitoring for localization of cerebral seizure focus by cable or radio, 16 or more channel telemetry, electroencephalographic (EEG) recording and interpretation, each 24 hours	3.08	12.39	12.39	0.47	15.94	15.94	XXX	
	26	A		3.08	1.35	1.35	0.11	4.54	4.54	XXX	
	TC	A		0.00	11.04	11.04	0.36	11.40	11.40	XXX	
95957		A	Digital analysis of electroencephalogram (EEG) (eg, for epileptic spike analysis)	1.98	2.52	2.52	0.17	4.67	4.67	XXX	
	26	A		1.98	0.90	0.90	0.07	2.95	2.95	XXX	
	TC	A		0.00	1.62	1.62	0.10	1.72	1.72	XXX	
95958		A	Wada activation test for hemispheric function, including electroencephalographic (EEG) monitoring	4.25	3.51	3.51	0.29	8.05	8.05	XXX	
	26	A		4.25	1.86	1.86	0.18	6.29	6.29	XXX	
	TC	A		0.00	1.65	1.65	0.11	1.76	1.76	XXX	
95961		A	Functional cortical and subcortical mapping by stimulation and/or recording of electrodes on brain surface, or of depth electrodes, to provoke seizures or identify vital brain structures; initial hour of physician attendance	2.97	2.67	2.67	0.24	5.88	5.88	XXX	
	26	A		2.97	1.43	1.43	0.18	4.58	4.58	XXX	
	TC	A		0.00	1.24	1.24	0.06	1.30	1.30	XXX	
95962		A	each additional hour of physician attendance (List separately in addition to code for primary procedure)	3.21	2.72	2.72	0.23	6.16	6.16	ZZZ	
	26	A		3.21	1.48	1.48	0.17	4.86	4.86	ZZZ	
	TC	A		0.00	1.24	1.24	0.06	1.30	1.30	ZZZ	
95965		C	Magnetoencephalography (MEG), recording and analysis; for spontaneous brain magnetic activity (eg, epileptic cerebral cortex localization)	0.00	0.00	0.00	0.00	0.00	0.00	XXX	
	26	A		8.00	3.19	3.19	0.20	11.39	11.39	XXX	
	TC	C		0.00	0.00	0.00	0.00	0.00	0.00	XXX	
95966		C	for evoked magnetic fields, single modality (eg, sensory, motor, language, or visual cortex localization)	0.00	0.00	0.00	0.00	0.00	0.00	XXX	
	26	A		4.00	1.60	1.60	0.18	5.78	5.78	XXX	
	TC	C		0.00	0.00	0.00	0.00	0.00	0.00	XXX	
95967		C	for evoked magnetic fields, each additional modality (eg, sensory, motor, language, or visual cortex localization) (List separately in addition to code for primary procedure)	0.00	0.00	0.00	0.00	0.00	0.00	ZZZ	
	26	A		3.50	1.40	1.40	0.17	5.07	5.07	ZZZ	
	TC	C		0.00	0.00	0.00	0.00	0.00	0.00	ZZZ	

■ RVU not developed by CMS. Gap-filled RVUs developed by Ingenix/CHEG.

Medicine

Code	M	S	Description	Work Value	Non-Fac PE	Fac PE	Mal-practice	Non-Fac Total	Fac Total	Global	Gap
95970		A	Electronic analysis of implanted neurostimulator pulse generator system (eg, rate, pulse amplitude and duration, configuration of wave form, battery status, electrode selectability, output modulation, cycling, impedance and patient compliance measurements); simple or complex brain, spinal cord, or peripheral (ie, cranial nerve, peripheral nerve, autonomic nerve, neuromuscular) neurostimulator pulse generator/transmitter, without reprogramming	0.45	0.18	0.16	0.03	0.66	0.64	XXX	
95971		A	simple brain, spinal cord, or peripheral (ie, peripheral nerve, autonomic nerve, neuromuscular) neurostimulator pulse generator/transmitter, with intraoperative or subsequent programming	0.78	0.28	0.24	0.06	1.12	1.08	XXX	
95972		A	complex brain, spinal cord, or peripheral (except cranial nerve) neurostimulator pulse generator/transmitter, with intraoperative or subsequent programming, first hour	1.50	0.62	0.51	0.17	2.29	2.18	XXX	
95973		A	complex brain, spinal cord, or peripheral (except cranial nerve) neurostimulator pulse generator/transmitter, with intraoperative or subsequent programming, each additional 30 minutes after first hour (List separately in addition to code for primary procedure)	0.92	0.42	0.36	0.07	1.41	1.35	ZZZ	
95974		A	complex cranial nerve neurostimulator pulse generator/transmitter, with intraoperative or subsequent programming, with or without nerve interface testing, first hour	3.00	1.37	1.37	0.15	4.52	4.52	XXX	
95975		A	complex cranial nerve neurostimulator pulse generator/transmitter, with intraoperative or subsequent programming, each additional 30 minutes after first hour (List separately in addition to code for primary procedure)	1.70	0.78	0.78	0.07	2.55	2.55	ZZZ	
95999		C	Unlisted neurological or neuromuscular diagnostic procedure	0.00	0.00	0.00	0.00	0.00	0.00	XXX	
96000		A	Comprehensive computer-based motion analysis by video-taping and 3-D kinematics;	1.80	0.72	0.72	0.02	2.54	2.54	XXX	
	26			0.00	0.00	0.00	0.00	0.00	0.00	XXX	■
	TC			1.80	0.72	0.72	0.02	2.54	2.54	XXX	■
96001		A	with dynamic plantar pressure measurements during walking	2.15	0.86	0.86	0.02	3.03	3.03	XXX	
	26			0.00	0.00	0.00	0.00	0.00	0.00	XXX	■
	TC			2.15	0.86	0.86	0.02	3.03	3.03	XXX	■
96002		A	Dynamic surface electromyography, during walking or other functional activities, 1-12 muscles	0.41	0.16	0.16	0.02	0.59	0.59	XXX	
	26			0.00	0.00	0.00	0.00	0.00	0.00	XXX	■
	TC			0.41	0.16	0.16	0.02	0.59	0.59	XXX	■

■ RVU not developed by CMS. Gap-filled RVUs developed by Ingenix/CHEG.

Code	M	S	Description	Work Value	Non-Fac PE	Fac PE	Mal-prac-tice	Non-Fac Total	Fac Total	Global	Gap
96003		A	Dynamic fine wire electromyography, during walking or other functional activities, 1 muscle	0.37	0.15	0.15	0.03	0.55	0.55	XXX	
	26			0.00	0.00	0.00	0.00	0.00	0.00	XXX	■
	TC			0.37	0.15	0.15	0.03	0.55	0.55	XXX	■
96004		A	Physician review and interpretation of comprehensive computer based motion analysis, dynamic plantar pressure measurements, dynamic surface electromyography during walking or other functional activities, and dynamic fine wire electromyography, with written report	1.80	0.72	0.72	0.08	2.60	2.60	XXX	
96100		A	Psychological testing (includes psychodiagnostic assessment of personality, psychopathology, emotionality, intellectual abilities, eg, WAIS-R, Rorschach, MMPI) with interpretation and report, per hour	0.00	1.67	1.67	0.15	1.82	1.82	XXX	
96105		A	Assessment of aphasia (includes assessment of expressive and receptive speech and language function, language comprehension, speech production ability, reading, spelling, writing, eg, by Boston Diagnostic Aphasia Examination) with interpretation and report, per hour	0.00	1.67	1.67	0.15	1.82	1.82	XXX	
96110		C	Developmental testing; limited (eg, Developmental Screening Test II, Early Language Milestone Screen), with interpretation and report	0.48	1.10	1.10	0.07	1.64	1.64	XXX	■
96111		A	extended (includes assessment of motor, language, social, adaptive and/or cognitive functioning by standardized developmental instruments, eg, Bayley Scales of Infant Development) with interpretation and report, per hour	0.00	1.67	1.67	0.15	1.82	1.82	XXX	
96115		A	Neurobehavorial status exam (clinical assessment of thinking, reasoning and judgment, eg, acquired knowledge, attention, memory, visual spatial abilities, language functions, planning) with interpretation and report, per hour	0.00	1.67	1.67	0.15	1.82	1.82	XXX	
96117		A	Neuropsychological testing battery (eg, Halstead-Reitan, Luria, WAIS-R) with interpretation and report, per hour	0.00	1.67	1.67	0.15	1.82	1.82	XXX	
96150		A	Health and behavior assessment (eg, health-focused clinical interview, behavioral observations, psychophysicological monitoring, health-oriented questionnaires), each 15 minutes face-to-face with the patient; initial assessment	0.50	0.21	0.20	0.02	0.73	0.72	XXX	
96151		A	re-assessment	0.48	0.21	0.19	0.02	0.71	0.69	XXX	
96152		A	Health and behavior intervention, each 15 minutes, face-to-face; individual	0.46	0.20	0.18	0.02	0.68	0.66	XXX	
96153		A	group (2 or more patients)	0.10	0.04	0.04	0.01	0.15	0.15	XXX	

■ RVU not developed by CMS. Gap-filled RVUs developed by Ingenix/CHEG.

Code	M	S	Description	Work Value	Non-Fac PE	Fac PE	Mal-practice	Non-Fac Total	Fac Total	Global	Gap
96154		A	family (with the patient present)	0.45	0.19	0.18	0.02	0.66	0.65	XXX	
96155		A	family (without the patient present)	0.44	0.18	0.18	0.02	0.64	0.64	XXX	
96400		A	Chemotherapy administration, subcutaneous or intramuscular, with or without local anesthesia	0.00	0.13	0.13	0.01	0.14	0.14	XXX	
96405		A	Chemotherapy administration, intralesional; up to and including 7 lesions	0.52	1.88	0.24	0.02	2.42	0.78	000	
96406		A	more than 7 lesions	0.80	2.94	0.41	0.02	3.76	1.23	000	
96408		A	Chemotherapy administration, intravenous; push technique	0.00	0.92	0.92	0.05	0.97	0.97	XXX	
96410		A	infusion technique, up to one hour	0.00	1.47	1.47	0.07	1.54	1.54	XXX	
96412		A	infusion technique, one to 8 hours, each additional hour (List separately in addition to code for primary procedure)	0.00	1.09	1.09	0.06	1.15	1.15	ZZZ	
96414		A	infusion technique, initiation of prolonged infusion (more than 8 hours), requiring the use of a portable or implantable pump	0.00	1.27	1.27	0.07	1.34	1.34	XXX	
96420		A	Chemotherapy administration, intra-arterial; push technique	0.00	1.18	1.18	0.07	1.25	1.25	XXX	
96422		A	infusion technique, up to one hour	0.00	1.17	1.17	0.07	1.24	1.24	XXX	
96423		A	infusion technique, one to 8 hours, each additional hour (List separately in addition to code for primary procedure)	0.00	0.46	0.46	0.02	0.48	0.48	ZZZ	
96425		A	infusion technique, initiation of prolonged infusion (more than 8 hours), requiring the use of a portable or implantable pump	0.00	1.36	1.36	0.07	1.43	1.43	XXX	
96440		A	Chemotherapy administration into pleural cavity, requiring and including thoracentesis	2.37	7.99	1.06	0.12	10.48	3.55	000	
96445		A	Chemotherapy administration into peritoneal cavity, requiring and including peritoneocentesis	2.20	8.74	1.08	0.07	11.01	3.35	000	
96450		A	Chemotherapy administration, into CNS (eg, intrathecal), requiring and including spinal puncture	1.89	6.79	0.95	0.06	8.74	2.90	000	
96520		A	Refilling and maintenance of portable pump	0.00	0.84	0.84	0.05	0.89	0.89	XXX	
96530		A	Refilling and maintenance of implantable pump or reservoir	0.00	1.01	1.01	0.05	1.06	1.06	XXX	
96542		A	Chemotherapy injection, subarachnoid or intraventricular via subcutaneous reservoir, single or multiple agents	1.42	4.70	0.55	0.05	6.17	2.02	XXX	
96545		B	Provision of chemotherapy agent	0.00	0.00	0.00	0.00	0.00	0.00	XXX	
96549		C	Unlisted chemotherapy procedure	0.00	0.00	0.00	0.00	0.00	0.00	XXX	

■ RVU not developed by CMS. Gap-filled RVUs developed by Ingenix/CHEG.

Code	M	S	Description	Work Value	Non-Fac PE	Fac PE	Mal-practice	Non-Fac Total	Fac Total	Global	Gap
96567		A	Photodynamic therapy by external application of light to destroy premalignant and/or malignant lesions of the skin and adjacent mucosa (eg, lip) by activation of photosensitive drug(s), each phototherapy exposure session	0.00	1.63	1.63	0.03	1.66	1.66	XXX	
96570		A	Photodynamic therapy by endoscopic application of light to ablate abnormal tissue via activation of photosensitive drug(s); first 30 minutes (List separately in addition to code for endoscopy or bronchoscopy procedures of lung and esophagus)	1.10	0.46	0.38	0.04	1.60	1.52	ZZZ	
96571		A	each additional 15 minutes (List separately in addition to code for endoscopy or bronchoscopy procedures of lung and esophagus)	0.55	0.22	0.20	0.02	0.79	0.77	ZZZ	
96900		A	Actinotherapy (ultraviolet light)	0.00	0.45	0.45	0.02	0.47	0.47	XXX	
96902		B	Microscopic examination of hairs plucked or clipped by the examiner (excluding hair collected by the patient) to determine telogen and anagen counts, or structural hair shaft abnormality	0.41	0.25	0.16	0.01	0.67	0.58	XXX	
96910		A	Photochemotherapy; tar and ultraviolet B (Goeckerman treatment) or petrolatum and ultraviolet B	0.00	1.37	1.37	0.03	1.40	1.40	XXX	
96912		A	psoralens and ultraviolet A (PUVA)	0.00	1.54	1.54	0.04	1.58	1.58	XXX	
96913		A	Photochemotherapy (Goeckerman and/or PUVA) for severe photoresponsive dermatoses requiring at least four to eight hours of care under direct supervision of the physician (includes application of medication and dressings)	0.00	2.26	2.26	0.08	2.34	2.34	XXX	
96999		C	Unlisted special dermatological service or procedure	0.00	0.00	0.00	0.00	0.00	0.00	XXX	
97001		A	Physical therapy evaluation	1.20	0.56	0.37	0.10	1.86	1.67	XXX	
97002		A	Physical therapy re-evaluation	0.60	0.35	0.27	0.04	0.99	0.91	XXX	
97003		A	Occupational therapy evaluation	1.20	0.69	0.32	0.05	1.94	1.57	XXX	
97004		A	Occupational therapy re-evaluation	0.60	0.69	0.12	0.02	1.31	0.74	XXX	
97005		I	Athletic training evaluation	0.44	1.02	1.02	0.06	1.52	1.52	XXX	■
97006		I	Athletic training re-evaluation	0.22	0.51	0.51	0.03	0.76	0.76	XXX	■
97010		B	Application of a modality to one or more areas; hot or cold packs	0.06	0.04	0.04	0.01	0.11	0.11	XXX	
97012		A	traction, mechanical	0.25	0.11	0.11	0.01	0.37	0.37	XXX	
97014		A	electrical stimulation (unattended)	0.18	0.19	0.19	0.01	0.38	0.38	XXX	

■ RVU not developed by CMS. Gap-filled RVUs developed by Ingenix/CHEG.

Medicine

Code	M	S	Description	Work Value	Non-Fac PE	Fac PE	Mal-practice	Non-Fac Total	Fac Total	Global	Gap
97016		A	vasopneumatic devices	0.18	0.14	0.14	0.01	0.33	0.33	XXX	
97018		A	paraffin bath	0.06	0.12	0.12	0.01	0.19	0.19	XXX	
97020		A	microwave	0.06	0.05	0.05	0.01	0.12	0.12	XXX	
97022		A	whirlpool	0.17	0.26	0.26	0.01	0.44	0.44	XXX	
97024		A	diathermy	0.06	0.05	0.05	0.01	0.12	0.12	XXX	
97026		A	infrared	0.06	0.05	0.05	0.01	0.12	0.12	XXX	
97028		A	ultraviolet	0.08	0.06	0.06	0.01	0.15	0.15	XXX	
97032		A	Application of a modality to one or more areas; electrical stimulation (manual), each 15 minutes	0.25	0.21	0.21	0.01	0.47	0.47	XXX	
97033		A	iontophoresis, each 15 minutes	0.26	0.12	0.12	0.02	0.40	0.40	XXX	
97034		A	contrast baths, each 15 minutes	0.21	0.14	0.14	0.01	0.36	0.36	XXX	
97035		A	ultrasound, each 15 minutes	0.21	0.08	0.08	0.01	0.30	0.30	XXX	
97036		A	Hubbard tank, each 15 minutes	0.28	0.34	0.34	0.01	0.63	0.63	XXX	
97039		A	Unlisted modality (specify type and time if constant attendance)	0.20	0.07	0.07	0.01	0.28	0.28	XXX	
97110		A	Therapeutic procedure, one or more areas, each 15 minutes; therapeutic exercises to develop strength and endurance, range of motion and flexibility	0.45	0.25	0.25	0.03	0.73	0.73	XXX	
97112		A	neuromuscular reeducation of movement, balance, coordination, kinesthetic sense, posture, and/or proprioception for sitting and/or standing activities	0.45	0.29	0.29	0.02	0.76	0.76	XXX	
97113		A	aquatic therapy with therapeutic exercises	0.44	0.33	0.33	0.03	0.80	0.80	XXX	
97116		A	gait training (includes stair climbing)	0.40	0.21	0.21	0.02	0.63	0.63	XXX	
97124		A	massage, including effleurage, petrissage and/or tapotement (stroking, compression, percussion)	0.35	0.21	0.21	0.01	0.57	0.57	XXX	
97139		A	unlisted therapeutic procedure (specify)	0.21	0.21	0.21	0.01	0.43	0.43	XXX	
97140		A	Manual therapy techniques (eg, mobilization/ manipulation, manual lymphatic drainage, manual traction), one or more regions, each 15 minutes	0.43	0.23	0.23	0.02	0.68	0.68	XXX	
97150		A	Therapeutic procedure(s), group (2 or more individuals)	0.27	0.20	0.20	0.02	0.49	0.49	XXX	
97504		A	Orthotic(s) fitting and training, upper extremity(ies), lower extremity(ies), and/or trunk, each 15 minutes	0.45	0.25	0.25	0.03	0.73	0.73	XXX	

■ RVU not developed by CMS. Gap-filled RVUs developed by Ingenix/CHEG.

Code	M	S	Description	Work Value	Non-Fac PE	Fac PE	Mal-practice	Non-Fac Total	Fac Total	Global	Gap
97520		**A**	Prosthetic training, upper and/or lower extremities, each 15 minutes	0.45	0.21	0.21	0.02	0.68	0.68	XXX	
97530		**A**	Therapeutic activities, direct (one on one) patient contact by the provider (use of dynamic activities to improve functional performance), each 15 minutes	0.44	0.45	0.45	0.02	0.91	0.91	XXX	
97532		**A**	Development of cognitive skills to improve attention, memory, problem solving, (includes compensatory training), direct (one-on-one) patient contact by the provider, each 15 minutes	0.44	0.17	0.17	0.01	0.62	0.62	XXX	
97533		**A**	Sensory integrative techniques to enhance sensory processing and promote adaptive responses to environmental demands, direct (one-on-one) patient contact by the provider, each 15 minutes	0.44	0.21	0.21	0.01	0.66	0.66	XXX	
97535		**A**	Self-care/home management training (eg, activities of daily living (ADL) and compensatory training, meal preparation, safety procedures, and instructions in use of assistive technology devices/adaptive equipment) direct one-on-one contact by provider, each 15 minutes	0.45	0.35	0.35	0.02	0.82	0.82	XXX	
97537		**A**	Community/work reintegration training (eg, shopping, transportation, money management, avocational activities and/or work environment/ modification analysis, work task analysis), direct one on one contact by provider, each 15 minutes	0.45	0.20	0.20	0.01	0.66	0.66	XXX	
97542		**A**	Wheelchair management/propulsion training, each 15 minutes	0.45	0.22	0.22	0.01	0.68	0.68	XXX	
97545		**R**	Work hardening/conditioning; initial 2 hours	1.06	2.44	2.44	0.15	3.64	3.64	XXX	■
97546		**R**	each additional hour (List separately in addition to code for primary procedure)	0.42	0.97	0.97	0.06	1.45	1.45	ZZZ	■
97601		**A**	Removal of devitalized tissue from wound(s); selective debridement, without anesthesia (eg, high pressure waterjet, sharp selective debridement with scissors, scalpel and tweezers), including topical application(s), wound assessment, and instruction(s) for ongoing care, per session	0.50	1.90	1.90	0.04	2.44	2.44	XXX	
97602		**B**	non-selective debridement, without anesthesia (eg, wet-to-moist dressings, enzymatic, abrasion), including topical application(s), wound assessment, and instruction(s) for ongoing care, per session	0.15	0.36	0.36	0.02	0.53	0.53	XXX	■
97703		**A**	Checkout for orthotic/prosthetic use, established patient, each 15 minutes	0.25	0.44	0.44	0.02	0.71	0.71	XXX	

Medicine

■ RVU not developed by CMS. Gap-filled RVUs developed by Ingenix/CHEG.

Code	M	S	Description	Work Value	Non-Fac PE	Fac PE	Mal-practice	Non-Fac Total	Fac Total	Global	Gap
97750		A	Physical performance test or measurement (eg, musculoskeletal, functional capacity), with written report, each 15 minutes	0.45	0.24	0.24	0.02	0.71	0.71	XXX	
97780		N	Acupuncture, one or more needles; without electrical stimulation	0.38	0.87	0.87	0.05	1.30	1.30	XXX	■
97781		N	with electrical stimulation	0.47	1.09	1.09	0.07	1.63	1.63	XXX	■
97799		C	Unlisted physical medicine/rehabilitation service or procedure	0.00	0.00	0.00	0.00	0.00	0.00	XXX	
97802		A	Medical nutrition therapy; initial assessment and intervention, individual, face-to-face with the patient, each 15 minutes	0.00	0.45	0.45	0.01	0.46	0.46	XXX	
97803		A	re-assessment and intervention, individual, face-to-face with the patient, each 15 minutes	0.00	0.45	0.45	0.01	0.46	0.46	XXX	
97804		A	group (2 or more individual(s)), each 30 minutes	0.00	0.17	0.17	0.01	0.18	0.18	XXX	
98925		A	Osteopathic manipulative treatment (OMT); one to two body regions involved	0.45	0.38	0.14	0.01	0.84	0.60	000	
98926		A	three to four body regions involved	0.65	0.44	0.25	0.02	1.11	0.92	000	
98927		A	five to six body regions involved	0.87	0.52	0.31	0.03	1.42	1.21	000	
98928		A	seven to eight body regions involved	1.03	0.59	0.38	0.03	1.65	1.44	000	
98929		A	nine to ten body regions involved	1.19	0.65	0.39	0.04	1.88	1.62	000	
98940		A	Chiropractic manipulative treatment (CMT); spinal, one to two regions	0.45	0.25	0.13	0.01	0.71	0.59	000	
98941		A	spinal, three to four regions	0.65	0.31	0.19	0.02	0.98	0.86	000	
98942		A	spinal, five regions	0.87	0.37	0.25	0.03	1.27	1.15	000	
98943		N	extraspinal, one or more regions	0.40	0.34	0.16	0.01	0.75	0.57	XXX	
99000		B	Handling and/or conveyance of specimen for transfer from the physician's office to a laboratory	0.07	0.16	0.16	0.01	0.24	0.24	XXX	■
99001		B	Handling and/or conveyance of specimen for transfer from the patient in other than a physician's office to a laboratory (distance may be indicated)	0.08	0.18	0.18	0.01	0.27	0.27	XXX	■
99002		B	Handling, conveyance, and/or any other service in connection with the implementation of an order involving devices (eg, designing, fitting, packaging, handling, delivery or mailing) when devices such as orthotics, protectives, prosthetics are fabricated by an outside laboratory or shop but which items have been designed, and are to be fitted and adjusted by the attending physician	0.11	0.26	0.26	0.02	0.39	0.39	XXX	■

■ RVU not developed by CMS. Gap-filled RVUs developed by Ingenix/CHEG.

Code	M	S	Description	Work Value	Non-Fac PE	Fac PE	Mal-prac-tice	Non-Fac Total	Fac Total	Global	Gap
99024		B	Postoperative follow-up visit, included in global service	0.00	0.00	0.00	0.00	0.00	0.00	XXX	
99025		B	Initial (new patient) visit when starred (*) surgical procedure constitutes major service at that visit	0.18	0.42	0.42	0.03	0.63	0.63	XXX	■
99050		B	Services requested after office hours in addition to basic service	0.21	0.48	0.48	0.03	0.72	0.72	XXX	■
99052		B	Services requested between 10:00 PM and 8:00 AM in addition to basic service	0.21	0.48	0.48	0.03	0.72	0.72	XXX	■
99054		B	Services requested on Sundays and holidays in addition to basic service	0.21	0.48	0.48	0.03	0.72	0.72	XXX	■
99056		B	Services provided at request of patient in a location other than physician's office which are normally provided in the office	0.27	0.63	0.63	0.04	0.94	0.94	XXX	■
99058		B	Office services provided on an emergency basis	0.28	0.65	0.65	0.04	0.97	0.97	XXX	■
99070		B	Supplies and materials (except spectacles), provided by the physician over and above those usually included with the office visit or other services rendered (list drugs, trays, supplies, or materials provided)	0.00	0.00	0.00	0.00	0.00	0.00	XXX	
99071		B	Educational supplies, such as books, tapes, and pamphlets, provided by the physician for the patient's education at cost to physician	0.00	0.00	0.00	0.00	0.00	0.00	XXX	
99075		N	Medical testimony	0.00	0.00	0.00	0.00	0.00	0.00	XXX	
99078		B	Physician educational services rendered to patients in a group setting (eg, prenatal, obesity, or diabetic instructions)	0.00	0.00	0.00	0.00	0.00	0.00	XXX	
99080		B	Special reports such as insurance forms, more than the information conveyed in the usual medical communications or standard reporting form	0.00	0.00	0.00	0.00	0.00	0.00	XXX	
99082		C	Unusual travel (eg, transportation and escort of patient)	0.00	0.00	0.00	0.00	0.00	0.00	XXX	
99090		B	Analysis of clinical data stored in computers (eg, ECGs, blood pressures, hematologic data)	0.00	0.00	0.00	0.00	0.00	0.00	XXX	
99091		B	Collection and interpretation of physiologic data (eg, ECG, blood pressure, glucose monitoring) digitally stored and/or transmitted by the patient and/or caregiver to the physician or other qualified health care professional, requiring a minimum of 30 minutes of time	0.00	0.00	0.00	0.00	0.00	0.00	XXX	
99100		B	Anesthesia for patient of extreme age, under one year and over seventy (List separately in addition to code for primary anesthesia procedure)	0.00	0.00	0.00	0.00	0.00	0.00	ZZZ	

Medicine

■ RVU not developed by CMS. Gap-filled RVUs developed by Ingenix/CHEG.

Code	M	S	Description	Work Value	Non-Fac PE	Fac PE	Mal-practice	Non-Fac Total	Fac Total	Global	Gap
99116		B	Anesthesia complicated by utilization of total body hypothermia (List separately in addition to code for primary anesthesia procedure)	0.00	0.00	0.00	0.00	0.00	0.00	ZZZ	
99135		B	Anesthesia complicated by utilization of controlled hypotension (List separately in addition to code for primary anesthesia procedure)	0.00	0.00	0.00	0.00	0.00	0.00	ZZZ	
99140		B	Anesthesia complicated by emergency conditions (specify) (List separately in addition to code for primary anesthesia procedure)	0.00	0.00	0.00	0.00	0.00	0.00	ZZZ	
99141		B	Sedation with or without analgesia (conscious sedation); intravenous, intramuscular or inhalation	0.80	2.12	0.39	0.04	2.96	1.23	XXX	
99142		B	oral, rectal and/or intranasal	0.60	1.24	0.31	0.03	1.87	0.94	XXX	
99170		A	Anogenital examination with colposcopic magnification in childhood for suspected trauma	1.75	2.02	0.55	0.07	3.84	2.37	000	
99172		N	Visual function screening, automated or semi-automated bilateral quantitative determination of visual acuity, ocular alignment, color vision by pseudoisochromatic plates, and field of vision (may include all or some screening of the determination(s) for contrast sensitivity, vision under glare)	0.15	0.36	0.36	0.02	0.53	0.53	XXX	■
	26			0.03	0.07	0.07	0.00	0.11	0.11	XXX	■
	TC			0.12	0.29	0.29	0.02	0.42	0.42	XXX	■
99173		N	Screening test of visual acuity, quantitative, bilateral	0.08	0.17	0.17	0.01	0.26	0.26	XXX	■
99175		A	Ipecac or similar administration for individual emesis and continued observation until stomach adequately emptied of poison	0.00	1.32	1.32	0.08	1.40	1.40	XXX	
99183		A	Physician attendance and supervision of hyperbaric oxygen therapy, per session	2.34	0.77	0.77	0.12	3.23	3.23	XXX	
99185		A	Hypothermia; regional	0.00	0.61	0.61	0.03	0.64	0.64	XXX	
	26			0.00	0.24	0.24	0.01	0.26	0.26	XXX	■
	TC			0.00	0.37	0.37	0.02	0.38	0.38	XXX	■
99186		A	total body	0.00	1.69	1.69	0.37	2.06	2.06	XXX	
	26			0.00	0.68	0.68	0.15	0.82	0.82	XXX	■
	TC			0.00	1.01	1.01	0.22	1.24	1.24	XXX	■
99190		X	Assembly and operation of pump with oxygenator or heat exchanger (with or without ECG and/or pressure monitoring); each hour	3.47	8.01	8.01	0.48	11.96	11.96	XXX	■
	26			0.00	0.00	0.00	0.00	0.00	0.00	XXX	■
	TC			3.47	8.01	8.01	0.48	11.96	11.96	XXX	■
99191		X	3/4 hour	2.60	6.00	6.00	0.36	8.96	8.96	XXX	■
	26			0.00	0.00	0.00	0.00	0.00	0.00	XXX	■
	TC			2.60	6.00	6.00	0.36	8.96	8.96	XXX	■
99192		X	1/2 hour	1.73	4.01	4.01	0.24	5.98	5.98	XXX	■
	26			0.00	0.00	0.00	0.00	0.00	0.00	XXX	■
	TC			1.73	4.01	4.01	0.24	5.98	5.98	XXX	■

■ RVU not developed by CMS. Gap-filled RVUs developed by Ingenix/CHEG.

Medicine

Code	M	S	Description	Work Value	Non-Fac PE	Fac PE	Mal-practice	Non-Fac Total	Fac Total	Global	Gap
99195		A	Phlebotomy, therapeutic (separate procedure)	0.00	0.42	0.42	0.02	0.44	0.44	XXX	
99199		C	Unlisted special service, procedure or report	0.00	0.00	0.00	0.00	0.00	0.00	XXX	
99500		I	Home visit for prenatal monitoring and assessment to include fetal heart rate, non-stress test, uterine monitoring, and gestational diabetes monitoring	0.00	0.00	0.00	0.00	0.00	0.00	XXX	
99501		I	Home visit for postnatal assessment and follow-up care	0.00	0.00	0.00	0.00	0.00	0.00	XXX	
99502		I	Home visit for newborn care and assessment	0.00	0.00	0.00	0.00	0.00	0.00	XXX	
99503		I	Home visit for respiratory therapy care (eg, bronchodilator, oxygen therapy, respiratory assessment, apnea evaluation)	0.00	0.00	0.00	0.00	0.00	0.00	XXX	
99504		I	Home visit for patients receiving mechanical ventilation	0.00	0.00	0.00	0.00	0.00	0.00	XXX	
99505		I	Home visit for stoma care and maintenance including colostomy and cystostomy	0.00	0.00	0.00	0.00	0.00	0.00	XXX	
99506		I	Home visit for intramuscular injections	0.00	0.00	0.00	0.00	0.00	0.00	XXX	
99507		I	Home visit for care and maintenance of catheter(s) (eg, urinary, drainage, and enteral)	0.00	0.00	0.00	0.00	0.00	0.00	XXX	
99508		I	Home visit for polysomnography and sleep studies	0.00	0.00	0.00	0.00	0.00	0.00	XXX	
99509		I	Home visit for assistance with activities of daily living and personal care	0.00	0.00	0.00	0.00	0.00	0.00	XXX	
99510		I	Home visit for individual, family, or marriage counseling	0.00	0.00	0.00	0.00	0.00	0.00	XXX	
99511		I	Home visit for fecal impaction management and enema administration	0.00	0.00	0.00	0.00	0.00	0.00	XXX	
99512		I	Home visit for hemodialysis, per diem	0.00	0.00	0.00	0.00	0.00	0.00	XXX	
99539		I	Unlisted home visit service or procedure	0.00	0.00	0.00	0.00	0.00	0.00	XXX	
99551		I	Home infusion for pain management (intravenous or subcutaneous), per diem	0.00	0.00	0.00	0.00	0.00	0.00	XXX	
99552		I	Home infusion for pain management (epidural or intrathecal), per diem	0.00	0.00	0.00	0.00	0.00	0.00	XXX	
99553		I	Home infusion for tocolytic therapy, per diem	0.00	0.00	0.00	0.00	0.00	0.00	XXX	
99554		I	Home infusion for hematopoietic hormones (eg, erythropoietin, G-CSF, CM-CSF) or platelets, per diem	0.00	0.00	0.00	0.00	0.00	0.00	XXX	
99555		I	Home infusion for chemotherapy, per diem	0.00	0.00	0.00	0.00	0.00	0.00	XXX	
99556		I	Home infusion for antibiotics/antifungals/antivirals, per diem	0.00	0.00	0.00	0.00	0.00	0.00	XXX	

■ RVU not developed by CMS. Gap-filled RVUs developed by Ingenix/CHEG.

Code	M	S	Description	Work Value	Non-Fac PE	Fac PE	Mal-practice	Non-Fac Total	Fac Total	Global	Gap
99557		I	Home infusion of continuous anticoagulant therapy (eg, heparin), per diem	0.00	0.00	0.00	0.00	0.00	0.00	XXX	
99558		I	Home infusion of immunotherapy, per diem	0.00	0.00	0.00	0.00	0.00	0.00	XXX	
99559		I	Home infusion of peritoneal dialysis, per diem	0.00	0.00	0.00	0.00	0.00	0.00	XXX	
99560		I	Home infusion of enteral nutrition, per diem	0.00	0.00	0.00	0.00	0.00	0.00	XXX	
99561		I	Home infusion of hydration therapy, per diem	0.00	0.00	0.00	0.00	0.00	0.00	XXX	
99562		I	Home infusion of total parenteral nutrition, per diem	0.00	0.00	0.00	0.00	0.00	0.00	XXX	
99563		I	Home administration of aerosolized pentamidine, per diem	0.00	0.00	0.00	0.00	0.00	0.00	XXX	
99564		I	Home infusion for anti-hemophilic agents (eg, Factor VIII), per diem	0.00	0.00	0.00	0.00	0.00	0.00	XXX	
99565		I	Home infusion of alpha-1-proteinase inhibitor (eg, Prolastin), per diem	0.00	0.00	0.00	0.00	0.00	0.00	XXX	
99566		I	Home infusion for uninterrupted, long-term intravenous treatment (eg, epoprostenol), per diem	0.00	0.00	0.00	0.00	0.00	0.00	XXX	
99567		I	Home infusion of sympathomimetic agents (eg, dobutamine), per diem	0.00	0.00	0.00	0.00	0.00	0.00	XXX	
99568		I	Home infusion of miscellaneous drugs, per diem	0.00	0.00	0.00	0.00	0.00	0.00	XXX	
99569		I	Home infusion, each additional therapy given on same day (List separately in addition to code for primary visit)	0.00	0.00	0.00	0.00	0.00	0.00	XXX	

■ RVU not developed by CMS. Gap-filled RVUs developed by Ingenix/CHEG.

Category III Codes

I. **General:** In 2001, the AMA began development of a set of temporary codes to allow collection of data for emerging technology, services, and procedures. The first set of these codes appear in *CPT 2002* in a new section titled Category III Codes. These five-character alphanumeric codes contain four numbers with one alpha character in the fifth place.

II. **Updating of Category III Codes:** Category III codes are temporary in nature. These codes may or may not be assigned a permanent Category I CPT code. If no permanent CPT code is assigned, the Category III code will be archived after 5 years unless it is demonstrated that a temporary code is still required. New Category III Codes are released semi-annually via the AMA/CPT internet site. The full set of codes will be published annually in the CPT book.

III. **CMS Status Code:** All Category III Codes have a status code of 'C' indicating that they are carrier priced codes. For status code 'C' services, individual carriers are responsible for assigning RVUs and establishing payment amounts. Services are generally priced on an individual, case-by-case basis. When reporting a Category III code, include a copy of the operative report or other pertinent documentation, including:

A. Complete description of the service or procedure

B. Pertinent clinical data

C. Descriptions of related services or procedures including CPT code

D. Relative values of related services and procedures

E. Suggested value of Category III service

Category III Values

Code	M	S	Description	Work Value	Non-Fac PE	Fac PE	Mal-practice	Non-Fac Total	Fac Total	Global	Gap
0001T		C	Endovascular repair of infrarenal abdominal aortic aneurysm or dissection; modular bifurcated prosthesis (two docking limbs)	0.00	0.00	0.00	0.00	0.00	0.00	XXX	
0002T		C	Endovascular repair of infrarenal abdominal aortic aneurysm or dissection; aorto-uni-iliac or aorto-unifemoral prosthesis	0.00	0.00	0.00	0.00	0.00	0.00	XXX	
0003T		C	Cervicography	0.00	0.00	0.00	0.00	0.00	0.00	XXX	
0005T		C	Transcatheter placement of extracranial cerebrovascular artery stent(s), percutaneous; initial vessel	0.00	0.00	0.00	0.00	0.00	0.00	XXX	
0006T		C	Transcatheter placement of extracranial cerebrovascular artery stent(s), percutaneous; each additional vessel (List separately in addition to code for primary procedure	0.00	0.00	0.00	0.00	0.00	0.00	XXX	
0007T		C	Transcatheter placement of extracranial cerebrovascular artery stent(s), percutaneous, radiological supervision and interpretation, each vessel	0.00	0.00	0.00	0.00	0.00	0.00	XXX	
0008T		C	Upper gastrointestinal endoscopy including esophagus, stomach, and either the duodenum and/or jejunum as appropriate; with suturing of the esophagogastric junction	0.00	0.00	0.00	0.00	0.00	0.00	XXX	
0009T		C	Endometrial cryoablation with ultrasonic guidance	0.00	0.00	0.00	0.00	0.00	0.00	XXX	
0010T		C	Tuberculosis test, cell mediated immunity measurement of gamma interferon antigen response	0.00	0.00	0.00	0.00	0.00	0.00	XXX	
0012T		C	Arthroscopy, knee, surgical, implantation of osteochondral graft(s) for treatment of articular surface defect; autografts	0.00	0.00	0.00	0.00	0.00	0.00	XXX	
0013T		C	Arthroscopy, knee, surgical, implantation of osteochondral graft(s) for treatment of articular surface defect; allografts	0.00	0.00	0.00	0.00	0.00	0.00	XXX	
0014T		C	Meniscal transplantation, medial or lateral, knee (any method)	0.00	0.00	0.00	0.00	0.00	0.00	XXX	
0016T		C	Destruction of localized lesion of choroid (eg, choroidal neovascularization), transpupillary thermotherapy	0.00	0.00	0.00	0.00	0.00	0.00	XXX	
0017T		C	Destruction of macular drusen, photocoagulation	0.00	0.00	0.00	0.00	0.00	0.00	XXX	
0018T		C	Delivery of high power, focal magnetic pulses for direct stimulation to cortical neurons	0.00	0.00	0.00	0.00	0.00	0.00	XXX	

Code	M	S	Description	Work Value	Non-Fac PE	Fac PE	Mal-prac-tice	Non-Fac Total	Fac Total	Global	Gap
0019T		C	Extracorporeal shock wave therapy; involving musculoskeletal system	0.00	0.00	0.00	0.00	0.00	0.00	XXX	
0020T		C	Extracorporeal shock wave therapy; involving plantar fascia	0.00	0.00	0.00	0.00	0.00	0.00	XXX	
0021T		C	Insertion of transcervical or transvaginal fetal oximetry sensor	0.00	0.00	0.00	0.00	0.00	0.00	XXX	
0023T		C	Infectious agent drug susceptibility phenotype prediction using genotypic comparison to known genotypic/phenotypic database, HIV 1	0.00	0.00	0.00	0.00	0.00	0.00	XXX	
0024T		C	Non-surgical septal reduction therapy (eg, alcohol ablation), for hypertrophic obstructive cardiomyopathy; with coronary arteriograms, with or without temporary pacemaker	0.00	0.00	0.00	0.00	0.00	0.00	XXX	
0025T		C	Determination of corneal thickness (eg, pachymetry) with interpretation and report, bilateral	0.00	0.00	0.00	0.00	0.00	0.00	XXX	
0026T		C	Lipoprotein, direct measurement, intermediate density lipoproteins (IDL) (remnant lipoproteins)	0.00	0.00	0.00	0.00	0.00	0.00	XXX	

Category III

■ RVU not developed by HCFA. Gap-filled RVUs developed by Ingenix/CHEG.

Evaluation and Management

The Introduction provides complete descriptions for the status column (abbreviated as S). If a relative value is not available for a procedure, it is indicated with a "0.00" in the individual units column.

I. **Glossary:** Visits, examinations, consultations, and similar services listed in this section reflect wide variations required in time and skill. The following alphabetical listing of definitions is included to aid in the determination of the correct code for the service provided. Documentation for each aspect of the service performed should be included in the patient record to substantiate the level of service. Listed values for each code group apply only when these services are performed by, or under the supervision of, a physician.

Chief Complaint: A concise statement describing the symptom, problem, condition, diagnosis or other factor that is the reason for the encounter.

Classification of Service: Each code in this section is grouped into a category. The groupings are defined by place (e.g., office, hospital, nursing home, etc.) and type of service (e.g., consultation, preventive, etc.). Some of the codes are grouped into subcategories (e.g., new patient, established patient, initial, etc.). Each code in the group represents a different level of service defined by the clinical components of a patient encounter for E/M. See Levels of Service.

Components: Each level of service recognizes seven components. The components include history, physical examination, medical decision making, counseling, coordination of care, nature of presenting problem, and time. See Levels of Service, Key Components, History, Physical Examination, Medical Decision Making, Counseling, Problem, and Time.

Concurrent Care: The provision of similar services (e.g., hospital visits) to the same patient by more than one physician on the same day. The CPT book does not require any special reporting for concurrent care.

Consultation: There are three categories for consultation: outpatient, inpatient, and confirmatory. Any physician may use an appropriate consultation code on any patient for any problem including one which has been previously evaluated by the consulting physician provided the following criteria are met:

- The attending physician or appropriate source requests that the physician render advice or opinion regarding the evaluation and/or management of a specific problem
- The need for the consultation, the consultant's opinion, and any services ordered or performed must be well documented in the patient's record
- The information is communicated to the requesting physician or appropriate source

Counseling: A discussion with the patient and/or family concerning one or more of the following:

- Diagnostic results, impressions, and/or recommended diagnostic studies
- Prognosis
- Risks and benefits of management options
- Instructions for management and/or follow-up
- Importance of compliance with chosen management
- Risk factor reduction

- Patient and family education

See *"Key Components"* and *"Time"*

Established Patient: A patient who has received professional services from a physician or another physician in the same specialty within the same group within the last three years. In the instance a physician is covering for or on call for another physician, the patient is classified as an established patient if the other physician or a member of the providing physician specialty group has provided services for the patient within the last three years.

Family History: A review of medical events in the patient's family that includes significant information about:

- Health status or cause of death of parents, siblings, and children
- Specific diseases related to problems identified in "Chief Complaint," "History of the Present Illness," and/or "System Review"
- Diseases of family members which may be hereditary or place the patient at risk

History: This key component relates to the type of history obtained during a patient encounter. The four types of history are defined as follows:

- Problem focused: brief history of present illness or problem as related to the chief complaint.
- Expanded problem focused: brief history of present illness relating to chief complaint and pertinent system review.
- Detailed: extended history of present illness related to chief complaint, an extended system review, and pertinent past, family and/or social history.
- Comprehensive: extended history of present illness related to chief complaint, complete system review and complete past, family and social history.

History of Present Illness: A chronological description of the development of the patient's present illness from the first sign and/or symptom to the present. This includes a description of location, quality, severity, timing, context, modifying factors, associated signs, and symptoms significantly related to the presenting problem(s).

Key Components: Those components which are used primarily to determine the appropriate code level. These components are history, medical decision making, and physical examination. Time is not considered a key component unless counseling constitutes more than 50 percent of the face-to-face patient/physician encounter. *See also "History," "Medical Decision Making," "Physical Examination," "Time," "Counseling."*

Levels of Service: Each category and subcategory contains three to five levels of service indicated by code. The services include examinations, evaluations, treatments, conferences with or concerning patients, preventative pediatric and adult health supervision, and similar services. Each level of service recognizes seven clinical components. Three of these components are considered key components, including history, medical decision making, and physical examination. Each level of service may be used by all physicians.

Medical Decision Making: The complexity of establishing a diagnosis or selecting a management option. Medical decision making is divided into four categories. The level of medical decision making is determined using documentation in the patient record for three subcategories including: number of possible diagnoses and or the number of management options considered; the amount and/or complexity of medical records, diagnostic tests, and/or other information which must be obtained, reviewed, and analyzed; and the risk of significant complications, morbidity and/or mortality, as well as comorbidities, associated with the patient's presenting problem(s), the diagnostic procedure(s), and/or the possible management options. The following four classifications for level of medical decision making are used in determining the proper code:

- Straightforward: minimal number of possible diagnoses or management options, minimal or no amount and/or complexity of data to be reviewed, and minimal risk of complications and/or morbidity or mortality.
- Low Complexity: limited number of possible diagnoses or management options, limited amount and/or complexity of data to be reviewed, and low risk of complications and/or morbidity or mortality.
- Moderate Complexity: multiple number of possible diagnoses or management options, moderate amount and/or complexity of data to be reviewed, and moderate risk of complications and/or morbidity or mortality.

- High Complexity: extensive number of possible diagnoses or management options, extensive amount and/or complexity of data to be reviewed, and high risk of complications and/or morbidity or mortality.

Nature of Presenting Problem: A presenting problem is a disease, condition, illness, injury, symptom, sign, finding, complaint, or other reason for encounter, with or without a diagnosis being established at the time of the encounter. The E/M codes recognize five types of presenting problems that are defined as follows:

- Minimal: A problem that may not require the presence of the physician, but service is provided under the physician's supervision.
- Self-limited or minor: A problem that runs a definite and prescribed course, is transient in nature, and is not likely to permanently alter health status OR has a good prognosis with management/compliance.
- Low severity: A problem where the risk of morbidity without treatment is low; there is little to no risk of mortality without treatment; full recovery without functional impairment is expected.
- Moderate severity: A problem where the risk of morbidity without treatment is moderate; there is moderate risk of mortality without treatment; uncertain prognosis OR increased probability of prolonged functional impairment.
- High severity: A problem where the risk of morbidity without treatment is high to extreme; there is a moderate to high risk of mortality without treatment OR high probability of severe, prolonged functional impairment.

New Patient: A patient who has not received any professional services from a physician or another physician in the same specialty within the same group within the past three years. In the instance where a physician is on call for or covering for another physician, the patient is classified as a new patient if the other physician or a member of the providing physicians specialty group has not provided any professional service for the patient within three years. *See also "Established Patient."*

Past History: A review of the patient's past experiences with illnesses, injuries, and treatments that include significant information about:

- Prior major illnesses and injuries
- Prior operations
- Prior hospitalizations
- Current medications
- Allergies (e.g., drug, food)
- Age appropriate immunization status
- Age appropriate feeding/dietary status

Physical Examination: This key component relates to the type of physical examination performed during a patient encounter. The four defined types of physical examination are:

- Problem focused: an examination limited to the affected body area or organ system
- Expanded problem focused: an examination of the affected body area or organ system and other symptomatic or related organ systems
- Detailed: an extended examination of the affected body area(s) and other symptomatic or related organ system(s)
- Comprehensive: a complete single system specialty examination or a complete multi-system examination

Problem: Describes the nature of the problem presented as the reason for the encounter. The problem is considered to be a contributing factor and therefore is not used as a primary factor in determining level of service. The problem includes the same five categories as "Nature of Presenting Problem."

Review of Systems: An inventory of body systems obtained through a series of questions seeking to identify signs and/or symptoms which the patient may be experiencing or has experienced. For the purposes of these CPT definitions, the following elements of a system review have been identified:

- Constitutional symptoms (fever, weight loss, etc.)
- Eyes
- Ears, Nose, Mouth, Throat
- Cardiovascular
- Respiratory
- Gastrointestinal
- Genitourinary
- Musculoskeletal
- Integumentary (skin and/or breast)
- Neurological
- Psychiatric
- Endocrine
- Hematologic/Lymphatic
- Allergic/Immunologic

Social History: An age appropriate review of past and current activities that includes significant information about:

- Marital status and/or living arrangements
- Current employment
- Occupational history
- Use of drugs, alcohol, and tobacco
- Level of education
- Sexual history
- Other relevant social factors

Time: Time for an outpatient is considered to be face-to-face time spent with the patient and does not include time spent in such activities as record review or dictation. The time for an inpatient is considered to be the time spent "on the floor" and does include record review, dictation, and other services rendered while in the hospital unit of the patient. Times given are considered to be an average and should not be used to determine the length of time spent in the encounter. Time is considered to be a contributory factor and as such is not used to define the level of service unless 50 percent or more of the service performed is spent in counseling or coordinating care. In cases where 50 percent of the service is counseling or coordinating care, time is used as the primary component for defining the level of service. Careful documentation of time is essential in cases where time is the defining component.

II. **Unusual Procedural Services:** A service may necessitate skills and time of the physician over and above listed services and values. If substantiated "By Report" (BR), additional values may be warranted. Use modifier -22 to indicate these procedures.

III. **Unlisted Service or Procedure:** When a service or procedure provided is not adequately identified, use of the unlisted procedure code for the related anatomical area is appropriate. Most codes of this type have "9" for the last digit. Value should be substantiated "By Report" (BR). *See "By Report."*

IV. Prolonged Evaluation and Management Service: When a service provided is prolonged or otherwise greater than that usually required for the E/M service, use of Modifier -21 or prolonged service codes is appropriate. Medicare will only pay for face-to-face prolonged care. A report may be required.

V. Unrelated E/M Service by the Same Physician During a Post-operative Period: If a service which is not related to the original procedure and is performed during the follow-up period for that period may be billed at 100 percent of the listed value. Use modifier -24 to indicate this service is unrelated.

VI. Significant, Separately Identifiable E/M Service by the Same Physician on the Same Day of a Procedure or Other Service: When an E/M service is performed on the same day of a procedure, separate reporting of the E/M service may be allowed. The E/M service must be for a condition that required services above and beyond the normal pre- and postoperative care associated with the procedure. In this case, the E/M service may be billed separately at 100 percent of the listed value. Services of this nature must be substantiated by report. Use modifier -25 to indicate this type of service. Medicare will pay for this service if it is used in conjunction with a same date procedure with a 0- or 10-day global period.

VII. E/M Service Resulting in Initial Decision for Surgery: If an evaluation and management encounter results in the initial decision to perform surgery, modifier -57 may be attached to the E/M service code. At such time as the decision for surgery is made, meaning recommended to the patient and agreed to by the patient, the pre-operative time begins and other E/M services related to the procedure are included in the global value of the procedure. The modifier does not reduce or increase the value of the service and should be billed at 100 percent of the listed value. Medicare will pay for this modifier if the service is provided on the day of or the day before a 90-day global procedure.

VIII. By Report: Value of a procedure should be established for any "by report" circumstance by identifying a similar service and justifying value difference. When a report is indicated, the report should include the following:

A. Accurate procedure definition or description

B. Operative report

C. Justification for procedural variance, when appropriate

D. Similar procedure and value

E. Justification for value difference

IX. Reduced Services: Under some circumstances, the value for a procedure may be reduced. Use modifier -52 to identify reduced value services.

X. Multiple Modifiers: If circumstances require the use of more than one modifier with any one procedure code, modifier -99 should be added to the procedure code. Other modifiers are then attached to the procedure code and listed separately with appropriate values for each.

XI. Materials Supplied by Physician: CPT code 99070 or the specific HCPCS Level II code may be used to identify materials provided by the physician (e.g., dressings, casting supplies, drugs, etc.) over and above those usually indicated with the office visit. Medicare no longer provides separate payment for a sterile supply tray when the service is provided in the physician's office as reimbursement for this type of supply is now included in the value of the non-facility practice expense component.

XII. Global Values: This column indicates the number of days in the global period for which services directly related to the procedure are included. The majority of codes have a numerical designation (i.e., 0, 10, or 90).

A. MMM codes describe services furnished in uncomplicated maternity care. This includes antepartum, delivery and postpartum care. The usual global surgical concept does not apply.

B. XXX codes indicate that the global surgery concept does not apply.

C. YYY codes indicate that the global period is to be set by the local carrier.

D. ZZZ codes indicate that the code is an add-on service and therefore is treated in the global period of the other procedure billed in conjunction with a ZZZ code. Do not bill these codes with modifier -51. They should not be reduced.

Evaluation and Management Values

Code	M	S	Description	Work Value	Non-Fac PE	Fac PE	Mal-practice	Non-Fac Total	Fac Total	Global	Gap
99201		A	Office or other outpatient visit for the evaluation and management of a new patient, which requires these three key components: a problem focused history; a problem focused examination; and straightforward medical decision making. Counseling and/or coordination of care with other providers or agencies are provided consistent with the nature of the problem(s) and the patient's and/or family's needs. Usually, the presenting problems are self limited or minor. Physicians typically spend 10 minutes face-to-face with the patient and/or family.	0.45	0.47	0.16	0.02	0.94	0.63	XXX	
99202		A	Office or other outpatient visit for the evaluation and management of a new patient, which requires these three key components: an expanded problem focused history; an expanded problem focused examination; and straightforward medical decision making. Counseling and/or coordination of care with other providers or agencies are provided consistent with the nature of the problem(s) and the patient's and/or family's needs. Usually, the presenting problem(s) are of low to moderate severity. Physicians typically spend 20 minutes face-to-face with the patient and/or family.	0.88	0.77	0.33	0.05	1.70	1.26	XXX	
99203		A	Office or other outpatient visit for the evaluation and management of a new patient, which requires these three key components: a detailed history; a detailed examination; and medical decision making of low complexity. Counseling and/or coordination of care with other providers or agencies are provided consistent with the nature of the problem(s) and the patient's and/or family's needs. Usually, the presenting problem(s) are of moderate severity. Physicians typically spend 30 minutes face-to-face with the patient and/or family.	1.34	1.12	0.50	0.08	2.54	1.92	XXX	
99204		A	Office or other outpatient visit for the evaluation and management of a new patient, which requires these three key components: a comprehensive history; a comprehensive examination; and medical decision making of moderate complexity. Counseling and/or coordination of care with other providers or agencies are provided consistent with the nature of the problem(s) and the patient's and/or family's needs. Usually, the presenting problem(s) are of moderate to high severity. Physicians typically spend 45 minutes face-to-face with the patient and/or family.	2.00	1.51	0.74	0.10	3.61	2.84	XXX	

E/M

■ RVU not developed by CMS. Gap-filled RVUs developed by Ingenix/CHEG.

Code	M	S	Description	Work Value	Non-Fac PE	Fac PE	Mal-practice	Non-Fac Total	Fac Total	Global	Gap
99205		A	Office or other outpatient visit for the evaluation and management of a new patient, which requires these three key components: a comprehensive history; a comprehensive examination; and medical decision making of high complexity. Counseling and/or coordination of care with other providers or agencies are provided consistent with the nature of the problem(s) and the patient's and/or family's needs. Usually, the presenting problem(s) are of moderate to high severity. Physicians typically spend 60 minutes face-to-face with the patient and/or family.	2.67	1.80	0.98	0.12	4.59	3.77	XXX	
99211		A	Office or other outpatient visit for the evaluation and management of an established patient, that may not require the presence of a physician. Usually, the presenting problem(s) are minimal. Typically, 5 minutes are spent performing or supervising these services.	0.17	0.38	0.06	0.01	0.56	0.24	XXX	
99212		A	Office or other outpatient visit for the evaluation and management of an established patient, which requires at least two of these three key components: a problem focused history; a problem focused examination; straightforward medical decision making. Counseling and/or coordination of care with other providers or agencies are provided consistent with the nature of the problem(s) and the patient's and/or family's needs. Usually, the presenting problem(s) are self limited or minor. Physicians typically spend 10 minutes face-to-face with the patient and/or family.	0.45	0.53	0.17	0.02	1.00	0.64	XXX	
99213		A	Office or other outpatient visit for the evaluation and management of an established patient, which requires at least two of these three key components: an expanded problem focused history; an expanded problem focused examination; medical decision making of low complexity. Counseling and coordination of care with other providers or agencies are provided consistent with the nature of the problem(s) and the patient's and/or family's needs. Usually, the presenting problem(s) are of low to moderate severity. Physicians typically spend 15 minutes face-to-face with the patient and/or family.	0.67	0.69	0.24	0.03	1.39	0.94	XXX	

E/M

■ RVU not developed by CMS. Gap-filled RVUs developed by Ingenix/CHEG.

Code	M	S	Description	Work Value	Non-Fac PE	Fac PE	Mal-practice	Non-Fac Total	Fac Total	Global	Gap
99214		A	Office or other outpatient visit for the evaluation and management of an established patient, which requires at least two of these three key components: a detailed history; a detailed examination; medical decision making of moderate complexity. Counseling and/or coordination of care with other providers or agencies are provided consistent with the nature of the problem(s) and the patient's and/or family's needs. Usually, the presenting problem(s) are of moderate to high severity. Physicians typically spend 25 minutes face-to-face with the patient and/or family.	1.10	1.04	0.41	0.04	2.18	1.55	XXX	
99215		A	Office or other outpatient visit for the evaluation and management of an established patient, which requires at least two of these three key components: a comprehensive history; a comprehensive examination; medical decision making of high complexity. Counseling and/or coordination of care with other providers or agencies are provided consistent with the nature of the problem(s) and the patient's and/or family's needs. Usually, the presenting problem(s) are of moderate to high severity. Physicians typically spend 40 minutes face-to-face with the patient and/or family.	1.77	1.36	0.66	0.07	3.20	2.50	XXX	
99217		A	Observation care discharge day management (This code is to be utilized by the physician to report all services provided to a patient on discharge from "observation status" if the discharge is on other than the initial date of "observation status." To report services to a patient designated as "observation status" or "inpatient status" and discharged on the same date, use the codes for Observation or Inpatient Care Services [including Admission and Discharge Services, 99234-99236 as appropriate.])	1.28	0.45	0.45	0.05	1.78	1.78	XXX	
99218		A	Initial observation care, per day, for the evaluation and management of a patient which requires these three key components: a detailed or comprehensive history; a detailed or comprehensive examination; and medical decision making that is straightforward or of low complexity. Counseling and/or coordination of care with other providers or agencies are provided consistent with the nature of the problem(s) and the patient's and/or family's needs. Usually, the problem(s) requiring admission to observation status are of low severity.	1.28	0.45	0.45	0.05	1.78	1.78	XXX	

E/M

■ RVU not developed by CMS. Gap-filled RVUs developed by Ingenix/CHEG.

Code	M	S	Description	Work Value	Non-Fac PE	Fac PE	Mal-prac-tice	Non-Fac Total	Fac Total	Global	Gap
99219		A	Initial observation care, per day, for the evaluation and management of a patient, which requires these three key components: a comprehensive history; a comprehensive examination; and medical decision making of moderate complexity. Counseling and/or coordination of care with other providers or agencies are provided consistent with the nature of the problem(s) and the patient's and/or family's needs. Usually, the problem(s) requiring admission to observation status are of moderate severity.	2.14	0.75	0.75	0.08	2.97	2.97	XXX	
99220		A	Initial observation care, per day, for the evaluation and management of a patient, which requires these three key components: a comprehensive history; a comprehensive examination; and medical decision making of high complexity. Counseling and/or coordination of care with other providers or agencies are provided consistent with the nature of the problem(s) and the patient's and/or family's needs. Usually, the problem(s) requiring admission to observation status are of high severity.	2.99	1.06	1.06	0.11	4.16	4.16	XXX	
99221		A	Initial hospital care, per day, for the evaluation and management of a patient which requires these three key components: a detailed or comprehensive history; a detailed or comprehensive examination; and medical decision making that is straightforward or of low complexity. Counseling and/or coordination of care with other providers or agencies are provided consistent with the nature of the problem(s) and the patient's and/or family's needs. Usually, the problem(s) requiring admission are of low severity. Physicians typically spend 30 minutes at the bedside and on the patient's hospital floor or unit.	1.28	0.47	0.47	0.05	1.80	1.80	XXX	
99222		A	Initial hospital care, per day, for the evaluation and management of a patient, which requires these three key components: a comprehensive history; a comprehensive examination; and medical decision making of moderate complexity. Counseling and/or coordination of care with other providers or agencies are provided consistent with the nature of the problem(s) and the patient's and/or family's needs. Usually, the problem(s) requiring admission are of moderate severity. Physicians typically spend 50 minutes at the bedside and on the patient's hospital floor or unit.	2.14	0.77	0.77	0.08	2.99	2.99	XXX	

E/M

■ RVU not developed by CMS. Gap-filled RVUs developed by Ingenix/CHEG.

Code	M	S	Description	Work Value	Non-Fac PE	Fac PE	Mal-practice	Non-Fac Total	Fac Total	Global	Gap
99223		A	Initial hospital care, per day, for the evaluation and management of a patient, which requires these three key components: a comprehensive history; a comprehensive examination; and medical decision making of high complexity. Counseling and/or coordination of care with other providers or agencies are provided consistent with the nature of the problem(s) and the patient's and/or family's needs. Usually, the problem(s) requiring admission are of high severity. Physicians typically spend 70 minutes at the bedside and on the patient's hospital floor or unit.	2.99	1.08	1.08	0.10	4.17	4.17	XXX	
99231		A	Subsequent hospital care, per day, for the evaluation and management of a patient, which requires at least two of these three key components: a problem focused interval history; a problem focused examination; medical decision making that is straightforward or of low complexity. Counseling and/or coordination of care with other providers or agencies are provided consistent with the nature of the problem(s) and the patient's and/or family's needs. Usually, the patient is stable, recovering or improving. Physicians typically spend 15 minutes at the bedside and on the patient's hospital floor or unit.	0.64	0.24	0.24	0.02	0.90	0.90	XXX	
99232		A	Subsequent hospital care, per day, for the evaluation and management of a patient, which requires at least two of these three key components: an expanded problem focused interval history; an expanded problem focused examination; medical decision making of moderate complexity. Counseling and/or coordination of care with other providers or agencies are provided consistent with the nature of the problem(s) and the patient's and/or family's needs. Usually, the patient is responding inadequately to therapy or has developed a minor complication. Physicians typically spend 25 minutes at the bedside and on the patient's hospital floor or unit.	1.06	0.39	0.39	0.03	1.48	1.48	XXX	
99233		A	Subsequent hospital care, per day, for the evaluation and management of a patient, which requires at least two of these three key components: a detailed interval history; a detailed examination; medical decision making of high complexity. Counseling and/or coordination of care with other providers or agencies are provided consistent with the nature of the problem(s) and the patient's and/or family's needs. Usually, the patient is unstable or has developed a significant complication or a significant new problem. Physicians typically spend 35 minutes at the bedside and on the patient's hospital floor or unit.	1.51	0.55	0.55	0.05	2.11	2.11	XXX	

E/M

■ RVU not developed by CMS. Gap-filled RVUs developed by Ingenix/CHEG.

Code	M	S	Description	Work Value	Non-Fac PE	Fac PE	Mal-practice	Non-Fac Total	Fac Total	Global	Gap
99234		A	Observation or inpatient hospital care, for the evaluation and management of a patient including admission and discharge on the same date which requires these three key components: a detailed or comprehensive history; a detailed or comprehensive examination; and medical decision making that is straightforward or of low complexity. Counseling and/or coordination of care with other providers or agencies are provided consistent with the nature of the problem(s) and the patient's and/or family's needs. Usually the presenting problem(s) requiring admission are of low severity.	2.56	0.93	0.93	0.11	3.60	3.60	XXX	
99235		A	Observation or inpatient hospital care, for the evaluation and management of a patient including admission and discharge on the same date which requires these three key components: a comprehensive history; a comprehensive examination; and medical decision making of moderate complexity. Counseling and/or coordination of care with other providers or agencies are provided consistent with the nature of the problem(s) and the patient's and/or family's needs. Usually the presenting problem(s) requiring admission are of moderate severity.	3.42	1.21	1.21	0.13	4.76	4.76	XXX	
99236		A	Observation or inpatient hospital care, for the evaluation and management of a patient including admission and discharge on the same date which requires these three key components: a comprehensive history; a comprehensive examination; and medical decision making of high complexity. Counseling and/or coordination of care with other providers or agencies are provided consistent with the nature of the problem(s) and the patient's and/or family's needs. Usually the presenting problem(s) requiring admission are of high severity.	4.27	1.49	1.49	0.17	5.93	5.93	XXX	
99238		A	Hospital discharge day management; 30 minutes or less	1.28	0.51	0.51	0.04	1.83	1.83	XXX	
99239		A	more than 30 minutes	1.75	0.71	0.71	0.05	2.51	2.51	XXX	
99241		A	Office consultation for a new or established patient, which requires these three key components: a problem focused history; a problem focused examination; and straightforward medical decision making. Counseling and/or coordination of care with other providers or agencies are provided consistent with the nature of the problem(s) and the patient's and/or family's needs. Usually, the presenting problem(s) are self limited or minor. Physicians typically spend 15 minutes face-to-face with the patient and/or family.	0.64	0.62	0.24	0.04	1.30	0.92	XXX	

■ RVU not developed by CMS. Gap-filled RVUs developed by Ingenix/CHEG.

Code	M	S	Description	Work Value	Non-Fac PE	Fac PE	Mal-practice	Non-Fac Total	Fac Total	Global	Gap
99242		A	Office consultation for a new or established patient, which requires these three key components: an expanded problem focused history; an expanded problem focused examination; and straightforward medical decision making. Counseling and/or coordination of care with other providers or agencies are provided consistent with the nature of the problem(s) and the patient's and/or family's needs. Usually, the presenting problem(s) are of low severity. Physicians typically spend 30 minutes face-to-face with the patient and/or family.	1.29	1.03	0.50	0.09	2.41	1.88	XXX	
99243		A	Office consultation for a new or established patient, which requires these three key components: a detailed history; a detailed examination; and medical decision making of low complexity. Counseling and/or coordination of care with other providers or agencies are provided consistent with the nature of the problem(s) and the patient's and/or family's needs. Usually, the presenting problem(s) are of moderate severity. Physicians typically spend 40 minutes face-to-face with the patient and/or family.	1.72	1.38	0.67	0.10	3.20	2.49	XXX	
99244		A	Office consultation for a new or established patient, which requires these three key components: a comprehensive history; a comprehensive examination; and medical decision making of moderate complexity. Counseling and/or coordination of care with other providers or agencies are provided consistent with the nature of the problem(s) and the patient's and/or family's needs. Usually, the presenting problem(s) are of moderate to high severity. Physicians typically spend 60 minutes face-to-face with the patient and/or family.	2.58	1.83	0.98	0.13	4.54	3.69	XXX	
99245		A	Office consultation for a new or established patient, which requires these three key components: a comprehensive history; a comprehensive examination; and medical decision making of high complexity. Counseling and/or coordination of care with other providers or agencies are provided consistent with the nature of the problem(s) and the patient's and/or family's needs. Usually, the presenting problem(s) are of moderate to high severity. Physicians typically spend 80 minutes face-to-face with the patient and/or family.	3.43	2.29	1.30	0.16	5.88	4.89	XXX	

■ RVU not developed by CMS. Gap-filled RVUs developed by Ingenix/CHEG.

Code	M	S	Description	Work Value	Non-Fac PE	Fac PE	Mal-practice	Non-Fac Total	Fac Total	Global	Gap
99251		A	Initial inpatient consultation for a new or established patient, which requires these three key components: a problem focused history; a problem focused examination; and straightforward medical decision making. Counseling and/or coordination of care with other providers or agencies are provided consistent with the nature of the problem(s) and the patient's and/or family's needs. Usually, the presenting problem(s) are self limited or minor. Physicians typically spend 20 minutes at the bedside and on the patient's hospital floor or unit.	0.66	0.26	0.26	0.04	0.96	0.96	XXX	
99252		A	Initial inpatient consultation for a new or established patient, which requires these three key components: an expanded problem focused history; an expanded problem focused examination; and straightforward medical decision making. Counseling and/or coordination of care with other providers or agencies are provided consistent with the nature of the problem(s) and the patient's and/or family's needs. Usually, the presenting problem(s) are of low severity. Physicians typically spend 40 minutes at the bedside and on the patient's hospital floor or unit.	1.32	0.53	0.53	0.08	1.93	1.93	XXX	
99253		A	Initial inpatient consultation for a new or established patient, which requires these three key components: a detailed history; a detailed examination; and medical decision making of low complexity. Counseling and/or coordination of care with other providers or agencies are provided consistent with the nature of the problem(s) and the patient's and/or family's needs. Usually, the presenting problem(s) are of moderate severity. Physicians typically spend 55 minutes at the bedside and on the patient's hospital floor or unit.	1.82	0.72	0.72	0.09	2.63	2.63	XXX	
99254		A	Initial inpatient consultation for a new or established patient, which requires three key components: a comprehensive history; a comprehensive examination; and medical decision making of moderate complexity. Counseling and/or coordination of care with other providers or agencies are provided consistent with the nature of the problem(s) and the patient's and/or family's needs. Usually, the presenting problem(s) are of moderate to high severity. Physicians typically spend 80 minutes at the bedside and on the patient's hospital floor or unit.	2.64	1.03	1.03	0.11	3.78	3.78	XXX	

■ RVU not developed by CMS. Gap-filled RVUs developed by Ingenix/CHEG.

Code	M	S	Description	Work Value	Non-Fac PE	Fac PE	Mal-practice	Non-Fac Total	Fac Total	Global	Gap
99255		A	Initial inpatient consultation for a new or established patient, which requires these three key components: a comprehensive history; a comprehensive examination; and medical decision making of high complexity. Counseling and/or coordination of care with other providers or agencies are provided consistent with the nature of the problem(s) and the patient's and/or family's needs. Usually, the presenting problem(s) are of moderate to high severity. Physicians typically spend 110 minutes at the bedside and on the patient's hospital floor or unit.	3.65	1.41	1.41	0.15	5.21	5.21	XXX	
99261		A	Follow-up inpatient consultation for an established patient, which requires at least two of these three key components: a problem focused interval history; a problem focused examination; medical decision making that is straightforward or of low complexity. Counseling and/or coordination of care with other providers or agencies are provided consistent with nature of the problem(s) and the patient's and/or family's needs. Usually, the patient is stable, recovering or improving. Physicians typically spend 10 minutes at the bedside and on the patient's hospital floor or unit.	0.42	0.16	0.16	0.02	0.60	0.60	XXX	
99262		A	Follow-up inpatient consultation for an established patient which requires at least two of these three key components: an expanded problem focused interval history; an expanded problem focused examination; medical decision making of moderate complexity. Counseling and/or coordination of care with other providers or agencies are provided consistent with the nature of the problem(s) and the patient's and/or family's needs. Usually, the patient is responding inadequately to therapy or has developed a minor complication. Physicians typically spend 20 minutes at the bedside and on the patient's hospital floor or unit.	0.85	0.32	0.32	0.03	1.20	1.20	XXX	
99263		A	Follow-up inpatient consultation for an established patient which requires at least two of these three key components: a detailed interval history; a detailed examination; medical decision making of high complexity. Counseling and/or coordination of care with other providers or agencies are provided consistent with the nature of the problem(s) and the patient's and/or family's needs. Usually, the patient is unstable or has developed a significant complication or a significant new problem. Physicians typically spend 30 minutes at the bedside and on the patient's hospital floor or unit.	1.27	0.48	0.48	0.04	1.79	1.79	XXX	

■ RVU not developed by CMS. Gap-filled RVUs developed by Ingenix/CHEG.

Code	M	S	Description	Work Value	Non-Fac PE	Fac PE	Mal-practice	Non-Fac Total	Fac Total	Global	Gap
99271		A	Confirmatory consultation for a new or established patient, which requires these three key components: a problem focused history; a problem focused examination; and straightforward medical decision making. Counseling and/or coordination of care with other providers or agencies are provided consistent with the nature of the problem(s) and the patient's and/or family's needs. Usually, the presenting problem(s) are self limited or minor.	0.45	0.67	0.17	0.03	1.15	0.65	XXX	
99272		A	Confirmatory consultation for a new or established patient, which requires these three key components: an expanded problem focused history; an expanded problem focused examination; and straightforward medical decision making. Counseling and/or coordination of care with other providers or agencies are provided consistent with the nature of the problem(s) and the patient's and/or family's needs. Usually, the presenting problem(s) are of low severity.	0.84	0.89	0.32	0.06	1.79	1.22	XXX	
99273		A	Confirmatory consultation for a new or established patient, which requires these three key components: a detailed history; a detailed examination; and medical decision making of low complexity. Counseling and/or coordination of care with other providers or agencies are provided consistent with the nature of the problem(s) and the patient's and/or family's needs. Usually, the presenting problem(s) are of moderate severity.	1.19	1.13	0.47	0.07	2.39	1.73	XXX	
99274		A	Confirmatory consultation for a new or established patient, which requires these three key components: a comprehensive history; a comprehensive examination; and medical decision making of moderate complexity. Counseling and/or coordination of care with other providers or agencies are provided consistent with the nature of the problem(s) and the patient's and/or family's needs. Usually, the presenting problem(s) are of moderate to high severity.	1.73	1.41	0.68	0.09	3.23	2.50	XXX	
99275		A	Confirmatory consultation for a new or established patient, which requires these three key components: a comprehensive history; a comprehensive examination; and medical decision making of high complexity. Counseling and/or coordination of care with other providers or agencies are provided consistent with the nature of the problem(s) and the patient's and/or family's needs. Usually, the presenting problem(s) are of moderate to high severity.	2.31	1.68	0.88	0.10	4.09	3.29	XXX	

■ RVU not developed by CMS. Gap-filled RVUs developed by Ingenix/CHEG.

Code	M	S	Description	Work Value	Non-Fac PE	Fac PE	Mal-practice	Non-Fac Total	Fac Total	Global	Gap
99281		A	Emergency department visit for the evaluation and management of a patient, which requires these three key components: a problem focused history; a problem focused examination; and straightforward medical decision making. Counseling and/or coordination of care with other providers or agencies are provided consistent with the nature of the problem(s) and the patient's and/or family's needs. Usually, the presenting problem(s) are self limited or minor.	0.33	0.09	0.09	0.02	0.44	0.44	XXX	
99282		A	Emergency department visit for the evaluation and management of a patient, which requires these three key components: an expanded problem focused history; an expanded problem focused examination; and medical decision making of low complexity. Counseling and/or coordination of care with other providers or agencies are provided consistent with the nature of the problem(s) and the patient's and/or family's needs. Usually, the presenting problem(s) are of low to moderate severity.	0.55	0.15	0.15	0.03	0.73	0.73	XXX	
99283		A	Emergency department visit for the evaluation and management of a patient, which requires these three key components: an expanded problem focused history; an expanded problem focused examination; and medical decision making of moderate complexity. Counseling and/or coordination of care with other providers or agencies are provided consistent with the nature of the problem(s) and the patient's and/or family's needs. Usually, the presenting problem(s) are of moderate severity.	1.24	0.32	0.32	0.08	1.64	1.64	XXX	
99284		A	Emergency department visit for the evaluation and management of a patient, which requires these three key components: a detailed history; a detailed examination; and medical decision making of moderate complexity. Counseling and/or coordination of care with other providers or agencies are provided consistent with the nature of the problem(s) and the patient's and/or family's needs. Usually, the presenting problem(s) are of high severity, and require urgent evaluation by the physician but do not pose an immediate significant threat to life or physiologic function.	1.95	0.49	0.49	0.12	2.56	2.56	XXX	

■ RVU not developed by CMS. Gap-filled RVUs developed by Ingenix/CHEG.

Code	M	S	Description	Work Value	Non-Fac PE	Fac PE	Mal-practice	Non-Fac Total	Fac Total	Global	Gap
99285		A	Emergency department visit for the evaluation and management of a patient, which requires these three key components within the constraints imposed by the urgency of the patient's clinical condition and/or mental status: a comprehensive history; a comprehensive examination; and medical decision making of high complexity. Counseling and/or coordination of care with other providers or agencies are provided consistent with the nature of the problem(s) and the patient's and/or family's needs. Usually, the presenting problem(s) are of high severity and pose an immediate significant threat to life or physiologic function.	3.06	0.75	0.75	0.19	4.00	4.00	XXX	
99288		B	Physician direction of emergency medical systems (EMS) emergency care, advanced life support	0.00	0.00	0.00	0.00	0.00	0.00	XXX	
99289		I	Physician constant attention of the critically ill or injured patient during an interfacility transport; first 30-74 minutes	0.00	0.00	0.00	0.00	0.00	0.00	XXX	
99290		I	each additional 30 minutes (List separately in addition to code for primary service)	0.00	0.00	0.00	0.00	0.00	0.00	ZZZ	
99291		A	Critical care, evaluation and management of the critically ill or critically injured patient; first 30-74 minutes	4.00	1.63	1.34	0.14	5.77	5.48	XXX	
99292		A	each additional 30 minutes (List separately in addition to code for primary service)	2.00	0.92	0.66	0.07	2.99	2.73	ZZZ	
99295		A	Initial neonatal intensive care, per day, for the evaluation and management of a critically ill neonate or infant This code is reserved for the date of admission for neonates who are critically ill. Critically ill neonates require cardiac and/or respiratory support (including ventilator or nasal CPAP when indicated), continuous or frequent vital sign monitoring, laboratory and blood gas interpretations, follow-up physician reevaluations, and constant observation by the health care team under direct physician supervision. Immediate preoperative evaluation and stabilization of neonates with life threatening surgical or cardiac conditions are included under this code.	16.00	4.53	4.53	0.70	21.23	21.23	XXX	

■ RVU not developed by CMS. Gap-filled RVUs developed by Ingenix/CHEG.

Code	M	S	Description	Work Value	Non-Fac PE	Fac PE	Mal-practice	Non-Fac Total	Fac Total	Global	Gap
99296		A	Subsequent neonatal intensive care, per day, for the evaluation and management of a critically ill and unstable neonate or infant A critically ill and unstable neonate will require cardiac and/or respiratory support (including ventilator or nasal CPAP when indicated), continuous or frequent vital sign monitoring, laboratory and blood gas interpretations, follow-up physician re-evaluations throughout a 24-hour period, and constant observation by the health care team under direct physician supervision. In addition, most will require frequent ventilator changes, intravenous fluid alterations, and/or early initiation of parenteral nutrition. Neonates in the immediate post-operative period or those who become critically ill and unstable during the hospital stay will commonly qualify for this level of care. This code encompasses intensive care provided on dates subsequent to the admission date.	8.00	2.58	2.58	0.23	10.81	10.81	XXX	
99297		A	Subsequent neonatal intensive care, per day, for the evaluation and management of a critically ill though stable neonate or infant Critically ill though stable neonates require cardiac and/or respiratory support (including ventilator and nasal CPAP when indicated), continuous or frequent vital sign monitoring, laboratory and blood gas interpretations, follow-up physician re-evaluations throughout a 24 hour period, and constant observation by the health care team under direct physician supervision. Neonates at this level of care would be expected to require less frequent changes in respiratory, cardiovascular and fluid and electrolyte therapy as those included under code 99296. This code encompasses intensive care provided on dates subsequent to the admission date.	4.00	1.32	1.32	0.12	5.44	5.44	XXX	
99298		A	Subsequent neonatal intensive care, per day, for the evaluation and management of the recovering very low birth weight infant (less than 1500 grams) Very low birth weight neonates who are no longer critically ill continue to require intensive cardiac and respiratory monitoring, continuous and/or frequent vital sign monitoring, heat maintenance, enteral and/or parenteral nutritional adjustments, laboratory and oxygen monitoring and constant observation by the health care team under direct physician supervision. Neonates of this level of care would be expected to require infrequent changes in respiratory, cardiovascular and/or fluid and electrolyte therapy as those induced under 99296 or 99297. This code encompasses intensive care provided on days subsequent to the admission date.	2.75	0.97	0.97	0.10	3.82	3.82	XXX	

E/M

■ RVU not developed by CMS. Gap-filled RVUs developed by Ingenix/CHEG.

Code	M	S	Description	Work Value	Non-Fac PE	Fac PE	Mal-practice	Non-Fac Total	Fac Total	Global	Gap
99301		A	Evaluation and management of a new or established patient involving an annual nursing facility assessment which requires these three key components: a detailed interval history; a comprehensive examination; and medical decision making that is straightforward or of low complexity. Counseling and/or coordination of care with other providers or agencies are provided consistent with the nature of the problem(s) and the patient's and/or family's needs. Usually, the patient is stable, recovering or improving. The review and affirmation of the medical plan of care is required. Physicians typically spend 30 minutes at the bedside and on the patient's facility floor or unit.	1.20	0.70	0.42	0.04	1.94	1.66	XXX	
99302		A	Evaluation and management of a new or established patient involving a nursing facility assessment which requires these three key components: a detailed interval history; a comprehensive examination; and medical decision making of moderate to high complexity. Counseling and/or coordination of care with other providers or agencies are provided consistent with the nature of the problem(s) and the patient's and/or family's needs. Usually, the patient has developed a significant complication or a significant new problem and has had a major permanent change in status. The creation of a new medical plan of care is required. Physicians typically spend 40 minutes at the bedside and on the patient's facility floor or unit.	1.61	0.98	0.57	0.05	2.64	2.23	XXX	
99303		A	Evaluation and management of a new or established patient involving a nursing facility assessment at the time of initial admission or readmission to the facility, which requires these three key components: a comprehensive history; a comprehensive examination; and medical decision making of moderate to high complexity. Counseling and/or coordination of care with other providers or agencies are provided consistent with the nature of the problem(s) and the patient's and/or family's needs. The creation of a medical plan of care is required. Physicians typically spend 50 minutes at the bedside and on the patient's facility floor or unit.	2.01	1.21	0.70	0.06	3.28	2.77	XXX	

■ RVU not developed by CMS. Gap-filled RVUs developed by Ingenix/CHEG.

Code	M	S	Description	Work Value	Non-Fac PE	Fac PE	Mal-prac-tice	Non-Fac Total	Fac Total	Global	Gap
99311		A	Subsequent nursing facility care, per day, for the evaluation and management of a new or established patient, which requires at least two of these three key components: a problem focused interval history; a problem focused examination; medical decision making that is straightforward or of low complexity. Counseling and/or coordination of care with other providers or agencies are provided consistent with the nature of the problem(s) and the patient's and/or family's needs. Usually, the patient is stable, recovering or improving. Physicians typically spend 15 minutes at the bedside and on the patient's facility floor or unit.	0.60	0.49	0.21	0.02	1.11	0.83	XXX	
99312		A	Subsequent nursing facility care, per day, for the evaluation and management of a new or established patient, which requires at least two of these three key components: an expanded problem focused interval history; an expanded problem focused examination; medical decision making of moderate complexity. Counseling and/or coordination of care with other providers or agencies are provided consistent with the nature of the problem(s) and the patient's and/or family's needs. Usually, the patient is responding inadequately to therapy or has developed a minor complication. Physicians typically spend 25 minutes at the bedside and on the patient's facility floor or unit.	1.00	0.68	0.35	0.03	1.71	1.38	XXX	
99313		A	Subsequent nursing facility care, per day, for the evaluation and management of a new or established patient, which requires at least two of these three key components: a detailed interval history; a detailed examination; medical decision making of moderate to high complexity. Counseling and/or coordination of care with other providers or agencies are provided consistent with the nature of the problem(s) and the patient's and/or family's needs. Usually, the patient has developed a significant complication or a significant new problem. Physicians typically spend 35 minutes at the bedside and on the patient's facility floor or unit.	1.42	0.87	0.50	0.04	2.33	1.96	XXX	
99315		A	Nursing facility discharge day management; 30 minutes or less	1.13	0.74	0.40	0.04	1.91	1.57	XXX	
99316		A	more than 30 minutes	1.50	0.95	0.53	0.05	2.50	2.08	XXX	

E/M

■ RVU not developed by CMS. Gap-filled RVUs developed by Ingenix/CHEG.

Code	M	S	Description	Work Value	Non-Fac PE	Fac PE	Mal-practice	Non-Fac Total	Fac Total	Global	Gap
99321		A	Domiciliary or rest home visit for the evaluation and management of a new patient which requires these three key components: a problem focused history; a problem focused examination; and medical decision making that is straightforward or of low complexity. Counseling and/or coordination of care with other providers or agencies are provided consistent with the nature of the problem(s) and the patient's and/or family's needs. Usually, the presenting problem(s) are of low severity.	0.71	0.49	0.49	0.02	1.22	1.22	XXX	
99322		A	Domiciliary or rest home visit for the evaluation and management of a new patient, which requires these three key components: an expanded problem focused history; an expanded problem focused examination; and medical decision making of moderate complexity. Counseling and/or coordination of care with other providers or agencies are provided consistent with the nature of the problem(s) and the patient's and/or family's needs. Usually, the presenting problem(s) are of moderate severity.	1.01	0.70	0.70	0.03	1.74	1.74	XXX	
99323		A	Domiciliary or rest home visit for the evaluation and management of a new patient, which requires these three key components: a detailed history; a detailed examination; and medical decision making of high complexity. Counseling and/or coordination of care with other providers or agencies are provided consistent with the nature of the problem(s) and the patient's and/or family's needs. Usually, the presenting problem(s) are of high complexity.	1.28	0.93	0.93	0.04	2.25	2.25	XXX	
99331		A	Domiciliary or rest home visit for the evaluation and management of an established patient, which requires at least two of these three key components: a problem focused interval history; a problem focused examination; medical decision making that is straightforward or of low complexity. Counseling and/or coordination of care with other providers or agencies are provided consistent with the nature of the problem(s) and the patient's and/or family's needs. Usually, the patient is stable, recovering or improving.	0.60	0.47	0.47	0.02	1.09	1.09	XXX	

■ RVU not developed by CMS. Gap-filled RVUs developed by Ingenix/CHEG.

Code	M	S	Description	Work Value	Non-Fac PE	Fac PE	Mal-practice	Non-Fac Total	Fac Total	Global	Gap
99332		A	Domiciliary or rest home visit for the evaluation and management of an established patient, which requires at least two of these three key components: an expanded problem focused interval history; an expanded problem focused examination; medical decision making of moderate complexity. Counseling and/or coordination of care with other providers or agencies are provided consistent with the nature of the problem(s) and the patient's and/or family's needs. Usually, the patient is responding inadequately to therapy or has developed a minor complication.	0.80	0.59	0.59	0.03	1.42	1.42	XXX	
99333		A	Domiciliary or rest home visit for the evaluation and management of an established patient, which requires at least two of these three key components: a detailed interval history; a detailed examination; medical decision making of high complexity. Counseling and/or coordination of care with other providers or agencies are provided consistent with the nature of the problem(s) and the patient's and/or family's needs. Usually, the patient is unstable or has developed a significant complication or a significant new problem.	1.00	0.73	0.73	0.03	1.76	1.76	XXX	
99341		A	Home visit for the evaluation and management of a new patient, which requires these three key components: a problem focused history; a problem focused examination; and straightforward medical decision making. Counseling and/or coordination of care with other providers or agencies are provided consistent with the nature of the problem(s) and the patient's and/or family's needs. Usually, the presenting problem(s) are of low severity. Physicians typically spend 20 minutes face-to-face with the patient and/or family.	1.01	0.56	0.56	0.05	1.62	1.62	XXX	
99342		A	Home visit for the evaluation and management of a new patient, which requires these three key components: an expanded problem focused history; an expanded problem focused examination; and medical decision making of low complexity. Counseling and/or coordination of care with other providers or agencies are provided consistent with the nature of the problem(s) and the patient's and/or family's needs. Usually, the presenting problem(s) are of moderate severity. Physicians typically spend 30 minutes face-to-face with the patient and/or family.	1.52	0.87	0.87	0.05	2.44	2.44	XXX	

■ RVU not developed by CMS. Gap-filled RVUs developed by Ingenix/CHEG.

Code	M	S	Description	Work Value	Non-Fac PE	Fac PE	Mal-prac-tice	Non-Fac Total	Fac Total	Global	Gap
99343		A	Home visit for the evaluation and management of a new patient, which requires these three key components: a detailed history; a detailed examination; and medical decision making of moderate complexity. Counseling and/or coordination of care with other providers or agencies are provided consistent with the nature of the problem(s) and the patient's and/or family's needs. Usually, the presenting problem(s) are of moderate to high severity. Physicians typically spend 45 minutes face-to-face with the patient and/or family.	2.27	1.29	1.29	0.07	3.63	3.63	XXX	
99344		A	Home visit for the evaluation and management of a new patient, which requires these three key components: a comprehensive history; a comprehensive examination; and medical decision making of moderate complexity. Counseling and/or coordination of care with other providers or agencies are provided consistent with the nature of the problem(s) and the patient's and/or family's needs. Usually, the presenting problem(s) are of high severity. Physicians typically spend 60 minutes face-to-face with the patient and/or family.	3.03	1.57	1.57	0.10	4.70	4.70	XXX	
99345		A	Home visit for the evaluation and management of a new patient, which requires these three key components: a comprehensive history; a comprehensive examination; and medical decision making of high complexity. Counseling and/or coordination of care with other providers or agencies are provided consistent with the nature of the problem(s) and the patient's and/or family's needs. Usually, the patient is unstable or has developed a significant new problem requiring immediate physician attention. Physicians typically spend 75 minutes face-to-face with the patient and/or family.	3.79	1.86	1.86	0.12	5.77	5.77	XXX	
99347		A	Home visit for the evaluation and management of an established patient, which requires at least two of these three key components: a problem focused interval history; a problem focused examination; straightforward medical decision making. Counseling and/or coordination of care with other providers or agencies are provided consistent with the nature of the problem(s) and the patient's and/or family's needs. Usually, the presenting problem(s) are self-limited or minor. Physicians typically spend 15 minutes face-to-face with the patient and/or family.	0.76	0.49	0.49	0.03	1.28	1.28	XXX	

■ RVU not developed by CMS. Gap-filled RVUs developed by Ingenix/CHEG.

Code	M	S	Description	Work Value	Non-Fac PE	Fac PE	Mal-practice	Non-Fac Total	Fac Total	Global	Gap
99348		A	Home visit for the evaluation and management of an established patient, which requires at least two of these three components: an expanded problem focused interval history; an expanded problem focused examination; medical decision making of low complexity. Counseling and/or coordination of care with other providers or agencies are provided consistent with the nature of the problem(s) and the patient's and/or family's needs. Usually, the presenting problem(s) are of low to moderate severity. Physicians typically spend 25 minutes face-to-face with the patient and/or family.	1.26	0.74	0.74	0.04	2.04	2.04	XXX	
99349		A	Home visit for the evaluation and management of an established patient, which requires at least two of these three key components: a detailed interval history; a detailed examination; medical decision making of moderate complexity. Counseling and/or coordination of care with other providers or agencies are provided consistent with the nature of the problem(s) and the patient's and/or family's needs. Usually, the presenting problem(s) are moderate to high severity. Physicians typically spend 40 minutes face-to-face with the patient and/or family.	2.02	1.08	1.08	0.06	3.16	3.16	XXX	
99350		A	Home visit for the evaluation and management of an established patient, which requires at least two of these three key components: a comprehensive interval history; a comprehensive examination; medical decision making of moderate to high complexity. Counseling and/or coordination of care with other providers or agencies are provided consistent with the nature of the problem(s) and the patient's and/or family's needs. Usually, the presenting problem(s) are of moderate to high severity. The patient may be unstable or may have developed a significant new problem requiring immediate physician attention. Physicians typically spend 60 minutes face-to-face with the patient and/or family.	3.03	1.47	1.47	0.10	4.60	4.60	XXX	
99354		A	Prolonged physician service in the office or other outpatient setting requiring direct (face-to-face) patient contact beyond the usual service (eg, prolonged care and treatment of an acute asthmatic patient in an outpatient setting); first hour (List separately in addition to code for office or other outpatient Evaluation and Management service)	1.77	1.46	0.66	0.06	3.29	2.49	ZZZ	
99355		A	each additional 30 minutes (List separately in addition to code for prolonged physician service)	1.77	1.24	0.65	0.06	3.07	2.48	ZZZ	

■ RVU not developed by CMS. Gap-filled RVUs developed by Ingenix/CHEG.

Code	M	S	Description	Work Value	Non-Fac PE	Fac PE	Mal-practice	Non-Fac Total	Fac Total	Global	Gap
99356		A	Prolonged physician service in the inpatient setting, requiring direct (face-to-face) patient contact beyond the usual service (eg, maternal fetal monitoring for high risk delivery or other physiological monitoring, prolonged care of an acutely ill inpatient); first hour (List separately in addition to code for inpatient Evaluation and Management service)	1.71	0.61	0.61	0.06	2.38	2.38	ZZZ	
99357		A	each additional 30 minutes (List separately in addition to code for prolonged physician service)	1.71	0.63	0.63	0.06	2.40	2.40	ZZZ	
99358		B	Prolonged evaluation and management service before and/or after direct (face-to-face) patient care (eg, review of extensive records and tests, communication with other professionals and/or the patient/family); first hour (List separately in addition to code(s) for other physician service(s) and/or inpatient or outpatient Evaluation and Management service)	2.66	1.50	1.50	0.10	4.26	4.26	ZZZ	■
99359		B	each additional 30 minutes (List separately in addition to code for prolonged physician service)	1.33	0.75	0.75	0.05	2.13	2.13	ZZZ	■
99360		X	Physician standby service, requiring prolonged physician attendance, each 30 minutes (eg, operative standby, standby for frozen section, for cesarean/high risk delivery, for monitoring EEG)	1.82	1.02	1.02	0.07	2.91	2.91	XXX	■
99361		B	Medical conference by a physician with interdisciplinary team of health professionals or representatives of community agencies to coordinate activities of patient care (patient not present); approximately 30 minutes	1.52	0.86	0.86	0.06	2.44	2.44	XXX	■
99362		B	approximately 60 minutes	2.66	1.50	1.50	0.10	4.26	4.26	XXX	■
99371		B	Telephone call by a physician to patient or for consultation or medical management or for coordinating medical management with other health care professionals (eg, nurses, therapists, social workers, nutritionists, physicians, pharmacists); simple or brief (eg, to report on tests and/or laboratory results, to clarify or alter previous instructions, to integrate new information from other health professionals into the medical treatment plan, or to adjust therapy)	0.24	0.14	0.14	0.01	0.39	0.39	XXX	■
99372		B	intermediate (eg, to provide advice to an established patient on a new problem, to initiate therapy that can be handled by telephone, to discuss test results in detail, to coordinate medical management of a new problem in an established patient, to discuss and evaluate new information and details, or to initiate new plan of care)	0.61	0.34	0.34	0.02	0.97	0.97	XXX	■

■ RVU not developed by CMS. Gap-filled RVUs developed by Ingenix/CHEG.

E/M

Code	M	S	Description	Work Value	Non-Fac PE	Fac PE	Mal-practice	Non-Fac Total	Fac Total	Global	Gap
99373		B	complex or lengthy (eg, lengthy counseling session with anxious or distraught patient, detailed or prolonged discussion with family members regarding seriously ill patient, lengthy communication necessary to coordinate complex services of several different health professionals working on different aspects of the total patient care plan)	1.21	0.68	0.68	0.05	1.94	1.94	XXX	■
99374		B	Physician supervision of a patient under care of home health agency (patient not present) in home, domiciliary or equivalent environment (eg, Alzheimer's facility) requiring complex and multidisciplinary care modalities involving regular physician development and/or revision of care plans, review of subsequent reports of patient status, review of related laboratory and other studies, communication (including telephone calls) for purposes of assessment or care decisions with health care professional(s), family member(s), surrogate decision maker(s) (eg, legal guardian) and/or key caregiver(s) involved in patient's care, integration of new information into the medical treatment plan and/or adjustment of medical therapy, within a calendar month; 15-29 minutes	1.10	1.47	0.44	0.04	2.61	1.58	XXX	
99375		G	Physician supervision of a patient under care of home health agency (patient not present) in home, domiciliary or equivalent environment (eg, Alzheimer's facility) requiring complex and multidisciplinary care modalities involving regular physician development and/or revision of care plans, review of subsequent reports of patient status, review of related laboratory and other studies, communication (including telephone calls) for purposes of assessment or care decisions with health care professional(s), family member(s), surrogate decision maker(s) (eg, legal guardian) and/or key caregiver(s) involved in patient's care, integration of new information into the medical treatment plan and/or adjustment of medical therapy, within a calendar month; 30 minutes or more **Note:** This code was omitted from the November 1, 2001, *Federal Register*. The values published here are from the August 2, 2001, *Federal Register/Proposed Rules*.	1.73	1.68	1.68	0.06	3.47	3.47	XXX	

E/M

■ RVU not developed by CMS. Gap-filled RVUs developed by Ingenix/CHEG.

Code	M	S	Description	Work Value	Non-Fac PE	Fac PE	Mal-practice	Non-Fac Total	Fac Total	Global	Gap
99377		B	Physician supervision of a hospice patient (patient not present) requiring complex and multidisciplinary care modalities involving regular physician development and/or revision of care plans, review of subsequent reports of patient status, review of related laboratory and other studies, communication (including telephone calls) for purposes of assessment or care decisions with health care professional(s), family member(s), surrogate decision maker(s) (eg, legal guardian) and/or key caregiver(s) involved in patient's care, integration of new information into the medical treatment plan and/or adjustment of medical therapy, within a calendar month; 15-29 minutes	1.10	1.47	0.44	0.04	2.61	1.58	XXX	
99378		G	Physician supervision of a hospice patient (patient not present) requiring complex and multidisciplinary care modalities involving regular physician development and/or revision of care plans, review of subsequent reports of patient status, review of related laboratory and other studies, communication (including telephone calls) for purposes of assessment or care decisions with health care professional(s), family member(s), surrogate decision maker(s) (eg, legal guardian) and/or key caregiver(s) involved in patient's care, integration of new information into the medical treatment plan and/or adjustment of medical therapy, within a calendar month; 30 minutes or more **Note:** This code was omitted from the November 1, 2001, *Federal Register*. The values published here are from the August 2, 2001, *Federal Register/Proposed Rules*.	1.73	1.68	1.68	0.06	3.47	3.47	XXX	
99379		B	Physician supervision of a nursing facility patient (patient not present) requiring complex and multidisciplinary care modalities involving regular physician development and/or revision of care plans, review of subsequent reports of patient status, review of related laboratory and other studies, communication (including telephone calls) for purposes of assessment or care decisions with health care professional(s), family member(s), surrogate decision maker(s) (eg, legal guardian) and/or key caregiver(s) involved in patient's care, integration of new information into the medical treatment plan and/or adjustment of medical therapy, within a calendar month; 15-29 minutes	1.10	1.47	0.44	0.03	2.60	1.57	XXX	
99380		B	30 minutes or more	1.73	1.72	0.69	0.05	3.50	2.47	XXX	

■ RVU not developed by CMS. Gap-filled RVUs developed by Ingenix/CHEG.

E/M

Code	M	S	Description	Work Value	Non-Fac PE	Fac PE	Mal-practice	Non-Fac Total	Fac Total	Global	Gap
99381		N	Initial comprehensive preventive medicine evaluation and management of an individual including an age and gender appropriate history, examination, counseling/anticipatory guidance/risk factor reduction interventions, and the ordering of appropriate immunization(s), laboratory/diagnostic procedures, new patient; infant (age under 1 year)	1.19	1.50	0.48	0.04	2.73	1.71	XXX	
99382		N	early childhood (age 1 through 4 years)	1.36	1.54	0.54	0.04	2.94	1.94	XXX	
99383		N	late childhood (age 5 through 11 years)	1.36	1.48	0.54	0.04	2.88	1.94	XXX	
99384		N	adolescent (age 12 through 17 years)	1.53	1.55	0.61	0.05	3.13	2.19	XXX	
99385		N	18-39 years	1.53	1.55	0.61	0.05	3.13	2.19	XXX	
99386		N	40-64 years	1.88	1.74	0.75	0.06	3.68	2.69	XXX	
99387		N	65 years and over	2.06	1.87	0.82	0.06	3.99	2.94	XXX	
99391		N	Periodic comprehensive preventive medicine reevaluation and management of an individual including an age and gender appropriate history, examination, counseling/anticipatory guidance/risk factor reduction interventions, and the ordering of appropriate immunization(s), laboratory/diagnostic procedures, established patient; infant (age under 1 year)	1.02	1.02	0.41	0.03	2.07	1.46	XXX	
99392		N	early childhood (age 1 through 4 years)	1.19	1.09	0.48	0.04	2.32	1.71	XXX	
99393		N	late childhood (age 5 through 11 years)	1.19	1.06	0.48	0.04	2.29	1.71	XXX	
99394		N	adolescent (age 12 through 17 years)	1.36	1.15	0.54	0.04	2.55	1.94	XXX	
99395		N	18-39 years	1.36	1.18	0.54	0.04	2.58	1.94	XXX	
99396		N	40-64 years	1.53	1.27	0.61	0.05	2.85	2.19	XXX	
99397		N	65 years and over	1.71	1.37	0.68	0.05	3.13	2.44	XXX	
99401		N	Preventive medicine counseling and/or risk factor reduction intervention(s) provided to an individual (separate procedure); approximately 15 minutes	0.48	0.62	0.19	0.01	1.11	0.68	XXX	
99402		N	approximately 30 minutes	0.98	0.86	0.39	0.02	1.86	1.39	XXX	
99403		N	approximately 45 minutes	1.46	1.10	0.58	0.03	2.59	2.07	XXX	
99404		N	approximately 60 minutes	1.95	1.35	0.78	0.04	3.34	2.77	XXX	
99411		N	Preventive medicine counseling and/or risk factor reduction intervention(s) provided to individuals in a group setting (separate procedure); approximately 30 minutes	0.15	0.18	0.06	0.01	0.34	0.22	XXX	
99412		N	approximately 60 minutes	0.25	0.24	0.10	0.01	0.5	0.36	XXX	

■ RVU not developed by CMS. Gap-filled RVUs developed by Ingenix/CHEG.

E/M

Code	M	S	Description	Work Value	Non-Fac PE	Fac PE	Mal-practice	Non-Fac Total	Fac Total	Global	Gap
99420		N	Administration and interpretation of health risk assessment instrument (eg, health hazard appraisal)	0.00	0.00	0.00	0.00	0.00	0.00	XXX	
99429		N	Unlisted preventive medicine service	0.00	0.00	0.00	0.00	0.00	0.00	XXX	
99431		A	History and examination of the normal newborn infant, initiation of diagnostic and treatment programs and preparation of hospital records. (This code should also be used for birthing room deliveries.)	1.17	0.39	0.39	0.04	1.60	1.60	XXX	
99432		A	Normal newborn care in other than hospital or birthing room setting, including physical examination of baby and conference(s) with parent(s)	1.26	1.12	0.50	0.06	2.44	1.82	XXX	
99433		A	Subsequent hospital care, for the evaluation and management of a normal newborn, per day	0.62	0.21	0.21	0.02	0.85	0.85	XXX	
99435		A	History and examination of the normal newborn infant, including the preparation of medical records (this code should only be used for newborns assessed and discharged from the hospital or birthing room on the same date)	1.50	0.54	0.54	0.05	2.09	2.09	XXX	
99436		A	Attendance at delivery (when requested by delivering physician) and initial stabilization of newborn	1.50	0.50	0.50	0.05	2.05	2.05	XXX	
99440		A	Newborn resuscitation: provision of positive pressure ventilation and/or chest compressions in the presence of acute inadequate ventilation and/or cardiac output	2.93	1.17	1.17	0.11	4.21	4.21	XXX	
99450		N	Basic life and/or disability examination that includes: measurement of height, weight and blood pressure; completion of a medical history following a life insurance pro forma; collection of blood sample and/or urinalysis complying with "chain of custody" protocols; and completion of necessary documentation/ certificates.	0.00	0.00	0.00	0.00	0.00	0.00	XXX	
99455		R	Work related or medical disability examination by the treating physician that includes: •completion of a medical history commensurate with the patient's condition; •performance of an examination commensurate with the patient's condition; •formulation of a diagnosis, assessment of capabilities and stability, and calculation of impairment; •development of future medical treatment plan; and •completion of necessary documentation/ certificates and report.	0.00	0.00	0.00	0.00	0.00	0.00	XXX	

E/M

■ RVU not developed by CMS. Gap-filled RVUs developed by Ingenix/CHEG.

Code	M	S	Description	Work Value	Non-Fac PE	Fac PE	Mal-practice	Non-Fac Total	Fac Total	Global	Gap
99456		R	Work related or medical disability examination by other than the treating physician that includes: •completion of a medical history commensurate with the patient's condition; •performance of an examination commensurate with the patient's condition; •formulation of a diagnosis, assessment of capabilities and stability, and calculation of impairment; •development of future medical treatment plan; and •completion of necessary documentation/ certificates and report.	0.00	0.00	0.00	0.00	0.00	0.00	XXX	
99499		C	Unlisted evaluation and management service	0.00	0.00	0.00	0.00	0.00	0.00	XXX	

E/M

■ RVU not developed by CMS. Gap-filled RVUs developed by Ingenix/CHEG.

HCPCS

Introduction

The Introduction provides a complete description for the status column (abbreviated as S). If a relative value is not available for a HCPCS code, it is indicated with a "0.00" in the individual units column.

General: Since HCPCS Level I codes (CPT) do not contain all the codes needed to report medical services and supplies, CMS (formerly HCFA) developed HCPCS Level II codes. Level II codes begin with a single letter (A through V, though not all the letters are used) followed by four numeric digits. They are grouped by the type of service or supply they represent and are updated annually by CMS. Check an official 2002 HCPCS Level II publication for the groupings as well as additional reporting guidelines related to the use of these codes.

HCPCS Level II codes are required for reporting most medical services and supplies provided to Medicare patients. Because of the greater specificity they provide, an increasing number of private insurance carriers also require the use of these codes.

Modifiers identify circumstances that alter or enhance the description of the service or supply. HCPCS Level II national modifiers differ from Level I (CPT), and are more specific and limited in their application. Only three modifiers are used in the Ingenix *RBRVS* but reporting of these services may require the use of additional modifiers so check an official 2002 HCPCS Level II publication for a complete list. The three modifiers included here are:

- **NU** New Equipment
- **RR** Rental Equipment
- **UE** Used Durable Medical Equipment (DME)

Valuation of HCPCS Level II Codes: HCPCS Level II codes are not valued in the Medicare Physician Fee Schedule nor does the *Federal Register* designate any relative values for these codes. Wherever possible, Ingenix has valued these codes using the same methodology that is detailed in the introduction of this book. However, in some cases, other methodology may be used to value these codes. This methodology may include information based on average wholesale price (AWP), the Clinical Laboratory Fee Schedule, the Durable Medical Equipment, Prosthetics, Orthotics and Supplies (DMEPOS) Fee Schedule or other relative value systems. Every effort has been made to value these codes consistently with other values in this book. However, please be aware that obtaining appropriate values for these codes may require additional analysis, and/or the application of a different conversion factor or several different conversion factors for the different types of services and supplies covered by HCPCS Level II codes in order for the values to approximate those that are customary in your area.

The J-codes, which are the codes developed for reporting drugs and biologicals, present unique problems for several reasons:

1. AWP is the primary method used to develop values for drugs and biologicals. However, there are multiple sources for AWP and these different sources sometimes provide different AWPs. Therefore, expect some variance when comparing these prices to your AWP source(s).

2. There is not always a one-to-one cross between the NDC codes for which AWP is provided and the J-codes. When there is not a one-to-one cross, the closest match or an average is used, depending on what the analyst believes will provide the most reliable data.

3. Drugs and biologicals are not always dispensed by the manufacturer in the same quantities described in the J-codes. For example, the J-code may specify a dosage amount as 10 mcg, but the AWP may provide the price based on a dosage amount of 1 ml. The value in the Ingenix *RBRVS* will be translated to match the J-code dosage description.

4. Values are dose specific and J-code descriptions are for specific dosages. This may require the reporting of multiple units when higher dosages than those specified in the J-code are required.

5. Prices for drugs and biologicals are not fixed. Therefore, prices may vary throughout the year or from location to location. Generally, physicians and facilities using larger quantities of these drugs and biologicals can negotiate lower prices (i.e., a volume discount) than those using smaller quantities. The conversion factor may need to be adjusted to reflect these variances.

HCPCS Values

Code	M	S	Description	Work Value	Non-Fac PE	Fac PE	Mal-practice	Non-Fac Total	Fac Total	Global	Gap
A0021		I	Ambulance service, outside state per mile, transport (Medicaid only)	0.00	0.18	0.18	0.00	0.18	0.18	XXX	■
A0080		I	Nonemergency transportation: per mile — volunteer, with no vested or personal interest	0.00	0.00	0.00	0.00	0.00	0.00	XXX	
A0090		I	Nonemergency transportation: per mile — volunteer, interested individual, neighbor	0.00	0.00	0.00	0.00	0.00	0.00	XXX	
A0100		I	Nonemergency transportation: taxi — intracity	0.00	0.00	0.00	0.00	0.00	0.00	XXX	
A0110		I	Nonemergency transportation and bus, intra- or interstate carrier	0.00	0.00	0.00	0.00	0.00	0.00	XXX	
A0120		I	Nonemergency transportation mini-bus, mountain area transports, other non-profit transportation systems	0.00	0.00	0.00	0.00	0.00	0.00	XXX	
A0130		I	Nonemergency transportation: wheelchair van	0.00	0.00	0.00	0.00	0.00	0.00	XXX	
A0140		I	Nonemergency transportation and air travel (private or commercial), intra- or interstate	0.00	0.00	0.00	0.00	0.00	0.00	XXX	
A0160		I	Nonemergency transportation: per mile — caseworker or social worker	0.00	0.01	0.01	0.00	0.01	0.01	XXX	■
A0170		I	Nonemergency transportation: ancillary: parking fees, tolls, other	0.00	0.00	0.00	0.00	0.00	0.00	XXX	
A0180		I	Nonemergency transportation: ancillary: lodging — recipient	0.00	0.00	0.00	0.00	0.00	0.00	XXX	
A0190		I	Nonemergency transportation: ancillary: meals — recipient	0.00	0.00	0.00	0.00	0.00	0.00	XXX	
A0200		I	Nonemergency transportation: ancillary: lodging — escort	0.00	0.00	0.00	0.00	0.00	0.00	XXX	
A0210		I	Nonemergency transportation: ancillary: meals — escort	0.00	0.00	0.00	0.00	0.00	0.00	XXX	
A0225			Ambulance service, neonatal transport, base rate, emergency transport, one way	0.00	5.96	5.96	0.00	5.96	5.96	XXX	■
A0380		X	BLS mileage (per mile)	0.00	0.15	0.15	0.00	0.15	0.15	XXX	■
A0382		X	BLS routine disposable supplies	0.00	0.15	0.15	0.00	0.15	0.15	XXX	■

■ RVU not developed by CMS. Gap-filled RVUs developed by CHEG.

Code	M	S	Description	Work Value	Non-Fac PE	Fac PE	Mal-practice	Non-Fac Total	Fac Total	Global	Gap
A0384		X	BLS specialized service disposable supplies; defibrillation (used by ALS ambulances and BLS ambulances in jurisdictions where defibrillation is permitted in BLS ambulances)	0.00	0.75	0.75	0.00	0.75	0.75	XXX	■
A0390		X	ALS mileage (per mile)	0.00	0.15	0.15	0.00	0.15	0.15	XXX	■
A0392		X	ALS specialized service disposable supplies; defibrillation (to be used only in jurisdictions where defibrillation cannot be performed by BLS ambulances)	0.00	0.75	0.75	0.00	0.75	0.75	XXX	■
A0394		X	ALS specialized service disposable supplies; IV drug therapy	0.00	0.36	0.36	0.00	0.36	0.36	XXX	■
A0396		X	ALS specialized service disposable supplies; esophageal intubation	0.00	0.60	0.60	0.00	0.60	0.60	XXX	■
A0398		X	ALS routine disposable supplies	0.00	0.15	0.15	0.00	0.15	0.15	XXX	■
A0420		X	Ambulance waiting time (ALS or BLS), one-half (1/2) hour increments	0.00	0.00	0.00	0.00	0.00	0.00	XXX	
A0422		X	Ambulance (ALS or BLS) oxygen and oxygen supplies, life sustaining situation	0.00	0.55	0.55	0.00	0.55	0.55	XXX	■
A0424		X	Extra ambulance attendant, ALS or BLS (requires medical review)	0.00	0.00	0.00	0.00	0.00	0.00	XXX	
A0425		X	Ground mileage, per statute mile	0.00	0.15	0.15	0.00	0.15	0.15	XXX	■
A0426		X	Ambulance service, advanced life support, non-emergency transport, level 1 (ALS 1)	0.00	4.52	4.52	0.00	4.52	4.52	XXX	■
A0427		X	Ambulance service, advanced life support, emergency transport, level 1 (ALS 1-emergency)	0.00	4.75	4.75	0.00	4.75	4.75	XXX	■
A0428		X	Ambulance service, basic life support, non-emergency transport (BLS)	0.00	3.98	3.98	0.00	3.98	3.98	XXX	■
A0429		X	Ambulance service, basic life support, emergency transport (BLS-emergency)	0.00	4.13	4.13	0.00	4.13	4.13	XXX	■
A0430		X	Ambulance service, conventional air services, transport, one way (fixed wing)	0.00	0.00	0.00	0.00	0.00	0.00	XXX	
A0431		X	Ambulance service, conventional air services, transport, one way (rotary wing)	0.00	0.00	0.00	0.00	0.00	0.00	XXX	
A0432		X	Paramedic intercept (PI), rural area, transport furnished by a volunteer ambulance company which is prohibited by state law from billing third party payers	0.00	0.00	0.00	0.00	0.00	0.00	XXX	
A0433		X	Advanced life support, level 2 (ALS 2)	0.00	0.00	0.00	0.00	0.00	0.00	XXX	
A0434		X	Specialty care transport (SCT)	0.00	0.00	0.00	0.00	0.00	0.00	XXX	
A0435		X	Fixed wing air mileage, per statute mile	0.00	0.00	0.00	0.00	0.00	0.00	XXX	
A0436		X	Rotary wing air mileage, per statute mile	0.00	0.00	0.00	0.00	0.00	0.00	XXX	

■ RVU not developed by CMS. Gap-filled RVUs developed by CHEG.

Code	M	S	Description	Work Value	Non-Fac PE	Fac PE	Mal-practice	Non-Fac Total	Fac Total	Global	Gap
A0888		N	Non-covered ambulance mileage, per mile (e.g., for miles traveled beyond closest appropriate facility)	0.00	0.00	0.00	0.00	0.00	0.00	XXX	
A0999		X	Unlisted ambulance service	0.00	0.00	0.00	0.00	0.00	0.00	XXX	
A4206		I	Syringe with needle, sterile 1 cc, each	0.00	0.01	0.01	0.00	0.01	0.01	XXX	■
A4207		I	Syringe with needle, sterile 2 cc, each	0.00	0.00	0.00	0.00	0.00	0.00	XXX	
A4208		I	Syringe with needle, sterile 3 cc, each	0.00	0.01	0.01	0.00	0.01	0.01	XXX	■
A4209		I	Syringe with needle, sterile 5 cc or greater, each	0.00	0.01	0.01	0.00	0.01	0.01	XXX	■
A4210		N	Needle-free injection device, each	0.00	31.03	31.03	0.00	31.03	31.03	XXX	■
A4211		P	Supplies for self-administered injections	0.00	0.00	0.00	0.00	0.00	0.00	XXX	
A4212		P	Non coring needle or stylet with or without catheter	0.00	0.30	0.30	0.00	0.30	0.30	XXX	■
A4213		I	Syringe, sterile, 20 cc or greater, each	0.00	0.03	0.03	0.00	0.03	0.03	XXX	■
A4214		P	Sterile saline or water, 30 cc vial	0.00	0.07	0.07	0.00	0.07	0.07	XXX	■
A4215		I	Needles only, sterile, any size, each	0.00	0.00	0.00	0.00	0.00	0.00	XXX	
A4220		P	Refill kit for implantable infusion pump	0.00	0.00	0.00	0.00	0.00	0.00	XXX	
A4221		X	Supplies for maintenance of drug infusion catheter, per week (list drug separately)	0.00	0.00	0.00	0.00	0.00	0.00	XXX	
A4222		X	Supplies for external drug infusion pump, per cassette or bag (list drug separately)	0.00	0.00	0.00	0.00	0.00	0.00	XXX	
A4230		X	Infusion set for external insulin pump, nonneedle cannula type	0.00	0.00	0.00	0.00	0.00	0.00	XXX	
A4231		X	Infusion set for external insulin pump, needle type	0.00	0.00	0.00	0.00	0.00	0.00	XXX	
A4232		X	Syringe with needle for external insulin pump, sterile, 3cc	0.00	0.00	0.00	0.00	0.00	0.00	XXX	
A4244		I	Alcohol or peroxide, per pint	0.00	0.03	0.03	0.00	0.03	0.03	XXX	■
A4245		I	Alcohol wipes, per box	0.00	0.10	0.10	0.00	0.10	0.10	XXX	■
A4246		I	Betadine or pHisoHex solution, per pint	0.00	0.11	0.11	0.00	0.11	0.11	XXX	■
A4247		I	Betadine or iodine swabs/wipes, per box	0.00	0.17	0.17	0.00	0.17	0.17	XXX	■
A4250		N	Urine test or reagent strips or tablets (100 tablets or strips)	0.00	0.63	0.63	0.00	0.63	0.63	XXX	■
A4253		P	Blood glucose test or reagent strips for home blood glucose monitor, per 50 strips	0.00	1.07	1.07	0.00	1.07	1.07	XXX	■
A4254		X	Replacement battery, any type, for use with medically necessary home blood glucose monitor owned by patient, each	0.00	0.20	0.20	0.00	0.20	0.20	XXX	■

■ RVU not developed by CMS. Gap-filled RVUs developed by CHEG.

Code	M	S	Description	Work Value	Non-Fac PE	Fac PE	Mal-practice	Non-Fac Total	Fac Total	Global	Gap
A4255		X	Platforms for home blood glucose monitor, 50 per box	0.00	0.06	0.06	0.00	0.06	0.06	XXX	■
A4256		P	Normal, low, and high calibrator solution/chips	0.00	0.34	0.34	0.00	0.34	0.34	XXX	■
A4257		X	Replacement lens shield cartridge for use with laser skin piercing device, each	0.00	0.00	0.00	0.00	0.00	0.00	XXX	
A4258		P	Spring-powered device for lancet, each	0.00	0.57	0.57	0.00	0.57	0.57	XXX	■
A4259		P	Lancets, per box of 100	0.00	0.24	0.24	0.00	0.24	0.24	XXX	■
A4260		N	Levonorgestrel (contraceptive) implants system, including implants and supplies	0.00	13.32	13.32	0.00	13.32	13.32	XXX	■
A4261		N	Cervical cap for contraceptive use	0.00	0.00	0.00	0.00	0.00	0.00	XXX	
A4262		B	Temporary, absorbable lacrimal duct implant, each	0.00	0.02	0.02	0.00	0.02	0.02	XXX	■
A4263		I	Permanent, long-term, nondissolvable lacrimal duct implant, each	0.00	1.44	1.44	0.00	1.44	1.44	XXX	■
A4265		P	Paraffin, per pound	0.00	0.08	0.08	0.00	0.08	0.08	XXX	■
A4270		B	Disposable endoscope sheath, each	0.00	0.00	0.00	0.00	0.00	0.00	XXX	
A4280		X	Adhesive skin support attachment for use with external breast prosthesis, each	0.00	0.18	0.18	0.00	0.18	0.18	XXX	■
A4290		X	Sacral nerve stimulation test lead, each	0.00	0.00	0.00	0.00	0.00	0.00	XXX	
A4300		B	Implantable access catheter, (e.g., venous, arterial, epidural subarachnoid, or peritoneal, etc.) external access	0.00	0.00	0.00	0.00	0.00	0.00	XXX	
A4301		P	Implantable access total system; catheter, port/reservoir (e.g., venous, arterial, epidural, or subarachnoid, etc.) percutaneous access	0.00	0.00	0.00	0.00	0.00	0.00	XXX	
A4305		P	Disposable drug delivery system, flow rate of 50 ml or greater per hour	0.00	0.47	0.47	0.00	0.47	0.47	XXX	■
A4306		P	Disposable drug delivery system, flow rate of 5 ml or less per hour	0.00	0.65	0.65	0.00	0.65	0.65	XXX	■
A4310		P	Insertion tray without drainage bag and without catheter (accessories only)	0.00	0.15	0.15	0.00	0.15	0.15	XXX	■
A4311		P	Insertion tray without drainage bag with indwelling catheter, Foley type, two-way latex with coating (Teflon, silicone, silicone elastomer or hydrophilic, etc.)	0.00	0.49	0.49	0.00	0.49	0.49	XXX	■
A4312		P	Insertion tray without drainage bag with indwelling catheter, Foley type, two-way, all silicone	0.00	0.60	0.60	0.00	0.60	0.60	XXX	■
A4313		P	Insertion tray without drainage bag with indwelling catheter, Foley type, three-way, for continuous irrigation	0.00	0.78	0.78	0.00	0.78	0.78	XXX	■

■ RVU not developed by CMS. Gap-filled RVUs developed by CHEG.

Code	M	S	Description	Work Value	Non-Fac PE	Fac PE	Mal-practice	Non-Fac Total	Fac Total	Global	Gap
A4314		P	Insertion tray with drainage bag with indwelling catheter, Foley type, two-way latex with coating (Teflon, silicone, silicone elastomer or hydrophilic, etc.)	0.00	0.52	0.52	0.00	0.52	0.52	XXX	■
A4315		P	Insertion tray with drainage bag with indwelling catheter, Foley type, two-way, all silicone	0.00	0.68	0.68	0.00	0.68	0.68	XXX	■
A4316		P	Insertion tray with drainage bag with indwelling catheter, Foley type, three-way, for continuous irrigation	0.00	0.95	0.95	0.00	0.95	0.95	XXX	■
A4319		X	Sterile water irrigation solution, 1000 ml	0.00	0.33	0.33	0.00	0.33	0.33	XXX	■
A4320		P	Irrigation tray with bulb or piston syringe, any purpose	0.00	0.11	0.11	0.00	0.11	0.11	XXX	■
A4321		X	Therapeutic agent for urinary catheter irrigation	0.00	0.00	0.00	0.00	0.00	0.00	XXX	
A4322		P	Irrigation syringe, bulb or piston, each	0.00	0.05	0.05	0.00	0.05	0.05	XXX	■
A4323		P	Sterile saline irrigation solution, 1000 ml	0.00	0.29	0.29	0.00	0.29	0.29	XXX	■
A4324		X	Male external catheter, with adhesive coating, each	0.00	0.06	0.06	0.00	0.06	0.06	XXX	■
A4325		X	Male external catheter, with adhesive strip, each	0.00	0.03	0.03	0.00	0.03	0.03	XXX	■
A4326		P	Male external catheter specialty type (e.g., inflatable, faceplate, etc.) each	0.00	0.00	0.00	0.00	0.00	0.00	XXX	
A4327		P	Female external urinary collection device; metal cup, each	0.00	0.00	0.00	0.00	0.00	0.00	XXX	
A4328		P	Female external urinary collection device; pouch, each	0.00	0.33	0.33	0.00	0.33	0.33	XXX	■
A4330		P	Perianal fecal collection pouch with adhesive, each	0.00	0.22	0.22	0.00	0.22	0.22	XXX	■
A4331		X	Extension drainage tubing, any type, any length, with connector/adaptor, for use with urinary leg bag or urostomy pouch, each	0.00	0.11	0.11	0.00	0.11	0.11	XXX	■
A4332		X	Lubricant, individual sterile packet, for insertion of urinary catheter, each	0.00	0.00	0.00	0.00	0.00	0.00	XXX	
A4333		X	Urinary catheter anchoring device, adhesive skin attachment, each	0.00	0.07	0.07	0.00	0.07	0.07	XXX	■
A4334		X	Urinary catheter anchoring device, leg strap, each	0.00	0.11	0.11	0.00	0.11	0.11	XXX	■
A4335		P	Incontinence supply; miscellaneous	0.00	0.00	0.00	0.00	0.00	0.00	XXX	
A4338		P	Indwelling catheter; Foley type, two-way latex with coating (Teflon, silicone, silicone elastomer, or hydrophilic, etc.), each	0.00	0.21	0.21	0.00	0.21	0.21	XXX	■

■ RVU not developed by CMS. Gap-filled RVUs developed by CHEG.

Code	M	S	Description	Work Value	Non-Fac PE	Fac PE	Mal-practice	Non-Fac Total	Fac Total	Global	Gap
A4340		P	Indwelling catheter; specialty type, (e.g., coudé, mushroom, wing, etc.), each	0.00	0.41	0.41	0.00	0.41	0.41	XXX	■
A4344		P	Indwelling catheter, Foley type, two-way, all silicone, each	0.00	0.36	0.36	0.00	0.36	0.36	XXX	■
A4346		P	Indwelling catheter; Foley type, three-way for continuous irrigation, each	0.00	0.62	0.62	0.00	0.62	0.62	XXX	■
A4347		P	Male external catheter with or without adhesive, with or without anti-reflux device; per dozen	0.00	0.47	0.47	0.00	0.47	0.47	XXX	■
A4348		X	Male external catheter with integral collection compartment, extended wear, each (e.g., 2 per month)	0.00	0.00	0.00	0.00	0.00	0.00	XXX	
A4351		P	Intermittent urinary catheter; straight tip, with or without coating (Teflon, silicone, silicone elastomer, or hydrophilic, etc.), each	0.00	0.06	0.06	0.00	0.06	0.06	XXX	■
A4352		P	Intermittent urinary catheter; coude (curved) tip, with or without coating (Teflon, silicone, silicone elastomeric, or hydrophilic, etc.), each	0.00	0.26	0.26	0.00	0.26	0.26	XXX	■
A4353		X	Intermittent urinary catheter, with insertion supplies	0.00	0.15	0.15	0.00	0.15	0.15	XXX	■
A4354		P	Insertion tray with drainage bag but without catheter	0.00	0.28	0.28	0.00	0.28	0.28	XXX	■
A4355		P	Irrigation tubing set for continuous bladder irrigation through a three-way indwelling Foley catheter, each	0.00	0.20	0.20	0.00	0.20	0.20	XXX	■
A4356		P	External urethral clamp or compression device (not to be used for catheter clamp), each	0.00	1.19	1.19	0.00	1.19	1.19	XXX	■
A4357		P	Bedside drainage bag, day or night, with or without anti-reflux device, with or without tube, each	0.00	0.17	0.17	0.00	0.17	0.17	XXX	■
A4358		P	Urinary drainage bag, leg or abdomen, vinyl, with or without tube, with straps, each	0.00	0.14	0.14	0.00	0.14	0.14	XXX	■
A4359		P	Urinary suspensory without leg bag, each	0.00	1.02	1.02	0.00	1.02	1.02	XXX	■
A4360		N	Adult incontinence garment (e.g., brief, diaper), each	0.00	0.03	0.03	0.00	0.03	0.03	XXX	■
A4361		P	Ostomy faceplate, each	0.00	0.51	0.51	0.00	0.51	0.51	XXX	■
A4362		P	Skin barrier; solid, four by four or equivalent; each	0.00	0.11	0.11	0.00	0.11	0.11	XXX	■
A4364		P	Adhesive, liquid, or equal, any type, per ounce	0.00	0.04	0.04	0.00	0.04	0.04	XXX	■
A4365		X	Adhesive remover wipes, any type, per 50	0.00	0.28	0.28	0.00	0.28	0.28	XXX	■
A4367		P	Ostomy belt, each	0.00	0.22	0.22	0.00	0.22	0.22	XXX	■
A4368		X	Ostomy filter, any type, each	0.00	0.02	0.02	0.00	0.02	0.02	XXX	■

■ RVU not developed by CMS. Gap-filled RVUs developed by CHEG.

Code	M	S	Description	Work Value	Non-Fac PE	Fac PE	Mal-practice	Non-Fac Total	Fac Total	Global	Gap
A4369		X	Ostomy skin barrier, liquid (spray, brush, etc), per oz	0.00	0.11	0.11	0.00	0.11	0.11	XXX	■
A4370		X	Ostomy skin barrier, paste, per oz	0.00	0.16	0.16	0.00	0.16	0.16	XXX	■
A4371		X	Ostomy skin barrier, powder, per oz	0.00	0.11	0.11	0.00	0.11	0.11	XXX	■
A4372		X	Ostomy skin barrier, solid 4x4 or equivalent, standard wear, with built-in convexity, each	0.00	0.12	0.12	0.00	0.12	0.12	XXX	■
A4373		X	Ostomy skin barrier, with flange (solid, flexible or accordion), standard wear, with built-in convexity, any size, each	0.00	0.21	0.21	0.00	0.21	0.21	XXX	■
A4374		X	Ostomy skin barrier, with flange (solid, flexible or accordion), extended wear, with built-in convexity, any size, each	0.00	0.00	0.00	0.00	0.00	0.00	XXX	
A4375		X	Ostomy pouch, drainable, with faceplate attached, plastic, each	0.00	0.00	0.00	0.00	0.00	0.00	XXX	
A4376		X	Ostomy pouch, drainable, with faceplate attached, rubber, each	0.00	0.00	0.00	0.00	0.00	0.00	XXX	
A4377		X	Ostomy pouch, drainable, for use on faceplate, plastic, each	0.00	0.00	0.00	0.00	0.00	0.00	XXX	
A4378		X	Ostomy pouch, drainable, for use on faceplate, rubber, each	0.00	0.00	0.00	0.00	0.00	0.00	XXX	
A4379		X	Ostomy pouch, urinary, with faceplate attached, plastic, each	0.00	0.00	0.00	0.00	0.00	0.00	XXX	
A4380		X	Ostomy pouch, urinary, with faceplate attached, rubber, each	0.00	0.00	0.00	0.00	0.00	0.00	XXX	
A4381		X	Ostomy pouch, urinary, for use on faceplate, plastic, each	0.00	0.00	0.00	0.00	0.00	0.00	XXX	
A4382		X	Ostomy pouch, urinary, for use on faceplate, heavy plastic, each	0.00	0.00	0.00	0.00	0.00	0.00	XXX	
A4383		X	Ostomy pouch, urinary, for use on faceplate, rubber, each	0.00	0.00	0.00	0.00	0.00	0.00	XXX	
A4384		X	Ostomy faceplate equivalent, silicone ring, each	0.00	0.00	0.00	0.00	0.00	0.00	XXX	
A4385		X	Ostomy skin barrier, solid 4x4 or equivalent, extended wear, without built-in convexity, each	0.00	0.13	0.13	0.00	0.13	0.13	XXX	■
A4386		X	Ostomy skin barrier, with flange (solid, flexible or accordion), extended wear, without built-in convexity, any size, each	0.00	0.18	0.18	0.00	0.18	0.18	XXX	■
A4387		X	Ostomy pouch closed, with standard wear barrier attached, with built-in convexity (1 piece), each	0.00	0.00	0.00	0.00	0.00	0.00	XXX	
A4388		X	Ostomy pouch, drainable, with extended wear barrier attached, without built-in convexity (1 piece)	0.00	0.09	0.09	0.00	0.09	0.09	XXX	■

■ RVU not developed by CMS. Gap-filled RVUs developed by CHEG.

Code	M	S	Description	Work Value	Non-Fac PE	Fac PE	Mal-practice	Non-Fac Total	Fac Total	Global	Gap
A4389		X	Ostomy pouch, drainable, with standard wear barrier attached, with built-in convexity (1 piece), each	0.00	0.09	0.09	0.00	0.09	0.09	XXX	■
A4390		X	Ostomy pouch, drainable, with extended wear barrier attached, with built-in convexity (1 piece), each	0.00	0.00	0.00	0.00	0.00	0.00	XXX	
A4391		X	Ostomy pouch, urinary, with extended wear barrier attached, without built-in convexity (1 piece), each	0.00	0.00	0.00	0.00	0.00	0.00	XXX	
A4392		X	Ostomy pouch, urinary, with standard wear barrier attached, with built-in convexity (1 piece), each	0.00	0.00	0.00	0.00	0.00	0.00	XXX	
A4393		X	Ostomy pouch, urinary, with extended wear barrier attached, with built-in convexity (1 piece), each	0.00	0.00	0.00	0.00	0.00	0.00	XXX	
A4394		X	Ostomy deodorant for use in ostomy pouch, liquid, per fluid ounce	0.00	0.10	0.10	0.00	0.10	0.10	XXX	■
A4395		X	Ostomy deodorant for use in ostomy pouch, solid, per tablet	0.00	0.00	0.00	0.00	0.00	0.00	XXX	
A4396		X	Ostomy belt with peristomal hernia support	0.00	0.22	0.22	0.00	0.22	0.22	XXX	■
A4397		P	Irrigation supply; sleeve, each	0.00	0.13	0.13	0.00	0.13	0.13	XXX	■
A4398		P	Ostomy irrigation supply; bag, each	0.00	0.15	0.15	0.00	0.15	0.15	XXX	■
A4399		P	Ostomy irrigation supply; cone/catheter, including brush	0.00	0.40	0.40	0.00	0.40	0.40	XXX	■
A4400		P	Ostomy irrigation set	0.00	1.09	1.09	0.00	1.09	1.09	XXX	■
A4402		P	Lubricant, per ounce	0.00	0.01	0.01	0.00	0.01	0.01	XXX	■
A4404		P	Ostomy ring, each	0.00	0.06	0.06	0.00	0.06	0.06	XXX	■
A4421		P	Ostomy supply; miscellaneous	0.00	0.00	0.00	0.00	0.00	0.00	XXX	
A4454		P	Tape, all types, all sizes	0.00	0.07	0.07	0.00	0.07	0.07	XXX	■
A4455		P	Adhesive remover or solvent (for tape, cement or other adhesive), per ounce	0.00	0.03	0.03	0.00	0.03	0.03	XXX	■
A4460		P	Elastic bandage, per roll (e.g., compression bandage)	0.00	0.13	0.13	0.00	0.13	0.13	XXX	■
A4462		X	Abdominal dressing holder/binder, each	0.00	0.43	0.43	0.00	0.43	0.43	XXX	■
A4464		N	Joint supportive device/garment, elastic or equal, each	0.00	0.00	0.00	0.00	0.00	0.00	XXX	
A4465		P	Nonelastic binder for extremity	0.00	0.33	0.33	0.00	0.33	0.33	XXX	■
A4470		P	Gravlee jet washer	0.00	0.23	0.23	0.00	0.23	0.23	XXX	■
A4480		P	VABRA aspirator	0.00	0.18	0.18	0.00	0.18	0.18	XXX	■

■ RVU not developed by CMS. Gap-filled RVUs developed by CHEG.

Code	M	S	Description	Work Value	Non-Fac PE	Fac PE	Mal-practice	Non-Fac Total	Fac Total	Global	Gap
A4481		X	Tracheostoma filter, any type, any size, each	0.00	0.00	0.00	0.00	0.00	0.00	XXX	
A4483	NU	X	Moisture exchanger, disposable, for use with invasive mechanical ventilation	0.00	0.00	0.00	0.00	0.00	0.00	XXX	
	RR			0.00	0.00	0.00	0.00	0.00	0.00	XXX	
	UE			0.00	0.00	0.00	0.00	0.00	0.00	XXX	
A4490		N	Surgical stocking above knee length, each	0.00	0.24	0.24	0.00	0.24	0.24	XXX	■
A4495		N	Surgical stocking thigh length, each	0.00	0.24	0.24	0.00	0.24	0.24	XXX	■
A4500		N	Surgical stocking below knee length, each	0.00	0.18	0.18	0.00	0.18	0.18	XXX	■
A4510		N	Surgical stocking full-length, each	0.00	0.44	0.44	0.00	0.44	0.44	XXX	■
A4550		I	Surgical trays	0.00	1.06	1.06	0.00	1.06	1.06	XXX	■
A4554		N	Disposable underpads, all sizes (e.g., Chux's)	0.00	0.11	0.11	0.00	0.11	0.11	XXX	■
A4556		P	Electrodes (e.g., Apnea monitor), per pair	0.00	0.27	0.27	0.00	0.27	0.27	XXX	■
A4557		P	Lead wires (e.g., Apnea monitor), per pair	0.00	0.28	0.28	0.00	0.28	0.28	XXX	■
A4558		P	Conductive paste or gel	0.00	0.12	0.12	0.00	0.12	0.12	XXX	■
A4561		X	Pessary, rubber, any type	0.00	0.61	0.61	0.00	0.61	0.61	XXX	■
A4562		X	Pessary, non rubber, any type	0.00	0.61	0.61	0.00	0.61	0.61	XXX	■
A4565		X	Slings	0.00	0.26	0.26	0.00	0.26	0.26	XXX	■
A4570		I	Splint	0.00	0.62	0.62	0.00	0.62	0.62	XXX	■
A4572		X	Rib belt	0.00	0.40	0.40	0.00	0.40	0.40	XXX	■
A4575		N	Topical hyperbaric oxygen chamber, disposable	0.00	0.00	0.00	0.00	0.00	0.00	XXX	
A4580		I	Cast supplies (e.g., plaster)	0.00	0.00	0.00	0.00	0.00	0.00	XXX	
A4590		I	Special casting material (e.g., fiberglass)	0.00	1.40	1.40	0.00	1.40	1.40	XXX	■
A4595		X	TENS supplies, 2 lead, per month	0.00	0.38	0.38	0.00	0.38	0.38	XXX	■
A4608		X	Transtracheal oxygen catheter, each	0.00	0.00	0.00	0.00	0.00	0.00	XXX	
A4611		X	Battery, heavy duty; replacement for patient-owned ventilator	0.00	6.31	6.31	0.00	6.31	6.31	XXX	■
A4612		X	Battery cables; replacement for patient-owned ventilator	0.00	2.63	2.63	0.00	2.63	2.63	XXX	■
A4613	NU	X	Battery charger; replacement for patient-owned ventilator	0.00	4.75	4.75	0.00	4.75	4.75	XXX	■
	RR			0.00	0.47	0.47	0.00	0.47	0.47	XXX	■
	UE			0.00	3.43	3.43	0.00	3.43	3.43	XXX	■
A4614		X	Peak expiratory flow rate meter, hand held	0.00	0.00	0.00	0.00	0.00	0.00	XXX	
A4615		X	Cannula, nasal	0.00	0.05	0.05	0.00	0.05	0.05	XXX	■
A4616		X	Tubing (oxygen), per foot	0.00	0.02	0.02	0.00	0.02	0.02	XXX	■

■ RVU not developed by CMS. Gap-filled RVUs developed by CHEG.

Code	M	S	Description	Work Value	Non-Fac PE	Fac PE	Mal-practice	Non-Fac Total	Fac Total	Global	Gap
A4617		X	Mouthpiece	0.00	0.29	0.29	0.00	0.29	0.29	XXX	■
A4618		X	Breathing circuits	0.00	0.28	0.28	0.00	0.28	0.28	XXX	■
A4619		X	Face tent	0.00	0.06	0.06	0.00	0.06	0.06	XXX	■
A4620		X	Variable concentration mask	0.00	0.10	0.10	0.00	0.10	0.10	XXX	■
A4621		X	Tracheostomy mask or collar	0.00	0.00	0.00	0.00	0.00	0.00	XXX	
A4622		X	Tracheostomy or laryngectomy tube	0.00	1.90	1.90	0.00	1.90	1.90	XXX	■
A4623		X	Tracheostomy, inner cannula (replacement only)	0.00	0.22	0.22	0.00	0.22	0.22	XXX	■
A4624		X	Tracheal suction catheter, any type, each	0.00	0.09	0.09	0.00	0.09	0.09	XXX	■
A4625		X	Tracheostomy care kit for new tracheostomy	0.00	0.22	0.22	0.00	0.22	0.22	XXX	■
A4626		X	Tracheostomy cleaning brush, each	0.00	0.11	0.11	0.00	0.11	0.11	XXX	■
A4627		N	Spacer, bag or reservoir, with or without mask, for use with metered dose inhaler	0.00	0.60	0.60	0.00	0.60	0.60	XXX	■
A4628		X	Oropharyngeal suction catheter, each	0.00	0.02	0.02	0.00	0.02	0.02	XXX	■
A4629		X	Tracheostomy care kit for established tracheostomy	0.00	0.15	0.15	0.00	0.15	0.15	XXX	■
A4630		X	Replacement batteries for medically necessary transcutaneous electrical nerve stimulator (TENS) owned by patient	0.00	0.15	0.15	0.00	0.15	0.15	XXX	■
A4631		X	Replacement batteries for medically necessary electronic wheelchair owned by patient	0.00	3.32	3.32	0.00	3.32	3.32	XXX	■
A4635		X	Underarm pad, crutch, replacement, each	0.00	0.14	0.14	0.00	0.14	0.14	XXX	■
A4636		X	Replacement, handgrip, cane, crutch, or walker, each	0.00	0.12	0.12	0.00	0.12	0.12	XXX	■
A4637		X	Replacement, tip, cane, crutch, walker, each	0.00	0.07	0.07	0.00	0.07	0.07	XXX	■
A4640		X	Replacement pad for use with medically necessary alternating pressure pad owned by patient	0.00	1.72	1.72	0.00	1.72	1.72	XXX	■
A4641		E	Supply of radiopharmaceutical diagnostic imaging agent, not otherwise classified	0.00	0.00	0.00	0.00	0.00	0.00	XXX	
A4642		E	Supply of satumomab pendetide, radiopharmaceutical diagnostic imaging agent, per dose	0.00	0.00	0.00	0.00	0.00	0.00	XXX	
A4643		E	Supply of additional high dose contrast material(s) during magnetic resonance imaging, e.g., gadoteridol injection	0.00	0.00	0.00	0.00	0.00	0.00	XXX	
A4644		E	Supply of low osmolar contrast material (100–199 mg of iodine)	0.00	0.00	0.00	0.00	0.00	0.00	XXX	

■ RVU not developed by CMS. Gap-filled RVUs developed by CHEG.

Code	M	S	Description	Work Value	Non-Fac PE	Fac PE	Mal-practice	Non-Fac Total	Fac Total	Global	Gap
A4645		E	Supply of low osmolar contrast material (200–299 mg of iodine)	0.00	0.00	0.00	0.00	0.00	0.00	XXX	
A4646		E	Supply of low osmolar contrast material (300–399 mg of iodine)	0.00	0.00	0.00	0.00	0.00	0.00	XXX	
A4647		B	Supply of paramagnetic contrast material (e.g., gadolinium)	0.00	3.29	3.29	0.00	3.29	3.29	XXX	■
A4649		P	Surgical supply; miscellaneous	0.00	0.00	0.00	0.00	0.00	0.00	XXX	
A4651		X	Calibrated microcapillary tube, each	0.00	0.00	0.00	0.00	0.00	0.00	XXX	
A4652		X	Microcapillary tube sealant	0.00	0.00	0.00	0.00	0.00	0.00	XXX	
A4656		X	Needle, any size, for dialysis, each	0.00	0.00	0.00	0.00	0.00	0.00	XXX	
A4657		X	Syringe, with or without needle, for dialysis, each	0.00	0.00	0.00	0.00	0.00	0.00	XXX	
A4660		X	Sphygmomanometer/blood pressure apparatus with cuff and stethoscope, for dialysis	0.00	0.48	0.48	0.00	0.48	0.48	XXX	■
A4663		X	Blood pressure cuff only, for dialysis	0.00	0.91	0.91	0.00	0.91	0.91	XXX	■
A4670		N	Automatic blood pressure monitor, for dialysis	0.00	2.34	2.34	0.00	2.34	2.34	XXX	■
A4680		X	Activated carbon filter for hemodialysis, each	0.00	2.37	2.37	0.00	2.37	2.37	XXX	■
A4690		X	Dialyzer (artificial kidneys), all types, all sizes, for hemodialysis, each	0.00	23.53	23.53	0.00	23.53	23.53	XXX	■
A4706		X	Bicarbonate concentrate, solution, for hemodialysis, per gallon	0.00	0.00	0.00	0.00	0.00	0.00	XXX	
A4707		X	Bicarbonate concentrate, powder, for hemodialysis, per packet	0.00	0.00	0.00	0.00	0.00	0.00	XXX	
A4708		X	Acetate concentrate solution, for hemodialysis, per gallon	0.00	0.00	0.00	0.00	0.00	0.00	XXX	
A4709		X	Acid concentrate, solution, for hemodialysis, per gallon	0.00	0.00	0.00	0.00	0.00	0.00	XXX	
A4712		X	Water, sterile, for injection for dialysis, per 10 ml	0.00	0.05	0.05	0.00	0.05	0.05	XXX	■
A4714		X	Treated water (deionized, distilled, or reverse osmosis) for peritoneal dialysis, per gallon	0.00	0.00	0.00	0.00	0.00	0.00	XXX	
A4719		X	Y set tubing for peritoneal dialysis	0.00	0.00	0.00	0.00	0.00	0.00	XXX	
A4720		X	Dialysate solution, any concentration of dextrose, fluid volume greater than 249 cc, but less than or equal to 999 cc, for peritoneal dialysis	0.00	0.00	0.00	0.00	0.00	0.00	XXX	
A4721		X	Dialysate solution, any concentration of dextrose, fluid volume greater than 999 cc, but less than or equal to 1999 cc, for peritoneal dialysis	0.00	0.00	0.00	0.00	0.00	0.00	XXX	

■ RVU not developed by CMS. Gap-filled RVUs developed by CHEG.

Code	M	S	Description	Work Value	Non-Fac PE	Fac PE	Mal-prac-tice	Non-Fac Total	Fac Total	Global	Gap
A4722		X	Dialysate solution, any concentration of dextrose, fluid volume greater than 1999 cc, but less than or equal to 2999 cc, for peritoneal dialysis	0.00	0.00	0.00	0.00	0.00	0.00	XXX	
A4723		X	Dialysate solution, any concentration of dextrose, fluid volume greater than 2999 cc, but less than or equal to 3999 cc, for peritoneal dialysis	0.00	0.00	0.00	0.00	0.00	0.00	XXX	
A4724		X	Dialysate solution, any concentration of dextrose, fluid volume greater than 3999 cc, but less than or equal to 4999 cc, for peritoneal dialysis	0.00	0.00	0.00	0.00	0.00	0.00	XXX	
A4725		X	Dialysate solution, any concentration of dextrose, fluid volume greater than 4999 cc, but less than or equal to 5999 cc, for peritoneal dialysis	0.00	0.00	0.00	0.00	0.00	0.00	XXX	
A4726		X	Dialysate solution, any concentration of dextrose, fluid volume greater than 5999 cc	0.00	0.00	0.00	0.00	0.00	0.00	XXX	
A4730		X	Fistula cannulation set for hemodialysis, each	0.00	0.00	0.00	0.00	0.00	0.00	XXX	
A4736		X	Topical anesthetic, for dialysis, per gm	0.00	0.00	0.00	0.00	0.00	0.00	XXX	
A4737		X	Injectable anesthetic, for dialysis, per 10 ml	0.00	0.00	0.00	0.00	0.00	0.00	XXX	
A4740		X	Shunt accessory, for hemodialysis, any type	0.00	0.00	0.00	0.00	0.00	0.00	XXX	
A4750		X	Blood tubing, arterial or venous, for hemodialysis, each	0.00	0.45	0.45	0.00	0.45	0.45	XXX	■
A4755		X	Blood tubing, arterial and venous combined, for hemodialysis, each	0.00	0.00	0.00	0.00	0.00	0.00	XXX	
A4760		X	Dialysate solution test kit, for peritoneal dialysis, any type, each	0.00	0.00	0.00	0.00	0.00	0.00	XXX	
A4765		X	Dialysate concentrate, powder, additive for peritoneal dialysis, per packet	0.00	0.00	0.00	0.00	0.00	0.00	XXX	
A4766		X	Dialysate concentrate, solution, additive for peritoneal dialysis, per 10 ml	0.00	0.00	0.00	0.00	0.00	0.00	XXX	
A4770		X	Blood collection tube, vacuum, for dialysis, per 50	0.00	0.00	0.00	0.00	0.00	0.00	XXX	
A4771		X	Serum clotting time tube, for dialysis, per 50	0.00	0.00	0.00	0.00	0.00	0.00	XXX	
A4772		X	Blood glucose test strips, for dialysis, per 50	0.00	0.95	0.95	0.00	0.95	0.95	XXX	■
A4773		X	Occult blood test strips, for dialysis, per 50	0.00	0.60	0.60	0.00	0.60	0.60	XXX	■
A4774		X	Ammonia test strips, for dialysis, per 50	0.00	0.00	0.00	0.00	0.00	0.00	XXX	
A4801		X	Heparin, any type, for hemodialysis, per 1000 units	0.00	0.07	0.07	0.00	0.07	0.07	XXX	■
A4802		X	Protamine sulfate, for hemodialysis, per 50 mg	0.00	0.17	0.17	0.00	0.17	0.17	XXX	■

■ RVU not developed by CMS. Gap-filled RVUs developed by CHEG.

Code	M	S	Description	Work Value	Non-Fac PE	Fac PE	Mal-practice	Non-Fac Total	Fac Total	Global	Gap
A4860		X	Disposable catheter tips for peritoneal dialysis, per 10	0.00	0.00	0.00	0.00	0.00	0.00	XXX	
A4870		X	Plumbing and/or electrical work for home hemodialysis equipment	0.00	0.00	0.00	0.00	0.00	0.00	XXX	
A4890		R	Contracts, repair and maintenance, for hemodialysis equipment	0.00	0.00	0.00	0.00	0.00	0.00	XXX	
A4911		X	Drain bag/bottle, for dialysis, each	0.00	0.00	0.00	0.00	0.00	0.00	XXX	
A4913		X	Miscellaneous dialysis supplies, not otherwise specified	0.00	0.00	0.00	0.00	0.00	0.00	XXX	
A4918		X	Venous pressure clamp, for hemodialysis, each	0.00	0.00	0.00	0.00	0.00	0.00	XXX	
A4927		X	Gloves, non-sterile, for dialysis, per 100	0.00	0.15	0.15	0.00	0.15	0.15	XXX	■
A4928		X	Surgical mask, for dialysis, per 20	0.00	0.00	0.00	0.00	0.00	0.00	XXX	
A4929		X	Tourniquet for dialysis, each	0.00	0.01	0.01	0.00	0.01	0.01	XXX	■
A5051		P	Pouch, closed; with barrier attached (one piece)	0.00	0.06	0.06	0.00	0.06	0.06	XXX	■
A5052		P	Pouch, closed; without barrier attached (one piece)	0.00	0.08	0.08	0.00	0.08	0.08	XXX	■
A5053		P	Pouch, closed; for use on faceplate	0.00	0.09	0.09	0.00	0.09	0.09	XXX	■
A5054		P	Pouch, closed; for use on barrier with flange (two piece)	0.00	0.03	0.03	0.00	0.03	0.03	XXX	■
A5055		P	Stoma cap	0.00	0.05	0.05	0.00	0.05	0.05	XXX	■
A5061		P	Pouch, drainable; with barrier attached (one piece)	0.00	0.09	0.09	0.00	0.09	0.09	XXX	■
A5062		P	Pouch, drainable; without barrier attached (one piece)	0.00	0.11	0.11	0.00	0.11	0.11	XXX	■
A5063		P	Pouch, drainable; for use on barrier with flange (two piece system)	0.00	0.06	0.06	0.00	0.06	0.06	XXX	■
A5071		P	Pouch, urinary; with barrier attached (one piece)	0.00	0.18	0.18	0.00	0.18	0.18	XXX	■
A5072		P	Pouch, urinary; without barrier attached (one piece)	0.00	0.11	0.11	0.00	0.11	0.11	XXX	■
A5073		P	Pouch, urinary; for use on barrier with flange (two piece)	0.00	0.12	0.12	0.00	0.12	0.12	XXX	■
A5081		P	Continent device; plug for continent stoma	0.00	0.06	0.06	0.00	0.06	0.06	XXX	■
A5082		P	Continent device; catheter for continent stoma	0.00	0.40	0.40	0.00	0.40	0.40	XXX	■
A5093		P	Ostomy accessory; convex insert	0.00	0.23	0.23	0.00	0.23	0.23	XXX	■
A5102		P	Bedside drainage bottle, with or without tubing, rigid or expandable, each	0.00	0.20	0.20	0.00	0.20	0.20	XXX	■

■ RVU not developed by CMS. Gap-filled RVUs developed by CHEG.

Code	M	S	Description	Work Value	Non-Fac PE	Fac PE	Mal-practice	Non-Fac Total	Fac Total	Global	Gap
A5105		P	Urinary suspensory; with leg bag, with or without tube	0.00	1.30	1.30	0.00	1.30	1.30	XXX	■
A5112		P	Urinary leg bag; latex	0.00	0.22	0.22	0.00	0.22	0.22	XXX	■
A5113		P	Leg strap; latex, replacement only, per set	0.00	0.18	0.18	0.00	0.18	0.18	XXX	■
A5114		P	Leg strap; foam or fabric, replacement only, per set	0.00	0.15	0.15	0.00	0.15	0.15	XXX	■
A5119		P	Skin barrier; wipes, box per 50	0.00	0.37	0.37	0.00	0.37	0.37	XXX	■
A5121		P	Skin barrier; solid, 6 x 6 or equivalent, each	0.00	0.22	0.22	0.00	0.22	0.22	XXX	■
A5122		P	Skin barrier; solid, 8 x 8 or equivalent, each	0.00	0.44	0.44	0.00	0.44	0.44	XXX	■
A5123		P	Skin barrier; with flange (solid, flexible or accordion), any size, each	0.00	0.18	0.18	0.00	0.18	0.18	XXX	■
A5126		P	Adhesive or non-adhesive; disk or foam pad	0.00	0.03	0.03	0.00	0.03	0.03	XXX	■
A5131		P	Appliance cleaner, incontinence and ostomy appliances, per 16 oz.	0.00	0.36	0.36	0.00	0.36	0.36	XXX	■
A5200		X	Percutaneous catheter/tube anchoring device, adhesive skin attachment	0.00	0.00	0.00	0.00	0.00	0.00	XXX	
A5500		X	For diabetics only, fitting (including follow-up) custom preparation and supply of off-the-shelf depth-inlay shoe manufactured to accommodate multi-density insert(s), per shoe	0.00	0.00	0.00	0.00	0.00	0.00	XXX	
A5501		X	For diabetics only, fitting (including follow-up) custom preparation and supply of shoe molded from cast(s) of patient's foot (custom molded shoe), per shoe	0.00	0.00	0.00	0.00	0.00	0.00	XXX	
A5503		X	For diabetics only, modification (including fitting) of off-the-shelf depth-inlay shoe or custom molded shoe with roller or rigid rocker bottom, per shoe	0.00	0.00	0.00	0.00	0.00	0.00	XXX	
A5504		X	For diabetics only, modification (including fitting) of off-the-shelf depth-inlay shoe or custom molded shoe with wedge(s), per shoe	0.00	0.00	0.00	0.00	0.00	0.00	XXX	
A5505		X	For diabetics only, modification (including fitting) of off-the-shelf depth-inlay shoe or custom molded shoe with metatarsal bar, per shoe	0.00	0.00	0.00	0.00	0.00	0.00	XXX	
A5506		X	For diabetics only, modification (including fitting) of off-the-shelf depth-inlay shoe or custom molded shoe with off-set heel(s), per shoe	0.00	0.00	0.00	0.00	0.00	0.00	XXX	
A5507		X	For diabetics only, not otherwise specified modification (including fitting) of off-the-shelf depth-inlay shoe or custom molded shoe, per shoe	0.00	0.00	0.00	0.00	0.00	0.00	XXX	

■ RVU not developed by CMS. Gap-filled RVUs developed by CHEG.

Code	M	S	Description	Work Value	Non-Fac PE	Fac PE	Mal-practice	Non-Fac Total	Fac Total	Global	Gap
A5508		X	For diabetics only, deluxe feature of off-the-shelf depth-inlay shoe or custom-molded shoe, per shoe	0.00	0.00	0.00	0.00	0.00	0.00	XXX	
A5509		X	For diabetics only, direct formed, molded to foot with external heat source (i.e. heat gun) multiple density insert(s), prefabricated, per shoe	0.00	0.00	0.00	0.00	0.00	0.00	XXX	
A5510		X	For diabetics only, direct formed, compression molded to patient's foot without external heat source, multiple-density insert(s) prefabricated, per shoe	0.00	0.00	0.00	0.00	0.00	0.00	XXX	
A5511		X	For diabetics only, custom-molded from model of patient's foot, multiple density insert(s), custom-fabricated, per shoe	0.00	0.00	0.00	0.00	0.00	0.00	XXX	
A6000		X	Non-contact wound warming wound cover for use with the non-contact wound warming device and warming card	0.00	0.00	0.00	0.00	0.00	0.00	XXX	
A6010		X	Collagen based wound filler, dry form, per gram of collagen	0.00	0.00	0.00	0.00	0.00	0.00	XXX	
A6020		D	Collagen based wound dressing, each dressing	0.00	0.00	0.00	0.00	0.00	0.00	XXX	
A6021		X	Collagen dressing, pad size 16 sq. in. or less, each	0.00	0.00	0.00	0.00	0.00	0.00	XXX	
A6022		X	Collagen dressing, pad size more than 16 sq. in. but less than or equal to 48 sq in, each	0.00	0.00	0.00	0.00	0.00	0.00	XXX	
A6023		X	Collagen dressing, pad size more than 48 sq. in., each	0.00	0.00	0.00	0.00	0.00	0.00	XXX	
A6024		X	Collagen dressing wound filler, per 6 in	0.00	0.00	0.00	0.00	0.00	0.00	XXX	
A6025		I	Silicone gel sheet, each	0.00	0.88	0.88	0.00	0.88	0.88	XXX	■
A6154		P	Wound pouch, each	0.00	0.23	0.23	0.00	0.23	0.23	XXX	■
A6196		P	Alginate or other fiber gelling dressing, wound cover, pad size 16 sq in or less, each dressing	0.00	0.26	0.26	0.00	0.26	0.26	XXX	■
A6197		P	Alginate or other fiber gelling dressing, wound cover, pad size more than 16 sq in but less than or equal to 48 sq in, each dressing	0.00	0.55	0.55	0.00	0.55	0.55	XXX	■
A6198		P	Alginate or other fiber gelling dressing, wound cover, pad size more than 48 sq in, each dressing	0.00	0.00	0.00	0.00	0.00	0.00	XXX	
A6199		P	Alginate or other fiber gelling dressing, wound filler, per 6 inches	0.00	0.18	0.18	0.00	0.18	0.18	XXX	■
A6200		X	Composite dressing, pad size 16 sq. in. or less, without adhesive border, each dressing	0.00	0.04	0.04	0.00	0.04	0.04	XXX	■
A6201		X	Composite dressing, pad size more than 16 sq. in. but less than or equal to 48 sq. in., without adhesive border, each dressing	0.00	0.07	0.07	0.00	0.07	0.07	XXX	■

■ RVU not developed by CMS. Gap-filled RVUs developed by CHEG.

Code	M	S	Description	Work Value	Non-Fac PE	Fac PE	Mal-practice	Non-Fac Total	Fac Total	Global	Gap
A6202		X	Composite dressing, pad size more than 48 sq. in., without adhesive border, each dressing	0.00	0.00	0.00	0.00	0.00	0.00	XXX	
A6203		P	Composite dressing, pad size 16 sq. in. or less, with any size adhesive border, each dressing	0.00	0.11	0.11	0.00	0.11	0.11	XXX	■
A6204		P	Composite dressing, pad size more than 16 sq. in. but less than or equal to 48 sq. in., with any size adhesive border, each dressing	0.00	0.15	0.15	0.00	0.15	0.15	XXX	■
A6205		P	Composite dressing, pad size more than 48 sq. in., with any size adhesive border, each dressing	0.00	0.00	0.00	0.00	0.00	0.00	XXX	
A6206		P	Contact layer, 16 sq. in. or less, each dressing	0.00	0.16	0.16	0.00	0.16	0.16	XXX	■
A6207		P	Contact layer, more than 16 sq. in. but less than or equal to 48 sq. in., each dressing	0.00	0.26	0.26	0.00	0.26	0.26	XXX	■
A6208		P	Contact layer, more than 48 sq. in., each dressing	0.00	0.00	0.00	0.00	0.00	0.00	XXX	
A6209		P	Foam dressing, wound cover, pad size 16 sq. in. or less, without adhesive border, each dressing	0.00	0.26	0.26	0.00	0.26	0.26	XXX	■
A6210		P	Foam dressing, wound cover, pad size more than 16 sq. in. but less than or equal to 48 sq. in., without adhesive border, each dressing	0.00	0.66	0.66	0.00	0.66	0.66	XXX	■
A6211		P	Foam dressing, wound cover, pad size more then 48 sq. in., without adhesive border, each dressing	0.00	0.95	0.95	0.00	0.95	0.95	XXX	■
A6212		P	Foam dressing, wound cover, pad size 16 sq. in. or less, with any size adhesive border, each dressing	0.00	0.33	0.33	0.00	0.33	0.33	XXX	■
A6213		P	Foam dressing, wound cover, pad size more than 16 sq. in. but less than or equal to 48 sq. in., with any size adhesive border, each dressing	0.00	0.77	0.77	0.00	0.77	0.77	XXX	■
A6214		P	Foam dressing, wound cover, pad size more than 48 sq. in., with any size adhesive border, each dressing	0.00	0.33	0.33	0.00	0.33	0.33	XXX	■
A6215		P	Foam dressing, wound filler, per gram	0.00	0.00	0.00	0.00	0.00	0.00	XXX	
A6216		P	Gauze, non-impregnated, non-sterile, pad size 16 sq. in. or less, without adhesive border, each dressing	0.00	0.01	0.01	0.00	0.01	0.01	XXX	■
A6217		P	Gauze, non-impregnated, non-sterile, pad size more than 16 sq. in. but less than or equal to 48 sq. in., without adhesive border, each dressing	0.00	0.01	0.01	0.00	0.01	0.01	XXX	■
A6218		P	Gauze, non-impregnated, non-sterile, pad size more than 48 sq. in., without adhesive border, each dressing	0.00	0.01	0.01	0.00	0.01	0.01	XXX	■
A6219		P	Gauze, non-impregnated, pad size 16 sq. in. or less, with any size adhesive border, each dressing	0.00	0.04	0.04	0.00	0.04	0.04	XXX	■

■ RVU not developed by CMS. Gap-filled RVUs developed by CHEG.

HCPCS

Code	M	S	Description	Work Value	Non-Fac PE	Fac PE	Mal-practice	Non-Fac Total	Fac Total	Global	Gap
A6220		P	Gauze, non-impregnated, pad size more than 16 sq. in. but less than or equal to 48 sq. in., with any size adhesive border, each dressing	0.00	0.07	0.07	0.00	0.07	0.07	XXX	■
A6221		P	Gauze, non-impregnated, pad size more than 48 sq. in., with any size adhesive border, each dressing	0.00	0.00	0.00	0.00	0.00	0.00	XXX	
A6222		P	Gauze, impregnated with other than water, normal saline, or hydrogel, pad size 16 sq. in. or less, without adhesive border, each dressing	0.00	0.02	0.02	0.00	0.02	0.02	XXX	■
A6223		P	Gauze, impregnated with other than water, normal saline, or hydrogel, pad size more than 16 sq. in. but less than or equal to 48 sq. in., without adhesive border, each dressing	0.00	0.07	0.07	0.00	0.07	0.07	XXX	■
A6224		P	Gauze, impregnated with other than water, normal saline, or hydrogel, pad size more than 48 sq. in., without adhesive border, each dressing	0.00	0.11	0.11	0.00	0.11	0.11	XXX	■
A6228		P	Gauze, impregnated, water or normal saline, pad size 16 sq. in. or less, without adhesive border, each dressing	0.00	0.07	0.07	0.00	0.07	0.07	XXX	■
A6229		P	Gauze, impregnated, water or normal saline, pad size more than 16 sq. in. but less than or equal to 48 sq. in., without adhesive border, each dressing	0.00	0.08	0.08	0.00	0.08	0.08	XXX	■
A6230		P	Gauze, impregnated, water or normal saline, pad size more than 48 sq. in., without adhesive border, each dressing	0.00	0.11	0.11	0.00	0.11	0.11	XXX	■
A6231		X	Gauze, impregnated, hydrogel, for direct wound contact, pad size 16 sq. in. or less, each dressing	0.00	0.00	0.00	0.00	0.00	0.00	XXX	
A6232		X	Gauze, impregnated, hydrogel, for direct wound contact, pad size greater than 16 sq. in., but less than or equal to 48 sq. in., each dressing	0.00	0.00	0.00	0.00	0.00	0.00	XXX	
A6233		X	Gauze, impregnated, hydrogel for direct wound contact, pad size more than 48 sq. in., each dressing	0.00	0.00	0.00	0.00	0.00	0.00	XXX	
A6234		P	Hydrocolloid dressing, wound cover, pad size 16 sq. in. or less, without adhesive border, each dressing	0.00	0.17	0.17	0.00	0.17	0.17	XXX	■
A6235		P	Hydrocolloid dressing, wound cover, pad size more than 16 sq. in. but less than or equal to 48 sq. in., without adhesive border, each dressing	0.00	0.38	0.38	0.00	0.38	0.38	XXX	■
A6236		P	Hydrocolloid dressing, wound cover, pad size more than 48 sq. in., without adhesive border, each dressing	0.00	0.63	0.63	0.00	0.63	0.63	XXX	■

■ RVU not developed by CMS. Gap-filled RVUs developed by CHEG.

Code	M	S	Description	Work Value	Non-Fac PE	Fac PE	Mal-practice	Non-Fac Total	Fac Total	Global	Gap
A6237		P	Hydrocolloid dressing, wound cover, pad size 16 sq. in. or less, with any size adhesive border, each dressing	0.00	0.21	0.21	0.00	0.21	0.21	XXX	■
A6238		P	Hydrocolloid dressing, wound cover, pad size more than 16 sq. in. but less than or equal to 48 sq. in., with any size adhesive border, each dressing	0.00	0.51	0.51	0.00	0.51	0.51	XXX	■
A6239		P	Hydrocolloid dressing, wound cover, pad size more than 48 sq. in., with any size adhesive border, each dressing	0.00	0.00	0.00	0.00	0.00	0.00	XXX	
A6240		P	Hydrocolloid dressing, wound filler, paste, per fluid ounce	0.00	0.40	0.40	0.00	0.40	0.40	XXX	■
A6241		P	Hydrocolloid dressing, wound filler, dry form, per gram	0.00	0.06	0.06	0.00	0.06	0.06	XXX	■
A6242		P	Hydrogel dressing, wound cover, pad size 16 sq. in. or less, without adhesive border, each dressing	0.00	0.18	0.18	0.00	0.18	0.18	XXX	■
A6243		P	Hydrogel dressing, wound cover, pad size more than 16 sq. in. but less than or equal to 48 sq. in., without adhesive border, each dressing	0.00	0.40	0.40	0.00	0.40	0.40	XXX	■
A6244		P	Hydrogel dressing, wound cover, pad size more than 48 sq. in., without adhesive border, each dressing	0.00	1.28	1.28	0.00	1.28	1.28	XXX	■
A6245		P	Hydrogel dressing, wound cover, pad size 16 sq. in. or less, with any size adhesive border, each dressing	0.00	0.19	0.19	0.00	0.19	0.19	XXX	■
A6246		P	Hydrogel dressing, wound cover, pad size more than 16 sq. in. but less than or equal to 48 sq. in., with any size adhesive border, each dressing	0.00	0.33	0.33	0.00	0.33	0.33	XXX	■
A6247		P	Hydrogel dressing, wound cover, pad size more than 48 sq. in., with any size adhesive border, each dressing	0.00	0.77	0.77	0.00	0.77	0.77	XXX	■
A6248		P	Hydrogel dressing, wound filler, gel, per fluid ounce	0.00	0.55	0.55	0.00	0.55	0.55	XXX	■
A6250		P	Skin sealants, protectants, moisturizers, ointments, any type, any size	0.00	0.00	0.00	0.00	0.00	0.00	XXX	
A6251		P	Specialty absorptive dressing, wound cover, pad size 16 sq. in. or less, without adhesive border, each dressing	0.00	0.07	0.07	0.00	0.07	0.07	XXX	■
A6252		P	Specialty absorptive dressing, wound cover, pad size more than 16 sq. in. but less than or equal to 48 sq. in., without adhesive border, each dressing	0.00	0.08	0.08	0.00	0.08	0.08	XXX	■
A6253		P	Specialty absorptive dressing, wound cover, pad size more than 48 sq. in., without adhesive border, each dressing	0.00	0.13	0.13	0.00	0.13	0.13	XXX	■

■ RVU not developed by CMS. Gap-filled RVUs developed by CHEG.

Code	M	S	Description	Work Value	Non-Fac PE	Fac PE	Mal-practice	Non-Fac Total	Fac Total	Global	Gap
A6254		P	Specialty absorptive dressing, wound cover, pad size 16 sq. in. or less, with any size adhesive border, each dressing	0.00	0.11	0.11	0.00	0.11	0.11	XXX	■
A6255		P	Specialty absorptive dressing, wound cover, pad size more than 16 sq. in. but less than or equal to 48 sq. in., with any size adhesive border, each dressing	0.00	0.00	0.00	0.00	0.00	0.00	XXX	
A6256		P	Specialty absorptive dressing, wound cover, pad size more than 48 sq. in., with any size adhesive border, each dressing	0.00	0.00	0.00	0.00	0.00	0.00	XXX	
A6257		P	Transparent film, 16 sq. in. or less, each dressing	0.00	0.08	0.08	0.00	0.08	0.08	XXX	■
A6258		P	Transparent film, more than 16 sq. in. but less than or equal to 48 sq. in., each dressing	0.00	0.15	0.15	0.00	0.15	0.15	XXX	■
A6259		P	Transparent film, more than 48 sq. in., each dressing	0.00	0.37	0.37	0.00	0.37	0.37	XXX	■
A6260		P	Wound cleansers, any type, any size	0.00	0.04	0.04	0.00	0.04	0.04	XXX	■
A6261		P	Wound filler, gel/paste, per fluid ounce, not elsewhere classified	0.00	0.15	0.15	0.00	0.15	0.15	XXX	■
A6262		P	Wound filler, dry form, per gram, not elsewhere classified	0.00	0.04	0.04	0.00	0.04	0.04	XXX	■
A6263		P	Gauze, elastic, non-sterile, all types, per linear yard	0.00	0.01	0.01	0.00	0.01	0.01	XXX	■
A6264		P	Gauze, non-elastic, non-sterile, per linear yard	0.00	0.02	0.02	0.00	0.02	0.02	XXX	■
A6265		P	Tape, all types, per 18 sq. in.	0.00	0.00	0.00	0.00	0.00	0.00	XXX	
A6266		P	Gauze, impregnated, other than water or normal saline, any width, per linear yard	0.00	0.06	0.06	0.00	0.06	0.06	XXX	■
A6402		P	Gauze, non-impregnated, sterile, pad size 16 sq. in. or less, without adhesive border, each dressing	0.00	0.01	0.01	0.00	0.01	0.01	XXX	■
A6403		P	Gauze, non-impregnated, sterile, pad size more than 16 sq. in. but less than or equal to 48 sq. in., without adhesive border, each dressing	0.00	0.01	0.01	0.00	0.01	0.01	XXX	■
A6404		P	Gauze, non-impregnated, sterile, pad size more than 48 sq. in., without adhesive border, each dressing	0.00	0.02	0.02	0.00	0.02	0.02	XXX	■
A6405		P	Gauze, elastic, sterile, all types, per linear yard	0.00	0.02	0.02	0.00	0.02	0.02	XXX	■
A6406		P	Gauze, non-elastic, sterile, all types, per linear yard	0.00	0.02	0.02	0.00	0.02	0.02	XXX	■
A7000		X	Canister, disposable, used with suction pump, each	0.00	0.33	0.33	0.00	0.33	0.33	XXX	■
A7001		X	Canister, non-disposable, used with suction pump, each	0.00	1.11	1.11	0.00	1.11	1.11	XXX	■

■ RVU not developed by CMS. Gap-filled RVUs developed by CHEG.

Code	M	S	Description	Work Value	Non-Fac PE	Fac PE	Mal-prac-tice	Non-Fac Total	Fac Total	Global	Gap
A7002		X	Tubing, used with suction pump, each	0.00	0.13	0.13	0.00	0.13	0.13	XXX	■
A7003		X	Administration set, with small volume nonfiltered pneumatic nebulizer, disposable	0.00	0.09	0.09	0.00	0.09	0.09	XXX	■
A7004		X	Small volume nonfiltered pneumatic nebulizer, disposable	0.00	0.06	0.06	0.00	0.06	0.06	XXX	■
A7005		X	Administration set, with small volume nonfiltered pneumatic nebulizer, non-disposable	0.00	1.05	1.05	0.00	1.05	1.05	XXX	■
A7006		X	Administration set, with small volume filtered pneumatic nebulizer	0.00	0.32	0.32	0.00	0.32	0.32	XXX	■
A7007		X	Large volume nebulizer, disposable, unfilled, used with aerosol compressor	0.00	0.16	0.16	0.00	0.16	0.16	XXX	■
A7008		X	Large volume nebulizer, disposable, prefilled, used with aerosol compressor	0.00	0.37	0.37	0.00	0.37	0.37	XXX	■
A7009		X	Reservoir bottle, non-disposable, used with large volume ultrasonic nebulizer	0.00	1.42	1.42	0.00	1.42	1.42	XXX	■
A7010		X	Corrugated tubing, disposable, used with large volume nebulizer, 100 feet	0.00	0.80	0.80	0.00	0.80	0.80	XXX	■
A7011		X	Corrugated tubing, non-disposable, used with large volume nebulizer, 10 feet	0.00	0.73	0.73	0.00	0.73	0.73	XXX	■
A7012		X	Water collection device, used with large volume nebulizer	0.00	0.13	0.13	0.00	0.13	0.13	XXX	■
A7013		X	Filter, disposable, used with aerosol compressor	0.00	0.03	0.03	0.00	0.03	0.03	XXX	■
A7014		X	Filter, non-disposable, used with aerosol compressor or ultrasonic generator	0.00	0.16	0.16	0.00	0.16	0.16	XXX	■
A7015		X	Aerosol mask, used with DME nebulizer	0.00	0.06	0.06	0.00	0.06	0.06	XXX	■
A7016		X	Dome and mouthpiece, used with small volume ultrasonic nebulizer	0.00	0.25	0.25	0.00	0.25	0.25	XXX	■
A7017		X	Nebulizer, durable, glass or autoclavable plastic, bottle type, not used with oxygen	0.00	0.00	0.00	0.00	0.00	0.00	XXX	
A7018		X	Water, distilled, used with large volume nebulizer, 1000 ml	0.00	0.02	0.02	0.00	0.02	0.02	XXX	■
A7019		X	Saline solution, per 10 ml, metered dose dispenser, for use with inhalation drugs	0.00	0.01	0.01	0.00	0.01	0.01	XXX	■
A7020		X	Sterile water or sterile saline, 1000 ml, used with large volume nebulizer	0.00	0.00	0.00	0.00	0.00	0.00	XXX	
A7501		X	Tracheostoma valve, including diaphragm, each	0.00	0.00	0.00	0.00	0.00	0.00	XXX	
A7502		X	Replacement diaphragm/faceplate for tracheostoma valve, each	0.00	0.00	0.00	0.00	0.00	0.00	XXX	

■ RVU not developed by CMS. Gap-filled RVUs developed by CHEG.

Code	M	S	Description	Work Value	Non-Fac PE	Fac PE	Mal-practice	Non-Fac Total	Fac Total	Global	Gap
A7503		X	Filter holder or filter cap, reusable, for use in a tracheostoma heat and moisture exchange system, each	0.00	0.00	0.00	0.00	0.00	0.00	XXX	
A7504		X	Filter for use in a tracheostoma heat and moisture exchange system, each	0.00	0.00	0.00	0.00	0.00	0.00	XXX	
A7505		X	Housing, reusable without adhesive, for use in a heat and moisture exchange system and/or with a tracheostoma valve, each	0.00	0.00	0.00	0.00	0.00	0.00	XXX	
A7506		X	Adhesive disc for use in a heat and moisture exchange system and/or with tracheostoma valve, any type each	0.00	0.00	0.00	0.00	0.00	0.00	XXX	
A7507		X	Filter holder and integrated filter without adhesive, for use in a tracheostoma heat and moisture exchange system, each	0.00	0.00	0.00	0.00	0.00	0.00	XXX	
A7508		X	Housing and integrated adhesive, for use in a tracheostoma heat and moisture exchange system and/or with a tracheostoma valve, each	0.00	0.00	0.00	0.00	0.00	0.00	XXX	
A7509		X	Filter holder and integrated filter housing, and adhesive, for use as a tracheostoma heat and moisture exchange system, each	0.00	0.00	0.00	0.00	0.00	0.00	XXX	
A9150		E	Nonprescription drug	0.00	0.00	0.00	0.00	0.00	0.00	XXX	
A9270		N	Noncovered item or service	0.00	0.00	0.00	0.00	0.00	0.00	XXX	
A9300		N	Exercise equipment	0.00	0.00	0.00	0.00	0.00	0.00	XXX	
A9500		E	Supply of radiopharmaceutical diagnostic imaging agent, technetium Tc 99m sestamibi, per dose	0.00	0.00	0.00	0.00	0.00	0.00	XXX	
A9502		X	Supply of radiopharmaceutical diagnostic imaging agent, technetium Tc 99m tetrofosmin, per unit dose	0.00	0.00	0.00	0.00	0.00	0.00	XXX	
A9503		E	Supply of radiopharmaceutical diagnostic imaging agent, technetium Tc 99m, medronate, up to 30 microcurie	0.00	0.00	0.00	0.00	0.00	0.00	XXX	
A9504		X	Supply of radiopharmaceutical diagnostic imaging agent, technetium Tc 99m apcitide	0.00	0.00	0.00	0.00	0.00	0.00	XXX	
A9505		E	Supply of radiopharmaceutical diagnostic imaging agent, thallous chloride TL-201, per microcurie	0.00	0.00	0.00	0.00	0.00	0.00	XXX	
A9507		X	Supply of radiopharmaceutical diagnostic imaging agent, indium IN 111 capromab pendetide, per dose	0.00	0.00	0.00	0.00	0.00	0.00	XXX	
A9508		X	Supply of radiopharmaceutical diagnostic imaging agent, iobenguane sulfate I-131, per 0.5 microcurie	0.00	0.00	0.00	0.00	0.00	0.00	XXX	

■ RVU not developed by CMS. Gap-filled RVUs developed by CHEG.

Code	M	S	Description	Work Value	Non-Fac PE	Fac PE	Mal-practice	Non-Fac Total	Fac Total	Global	Gap
A9510		X	Supply of radiopharmaceutical diagnostic imaging agent, technetium Tc 99m disofenin, per vial	0.00	0.00	0.00	0.00	0.00	0.00	XXX	
A9511		X	Supply of radiopharmaceutical diagnostic imaging agent, technetium Tc 99m, Depreotide, per microcurie	0.00	0.00	0.00	0.00	0.00	0.00	XXX	
A9600		X	Supply of therapeutic radiopharmaceutical, strontium-89 chloride, per microcurie	0.00	21.25	21.25	0.00	21.25	21.25	XXX	■
A9605		X	Supply of therapeutic radiopharmaceutical, samarium sm 153 lexidronamm, 50 microcurie	0.00	0.00	0.00	0.00	0.00	0.00	XXX	
A9700		X	Supply of injectable contrast material for use in echocardiography, per study	0.00	0.00	0.00	0.00	0.00	0.00	XXX	
A9900		X	Miscellaneous DME supply, accessory, and/or service component of another HCPCS code	0.00	0.00	0.00	0.00	0.00	0.00	XXX	
A9901		X	DME delivery, set up, and/or dispensing service component of another HCPCS code	0.00	0.00	0.00	0.00	0.00	0.00	XXX	
B4034			Enteral feeding supply kit; syringe, per day	0.00	0.00	0.00	0.00	0.00	0.00	XXX	
B4035			Enteral feeding supply kit; pump fed, per day	0.00	0.00	0.00	0.00	0.00	0.00	XXX	
B4036			Enteral feeding supply kit; gravity fed, per day	0.00	0.00	0.00	0.00	0.00	0.00	XXX	
B4081			Nasogastric tubing with stylet	0.00	0.75	0.75	0.00	0.75	0.75	XXX	■
B4082			Nasogastric tubing without stylet	0.00	0.39	0.39	0.00	0.39	0.39	XXX	■
B4083			Stomach tube — Levine type	0.00	0.10	0.10	0.00	0.10	0.10	XXX	■
B4086			Gastrostomy/jejunostomy tube, any material, any type, (standard or low profile), each	0.00	0.00	0.00	0.00	0.00	0.00	XXX	
B4150			Enteral formulae; category I; semi-synthetic intact protein/protein isolates, administered through an enteral feeding tube, 100 calories = 1 unit	0.00	0.08	0.08	0.00	0.08	0.08	XXX	■
B4151			Enteral formulae; category I: natural intact protein/protein isolates, administered through an enteral feeding tube, 100 calories = 1 unit	0.00	0.08	0.08	0.00	0.08	0.08	XXX	■
B4152			Enteral formulae; category II: intact protein/protein isolates (calorically dense), administered through an enteral feeding tube, 100 calories = 1 unit	0.00	0.08	0.08	0.00	0.08	0.08	XXX	■
B4153			Enteral formulae; category III: hydrolized protein/amino acids, administered through an enteral feeding tube, 100 calories = 1 unit	0.00	0.28	0.28	0.00	0.28	0.28	XXX	■
B4154			Enteral formulae; category IV: defined formula for special metabolic need, administered through an enteral feeding tube, 100 calories = 1 unit	0.00	0.38	0.38	0.00	0.38	0.38	XXX	■

■ RVU not developed by CMS. Gap-filled RVUs developed by CHEG.

Code	M	S	Description	Work Value	Non-Fac PE	Fac PE	Mal-practice	Non-Fac Total	Fac Total	Global	Gap
B4155			Enteral formulae; category V: modular components, administered through an enteral feeding tube, 100 calories = 1 unit	0.00	0.71	0.71	0.00	0.71	0.71	XXX	■
B4156			Enteral formulae; category VI: standardized nutrients, administered through an enteral feeding tube, 100 calories = 1 unit	0.00	0.27	0.27	0.00	0.27	0.27	XXX	■
B4164			Parenteral nutrition solution; carbohydrates (dextrose), 50% or less (500 ml = 1 unit) — home mix	0.00	0.81	0.81	0.00	0.81	0.81	XXX	■
B4168			Parenteral nutrition solution; amino acid, 3.5%, (500 ml = 1 unit) — home mix	0.00	1.55	1.55	0.00	1.55	1.55	XXX	■
B4172			Parenteral nutrition solution; amino acid, 5.5% through 7%, (500 ml = 1 unit) — home mix	0.00	2.33	2.33	0.00	2.33	2.33	XXX	■
B4176			Parenteral nutrition solution; amino acid, 7% through 8.5%, (500 ml = 1 unit) — home mix	0.00	2.65	2.65	0.00	2.65	2.65	XXX	■
B4178			Parenteral nutrition solution; amino acid, greater than 8.5% (500 ml = 1 unit) — home mix	0.00	3.37	3.37	0.00	3.37	3.37	XXX	■
B4180			Parenteral nutrition solution; carbohydrates (dextrose), greater than 50% (500 ml = 1 unit) — home mix	0.00	1.11	1.11	0.00	1.11	1.11	XXX	■
B4184			Parenteral nutrition solution; lipids, 10% with administration set (500 ml = 1 unit)	0.00	2.45	2.45	0.00	2.45	2.45	XXX	■
B4186			Parenteral nutrition solution; lipids, 20% with administration set (500 ml = 1 unit)	0.00	3.22	3.22	0.00	3.22	3.22	XXX	■
B4189			Parenteral nutrition solution; compounded amino acid and carbohydrates with electrolytes, trace elements, and vitamins, including preparation, any strength, 10 to 51 grams of protein — premix	0.00	3.87	3.87	0.00	3.87	3.87	XXX	■
B4193			Parenteral nutrition solution; compounded amino acid and carbohydrates with electrolytes, trace elements, and vitamins, including preparation, any strength, 52 to 73 grams of protein — premix	0.00	4.18	4.18	0.00	4.18	4.18	XXX	■
B4197			Parenteral nutrition solution; compounded amino acid and carbohydrates with electrolytes, trace elements and vitamins, including preparation, any strength, 74 to 100 grams of protein — premix	0.00	4.34	4.34	0.00	4.34	4.34	XXX	■
B4199			Parenteral nutrition solution; compounded amino acid and carbohydrates with electrolytes, trace elements and vitamins, including preparation, any strength, over 100 grams of protein — premix	0.00	4.58	4.58	0.00	4.58	4.58	XXX	■
B4216			Parenteral nutrition; additives (vitamins, trace elements, heparin, electrolytes) — home mix, per day	0.00	0.00	0.00	0.00	0.00	0.00	XXX	

■ RVU not developed by CMS. Gap-filled RVUs developed by CHEG.

Code	M	S	Description	Work Value	Non-Fac PE	Fac PE	Mal-practice	Non-Fac Total	Fac Total	Global	Gap
B4220			Parenteral nutrition supply kit; premix, per day	0.00	0.00	0.00	0.00	0.00	0.00	XXX	
B4222			Parenteral nutrition supply kit; home mix, per day	0.00	0.00	0.00	0.00	0.00	0.00	XXX	
B4224			Parenteral nutrition administration kit, per day	0.00	0.71	0.71	0.00	0.71	0.71	XXX	■
B5000			Parenteral nutrition solution; compounded amino acid and carbohydrates with electrolytes, trace elements, and vitamins, including preparation, any strength, renal — amirosyn RF, nephramine, renamine — premix	0.00	2.51	2.51	0.00	2.51	2.51	XXX	■
B5100			Parenteral nutrition solution; compounded amino acid and carbohydrates with electrolytes, trace elements, and vitamins, including preparation, any strength, hepatic — freamine HBC, hepatamine — premix	0.00	3.11	3.11	0.00	3.11	3.11	XXX	■
B5200			Parenteral nutrition solution; compounded amino acid and carbohydrates with electrolytes, trace elements, and vitamins, including preparation, any strength, stress — branch chain amino acids — premix	0.00	0.00	0.00	0.00	0.00	0.00	XXX	
B9000	NU		Enteral nutrition infusion pump — without alarm	0.00	28.29	28.29	0.00	28.29	28.29	XXX	■
	RR			0.00	2.74	2.74	0.00	2.74	2.74	XXX	■
	UE			0.00	18.14	18.14	0.00	18.14	18.14	XXX	■
B9002	NU		Enteral nutrition infusion pump — with alarm	0.00	30.44	30.44	0.00	30.44	30.44	XXX	■
	RR			0.00	3.74	3.74	0.00	3.74	3.74	XXX	■
B9004	NU		Parenteral nutrition infusion pump, portable	0.00	0.00	0.00	0.00	0.00	0.00	XXX	
	RR			0.00	0.63	0.63	0.00	0.63	0.63	XXX	■
	UE			0.00	0.00	0.00	0.00	0.00	0.00	XXX	
B9006	NU		Parenteral nutrition infusion pump, stationary	0.00	0.00	0.00	0.00	0.00	0.00	XXX	
	RR			0.00	0.37	0.37	0.00	0.37	0.37	XXX	■
	UE			0.00	0.00	0.00	0.00	0.00	0.00	XXX	
B9998			NOC for enteral supplies	0.00	0.00	0.00	0.00	0.00	0.00	XXX	
B9999			NOC for parenteral supplies	0.00	0.00	0.00	0.00	0.00	0.00	XXX	
C1010			Blood, leukoreduced CMV-negative, each unit	0.00	0.00	0.00	0.00	0.00	0.00	XXX	
C1011			Platelet, HLA-matched leukoreduced, apheresis/pheresis, each unit	0.00	0.00	0.00	0.00	0.00	0.00	XXX	
C1012			Platelet concentrate, leukoreduced, irradiated, each unit	0.00	0.00	0.00	0.00	0.00	0.00	XXX	
C1013			Platelet concentrate, leukoreduced, each unit	0.00	0.00	0.00	0.00	0.00	0.00	XXX	
C1014			Platelet, leukoreduced, apheresis/pheresis, each unit	0.00	0.00	0.00	0.00	0.00	0.00	XXX	
C1016			Blood, leukoreduced, frozen/deglycerol/washed, each unit	0.00	0.00	0.00	0.00	0.00	0.00	XXX	

■ RVU not developed by CMS. Gap-filled RVUs developed by CHEG.

Code	M	S	Description	Work Value	Non-Fac PE	Fac PE	Mal-practice	Non-Fac Total	Fac Total	Global	Gap
C1017			Platelet, leukoreduced, CMV-negative, apheresis/pheresis, each unit	0.00	0.00	0.00	0.00	0.00	0.00	XXX	
C1018			Blood, leukoreduced, irradiated, each unit	0.00	0.00	0.00	0.00	0.00	0.00	XXX	
C1031			Electrode, needle, ablation, MR Compatible Leveen, modified Leveen needle electrode	0.00	0.00	0.00	0.00	0.00	0.00	XXX	
C1045			Supply of radiopharmaceutical diagnostic imaging agent, I-131 MIBG [iobenguane sulfate I-131], per 0.5 microcurie	0.00	0.00	0.00	0.00	0.00	0.00	XXX	
C1058			Supply of radiopharmaceutical diagnostic imaging agent, Technetium TC 99m Oxidronate, per vial	0.00	0.00	0.00	0.00	0.00	0.00	XXX	
C1064			Supply of radiopharmaceutical therapeutic imaging agent, Sodium Iodide I-131, capsule, each additional microcurie	0.00	0.00	0.00	0.00	0.00	0.00	XXX	
C1065			Supply of radiopharmacuetical therapeutic imaging agent, Sodium Iodide I-131, solution, each additional microcurie	0.00	0.00	0.00	0.00	0.00	0.00	XXX	
C1066			Supply of radiopharmaceutical diagnostic imaging agent, Indium 111 satumomab pendetide, per vial	0.00	0.00	0.00	0.00	0.00	0.00	XXX	
C1079			Supply of radiopharmaceutical diagnostic imaging agent, cyanocobalamin co 57/58, per 0.5 microcurie	0.00	0.00	0.00	0.00	0.00	0.00	XXX	
C1087			Supply of radiopharmaceutical diagnostic imaging agent, sodium iodide 1-123 per 100 microcurie	0.00	0.00	0.00	0.00	0.00	0.00	XXX	
C1088			Laser optic treatment system, Indigo Laseroptic Treatment System	0.00	0.00	0.00	0.00	0.00	0.00	XXX	
C1089			Supply of radiopharmaceutical diagnostic imaging agent, cyanocobalamin Co 57, 0.5 microcurie, capsule	0.00	0.00	0.00	0.00	0.00	0.00	XXX	
C1091			Supply of radiopharmaceutical diagnostic imaging agent, indium 111 oxyquinoline, per 0.5 millicurie	0.00	0.00	0.00	0.00	0.00	0.00	XXX	
C1092			Supply of radiopharmaceutical diagnostic imaging agent, indium 111 pentetate, per 0.5 millicurie	0.00	0.00	0.00	0.00	0.00	0.00	XXX	
C1094			Supply of radiopharmaceutical diagnostic imaging agent, technetium tc 99m albumin aggregated, per 1.0 millicurie	0.00	0.00	0.00	0.00	0.00	0.00	XXX	
C1096			Supply of radiopharmaceutical diagnostic imaging agent, technetium Tc 99m exametazime, per dose	0.00	0.00	0.00	0.00	0.00	0.00	XXX	
C1097			Supply of radiopharmaceutical diagnostic imaging agent, technetium Tc 99m mebrofenin, per vial	0.00	0.00	0.00	0.00	0.00	0.00	XXX	

■ RVU not developed by CMS. Gap-filled RVUs developed by CHEG.

Code	M	S	Description	Work Value	Non-Fac PE	Fac PE	Mal-practice	Non-Fac Total	Fac Total	Global	Gap
C1098			Supply of radiopharmaceutical diagnostic imaging agent, technetium Tc 99m pentetate, per vial	0.00	0.00	0.00	0.00	0.00	0.00	XXX	
C1099			Supply of radiopharmaceutical diagnostic imaging agent, technetium Tc 99m pyrophosphate, per vial	0.00	0.00	0.00	0.00	0.00	0.00	XXX	
C1122			Supply of radiopharmaceutical diagnostic imaging agent, technetium Tc 99m arcitumomab, per vial	0.00	0.00	0.00	0.00	0.00	0.00	XXX	
C1146			Endotracheal tube, Vett Tracheobronchial Tube	0.00	0.00	0.00	0.00	0.00	0.00	XXX	
C1166			Injection, cytarabine liposome, 10 mg, depocyt/ liposomal cytarabine	0.00	0.00	0.00	0.00	0.00	0.00	XXX	
C1167			Injection, epirubicin hydrochloride, 2 mg	0.00	0.00	0.00	0.00	0.00	0.00	XXX	
C1170			Biopsy device, breast, abbi device	0.00	0.00	0.00	0.00	0.00	0.00	XXX	
C1175			Biopsy device, MIBB device	0.00	0.00	0.00	0.00	0.00	0.00	XXX	
C1176			Biopsy device, Mammotome HH Hand-Held Probe with Smartvac Vacuum System	0.00	0.00	0.00	0.00	0.00	0.00	XXX	
C1177			Biopsy Device, 11-Gauge Mammotome Probe with Vacuum Cannister	0.00	0.00	0.00	0.00	0.00	0.00	XXX	
C1178			Injection, busulfan (busulfex IV) per 6 mg	0.00	0.00	0.00	0.00	0.00	0.00	XXX	
C1179			Biopsy device, 14-Gauge Mammotome Probe With Vacuum Cannister	0.00	0.00	0.00	0.00	0.00	0.00	XXX	
C1188			Supply of radiopharmaceutical therapeutic imaging agent, sodium iodide I-131, capsule, per initial 1-5 microcurie	0.00	0.00	0.00	0.00	0.00	0.00	XXX	
C1200			Supply of radiopharmaceutical diagnostic imaging agent, technetium Tc 99m sodium glucoheptonate, per vial	0.00	0.00	0.00	0.00	0.00	0.00	XXX	
C1201			Supply of radiopharmaceutical diagnostic imaging agent, technetium Tc 99m succimer, per vial	0.00	0.00	0.00	0.00	0.00	0.00	XXX	
C1202			Supply of radiopharmaceutical diagnostic imaging agent, technetium Tc 99m sulfur colloid, per dose	0.00	0.00	0.00	0.00	0.00	0.00	XXX	
C1207			Octreotide acetate, 1 mg	0.00	0.00	0.00	0.00	0.00	0.00	XXX	
C1300			Hyperbaric oxygen under pressure, full body chamber, per 30 minute interval	0.00	0.00	0.00	0.00	0.00	0.00	XXX	
C1305			Apligraf, per 44 sq cm	0.00	0.00	0.00	0.00	0.00	0.00	XXX	
C1321			Electrode, disposable, Palate Somnoplasty Coagulating Electrode, Base Of Tongue Somnoplasty Coagulating Electrode	0.00	0.00	0.00	0.00	0.00	0.00	XXX	

■ RVU not developed by CMS. Gap-filled RVUs developed by CHEG.

Code	M	S	Description	Work Value	Non-Fac PE	Fac PE	Mal-practice	Non-Fac Total	Fac Total	Global	Gap
C1322			Electrode, disposable, Turbinate Somnoplasty Coagulating Electrode	0.00	0.00	0.00	0.00	0.00	0.00	XXX	
C1323			Electrode, disposable, VAPR Electrode, VAPR T Thermal Electrode	0.00	0.00	0.00	0.00	0.00	0.00	XXX	
C1324			Electrode, disposable, Ligasure Disposable Electrode	0.00	0.00	0.00	0.00	0.00	0.00	XXX	
C1329			Electrode, disposable, Gynecare Versapoint Resectoscopic System Bipolar Electrode	0.00	0.00	0.00	0.00	0.00	0.00	XXX	
C1348			Supply of radiopharmaceutical therapeutic imaging agent, sodium iodide I-131, solution, per initial 1-6 microcurie	0.00	0.00	0.00	0.00	0.00	0.00	XXX	
C1360			Ocular photodynamic therapy	0.00	0.00	0.00	0.00	0.00	0.00	XXX	
C1368			Infusion System, On-Q Pain Management System, On-Q Soaker Pain Management System, and Painbuster Pain Management System	0.00	0.00	0.00	0.00	0.00	0.00	XXX	
C1713			Anchor/screw for opposing bone-to-bone or soft tissue-to-bone (implantable)	0.00	0.00	0.00	0.00	0.00	0.00	XXX	
C1714			Catheter, transluminal atherectomy, directional	0.00	0.00	0.00	0.00	0.00	0.00	XXX	
C1715			Brachytherapy needle	0.00	0.00	0.00	0.00	0.00	0.00	XXX	
C1716			Brachytherapy seed, Gold 198	0.00	0.00	0.00	0.00	0.00	0.00	XXX	
C1717			Brachytherapy seed, high dose rate iridium 192	0.00	0.00	0.00	0.00	0.00	0.00	XXX	
C1718			Brachytherapy seed, Iodine 125	0.00	0.00	0.00	0.00	0.00	0.00	XXX	
C1719			Brachytherapy seed, non-high dose rate Iridium 192	0.00	0.00	0.00	0.00	0.00	0.00	XXX	
C1720			Brachytherapy seed, palladium 103	0.00	0.00	0.00	0.00	0.00	0.00	XXX	
C1721			Cardioverter-defibrillator, dual chamber (implantable)	0.00	0.00	0.00	0.00	0.00	0.00	XXX	
C1722			Cardioverter-defibrillator, single chamber (implantable)	0.00	0.00	0.00	0.00	0.00	0.00	XXX	
C1724			Catheter, transluminal atherectomy, rotational	0.00	0.00	0.00	0.00	0.00	0.00	XXX	
C1725			Catheter, transluminal angioplasty, non-laser (may include guidance, infusion/perfusion capability)	0.00	0.00	0.00	0.00	0.00	0.00	XXX	
C1726			Catheter, balloon dilatation, non-vascular	0.00	0.00	0.00	0.00	0.00	0.00	XXX	
C1727			Catheter, balloon tissue dissector, non-vascular (insertable)	0.00	0.00	0.00	0.00	0.00	0.00	XXX	
C1728			Catheter, brachytherapy seed administration	0.00	0.00	0.00	0.00	0.00	0.00	XXX	
C1729			Catheter, drainage	0.00	0.00	0.00	0.00	0.00	0.00	XXX	

■ RVU not developed by CMS. Gap-filled RVUs developed by CHEG.

Code	M	S	Description	Work Value	Non-Fac PE	Fac PE	Mal-prac-tice	Non-Fac Total	Fac Total	Global	Gap
C1730			Catheter, electrophysiology, diagnostic, other than 3D mapping (19 or fewer electrodes)	0.00	0.00	0.00	0.00	0.00	0.00	XXX	
C1731			Catheter, electrophysiology, diagnostic, other than 3D mapping (20 or more electrodes)	0.00	0.00	0.00	0.00	0.00	0.00	XXX	
C1732			Catheter, electrophysiology, diagnostic/ ablation, 3D or vector mapping	0.00	0.00	0.00	0.00	0.00	0.00	XXX	
C1733			Catheter, electrophysiology, diagnostic/ ablation, other than 3D or vector mapping, other than cool-tip	0.00	0.00	0.00	0.00	0.00	0.00	XXX	
C1750			Catheter, hemodialysis, long-term	0.00	0.00	0.00	0.00	0.00	0.00	XXX	
C1751			Catheter, infusion, inserted peripherally, centrally or midline (other than hemodialysis)	0.00	0.00	0.00	0.00	0.00	0.00	XXX	
C1752			Catheter, hemodialysis, short-term	0.00	0.00	0.00	0.00	0.00	0.00	XXX	
C1753			Catheter, intravascular ultrasound	0.00	0.00	0.00	0.00	0.00	0.00	XXX	
C1754			Catheter, intradiscal	0.00	0.00	0.00	0.00	0.00	0.00	XXX	
C1755			Catheter, intraspinal	0.00	0.00	0.00	0.00	0.00	0.00	XXX	
C1756			Catheter, pacing, transesophageal	0.00	0.00	0.00	0.00	0.00	0.00	XXX	
C1757			Catheter, thrombectomy/embolectomy	0.00	0.00	0.00	0.00	0.00	0.00	XXX	
C1758			Catheter, ureteral	0.00	0.00	0.00	0.00	0.00	0.00	XXX	
C1759			Catheter, intracardiac echocardiography	0.00	0.00	0.00	0.00	0.00	0.00	XXX	
C1760			Closure device, vascular (implantable/ insertable)	0.00	0.00	0.00	0.00	0.00	0.00	XXX	
C1762			Connective tissue, human (includes fascia lata)	0.00	0.00	0.00	0.00	0.00	0.00	XXX	
C1763			Connective tissue, non-human (includes synthetic)	0.00	0.00	0.00	0.00	0.00	0.00	XXX	
C1764			Event recorder, cardiac (implantable)	0.00	0.00	0.00	0.00	0.00	0.00	XXX	
C1765			Adhesion barrier	0.00	0.00	0.00	0.00	0.00	0.00	XXX	
C1766			Introducer/sheath, guiding, intracardiac electrophysiological, steerable, other than peel-away	0.00	0.00	0.00	0.00	0.00	0.00	XXX	
C1767			Generator, neurostimulator (implantable)	0.00	0.00	0.00	0.00	0.00	0.00	XXX	
C1768			Graft, vascular	0.00	0.00	0.00	0.00	0.00	0.00	XXX	
C1769			Guide wire	0.00	0.00	0.00	0.00	0.00	0.00	XXX	
C1770			Imaging coil, magnetic resonance (insertable)	0.00	0.00	0.00	0.00	0.00	0.00	XXX	
C1771			Repair device, urinary, incontinence, with sling graft	0.00	0.00	0.00	0.00	0.00	0.00	XXX	

Code	M	S	Description	Work Value	Non-Fac PE	Fac PE	Mal-prac-tice	Non-Fac Total	Fac Total	Global	Gap
C1772			Infusion pump, programmable (implantable)	0.00	0.00	0.00	0.00	0.00	0.00	XXX	
C1773			Retrieval device, insertable (used to retrieve fractured medical devices)	0.00	0.00	0.00	0.00	0.00	0.00	XXX	
C1776			Joint device (implantable)	0.00	0.00	0.00	0.00	0.00	0.00	XXX	
C1777			Lead, cardioverter-defibrillator, endocardial single coil (implantable)	0.00	0.00	0.00	0.00	0.00	0.00	XXX	
C1778			Lead, neurostimulator (implantable)	0.00	0.00	0.00	0.00	0.00	0.00	XXX	
C1779			Lead, pacemaker, transvenous VDD single pass	0.00	0.00	0.00	0.00	0.00	0.00	XXX	
C1780			Lens, intraocular (new technology)	0.00	0.00	0.00	0.00	0.00	0.00	XXX	
C1781			Mesh (implantable)	0.00	0.00	0.00	0.00	0.00	0.00	XXX	
C1782			Morcellator	0.00	0.00	0.00	0.00	0.00	0.00	XXX	
C1784			Ocular device, intraoperative, detached retina	0.00	0.00	0.00	0.00	0.00	0.00	XXX	
C1785			Pacemaker, dual chamber, rate-responsive (implantable)	0.00	0.00	0.00	0.00	0.00	0.00	XXX	
C1786			Pacemaker, single chamber, rate-responsive (implantable)	0.00	0.00	0.00	0.00	0.00	0.00	XXX	
C1787			Patient programmer, neurostimulator	0.00	0.00	0.00	0.00	0.00	0.00	XXX	
C1788			Port, indwelling (implantable)	0.00	0.00	0.00	0.00	0.00	0.00	XXX	
C1789			Prosthesis, breast (implantable)	0.00	0.00	0.00	0.00	0.00	0.00	XXX	
C1813			Prosthesis, penile, inflatable	0.00	0.00	0.00	0.00	0.00	0.00	XXX	
C1815			Prosthesis, urinary sphincter (implantable)	0.00	0.00	0.00	0.00	0.00	0.00	XXX	
C1816			Receiver and/or transmitter, neurostimulator (implantable)	0.00	0.00	0.00	0.00	0.00	0.00	XXX	
C1817			Septal defect implant system, intracardiac	0.00	0.00	0.00	0.00	0.00	0.00	XXX	
C1874			Stent, coated/covered, with delivery system	0.00	0.00	0.00	0.00	0.00	0.00	XXX	
C1875			Stent, coated/covered, without delivery system	0.00	0.00	0.00	0.00	0.00	0.00	XXX	
C1876			Stent, non-coated/non-covered, with delivery system	0.00	0.00	0.00	0.00	0.00	0.00	XXX	
C1877			Stent, non-coated/non-covered, without delivery system	0.00	0.00	0.00	0.00	0.00	0.00	XXX	
C1878			Material for vocal cord medialization, synthetic (implantable)	0.00	0.00	0.00	0.00	0.00	0.00	XXX	
C1879			Tissue marker (implantable)	0.00	0.00	0.00	0.00	0.00	0.00	XXX	
C1880			Vena cava filter	0.00	0.00	0.00	0.00	0.00	0.00	XXX	
C1881			Dialysis access system (implantable)	0.00	0.00	0.00	0.00	0.00	0.00	XXX	

■ RVU not developed by CMS. Gap-filled RVUs developed by CHEG.

Code	M	S	Description	Work Value	Non-Fac PE	Fac PE	Mal-practice	Non-Fac Total	Fac Total	Global	Gap
C1882			Cardioverter-defibrillator, other than single or dual chamber (implantable)	0.00	0.00	0.00	0.00	0.00	0.00	XXX	
C1883			Adaptor/extension, pacing lead or neurostimulator lead (implantable)	0.00	0.00	0.00	0.00	0.00	0.00	XXX	
C1885			Catheter, transluminal angioplasty, laser	0.00	0.00	0.00	0.00	0.00	0.00	XXX	
C1887			Catheter, guiding (may include infusion/ perfusion capability)	0.00	0.00	0.00	0.00	0.00	0.00	XXX	
C1891			Infusion pump, non-programmable, permanent (implantable)	0.00	0.00	0.00	0.00	0.00	0.00	XXX	
C1892			Introducer/sheath, guiding, intracardiac electrophysiological, fixed-curve, peel-away	0.00	0.00	0.00	0.00	0.00	0.00	XXX	
C1893			Introducer/sheath, guiding, intracardiac electrophysiological, fixed-curve, other than peel-away	0.00	0.00	0.00	0.00	0.00	0.00	XXX	
C1894			Introducer/sheath, other than guiding, intracardiac electrophysiological, non-laser	0.00	0.00	0.00	0.00	0.00	0.00	XXX	
C1895			Lead, cardioverter-defibrillator, endocardial dual coil (implantable)	0.00	0.00	0.00	0.00	0.00	0.00	XXX	
C1896			Lead, cardioverter-defibrillator, other than endocardial single or dual coil (implantable)	0.00	0.00	0.00	0.00	0.00	0.00	XXX	
C1897			Lead, neurostimulator test kit (implantable)	0.00	0.00	0.00	0.00	0.00	0.00	XXX	
C1898			Lead, pacemaker, other than transvenous vdd single pass	0.00	0.00	0.00	0.00	0.00	0.00	XXX	
C1899			Lead, pacemaker/cardioverter-defibrillator combination (implantable)	0.00	0.00	0.00	0.00	0.00	0.00	XXX	
C2600			Catheter, gold probe single-use electrohemostatis catheter	0.00	0.00	0.00	0.00	0.00	0.00	XXX	
C2615			Sealant, pulmonary, liquid	0.00	0.00	0.00	0.00	0.00	0.00	XXX	
C2616			Brachytherapy seed, yttrium-90	0.00	0.00	0.00	0.00	0.00	0.00	XXX	
C2617			Stent, non-coronary, temporary, without delivery system	0.00	0.00	0.00	0.00	0.00	0.00	XXX	
C2618			Probe, cryoablation	0.00	0.00	0.00	0.00	0.00	0.00	XXX	
C2619			Pacemaker, dual chamber, non-rate-responsive (implantable)	0.00	0.00	0.00	0.00	0.00	0.00	XXX	
C2620			Pacemaker, single chamber, non-rate-responsive (implantable)	0.00	0.00	0.00	0.00	0.00	0.00	XXX	
C2621			Pacemaker, other than single or dual chamber (implantable)	0.00	0.00	0.00	0.00	0.00	0.00	XXX	
C2622			Prosthesis, penile, non-inflatable	0.00	0.00	0.00	0.00	0.00	0.00	XXX	

■ RVU not developed by CMS. Gap-filled RVUs developed by CHEG.

Code	M	S	Description	Work Value	Non-Fac PE	Fac PE	Mal-practice	Non-Fac Total	Fac Total	Global	Gap
C2625			Stent, non-coronary, temporary, with delivery system	0.00	0.00	0.00	0.00	0.00	0.00	XXX	
C2626			Infusion pump, non-programmable, temporary (implantable)	0.00	0.00	0.00	0.00	0.00	0.00	XXX	
C2627			Catheter, suprapubic/cystoscopic	0.00	0.00	0.00	0.00	0.00	0.00	XXX	
C2628			Catheter, occlusion	0.00	0.00	0.00	0.00	0.00	0.00	XXX	
C2629			Introducer/sheath, other than guiding, intracardiac electrophysiological, laser	0.00	0.00	0.00	0.00	0.00	0.00	XXX	
C2630			Catheter, electrophysiology, diagnostic/ ablation, other than 3D or vector mapping, cool-tip	0.00	0.00	0.00	0.00	0.00	0.00	XXX	
C2631			Repair device, urinary, incontinence, without sling graft	0.00	0.00	0.00	0.00	0.00	0.00	XXX	
C8103			Capio Suture Capturing Device, standard or open access	0.00	0.00	0.00	0.00	0.00	0.00	XXX	
C8900			Magnetic resonance angiography with contrast, abdomen	0.00	0.00	0.00	0.00	0.00	0.00	XXX	
C8901			Magnetic resonance angiography without contrast, abdomen	0.00	0.00	0.00	0.00	0.00	0.00	XXX	
C8902			Magnetic resonance angiography without contrast followed by with contrast, abdomen	0.00	0.00	0.00	0.00	0.00	0.00	XXX	
C8903			Magnetic resonance imaging with contrast, breast; unilateral	0.00	0.00	0.00	0.00	0.00	0.00	XXX	
C8904			Magnetic resonance imaging without contrast, breast; unilateral	0.00	0.00	0.00	0.00	0.00	0.00	XXX	
C8905			Magnetic resonance imaging without contrast followed by with contrast, breast; unilateral	0.00	0.00	0.00	0.00	0.00	0.00	XXX	
C8906			Magnetic resonance imaging with contrast, breast; bilateral	0.00	0.00	0.00	0.00	0.00	0.00	XXX	
C8907			Magnetic resonance imaging without contrast, breast; bilateral	0.00	0.00	0.00	0.00	0.00	0.00	XXX	
C8908			Magnetic resonance imaging without contrast followed by with contrast, breast; bilateral	0.00	0.00	0.00	0.00	0.00	0.00	XXX	
C8909			Magnetic resonance angiography with contrast, chest (excluding myocardium)	0.00	0.00	0.00	0.00	0.00	0.00	XXX	
C8910			Magnetic resonance angiography without contrast, chest (excluding myocardium)	0.00	0.00	0.00	0.00	0.00	0.00	XXX	
C8911			Magnetic resonance angiography without contrast followed by with contrast, chest (excluding myocardium)	0.00	0.00	0.00	0.00	0.00	0.00	XXX	
C8912			Magnetic resonance angiography with contrast, lower extremity	0.00	0.00	0.00	0.00	0.00	0.00	XXX	

■ RVU not developed by CMS. Gap-filled RVUs developed by CHEG.

Code	M	S	Description	Work Value	Non-Fac PE	Fac PE	Mal-prac-tice	Non-Fac Total	Fac Total	Global	Gap
C8913			Magnetic resonance angiography without contrast, lower extremity	0.00	0.00	0.00	0.00	0.00	0.00	XXX	
C8914			Magnetic resonance angiography without contrast followed by with contrast, lower extremity	0.00	0.00	0.00	0.00	0.00	0.00	XXX	
C9000			Injection, sodium chromate Cr51, per 0.25 microcurie	0.00	0.00	0.00	0.00	0.00	0.00	XXX	
C9003			Palivizumab-rsv-igm, per 50 mg	0.00	0.00	0.00	0.00	0.00	0.00	XXX	
C9007			Baclofen Intrathecal Screening Kit (1 amp)	0.00	0.00	0.00	0.00	0.00	0.00	XXX	
C9008			Baclofen Intrathecal Refill Kit, per 500 mcg	0.00	0.00	0.00	0.00	0.00	0.00	XXX	
C9009			Baclofen Refill Kit, per 2000 mcg	0.00	0.00	0.00	0.00	0.00	0.00	XXX	
C9010			Baclofen Intrathecal Refill Kit, per 4000 mcg	0.00	0.00	0.00	0.00	0.00	0.00	XXX	
C9013			Supply of CO 57 cobaltous chloride, radiopharmaceutical diagnostic imaging agent	0.00	0.00	0.00	0.00	0.00	0.00	XXX	
C9019			Injection, caspofungin acetate, 5 mg	0.00	0.00	0.00	0.00	0.00	0.00	XXX	
C9020			Sirolimus tablet, 1 mg	0.00	0.00	0.00	0.00	0.00	0.00	XXX	
C9100			Supply of radiopharmaceutical diagnostic imaging agent, iodinated I-131 albumin, per microcurie	0.00	0.00	0.00	0.00	0.00	0.00	XXX	
C9102			Supply of radiopharmaceutical diagnostic imaging agent, 51 sodium chromate, per 50 microcurie	0.00	0.00	0.00	0.00	0.00	0.00	XXX	
C9103			Supply of radiopharmaceutical diagnostic imaging agent, sodium iothalamate I-125 injection, per 10 uCi	0.00	0.00	0.00	0.00	0.00	0.00	XXX	
C9105			Injection, hepatitis B immune globulin, per 1 ml	0.00	0.00	0.00	0.00	0.00	0.00	XXX	
C9108			Injection, thyrotropin alpha, 1.1 mg	0.00	0.00	0.00	0.00	0.00	0.00	XXX	
C9109			Injection, tirofiban hydrochloride, 6.25 mg	0.00	0.00	0.00	0.00	0.00	0.00	XXX	
C9110			Alemtuzumab, per 10 mg/ ml	0.00	0.00	0.00	0.00	0.00	0.00	XXX	
C9111			Injection, bivalirudin, 250 mg per vial	0.00	0.00	0.00	0.00	0.00	0.00	XXX	
C9112			Injection, perflutren lipid microsphere, per 2 ml vial	0.00	0.00	0.00	0.00	0.00	0.00	XXX	
C9113			Injection, pantoprazole sodium, per vial	0.00	0.00	0.00	0.00	0.00	0.00	XXX	
C9114			Injection, nesiritide, per 1.5 mg vial	0.00	0.00	0.00	0.00	0.00	0.00	XXX	
C9115			Injection, zoledronic acid, per 2 mg	0.00	0.00	0.00	0.00	0.00	0.00	XXX	
C9200			Orcel, per 36 sq cm	0.00	0.00	0.00	0.00	0.00	0.00	XXX	

■ RVU not developed by CMS. Gap-filled RVUs developed by CHEG.

Code	M	S	Description	Work Value	Non-Fac PE	Fac PE	Mal-practice	Non-Fac Total	Fac Total	Global	Gap
C9201			Dermagraft, per 37.5 sq cm	0.00	0.00	0.00	0.00	0.00	0.00	XXX	
C9503			Fresh frozen plasma, donor retested, each unit	0.00	0.00	0.00	0.00	0.00	0.00	XXX	
C9701			Stretta System	0.00	0.00	0.00	0.00	0.00	0.00	XXX	
C9703			Bard Endoscopic Suturing System	0.00	0.00	0.00	0.00	0.00	0.00	XXX	
C9708			Preview treatment planning software	0.00	0.00	0.00	0.00	0.00	0.00	XXX	
C9711			H.E.L.P. apheresis system	0.00	0.00	0.00	0.00	0.00	0.00	XXX	
D0120		N	Periodic oral examination	0.29	0.16	0.16	0.01	0.46	0.46	XXX	■
D0140		N	Limited oral evaluation — problem focused	0.48	0.27	0.27	0.02	0.77	0.77	XXX	■
D0150		R	Comprehensive oral evaluation	0.50	0.28	0.28	0.02	0.80	0.80	YYY	■
D0160		N	Detailed and extensive oral evaluation — problem focused, by report	1.40	0.79	0.79	0.05	2.24	2.24	XXX	■
D0170		N	Re-evaluation — limited, problem focused (Established patient; not post-operative visit)	0.35	0.20	0.20	0.01	0.56	0.56	XXX	■
D0210		I	Intraoral — complete series (including bitewings). See also code 70320.	0.21	1.13	1.13	0.06	1.40	1.40	XXX	■
D0220		I	Intraoral — periapical, first film. See also code 70300.	0.04	0.22	0.22	0.01	0.27	0.27	XXX	■
D0230		I	Intraoral — periapical, each additional film. See also code 70310.	0.03	0.17	0.17	0.01	0.21	0.21	XXX	■
D0240		R	Intraoral — occlusal film	0.06	0.32	0.32	0.02	0.39	0.39	YYY	■
D0250		R	Extraoral — first film	0.08	0.43	0.43	0.02	0.53	0.53	YYY	■
D0260		R	Extraoral — each additional film	0.08	0.42	0.42	0.02	0.52	0.52	YYY	■
D0270		R	Bitewing — single film	0.04	0.23	0.23	0.01	0.29	0.29	YYY	■
D0272		R	Bitewings — two films	0.07	0.36	0.36	0.02	0.45	0.45	YYY	■
D0274		R	Bitewings — four films	0.10	0.51	0.51	0.03	0.63	0.63	YYY	■
D0277		R	Vertical bitewings — 7 to 8 films	0.15	0.79	0.79	0.04	0.98	0.98	XXX	■
D0290		I	Posterior-anterior or lateral skull and facial bone survey film. See also code 70150.	0.33	1.76	1.76	0.09	2.17	2.17	XXX	■
D0310		I	Sialography. See also code 70390.	0.84	4.48	4.48	0.22	5.54	5.54	XXX	■
D0320		I	Temporomandibular joint arthrogram, including injection. See also code 70332.	1.43	7.68	7.68	0.38	9.49	9.49	XXX	■
D0321		I	Other temporomandibular joint films, by report. See also code 76499.	0.00	0.00	0.00	0.00	0.00	0.00	XXX	
D0322		I	Tomographic survey. See also CPT.	1.15	6.16	6.16	0.30	7.61	7.61	XXX	■
D0330		I	Panoramic film. See also code 70320.	0.20	1.05	1.05	0.05	1.30	1.30	XXX	■

■ RVU not developed by CMS. Gap-filled RVUs developed by CHEG.

Code	M	S	Description	Work Value	Non-Fac PE	Fac PE	Mal-practice	Non-Fac Total	Fac Total	Global	Gap
D0340		I	Cephalometric film. See also code 70350.	0.24	1.30	1.30	0.06	1.61	1.61	XXX	■
D0350		I	Oral/facial images (includes intra and extraoral images)	0.11	0.57	0.57	0.03	0.70	0.70	XXX	■
D0415		N	Bacteriologic studies for determination of pathologic agents	0.17	0.31	0.31	0.01	0.49	0.49	XXX	■
D0425		N	Caries susceptibility tests	0.11	0.20	0.20	0.01	0.32	0.32	XXX	■
D0460		R	Pulp vitality tests	0.19	0.36	0.36	0.01	0.56	0.56	YYY	■
D0470		N	Diagnostic casts	0.41	0.75	0.75	0.02	1.19	1.19	XXX	■
D0472		R	Accession of tissue, gross examination, preparation and transmission of written report	0.29	0.53	0.53	0.02	0.84	0.84	XXX	■
D0473		R	Accession of tissue, gross and microscopic examination, preparation and transmission of written report	0.56	1.03	1.03	0.03	1.63	1.63	XXX	■
D0474		R	Accession of tissue, gross and microscopic examination, including assessment of surgical margins for presence of disease, preparation and transmission of written report	0.68	1.24	1.24	0.04	1.96	1.96	XXX	■
D0480		R	Processing and interpretation of cytologic smears, including the preparation and transmission of written report	0.41	0.75	0.75	0.02	1.19	1.19	XXX	■
D0501		R	Histopathologic examinations	0.53	0.98	0.98	0.03	1.54	1.54	YYY	■
D0502		R	Other oral pathology procedures, by report	0.00	0.00	0.00	0.00	0.00	0.00	YYY	
D0999		R	Unspecified diagnostic procedure, by report	0.00	0.00	0.00	0.00	0.00	0.00	YYY	
D1110		N	Prophylaxis — adult	0.52	0.41	0.41	0.06	0.99	0.99	XXX	■
D1120		N	Prophylaxis — child	0.36	0.29	0.29	0.04	0.69	0.69	XXX	■
D1201		N	Topical application of fluoride (including prophylaxis) — child	0.52	0.41	0.41	0.05	0.98	0.98	XXX	■
D1203		N	Topical application of fluoride (prophylaxis not included) — child	0.21	0.16	0.16	0.02	0.39	0.39	XXX	■
D1204		N	Topical application of fluoride (prophylaxis not included) — adult	0.22	0.17	0.17	0.02	0.41	0.41	XXX	■
D1205		N	Topical application of fluoride (including prophylaxis) — adult	0.60	0.48	0.48	0.06	1.15	1.15	XXX	■
D1310		N	Nutritional counseling for control of dental disease	0.28	0.22	0.22	0.03	0.53	0.53	XXX	■
D1320		N	Tobacco counseling for the control and prevention of oral disease	0.26	0.20	0.20	0.03	0.49	0.49	XXX	■
D1330		N	Oral hygiene instructions	0.37	0.30	0.30	0.04	0.71	0.71	XXX	■
D1351		N	Sealant — per tooth	0.29	0.23	0.23	0.03	0.55	0.55	XXX	■

■ RVU not developed by CMS. Gap-filled RVUs developed by CHEG.

Code	M	S	Description	Work Value	Non-Fac PE	Fac PE	Mal-practice	Non-Fac Total	Fac Total	Global	Gap
D1510		R	Space maintainer — fixed-unilateral	1.84	1.46	1.46	0.20	3.50	3.50	YYY	■
D1515		R	Space maintainer — fixed-bilateral	2.43	1.93	1.93	0.26	4.62	4.62	YYY	■
D1520		R	Space maintainer — removable-unilateral	2.28	1.81	1.81	0.24	4.34	4.34	YYY	■
D1525		R	Space maintainer — removable-bilateral	3.13	2.49	2.49	0.33	5.96	5.96	YYY	■
D1550		R	Recementation of space maintainer	0.40	0.32	0.32	0.04	0.76	0.76	YYY	■
D2110		N	Amalgam — one surface, primary	0.57	0.45	0.45	0.06	1.08	1.08	XXX	■
D2120		N	Amalgam — two surfaces, primary	0.72	0.57	0.57	0.08	1.37	1.37	XXX	■
D2130		N	Amalgam — three surfaces, primary	0.87	0.69	0.69	0.09	1.65	1.65	XXX	■
D2131		N	Amalgam — four or more surfaces, primary	1.03	0.82	0.82	0.11	1.96	1.96	XXX	■
D2140		N	Amalgam — one surface, permanent	0.63	0.50	0.50	0.07	1.19	1.19	XXX	■
D2150		N	Amalgam — two surfaces, permanent	0.81	0.64	0.64	0.09	1.54	1.54	XXX	■
D2160		N	Amalgam — three surfaces, permanent	0.98	0.78	0.78	0.10	1.86	1.86	XXX	■
D2161		N	Amalgam — four or more surfaces, permanent	1.19	0.95	0.95	0.13	2.27	2.27	XXX	■
D2330		N	Resin-based composite — one surface, anterior	0.77	0.61	0.61	0.08	1.47	1.47	XXX	■
D2331		N	Resin-based composite — two surfaces, anterior	0.99	0.79	0.79	0.11	1.88	1.88	XXX	■
D2332		N	Resin-based composite — three surfaces, anterior	1.21	0.96	0.96	0.13	2.30	2.30	XXX	■
D2335		N	Resin-based composite — four or more surfaces or involving incisal angle (anterior)	1.43	1.14	1.14	0.15	2.72	2.72	XXX	■
D2336		N	Resin-based composite crown, anterior — primary	1.55	1.23	1.23	0.16	2.94	2.94	XXX	■
D2337		N	Resin-based composite crown, anterior — permanent	1.70	1.35	1.35	0.18	3.24	3.24	XXX	■
D2380		N	Resin-based composite — one surface, posterior — primary	0.88	0.70	0.70	0.09	1.68	1.68	XXX	■
D2381		N	Resin-based composite — two surfaces, posterior — primary	1.03	0.82	0.82	0.11	1.96	1.96	XXX	■
D2382		N	Resin-based composite — three or more surfaces, posterior — primary	1.25	0.99	0.99	0.13	2.38	2.38	XXX	■
D2385		N	Resin-based composite — one surface, posterior — permanent	0.87	0.69	0.69	0.09	1.65	1.65	XXX	■
D2386		N	Resin-based composite — two surfaces, posterior — permanent	1.20	0.95	0.95	0.13	2.28	2.28	XXX	■
D2387		N	Resin-based composite — three surfaces, posterior — permanent	1.49	1.19	1.19	0.16	2.84	2.84	XXX	■

■ RVU not developed by CMS. Gap-filled RVUs developed by CHEG.

Code	M	S	Description	Work Value	Non-Fac PE	Fac PE	Mal-prac-tice	Non-Fac Total	Fac Total	Global	Gap
D2388		N	Resin-based composite — four or more surfaces, posterior — permanent	1.79	1.43	1.43	0.19	3.41	3.41	XXX	■
D2410		N	Gold foil — one surface	1.66	1.32	1.32	0.18	3.15	3.15	XXX	■
D2420		N	Gold foil — two surfaces	2.76	2.19	2.19	0.29	5.25	5.25	XXX	■
D2430		N	Gold foil — three surfaces	4.79	3.81	3.81	0.51	9.11	9.11	XXX	■
D2510		N	Inlay — metallic — one surface	4.39	3.49	3.49	0.47	8.34	8.34	XXX	■
D2520		N	Inlay — metallic — two surfaces	4.98	3.95	3.95	0.53	9.46	9.46	XXX	■
D2530		N	Inlay — metallic — three or more surfaces	5.73	4.56	4.56	0.61	10.90	10.90	XXX	■
D2542		N	Onlay — metallic — two surfaces	5.62	4.47	4.47	0.60	10.69	10.69	XXX	■
D2543		N	Onlay — metallic — three surfaces	5.88	4.67	4.67	0.63	11.18	11.18	XXX	■
D2544		N	Onlay — metallic — four or more surfaces	6.12	4.86	4.86	0.65	11.63	11.63	XXX	■
D2610		N	Inlay — porcelain/ceramic — one surface	5.16	4.10	4.10	0.55	9.81	9.81	XXX	■
D2620		N	Inlay — porcelain/ceramic — two surfaces	5.45	4.33	4.33	0.58	10.36	10.36	XXX	■
D2630		N	Inlay — porcelain/ceramic — three or more surfaces	5.80	4.61	4.61	0.62	11.03	11.03	XXX	■
D2642		N	Onlay — porcelain/ceramic — two surfaces	5.64	4.48	4.48	0.60	10.72	10.72	XXX	■
D2643		N	Onlay — porcelain/ceramic — three surfaces	6.08	4.83	4.83	0.65	11.56	11.56	XXX	■
D2644		N	Onlay — porcelain/ceramic — four or more surfaces	6.45	5.12	5.12	0.69	12.26	12.26	XXX	■
D2650		N	Inlay — resin-based composite composite/resin — one surface	3.39	2.70	2.70	0.36	6.45	6.45	XXX	■
D2651		N	Inlay — resin-based composite composite/resin — two surfaces	4.04	3.21	3.21	0.43	7.68	7.68	XXX	■
D2652		N	Inlay — resin-based composite composite/resin — three or more surfaces	4.24	3.37	3.37	0.45	8.07	8.07	XXX	■
D2662		N	Onlay — resin-based composite composite/ resin — two surfaces	3.69	2.93	2.93	0.39	7.01	7.01	XXX	■
D2663		N	Onlay — resin-based composite composite/ resin — three surfaces	4.33	3.44	3.44	0.46	8.24	8.24	XXX	■
D2664		N	Onlay — resin-based composite composite/ resin — four or more surfaces	4.64	3.69	3.69	0.49	8.83	8.83	XXX	■
D2710		N	Crown — resin (laboratory)	2.61	2.08	2.08	0.28	4.97	4.97	XXX	■
D2720		N	Crown — resin with high noble metal	6.45	5.12	5.12	0.69	12.26	12.26	XXX	■
D2721		N	Crown — resin with predominantly base metal	6.04	4.80	4.80	0.64	11.49	11.49	XXX	■
D2722		N	Crown — resin with noble metal	6.18	4.91	4.91	0.66	11.74	11.74	XXX	■

■ RVU not developed by CMS. Gap-filled RVUs developed by CHEG.

Code	M	S	Description	Work Value	Non-Fac PE	Fac PE	Mal-practice	Non-Fac Total	Fac Total	Global	Gap
D2740		N	Crown — porcelain/ceramic substrate	6.62	5.26	5.26	0.70	12.58	12.58	XXX	■
D2750		N	Crown — porcelain fused to high noble metal	6.53	5.19	5.19	0.70	12.42	12.42	XXX	■
D2751		N	Crown — porcelain fused to predominantly base metal	6.08	4.83	4.83	0.65	11.56	11.56	XXX	■
D2752		N	Crown — porcelain fused to noble metal	6.23	4.95	4.95	0.66	11.84	11.84	XXX	■
D2780		N	Crown — 3/4 cast high noble metal	6.26	4.98	4.98	0.67	11.91	11.91	XXX	■
D2781		N	Crown — 3/4 cast predominately base metal	5.90	4.69	4.69	0.63	11.21	11.21	XXX	■
D2782		N	Crown — 3/4 cast noble metal	6.09	4.84	4.84	0.65	11.57	11.57	XXX	■
D2783		N	Crown — 3/4 porcelain/ceramic	6.44	5.12	5.12	0.69	12.25	12.25	XXX	■
D2790		N	Crown — full cast high noble metal	6.30	5.01	5.01	0.67	11.98	11.98	XXX	■
D2791		N	Crown — full cast predominantly base metal	5.97	4.74	4.74	0.64	11.35	11.35	XXX	■
D2792		N	Crown — full cast noble metal	6.08	4.83	4.83	0.65	11.56	11.56	XXX	■
D2799		N	Provisional crown	2.61	2.08	2.08	0.28	4.97	4.97	XXX	■
D2910		N	Recement inlay	0.52	0.41	0.41	0.05	0.98	0.98	XXX	■
D2920		N	Recement crown	0.54	0.43	0.43	0.06	1.02	1.02	XXX	■
D2930		N	Prefabricated stainless steel crown — primary tooth	1.47	1.17	1.17	0.16	2.79	2.79	XXX	■
D2931		N	Prefabricated stainless steel crown — permanent tooth	1.66	1.32	1.32	0.18	3.15	3.15	XXX	■
D2932		N	Prefabricated resin crown	1.80	1.43	1.43	0.19	3.43	3.43	XXX	■
D2933		N	Prefabricated stainless steel crown with resin window	2.03	1.61	1.61	0.22	3.85	3.85	XXX	■
D2940		N	Sedative filling	0.56	0.44	0.44	0.06	1.06	1.06	XXX	■
D2950		N	Core buildup, including any pins	1.40	1.11	1.11	0.15	2.66	2.66	XXX	■
D2951		N	Pin retention — per tooth, in addition to restoration	0.29	0.23	0.23	0.03	0.56	0.56	XXX	■
D2952		N	Cast post and core in addition to crown	2.14	1.70	1.70	0.23	4.06	4.06	XXX	■
D2953		N	Each additional cast post — same tooth	1.07	0.85	0.85	0.11	2.03	2.03	XXX	■
D2954		N	Prefabricated post and core in addition to crown	1.77	1.40	1.40	0.19	3.36	3.36	XXX	■
D2955		N	Post removal (not in conjunction with endodontic therapy)	1.33	1.05	1.05	0.14	2.52	2.52	XXX	■
D2957		N	Each additional prefabricated post — same tooth	0.88	0.70	0.70	0.09	1.68	1.68	XXX	■
D2960		N	Labial veneer (resin laminate) — chairside	4.33	3.44	3.44	0.46	8.24	8.24	XXX	■

■ RVU not developed by CMS. Gap-filled RVUs developed by CHEG.

Code	M	S	Description	Work Value	Non-Fac PE	Fac PE	Mal-practice	Non-Fac Total	Fac Total	Global	Gap
D2961		N	Labial veneer (resin laminate) — laboratory	4.85	3.85	3.85	0.52	9.22	9.22	XXX	■
D2962		N	Labial veneer (porcelain laminate) — laboratory	5.27	4.19	4.19	0.56	10.02	10.02	XXX	■
D2970		R	Temporary crown (fractured tooth)	1.25	0.99	0.99	0.13	2.38	2.38	YYY	■
D2980		N	Crown repair, by report	0.00	0.00	0.00	0.00	0.00	0.00	XXX	
D2999		R	Unspecified restorative procedure, by report	0.00	0.00	0.00	0.00	0.00	0.00	YYY	
D3110		N	Pulp cap — direct (excluding final restoration)	0.38	0.31	0.31	0.04	0.73	0.73	XXX	■
D3120		N	Pulp cap — indirect (excluding final restoration)	0.30	0.24	0.24	0.03	0.57	0.57	XXX	■
D3220		N	Therapeutic pulpotomy (excluding final restoration) — removal of pulp coronal to the dentinocemental junction and application of medicament	0.90	0.72	0.72	0.10	1.72	1.72	XXX	■
D3221		N	Gross pulpal debridement, primary and permanent teeth	0.99	0.79	0.79	0.11	1.89	1.89	XXX	■
D3230		N	Pulpal therapy (resorbable filling) — anterior, primary tooth (excluding final restoration)	0.96	0.76	0.76	0.10	1.82	1.82	XXX	■
D3240		N	Pulpal therapy (resorbable filling) — posterior, primary tooth (excluding final restoration)	1.03	0.82	0.82	0.11	1.96	1.96	XXX	■
D3310		N	Anterior (excluding final restoration)	3.83	3.05	3.05	0.41	7.29	7.29	XXX	■
D3320		N	Bicuspid (excluding final restoration)	4.68	3.72	3.72	0.50	8.90	8.90	XXX	■
D3330		N	Molar (excluding final restoration)	6.04	4.80	4.80	0.64	11.49	11.49	XXX	■
D3331		N	Treatment of root canal obstruction; non-surgical access	1.29	1.02	1.02	0.14	2.45	2.45	XXX	■
D3332		N	Incomplete endodontic therapy; inoperable or fractured tooth	3.32	2.64	2.64	0.35	6.31	6.31	XXX	■
D3333		N	Internal root repair of perforation defects	1.10	0.88	0.88	0.12	2.10	2.10	XXX	■
D3346		N	Retreatment of previous root canal therapy — anterior	5.16	4.10	4.10	0.55	9.81	9.81	XXX	■
D3347		N	Retreatment of previous root canal therapy — bicuspid	6.08	4.83	4.83	0.65	11.56	11.56	XXX	■
D3348		N	Retreatment of previous root canal therapy — molar	7.31	5.81	5.81	0.78	13.90	13.90	XXX	■
D3351		N	Apexification/recalcification — initial visit (apical closure/calcific repair of perforations, root resorption, etc.)	2.17	1.73	1.73	0.23	4.13	4.13	XXX	■
D3352		N	Apexification/recalcification — interim medication replacement (apical closure/calcific repair of perforations, root resorption, etc.)	0.95	0.76	0.76	0.10	1.81	1.81	XXX	■

■ RVU not developed by CMS. Gap-filled RVUs developed by CHEG.

Code	M	S	Description	Work Value	Non-Fac PE	Fac PE	Mal-prac-tice	Non-Fac Total	Fac Total	Global	Gap
D3353		N	Apexification/recalcification – final visit (includes completed root canal therapy — apical closure/calcific repair of perforations, root resorption, etc.)	3.21	2.55	2.55	0.34	6.10	6.10	XXX	■
D3410		N	Apicoectomy/periradicular surgery — anterior	4.39	3.49	3.49	0.47	8.34	8.34	XXX	■
D3421		N	Apicoectomy/periradicular surgery — bicuspid (first root)	4.79	3.81	3.81	0.51	9.11	9.11	XXX	■
D3425		N	Apicoectomy/periradicular surgery — molar (first root)	5.42	4.31	4.31	0.58	10.30	10.30	XXX	■
D3426		N	Apicoectomy/periradicular surgery (each additional root)	1.80	1.43	1.43	0.19	3.43	3.43	XXX	■
D3430		N	Retrograde filling — per root	1.33	1.05	1.05	0.14	2.52	2.52	XXX	■
D3450		N	Root amputation — per root	2.69	2.14	2.14	0.29	5.11	5.11	XXX	■
D3460		R	Endodontic endosseous implant	12.91	10.26	10.26	1.37	24.55	24.55	YYY	■
D3470		N	Intentional reimplantation (including necessary splinting)	5.37	4.26	4.26	0.57	10.20	10.20	XXX	■
D3910		N	Surgical procedure for isolation of tooth with rubber dam	0.70	0.56	0.56	0.07	1.33	1.33	XXX	■
D3920		N	Hemisection (including any root removal), not including root canal therapy	2.10	1.67	1.67	0.22	3.99	3.99	XXX	■
D3950		N	Canal preparation and fitting of preformed dowel or post	0.96	0.76	0.76	0.10	1.82	1.82	XXX	■
D3999		R	Unspecified endodontic procedure, by report	0.00	0.00	0.00	0.00	0.00	0.00	YYY	
D4210		I	Gingivectomy or gingivoplasty — per quadrant. See also code 41820.	3.72	2.96	2.96	0.40	7.08	7.08	XXX	■
D4211		I	Gingivectomy or gingivoplasty — per tooth. See also code 41820 or 41872.	0.99	0.79	0.79	0.11	1.89	1.89	XXX	■
D4220		N	Gingival curettage, surgical — per quadrant, by report	1.33	1.05	1.05	0.14	2.52	2.52	XXX	■
D4240		N	Gingival flap procedure, including root planing — per quadrant	4.39	3.49	3.49	0.47	8.34	8.34	XXX	■
D4245		N	Apically positioned flap	3.16	2.51	2.51	0.34	6.00	6.00	XXX	■
D4249		N	Clinical crown lengthening — hard tissue	5.00	3.98	3.98	0.53	9.51	9.51	XXX	■
D4260		R	Osseous surgery (including flap entry and closure) — per quadrant	7.07	5.62	5.62	0.75	13.45	13.45	YYY	■
D4263		R	Bone replacement graft — first site in quadrant	2.14	1.70	1.70	0.23	4.06	4.06	YYY	■
D4264		R	Bone replacement graft — each additional site in quadrant (use if performed on same date of service as D4263)	1.07	0.85	0.85	0.11	2.03	2.03	YYY	■

■ RVU not developed by CMS. Gap-filled RVUs developed by CHEG.

Code	M	S	Description	Work Value	Non-Fac PE	Fac PE	Mal-prac-tice	Non-Fac Total	Fac Total	Global	Gap
D4266		N	Guided tissue regeneration — resorbable barrier, per site	2.58	2.05	2.05	0.27	4.90	4.90	XXX	■
D4267		N	Guided tissue regeneration — nonresorbable barrier, per site (includes membrane removal)	3.32	2.64	2.64	0.35	6.31	6.31	XXX	■
D4268		R	Surgical revision procedure, per tooth	0.00	0.00	0.00	0.00	0.00	0.00	XXX	
D4270		R	Pedicle soft tissue graft procedure	5.23	4.16	4.16	0.56	9.95	9.95	YYY	■
D4271		R	Free soft tissue graft procedure (including donor site surgery)	5.38	4.28	4.28	0.57	10.23	10.23	YYY	■
D4273		R	Subepithelial connective tissue graft procedure (including donor site surgery)	5.74	4.56	4.56	0.61	10.92	10.92	YYY	■
D4274		N	Distal or proximal wedge procedure (when not performed in conjunction with surgical procedures in the same anatomical area)	1.62	1.29	1.29	0.17	3.08	3.08	XXX	■
D4320		N	Provisional splinting — intracoronal	2.65	2.11	2.11	0.28	5.04	5.04	XXX	■
D4321		N	Provisional splinting — extracoronal	2.32	1.84	1.84	0.25	4.41	4.41	XXX	■
D4341		N	Periodontal scaling and root planing, per quadrant	1.44	1.14	1.14	0.15	2.73	2.73	XXX	■
D4355		R	Full mouth debridement to enable comprehensive periodontal evaluation and diagnosis	0.96	0.76	0.76	0.10	1.82	1.82	YYY	■
D4381		R	Localized delivery of chemotherapeutic agents via a controlled release vehicle into diseased crevicular tissue, per tooth, by report	0.00	0.00	0.00	0.00	0.00	0.00	YYY	
D4910		N	Periodontal maintenance procedures (following active therapy)	0.86	0.69	0.69	0.09	1.64	1.64	XXX	■
D4920		N	Unscheduled dressing change (by someone other than treating dentist)	0.74	0.59	0.59	0.08	1.40	1.40	XXX	■
D4999		N	Unspecified periodontal procedure, by report	0.00	0.00	0.00	0.00	0.00	0.00	XXX	
D5110		N	Complete denture — maxillary	8.08	6.42	6.42	0.86	15.36	15.36	XXX	■
D5120		N	Complete denture — mandibular	8.08	6.42	6.42	0.86	15.36	15.36	XXX	■
D5130		N	Immediate denture — maxillary	8.81	7.00	7.00	0.94	16.75	16.75	XXX	■
D5140		N	Immediate denture — mandibular	8.81	7.00	7.00	0.94	16.75	16.75	XXX	■
D5211		N	Maxillary partial denture — resin base (including any conventional clasps, rests and teeth)	6.82	5.42	5.42	0.73	12.96	12.96	XXX	■
D5212		N	Mandibular partial denture — resin base (including any conventional clasps, rests and teeth)	7.92	6.30	6.30	0.84	15.06	15.06	XXX	■
D5213		N	Maxillary partial denture — cast metal framework with resin denture bases (including any conventional clasps, rests and teeth)	8.93	7.09	7.09	0.95	16.97	16.97	XXX	■

■ RVU not developed by CMS. Gap-filled RVUs developed by CHEG.

HCPCS

Code	M	S	Description	Work Value	Non-Fac PE	Fac PE	Mal-practice	Non-Fac Total	Fac Total	Global	Gap
D5214		N	Mandibular partial denture— cast metal framework with resin denture bases (including any conventional clasps, rests and teeth)	8.93	7.09	7.09	0.95	16.97	16.97	XXX	■
D5281		N	Removable unilateral partial denture — one piece cast metal (including clasps and teeth)	5.20	4.13	4.13	0.55	9.89	9.89	XXX	■
D5410		N	Adjust complete denture — maxillary	0.44	0.35	0.35	0.05	0.84	0.84	XXX	■
D5411		N	Adjust complete denture — mandibular	0.44	0.35	0.35	0.05	0.84	0.84	XXX	■
D5421		N	Adjust partial denture — maxillary	0.44	0.35	0.35	0.05	0.84	0.84	XXX	■
D5422		N	Adjust partial denture — mandibular	0.44	0.35	0.35	0.05	0.84	0.84	XXX	■
D5510		N	Repair broken complete denture base	0.88	0.70	0.70	0.09	1.68	1.68	XXX	■
D5520		N	Replace missing or broken teeth — complete denture (each tooth)	0.74	0.59	0.59	0.08	1.40	1.40	XXX	■
D5610		N	Repair resin denture base	0.96	0.76	0.76	0.10	1.82	1.82	XXX	■
D5620		N	Repair cast framework	1.03	0.82	0.82	0.11	1.96	1.96	XXX	■
D5630		N	Repair or replace broken clasp	1.25	0.99	0.99	0.13	2.38	2.38	XXX	■
D5640		N	Replace broken teeth — per tooth	0.81	0.64	0.64	0.09	1.54	1.54	XXX	■
D5650		N	Add tooth to existing partial denture	1.10	0.88	0.88	0.12	2.10	2.10	XXX	■
D5660		N	Add clasp to existing partial denture	1.33	1.05	1.05	0.14	2.52	2.52	XXX	■
D5710		N	Rebase complete maxillary denture	3.28	2.61	2.61	0.35	6.24	6.24	XXX	■
D5711		N	Rebase complete mandibular denture	3.13	2.49	2.49	0.33	5.96	5.96	XXX	■
D5720		N	Rebase maxillary partial denture	3.10	2.46	2.46	0.33	5.89	5.89	XXX	■
D5721		N	Rebase mandibular partial denture	3.10	2.46	2.46	0.33	5.89	5.89	XXX	■
D5730		N	Reline complete maxillary denture (chairside)	1.85	1.47	1.47	0.20	3.52	3.52	XXX	■
D5731		N	Reline complete mandibular denture (chairside)	1.85	1.47	1.47	0.20	3.52	3.52	XXX	■
D5740		N	Reline maxillary partial denture (chairside)	1.69	1.35	1.35	0.18	3.22	3.22	XXX	■
D5741		N	Reline mandibular partial denture (chairside)	1.69	1.35	1.35	0.18	3.22	3.22	XXX	■
D5750		N	Reline complete maxillary denture (laboratory)	2.47	1.96	1.96	0.26	4.69	4.69	XXX	■
D5751		N	Reline complete mandibular denture (laboratory)	2.47	1.96	1.96	0.26	4.69	4.69	XXX	■
D5760		N	Reline maxillary partial denture (laboratory)	2.43	1.93	1.93	0.26	4.62	4.62	XXX	■
D5761		N	Reline mandibular partial denture (laboratory)	2.43	1.93	1.93	0.26	4.62	4.62	XXX	■
D5810		N	Interim complete denture (maxillary)	3.91	3.11	3.11	0.42	7.43	7.43	XXX	■
D5811		N	Interim complete denture (mandibular)	4.20	3.34	3.34	0.45	7.99	7.99	XXX	■

■ RVU not developed by CMS. Gap-filled RVUs developed by CHEG.

Code	M	S	Description	Work Value	Non-Fac PE	Fac PE	Mal-practice	Non-Fac Total	Fac Total	Global	Gap
D5820		N	Interim partial denture (maxillary)	3.02	2.40	2.40	0.32	5.75	5.75	XXX	■
D5821		N	Interim partial denture (mandibular)	3.21	2.55	2.55	0.34	6.10	6.10	XXX	■
D5850		N	Tissue conditioning, maxillary	0.77	0.61	0.61	0.08	1.47	1.47	XXX	■
D5851		N	Tissue conditioning, mandibular	0.77	0.61	0.61	0.08	1.47	1.47	XXX	■
D5860		N	Overdenture — complete, by report	0.00	0.00	0.00	0.00	0.00	0.00	XXX	
D5861		N	Overdenture — partial, by report	0.00	0.00	0.00	0.00	0.00	0.00	XXX	
D5862		N	Precision attachment, by report	0.00	0.00	0.00	0.00	0.00	0.00	XXX	
D5867		N	Replacement of replaceable part of semi-precision or precision attachment (male or female component)	0.00	0.00	0.00	0.00	0.00	0.00	XXX	
D5875		N	Modification of removable prosthesis following implant surgery	0.00	0.00	0.00	0.00	0.00	0.00	XXX	
D5899		N	Unspecified removable prosthodontic procedure, by report	0.00	0.00	0.00	0.00	0.00	0.00	XXX	
D5911		R	Facial moulage (sectional)	2.05	1.63	1.63	0.22	3.90	3.90	YYY	■
D5912		R	Facial moulage (complete)	2.05	1.63	1.63	0.22	3.90	3.90	YYY	■
D5913		I	Nasal prosthesis. See also code 21087.	43.15	34.29	34.29	4.59	82.03	82.03	XXX	■
D5914		I	Auricular prosthesis. See also code 21086.	43.15	34.29	34.29	4.59	82.03	82.03	XXX	■
D5915		I	Orbital prosthesis. See also code L8611.	58.39	46.40	46.40	6.22	111.01	111.01	XXX	■
D5916		I	Ocular prosthesis. See also code V2623, V2629 and CPT.	15.57	12.38	12.38	1.66	29.61	29.61	XXX	■
D5919		I	Facial prosthesis. See also code 21088.	0.00	0.00	0.00	0.00	0.00	0.00	XXX	
D5922		I	Nasal septal prosthesis. See also code 30220.	0.00	0.00	0.00	0.00	0.00	0.00	XXX	
D5923		I	Ocular prosthesis, interim. See also code 92330.	0.00	0.00	0.00	0.00	0.00	0.00	XXX	
D5924		I	Cranial prosthesis. See also code 62143.	0.00	0.00	0.00	0.00	0.00	0.00	XXX	
D5925		I	Facial augmentation implant prosthesis. See also code 21208.	0.00	0.00	0.00	0.00	0.00	0.00	XXX	
D5926		I	Nasal prosthesis, replacement. See also code 21087.	0.00	0.00	0.00	0.00	0.00	0.00	XXX	
D5927		I	Auricular prosthesis, replacement. See also code 21086.	0.00	0.00	0.00	0.00	0.00	0.00	XXX	
D5928		I	Orbital prosthesis, replacement. See also code 67550.	0.00	0.00	0.00	0.00	0.00	0.00	XXX	
D5929		I	Facial prosthesis, replacement. See also code 21088.	0.00	0.00	0.00	0.00	0.00	0.00	XXX	

■ RVU not developed by CMS. Gap-filled RVUs developed by CHEG.

Code	M	S	Description	Work Value	Non-Fac PE	Fac PE	Mal-practice	Non-Fac Total	Fac Total	Global	Gap
D5931		I	Obturator prosthesis, surgical. See also code 21079.	23.23	18.46	18.46	2.47	44.17	44.17	XXX	■
D5932		I	Obturator prosthesis, definitive. See also code 21080.	43.45	34.53	34.53	4.63	82.61	82.61	XXX	■
D5933		I	Obturator prosthesis, modification. See also code 21080.	0.00	0.00	0.00	0.00	0.00	0.00	XXX	
D5934		I	Mandibular resection prosthesis with guide flange. See also code 21081.	39.60	31.47	31.47	4.22	75.29	75.29	XXX	■
D5935		I	Mandibular resection prosthesis without guide flange. See also code 21081.	34.46	27.38	27.38	3.67	65.51	65.51	XXX	■
D5936		I	Obturator/prosthesis, interim. See also code 21079.	38.70	30.76	30.76	4.12	73.58	73.58	XXX	■
D5937		I	Trismus appliance (not for TMD treatment)	4.87	3.87	3.87	0.52	9.25	9.25	XXX	■
D5951		R	Feeding aid	6.32	5.02	5.02	0.67	12.02	12.02	YYY	■
D5952		I	Speech aid prosthesis, pediatric. See also code 21084.	20.54	16.32	16.32	2.19	39.04	39.04	XXX	■
D5953		I	Speech aid prosthesis, adult. See also code 21084.	39.00	30.99	30.99	4.15	74.14	74.14	XXX	■
D5954		I	Palatal augmentation prosthesis. See also code 21082.	36.14	28.72	28.72	3.85	68.71	68.71	XXX	■
D5955		I	Palatal lift prosthesis, definitive. See also code 21083.	33.43	26.56	26.56	3.56	63.55	63.55	XXX	■
D5958		I	Palatal lift prosthesis, interim. See also code 21083.	0.00	0.00	0.00	0.00	0.00	0.00	XXX	
D5959		I	Palatal lift prosthesis, modification. See also code 21083.	0.00	0.00	0.00	0.00	0.00	0.00	XXX	
D5960		I	Speech aid prosthesis, modification. See also code 21084.	0.00	0.00	0.00	0.00	0.00	0.00	XXX	
D5982		I	Surgical stent. See also code 21085.	4.02	3.19	3.19	0.43	7.64	7.64	XXX	■
D5983		R	Radiation carrier	9.73	7.73	7.73	1.04	18.50	18.50	YYY	■
D5984		R	Radiation shield	9.73	7.73	7.73	1.04	18.50	18.50	YYY	■
D5985		R	Radiation cone locator	9.73	7.73	7.73	1.04	18.50	18.50	YYY	■
D5986		N	Fluoride gel carrier	0.83	0.66	0.66	0.09	1.57	1.57	XXX	■
D5987		R	Commissure splint	14.60	11.60	11.60	1.55	27.76	27.76	YYY	■
D5988		I	Surgical splint. See also CPT.	0.00	0.00	0.00	0.00	0.00	0.00	XXX	
D5999		I	Unspecified maxillofacial prosthesis, by report. See also CPT.	0.00	0.00	0.00	0.00	0.00	0.00	XXX	
D6010		I	Surgical placement of implant body: endosteal implant. See also code 21248.	13.50	10.73	10.73	1.44	25.66	25.66	XXX	■

■ RVU not developed by CMS. Gap-filled RVUs developed by CHEG.

Code	M	S	Description	Work Value	Non-Fac PE	Fac PE	Mal-practice	Non-Fac Total	Fac Total	Global	Gap
D6020		I	Abutment placement or substitution: endosteal implant. See also code 21248.	1.65	1.31	1.31	0.18	3.14	3.14	XXX	■
D6040		I	Surgical placement: eposteal implant. See also code 21245.	62.08	49.33	49.33	6.61	118.02	118.02	XXX	■
D6050		I	Surgical placement: transosteal implant. See also code 21244.	38.53	30.62	30.62	4.10	73.25	73.25	XXX	■
D6055		I	Dental implant supported connecting bar	3.43	2.73	2.73	0.37	6.52	6.52	XXX	■
D6056		N	Prefabricated abutment	0.00	0.00	0.00	0.00	0.00	0.00	XXX	
D6057		N	Custom abutment	0.00	0.00	0.00	0.00	0.00	0.00	XXX	
D6058		N	Abutment supported porcelain/ceramic crown	7.77	6.17	6.17	0.83	14.77	14.77	XXX	■
D6059		N	Abutment supported porcelain fused to metal crown (high noble metal)	7.66	6.09	6.09	0.82	14.57	14.57	XXX	■
D6060		N	Abutment supported porcelain fused to metal crown (predominantly base metal)	7.24	5.76	5.76	0.77	13.77	13.77	XXX	■
D6061		N	Abutment supported porcelain fused to metal crown (noble metal)	7.40	5.88	5.88	0.79	14.06	14.06	XXX	■
D6062		N	Abutment supported cast metal crown (high noble metal)	7.36	5.85	5.85	0.78	14.00	14.00	XXX	■
D6063		N	Abutment supported cast metal crown (predominantly base metal)	6.32	5.02	5.02	0.67	12.02	12.02	XXX	■
D6064		N	Abutment supported cast metal crown (noble metal)	6.70	5.33	5.33	0.71	12.74	12.74	XXX	■
D6065		N	Implant supported porcelain/ceramic crown	7.64	6.07	6.07	0.81	14.53	14.53	XXX	■
D6066		N	Implant supported porcelain fused to metal crown (titanium, titanium alloy, high noble metal)	7.44	5.91	5.91	0.79	14.15	14.15	XXX	■
D6067		N	Implant supported metal crown (titanium, titanium alloy, high noble metal)	7.22	5.74	5.74	0.77	13.73	13.73	XXX	■
D6068		N	Abutment supported retainer for porcelain/ ceramic FPD	7.77	6.17	6.17	0.83	14.77	14.77	XXX	■
D6069		N	Abutment supported retainer for porcelain fused to metal FPD (high noble metal)	7.66	6.09	6.09	0.82	14.57	14.57	XXX	■
D6070		N	Abutment supported retainer for porcelain fused to metal FPD (predominately base metal)	7.24	5.76	5.76	0.77	13.77	13.77	XXX	■
D6071		N	Abutment supported retainer for porcelain fused to metal FPD (noble metal)	7.40	5.88	5.88	0.79	14.06	14.06	XXX	■
D6072		N	Abutment supported retainer for cast metal FPD (high noble metal)	7.55	6.00	6.00	0.80	14.35	14.35	XXX	■
D6073		N	Abutment supported retainer for cast metal FPD (predominately base metal)	6.83	5.43	5.43	0.73	12.99	12.99	XXX	■

■ RVU not developed by CMS. Gap-filled RVUs developed by CHEG.

HCPCS

Code	M	S	Description	Work Value	Non-Fac PE	Fac PE	Mal-practice	Non-Fac Total	Fac Total	Global	Gap
D6074		N	Abutment supported retainer for cast metal FPD (noble metal)	7.36	5.85	5.85	0.78	14.00	14.00	XXX	■
D6075		N	Implant supported retainer for ceramic FPD	7.64	6.07	6.07	0.81	14.53	14.53	XXX	■
D6076		N	Implant supported retainer for porcelain fused to metal FPD (titanium, titanium alloy, or high noble metal)	7.44	5.91	5.91	0.79	14.15	14.15	XXX	■
D6077		N	Implant supported retainer for cast metal FPD (titanium, titanium alloy, or high noble metal)	7.22	5.74	5.74	0.77	13.73	13.73	XXX	■
D6078		N	Implant/abutment supported fixed denture for completely edentulous arch	0.00	0.00	0.00	0.00	0.00	0.00	XXX	
D6079		N	Implant/abutment supported fixed denture for partially edentulous arch	0.00	0.00	0.00	0.00	0.00	0.00	XXX	
D6080		I	Implant maintenance procedures, including removal of prosthesis, cleansing of prosthesis and abutments, reinsertion of prosthesis	0.70	0.56	0.56	0.07	1.33	1.33	XXX	■
D6090		I	Repair implant supported prosthesis, by report. See also code 21299.	0.00	0.00	0.00	0.00	0.00	0.00	XXX	
D6095		I	Repair implant abutment, by report. See also code 21299.	0.00	0.00	0.00	0.00	0.00	0.00	XXX	
D6100		I	Implant removal, by report. See also code 21299.	0.00	0.00	0.00	0.00	0.00	0.00	XXX	
D6199		I	Unspecified implant procedure, by report. See also code 21299.	0.00	0.00	0.00	0.00	0.00	0.00	XXX	
D6210		N	Pontic — cast high noble metal	5.86	4.66	4.66	0.62	11.14	11.14	XXX	■
D6211		N	Pontic — cast predominantly base metal	5.49	4.36	4.36	0.58	10.44	10.44	XXX	■
D6212		N	Pontic — cast noble metal	5.71	4.54	4.54	0.61	10.86	10.86	XXX	■
D6240		N	Pontic — porcelain fused to high noble metal	5.79	4.60	4.60	0.62	11.00	11.00	XXX	■
D6241		N	Pontic — porcelain fused to predominantly base metal	5.34	4.25	4.25	0.57	10.16	10.16	XXX	■
D6242		N	Pontic — porcelain fused to noble metal	5.64	4.48	4.48	0.60	10.72	10.72	XXX	■
D6245		N	Pontic — porcelain/ceramic	5.97	4.74	4.74	0.64	11.35	11.35	XXX	■
D6250		N	Pontic — resin with high noble metal	5.71	4.54	4.54	0.61	10.86	10.86	XXX	■
D6251		N	Pontic — resin with predominantly base metal	5.27	4.19	4.19	0.56	10.02	10.02	XXX	■
D6252		N	Pontic — resin with noble metal	5.44	4.32	4.32	0.58	10.34	10.34	XXX	■
D6519		N	Inlay/onlay — porcelain/ceramic	5.42	4.31	4.31	0.58	10.30	10.30	XXX	■
D6520		N	Inlay — metallic — two surfaces	5.05	4.01	4.01	0.54	9.60	9.60	XXX	■
D6530		N	Inlay — metallic — three or more surfaces	5.79	4.60	4.60	0.62	11.00	11.00	XXX	■

■ RVU not developed by CMS. Gap-filled RVUs developed by CHEG.

Code	M	S	Description	Work Value	Non-Fac PE	Fac PE	Mal-practice	Non-Fac Total	Fac Total	Global	Gap
D6543		N	Onlay — metallic — three surfaces	5.93	4.72	4.72	0.63	11.28	11.28	XXX	■
D6544		N	Onlay — metallic — four or more surfaces	6.19	4.92	4.92	0.66	11.77	11.77	XXX	■
D6545		N	Retainer — cast metal for resin bonded fixed prosthesis	2.43	1.93	1.93	0.26	4.62	4.62	XXX	■
D6548		N	Retainer — porcelain/ceramic for resin bonded fixed prosthesis	2.68	2.13	2.13	0.29	5.09	5.09	XXX	■
D6720		N	Crown — resin with high noble metal	6.45	5.12	5.12	0.69	12.26	12.26	XXX	■
D6721		N	Crown — resin with predominantly base metal	6.12	4.86	4.86	0.65	11.63	11.63	XXX	■
D6722		N	Crown — resin with noble metal	6.23	4.95	4.95	0.66	11.84	11.84	XXX	■
D6740		N	Crown — porcelain/ceramic	6.78	5.39	5.39	0.72	12.89	12.89	XXX	■
D6750		N	Crown — porcelain fused to high noble metal	6.61	5.25	5.25	0.70	12.56	12.56	XXX	■
D6751		N	Crown — porcelain fused to predominantly base metal	6.16	4.89	4.89	0.66	11.71	11.71	XXX	■
D6752		N	Crown — porcelain fused to noble metal	6.31	5.02	5.02	0.67	12.00	12.00	XXX	■
D6780		N	Crown — 3/4 cast high noble metal	6.23	4.95	4.95	0.66	11.84	11.84	XXX	■
D6781		N	Crown — 3/4 cast predominately based metal	6.23	4.95	4.95	0.66	11.84	11.84	XXX	■
D6782		N	Crown — 3/4 cast noble metal	5.79	4.60	4.60	0.62	11.00	11.00	XXX	■
D6783		N	Crown — 3/4 porcelain/ceramic	6.41	5.10	5.10	0.68	12.19	12.19	XXX	■
D6790		N	Crown — full cast high noble metal	6.38	5.07	5.07	0.68	12.12	12.12	XXX	■
D6791		N	Crown — full cast predominantly base metal	6.04	4.80	4.80	0.64	11.49	11.49	XXX	■
D6792		N	Crown — full cast noble metal	6.26	4.98	4.98	0.67	11.91	11.91	XXX	■
D6920		R	Connector bar	1.10	0.88	0.88	0.12	2.10	2.10	YYY	■
D6930		N	Recement fixed partial denture	0.77	0.61	0.61	0.08	1.47	1.47	XXX	■
D6940		N	Stress breaker	1.76	1.40	1.40	0.19	3.34	3.34	XXX	■
D6950		N	Precision attachment	3.43	2.73	2.73	0.37	6.52	6.52	XXX	■
D6970		N	Cast post and core in addition to fixed partial denture retainer	2.14	1.70	1.70	0.23	4.06	4.06	XXX	■
D6971		N	Cast post as part of fixed partial denture retainer	1.88	1.49	1.49	0.20	3.57	3.57	XXX	■
D6972		N	Prefabricated post and core in addition to fixed partial denture retainer	1.74	1.38	1.38	0.19	3.31	3.31	XXX	■
D6973		N	Core build up for retainer, including any pins	1.40	1.11	1.11	0.15	2.66	2.66	XXX	■
D6975		N	Coping — metal	3.83	3.05	3.05	0.41	7.29	7.29	XXX	■
D6976		N	Each additional cast post — same tooth	0.90	0.72	0.72	0.10	1.72	1.72	XXX	■

■ RVU not developed by CMS. Gap-filled RVUs developed by CHEG.

Code	M	S	Description	Work Value	Non-Fac PE	Fac PE	Mal-prac-tice	Non-Fac Total	Fac Total	Global	Gap
D6977		N	Each additional prefabricated post — same tooth	0.87	0.69	0.69	0.09	1.65	1.65	XXX	■
D6980		N	Fixed partial denture repair, by report	0.00	0.00	0.00	0.00	0.00	0.00	XXX	
D6999		N	Unspecified, fixed prosthodontic procedure, by report	0.00	0.00	0.00	0.00	0.00	0.00	XXX	
D7110		R	Extraction — single tooth	0.75	0.60	0.60	0.08	1.43	1.43	YYY	■
D7120		R	Extraction — each additional tooth	0.71	0.56	0.56	0.08	1.35	1.35	YYY	■
D7130		R	Root removal — exposed roots	0.96	0.76	0.76	0.10	1.82	1.82	YYY	■
D7210		R	Surgical removal of erupted tooth requiring elevation of mucoperiosteal flap and removal of bone and/or section of tooth	1.42	1.13	1.13	0.15	2.70	2.70	YYY	■
D7220		R	Removal of impacted tooth — soft tissue	1.78	1.42	1.42	0.19	3.39	3.39	YYY	■
D7230		R	Removal of impacted tooth — partially bony	2.37	1.89	1.89	0.25	4.51	4.51	YYY	■
D7240		R	Removal of impacted tooth — completely bony	2.79	2.22	2.22	0.30	5.30	5.30	YYY	■
D7241		R	Removal of impacted tooth — completely bony, with unusual surgical complications	3.50	2.78	2.78	0.37	6.66	6.66	YYY	■
D7250		R	Surgical removal of residual tooth roots (cutting procedure)	1.50	1.20	1.20	0.16	2.86	2.86	YYY	■
D7260		R	Orolantral fistula closure	14.75	11.72	11.72	1.57	28.05	28.05	YYY	■
D7270		N	Tooth reimplantation and/or stabilization of accidentally evulsed or displaced tooth and/or alveolus	3.06	2.43	2.43	0.33	5.82	5.82	XXX	■
D7272		N	Tooth transplantation (includes reimplantation from one site to another and splinting and/or stabilization)	4.35	3.46	3.46	0.46	8.27	8.27	XXX	■
D7280		N	Surgical exposure of impacted or unerupted tooth for orthodontic reasons (including orthodontic attachments)	3.36	2.67	2.67	0.36	6.38	6.38	XXX	■
D7281		N	Surgical exposure of impacted or unerupted tooth to aid eruption	2.84	2.26	2.26	0.30	5.40	5.40	XXX	■
D7285		I	Biopsy of oral tissue — hard (bone, tooth) See also codes 20220, 20225, 20240, 20245.	5.93	4.72	4.72	0.63	11.28	11.28	XXX	■
D7286		I	Biopsy of oral tissue — soft (all others) See also code 40808.	2.43	1.93	1.93	0.26	4.62	4.62	XXX	■
D7290		N	Surgical repositioning of teeth	2.76	2.19	2.19	0.29	5.25	5.25	XXX	■
D7291		R	Transseptal fiberotomy, by report	0.00	0.00	0.00	0.00	0.00	0.00	YYY	
D7310		I	Alveoloplasty in conjunction with extractions — per quadrant. See also code 41874.	1.66	1.32	1.32	0.18	3.15	3.15	XXX	■

■ RVU not developed by CMS. Gap-filled RVUs developed by CHEG.

Code	M	S	Description	Work Value	Non-Fac PE	Fac PE	Mal-practice	Non-Fac Total	Fac Total	Global	Gap
D7320		I	Alveoloplasty not in conjunction with extractions — per quadrant. See also code 41870.	7.41	5.89	5.89	0.79	14.08	14.08	XXX	■
D7340		I	Vestibuloplasty — ridge extension (second epithelialization), See also codes 40840, 40842, 40843, 40844.	13.27	10.54	10.54	1.41	25.22	25.22	XXX	■
D7350		I	Vestibuloplasty — ridge extension (including soft tissue grafts, muscle reattachments, revision of soft tissue attachment and management of hypertrophied and hyperplastic tissue). See also code 40845.	41.46	32.95	32.95	4.41	78.82	78.82	XXX	■
D7410		I	Radical excision — lesion diameter up to 1.25 cm. See also CPT.	9.22	7.32	7.32	0.98	17.52	17.52	XXX	■
D7420		I	Radical excision — lesion diameter greater than 1.25 cm. See also CPT.	8.29	6.59	6.59	0.88	15.76	15.76	XXX	■
D7430		I	Excision of benign tumor – lesion diameter up to 1.25 cm. See also CPT.	5.29	4.20	4.20	0.56	10.05	10.05	XXX	■
D7431		I	Excision of benign tumor – lesion diameter greater than 1.25 cm. See also CPT.	9.03	7.18	7.18	0.96	17.17	17.17	XXX	■
D7440		I	Excision of malignant tumor – lesion diameter up to 1.25 cm. See also CPT.	9.33	7.42	7.42	0.99	17.74	17.74	XXX	■
D7441		I	Excision of malignant tumor – lesion diameter greater than 1.25 cm. See also CPT.	14.51	11.53	11.53	1.54	27.58	27.58	XXX	■
D7450		I	Removal of odontogenic cyst or tumor – lesion diameter up to 1.25 cm. See also CPT.	5.29	4.20	4.20	0.56	10.05	10.05	XXX	■
D7451		I	Removal of odontogenic cyst or tumor – lesion diameter greater than 1.25 cm. See also CPT.	8.30	6.60	6.60	0.88	15.78	15.78	XXX	■
D7460		I	Removal of nonodontogenic cyst or tumor – lesion diameter up to 1.25 cm. See also CPT.	5.29	4.20	4.20	0.56	10.05	10.05	XXX	■
D7461		I	Removal of nonodontogenic cyst or tumor – lesion diameter greater than 1.25 cm. See also CPT.	8.52	6.77	6.77	0.91	16.19	16.19	XXX	■
D7465		I	Destruction of lesion(s) by physical or chemical method, by report. See also code 41850.	3.01	2.40	2.40	0.32	5.73	5.73	XXX	■
D7471		I	Removal of exostosis — per site	5.48	4.35	4.35	0.58	10.41	10.41	XXX	■
D7480		I	Partial ostectomy (guttering or saucerization). See also code 21025.	7.24	5.76	5.76	0.77	13.77	13.77	XXX	■
D7490		I	Radical resection of mandible with bone graft. See also code 21095.	44.23	35.15	35.15	4.71	84.08	84.08	XXX	■
D7510		I	Incision and drainage of abscess – intraoral soft tissue. See also code 41800.	1.58	1.26	1.26	0.17	3.01	3.01	XXX	■
D7520		I	Incision and drainage of abscess – extraoral soft tissue. See also code 40800.	7.55	6.00	6.00	0.80	14.35	14.35	XXX	■

Code	M	S	Description	Work Value	Non-Fac PE	Fac PE	Mal-practice	Non-Fac Total	Fac Total	Global	Gap
D7530		I	Removal of foreign body, skin, or subcutaneous alveolar tissue. See also codes 41805, 41828.	2.72	2.16	2.16	0.29	5.17	5.17	XXX	■
D7540		I	Removal of reaction-producing foreign bodies, musculoskeletal system. See also codes 20520, 41800, 41806.	3.01	2.40	2.40	0.32	5.73	5.73	XXX	■
D7550		I	Sequestrectomy for osteomyelitis. See also code 20999.	1.88	1.49	1.49	0.20	3.57	3.57	XXX	■
D7560		I	Maxillary sinusotomy for removal of tooth fragment or foreign body. See also code 31020.	14.93	11.86	11.86	1.59	28.38	28.38	XXX	■
D7610		I	Maxilla — open reduction (teeth immobilized, if present). See also CPT.	24.14	19.18	19.18	2.57	45.89	45.89	XXX	■
D7620		I	Maxilla — closed reduction (teeth immobilized, if present). See also CPT.	18.10	14.39	14.39	1.93	34.42	34.42	XXX	■
D7630		I	Mandible — open reduction (teeth immobilized, if present). See also CPT.	31.39	24.94	24.94	3.34	59.67	59.67	XXX	■
D7640		I	Mandible — closed reduction (teeth immobilized, if present). See also CPT.	19.91	15.83	15.83	2.12	37.86	37.86	XXX	■
D7650		I	Malar and/or zygomatic arch — open reduction. See also CPT.	15.09	11.99	11.99	1.61	28.68	28.68	XXX	■
D7660		I	Malar and/or zygomatic arch — closed reduction. See also CPT.	8.89	7.07	7.07	0.95	16.91	16.91	XXX	■
D7670		I	Alveolus — stabilization of teeth, closed reduction splinting. See also CPT.	6.94	5.52	5.52	0.74	13.20	13.20	XXX	■
D7680		I	Facial bones — complicated reduction with fixation and multiple surgical approaches. See also CPT.	45.26	35.97	35.97	4.82	86.05	86.05	XXX	■
D7710		I	Maxilla — open reduction. See also code 21346.	28.37	22.55	22.55	3.02	53.94	53.94	XXX	■
D7720		I	Maxilla — closed reduction. See also code 21345.	19.91	15.83	15.83	2.12	37.86	37.86	XXX	■
D7730		I	Mandible — open reduction. See also codes 21461, 21462.	41.04	32.61	32.61	4.37	78.02	78.02	XXX	■
D7740		I	Mandible — closed reduction. See also code 21455.	20.31	16.14	16.14	2.16	38.61	38.61	XXX	■
D7750		I	Malar and/or zygomatic arch — open reduction. See also codes 21360, 21365.	25.83	20.52	20.52	2.75	49.10	49.10	XXX	■
D7760		I	Malar and/or zygomatic arch — closed reduction. See also code 21355.	10.36	8.23	8.23	1.10	19.70	19.70	XXX	■
D7770		I	Alveolus — stabilization of teeth, open reduction splinting. See also code 21422.	14.04	11.16	11.16	1.49	26.69	26.69	XXX	■
D7780		I	Facial bones — complicated reduction with fixation and multiple surgical approaches. See also codes 21433, 21435, 21436.	60.35	47.96	47.96	6.43	114.74	114.74	XXX	■

■ RVU not developed by CMS. Gap-filled RVUs developed by CHEG.

Code	M	S	Description	Work Value	Non-Fac PE	Fac PE	Mal-practice	Non-Fac Total	Fac Total	Global	Gap
D7810		I	Open reduction of dislocation. See also code 21490.	26.55	21.10	21.10	2.83	50.47	50.47	XXX	■
D7820		I	Closed reduction of dislocation. See also code 21480.	4.35	3.46	3.46	0.46	8.27	8.27	XXX	■
D7830		I	Manipulation under anesthesia. See also code 00190.	2.49	1.98	1.98	0.27	4.74	4.74	XXX	■
D7840		I	Condylectomy. See also code 21050.	36.19	28.76	28.76	3.85	68.80	68.80	XXX	■
D7850		I	Surgical discectomy, with/without implant. See also code 21060.	31.25	24.84	24.84	3.33	59.42	59.42	XXX	■
D7852		I	Disc repair. See also code 21299.	35.78	28.44	28.44	3.81	68.03	68.03	XXX	■
D7854		I	Synovectomy. See also code 21299.	36.93	29.35	29.35	3.93	70.21	70.21	XXX	■
D7856		I	Myotomy. See also code 21299.	26.21	20.82	20.82	2.79	49.82	49.82	XXX	■
D7858		I	Joint reconstruction. See also codes 21242, 21243.	74.69	59.35	59.35	7.95	141.99	141.99	XXX	■
D7860		I	Arthrotomy	31.83	25.30	25.30	3.39	60.52	60.52	XXX	■
D7865		I	Arthroplasty. See also code 21240.	51.30	40.77	40.77	5.46	97.53	97.53	XXX	■
D7870		I	Arthrocentesis. See also code 21060.	1.69	1.35	1.35	0.18	3.22	3.22	XXX	■
D7871		N	Non-arthroscopic lysis and lavage	3.39	2.70	2.70	0.36	6.45	6.45	XXX	■
D7872		I	Arthroscopy — diagnosis, with or without biopsy. See also code 29800.	18.09	14.38	14.38	1.93	34.40	34.40	XXX	■
D7873		I	Arthroscopy — surgical: lavage and lysis of adhesions. See also code 29804.	21.79	17.31	17.31	2.32	41.42	41.42	XXX	■
D7874		I	Arthroscopy — surgical: disc repositioning and stabilization. See also code 29804.	31.25	24.84	24.84	3.33	59.42	59.42	XXX	■
D7875		I	Arthroscopy — surgical: synovectomy. See also code 29804.	34.24	27.21	27.21	3.65	65.09	65.09	XXX	■
D7876		I	Arthroscopy — surgical: discectomy. See also code 29804.	36.91	29.34	29.34	3.93	70.18	70.18	XXX	■
D7877		I	Arthroscopy — surgical: debridement. See also code 29804.	32.58	25.89	25.89	3.47	61.94	61.94	XXX	■
D7880		I	Occlusal orthotic device, by report. See also code 21499.	4.07	3.24	3.24	0.43	7.74	7.74	XXX	■
D7899		I	Unspecified TMD therapy, by report. See also code 21499.	0.00	0.00	0.00	0.00	0.00	0.00	XXX	
D7910		I	Suture of recent small wounds up to 5 cm. See also codes 12011, 12013.	2.42	1.92	1.92	0.26	4.60	4.60	XXX	■
D7911		I	Complicated suture — up to 5 cm. See also codes 12051, 12052.	6.04	4.80	4.80	0.64	11.48	11.48	XXX	■

■ RVU not developed by CMS. Gap-filled RVUs developed by CHEG.

Code	M	S	Description	Work Value	Non-Fac PE	Fac PE	Mal-practice	Non-Fac Total	Fac Total	Global	Gap
D7912		I	Complicated suture — greater than 5 cm. See also code 13132.	10.87	8.64	8.64	1.16	20.66	20.66	XXX	■
D7920		I	Skin graft (identify defect covered, location and type of graft). See also CPT.	17.80	14.15	14.15	1.90	33.84	33.84	XXX	■
D7940		R	Osteoplasty — for orthognathic deformities	0.00	0.00	0.00	0.00	0.00	0.00	YYY	
D7941		I	Osteotomy — mandibular rami. See also codes 21193, 21195, 21196.	53.29	42.35	42.35	5.67	101.31	101.31	XXX	■
D7943		I	Osteotomy — mandibular rami with bone graft; includes obtaining the graft. See also code 21194.	55.50	44.11	44.11	5.91	105.52	105.52	XXX	■
D7944		I	Osteotomy — segmented or subapical — per sextant or quadrant. See also codes 21198, 21206.	49.49	39.33	39.33	5.27	94.08	94.08	XXX	■
D7945		I	Osteotomy — body of mandible. See also codes 21193, 21194, 21195, 21196.	54.91	43.64	43.64	5.85	104.40	104.40	XXX	■
D7946		I	LeFort I (maxilla — total). See also code 21147.	67.85	53.92	53.92	7.22	129.00	129.00	XXX	■
D7947		I	LeFort I (maxilla — segmented). See also codes 21145, 21146.	57.16	45.42	45.42	6.09	108.67	108.67	XXX	■
D7948		I	LeFort II or LeFort III (osteoplasty of facial bones for midface hypoplasia or retrusion) — without bone graft. See also code 21150.	89.02	70.74	70.74	9.48	169.24	169.24	XXX	■
D7949		I	LeFort II or LeFort III — with bone graft. See also CPT.	125.23	99.52	99.52	13.33	238.08	238.08	XXX	■
D7950		I	Osseous, osteoperiosteal, or cartilage graft of the mandible or facial bones— autogenous or nonautogenous, by report. See also code 21247.	0.00	0.00	0.00	0.00	0.00	0.00	XXX	
D7955		I	Repair of maxillofacial soft and hard tissue defect. See also code 21299.	0.00	0.00	0.00	0.00	0.00	0.00	XXX	
D7960		I	Frenulectomy (frenectomy or frenotomy) — separate procedure. See also codes 40819, 41010, 41115.	3.49	2.77	2.77	0.37	6.63	6.63	XXX	■
D7970		I	Excision of hyperplastic tissue — per arch. See also CPT.	3.60	2.86	2.86	0.38	6.84	6.84	XXX	■
D7971		I	Excision of pericoronal gingiva. See also code 41821.	1.14	0.91	0.91	0.12	2.17	2.17	XXX	■
D7980		I	Sialolithotomy. See also codes 42330, 42335, 42340.	5.12	4.07	4.07	0.55	9.74	9.74	XXX	■
D7981		I	Excision of salivary gland, by report. See also code 42408.	0.00	0.00	0.00	0.00	0.00	0.00	XXX	
D7982		I	Sialodochoplasty. See also code 42500.	13.78	10.95	10.95	1.47	26.20	26.20	XXX	■
D7983		I	Closure of salivary fistula. See also code 42600.	13.16	10.45	10.45	1.40	25.01	25.01	XXX	■

■ RVU not developed by CMS. Gap-filled RVUs developed by CHEG.

Code	M	S	Description	Work Value	Non-Fac PE	Fac PE	Mal-practice	Non-Fac Total	Fac Total	Global	Gap
D7990		I	Emergency tracheotomy. See also codes 31603, 31605.	12.07	9.59	9.59	1.28	22.94	22.94	XXX	■
D7991		I	Coronoidectomy. See also code 21070.	29.87	23.74	23.74	3.18	56.79	56.79	XXX	■
D7995		I	Synthetic graft — mandible or facial bones, by report. See also code 21299.	0.00	0.00	0.00	0.00	0.00	0.00	XXX	
D7996		I	Implant — mandible for augmentation purposes (excluding alveolar ridge), by report. See also code 21299.	0.00	0.00	0.00	0.00	0.00	0.00	XXX	
D7997		N	Appliance removal (not by dentist who placed appliance), includes removal of archbar	1.85	1.47	1.47	0.20	3.52	3.52	XXX	■
D7999		I	Unspecified oral surgery procedure, by report. See also code 21299.	0.00	0.00	0.00	0.00	0.00	0.00	XXX	
D8010		N	Limited orthodontic treatment of the primary dentition	0.00	0.00	0.00	0.00	0.00	0.00	XXX	
D8020		N	Limited orthodontic treatment of the transitional dentition	0.00	0.00	0.00	0.00	0.00	0.00	XXX	
D8030		N	Limited orthodontic treatment of the adolescent dentition	0.00	0.00	0.00	0.00	0.00	0.00	XXX	
D8040		N	Limited orthodontic treatment of the adult dentition	0.00	0.00	0.00	0.00	0.00	0.00	XXX	
D8050		N	Interceptive orthodontic treatment of the primary dentition	0.00	0.00	0.00	0.00	0.00	0.00	XXX	
D8060		N	Interceptive orthodontic treatment of the transitional dentition	0.00	0.00	0.00	0.00	0.00	0.00	XXX	
D8070		N	Comprehensive orthodontic treatment of the transitional dentition	0.00	0.00	0.00	0.00	0.00	0.00	XXX	
D8080		N	Comprehensive orthodontic treatment of the adolescent dentition	0.00	0.00	0.00	0.00	0.00	0.00	XXX	
D8090		N	Comprehensive orthodontic treatment of the adult dentition	0.00	0.00	0.00	0.00	0.00	0.00	XXX	
D8210		N	Removable appliance therapy	0.00	0.00	0.00	0.00	0.00	0.00	XXX	
D8220		N	Fixed appliance therapy	0.00	0.00	0.00	0.00	0.00	0.00	XXX	
D8660		N	Pre-orthodontic treatment visit	0.22	0.52	0.52	0.03	0.77	0.77	XXX	■
D8670		N	Periodic orthodontic treatment visit (as part of contract)	1.08	2.49	2.49	0.15	3.71	3.71	XXX	■
D8680		N	Orthodontic retention (removal of appliances, construction and placement of retainer(s))	2.37	5.47	5.47	0.33	8.16	8.16	XXX	■
D8690		N	Orthodontic treatment (alternative billing to a contract fee)	1.12	2.58	2.58	0.15	3.85	3.85	XXX	■
D8691		N	Repair of orthodontic appliance	0.59	1.35	1.35	0.08	2.02	2.02	XXX	■

■ RVU not developed by CMS. Gap-filled RVUs developed by CHEG.

Code	M	S	Description	Work Value	Non-Fac PE	Fac PE	Mal-practice	Non-Fac Total	Fac Total	Global	Gap
D8692		N	Replacement of lost or broken retainer	1.17	2.71	2.71	0.16	4.04	4.04	XXX	■
D8999		N	Unspecified orthodontic procedure, by report	0.00	0.00	0.00	0.00	0.00	0.00	XXX	
D9110		R	Palliative (emergency) treatment of dental pain — minor procedure	0.31	0.72	0.72	0.04	1.08	1.08	YYY	■
D9210		I	Local anesthesia not in conjunction with operative or surgical procedures. See also code 90784.	0.10	0.23	0.23	0.01	0.34	0.34	XXX	■
D9211		I	Regional block anesthesia. See also code 01995.	0.14	0.33	0.33	0.02	0.49	0.49	XXX	■
D9212		I	Trigeminal division block anesthesia. See also code 64400.	0.28	0.66	0.66	0.04	0.98	0.98	XXX	■
D9215		I	Local anesthesia. See also code 90784.	0.10	0.23	0.23	0.01	0.34	0.34	XXX	■
D9220		I	General anesthesia — first 30 minutes. See also CPT.	1.26	2.91	2.91	0.17	4.34	4.34	XXX	■
D9221		I	General anesthesia — each additional 15 minutes	0.53	1.22	1.22	0.07	1.82	1.82	XXX	■
D9230		R	Analgesia, anxiolysis, inhalation of nitrous oxide	0.17	0.40	0.40	0.02	0.59	0.59	YYY	■
D9241		I	Intravenous sedation/analgesia — first 30 minutes	0.99	2.29	2.29	0.14	3.42	3.42	XXX	■
D9242		I	Intravenous sedation/analgesia — each additional 15 minutes	0.41	0.96	0.96	0.06	1.43	1.43	XXX	■
D9248		R	Non-intravenous conscious sedation	0.21	0.49	0.49	0.03	0.73	0.73	XXX	■
D9310		I	Consultation (diagnostic service provided by dentist or physician other than practitioner providing treatment). See also CPT.	0.66	1.53	1.53	0.09	2.28	2.28	XXX	■
D9410		I	House/extrended care facility call. See also CPT.	0.87	2.02	2.02	0.12	3.01	3.01	XXX	■
D9420		I	Hospital call. See also CPT.	1.20	2.78	2.78	0.17	4.15	4.15	XXX	■
D9430		I	Office visit for observation (during regularly scheduled hours) — no other services performed. See also CPT.	0.22	0.52	0.52	0.03	0.77	0.77	XXX	■
D9440		I	Office visit — after regularly scheduled hours. See also code 99050.	0.40	0.93	0.93	0.06	1.39	1.39	XXX	■
D9610		I	Therapeutic drug injection, by report. See also codes 90784, 90788.	0.00	0.00	0.00	0.00	0.00	0.00	XXX	
D9630		R	Other drugs and/or medicaments, by report	0.00	0.00	0.00	0.00	0.00	0.00	YYY	
D9910		N	Application of desensitizing medicament	0.14	0.33	0.33	0.02	0.49	0.49	XXX	■
D9911		N	Application of desensitizing resin for cervical and/or root surface, per tooth	0.22	0.52	0.52	0.03	0.77	0.77	XXX	■
D9920		N	Behavior management, by report	0.00	0.00	0.00	0.00	0.00	0.00	XXX	

■ RVU not developed by CMS. Gap-filled RVUs developed by CHEG.

Code	M	S	Description	Work Value	Non-Fac PE	Fac PE	Mal-practice	Non-Fac Total	Fac Total	Global	Gap
D9930		R	Treatment of complications (post-surgical) — unusual circumstances, by report	0.00	0.00	0.00	0.00	0.00	0.00	YYY	
D9940		R	Occlusal guard, by report	0.00	0.00	0.00	0.00	0.00	0.00	YYY	
D9941		N	Fabrication of athletic mouthguard. See also code 21089.	0.50	1.15	1.15	0.07	1.72	1.72	XXX	■
D9950		R	Occlusion analysis — mounted case	0.88	2.03	2.03	0.12	3.03	3.03	YYY	■
D9951		R	Occlusal adjustment — limited	0.40	0.92	0.92	0.05	1.37	1.37	YYY	■
D9952		R	Occlusal adjustment — complete	2.24	5.19	5.19	0.31	7.74	7.74	YYY	■
D9970		N	Enamel microabrasion	0.15	0.36	0.36	0.02	0.53	0.53	XXX	■
D9971		N	Odontoplasty 1–2 teeth; includes removal of enamel projections	0.21	0.50	0.50	0.03	0.74	0.74	XXX	■
D9972		N	External bleaching — per arch	0.99	2.28	2.28	0.14	3.41	3.41	XXX	■
D9973		N	External bleaching — per tooth	0.11	0.25	0.25	0.02	0.38	0.38	XXX	■
D9974		N	Internal bleaching — per tooth	0.84	1.94	1.94	0.12	2.90	2.90	XXX	■
D9999		I	Unspecified adjunctive procedure, by report	0.00	0.00	0.00	0.00	0.00	0.00	XXX	
E0100	NU		Cane, includes canes of all materials, adjustable or fixed, with tip	0.00	0.48	0.48	0.00	0.48	0.48	XXX	■
	RR			0.00	0.19	0.19	0.00	0.19	0.19	XXX	■
	UE			0.00	0.38	0.38	0.00	0.38	0.38	XXX	■
E0105	NU		Cane, quad or three-prong, includes canes of all materials, adjustable or fixed, with tips	0.00	0.76	0.76	0.00	0.76	0.76	XXX	■
	RR			0.00	0.25	0.25	0.00	0.25	0.25	XXX	■
	UE			0.00	0.68	0.68	0.00	0.68	0.68	XXX	■
E0110	NU		Crutches, forearm, includes crutches of various materials, adjustable or fixed, pair, complete with tips and handgrips	0.00	1.30	1.30	0.00	1.30	1.30	XXX	■
	RR			0.00	0.50	0.50	0.00	0.50	0.50	XXX	■
	UE			0.00	1.17	1.17	0.00	1.17	1.17	XXX	■
E0111	NU		Crutch, forearm, includes crutches of various materials, adjustable or fixed, each, with tip and handgrip	0.00	1.43	1.43	0.00	1.43	1.43	XXX	■
	RR			0.00	0.33	0.33	0.00	0.33	0.33	XXX	■
	UE			0.00	1.10	1.10	0.00	1.10	1.10	XXX	■
E0112	NU		Crutches, underarm, wood, adjustable or fixed, pair, with pads, tips and handgrips	0.00	0.35	0.35	0.00	0.35	0.35	XXX	■
	RR			0.00	0.31	0.31	0.00	0.31	0.31	XXX	■
	UE			0.00	0.32	0.32	0.00	0.32	0.32	XXX	■
E0113	NU		Crutch, underarm, wood, adjustable or fixed, each, with pad, tip and handgrip	0.00	0.66	0.66	0.00	0.66	0.66	XXX	■
	RR			0.00	0.15	0.15	0.00	0.15	0.15	XXX	■
	UE			0.00	0.42	0.42	0.00	0.42	0.42	XXX	■
E0114	NU		Crutches, underarm, other than wood, adjustable or fixed, pair, with pads, tips and handgrips	0.00	0.73	0.73	0.00	0.73	0.73	XXX	■
	RR			0.00	0.33	0.33	0.00	0.33	0.33	XXX	■
	UE			0.00	0.66	0.66	0.00	0.66	0.66	XXX	■
E0116	NU		Crutch, underarm, other than wood, adjustable or fixed, each, with pad, tip and handgrip	0.00	0.89	0.89	0.00	0.89	0.89	XXX	■
	RR			0.00	0.24	0.24	0.00	0.24	0.24	XXX	■
	UE			0.00	0.66	0.66	0.00	0.66	0.66	XXX	■

■ RVU not developed by CMS. Gap-filled RVUs developed by CHEG.

Code	M	S	Description	Work Value	Non-Fac PE	Fac PE	Mal-practice	Non-Fac Total	Fac Total	Global	Gap
E0130	NU		Walker, rigid (pickup), adjustable or fixed height	0.00	1.95	1.95	0.00	1.95	1.95	XXX	■
	RR			0.00	0.51	0.51	0.00	0.51	0.51	XXX	■
	UE			0.00	1.56	1.56	0.00	1.56	1.56	XXX	■
E0135	NU		Walker, folding (pickup), adjustable or fixed height	0.00	1.37	1.37	0.00	1.37	1.37	XXX	■
	RR			0.00	0.54	0.54	0.00	0.54	0.54	XXX	■
	UE			0.00	1.07	1.07	0.00	1.07	1.07	XXX	■
E0141	NU		Rigid walker, wheeled, without seat	0.00	0.89	0.89	0.00	0.89	0.89	XXX	■
	RR			0.00	0.61	0.61	0.00	0.61	0.61	XXX	■
	UE			0.00	0.59	0.59	0.00	0.59	0.59	XXX	■
E0142	NU		Rigid walker, wheeled, with seat	0.00	3.82	3.82	0.00	3.82	3.82	XXX	■
	RR			0.00	0.72	0.72	0.00	0.72	0.72	XXX	■
	UE			0.00	3.05	3.05	0.00	3.05	3.05	XXX	■
E0143	NU		Folding walker, wheeled, without seat	0.00	3.31	3.31	0.00	3.31	3.31	XXX	■
	RR			0.00	0.68	0.68	0.00	0.68	0.68	XXX	■
	UE			0.00	2.64	2.64	0.00	2.64	2.64	XXX	■
E0144			Enclosed, framed folding walker, wheeled, with posterior seat	0.00	0.00	0.00	0.00	0.00	0.00	XXX	
E0145	NU		Walker, wheeled, with seat and crutch attachments	0.00	4.47	4.47	0.00	4.47	4.47	XXX	■
	RR			0.00	0.65	0.65	0.00	0.65	0.65	XXX	■
	UE			0.00	3.58	3.58	0.00	3.58	3.58	XXX	■
E0146	NU		Folding walker, wheeled, with seat	0.00	4.25	4.25	0.00	4.25	4.25	XXX	■
	RR			0.00	0.45	0.45	0.00	0.45	0.45	XXX	■
	UE			0.00	3.40	3.40	0.00	3.40	3.40	XXX	■
E0147	NU		Heavy duty, multiple breaking system, variable wheel resistance walker	0.00	10.73	10.73	0.00	10.73	10.73	XXX	■
	RR			0.00	1.18	1.18	0.00	1.18	1.18	XXX	■
	UE			0.00	8.58	8.58	0.00	8.58	8.58	XXX	■
E0148	NU		Walker, heavy duty, without wheels, rigid or folding, any type, each	0.00	3.07	3.07	0.00	3.07	3.07	XXX	■
	RR			0.00	0.30	0.30	0.00	0.30	0.30	XXX	■
	UE			0.00	2.29	2.29	0.00	2.29	2.29	XXX	■
E0149	NU		Walker, heavy duty, wheeled, rigid or folding, any type, each	0.00	5.39	5.39	0.00	5.39	5.39	XXX	■
	RR			0.00	0.54	0.54	0.00	0.54	0.54	XXX	■
	UE			0.00	4.05	4.05	0.00	4.05	4.05	XXX	■
E0153	NU		Platform attachment, forearm crutch, each	0.00	1.94	1.94	0.00	1.94	1.94	XXX	■
	RR			0.00	0.21	0.21	0.00	0.21	0.21	XXX	■
	UE			0.00	1.34	1.34	0.00	1.34	1.34	XXX	■
E0154	NU		Platform attachment, walker, each	0.00	1.95	1.95	0.00	1.95	1.95	XXX	■
	RR			0.00	0.24	0.24	0.00	0.24	0.24	XXX	■
	UE			0.00	1.56	1.56	0.00	1.56	1.56	XXX	■
E0155	NU		Wheel attachment, rigid pick-up walker, per pair seat attachment, walker	0.00	0.99	0.99	0.00	0.99	0.99	XXX	■
	RR			0.00	0.12	0.12	0.00	0.12	0.12	XXX	■
	UE			0.00	0.75	0.75	0.00	0.75	0.75	XXX	■
E0156	NU		Seat attachment, walker	0.00	0.75	0.75	0.00	0.75	0.75	XXX	■
	RR			0.00	0.13	0.13	0.00	0.13	0.13	XXX	■
	UE			0.00	0.60	0.60	0.00	0.60	0.60	XXX	■

■ RVU not developed by CMS. Gap-filled RVUs developed by CHEG.

Code	M	S	Description	Work Value	Non-Fac PE	Fac PE	Mal-practice	Non-Fac Total	Fac Total	Global	Gap
E0157	NU		Crutch attachment, walker, each	0.00	2.24	2.24	0.00	2.24	2.24	XXX	■
	RR			0.00	0.24	0.24	0.00	0.24	0.24	XXX	■
	UE			0.00	1.79	1.79	0.00	1.79	1.79	XXX	■
E0158	NU		Leg extensions for walker, per set of four (4)	0.00	0.80	0.80	0.00	0.80	0.80	XXX	■
	RR			0.00	0.08	0.08	0.00	0.08	0.08	XXX	■
	UE			0.00	0.60	0.60	0.00	0.60	0.60	XXX	■
E0159			Brake attachment for wheeled walker, replacement, each	0.00	0.71	0.71	0.00	0.71	0.71	XXX	■
E0160	NU		Sitz type bath or equipment, portable, used with or without commode	0.00	0.91	0.91	0.00	0.91	0.91	XXX	■
	RR			0.00	0.12	0.12	0.00	0.12	0.12	XXX	■
	UE			0.00	0.73	0.73	0.00	0.73	0.73	XXX	■
E0161	NU		Sitz type bath or equipment, portable, used with or without commode, with faucet attachment/s	0.00	0.72	0.72	0.00	0.72	0.72	XXX	■
	RR			0.00	0.09	0.09	0.00	0.09	0.09	XXX	■
	UE			0.00	0.57	0.57	0.00	0.57	0.57	XXX	■
E0162	NU		Sitz bath chair	0.00	4.17	4.17	0.00	4.17	4.17	XXX	■
	RR			0.00	0.42	0.42	0.00	0.42	0.42	XXX	■
	UE			0.00	3.34	3.34	0.00	3.34	3.34	XXX	■
E0163	NU		Commode chair, stationary, with fixed arms	0.00	3.28	3.28	0.00	3.28	3.28	XXX	■
	RR			0.00	0.77	0.77	0.00	0.77	0.77	XXX	■
	UE			0.00	2.38	2.38	0.00	2.38	2.38	XXX	■
E0164	NU		Commode chair, mobile, with fixed arms	0.00	5.67	5.67	0.00	5.67	5.67	XXX	■
	RR			0.00	0.83	0.83	0.00	0.83	0.83	XXX	■
	UE			0.00	4.25	4.25	0.00	4.25	4.25	XXX	■
E0165	NU		Commode chair, stationary, with detachable arms	0.00	5.04	5.04	0.00	5.04	5.04	XXX	■
	RR			0.00	0.58	0.58	0.00	0.58	0.58	XXX	■
	UE			0.00	4.02	4.02	0.00	4.02	4.02	XXX	■
E0166	NU		Commode chair, mobile, with detachable arms	0.00	6.91	6.91	0.00	6.91	6.91	XXX	■
	RR			0.00	0.83	0.83	0.00	0.83	0.83	XXX	■
	UE			0.00	5.51	5.51	0.00	5.51	5.51	XXX	■
E0167	NU		Pail or pan for use with commode chair	0.00	0.37	0.37	0.00	0.37	0.37	XXX	■
	RR			0.00	0.06	0.06	0.00	0.06	0.06	XXX	■
	UE			0.00	0.28	0.28	0.00	0.28	0.28	XXX	■
E0168	NU		Commode chair, extra wide and/or heavy duty, stationary or mobile, with or without arms, any type, each	0.00	3.64	3.64	0.00	3.64	3.64	XXX	■
	RR			0.00	0.36	0.36	0.00	0.36	0.36	XXX	■
	UE			0.00	2.73	2.73	0.00	2.73	2.73	XXX	■
E0169	NU		Commode chair with seat lift mechanism	0.00	9.69	9.69	0.00	9.69	9.69	XXX	■
	RR			0.00	1.49	1.49	0.00	1.49	1.49	XXX	■
	UE			0.00	7.24	7.24	0.00	7.24	7.24	XXX	■
E0175	NU		Foot rest, for use with commode chair, each	0.00	2.07	2.07	0.00	2.07	2.07	XXX	■
	RR			0.00	0.21	0.21	0.00	0.21	0.21	XXX	■
	UE			0.00	1.53	1.53	0.00	1.53	1.53	XXX	■
E0176	NU		Air pressure pad or cushion, nonpositioning	0.00	2.98	2.98	0.00	2.98	2.98	XXX	■
	RR			0.00	0.45	0.45	0.00	0.45	0.45	XXX	■
	UE			0.00	2.38	2.38	0.00	2.38	2.38	XXX	■

■ RVU not developed by CMS. Gap-filled RVUs developed by CHEG.

HCPCS

Code	M	S	Description	Work Value	Non-Fac PE	Fac PE	Mal-practice	Non-Fac Total	Fac Total	Global	Gap
E0177	NU		Water pressure pad or cushion, nonpositioning	0.00	2.92	2.92	0.00	2.92	2.92	XXX	■
	RR			0.00	0.45	0.45	0.00	0.45	0.45	XXX	■
	UE			0.00	2.24	2.24	0.00	2.24	2.24	XXX	■
E0178	NU		Gel or gel-like pressure pad or cushion, nonpositioning	0.00	3.73	3.73	0.00	3.73	3.73	XXX	■
	RR			0.00	0.48	0.48	0.00	0.48	0.48	XXX	■
	UE			0.00	2.53	2.53	0.00	2.53	2.53	XXX	■
E0179	NU		Dry pressure pad or cushion, nonpositioning	0.00	0.45	0.45	0.00	0.45	0.45	XXX	■
	RR			0.00	0.04	0.04	0.00	0.04	0.04	XXX	■
	UE			0.00	0.30	0.30	0.00	0.30	0.30	XXX	■
E0180	NU		Pressure pad, alternating with pump	0.00	10.43	10.43	0.00	10.43	10.43	XXX	■
	RR			0.00	1.15	1.15	0.00	1.15	1.15	XXX	■
	UE			0.00	6.56	6.56	0.00	6.56	6.56	XXX	■
E0181	NU		Pressure pad, alternating with pump, heavy duty	0.00	7.81	7.81	0.00	7.81	7.81	XXX	■
	RR			0.00	0.72	0.72	0.00	0.72	0.72	XXX	■
	UE			0.00	6.23	6.23	0.00	6.23	6.23	XXX	■
E0182	NU		Pump for alternating pressure pad	0.00	7.45	7.45	0.00	7.45	7.45	XXX	■
	RR			0.00	0.72	0.72	0.00	0.72	0.72	XXX	■
	UE			0.00	6.14	6.14	0.00	6.14	6.14	XXX	■
E0184	NU		Dry pressure mattress	0.00	5.96	5.96	0.00	5.96	5.96	XXX	■
	RR			0.00	0.77	0.77	0.00	0.77	0.77	XXX	■
	UE			0.00	4.47	4.47	0.00	4.47	4.47	XXX	■
E0185	NU		Gel or gel-like pressure pad for mattress, standard mattress length and width	0.00	9.69	9.69	0.00	9.69	9.69	XXX	■
	RR			0.00	1.25	1.25	0.00	1.25	1.25	XXX	■
	UE			0.00	6.85	6.85	0.00	6.85	6.85	XXX	■
E0186	NU		Air pressure mattress	0.00	5.22	5.22	0.00	5.22	5.22	XXX	■
	RR			0.00	0.45	0.45	0.00	0.45	0.45	XXX	■
	UE			0.00	2.59	2.59	0.00	2.59	2.59	XXX	■
E0187	NU		Water pressure mattress	0.00	5.96	5.96	0.00	5.96	5.96	XXX	■
	RR			0.00	0.60	0.60	0.00	0.60	0.60	XXX	■
	UE			0.00	5.07	5.07	0.00	5.07	5.07	XXX	■
E0188			Synthetic sheepskin pad	0.00	1.22	1.22	0.00	1.22	1.22	XXX	■
E0189			Lambswool sheepskin pad, any size	0.00	0.00	0.00	0.00	0.00	0.00	XXX	
E0191	NU		Heel or elbow protector, each	0.00	0.16	0.16	0.00	0.16	0.16	XXX	■
	RR			0.00	0.04	0.04	0.00	0.04	0.04	XXX	■
E0192	NU		Low pressure and positioning equalization pad, for wheelchair	0.00	10.43	10.43	0.00	10.43	10.43	XXX	■
	RR			0.00	1.37	1.37	0.00	1.37	1.37	XXX	■
	UE			0.00	8.20	8.20	0.00	8.20	8.20	XXX	■
E0193	RR		Powered air flotation bed (low air loss therapy)	0.00	33.87	33.87	0.00	33.87	33.87	XXX	■
E0194	NU		Air fluidized bed	0.00	0.00	0.00	0.00	0.00	0.00	XXX	
	RR			0.00	89.40	89.40	0.00	89.40	89.40	XXX	■
	UE			0.00	0.00	0.00	0.00	0.00	0.00	XXX	

■ RVU not developed by CMS. Gap-filled RVUs developed by CHEG.

Code	M	S	Description	Work Value	Non-Fac PE	Fac PE	Mal-prac-tice	Non-Fac Total	Fac Total	Global	Gap
E0196	NU		Gel pressure mattress	0.00	8.94	8.94	0.00	8.94	8.94	XXX	■
	RR			0.00	0.89	0.89	0.00	0.89	0.89	XXX	■
	UE			0.00	6.71	6.71	0.00	6.71	6.71	XXX	■
E0197	NU		Air pressure pad for mattress, standard mattress length and width	0.00	5.96	5.96	0.00	5.96	5.96	XXX	■
	RR			0.00	0.83	0.83	0.00	0.83	0.83	XXX	■
	UE			0.00	5.22	5.22	0.00	5.22	5.22	XXX	■
E0198	NU		Water pressure pad for mattress, standard mattress length and width	0.00	6.56	6.56	0.00	6.56	6.56	XXX	■
	RR			0.00	0.72	0.72	0.00	0.72	0.72	XXX	■
	UE			0.00	4.62	4.62	0.00	4.62	4.62	XXX	■
E0199	NU		Dry pressure pad for mattress, standard mattress length and width	0.00	1.04	1.04	0.00	1.04	1.04	XXX	■
	RR			0.00	0.12	0.12	0.00	0.12	0.12	XXX	■
	UE			0.00	0.75	0.75	0.00	0.75	0.75	XXX	■
E0200	NU		Heat lamp, without stand (table model), includes bulb, or infrared element	0.00	2.91	2.91	0.00	2.91	2.91	XXX	■
	RR			0.00	0.39	0.39	0.00	0.39	0.39	XXX	■
	UE			0.00	2.19	2.19	0.00	2.19	2.19	XXX	■
E0202	RR		Phototherapy (bilirubin) light with photometer	0.00	2.85	2.85	0.00	2.85	2.85	XXX	■
E0205	NU		Heat lamp, with stand, includes bulb, or infrared element	0.00	5.36	5.36	0.00	5.36	5.36	XXX	■
	RR			0.00	0.66	0.66	0.00	0.66	0.66	XXX	■
	UE			0.00	4.17	4.17	0.00	4.17	4.17	XXX	■
E0210	NU		Electric heat pad, standard	0.00	0.86	0.86	0.00	0.86	0.86	XXX	■
	RR			0.00	0.11	0.11	0.00	0.11	0.11	XXX	■
	UE			0.00	0.66	0.66	0.00	0.66	0.66	XXX	■
E0215	NU		Electric heat pad, moist	0.00	1.97	1.97	0.00	1.97	1.97	XXX	■
	RR			0.00	0.24	0.24	0.00	0.24	0.24	XXX	■
	UE			0.00	1.62	1.62	0.00	1.62	1.62	XXX	■
E0217	NU		Water circulating heat pad with pump	0.00	10.06	10.06	0.00	10.06	10.06	XXX	■
	RR			0.00	1.16	1.16	0.00	1.16	1.16	XXX	■
	UE			0.00	7.54	7.54	0.00	7.54	7.54	XXX	■
E0218	NU		Water circulating cold pad with pump	0.00	10.06	10.06	0.00	10.06	10.06	XXX	■
	RR			0.00	1.16	1.16	0.00	1.16	1.16	XXX	■
	UE			0.00	7.54	7.54	0.00	7.54	7.54	XXX	■
E0220	NU		Hot water bottle	0.00	0.27	0.27	0.00	0.27	0.27	XXX	■
	RR			0.00	0.03	0.03	0.00	0.03	0.03	XXX	■
	UE			0.00	0.20	0.20	0.00	0.20	0.20	XXX	■
E0221			Infrared heating pad system	0.00	0.00	0.00	0.00	0.00	0.00	XXX	
E0225	NU		Hydrocollator unit, includes pads	0.00	10.46	10.46	0.00	10.46	10.46	XXX	■
	RR			0.00	1.05	1.05	0.00	1.05	1.05	XXX	■
	UE			0.00	7.84	7.84	0.00	7.84	7.84	XXX	■
E0230	NU		Ice cap or collar	0.00	0.27	0.27	0.00	0.27	0.27	XXX	■
	RR			0.00	0.05	0.05	0.00	0.05	0.05	XXX	■
	UE			0.00	0.22	0.22	0.00	0.22	0.22	XXX	■

■ RVU not developed by CMS. Gap-filled RVUs developed by CHEG.

Code	M	S	Description	Work Value	Non-Fac PE	Fac PE	Mal-practice	Non-Fac Total	Fac Total	Global	Gap
E0231			Non-contact wound warming device (temperature control unit, AC adapter and power cord) for use with warming card and wound cover	0.00	0.00	0.00	0.00	0.00	0.00	XXX	
E0232			Warming card for use with the non-contact wound warming device and non-contact wound warming wound cover	0.00	0.00	0.00	0.00	0.00	0.00	XXX	
E0235	NU		Paraffin bath unit, portable (see medical supply code A4265 for paraffin)	0.00	6.35	6.35	0.00	6.35	6.35	XXX	■
	RR			0.00	0.63	0.63	0.00	0.63	0.63	XXX	■
	UE			0.00	4.76	4.76	0.00	4.76	4.76	XXX	■
E0236	NU		Pump for water circulating pad	0.00	8.37	8.37	0.00	8.37	8.37	XXX	■
	RR			0.00	1.62	1.62	0.00	1.62	1.62	XXX	■
	UE			0.00	6.71	6.71	0.00	6.71	6.71	XXX	■
E0238	NU		Nonelectric heat pad, moist	0.00	0.81	0.81	0.00	0.81	0.81	XXX	■
	RR			0.00	0.16	0.16	0.00	0.16	0.16	XXX	■
	UE			0.00	0.65	0.65	0.00	0.65	0.65	XXX	■
E0239	NU		Hydrocollator unit, portable	0.00	12.07	12.07	0.00	12.07	12.07	XXX	■
	RR			0.00	1.22	1.22	0.00	1.22	1.22	XXX	■
	UE			0.00	9.06	9.06	0.00	9.06	9.06	XXX	■
E0241			Bathtub wall rail, each	0.00	0.70	0.70	0.00	0.70	0.70	XXX	■
E0242			Bathtub rail, floor base	0.00	1.59	1.59	0.00	1.59	1.59	XXX	■
E0243			Toilet rail, each	0.00	1.26	1.26	0.00	1.26	1.26	XXX	■
E0244			Raised toilet seat	0.00	0.95	0.95	0.00	0.95	0.95	XXX	■
E0245			Tub stool or bench	0.00	1.57	1.57	0.00	1.57	1.57	XXX	■
E0246			Transfer tub rail attachment	0.00	2.15	2.15	0.00	2.15	2.15	XXX	■
E0249	NU		Pad for water circulating heat unit	0.00	2.68	2.68	0.00	2.68	2.68	XXX	■
	RR			0.00	0.34	0.34	0.00	0.34	0.34	XXX	■
	UE			0.00	2.00	2.00	0.00	2.00	2.00	XXX	■
E0250	NU		Hospital bed, fixed height, with any type side rails, with mattress	0.00	35.76	35.76	0.00	35.76	35.76	XXX	■
	RR			0.00	2.68	2.68	0.00	2.68	2.68	XXX	■
	UE			0.00	23.16	23.16	0.00	23.16	23.16	XXX	■
E0251	NU		Hospital bed, fixed height, with any type side rails, without mattress	0.00	19.97	19.97	0.00	19.97	19.97	XXX	■
	RR			0.00	2.00	2.00	0.00	2.00	2.00	XXX	■
	UE			0.00	15.97	15.97	0.00	15.97	15.97	XXX	■
E0255	NU		Hospital bed, variable height, hi-lo, with any type side rails, with mattress	0.00	37.25	37.25	0.00	37.25	37.25	XXX	■
	RR			0.00	3.25	3.25	0.00	3.25	3.25	XXX	■
	UE			0.00	27.89	27.89	0.00	27.89	27.89	XXX	■
E0256	NU		Hospital bed, variable height, hi-lo, with any type side rails, without mattress	0.00	22.35	22.35	0.00	22.35	22.35	XXX	■
	RR			0.00	2.24	2.24	0.00	2.24	2.24	XXX	■
	UE			0.00	17.88	17.88	0.00	17.88	17.88	XXX	■
E0260	NU		Hospital bed, semi-electric (head and foot adjustment), with any type side rails, with mattress	0.00	38.74	38.74	0.00	38.74	38.74	XXX	■
	RR			0.00	4.77	4.77	0.00	4.77	4.77	XXX	■
	UE			0.00	29.92	29.92	0.00	29.92	29.92	XXX	■

■ RVU not developed by CMS. Gap-filled RVUs developed by CHEG.

Code	M	S	Description	Work Value	Non-Fac PE	Fac PE	Mal-practice	Non-Fac Total	Fac Total	Global	Gap
E0261	NU		Hospital bed, semi-electric (head and foot adjustment), with any type side rails, without mattress	0.00	35.76	35.76	0.00	35.76	35.76	XXX	■
	RR			0.00	3.73	3.73	0.00	3.73	3.73	XXX	■
	UE			0.00	23.84	23.84	0.00	23.84	23.84	XXX	■
E0265	NU		Hospital bed, total electric (head, foot, and height adjustments), with any type side rails, with mattress	0.00	46.04	46.04	0.00	46.04	46.04	XXX	■
	RR			0.00	5.54	5.54	0.00	5.54	5.54	XXX	■
	UE			0.00	29.80	29.80	0.00	29.80	29.80	XXX	■
E0266	NU		Hospital bed, total electric (head, foot, and height adjustments), with any type side rails, without mattress	0.00	47.68	47.68	0.00	47.68	47.68	XXX	■
	RR			0.00	4.77	4.77	0.00	4.77	4.77	XXX	■
	UE			0.00	32.78	32.78	0.00	32.78	32.78	XXX	■
E0270	NU		Hospital bed, institutional type includes: oscillating, circulating and stryker frame, with mattress	0.00	0.00	0.00	0.00	0.00	0.00	XXX	
	RR			0.00	0.00	0.00	0.00	0.00	0.00	XXX	
	UE			0.00	0.00	0.00	0.00	0.00	0.00	XXX	
E0271	NU		Mattress, inner spring	0.00	5.96	5.96	0.00	5.96	5.96	XXX	■
	RR			0.00	0.63	0.63	0.00	0.63	0.63	XXX	■
	UE			0.00	4.65	4.65	0.00	4.65	4.65	XXX	■
E0272	NU		Mattress, foam rubber	0.00	5.42	5.42	0.00	5.42	5.42	XXX	■
	RR			0.00	0.57	0.57	0.00	0.57	0.57	XXX	■
	UE			0.00	4.05	4.05	0.00	4.05	4.05	XXX	■
E0273	NU		Bed board	0.00	0.76	0.76	0.00	0.76	0.76	XXX	■
	RR			0.00	0.30	0.30	0.00	0.30	0.30	XXX	■
	UE			0.00	0.60	0.60	0.00	0.60	0.60	XXX	■
E0274	NU		Over-bed table	0.00	1.22	1.22	0.00	1.22	1.22	XXX	■
	RR			0.00	0.54	0.54	0.00	0.54	0.54	XXX	■
	UE			0.00	0.98	0.98	0.00	0.98	0.98	XXX	■
E0275	NU		Bed pan, standard, metal or plastic	0.00	0.33	0.33	0.00	0.33	0.33	XXX	■
	RR			0.00	0.06	0.06	0.00	0.06	0.06	XXX	■
	UE			0.00	0.25	0.25	0.00	0.25	0.25	XXX	■
E0276	NU		Bed pan, fracture, metal or plastic	0.00	0.31	0.31	0.00	0.31	0.31	XXX	■
	RR			0.00	0.06	0.06	0.00	0.06	0.06	XXX	■
	UE			0.00	0.30	0.30	0.00	0.30	0.30	XXX	■
E0277	NU		Powered pressure-reducing air mattress	0.00	0.00	0.00	0.00	0.00	0.00	XXX	
	RR			0.00	22.05	22.05	0.00	22.05	22.05	XXX	■
	UE			0.00	0.00	0.00	0.00	0.00	0.00	XXX	
E0280	NU		Bed cradle, any type	0.00	1.07	1.07	0.00	1.07	1.07	XXX	■
	RR			0.00	0.12	0.12	0.00	0.12	0.12	XXX	■
	UE			0.00	0.83	0.83	0.00	0.83	0.83	XXX	■
E0290	NU		Hospital bed, fixed height, without side rails, with mattress	0.00	20.86	20.86	0.00	20.86	20.86	XXX	■
	RR			0.00	2.03	2.03	0.00	2.03	2.03	XXX	■
	UE			0.00	16.69	16.69	0.00	16.69	16.69	XXX	■
E0291	NU		Hospital bed, fixed height, without side rails, without mattress	0.00	14.90	14.90	0.00	14.90	14.90	XXX	■
	RR			0.00	1.49	1.49	0.00	1.49	1.49	XXX	■
	UE			0.00	11.03	11.03	0.00	11.03	11.03	XXX	■
E0292	NU		Hospital bed, variable height, hi-lo, without side rails, with mattress	0.00	22.65	22.65	0.00	22.65	22.65	XXX	■
	RR			0.00	2.26	2.26	0.00	2.26	2.26	XXX	■
	UE			0.00	18.12	18.12	0.00	18.12	18.12	XXX	■

■ RVU not developed by CMS. Gap-filled RVUs developed by CHEG.

Code	M	S	Description	Work Value	Non-Fac PE	Fac PE	Mal-practice	Non-Fac Total	Fac Total	Global	Gap
E0293	NU		Hospital bed, variable height, hi-lo, without side rails, without mattress	0.00	19.37	19.37	0.00	19.37	19.37	XXX	■
	RR			0.00	1.94	1.94	0.00	1.94	1.94	XXX	■
	UE			0.00	14.16	14.16	0.00	14.16	14.16	XXX	■
E0294	NU		Hospital bed, semi-electric (head and foot adjustment), without side rails, with mattress	0.00	34.69	34.69	0.00	34.69	34.69	XXX	■
	RR			0.00	3.58	3.58	0.00	3.58	3.58	XXX	■
	UE			0.00	23.84	23.84	0.00	23.84	23.84	XXX	■
E0295	NU		Hospital bed, semi-electric (head and foot adjustment), without side rails, without mattress	0.00	32.15	32.15	0.00	32.15	32.15	XXX	■
	RR			0.00	3.52	3.52	0.00	3.52	3.52	XXX	■
	UE			0.00	20.86	20.86	0.00	20.86	20.86	XXX	■
E0296	NU		Hospital bed, total electric (head, foot, and height adjustments), without side rails, with mattress	0.00	44.10	44.10	0.00	44.10	44.10	XXX	■
	RR			0.00	4.41	4.41	0.00	4.41	4.41	XXX	■
	UE			0.00	35.28	35.28	0.00	35.28	35.28	XXX	■
E0297	NU		Hospital bed, total electric (head, foot, and height adjustments), without side rails, without mattress	0.00	37.85	37.85	0.00	37.85	37.85	XXX	■
	RR			0.00	3.78	3.78	0.00	3.78	3.78	XXX	■
	UE			0.00	25.33	25.33	0.00	25.33	25.33	XXX	■
E0305	NU		Bedside rails, half-length	0.00	4.77	4.77	0.00	4.77	4.77	XXX	■
	RR			0.00	0.48	0.48	0.00	0.48	0.48	XXX	■
	UE			0.00	3.43	3.43	0.00	3.43	3.43	XXX	■
E0310	NU		Bedside rails, full-length	0.00	5.36	5.36	0.00	5.36	5.36	XXX	■
	RR			0.00	0.63	0.63	0.00	0.63	0.63	XXX	■
	UE			0.00	4.11	4.11	0.00	4.11	4.11	XXX	■
E0315			Bed accessory: board, table, or support device, any type	0.00	0.00	0.00	0.00	0.00	0.00	XXX	
E0316			Safety enclosure frame/canopy for use with hospital bed, any type	0.00	0.00	0.00	0.00	0.00	0.00	XXX	
E0325	NU		Urinal; male, jug-type, any material	0.00	0.22	0.22	0.00	0.22	0.22	XXX	■
	RR			0.00	0.09	0.09	0.00	0.09	0.09	XXX	■
	UE			0.00	0.15	0.15	0.00	0.15	0.15	XXX	■
E0326	NU		Urinal; female, jug-type, any material	0.00	0.30	0.30	0.00	0.30	0.30	XXX	■
	RR			0.00	0.09	0.09	0.00	0.09	0.09	XXX	■
	UE			0.00	0.18	0.18	0.00	0.18	0.18	XXX	■
E0350	NU		Control unit for electronic bowel irrigation/evacuation system	0.00	0.00	0.00	0.00	0.00	0.00	XXX	
	RR			0.00	0.00	0.00	0.00	0.00	0.00	XXX	
	UE			0.00	0.00	0.00	0.00	0.00	0.00	XXX	
E0352			Disposable pack (water reservoir bag, speculum, valving mechanism and collection bag/box) for use with the electronic bowel irrigation/evacuation system	0.00	0.00	0.00	0.00	0.00	0.00	XXX	
E0370			Air pressure elevator for heel	0.00	0.00	0.00	0.00	0.00	0.00	XXX	
E0371			Nonpowered advanced pressure reducing overlay for mattress, standard mattress length and width	0.00	0.00	0.00	0.00	0.00	0.00	XXX	
E0372			Powered air overlay for mattress, standard mattress length and width	0.00	0.00	0.00	0.00	0.00	0.00	XXX	

■ RVU not developed by CMS. Gap-filled RVUs developed by CHEG.

Code	M	S	Description	Work Value	Non-Fac PE	Fac PE	Mal-prac-tice	Non-Fac Total	Fac Total	Global	Gap
E0373			Nonpowered advanced pressure reducing mattress	0.00	0.00	0.00	0.00	0.00	0.00	XXX	
E0424	RR		Stationary compressed gaseous oxygen system, rental; includes container, contents, regulator, flowmeter, humidifier, nebulizer, cannula or mask, and tubing	0.00	7.57	7.57	0.00	7.57	7.57	XXX	■
E0425	NU		Stationary compressed gas system, purchase; includes regulator, flowmeter, humidifier, nebulizer, cannula or mask, and tubing	0.00	94.76	94.76	0.00	94.76	94.76	XXX	■
	UE			0.00	71.52	71.52	0.00	71.52	71.52	XXX	■
E0430	NU		Portable gaseous oxygen system, purchase; includes regulator, flowmeter, humidifier, cannula or mask, and tubing	0.00	42.91	42.91	0.00	42.91	42.91	XXX	■
	UE			0.00	32.18	32.18	0.00	32.18	32.18	XXX	■
E0431	RR		Portable gaseous oxygen system, rental; includes portable container, regulator, flowmeter, humidifier, cannula or mask, and tubing	0.00	1.24	1.24	0.00	1.24	1.24	XXX	■
E0434	RR		Portable liquid oxygen system, rental; includes portable container, supply reservoir, humidifier, flowmeter, refill adaptor, contents gauge, cannula or mask, and tubing	0.00	1.24	1.24	0.00	1.24	1.24	XXX	■
E0435	NU		Portable liquid oxygen system, purchase; includes portable container, supply reservoir, flowmeter, humidifier, contents gauge, cannula or mask, tubing, and refill adapter	0.00	29.50	29.50	0.00	29.50	29.50	XXX	■
	UE			0.00	22.13	22.13	0.00	22.13	22.13	XXX	■
E0439	RR		Stationary liquid oxygen system, rental; includes container, contents, regulator, flowmeter, humidifier, nebulizer, cannula or mask, and tubing	0.00	7.57	7.57	0.00	7.57	7.57	XXX	■
E0440	NU		Stationary liquid oxygen system, purchase; includes use of reservoir, contents indicator, regulator, flowmeter, humidifier, nebulizer, cannula or mask, and tubing	0.00	59.90	59.90	0.00	59.90	59.90	XXX	■
	UE			0.00	44.92	44.92	0.00	44.92	44.92	XXX	■
E0441			Oxygen contents, gaseous (for use with owned gaseous stationary systems or when both a stationary and portable gaseous system are owned)	0.00	0.75	0.75	0.00	0.75	0.75	XXX	■
E0442			Oxygen contents, liquid (for use with owned liquid stationary systems or when both a stationary and portable liquid system are owned)	0.00	0.05	0.05	0.00	0.05	0.05	XXX	■
E0443			Portable oxygen contents, gaseous (for use only with portable gaseous systems when no stationary gas or liquid system is used)	0.00	0.42	0.42	0.00	0.42	0.42	XXX	■
E0444			Portable oxygen contents, liquid (for use only with portable liquid systems when no stationary gas or liquid system is used)	0.00	0.05	0.05	0.00	0.05	0.05	XXX	■
E0450	NU		Volume ventilator, stationary or portable, with backup rate feature, used with invasive interface (e.g., tracheostomy tube)	0.00	0.00	0.00	0.00	0.00	0.00	XXX	
	RR			0.00	0.00	0.00	0.00	0.00	0.00	XXX	
	UE			0.00	0.00	0.00	0.00	0.00	0.00	XXX	

■ RVU not developed by CMS. Gap-filled RVUs developed by CHEG.

Code	M	S	Description	Work Value	Non-Fac PE	Fac PE	Mal-practice	Non-Fac Total	Fac Total	Global	Gap
E0455	NU		Oxygen tent, excluding croup or pediatric tents	0.00	0.00	0.00	0.00	0.00	0.00	XXX	
	RR			0.00	0.00	0.00	0.00	0.00	0.00	XXX	
	UE			0.00	0.00	0.00	0.00	0.00	0.00	XXX	
E0457	NU		Chest shell (cuirass)	0.00	21.47	21.47	0.00	21.47	21.47	XXX	■
	RR			0.00	2.15	2.15	0.00	2.15	2.15	XXX	■
	UE			0.00	16.11	16.11	0.00	16.11	16.11	XXX	■
E0459	NU		Chest wrap	0.00	15.91	15.91	0.00	15.91	15.91	XXX	■
	RR			0.00	1.59	1.59	0.00	1.59	1.59	XXX	■
	UE			0.00	11.93	11.93	0.00	11.93	11.93	XXX	■
E0460	NU		Negative pressure ventilator; portable or stationary	0.00	0.00	0.00	0.00	0.00	0.00	XXX	
	RR			0.00	0.00	0.00	0.00	0.00	0.00	XXX	
	UE			0.00	0.00	0.00	0.00	0.00	0.00	XXX	
E0462	NU		Rocking bed, with or without side rails	0.00	91.10	91.10	0.00	91.10	91.10	XXX	■
	RR			0.00	9.11	9.11	0.00	9.11	9.11	XXX	■
	UE			0.00	68.32	68.32	0.00	68.32	68.32	XXX	■
E0480	NU		Percussor, electric or pneumatic, home model	0.00	12.90	12.90	0.00	12.90	12.90	XXX	■
	RR			0.00	1.34	1.34	0.00	1.34	1.34	XXX	■
	UE			0.00	11.32	11.32	0.00	11.32	11.32	XXX	■
E0481			Intrapulmonary percussive ventilation system and related accessories	0.00	0.00	0.00	0.00	0.00	0.00	XXX	
E0482			Cough stimulating device, alternating positive and negative airway pressure	0.00	0.00	0.00	0.00	0.00	0.00	XXX	
E0500	NU		IPPB machine, all types, with built-in nebulization; manual or automatic valves; internal or external power source	0.00	32.78	32.78	0.00	32.78	32.78	XXX	■
	RR			0.00	2.98	2.98	0.00	2.98	2.98	XXX	■
	UE			0.00	21.61	21.61	0.00	21.61	21.61	XXX	■
E0550	NU		Humidifier, durable for extensive supplemental humidification during IPPB treatments or oxygen delivery	0.00	8.34	8.34	0.00	8.34	8.34	XXX	■
	RR			0.00	1.37	1.37	0.00	1.37	1.37	XXX	■
	UE			0.00	6.68	6.68	0.00	6.68	6.68	XXX	■
E0555	NU		Humidifier, durable, glass or autoclavable plastic bottle type, for use with regulator or flowmeter	0.00	0.21	0.21	0.00	0.21	0.21	XXX	■
	RR			0.00	0.15	0.15	0.00	0.15	0.15	XXX	■
	UE			0.00	0.18	0.18	0.00	0.18	0.18	XXX	■
E0560	NU		Humidifier, durable for supplemental humidification during IPPB treatment or oxygen delivery	0.00	4.62	4.62	0.00	4.62	4.62	XXX	■
	RR			0.00	0.65	0.65	0.00	0.65	0.65	XXX	■
	UE			0.00	4.08	4.08	0.00	4.08	4.08	XXX	■
E0565	NU		Compressor, air power source for equipment which is not self-contained or cylinder driven	0.00	16.09	16.09	0.00	16.09	16.09	XXX	■
	RR			0.00	1.61	1.61	0.00	1.61	1.61	XXX	■
	UE			0.00	11.32	11.32	0.00	11.32	11.32	XXX	■
E0570	NU		Nebulizer, with compressor	0.00	4.87	4.87	0.00	4.87	4.87	XXX	■
	RR			0.00	0.54	0.54	0.00	0.54	0.54	XXX	■
	UE			0.00	1.95	1.95	0.00	1.95	1.95	XXX	■
E0571			Aerosol compressor, battery powered, for use with small volume nebulizer	0.00	0.00	0.00	0.00	0.00	0.00	XXX	
E0572			Aerosol compressor, adjustable pressure, light duty for intermittent use	0.00	0.00	0.00	0.00	0.00	0.00	XXX	

■ RVU not developed by CMS. Gap-filled RVUs developed by CHEG.

Code	M	S	Description	Work Value	Non-Fac PE	Fac PE	Mal-practice	Non-Fac Total	Fac Total	Global	Gap
E0574			Ultrasonic generator with small volume ultrasonic nebulizer	0.00	0.00	0.00	0.00	0.00	0.00	XXX	
E0575	NU		Nebulizer, ultrasonic, large volume	0.00	12.81	12.81	0.00	12.81	12.81	XXX	■
	RR			0.00	1.28	1.28	0.00	1.28	1.28	XXX	■
	UE			0.00	8.34	8.34	0.00	8.34	8.34	XXX	■
E0580	NU		Nebulizer, durable, glass or autoclavable plastic, bottle type, for use with regulator or flowmeter	0.00	0.60	0.60	0.00	0.60	0.60	XXX	■
	RR			0.00	0.54	0.54	0.00	0.54	0.54	XXX	■
	UE			0.00	0.57	0.57	0.00	0.57	0.57	XXX	■
E0585	NU		Nebulizer, with compressor and heater	0.00	9.24	9.24	0.00	9.24	9.24	XXX	■
	RR			0.00	0.92	0.92	0.00	0.92	0.92	XXX	■
	UE			0.00	5.96	5.96	0.00	5.96	5.96	XXX	■
E0590			Dispensing fee covered drug administered through DME nebulizer suction pump, home model, portable	0.00	0.00	0.00	0.00	0.00	0.00	XXX	
E0600	NU		Respiratory suction pump, home model, portable or stationary, electric	0.00	11.32	11.32	0.00	11.32	11.32	XXX	■
	RR			0.00	1.25	1.25	0.00	1.25	1.25	XXX	■
	UE			0.00	6.79	6.79	0.00	6.79	6.79	XXX	■
E0601	NU		Continuous airway pressure (CPAP) device	0.00	32.36	32.36	0.00	32.36	32.36	XXX	■
	RR			0.00	3.52	3.52	0.00	3.52	3.52	XXX	■
	UE			0.00	19.37	19.37	0.00	19.37	19.37	XXX	■
E0602			Breast pump, manual, any type	0.00	0.69	0.69	0.00	0.69	0.69	XXX	■
E0603	NU		Breast pump, electric (AC and/or DC), any type	0.00	2.24	2.24	0.00	2.24	2.24	XXX	■
	RR			0.00	0.75	0.75	0.00	0.75	0.75	XXX	■
	UE			0.00	1.79	1.79	0.00	1.79	1.79	XXX	■
E0604	NU		Breast pump, heavy duty, hospital grade, piston operated, pulsatile vacuum suction/release cycles, vacuum regulator, supplies, transformer, electric (AC and/or DC)	0.00	6.44	6.44	0.00	6.44	6.44	XXX	■
	RR			0.00	2.47	2.47	0.00	2.47	2.47	XXX	■
	UE			0.00	4.83	4.83	0.00	4.83	4.83	XXX	■
E0605	NU		Vaporizer, room type	0.00	0.87	0.87	0.00	0.87	0.87	XXX	■
	RR			0.00	0.10	0.10	0.00	0.10	0.10	XXX	■
	UE			0.00	0.68	0.68	0.00	0.68	0.68	XXX	■
E0606	NU		Postural drainage board	0.00	7.17	7.17	0.00	7.17	7.17	XXX	■
	RR			0.00	0.72	0.72	0.00	0.72	0.72	XXX	■
	UE			0.00	5.38	5.38	0.00	5.38	5.38	XXX	■
E0607	NU		Home blood glucose monitor	0.00	1.43	1.43	0.00	1.43	1.43	XXX	■
	RR			0.00	0.14	0.14	0.00	0.14	0.14	XXX	■
	UE			0.00	1.29	1.29	0.00	1.29	1.29	XXX	■
E0608	RR		Apnea monitor	0.00	8.14	8.14	0.00	8.14	8.14	XXX	■
E0610	NU		Pacemaker monitor, self-contained, checks battery depletion, includes audible and visible check systems	0.00	7.15	7.15	0.00	7.15	7.15	XXX	■
	RR			0.00	0.72	0.72	0.00	0.72	0.72	XXX	■
	UE			0.00	4.92	4.92	0.00	4.92	4.92	XXX	■
E0615	NU		Pacemaker monitor, self-contained, checks battery depletion and other pacemaker components, includes digital/visible check systems	0.00	12.93	12.93	0.00	12.93	12.93	XXX	■
	RR			0.00	1.64	1.64	0.00	1.64	1.64	XXX	■
	UE			0.00	9.69	9.69	0.00	9.69	9.69	XXX	■

■ RVU not developed by CMS. Gap-filled RVUs developed by CHEG.

Code	M	S	Description	Work Value	Non-Fac PE	Fac PE	Mal-practice	Non-Fac Total	Fac Total	Global	Gap
E0616			Implantable cardiac event recorder with memory, activator and programmer	0.00	0.00	0.00	0.00	0.00	0.00	XXX	
E0617			External defibrillator with integrated electrocardiogram analysis	0.00	0.00	0.00	0.00	0.00	0.00	XXX	
E0620			Skin piercing device for collection of capillary blood, laser, each	0.00	0.00	0.00	0.00	0.00	0.00	XXX	
E0621	NU		Sling or seat, patient lift, canvas or nylon	0.00	2.62	2.62	0.00	2.62	2.62	XXX	■
	RR			0.00	0.27	0.27	0.00	0.27	0.27	XXX	■
	UE			0.00	2.00	2.00	0.00	2.00	2.00	XXX	■
E0625	NU		Patient lift, Kartop, bathroom or toilet	0.00	0.00	0.00	0.00	0.00	0.00	XXX	
	RR			0.00	0.00	0.00	0.00	0.00	0.00	XXX	
	UE			0.00	0.00	0.00	0.00	0.00	0.00	XXX	
E0627	NU		Seat lift mechanism incorporated into a combination lift-chair mechanism	0.00	12.14	12.14	0.00	12.14	12.14	XXX	■
	RR			0.00	1.21	1.21	0.00	1.21	1.21	XXX	■
	UE			0.00	9.11	9.11	0.00	9.11	9.11	XXX	■
E0628	NU		Separate seat lift mechanism for use with patient owned furniture — electric	0.00	12.14	12.14	0.00	12.14	12.14	XXX	■
	RR			0.00	1.21	1.21	0.00	1.21	1.21	XXX	■
	UE			0.00	9.11	9.11	0.00	9.11	9.11	XXX	■
E0629	NU		Separate seat lift mechanism for use with patient owned furniture — nonelectric	0.00	12.14	12.14	0.00	12.14	12.14	XXX	■
	RR			0.00	1.21	1.21	0.00	1.21	1.21	XXX	■
	UE			0.00	9.11	9.11	0.00	9.11	9.11	XXX	■
E0630	NU		Patient lift, hydraulic, with seat or sling	0.00	30.40	30.40	0.00	30.40	30.40	XXX	■
	RR			0.00	2.83	2.83	0.00	2.83	2.83	XXX	■
	UE			0.00	21.61	21.61	0.00	21.61	21.61	XXX	■
E0635	NU		Patient lift, electric, with seat or sling	0.00	44.10	44.10	0.00	44.10	44.10	XXX	■
	RR			0.00	4.41	4.41	0.00	4.41	4.41	XXX	■
	UE			0.00	30.10	30.10	0.00	30.10	30.10	XXX	■
E0650	NU		Pneumatic compressor, nonsegmental home model	0.00	22.38	22.38	0.00	22.38	22.38	XXX	■
	RR			0.00	2.58	2.58	0.00	2.58	2.58	XXX	■
	UE			0.00	14.60	14.60	0.00	14.60	14.60	XXX	■
E0651	NU		Pneumatic compressor, segmental home model without calibrated gradient pressure	0.00	24.88	24.88	0.00	24.88	24.88	XXX	■
	RR			0.00	2.68	2.68	0.00	2.68	2.68	XXX	■
	UE			0.00	18.92	18.92	0.00	18.92	18.92	XXX	■
E0652	NU		Pneumatic compressor, segmental home model with calibrated gradient pressure	0.00	154.87	154.87	0.00	154.87	154.87	XXX	■
	RR			0.00	14.90	14.90	0.00	14.90	14.90	XXX	■
	UE			0.00	104.30	104.30	0.00	104.30	104.30	XXX	■
E0655	NU		Nonsegmental pneumatic appliance for use with pneumatic compressor, half arm	0.00	3.04	3.04	0.00	3.04	3.04	XXX	■
	RR			0.00	0.36	0.36	0.00	0.36	0.36	XXX	■
	UE			0.00	2.32	2.32	0.00	2.32	2.32	XXX	■
E0660	NU		Nonsegmental pneumatic appliance for use with pneumatic compressor, full leg	0.00	4.38	4.38	0.00	4.38	4.38	XXX	■
	RR			0.00	0.54	0.54	0.00	0.54	0.54	XXX	■
	UE			0.00	3.34	3.34	0.00	3.34	3.34	XXX	■

■ RVU not developed by CMS. Gap-filled RVUs developed by CHEG.

Code	M	S	Description	Work Value	Non-Fac PE	Fac PE	Mal-practice	Non-Fac Total	Fac Total	Global	Gap
E0665	NU		Nonsegmental pneumatic appliance for use with pneumatic compressor, full arm	0.00	3.73	3.73	0.00	3.73	3.73	XXX	■
	RR			0.00	0.42	0.42	0.00	0.42	0.42	XXX	■
	UE			0.00	2.83	2.83	0.00	2.83	2.83	XXX	■
E0666	NU		Nonsegmental pneumatic appliance for use with pneumatic compressor, half leg	0.00	3.87	3.87	0.00	3.87	3.87	XXX	■
	RR			0.00	0.45	0.45	0.00	0.45	0.45	XXX	■
	UE			0.00	2.92	2.92	0.00	2.92	2.92	XXX	■
E0667	NU		Segmental pneumatic appliance for use with pneumatic compressor, full leg	0.00	13.35	13.35	0.00	13.35	13.35	XXX	■
	RR			0.00	1.07	1.07	0.00	1.07	1.07	XXX	■
	UE			0.00	8.46	8.46	0.00	8.46	8.46	XXX	■
E0668	NU		Segmental pneumatic appliance for use with pneumatic compressor, full arm	0.00	12.07	12.07	0.00	12.07	12.07	XXX	■
	RR			0.00	1.28	1.28	0.00	1.28	1.28	XXX	■
	UE			0.00	9.18	9.18	0.00	9.18	9.18	XXX	■
E0669	NU		Segmental pneumatic appliance for use with pneumatic compressor, half leg	0.00	5.07	5.07	0.00	5.07	5.07	XXX	■
	RR			0.00	0.60	0.60	0.00	0.60	0.60	XXX	■
	UE			0.00	3.81	3.81	0.00	3.81	3.81	XXX	■
E0671			Segmental gradient pressure pneumatic appliance, full leg	0.00	0.00	0.00	0.00	0.00	0.00	XXX	
E0672			Segmental gradient pressure pneumatic appliance, full arm	0.00	0.00	0.00	0.00	0.00	0.00	XXX	
E0673			Segmental gradient pressure pneumatic appliance, half leg	0.00	0.00	0.00	0.00	0.00	0.00	XXX	
E0690	NU		Ultraviolet cabinet, appropriate for home use	0.00	36.80	36.80	0.00	36.80	36.80	XXX	■
	RR			0.00	3.87	3.87	0.00	3.87	3.87	XXX	■
	UE			0.00	27.57	27.57	0.00	27.57	27.57	XXX	■
E0700			Safety equipment (e.g., belt, harness or vest)	0.00	0.00	0.00	0.00	0.00	0.00	XXX	
E0710			Restraint, any type (body, chest, wrist or ankle)	0.00	0.00	0.00	0.00	0.00	0.00	XXX	
E0720	NU		TENS, two lead, localized stimulation	0.00	6.57	6.57	0.00	6.57	6.57	XXX	■
	RR			0.00	1.89	1.89	0.00	1.89	1.89	XXX	■
	UE			0.00	3.61	3.61	0.00	3.61	3.61	XXX	■
E0730	NU		TENS, four lead, larger area/multiple nerve stimulation	0.00	6.76	6.76	0.00	6.76	6.76	XXX	■
	RR			0.00	2.30	2.30	0.00	2.30	2.30	XXX	■
	UE			0.00	3.73	3.73	0.00	3.73	3.73	XXX	■
E0731	NU		Form-fitting conductive garment for delivery of TENS or NMES (with conductive fibers separated from the patient's skin by layers of fabric)	0.00	0.00	0.00	0.00	0.00	0.00	XXX	
	RR			0.00	0.00	0.00	0.00	0.00	0.00	XXX	
	UE			0.00	0.00	0.00	0.00	0.00	0.00	XXX	
E0740			Incontinence treatment system, pelvic floor stimulator, monitor, sensor and/or trainer	0.00	0.00	0.00	0.00	0.00	0.00	XXX	
E0744	NU		Neuromuscular stimulator for scoliosis	0.00	15.94	15.94	0.00	15.94	15.94	XXX	■
	RR			0.00	2.38	2.38	0.00	2.38	2.38	XXX	■
	UE			0.00	14.45	14.45	0.00	14.45	14.45	XXX	■
E0745	NU		Neuromuscular stimulator, electronic shock unit	0.00	10.03	10.03	0.00	10.03	10.03	XXX	■
	RR			0.00	3.37	3.37	0.00	3.37	3.37	XXX	■
	UE			0.00	8.02	8.02	0.00	8.02	8.02	XXX	■

■ RVU not developed by CMS. Gap-filled RVUs developed by CHEG.

Code	M	S	Description	Work Value	Non-Fac PE	Fac PE	Mal-practice	Non-Fac Total	Fac Total	Global	Gap
E0746	NU		Electromyography (EMG), biofeedback device	0.00	0.00	0.00	0.00	0.00	0.00	XXX	
	RR			0.00	0.00	0.00	0.00	0.00	0.00	XXX	
	UE			0.00	0.00	0.00	0.00	0.00	0.00	XXX	
E0747	NU		Osteogenesis stimulator, electrical, noninvasive, other than spinal applications	0.00	129.73	129.73	0.00	129.73	129.73	XXX	■
	RR			0.00	12.89	12.89	0.00	12.89	12.89	XXX	■
	UE			0.00	96.38	96.38	0.00	96.38	96.38	XXX	■
E0748			Osteogenesis stimulator, electrical, noninvasive, spinal applications	0.00	0.00	0.00	0.00	0.00	0.00	XXX	
E0749			Osteogenesis stimulator, electrical, surgically implanted	0.00	94.21	94.21	0.00	94.21	94.21	XXX	■
E0752			Implantable neurostimulator electrode, each	0.00	0.00	0.00	0.00	0.00	0.00	XXX	
E0754			Patient programmer (external) for use with implantable programmable neurostimulator pulse generator	0.00	0.00	0.00	0.00	0.00	0.00	XXX	
E0755			Electronic salivary reflex stimulator (intraoral/ noninvasive)	0.00	0.00	0.00	0.00	0.00	0.00	XXX	
E0756			Implantable neurostimulator pulse generator	0.00	0.00	0.00	0.00	0.00	0.00	XXX	
E0757			Implantable neurostimulator radiofrequency receiver	0.00	0.00	0.00	0.00	0.00	0.00	XXX	
E0758			Radiofrequency transmitter (external) for use with implantable neurostimulator radiofrequency receiver	0.00	0.00	0.00	0.00	0.00	0.00	XXX	
E0759			Rediofrequency transmitter (external) for use with implantable sacral root neurostimulator receiver for bowel and bladder management, replacement	0.00	0.00	0.00	0.00	0.00	0.00	XXX	
E0760			Osteogenesis stimulator, low intensity ultrasound, non-invasive	0.00	0.00	0.00	0.00	0.00	0.00	XXX	
E0765			FDA approved nerve stimulator, with replaceable batteries, for treatment of nausea and vomiting	0.00	0.00	0.00	0.00	0.00	0.00	XXX	
E0776	NU		IV pole	0.00	3.93	3.93	0.00	3.93	3.93	XXX	■
	RR			0.00	0.60	0.60	0.00	0.60	0.60	XXX	■
	UE			0.00	2.92	2.92	0.00	2.92	2.92	XXX	■
E0779			Ambulatory infusion pump, mechanical, reusable, for infusion 8 hours or greater	0.00	0.00	0.00	0.00	0.00	0.00	XXX	
E0780			Ambulatory infusion pump, mechanical, reusable, for infusion less than 8 hours	0.00	0.00	0.00	0.00	0.00	0.00	XXX	
E0781	RR		Ambulatory infusion pump, single or multiple channels, electric or battery operated, with administrative equipment, worn by patient	0.00	6.41	6.41	0.00	6.41	6.41	XXX	■
E0782			Infusion pump, implantable, non-programmable	0.00	126.87	126.87	0.00	126.87	126.87	XXX	■

■ RVU not developed by CMS. Gap-filled RVUs developed by CHEG.

Code	M S	Description	Work Value	Non-Fac PE	Fac PE	Mal-practice	Non-Fac Total	Fac Total	Global	Gap
E0783		Infusion pump system, implantable, programmable (includes all components, e.g., pump, catheter, connectors, etc.)	0.00	0.00	0.00	0.00	0.00	0.00	XXX	
E0784		External ambulatory infusion pump, insulin	0.00	83.44	83.44	0.00	83.44	83.44	XXX	■
E0785		Implantable intraspinal (epidural/intrathecal) catheter used with implantable infusion pump, replacement	0.00	0.00	0.00	0.00	0.00	0.00	XXX	
E0786		Implantable programmable infusion pump, replacement (excludes implantable intraspinal catheter)	0.00	0.00	0.00	0.00	0.00	0.00	XXX	
E0791	NU	Parenteral infusion pump, stationary, single or multichannel	0.00	0.00	0.00	0.00	0.00	0.00	XXX	
	RR		0.00	0.00	0.00	0.00	0.00	0.00	XXX	
	UE		0.00	0.00	0.00	0.00	0.00	0.00	XXX	
E0830		Ambulatory traction device, all types, each	0.00	0.00	0.00	0.00	0.00	0.00	XXX	
E0840	NU	Traction frame, attached to headboard, cervical traction	0.00	2.15	2.15	0.00	2.15	2.15	XXX	■
	RR		0.00	0.51	0.51	0.00	0.51	0.51	XXX	■
	UE		0.00	1.55	1.55	0.00	1.55	1.55	XXX	■
E0850	NU	Traction stand, freestanding, cervical traction	0.00	3.29	3.29	0.00	3.29	3.29	XXX	■
	RR		0.00	0.48	0.48	0.00	0.48	0.48	XXX	■
	UE		0.00	2.47	2.47	0.00	2.47	2.47	XXX	■
E0855	NU	Cervical traction equipment not requiring additional stand or frame	0.00	11.92	11.92	0.00	11.92	11.92	XXX	■
	RR		0.00	1.19	1.19	0.00	1.19	1.19	XXX	■
	UE		0.00	8.94	8.94	0.00	8.94	8.94	XXX	■
E0860	NU	Traction equipment, overdoor, cervical	0.00	0.82	0.82	0.00	0.82	0.82	XXX	■
	RR		0.00	0.27	0.27	0.00	0.27	0.27	XXX	■
	UE		0.00	0.74	0.74	0.00	0.74	0.74	XXX	■
E0870	NU	Traction frame, attached to footboard, extremity traction (e.g., Buck's)	0.00	3.22	3.22	0.00	3.22	3.22	XXX	■
	RR		0.00	0.48	0.48	0.00	0.48	0.48	XXX	■
	UE		0.00	2.50	2.50	0.00	2.50	2.50	XXX	■
E0880	NU	Traction stand, freestanding, extremity traction (e.g., Buck's)	0.00	3.52	3.52	0.00	3.52	3.52	XXX	■
	RR		0.00	0.66	0.66	0.00	0.66	0.66	XXX	■
	UE		0.00	2.68	2.68	0.00	2.68	2.68	XXX	■
E0890	NU	Traction frame, attached to footboard, pelvic traction	0.00	3.52	3.52	0.00	3.52	3.52	XXX	■
	RR		0.00	1.21	1.21	0.00	1.21	1.21	XXX	■
	UE		0.00	2.89	2.89	0.00	2.89	2.89	XXX	■
E0900	NU	Traction stand, freestanding, pelvic traction (e.g., Buck's)	0.00	1.89	1.89	0.00	1.89	1.89	XXX	■
	RR		0.00	1.01	1.01	0.00	1.01	1.01	XXX	■
	UE		0.00	1.67	1.67	0.00	1.67	1.67	XXX	■
E0910	NU	Trapeze bars, also known as Patient Helper, attached to bed, with grab bar	0.00	6.91	6.91	0.00	6.91	6.91	XXX	■
	RR		0.00	0.69	0.69	0.00	0.69	0.69	XXX	■
	UE		0.00	5.18	5.18	0.00	5.18	5.18	XXX	■
E0920	NU	Fracture frame, attached to bed, includes weights	0.00	13.11	13.11	0.00	13.11	13.11	XXX	■
	RR		0.00	1.31	1.31	0.00	1.31	1.31	XXX	■
	UE		0.00	10.88	10.88	0.00	10.88	10.88	XXX	■

■ RVU not developed by CMS. Gap-filled RVUs developed by CHEG.

Code	M	S	Description	Work Value	Non-Fac PE	Fac PE	Mal-practice	Non-Fac Total	Fac Total	Global	Gap
E0930	NU		Fracture frame, freestanding, includes weights	0.00	12.52	12.52	0.00	12.52	12.52	XXX	■
	RR			0.00	1.25	1.25	0.00	1.25	1.25	XXX	■
	UE			0.00	9.21	9.21	0.00	9.21	9.21	XXX	■
E0935	RR		Passive motion exercise device	0.00	0.00	0.00	0.00	0.00	0.00	XXX	
E0940	NU		Trapeze bar, freestanding, complete with grab bar	0.00	9.77	9.77	0.00	9.77	9.77	XXX	■
	RR			0.00	1.04	1.04	0.00	1.04	1.04	XXX	■
	UE			0.00	6.91	6.91	0.00	6.91	6.91	XXX	■
E0941	NU		Gravity assisted traction device, any type	0.00	12.22	12.22	0.00	12.22	12.22	XXX	■
	RR			0.00	1.22	1.22	0.00	1.22	1.22	XXX	■
	UE			0.00	9.24	9.24	0.00	9.24	9.24	XXX	■
E0942	NU		Cervical head harness/halter	0.00	0.62	0.62	0.00	0.62	0.62	XXX	■
	RR			0.00	0.07	0.07	0.00	0.07	0.07	XXX	■
	UE			0.00	0.46	0.46	0.00	0.46	0.46	XXX	■
E0943	NU		Cervical pillow	0.00	0.95	0.95	0.00	0.95	0.95	XXX	■
	RR			0.00	0.10	0.10	0.00	0.10	0.10	XXX	■
	UE			0.00	0.80	0.80	0.00	0.80	0.80	XXX	■
E0944	NU		Pelvic belt/harness/boot	0.00	0.63	0.63	0.00	0.63	0.63	XXX	■
	RR			0.00	0.14	0.14	0.00	0.14	0.14	XXX	■
	UE			0.00	0.57	0.57	0.00	0.57	0.57	XXX	■
E0945	NU		Extremity belt/harness	0.00	1.39	1.39	0.00	1.39	1.39	XXX	■
	RR			0.00	0.14	0.14	0.00	0.14	0.14	XXX	■
	UE			0.00	1.07	1.07	0.00	1.07	1.07	XXX	■
E0946	NU		Fracture, frame, dual with cross bars, attached to bed (e.g., Balken, Four Poster)	0.00	18.49	18.49	0.00	18.49	18.49	XXX	■
	RR			0.00	1.85	1.85	0.00	1.85	1.85	XXX	■
	UE			0.00	13.87	13.87	0.00	13.87	13.87	XXX	■
E0947	NU		Fracture frame, attachments for complex pelvic traction	0.00	17.88	17.88	0.00	17.88	17.88	XXX	■
	RR			0.00	1.79	1.79	0.00	1.79	1.79	XXX	■
	UE			0.00	13.41	13.41	0.00	13.41	13.41	XXX	■
E0948	NU		Fracture frame, attachments for complex cervical traction	0.00	16.99	16.99	0.00	16.99	16.99	XXX	■
	RR			0.00	1.70	1.70	0.00	1.70	1.70	XXX	■
	UE			0.00	11.77	11.77	0.00	11.77	11.77	XXX	■
E0950	NU		Tray	0.00	3.25	3.25	0.00	3.25	3.25	XXX	■
	RR			0.00	0.36	0.36	0.00	0.36	0.36	XXX	■
	UE			0.00	2.44	2.44	0.00	2.44	2.44	XXX	■
E0951	NU		Loop heel, each	0.00	0.59	0.59	0.00	0.59	0.59	XXX	■
	RR			0.00	0.06	0.06	0.00	0.06	0.06	XXX	■
	UE			0.00	0.44	0.44	0.00	0.44	0.44	XXX	■
E0952	NU		Loop toe, each	0.00	0.69	0.69	0.00	0.69	0.69	XXX	■
	RR			0.00	0.07	0.07	0.00	0.07	0.07	XXX	■
	UE			0.00	0.52	0.52	0.00	0.52	0.52	XXX	■
E0953	NU		Pneumatic tire, each	0.00	1.33	1.33	0.00	1.33	1.33	XXX	■
	RR			0.00	0.13	0.13	0.00	0.13	0.13	XXX	■
	UE			0.00	0.99	0.99	0.00	0.99	0.99	XXX	■

■ RVU not developed by CMS. Gap-filled RVUs developed by CHEG.

Code	M	S	Description	Work Value	Non-Fac PE	Fac PE	Mal-practice	Non-Fac Total	Fac Total	Global	Gap
E0954	NU		Semi-pneumatic caster, each	0.00	1.34	1.34	0.00	1.34	1.34	XXX	■
	RR			0.00	0.17	0.17	0.00	0.17	0.17	XXX	■
	UE			0.00	0.77	0.77	0.00	0.77	0.77	XXX	■
E0958	NU		Wheelchair attachment to convert any wheelchair to one arm drive	0.00	16.05	16.05	0.00	16.05	16.05	XXX	■
	RR			0.00	1.60	1.60	0.00	1.60	1.60	XXX	■
	UE			0.00	12.04	12.04	0.00	12.04	12.04	XXX	■
E0959	NU		Amputee adapter (device used to compensate for transfer of weight due to lost limbs to maintain proper balance)	0.00	2.68	2.68	0.00	2.68	2.68	XXX	■
	RR			0.00	0.33	0.33	0.00	0.33	0.33	XXX	■
	UE			0.00	2.09	2.09	0.00	2.09	2.09	XXX	■
E0961	NU		Brake extension, for wheelchair	0.00	1.10	1.10	0.00	1.10	1.10	XXX	■
	RR			0.00	0.12	0.12	0.00	0.12	0.12	XXX	■
	UE			0.00	0.82	0.82	0.00	0.82	0.82	XXX	■
E0962	NU		One-inch cushion, for wheelchair	0.00	1.92	1.92	0.00	1.92	1.92	XXX	■
	RR			0.00	0.22	0.22	0.00	0.22	0.22	XXX	■
	UE			0.00	1.43	1.43	0.00	1.43	1.43	XXX	■
E0963	NU		Two-inch cushion, for wheelchair	0.00	2.28	2.28	0.00	2.28	2.28	XXX	■
	RR			0.00	0.27	0.27	0.00	0.27	0.27	XXX	■
	UE			0.00	1.71	1.71	0.00	1.71	1.71	XXX	■
E0964	NU		Three-inch cushion, for wheelchair	0.00	2.24	2.24	0.00	2.24	2.24	XXX	■
	RR			0.00	0.29	0.29	0.00	0.29	0.29	XXX	■
	UE			0.00	1.73	1.73	0.00	1.73	1.73	XXX	■
E0965	NU		Four-inch cushion, for wheelchair	0.00	2.62	2.62	0.00	2.62	2.62	XXX	■
	RR			0.00	0.31	0.31	0.00	0.31	0.31	XXX	■
	UE			0.00	1.88	1.88	0.00	1.88	1.88	XXX	■
E0966	NU		Hook on headrest extension	0.00	2.09	2.09	0.00	2.09	2.09	XXX	■
	RR			0.00	0.21	0.21	0.00	0.21	0.21	XXX	■
	UE			0.00	1.43	1.43	0.00	1.43	1.43	XXX	■
E0967	NU		Wheelchair hand rims with eight vertical rubber-tipped projections, pair	0.00	4.23	4.23	0.00	4.23	4.23	XXX	■
	RR			0.00	0.43	0.43	0.00	0.43	0.43	XXX	■
	UE			0.00	2.92	2.92	0.00	2.92	2.92	XXX	■
E0968	NU		Commode seat, wheelchair	0.00	5.61	5.61	0.00	5.61	5.61	XXX	■
	RR			0.00	0.56	0.56	0.00	0.56	0.56	XXX	■
	UE			0.00	3.58	3.58	0.00	3.58	3.58	XXX	■
E0969	NU		Narrowing device, wheelchair	0.00	4.89	4.89	0.00	4.89	4.89	XXX	■
	RR			0.00	0.48	0.48	0.00	0.48	0.48	XXX	■
	UE			0.00	3.67	3.67	0.00	3.67	3.67	XXX	■
E0970	NU		No. 2 footplates, except for elevating legrest	0.00	1.50	1.50	0.00	1.50	1.50	XXX	■
	RR			0.00	0.13	0.13	0.00	0.13	0.13	XXX	■
	UE			0.00	1.13	1.13	0.00	1.13	1.13	XXX	■
E0971	NU		Anti-tipping device, wheelchair	0.00	2.03	2.03	0.00	2.03	2.03	XXX	■
	RR			0.00	0.28	0.28	0.00	0.28	0.28	XXX	■
	UE			0.00	1.34	1.34	0.00	1.34	1.34	XXX	■
E0972	NU		Transfer board or device	0.00	1.61	1.61	0.00	1.61	1.61	XXX	■
	RR			0.00	0.21	0.21	0.00	0.21	0.21	XXX	■
	UE			0.00	1.19	1.19	0.00	1.19	1.19	XXX	■

■ RVU not developed by CMS. Gap-filled RVUs developed by CHEG.

Code	M	S	Description	Work Value	Non-Fac PE	Fac PE	Mal-practice	Non-Fac Total	Fac Total	Global	Gap
E0973	NU		Adjustable height detachable arms, desk or full-length, wheelchair	0.00	3.22	3.22	0.00	3.22	3.22	XXX	■
	RR			0.00	0.31	0.31	0.00	0.31	0.31	XXX	■
	UE			0.00	2.32	2.32	0.00	2.32	2.32	XXX	■
E0974	NU		"Grade-aid" (device to prevent rolling back on an incline) for wheelchair	0.00	2.47	2.47	0.00	2.47	2.47	XXX	■
	RR			0.00	0.26	0.26	0.00	0.26	0.26	XXX	■
	UE			0.00	1.86	1.86	0.00	1.86	1.86	XXX	■
E0975	NU		Reinforced seat upholstery, wheelchair	0.00	1.59	1.59	0.00	1.59	1.59	XXX	■
	RR			0.00	0.16	0.16	0.00	0.16	0.16	XXX	■
	UE			0.00	1.19	1.19	0.00	1.19	1.19	XXX	■
E0976	NU		Reinforced back, wheelchair, upholstery or other material	0.00	1.36	1.36	0.00	1.36	1.36	XXX	■
	RR			0.00	0.16	0.16	0.00	0.16	0.16	XXX	■
	UE			0.00	1.19	1.19	0.00	1.19	1.19	XXX	■
E0977	NU		Wedge cushion, wheelchair	0.00	1.94	1.94	0.00	1.94	1.94	XXX	■
	RR			0.00	0.23	0.23	0.00	0.23	0.23	XXX	■
	UE			0.00	1.49	1.49	0.00	1.49	1.49	XXX	■
E0978	NU		Belt, safety with airplane buckle, wheelchair	0.00	1.45	1.45	0.00	1.45	1.45	XXX	■
	RR			0.00	0.15	0.15	0.00	0.15	0.15	XXX	■
	UE			0.00	1.09	1.09	0.00	1.09	1.09	XXX	■
E0979	NU		Belt, safety with Velcro closure, wheelchair	0.00	1.06	1.06	0.00	1.06	1.06	XXX	■
	RR			0.00	0.10	0.10	0.00	0.10	0.10	XXX	■
	UE			0.00	0.79	0.79	0.00	0.79	0.79	XXX	■
E0980	NU		Safety vest, wheelchair	0.00	1.04	1.04	0.00	1.04	1.04	XXX	■
	RR			0.00	0.10	0.10	0.00	0.10	0.10	XXX	■
	UE			0.00	0.77	0.77	0.00	0.77	0.77	XXX	■
E0990	NU		Elevating leg rest, each	0.00	3.58	3.58	0.00	3.58	3.58	XXX	■
	RR			0.00	0.42	0.42	0.00	0.42	0.42	XXX	■
	UE			0.00	2.83	2.83	0.00	2.83	2.83	XXX	■
E0991	NU		Upholstery seat	0.00	1.43	1.43	0.00	1.43	1.43	XXX	■
	RR			0.00	0.16	0.16	0.00	0.16	0.16	XXX	■
	UE			0.00	1.07	1.07	0.00	1.07	1.07	XXX	■
E0992	NU		Solid seat insert	0.00	2.98	2.98	0.00	2.98	2.98	XXX	■
	RR			0.00	0.30	0.30	0.00	0.30	0.30	XXX	■
	UE			0.00	1.91	1.91	0.00	1.91	1.91	XXX	■
E0993	NU		Back, upholstery	0.00	1.34	1.34	0.00	1.34	1.34	XXX	■
	RR			0.00	0.15	0.15	0.00	0.15	0.15	XXX	■
	UE			0.00	1.01	1.01	0.00	1.01	1.01	XXX	■
E0994	NU		Armrest, each	0.00	0.61	0.61	0.00	0.61	0.61	XXX	■
	RR			0.00	0.06	0.06	0.00	0.06	0.06	XXX	■
	UE			0.00	0.45	0.45	0.00	0.45	0.45	XXX	■
E0995	NU		Calf rest, each	0.00	0.95	0.95	0.00	0.95	0.95	XXX	■
	RR			0.00	0.11	0.11	0.00	0.11	0.11	XXX	■
	UE			0.00	0.83	0.83	0.00	0.83	0.83	XXX	■
E0996	NU		Tire, solid, each	0.00	0.89	0.89	0.00	0.89	0.89	XXX	■
	RR			0.00	0.10	0.10	0.00	0.10	0.10	XXX	■
	UE			0.00	0.69	0.69	0.00	0.69	0.69	XXX	■

■ RVU not developed by CMS. Gap-filled RVUs developed by CHEG.

Code	M S	Description	Work Value	Non-Fac PE	Fac PE	Mal-practice	Non-Fac Total	Fac Total	Global	Gap
E0997	NU	Caster with fork	0.00	2.09	2.09	0.00	2.09	2.09	XXX	■
	RR		0.00	0.21	0.21	0.00	0.21	0.21	XXX	■
	UE		0.00	1.49	1.49	0.00	1.49	1.49	XXX	■
E0998	NU	Caster without fork	0.00	1.07	1.07	0.00	1.07	1.07	XXX	■
	RR		0.00	0.13	0.13	0.00	0.13	0.13	XXX	■
	UE		0.00	0.83	0.83	0.00	0.83	0.83	XXX	■
E0999	NU	Pneumatic tire with wheel	0.00	3.28	3.28	0.00	3.28	3.28	XXX	■
	RR		0.00	0.36	0.36	0.00	0.36	0.36	XXX	■
	UE		0.00	2.53	2.53	0.00	2.53	2.53	XXX	■
E1000	NU	Tire, pneumatic caster	0.00	1.13	1.13	0.00	1.13	1.13	XXX	■
	RR		0.00	0.15	0.15	0.00	0.15	0.15	XXX	■
	UE		0.00	0.85	0.85	0.00	0.85	0.85	XXX	■
E1001	NU	Wheel, single	0.00	2.92	2.92	0.00	2.92	2.92	XXX	■
	RR		0.00	0.32	0.32	0.00	0.32	0.32	XXX	■
	UE		0.00	2.35	2.35	0.00	2.35	2.35	XXX	■
E1031	NU	Rollabout chair, any and all types with casters five inches or greater	0.00	15.79	15.79	0.00	15.79	15.79	XXX	■
	RR		0.00	1.58	1.58	0.00	1.58	1.58	XXX	■
	UE		0.00	11.85	11.85	0.00	11.85	11.85	XXX	■
E1035		Multi-positional patient transfer system, with integrated seat, operated by care giver	0.00	0.00	0.00	0.00	0.00	0.00	XXX	
E1050	NU	Fully reclining wheelchair; fixed full-length arms, swing-away, detachable, elevating legrests	0.00	37.45	37.45	0.00	37.45	37.45	XXX	■
	RR		0.00	3.34	3.34	0.00	3.34	3.34	XXX	■
	UE		0.00	28.09	28.09	0.00	28.09	28.09	XXX	■
E1060	NU	Fully reclining wheelchair; detachable arms, desk or full-length, swing-away, detachable, elevating legrests	0.00	40.28	40.28	0.00	40.28	40.28	XXX	■
	RR		0.00	3.40	3.40	0.00	3.40	3.40	XXX	■
	UE		0.00	30.21	30.21	0.00	30.21	30.21	XXX	■
E1065	NU	Power attachment (to convert any wheelchair to motorized wheelchair, e.g., Solo)	0.00	90.88	90.88	0.00	90.88	90.88	XXX	■
	RR		0.00	8.26	8.26	0.00	8.26	8.26	XXX	■
	UE		0.00	68.16	68.16	0.00	68.16	68.16	XXX	■
E1066	NU	Battery charger	0.00	8.34	8.34	0.00	8.34	8.34	XXX	■
	RR		0.00	0.83	0.83	0.00	0.83	0.83	XXX	■
	UE		0.00	5.81	5.81	0.00	5.81	5.81	XXX	■
E1069	NU	Deep cycle battery	0.00	3.06	3.06	0.00	3.06	3.06	XXX	■
	RR		0.00	0.42	0.42	0.00	0.42	0.42	XXX	■
	UE		0.00	2.68	2.68	0.00	2.68	2.68	XXX	■
E1070	NU	Fully reclining wheelchair; detachable arms, desk or full-length, swing-away, detachable footrests	0.00	40.28	40.28	0.00	40.28	40.28	XXX	■
	RR		0.00	3.28	3.28	0.00	3.28	3.28	XXX	■
	UE		0.00	30.21	30.21	0.00	30.21	30.21	XXX	■
E1083	NU	Hemi-wheelchair; fixed full-length arms, swing-away, detachable, elevating legrests	0.00	25.93	25.93	0.00	25.93	25.93	XXX	■
	RR		0.00	2.59	2.59	0.00	2.59	2.59	XXX	■
	UE		0.00	18.92	18.92	0.00	18.92	18.92	XXX	■
E1084	NU	Hemi-wheelchair; detachable arms, desk or full-length, swing-away, detachable, elevating legrests	0.00	31.29	31.29	0.00	31.29	31.29	XXX	■
	RR		0.00	2.56	2.56	0.00	2.56	2.56	XXX	■
	UE		0.00	22.35	22.35	0.00	22.35	22.35	XXX	■

■ RVU not developed by CMS. Gap-filled RVUs developed by CHEG.

Code	M	S	Description	Work Value	Non-Fac PE	Fac PE	Mal-prac-tice	Non-Fac Total	Fac Total	Global	Gap
E1085	NU		Hemi-wheelchair; fixed full-length arms, swing-away, detachable footrests	0.00	23.24	23.24	0.00	23.24	23.24	XXX	■
	RR			0.00	2.32	2.32	0.00	2.32	2.32	XXX	■
	UE			0.00	16.69	16.69	0.00	16.69	16.69	XXX	■
E1086	NU		Hemi-wheelchair; detachable arms, desk or full-length, swing-away, detachable footrests	0.00	28.31	28.31	0.00	28.31	28.31	XXX	■
	RR			0.00	2.58	2.58	0.00	2.58	2.58	XXX	■
	UE			0.00	20.56	20.56	0.00	20.56	20.56	XXX	■
E1087	NU		High-strength lightweight wheelchair; fixed full-length arms, swing-away, detachable, elevating legrests	0.00	35.76	35.76	0.00	35.76	35.76	XXX	■
	RR			0.00	3.58	3.58	0.00	3.58	3.58	XXX	■
	UE			0.00	26.08	26.08	0.00	26.08	26.08	XXX	■
E1088	NU		High-strength lightweight wheelchair; detachable arms, desk or full-length, swing-away, detachable, elevating legrests	0.00	41.27	41.27	0.00	41.27	41.27	XXX	■
	RR			0.00	4.11	4.11	0.00	4.11	4.11	XXX	■
	UE			0.00	28.31	28.31	0.00	28.31	28.31	XXX	■
E1089	NU		High-strength lightweight wheelchair; fixed-length arms, swing-away, detachable footrests	0.00	37.58	37.58	0.00	37.58	37.58	XXX	■
	RR			0.00	3.75	3.75	0.00	3.75	3.75	XXX	■
	UE			0.00	28.18	28.18	0.00	28.18	28.18	XXX	■
E1090	NU		High-strength lightweight wheelchair; detachable arms, desk or full-length, swing-away, detachable footrests	0.00	38.74	38.74	0.00	38.74	38.74	XXX	■
	RR			0.00	3.75	3.75	0.00	3.75	3.75	XXX	■
	UE			0.00	28.31	28.31	0.00	28.31	28.31	XXX	■
E1091			Youth wheelchair; any type	0.00	0.00	0.00	0.00	0.00	0.00	XXX	
E1092	NU		Wide, heavy-duty wheelchair; detachable arms, desk or full-length, swing-away, detachable, elevating legrests	0.00	38.74	38.74	0.00	38.74	38.74	XXX	■
	RR			0.00	3.52	3.52	0.00	3.52	3.52	XXX	■
	UE			0.00	28.31	28.31	0.00	28.31	28.31	XXX	■
E1093	NU		Wide, heavy-duty wheelchair; detachable arms, desk or full-length arms, swing-away, detachable footrests	0.00	32.04	32.04	0.00	32.04	32.04	XXX	■
	RR			0.00	3.28	3.28	0.00	3.28	3.28	XXX	■
	UE			0.00	23.84	23.84	0.00	23.84	23.84	XXX	■
E1100	NU		Semi-reclining wheelchair; fixed full-length arms, swing-away, detachable, elevating legrests	0.00	34.46	34.46	0.00	34.46	34.46	XXX	■
	RR			0.00	3.45	3.45	0.00	3.45	3.45	XXX	■
	UE			0.00	25.85	25.85	0.00	25.85	25.85	XXX	■
E1110	NU		Semi-reclining wheelchair; detachable arms, desk or full-length, elevating legrest	0.00	29.50	29.50	0.00	29.50	29.50	XXX	■
	RR			0.00	2.95	2.95	0.00	2.95	2.95	XXX	■
	UE			0.00	21.46	21.46	0.00	21.46	21.46	XXX	■
E1130	NU		Standard wheelchair; fixed full-length arms, fixed or swing-away, detachable footrests	0.00	14.90	14.90	0.00	14.90	14.90	XXX	■
	RR			0.00	1.49	1.49	0.00	1.49	1.49	XXX	■
	UE			0.00	11.32	11.32	0.00	11.32	11.32	XXX	■
E1140	NU		Wheelchair; detachable arms, desk or full-length, swing-away, detachable footrests	0.00	21.46	21.46	0.00	21.46	21.46	XXX	■
	RR			0.00	2.15	2.15	0.00	2.15	2.15	XXX	■
	UE			0.00	15.20	15.20	0.00	15.20	15.20	XXX	■
E1150	NU		Wheelchair; detachable arms, desk or full-length, swing-away, detachable, elevating legrests	0.00	22.50	22.50	0.00	22.50	22.50	XXX	■
	RR			0.00	2.18	2.18	0.00	2.18	2.18	XXX	■
	UE			0.00	14.90	14.90	0.00	14.90	14.90	XXX	■
E1160	NU		Wheelchair; fixed full-length arms, swing-away, detachable, elevating legrests	0.00	18.77	18.77	0.00	18.77	18.77	XXX	■
	RR			0.00	1.71	1.71	0.00	1.71	1.71	XXX	■
	UE			0.00	13.11	13.11	0.00	13.11	13.11	XXX	■

■ RVU not developed by CMS. Gap-filled RVUs developed by CHEG.

Code	M S	Description	Work Value	Non-Fac PE	Fac PE	Mal-practice	Non-Fac Total	Fac Total	Global	Gap
E1170	NU	Amputee wheelchair; fixed full-length arms, swing-away, detachable, elevating legrests	0.00	27.92	27.92	0.00	27.92	27.92	XXX	■
	RR		0.00	2.79	2.79	0.00	2.79	2.79	XXX	■
	UE		0.00	20.94	20.94	0.00	20.94	20.94	XXX	■
E1171	NU	Amputee wheelchair; fixed full-length arms, without footrests or legrests	0.00	29.48	29.48	0.00	29.48	29.48	XXX	■
	RR		0.00	2.95	2.95	0.00	2.95	2.95	XXX	■
	UE		0.00	22.11	22.11	0.00	22.11	22.11	XXX	■
E1172	NU	Amputee wheelchair; detachable arms, desk or full-length, without footrests or legrests	0.00	36.02	36.02	0.00	36.02	36.02	XXX	■
	RR		0.00	3.61	3.61	0.00	3.61	3.61	XXX	■
	UE		0.00	27.01	27.01	0.00	27.01	27.01	XXX	■
E1180	NU	Amputee wheelchair; detachable arms, desk or full-length, swing-away, detachable footrests	0.00	31.68	31.68	0.00	31.68	31.68	XXX	■
	RR		0.00	3.17	3.17	0.00	3.17	3.17	XXX	■
	UE		0.00	23.76	23.76	0.00	23.76	23.76	XXX	■
E1190	NU	Amputee wheelchair; detachable arms, desk or full-length, swing-away, detachable, elevating legrests	0.00	34.27	34.27	0.00	34.27	34.27	XXX	■
	RR		0.00	3.43	3.43	0.00	3.43	3.43	XXX	■
	UE		0.00	25.03	25.03	0.00	25.03	25.03	XXX	■
E1195	NU	Heavy duty wheelchair; fixed full-length arms, swing-away, detachable, elevating legrests	0.00	42.54	42.54	0.00	42.54	42.54	XXX	■
	RR		0.00	4.25	4.25	0.00	4.25	4.25	XXX	■
	UE		0.00	31.91	31.91	0.00	31.91	31.91	XXX	■
E1200	NU	Amputee wheelchair; fixed full-length arms, swing-away, detachable footrests	0.00	30.74	30.74	0.00	30.74	30.74	XXX	■
	RR		0.00	3.08	3.08	0.00	3.08	3.08	XXX	■
	UE		0.00	23.05	23.05	0.00	23.05	23.05	XXX	■
E1210	NU	Motorized wheelchair; fixed full-length arms, swing-away, detachable, elevating legrests	0.00	128.45	128.45	0.00	128.45	128.45	XXX	■
	RR		0.00	12.84	12.84	0.00	12.84	12.84	XXX	■
	UE		0.00	96.34	96.34	0.00	96.34	96.34	XXX	■
E1211	NU	Motorized wheelchair; detachable arms, desk or full-length, swing-away, detachable, elevating legrests	0.00	130.83	130.83	0.00	130.83	130.83	XXX	■
	RR		0.00	13.08	13.08	0.00	13.08	13.08	XXX	■
	UE		0.00	98.12	98.12	0.00	98.12	98.12	XXX	■
E1212	NU	Motorized wheelchair; fixed full-length arms, swing-away, detachable footrests	0.00	126.81	126.81	0.00	126.81	126.81	XXX	■
	RR		0.00	12.68	12.68	0.00	12.68	12.68	XXX	■
	UE		0.00	95.10	95.10	0.00	95.10	95.10	XXX	■
E1213	NU	Motorized wheelchair; detachable arms, desk or full-length, swing-away, detachable footrests	0.00	136.37	136.37	0.00	136.37	136.37	XXX	■
	RR		0.00	13.63	13.63	0.00	13.63	13.63	XXX	■
	UE		0.00	102.27	102.27	0.00	102.27	102.27	XXX	■
E1220		Wheelchair; specially sized or constructed (indicate brand name, model number, if any, and justification)	0.00	0.00	0.00	0.00	0.00	0.00	XXX	
E1221	NU	Wheelchair with fixed arm, footrests	0.00	14.86	14.86	0.00	14.86	14.86	XXX	■
	RR		0.00	1.48	1.48	0.00	1.48	1.48	XXX	■
	UE		0.00	11.15	11.15	0.00	11.15	11.15	XXX	■
E1222	NU	Wheelchair with fixed arm, elevating legrests	0.00	19.97	19.97	0.00	19.97	19.97	XXX	■
	RR		0.00	2.00	2.00	0.00	2.00	2.00	XXX	■
	UE		0.00	14.36	14.36	0.00	14.36	14.36	XXX	■
E1223	NU	Wheelchair with detachable arms, footrests	0.00	21.46	21.46	0.00	21.46	21.46	XXX	■
	RR		0.00	2.15	2.15	0.00	2.15	2.15	XXX	■
	UE		0.00	15.35	15.35	0.00	15.35	15.35	XXX	■

■ RVU not developed by CMS. Gap-filled RVUs developed by CHEG.

Code	M	S	Description	Work Value	Non-Fac PE	Fac PE	Mal-practice	Non-Fac Total	Fac Total	Global	Gap
E1224	NU		Wheelchair with detachable arms, elevating legrests	0.00	24.44	24.44	0.00	24.44	24.44	XXX	■
	RR			0.00	2.32	2.32	0.00	2.32	2.32	XXX	■
	UE			0.00	16.39	16.39	0.00	16.39	16.39	XXX	■
E1225	NU		Semi-reclining back for customized wheelchair	0.00	14.97	14.97	0.00	14.97	14.97	XXX	■
	RR			0.00	1.50	1.50	0.00	1.50	1.50	XXX	■
	UE			0.00	11.23	11.23	0.00	11.23	11.23	XXX	■
E1226	NU		Full reclining back for customized wheelchair	0.00	16.39	16.39	0.00	16.39	16.39	XXX	■
	RR			0.00	1.64	1.64	0.00	1.64	1.64	XXX	■
	UE			0.00	11.62	11.62	0.00	11.62	11.62	XXX	■
E1227	NU		Special height arms for wheelchair	0.00	8.67	8.67	0.00	8.67	8.67	XXX	■
	RR			0.00	0.86	0.86	0.00	0.86	0.86	XXX	■
	UE			0.00	6.50	6.50	0.00	6.50	6.50	XXX	■
E1228	NU		Special back height for wheelchair	0.00	9.48	9.48	0.00	9.48	9.48	XXX	■
	RR			0.00	0.95	0.95	0.00	0.95	0.95	XXX	■
	UE			0.00	7.11	7.11	0.00	7.11	7.11	XXX	■
E1230	NU		Power operated vehicle (three- or four-wheel nonhighway), specify brand name and model number	0.00	73.86	73.86	0.00	73.86	73.86	XXX	■
	RR			0.00	7.38	7.38	0.00	7.38	7.38	XXX	■
	UE			0.00	65.79	65.79	0.00	65.79	65.79	XXX	■
E1240	NU		Lightweight wheelchair; detachable arms, desk or full-length, swing-away, detachable, elevating legrest	0.00	28.31	28.31	0.00	28.31	28.31	XXX	■
	RR			0.00	2.83	2.83	0.00	2.83	2.83	XXX	■
	UE			0.00	20.26	20.26	0.00	20.26	20.26	XXX	■
E1250	NU		Lightweight wheelchair; fixed full-length arms, swing-away, detachable footrests	0.00	22.95	22.95	0.00	22.95	22.95	XXX	■
	RR			0.00	2.09	2.09	0.00	2.09	2.09	XXX	■
	UE			0.00	18.18	18.18	0.00	18.18	18.18	XXX	■
E1260	NU		Lightweight wheelchair; detachable arms, desk or full-length, swing-away, detachable footrests	0.00	26.82	26.82	0.00	26.82	26.82	XXX	■
	RR			0.00	2.68	2.68	0.00	2.68	2.68	XXX	■
	UE			0.00	21.16	21.16	0.00	21.16	21.16	XXX	■
E1270	NU		Lightweight wheelchair; fixed full-length arms, swing-away, detachable elevating legrests	0.00	23.54	23.54	0.00	23.54	23.54	XXX	■
	RR			0.00	2.35	2.35	0.00	2.35	2.35	XXX	■
	UE			0.00	17.28	17.28	0.00	17.28	17.28	XXX	■
E1280	NU		Heavy-duty wheelchair; detachable arms, desk or full-length, elevating legrests	0.00	35.76	35.76	0.00	35.76	35.76	XXX	■
	RR			0.00	3.58	3.58	0.00	3.58	3.58	XXX	■
	UE			0.00	25.63	25.63	0.00	25.63	25.63	XXX	■
E1285	NU		Heavy-duty wheelchair; fixed full-length arms, swing-away, detachable footrests	0.00	34.57	34.57	0.00	34.57	34.57	XXX	■
	RR			0.00	3.46	3.46	0.00	3.46	3.46	XXX	■
	UE			0.00	25.33	25.33	0.00	25.33	25.33	XXX	■
E1290	NU		Heavy-duty wheelchair; detachable arms, desk or full-length, swing-away, detachable footrests	0.00	35.76	35.76	0.00	35.76	35.76	XXX	■
	RR			0.00	3.58	3.58	0.00	3.58	3.58	XXX	■
	UE			0.00	26.08	26.08	0.00	26.08	26.08	XXX	■
E1295	NU		Heavy-duty wheelchair; fixed full-length arms, elevating legrests	0.00	34.87	34.87	0.00	34.87	34.87	XXX	■
	RR			0.00	3.49	3.49	0.00	3.49	3.49	XXX	■
	UE			0.00	25.33	25.33	0.00	25.33	25.33	XXX	■
E1296	NU		Special wheelchair seat height from floor	0.00	14.90	14.90	0.00	14.90	14.90	XXX	■
	RR			0.00	1.49	1.49	0.00	1.49	1.49	XXX	■
	UE			0.00	10.43	10.43	0.00	10.43	10.43	XXX	■

■ RVU not developed by CMS. Gap-filled RVUs developed by CHEG.

Code	M	S	Description	Work Value	Non-Fac PE	Fac PE	Mal-practice	Non-Fac Total	Fac Total	Global	Gap
E1297	NU		Special wheelchair seat depth, by upholstery	0.00	3.04	3.04	0.00	3.04	3.04	XXX	■
	RR			0.00	0.36	0.36	0.00	0.36	0.36	XXX	■
	UE			0.00	2.38	2.38	0.00	2.38	2.38	XXX	■
E1298	NU		Special wheelchair seat depth and/or width, by construction	0.00	11.92	11.92	0.00	11.92	11.92	XXX	■
	RR			0.00	1.31	1.31	0.00	1.31	1.31	XXX	■
	UE			0.00	8.94	8.94	0.00	8.94	8.94	XXX	■
E1300	NU		Whirlpool, portable (overtub type)	0.00	0.00	0.00	0.00	0.00	0.00	XXX	
	RR			0.00	0.00	0.00	0.00	0.00	0.00	XXX	
	UE			0.00	0.00	0.00	0.00	0.00	0.00	XXX	
E1310	NU		Whirlpool, nonportable (built-in type)	0.00	70.03	70.03	0.00	70.03	70.03	XXX	■
	RR			0.00	5.22	5.22	0.00	5.22	5.22	XXX	■
	UE			0.00	52.15	52.15	0.00	52.15	52.15	XXX	■
E1340			Repair or nonroutine service for durable medical equipment requiring the skill of a technician, labor component, per 15 minutes	0.00	0.00	0.00	0.00	0.00	0.00	XXX	
E1353	NU		Regulator	0.00	2.24	2.24	0.00	2.24	2.24	XXX	■
	RR			0.00	0.12	0.12	0.00	0.12	0.12	XXX	■
	UE			0.00	1.79	1.79	0.00	1.79	1.79	XXX	■
E1355	NU		Stand/rack	0.00	1.52	1.52	0.00	1.52	1.52	XXX	■
	RR			0.00	0.18	0.18	0.00	0.18	0.18	XXX	■
	UE			0.00	1.22	1.22	0.00	1.22	1.22	XXX	■
E1372	NU		Immersion external heater for nebulizer	0.00	4.92	4.92	0.00	4.92	4.92	XXX	■
	RR			0.00	0.77	0.77	0.00	0.77	0.77	XXX	■
	UE			0.00	3.67	3.67	0.00	3.67	3.67	XXX	■
E1390	NU		Oxygen concentrator, capable of delivering 85 percent or greater oxygen concentration at the prescribed flow rate	0.00	54.83	54.83	0.00	54.83	54.83	XXX	■
	RR			0.00	7.21	7.21	0.00	7.21	7.21	XXX	■
E1399			Durable medical equipment, miscellaneous	0.00	0.00	0.00	0.00	0.00	0.00	XXX	
E1405	NU		Oxygen and water vapor enriching system with heated delivery	0.00	0.00	0.00	0.00	0.00	0.00	XXX	
	RR			0.00	7.15	7.15	0.00	7.15	7.15	XXX	■
	UE			0.00	0.00	0.00	0.00	0.00	0.00	XXX	
E1406	NU		Oxygen and water vapor enriching system without heated delivery	0.00	0.00	0.00	0.00	0.00	0.00	XXX	
	RR			0.00	2.98	2.98	0.00	2.98	2.98	XXX	■
	UE			0.00	0.00	0.00	0.00	0.00	0.00	XXX	
E1500			Centrifuge, for dialysis	0.00	0.00	0.00	0.00	0.00	0.00	XXX	
E1510	NU		Kidney, dialysate delivery system kidney machine, pump recirculating, air removal system, flowrate meter, power off, heater and temp control with alarm, IV poles, pressure gauge, concentrate container	0.00	0.00	0.00	0.00	0.00	0.00	XXX	
	RR			0.00	0.00	0.00	0.00	0.00	0.00	XXX	
	UE			0.00	0.00	0.00	0.00	0.00	0.00	XXX	
E1520	NU		Heparin infusion pump for hemodialysis	0.00	0.00	0.00	0.00	0.00	0.00	XXX	
	RR			0.00	0.00	0.00	0.00	0.00	0.00	XXX	
	UE			0.00	0.00	0.00	0.00	0.00	0.00	XXX	

■ RVU not developed by CMS. Gap-filled RVUs developed by CHEG.

Code	M	S	Description	Work Value	Non-Fac PE	Fac PE	Mal-practice	Non-Fac Total	Fac Total	Global	Gap
E1530	NU		Air bubble detector for hemodialysis, each, replacement	0.00	0.00	0.00	0.00	0.00	0.00	XXX	
	RR			0.00	0.00	0.00	0.00	0.00	0.00	XXX	
	UE			0.00	0.00	0.00	0.00	0.00	0.00	XXX	
E1540	NU		Pressure alarm for hemodialysis, each, replacement	0.00	0.00	0.00	0.00	0.00	0.00	XXX	
	RR			0.00	0.00	0.00	0.00	0.00	0.00	XXX	
	UE			0.00	0.00	0.00	0.00	0.00	0.00	XXX	
E1550	NU		Bath conductivity meter for hemodialysis, each	0.00	0.00	0.00	0.00	0.00	0.00	XXX	
	RR			0.00	0.00	0.00	0.00	0.00	0.00	XXX	
	UE			0.00	0.00	0.00	0.00	0.00	0.00	XXX	
E1560	NU		Blood leak detector for hemodialysis, each, replacement	0.00	0.00	0.00	0.00	0.00	0.00	XXX	
	RR			0.00	0.00	0.00	0.00	0.00	0.00	XXX	
	UE			0.00	0.00	0.00	0.00	0.00	0.00	XXX	
E1570	NU		Adjustable chair, for ESRD patients	0.00	0.00	0.00	0.00	0.00	0.00	XXX	
	RR			0.00	0.00	0.00	0.00	0.00	0.00	XXX	
	UE			0.00	0.00	0.00	0.00	0.00	0.00	XXX	
E1575	NU		Transducer protectors/fluid barriers, for hemodialysis, any size, per 10	0.00	0.00	0.00	0.00	0.00	0.00	XXX	
	RR			0.00	0.00	0.00	0.00	0.00	0.00	XXX	
	UE			0.00	0.00	0.00	0.00	0.00	0.00	XXX	
E1580	NU		Unipuncture control system for hemodialysis	0.00	0.00	0.00	0.00	0.00	0.00	XXX	
	RR			0.00	0.00	0.00	0.00	0.00	0.00	XXX	
	UE			0.00	0.00	0.00	0.00	0.00	0.00	XXX	
E1590	NU		Hemodialysis machine	0.00	0.00	0.00	0.00	0.00	0.00	XXX	
	RR			0.00	0.00	0.00	0.00	0.00	0.00	XXX	
	UE			0.00	0.00	0.00	0.00	0.00	0.00	XXX	
E1592	NU		Automatic intermittent peritoneal dialysis system	0.00	0.00	0.00	0.00	0.00	0.00	XXX	
	RR			0.00	0.00	0.00	0.00	0.00	0.00	XXX	
	UE			0.00	0.00	0.00	0.00	0.00	0.00	XXX	
E1594	NU		Cycler dialysis machine for peritoneal dialysis	0.00	0.00	0.00	0.00	0.00	0.00	XXX	
	RR			0.00	0.00	0.00	0.00	0.00	0.00	XXX	
	UE			0.00	0.00	0.00	0.00	0.00	0.00	XXX	
E1600	NU		Delivery and/or installation charges for hemodialysis equipment	0.00	0.00	0.00	0.00	0.00	0.00	XXX	
	RR			0.00	0.00	0.00	0.00	0.00	0.00	XXX	
	UE			0.00	0.00	0.00	0.00	0.00	0.00	XXX	
E1610	NU		Reverse osmosis water purification system, for hemodialysis	0.00	0.00	0.00	0.00	0.00	0.00	XXX	
	RR			0.00	0.00	0.00	0.00	0.00	0.00	XXX	
	UE			0.00	0.00	0.00	0.00	0.00	0.00	XXX	
E1615	NU		Deionizer water purification system, for hemodialysis	0.00	0.00	0.00	0.00	0.00	0.00	XXX	
	RR			0.00	0.00	0.00	0.00	0.00	0.00	XXX	
	UE			0.00	0.00	0.00	0.00	0.00	0.00	XXX	
E1620	NU		Blood pump for hemodialysis, replacement	0.00	0.00	0.00	0.00	0.00	0.00	XXX	
	RR			0.00	0.00	0.00	0.00	0.00	0.00	XXX	
	UE			0.00	0.00	0.00	0.00	0.00	0.00	XXX	
E1625	NU		Water softening system, for hemodialysis	0.00	0.00	0.00	0.00	0.00	0.00	XXX	
	RR			0.00	0.00	0.00	0.00	0.00	0.00	XXX	
	UE			0.00	0.00	0.00	0.00	0.00	0.00	XXX	

■ RVU not developed by CMS. Gap-filled RVUs developed by CHEG.

Code	M	S	Description	Work Value	Non-Fac PE	Fac PE	Mal-practice	Non-Fac Total	Fac Total	Global	Gap
E1630	NU		Reciprocating peritoneal dialysis system	0.00	0.00	0.00	0.00	0.00	0.00	XXX	
	RR			0.00	0.00	0.00	0.00	0.00	0.00	XXX	
	UE			0.00	0.00	0.00	0.00	0.00	0.00	XXX	
E1632	NU		Wearable artificial kidney, each	0.00	0.00	0.00	0.00	0.00	0.00	XXX	
	RR			0.00	0.00	0.00	0.00	0.00	0.00	XXX	
	UE			0.00	0.00	0.00	0.00	0.00	0.00	XXX	
E1635	NU		Compact (portable) travel hemodialyzer system	0.00	0.00	0.00	0.00	0.00	0.00	XXX	
	RR			0.00	0.00	0.00	0.00	0.00	0.00	XXX	
	UE			0.00	0.00	0.00	0.00	0.00	0.00	XXX	
E1636	NU		Sorbent cartridges, for hemodialysis, per 10	0.00	0.00	0.00	0.00	0.00	0.00	XXX	
	RR			0.00	0.00	0.00	0.00	0.00	0.00	XXX	
	UE			0.00	0.00	0.00	0.00	0.00	0.00	XXX	
E1637			Hemostats, for dialysis, each	0.00	0.00	0.00	0.00	0.00	0.00	XXX	
E1638			Heating pad, for peritoneal dialysis, any size, each	0.00	0.00	0.00	0.00	0.00	0.00	XXX	
E1639			Scale, for dialysis, each	0.00	0.00	0.00	0.00	0.00	0.00	XXX	
E1699			Dialysis equipment, not otherwise specified	0.00	0.00	0.00	0.00	0.00	0.00	XXX	
E1700	NU		Jaw motion rehabilitation system	0.00	10.78	10.78	0.00	10.78	10.78	XXX	■
	RR			0.00	1.06	1.06	0.00	1.06	1.06	XXX	■
	UE			0.00	8.08	8.08	0.00	8.08	8.08	XXX	■
E1701			Replacement cushions for jaw motion rehabilitation system, package of six	0.00	0.39	0.39	0.00	0.39	0.39	XXX	■
E1702			Replacement measuring scales for jaw motion rehabilitation system, package of 200	0.00	0.71	0.71	0.00	0.71	0.71	XXX	■
E1800			Dynamic adjustable elbow extension/flexion device, includes soft interface material	0.00	0.00	0.00	0.00	0.00	0.00	XXX	
E1801			Bi-directional static progressive stretch elbow device with range of motion adjustment, includes cuffs	0.00	0.00	0.00	0.00	0.00	0.00	XXX	
E1805			Dynamic adjustable wrist extension/flexion device, includes soft interface material	0.00	0.00	0.00	0.00	0.00	0.00	XXX	
E1806			Bi-directional static progressive stretch wrist device with range of motion adjustment, includes cuffs	0.00	0.00	0.00	0.00	0.00	0.00	XXX	
E1810			Dynamic adjustable knee extension/flexion device, includes soft interface material	0.00	0.00	0.00	0.00	0.00	0.00	XXX	
E1811			Bi-directional progressive stretch knee device with range of motion adjustment, includes cuffs	0.00	0.00	0.00	0.00	0.00	0.00	XXX	
E1815			Dynamic adjustable ankle extension/flexion, includes soft interface material	0.00	0.00	0.00	0.00	0.00	0.00	XXX	
E1816			Bi-directional static progressive stretch ankle device with range of motion adjustment, includes cuffs	0.00	0.00	0.00	0.00	0.00	0.00	XXX	

■ RVU not developed by CMS. Gap-filled RVUs developed by CHEG.

Code	M	S	Description	Work Value	Non-Fac PE	Fac PE	Mal-practice	Non-Fac Total	Fac Total	Global	Gap
E1818			Bi-directional static progressive stretch forearm pronation/supination device with range of motion adjustment, includes cuffs	0.00	0.00	0.00	0.00	0.00	0.00	XXX	
E1820			Replacement soft interface material, dynamic adjustable extension/flexion device	0.00	0.00	0.00	0.00	0.00	0.00	XXX	
E1821			Replacement soft interface material/cuffs for bi-directional static progressive stretch device	0.00	0.00	0.00	0.00	0.00	0.00	XXX	
E1825			Dynamic adjustable finger extension/flexion device, includes soft interface material	0.00	0.00	0.00	0.00	0.00	0.00	XXX	
E1830			Dynamic adjustable toe extension/flexion device, includes soft interface material	0.00	0.00	0.00	0.00	0.00	0.00	XXX	
E1840			Dynamic adjustable shoulder flexion/ abduction/rotation device, includes soft interface material	0.00	0.00	0.00	0.00	0.00	0.00	XXX	
E1902			Communication board, non-electronic augmentative or alternative communication device	0.00	0.00	0.00	0.00	0.00	0.00	XXX	
E2000			Gastric suction pump, home model, portable or stationary, electric	0.00	0.00	0.00	0.00	0.00	0.00	XXX	
E2100			Blood glucose monitor with integrated voice synthesizer	0.00	0.00	0.00	0.00	0.00	0.00	XXX	
E2101			Blood glucose monitor with integrated lancing/ blood sample	0.00	0.00	0.00	0.00	0.00	0.00	XXX	
G0001		X	Routine venipuncture for collection of specimen(s)	0.00	0.17	0.17	0.00	0.17	0.17	XXX	■
G0002		A	Office procedure, insertion of temporary indwelling catheter, Foley type (separate procedure)	0.50	3.32	0.17	0.03	3.85	0.70	XXX	
G0004		A	Patient demand single or multiple event recording with presymptom memory loop and 24-hour attended monitoring, per 30-day period; includes transmission, physician review and interpretation	0.52	7.10	7.10	0.45	8.07	8.07	XXX	
G0005		A	Patient demand single or multiple event recording with presymptom memory loop and 24-hour attended monitoring, per 30-day period; recording (includes hookup, recording and disconnection)	0.00	1.18	1.18	0.07	1.25	1.25	XXX	
G0006		A	Patient demand single or multiple event recording with presymptom memory loop and 24-hour attended monitoring, per 30-day period; 24-hour attended monitoring, receipt of transmissions, and analysis	0.00	5.71	5.71	0.36	6.07	6.07	XXX	

■ RVU not developed by CMS. Gap-filled RVUs developed by CHEG.

Code	M	S	Description	Work Value	Non-Fac PE	Fac PE	Mal-prac-tice	Non-Fac Total	Fac Total	Global	Gap
G0007		A	Patient demand single or multiple event recording with presymptom memory loop and 24-hour attended monitoring, per 30-day period; physician review and interpretation only	0.52	0.21	0.21	0.02	0.75	0.75	XXX	
G0008		X	Administration of influenza virus vaccine when no physician fee schedule service on the same day	0.00	0.24	0.24	0.00	0.24	0.24	XXX	■
G0009		X	Administration of pneumococcal vaccine when no physician fee schedule service on the same day	0.00	0.24	0.24	0.00	0.24	0.24	XXX	■
G0010		X	Administration of hepatitis B vaccine when no physician fee schedule service on the same day	0.00	0.24	0.24	0.00	0.24	0.24	XXX	■
G0015		A	Post-symptom telephonic transmission of electrocardiogram rhythm strip(s) and 24-hour attended monitoring, per 30-day period: Tracing only	0.00	5.71	5.71	0.36	6.07	6.07	XXX	
G0025		I	Collagen skin test kit	0.00	1.00	1.00	0.00	1.00	1.00	XXX	■
G0026		X	Fecal leukocyte examination	0.00	0.30	0.30	0.00	0.30	0.30	XXX	■
G0027		X	Semen analysis; presence and/or motility of sperm excluding Huhner test	0.00	0.55	0.55	0.00	0.55	0.55	XXX	■
G0030		C	PET myocardial perfusion imaging, (following previous PET, G0030–G0047); single study, rest or stress (exercise and/or pharmacologic)	0.00	0.00	0.00	0.00	0.00	0.00	XXX	
	26	A		1.50	0.52	0.52	0.04	2.06	2.06	XXX	
	TC	C		0.00	0.00	0.00	0.00	0.00	0.00	XXX	
G0031		C	PET myocardial perfusion imaging, (following previous PET, G0030–G0047); multiple studies, rest or stress (exercise and/or pharmacologic)	0.00	0.00	0.00	0.00	0.00	0.00	XXX	
	26	A		1.87	0.70	0.70	0.06	2.63	2.63	XXX	
	TC	C		0.00	0.00	0.00	0.00	0.00	0.00	XXX	
G0032		C	PET myocardial perfusion imaging, (following rest SPECT, 78464); single study, rest or stress (exercise and/or pharmacologic)	0.00	0.00	0.00	0.00	0.00	0.00	XXX	
	26	A		1.50	0.52	0.52	0.05	2.07	2.07	XXX	
	TC	C		0.00	0.00	0.00	0.00	0.00	0.00	XXX	
G0033		C	PET myocardial perfusion imaging, (following rest SPECT, 78464); multiple studies, rest or stress (exercise and/or pharmacologic)	0.00	0.00	0.00	0.00	0.00	0.00	XXX	
	26	A		1.87	0.70	0.70	0.06	2.63	2.63	XXX	
	TC	C		0.00	0.00	0.00	0.00	0.00	0.00	XXX	
G0034		C	PET myocardial perfusion imaging, (following stress SPECT, 78465); single study, rest or stress (exercise and/or pharmacologic)	0.00	0.00	0.00	0.00	0.00	0.00	XXX	
	26	A		1.50	0.52	0.52	0.05	2.07	2.07	XXX	
	TC	C		0.00	0.00	0.00	0.00	0.00	0.00	XXX	
G0035		C	PET myocardial perfusion imaging, (following stress SPECT, 78465); multiple studies, rest or stress (exercise and/or pharmacologic)	0.00	0.00	0.00	0.00	0.00	0.00	XXX	
	26	A		1.87	0.70	0.70	0.06	2.63	2.63	XXX	
	TC	C		0.00	0.00	0.00	0.00	0.00	0.00	XXX	
G0036		C	PET myocardial perfusion imaging, (following coronary angiography, 93510–93529); single study, rest or stress (exercise and/or pharmacologic)	0.00	0.00	0.00	0.00	0.00	0.00	XXX	
	26	A		1.50	0.52	0.52	0.04	2.06	2.06	XXX	
	TC	C		0.00	0.00	0.00	0.00	0.00	0.00	XXX	

■ RVU not developed by CMS. Gap-filled RVUs developed by CHEG.

Code	M	S	Description	Work Value	Non-Fac PE	Fac PE	Mal-practice	Non-Fac Total	Fac Total	Global	Gap
G0037		C	PET myocardial perfusion imaging, (following coronary angiography, 93510–93529); multiple studies, rest or stress (exercise and/or pharmacologic)	0.00	0.00	0.00	0.00	0.00	0.00	XXX	
	26	A		1.87	0.70	0.70	0.06	2.63	2.63	XXX	
	TC	C		0.00	0.00	0.00	0.00	0.00	0.00	XXX	
G0038		C	PET myocardial perfusion imaging, (following stress planar myocardial perfusion, 78460); single study, rest or stress (exercise and/or pharmacologic)	0.00	0.00	0.00	0.00	0.00	0.00	XXX	
	26	A		1.50	0.52	0.52	0.04	2.06	2.06	XXX	
	TC	C		0.00	0.00	0.00	0.00	0.00	0.00	XXX	
G0039		C	PET myocardial perfusion imaging, (following stress planar myocardial perfusion, 78460); multiple studies, rest or stress (exercise and/or pharmacologic)	0.00	0.00	0.00	0.00	0.00	0.00	XXX	
	26	A		1.87	0.70	0.70	0.07	2.64	2.64	XXX	
	TC	C		0.00	0.00	0.00	0.00	0.00	0.00	XXX	
G0040		C	PET myocardial perfusion imaging, (following stress echocardiogram, 93350); single study, rest or stress (exercise and/or pharmacologic)	0.00	0.00	0.00	0.00	0.00	0.00	XXX	
	26	A		1.50	0.52	0.52	0.04	2.06	2.06	XXX	
	TC	C		0.00	0.00	0.00	0.00	0.00	0.00	XXX	
G0041		C	PET myocardial perfusion imaging, (following stress echocardiogram, 93350); multiple studies, rest or stress (exercise and/or pharmacologic)	0.00	0.00	0.00	0.00	0.00	0.00	XXX	
	26	A		1.87	0.70	0.70	0.05	2.62	2.62	XXX	
	TC	C		0.00	0.00	0.00	0.00	0.00	0.00	XXX	
G0042		C	PET myocardial perfusion imaging, (following stress nuclear ventriculogram, 78481 or 78483); single study, rest or stress (exercise and/or pharmacologic)	0.00	0.00	0.00	0.00	0.00	0.00	XXX	
	26	A		1.50	0.52	0.52	0.04	2.06	2.06	XXX	
	TC	C		0.00	0.00	0.00	0.00	0.00	0.00	XXX	
G0043		C	PET myocardial perfusion imaging, (following stress nuclear ventriculogram, 78481 or 78483); multiple studies, rest or stress (exercise and/or pharmacologic)	0.00	0.00	0.00	0.00	0.00	0.00	XXX	
	26	A		1.87	0.70	0.70	0.06	2.63	2.63	XXX	
	TC	C		0.00	0.00	0.00	0.00	0.00	0.00	XXX	
G0044		C	PET myocardial perfusion imaging, (following rest ECG, 93000); single study, rest or stress (exercise and/or pharmacologic)	0.00	0.00	0.00	0.00	0.00	0.00	XXX	
	26	A		1.50	0.52	0.52	0.04	2.06	2.06	XXX	
	TC	C		0.00	0.00	0.00	0.00	0.00	0.00	XXX	
G0045		C	PET myocardial perfusion imaging, (following rest ECG, 93000); multiple studies, rest or stress (exercise and/or pharmacologic)	0.00	0.00	0.00	0.00	0.00	0.00	XXX	
	26	A		1.87	0.70	0.70	0.06	2.63	2.63	XXX	
	TC	C		0.00	0.00	0.00	0.00	0.00	0.00	XXX	
G0046		C	PET myocardial perfusion imaging, (following stress ECG, 93015); single study, rest or stress (exercise and/or pharmacologic)	0.00	0.00	0.00	0.00	0.00	0.00	XXX	
	26	A		1.50	0.52	0.52	0.04	2.06	2.06	XXX	
	TC	C		0.00	0.00	0.00	0.00	0.00	0.00	XXX	
G0047		C	PET myocardial perfusion imaging, (following stress ECG, 93015); multiple studies, rest or stress (exercise and/or pharmacologic)	0.00	0.00	0.00	0.00	0.00	0.00	XXX	
	26	A		1.87	0.70	0.70	0.06	2.63	2.63	XXX	
	TC	C		0.00	0.00	0.00	0.00	0.00	0.00	XXX	
G0050		A	Measurement of post-voiding residual urine and/or bladder capacity by ultrasound	0.00	0.81	0.81	0.04	0.85	0.85	XXX	
G0101		A	Cervical or vaginal cancer screening; pelvic and clinical breast examination	0.45	0.52	0.18	0.01	0.98	0.64	XXX	
G0102		A	Prostate cancer screening; digital rectal examination	0.17	0.38	0.06	0.01	0.56	0.24	XXX	
G0103		X	Prostate cancer screening; prostate specific antigen test (PSA), total	0.00	1.52	1.52	0.00	1.52	1.52	XXX	■

■ RVU not developed by CMS. Gap-filled RVUs developed by CHEG.

Code	M	S	Description	Work Value	Non-Fac PE	Fac PE	Mal-practice	Non-Fac Total	Fac Total	Global	Gap
G0104		A	Colorectal cancer screening; flexible sigmoidoscopy	0.96	1.92	0.53	0.05	2.93	1.54	XXX	
G0105		A	Colorectal cancer screening; colonoscopy on individual at high risk	3.70	8.79	1.77	0.20	12.69	5.67	XXX	
G0106		A	Colorectal cancer screening; alternative to G0104, screening sigmoidoscopy, barium enema	0.99	2.47	2.47	0.15	3.61	3.61	XXX	
	26	A		0.99	0.35	0.35	0.04	1.38	1.38	XXX	
	TC	A		0.00	2.12	2.12	0.11	2.23	2.23	XXX	
G0107		X	Colorectal cancer screening; fecal-occult blood test, 1-3 simultaneous determinations	0.00	0.30	0.30	0.00	0.30	0.30	XXX	■
G0108		A	Diabetes outpatient self-management training services, individual, per 30 minutes	0.00	1.64	1.64	0.01	1.65	1.65	XXX	
G0109		A	Diabetes self-management training services, group session (2 or more), per 30 minutes	0.00	0.96	0.96	0.01	0.97	0.97	XXX	
G0110		R	NETT pulmonary rehabilitation; education/ skills training, individual	0.90	0.67	0.36	0.03	1.60	1.29	XXX	
G0111		R	NETT pulmonary rehabilitation; education/ skills, group	0.27	0.29	0.11	0.01	0.57	0.39	XXX	
G0112		R	NETT pulmonary rehabilitation; nutritional guidance, initial	1.72	1.24	0.69	0.05	3.01	2.46	XXX	
G0113		R	NETT pulmonary rehabilitation; nutritional guidance, subsequent	1.29	0.97	0.51	0.04	2.30	1.84	XXX	
G0114		R	NETT pulmonary rehabilitation; psychosocial consultation	1.20	0.49	0.48	0.03	1.72	1.71	XXX	
G0115		R	NETT pulmonary rehabilitation; psychological testing	1.20	0.57	0.48	0.04	1.81	1.72	XXX	
G0116		R	NETT pulmonary rehabilitation; psychosocial counselling	1.11	0.69	0.44	0.04	1.84	1.59	XXX	
G0117		T	Glaucoma screening for high risk patients furnished by an optometrist or ophthalmologist	0.45	0.97	0.22	0.02	1.44	0.69	XXX	
G0118		T	Glaucoma screening for high risk patient furnished under the direct supervision of an optometrist or ophthalomologist	0.17	0.84	0.08	0.01	1.02	0.26	XXX	
G0120		A	Colorectal cancer screening; alternative to G0105, screening colonoscopy, barium enema	0.99	2.47	2.47	0.15	3.61	3.61	XXX	
	26	A		0.99	0.35	0.35	0.04	1.38	1.38	XXX	
	TC	A		0.00	2.12	2.12	0.11	2.23	2.23	XXX	
G0121		A	Colorectal cancer screening; colonoscopy on individual not meeting criteria for high risk	3.70	8.79	1.77	0.20	12.69	5.67	XXX	
G0122		N	Colorectal cancer screening; barium enema	0.99	2.52	2.52	0.15	3.66	3.66	XXX	
	26	N		0.99	0.40	0.40	0.04	1.43	1.43	XXX	
	TC	N		0.00	2.12	2.12	0.11	2.23	2.23	XXX	

■ RVU not developed by CMS. Gap-filled RVUs developed by CHEG.

Code	M	S	Description	Work Value	Non-Fac PE	Fac PE	Mal-prac-tice	Non-Fac Total	Fac Total	Global	Gap
G0123		X	Screening cytopathology, cervical or vaginal (any reporting system), collected in preservative fluid, automated thin layer preparation, screening by cytotechnologist under physician supervision	0.00	0.39	0.39	0.00	0.39	0.39	XXX	■
G0124		A	Screening cytopathology, cervical or vaginal (any reporting system), collected in preservative fluid, automated thin layer preparation, requiring interpretation by physician	0.42	0.19	0.19	0.01	0.62	0.62	XXX	
G0125		A	PET imaging regional or whole body; single pulmonary nodule; full- and partial-ring PET scanners only	1.50	56.10	56.10	2.00	59.60	59.60	XXX	
	26	A		1.50	0.52	0.52	0.05	2.07	2.07	XXX	
	TC	A		0.00	55.58	55.58	1.95	57.53	57.53	XXX	
G0127		R	Trimming of dystrophic nails, any number	0.17	0.26	0.07	0.01	0.44	0.25	XXX	
G0128		R	Direct (face-to-face with patient) skilled nursing services of a registered nurse provided in a comprehensive outpatient rehabilitation facility, each 10 minutes beyond the first 5 minutes	0.08	0.03	0.03	0.01	0.12	0.12	XXX	
G0129			Occupational therapy requiring the skills of a qualified occupational therapist, furnished as a component of a partial hospitalization treatment program, per day	0.00	0.00	0.00	0.00	0.00	0.00	XXX	
G0130		A	Single energy x-ray absorptiometry (SEXA) bone density study, one or more sites; appendicular skeleton (peripheral) (e.g., radius, wrist, heel)	0.22	0.90	0.90	0.05	1.17	1.17	XXX	
	26	A		0.22	0.11	0.11	0.01	0.34	0.34	XXX	
	TC	A		0.00	0.79	0.79	0.04	0.83	0.83	XXX	
G0131		A	Computerized tomography bone mineral density study, one or more sites; axial skeleton (e.g., hips, pelvis, spine)	0.25	3.18	3.18	0.14	3.57	3.57	XXX	
	26	A		0.25	0.13	0.13	0.01	0.39	0.39	XXX	
	TC	A		0.00	3.05	3.05	0.13	3.18	3.18	XXX	
G0132		A	Computerized tomography bone mineral density study, one or more sites; appendicular skeleton (peripheral) (e.g., radius, wrist, heel)	0.22	0.90	0.90	0.05	1.17	1.17	XXX	
	26	A		0.22	0.11	0.11	0.01	0.34	0.34	XXX	
	TC	A		0.00	0.79	0.79	0.04	0.83	0.83	XXX	
G0141		A	Screening cytopathology smears, cervical or vaginal, performed by automated system, with manual rescreening, requiring interpretation by physician	0.42	0.19	0.19	0.01	0.62	0.62	XXX	
G0143		X	Screening cytopathology, cervical or vaginal (any reporting system), collected in preservative fluid, automated thin layer preparation, with manual screening and rescreening by cytotechnologist under physician supervision	0.00	0.54	0.54	0.00	0.54	0.54	XXX	■
G0144		X	Screening cytopathology, cervical or vaginal (any reporting system), collected in preservative fluid, automated thin layer preparation, with manual screening and computer-assisted rescreening by cytotechnologist under physician supervision	0.00	0.52	0.52	0.00	0.52	0.52	XXX	■

■ RVU not developed by CMS. Gap-filled RVUs developed by CHEG.

Code	M	S	Description	Work Value	Non-Fac PE	Fac PE	Mal-prac-tice	Non-Fac Total	Fac Total	Global	Gap
G0145		X	Screening cytopathology, cervical or vaginal (any reporting system), collected in preservative fluid, automated thin layer preparation, with manual screening and computer-assisted rescreening using cell selection and review under physician supervision	0.00	0.56	0.56	0.00	0.56	0.56	XXX	■
G0147		X	Screening cytopathology smears, cervical or vaginal, performed by automated system under physician supervision	0.00	0.52	0.52	0.00	0.52	0.52	XXX	■
G0148		X	Screening cytopathology smears, cervical or vaginal, performed by automated system with manual rescreening	0.00	0.54	0.54	0.00	0.54	0.54	XXX	■
G0151			Services of physical therapist in home health setting, each 15 minutes	0.00	0.00	0.00	0.00	0.00	0.00	XXX	
G0152			Services of occupational therapist in home health setting, each 15 minutes	0.00	0.00	0.00	0.00	0.00	0.00	XXX	
G0153			Services of speech and language pathologist in home health setting, each 15 minutes	0.00	0.00	0.00	0.00	0.00	0.00	XXX	
G0154			Services of skilled nurse in home health setting, each 15 minutes	0.00	0.00	0.00	0.00	0.00	0.00	XXX	
G0155			Services of clinical social worker in home health setting, each 15 minutes	0.00	0.00	0.00	0.00	0.00	0.00	XXX	
G0156			Services of home health aide in home health setting, each 15 minutes	0.00	0.00	0.00	0.00	0.00	0.00	XXX	
G0166		A	External counterpulsation, per treatment session	0.07	4.17	0.03	0.01	4.25	0.11	XXX	
G0167		C	Hyperbaric oxygen treatment not requiring physician attendance, per treatment session	0.00	0.00	0.00	0.00	0.00	0.00	XXX	
G0168		A	Wound closure utilizing tissue adhesive(s) only	0.45	2.33	0.19	0.01	2.79	0.65	XXX	
G0173		X	Stereotactic radiosurgery, complete course of therapy in one session	0.00	0.00	0.00	0.00	0.00	0.00	XXX	
G0175		X	Scheduled interdisciplinary team conference (minimum of three exclusive of patient care nursing staff) with patient present	0.00	0.00	0.00	0.00	0.00	0.00	XXX	
G0176		X	Activity therapy, such as music, dance, art or play therapies not for recreation, related to the care and treatment of patient's disabling mental health problems, per session (45 minutes or more)	0.00	0.00	0.00	0.00	0.00	0.00	XXX	
G0177		X	Training and educational services related to the care and treatment of patient's disabling mental health problems per session (45 minutes or more)	0.00	0.00	0.00	0.00	0.00	0.00	XXX	

■ RVU not developed by CMS. Gap-filled RVUs developed by CHEG.

Code	M	S	Description	Work Value	Non-Fac PE	Fac PE	Mal-practice	Non-Fac Total	Fac Total	Global	Gap
G0179		A	Physician recertifiction services for Medicare-covered services, provided by a participating home health agency (patient not present) including review of subsequent reports of patient status, review or patient's responses to the OASIS assessment instrument, contact with the home health agency to ascecrtain the follow-up implementation plan of care, and documentation in the patient's office record, per certification period	0.45	1.21	1.21	0.01	1.67	1.67	XXX	
G0180		A	Physician certification services for Medicare-covered services provided by a participating home health agency (patient not present), including review of initial or subsequent reports of patient status, review of patient's responses to the Oasis assessment instrument, contact with the home health agency to ascertain the initial implementation plan of care, and documentation in the patient's office record, per certification period	0.67	1.29	1.29	0.02	1.98	1.98	XXX	
G0181		A	Physician supervision of a patient receiving Medicare-covered services provided by a participatient home health agency (patient not present) requiring complex and multidisciplinary care modalities involving regular physician development and/or revision of care plans, review of subsequent reports of patient status, review of laboratory and other studies, communication (including telephone calls) with other health care professionals involved in the patient's care, integration of new information into the medical treatment plan and/or adjustment of medical therapy, within a calendar month, 30 minutes or more	1.73	1.57	1.57	0.06	3.36	3.36	XXX	
G0182		A	Physician supervision of a patient under a Medicare-approved hospice (patient not present) requiring complex and multidisciplinary care modalities involving regular physician development and/or revision of care plans, review of subsequent reports of patient status, review of laboratory and other studies, communication (including telephone calls) with other health care professionals involved in the patient's care, integration of new information into the medical treatment plan and/or adjustment of medical therapy, within a calendar month, 30 minutes or more	1.73	1.97	1.97	0.06	3.76	3.76	XXX	
G0185		C	Destruction of localized lesion of choroid (for example, choroidal neovascularization); transpupillary thermotherapy (one or more sessions)	0.00	0.00	0.00	0.00	0.00	0.00	YYY	
G0186		C	Destruction of localized lesion of choroid (for example, choroidal neovascularization); photocoagulation, feeder vessel technique (one or more sessions)	0.00	0.00	0.00	0.00	0.00	0.00	YYY	

■ RVU not developed by CMS. Gap-filled RVUs developed by CHEG.

Code	M	S	Description	Work Value	Non-Fac PE	Fac PE	Mal-practice	Non-Fac Total	Fac Total	Global	Gap
G0187		C	Destruction of macular drusen, photocoagulation (one or more sessions)	0.00	0.00	0.00	0.00	0.00	0.00	YYY	
G0192		N	Intranasal or oral administration; one vaccine (single or combination vaccine/toxoid)	0.00	0.00	0.00	0.00	0.00	0.00	XXX	
G0193		C	Endoscopic study of swallowing function (also fiberoptic endoscopic evaluation of swallowing) (FEES)	0.00	0.00	0.00	0.00	0.00	0.00	XXX	
G0194		C	Sensory testing during endoscopic study of swallowing (add on code) referred to as fiberoptic endoscopic evaluation of swallowing with sensory testing (FEEST)	0.00	0.00	0.00	0.00	0.00	0.00	XXX	
G0195		A	Clinical evaluation of swallowing function (not involving interpretation of dynamic radiological studies or endoscopic study of swallowing)	1.50	1.95	0.76	0.07	3.52	2.33	XXX	
G0196		A	Evaluation of swallowing involving swallowing of radio-opaque materials	1.50	1.95	0.76	0.07	3.52	2.33	XXX	
G0197		A	Evaluation of patient for prescription of speech generating devices	1.35	2.11	0.75	0.04	3.50	2.14	XXX	
G0198		A	Patient adaptation and training for use of speech generating devices	0.99	1.14	0.58	0.03	2.16	1.60	XXX	
G0199		A	Re-evaluation of patient using speech generating devices	1.01	1.92	0.56	0.03	2.96	1.60	XXX	
G0200		A	Evaluation of patient for prescription of voice prosthetic	1.35	2.11	0.75	0.04	3.50	2.14	XXX	
G0201		A	Modification or training in use of voice prosthetic	0.99	1.14	0.58	0.03	2.16	1.60	XXX	
G0202		A	Screening mammography, producing direct digital image, bilateral, all views	0.70	2.70	2.70	0.09	3.49	3.49	XXX	
	26	A		0.70	0.28	0.28	0.03	1.01	1.01	XXX	
	TC	A		0.00	2.42	2.42	0.06	2.48	2.48	XXX	
G0204		A	Diagnostic mammography, producing direct digital image, bilateral, all views	0.87	2.73	2.73	0.09	3.69	3.69	XXX	
	26	A		0.87	0.35	0.35	0.03	1.25	1.25	XXX	
	TC	A		0.00	2.38	2.38	0.06	2.44	2.44	XXX	
G0206		A	Diagnostic mammography, producing direct digital image, unilateral, all views	0.70	2.20	2.20	0.08	2.98	2.98	XXX	
	26	A		0.70	0.28	0.28	0.03	1.01	1.01	XXX	
	TC	A		0.00	1.92	1.92	0.05	1.97	1.97	XXX	
G0210		C	PET imaging whole body; full- and partial-ring PET scanners only, diagnosis; lung cancer, non-small cell	0.00	0.00	0.00	0.00	0.00	0.00	XXX	
	26	A		1.50	0.60	0.60	0.04	2.14	2.14	XXX	
	TC	C		0.00	0.00	0.00	0.00	0.00	0.00	XXX	
G0211		C	PET imaging whole body; full- and partial-ring PET scanners only, intial staging; lung cancer; non-small cell	0.00	0.00	0.00	0.00	0.00	0.00	XXX	
	26	A		1.50	0.60	0.60	0.04	2.14	2.14	XXX	
	TC	C		0.00	0.00	0.00	0.00	0.00	0.00	XXX	
G0212		C	PET imaging whole body; full- and partial-ring PET scanners only, restaging; lung cancer; non-small cell	0.00	0.00	0.00	0.00	0.00	0.00	XXX	
	26	A		1.50	0.60	0.60	0.04	2.14	2.14	XXX	
	TC	C		0.00	0.00	0.00	0.00	0.00	0.00	XXX	

■ RVU not developed by CMS. Gap-filled RVUs developed by CHEG.

Code	M	S	Description	Work Value	Non-Fac PE	Fac PE	Mal-practice	Non-Fac Total	Fac Total	Global	Gap
G0213		C	PET imaging whole body; full- and partial ring PET scanners only, diagnosis; colorectal cancer	0.00	0.00	0.00	0.00	0.00	0.00	XXX	
	26	A		1.50	0.60	0.60	0.04	2.14	2.14	XXX	
	TC	C		0.00	0.00	0.00	0.00	0.00	0.00	XXX	
G0214		C	PET imaging whole body; full- and partial-ring PET scanners only, initial staging; colorectal cancer	0.00	0.00	0.00	0.00	0.00	0.00	XXX	
	26	A		1.50	0.60	0.60	0.04	2.14	2.14	XXX	
	TC	C		0.00	0.00	0.00	0.00	0.00	0.00	XXX	
G0215		C	PET imaging whole body; full- and partial-ring PET scanners only, restaging; colorectal cancer	0.00	0.00	0.00	0.00	0.00	0.00	XXX	
	26	A		1.50	0.60	0.60	0.04	2.14	2.14	XXX	
	TC	C		0.00	0.00	0.00	0.00	0.00	0.00	XXX	
G0216		C	PET imaging whole body; full- and partial-ring PET scanners only, diagnosis; melanoma	0.00	0.00	0.00	0.00	0.00	0.00	XXX	
	26	A		1.50	0.60	0.60	0.04	2.14	2.14	XXX	
	TC	C		0.00	0.00	0.00	0.00	0.00	0.00	XXX	
G0217		C	PET imaging whole body; full- and partial-staging PET scanners only, initial staging; melanoma	0.00	0.00	0.00	0.00	0.00	0.00	XXX	
	26	A		1.50	0.60	0.60	0.04	2.14	2.14	XXX	
	TC	C		0.00	0.00	0.00	0.00	0.00	0.00	XXX	
G0218		C	PET imaging whole body; full- and partial-ring PET scanners only, restaging; melanoma (replaces G0165)	0.00	0.00	0.00	0.00	0.00	0.00	XXX	
	26	A		1.50	0.60	0.60	0.04	2.14	2.14	XXX	
	TC	C		0.00	0.00	0.00	0.00	0.00	0.00	XXX	
G0219		N	PET imaging whole body; full- and partial-ring PET scanners only, non-covered individual (replaces G0165)	1.50	0.60	0.60	0.04	2.14	2.14	XXX	
	26	N		1.50	0.60	0.60	0.04	2.14	2.14	XXX	
	TC	N		0.00	0.00	0.00	0.00	0.00	0.00	XXX	
G0220		C	PET imaging whole body; full- and partial-ring PET scanners only, diagnosis; lymphoma	0.00	0.00	0.00	0.00	0.00	0.00	XXX	
	26	A		1.50	0.60	0.60	0.04	2.14	2.14	XXX	
	TC	C		0.00	0.00	0.00	0.00	0.00	0.00	XXX	
G0221		C	PET imaging whole body; full- and partial-ring PET scanners only, initial staging; lymphoma (replaces G0164)	0.00	0.00	0.00	0.00	0.00	0.00	XXX	
	26	A		1.50	0.60	0.60	0.04	2.14	2.14	XXX	
	TC	C		0.00	0.00	0.00	0.00	0.00	0.00	XXX	
G0222		C	PET imaging whole body; full- and partial-ring PET scanners only, restaging; lymphoma (replaces G0164)	0.00	0.00	0.00	0.00	0.00	0.00	XXX	
	26	A		1.50	0.60	0.60	0.04	2.14	2.14	XXX	
	TC	C		0.00	0.00	0.00	0.00	0.00	0.00	XXX	
G0223		C	PET imaging whole body or regional; full- and partial-ring PET scanners only, diagnosis; head and neck cancer; excluding thyroid and CNS cancers	0.00	0.00	0.00	0.00	0.00	0.00	XXX	
	26	A		1.50	0.60	0.60	0.04	2.14	2.14	XXX	
	TC	C		0.00	0.00	0.00	0.00	0.00	0.00	XXX	
G0224		C	PET imaging whole body or regional; full- and partial-ring PET scanners only, initial staging; head and neck cancer; excluding thyroid and CNS cancers	0.00	0.00	0.00	0.00	0.00	0.00	XXX	
	26	A		1.50	0.60	0.60	0.04	2.14	2.14	XXX	
	TC	C		0.00	0.00	0.00	0.00	0.00	0.00	XXX	
G0225		C	PET imaging whole body or regional; full-and partial-ring PET scanners only, restaging; head and neck cancer, excluding thyroid and CNS cancers	0.00	0.00	0.00	0.00	0.00	0.00	XXX	
	26	A		1.50	0.60	0.60	0.04	2.14	2.14	XXX	
	TC	C		0.00	0.00	0.00	0.00	0.00	0.00	XXX	
G0226		C	PET imaging whole body; full- and partial-ring PET scanners only, diagnostic; esophageal cancer	0.00	0.00	0.00	0.00	0.00	0.00	XXX	
	26	A		1.50	0.60	0.60	0.04	2.14	2.14	XXX	
	TC	C		0.00	0.00	0.00	0.00	0.00	0.00	XXX	

Code	M	S	Description	Work Value	Non-Fac PE	Fac PE	Mal-practice	Non-Fac Total	Fac Total	Global	Gap
G0227		C	PET imaging whole body; full- and partial-ring PET scanners only, initial staging; esophageal cancer	0.00	0.00	0.00	0.00	0.00	0.00	XXX	
	26	A		1.50	0.60	0.60	0.04	2.14	2.14	XXX	
	TC	C		0.00	0.00	0.00	0.00	0.00	0.00	XXX	
G0228		C	PET imaging whole body; full- and partial-ring PET scanners only, restaging; esophageal cancer	0.00	0.00	0.00	0.00	0.00	0.00	XXX	
	26	A		1.50	0.60	0.60	0.04	2.14	2.14	XXX	
	TC	C		0.00	0.00	0.00	0.00	0.00	0.00	XXX	
G0229		C	PET imaging; metabolic brain imaging for pre-surgical evaluation of refractory seizures; full- and partial-ring PET scanners only	0.00	0.00	0.00	0.00	0.00	0.00	XXX	
	26	A		1.50	0.60	0.60	0.04	2.14	2.14	XXX	
	TC	C		0.00	0.00	0.00	0.00	0.00	0.00	XXX	
G0230		C	PET imaging; metabolic assessment for myocardial viability following inconclusive spect study; full- and partial-ring PET scanners only	0.00	0.00	0.00	0.00	0.00	0.00	XXX	
	26	A		1.50	0.60	0.60	0.04	2.14	2.14	XXX	
	TC	C		0.00	0.00	0.00	0.00	0.00	0.00	XXX	
G0231		C	PET, whole body, for recurrence of colorectal or colorectal metastatic cancer; gamma cameras only	0.00	0.00	0.00	0.00	0.00	0.00	XXX	
	26	A		1.50	0.60	0.60	0.04	2.14	2.14	XXX	
	TC	C		0.00	0.00	0.00	0.00	0.00	0.00	XXX	
G0232		C	PET, whole body, for recurrence of lymphoma; gamma cameras only	0.00	0.00	0.00	0.00	0.00	0.00	XXX	
	26	A		1.50	0.60	0.60	0.04	2.14	2.14	XXX	
	TC	C		0.00	0.00	0.00	0.00	0.00	0.00	XXX	
G0233		C	PET, whole body, for recurrence of melanoma; gamma cameras only	0.00	0.00	0.00	0.00	0.00	0.00	XXX	
	26	A		1.50	0.60	0.60	0.04	2.14	2.14	XXX	
	TC	C		0.00	0.00	0.00	0.00	0.00	0.00	XXX	
G0234		C	PET, regional or whole body, for solitary pulmonary nodule following CT or for initial staging of pathologically diagnosed nonsmall cell lung cancer; gamma cameras only	0.00	0.00	0.00	0.00	0.00	0.00	XXX	
	26	A		1.50	0.60	0.60	0.04	2.14	2.14	XXX	
	TC	C		0.00	0.00	0.00	0.00	0.00	0.00	XXX	
G0236		A	Digitization of film radiographic images with computer analysis for lesion detection and further physician review for interpretation, diagnostic mammography(list separately in addition to code for primary procedure)	0.06	0.31	0.31	0.02	0.39	0.39	ZZZ	
	26	A		0.06	0.02	0.02	0.01	0.09	0.09	ZZZ	
	TC	A		0.00	0.29	0.29	0.01	0.30	0.30	ZZZ	
G0237		A	Therapeutic procedures to increase strength or endurance of respiratory muscles, face to face, one on one, each 15 minutes (includes monitoring)	0.00	0.45	0.45	0.02	0.47	0.47	XXX	
G0238		C	Therapeutic procedures to improve respiratory function, other than described by g0237, one on one, face to face, per 15 minutes (includes monitoring)	0.00	0.00	0.00	0.00	0.00	0.00	XXX	
G0239		C	Therapeutic procedures to improve respiratory function, other than services described by G0237, two or more (includes monitoring)	0.00	0.00	0.00	0.00	0.00	0.00	XXX	
G0240		A	Critical care service delivered by a physician, face to face; during interfacility transport of a critically ill or critically injured patient; first 30-74 minutes of active transport	4.00	1.60	1.60	0.14	5.74	5.74	XXX	
G0241		A	Each additional 30 minutes (list separately in addition to G0240)	2.00	0.80	0.80	0.07	2.87	2.87	ZZZ	

■ RVU not developed by CMS. Gap-filled RVUs developed by CHEG.

Code	M	S	Description	Work Value	Non-Fac PE	Fac PE	Mal-practice	Non-Fac Total	Fac Total	Global	Gap
G0242		X	Multi-source photon stereotactic radiosurgery (cobalt 60 multi-source converging beams) plan, including dose volume histograms for target and critical structure tolerances, plan optimization performed for highly conformal distributions, plan positional a ccuracy and dose verification, all lesions treated, per course of treatment	0.00	0.00	0.00	0.00	0.00	0.00	XXX	
G0243		X	Multi-source photon stereotactic radiosurgery, delivery including collimator changes and custom plugging, complete course of treatment, all lesions	0.00	0.00	0.00	0.00	0.00	0.00	XXX	
G0244		X	Observation care provided by a facility to a patient with CHF, chest pain, or asthma, minimum eight hours, maximum forty eight hours	0.00	0.00	0.00	0.00	0.00	0.00	XXX	
G9001		X	Coordinated care fee, initial rate	0.00	0.00	0.00	0.00	0.00	0.00	XXX	
G9002		X	Coordinated care fee, maintenance rate	0.00	0.00	0.00	0.00	0.00	0.00	XXX	
G9003		X	Coordinated care fee, risk adjusted high, initial	0.00	0.00	0.00	0.00	0.00	0.00	XXX	
G9004		X	Coordinated care fee, risk adjusted low, initial	0.00	0.00	0.00	0.00	0.00	0.00	XXX	
G9005		X	Coordinated care fee, risk adjusted maintenance	0.00	0.00	0.00	0.00	0.00	0.00	XXX	
G9006		X	Coordinated care fee, home monitoring	0.00	0.00	0.00	0.00	0.00	0.00	XXX	
G9007		X	Coordinated care fee, schedule team conference	0.00	0.00	0.00	0.00	0.00	0.00	XXX	
G9008		X	Coordinated care fee, physician coordinated care oversight services	0.00	0.00	0.00	0.00	0.00	0.00	XXX	
G9009		X	Coordinated care fee, risk adjusted maintenance, level 3	0.00	0.00	0.00	0.00	0.00	0.00	XXX	
G9010		X	Coordinated care fee, risk adjusted maintenance, level 4	0.00	0.00	0.00	0.00	0.00	0.00	XXX	
G9011		X	Coordinated care fee, risk adjusted maintenance, level 5	0.00	0.00	0.00	0.00	0.00	0.00	XXX	
G9012		X	Coordinated care fee, risk adjusted maintenance, level 3	0.00	0.00	0.00	0.00	0.00	0.00	XXX	
G9016		N	Smoking cessation counseling, individual, in the absence of or in addition to any other evaluation and management service, per session (6-10 minutes) [demo project code only]	0.00	0.00	0.00	0.00	0.00	0.00	XXX	
H0001		I	Alcohol and/or drug assessment	0.00	0.00	0.00	0.00	0.00	0.00	XXX	
H0002		I	Alcohol and/or drug screening to determine eligibility for admission to treatment program	0.00	0.00	0.00	0.00	0.00	0.00	XXX	
H0003		I	Alcohol and/or drug screening; laboratory analysis of specimens for presence of alcohol and/or drugs	0.00	0.00	0.00	0.00	0.00	0.00	XXX	

■ RVU not developed by CMS. Gap-filled RVUs developed by CHEG.

Code	M	S	Description	Work Value	Non-Fac PE	Fac PE	Mal-practice	Non-Fac Total	Fac Total	Global	Gap
H0004		I	Alcohol and/or drug services; individual counseling by a clinician	0.00	0.00	0.00	0.00	0.00	0.00	XXX	
H0005		I	Alcohol and/or drug services; group counseling by a clinician	0.00	0.00	0.00	0.00	0.00	0.00	XXX	
H0006		I	Alcohol and/or drug services; case management	0.00	0.00	0.00	0.00	0.00	0.00	XXX	
H0007		I	Alcohol and/or drug services; crisis intervention (outpatient)	0.00	0.00	0.00	0.00	0.00	0.00	XXX	
H0008		I	Alcohol and/or drug services; sub-acute detoxification (hospital inpatient)	0.00	0.00	0.00	0.00	0.00	0.00	XXX	
H0009		I	Alcohol and/or drug services; acute detoxification (hospital inpatient)	0.00	0.00	0.00	0.00	0.00	0.00	XXX	
H0010		I	Alcohol and/or drug services; sub-acute detoxification (residential addiction program inpatient)	0.00	0.00	0.00	0.00	0.00	0.00	XXX	
H0011		I	Alcohol and/or drug services; acute detoxification (residential addiction program inpatient)	0.00	0.00	0.00	0.00	0.00	0.00	XXX	
H0012		I	Alcohol and/or drug services; sub-acute detoxification (residential addiction program outpatient)	0.00	0.00	0.00	0.00	0.00	0.00	XXX	
H0013		I	Alcohol and/or drug services; acute detoxification (residential addiction program outpatient)	0.00	0.00	0.00	0.00	0.00	0.00	XXX	
H0014		I	Alcohol and/or drug services; ambulatory detoxification	0.00	0.00	0.00	0.00	0.00	0.00	XXX	
H0015		I	Alcohol and/or drug services; intensive outpatient (treatment program that operates at least 3 hours/day and at least 3 days/week and is based on an individualized treatment plan), including assessment, counseling; crisis intervention, and activity therapies or education	0.00	0.00	0.00	0.00	0.00	0.00	XXX	
H0016		I	Alcohol and/or drug services; medical/somatic (medical intervention in ambulatory setting)	0.00	0.00	0.00	0.00	0.00	0.00	XXX	
H0017		I	Alcohol and/or drug services; residential (hospital residential treatment program)	0.00	0.00	0.00	0.00	0.00	0.00	XXX	
H0018		I	Alcohol and/or drug services; short-term residential (non-hospital residential treatment program)	0.00	0.00	0.00	0.00	0.00	0.00	XXX	
H0019		I	Alcohol and/or drug services; long-term residential (non-medical, non-acute care in residential treatment program where stay is typically longer than 30 days)	0.00	0.00	0.00	0.00	0.00	0.00	XXX	
H0020		I	Alcohol and/or drug services; methadone administration and/or service (provision of the drug by a licensed program)	0.00	0.00	0.00	0.00	0.00	0.00	XXX	

■ RVU not developed by CMS. Gap-filled RVUs developed by CHEG.

Code	M	S	Description	Work Value	Non-Fac PE	Fac PE	Mal-practice	Non-Fac Total	Fac Total	Global	Gap
H0021		I	Alcohol and/or drug training service (for staff and personnel not employed by providers)	0.00	0.00	0.00	0.00	0.00	0.00	XXX	
H0022		I	Alcohol and/or drug intervention service (planned facilitation)	0.00	0.00	0.00	0.00	0.00	0.00	XXX	
H0023		I	Alcohol and/or drug outreach service (planned approach to reach a target population)	0.00	0.00	0.00	0.00	0.00	0.00	XXX	
H0024		I	Alcohol and/or drug prevention information dissemination service (one-way direct or non-direct contact with service audiences to affect knowledge or attitude)	0.00	0.00	0.00	0.00	0.00	0.00	XXX	
H0025		I	Alcohol and/or drug prevention education service (delivery of services with target population to affect knowledge, attitude and/or behavior)	0.00	0.00	0.00	0.00	0.00	0.00	XXX	
H0026		I	Alcohol and/or drug prevention process service, community-based (delivery of services to develop skills of impactors)	0.00	0.00	0.00	0.00	0.00	0.00	XXX	
H0027		I	Alcohol and/or drug prevention environmental service (broad range of external activities geared toward modifying systems in order to mainstream prevention through policy and law)	0.00	0.00	0.00	0.00	0.00	0.00	XXX	
H0028		I	Alcohol and/or drug prevention problem identification and referral service (e.g., student assistance and employee assistance programs), does not include assessment	0.00	0.00	0.00	0.00	0.00	0.00	XXX	
H0029		I	Alcohol and/or drug prevention alternatives service (services for populations that exclude alcohol and other drug use e.g., alcohol free social events)	0.00	0.00	0.00	0.00	0.00	0.00	XXX	
H0030		I	Alcohol and/or drug hotline service	0.00	0.00	0.00	0.00	0.00	0.00	XXX	
H1000		I	Prenatal care, at-risk assessment	0.00	0.00	0.00	0.00	0.00	0.00	XXX	
H1001		I	Prenatal care, at-risk enhanced service; antepartum management	0.00	0.00	0.00	0.00	0.00	0.00	XXX	
H1002		I	Prenatal care, at risk enhanced service; care coordination	0.00	0.00	0.00	0.00	0.00	0.00	XXX	
H1003		I	Prenatal care, at-risk enhanced service; education	0.00	0.00	0.00	0.00	0.00	0.00	XXX	
H1004		I	Prenatal care, at-risk enhanced service; follow-up home visit	0.00	0.00	0.00	0.00	0.00	0.00	XXX	
H1005		I	Prenatal care, at-risk enhanced service package (includes H1001-H1004)	0.00	0.00	0.00	0.00	0.00	0.00	XXX	
J0120		E	Injection, tetracycline, up to 250 mg	0.00	0.00	0.00	0.00	0.00	0.00	XXX	
J0130		E	Injection abciximab, 10 mg	0.00	20.86	20.86	0.00	20.86	20.86	XXX	■

■ RVU not developed by CMS. Gap-filled RVUs developed by CHEG.

Code	M	S	Description	Work Value	Non-Fac PE	Fac PE	Mal-practice	Non-Fac Total	Fac Total	Global	Gap
J0150		E	Injection, adenosine, 6 mg (not to be used to report any adenosine phosphate compounds; instead use A9270)	0.00	1.33	1.33	0.00	1.33	1.33	XXX	■
J0151		E	Injection, adenosine, 90 mg (not to be used to report any adenosine phosphate compounds; instead use A9270)	0.00	8.44	8.44	0.00	8.44	8.44	XXX	■
J0170		E	Injection, adrenalin, epinephrine, up to 1 ml ampule	0.00	0.08	0.08	0.00	0.08	0.08	XXX	■
J0190		E	Injection, biperiden lactate, per 5 mg	0.00	0.00	0.00	0.00	0.00	0.00	XXX	
J0200		E	Injection, alatrofloxacin mesylate, 100 mg	0.00	0.72	0.72	0.00	0.72	0.72	XXX	■
J0205		E	Injection, alglucerase, per 10 units	0.00	1.64	1.64	0.00	1.64	1.64	XXX	■
J0207		E	Injection, amifostine, 500 mg	0.00	15.21	15.21	0.00	15.21	15.21	XXX	■
J0210		E	Injection, methyldopate HCl, up to 250 mg	0.00	0.40	0.40	0.00	0.40	0.40	XXX	■
J0256		E	Injection, alpha 1-proteinase inhibitor — human, 10 mg	0.00	0.01	0.01	0.00	0.01	0.01	XXX	■
J0270		E	Injection, alprostadil, 1.25 mcg (code may be used for Medicare when drug administered under direct supervision of a physician, not for use when drug is self-administered)	0.00	0.09	0.09	0.00	0.09	0.09	XXX	■
J0275		E	Alprostadil urethral suppository (code may be used for Medicare when drug administered under direct supervision of a physician, not for use when drug is self-administered)	0.00	0.00	0.00	0.00	0.00	0.00	XXX	
J0280		E	Injection, aminophyllin, up to 250 mg	0.00	0.08	0.08	0.00	0.08	0.08	XXX	■
J0282		E	Injection, amiodarone hydrochloride, 30 mg	0.00	3.25	3.25	0.00	3.25	3.25	XXX	■
J0285		E	Injection, amphotericin B, 50 mg	0.00	0.69	0.69	0.00	0.69	0.69	XXX	■
J0286		E	Injection, amphotericin B, any lipid formulation, 50 mg	0.00	4.60	4.60	0.00	4.60	4.60	XXX	■
J0290		E	Injection, ampicillin sodium, 500 mg	0.00	0.06	0.06	0.00	0.06	0.06	XXX	■
J0295		E	Injection, ampicillin sodium/sulbactam sodium, per 1.5 g	0.00	0.31	0.31	0.00	0.31	0.31	XXX	■
J0300		E	Injection, amobarbital, up to 125 mg	0.00	0.16	0.16	0.00	0.16	0.16	XXX	■
J0330		E	Injection, succinylcholine chloride, up to 20 mg	0.00	0.01	0.01	0.00	0.01	0.01	XXX	■
J0350		E	Injection, anistreplase, per 30 units	0.00	0.00	0.00	0.00	0.00	0.00	XXX	
J0360		E	Injection, hydralazine HCl, up to 20 mg	0.00	0.69	0.69	0.00	0.69	0.69	XXX	■
J0380		E	Injection, metaraminol bitartrate, per 10 mg	0.00	0.05	0.05	0.00	0.05	0.05	XXX	■
J0390		E	Injection, chloroquine HCl, up to 250 mg	0.00	0.73	0.73	0.00	0.73	0.73	XXX	■

■ RVU not developed by CMS. Gap-filled RVUs developed by CHEG.

Code	M	S	Description	Work Value	Non-Fac PE	Fac PE	Mal-practice	Non-Fac Total	Fac Total	Global	Gap
J0395		E	Injection, arbutamine HCl, 1 mg	0.00	0.71	0.71	0.00	0.71	0.71	XXX	■
J0456		E	Injection, azithromycin, 500 mg	0.00	0.89	0.89	0.00	0.89	0.89	XXX	■
J0460		E	Injection, atropine sulfate, up to 0.3 mg	0.00	0.21	0.21	0.00	0.21	0.21	XXX	■
J0470		E	Injection, dimercaprol, per 100 mg	0.00	0.00	0.00	0.00	0.00	0.00	XXX	
J0475		E	Injection, baclofen, 10 mg	0.00	0.00	0.00	0.00	0.00	0.00	XXX	
J0476		E	Injection, baclofen, 50 mcg for intrathecal trial	0.00	3.10	3.10	0.00	3.10	3.10	XXX	■
J0500		E	Injection, dicyclomine HCl, up to 20 mg	0.00	0.08	0.08	0.00	0.08	0.08	XXX	■
J0515		E	Injection, benztropine mesylate, per 1 mg	0.00	0.30	0.30	0.00	0.30	0.30	XXX	■
J0520		E	Injection, bethanechol chloride, mytonachol or urecholine, up to 5 mg	0.00	0.00	0.00	0.00	0.00	0.00	XXX	
J0530		E	Injection, penicillin G benzathine and penicillin G procaine, up to 600,000 units	0.00	0.34	0.34	0.00	0.34	0.34	XXX	■
J0540		E	Injection, penicillin G benzathine and penicillin G procaine, up to 1,200,000 units	0.00	0.67	0.67	0.00	0.67	0.67	XXX	■
J0550		E	Injection, penicillin G benzathine and penicillin G procaine, up to 2,400,000 units	0.00	1.44	1.44	0.00	1.44	1.44	XXX	■
J0560		E	Injection, penicillin G benzathine, up to 600,000 units	0.00	0.48	0.48	0.00	0.48	0.48	XXX	■
J0570		E	Injection, penicillin G benzathine, up to 1,200,000 units	0.00	0.84	0.84	0.00	0.84	0.84	XXX	■
J0580		E	Injection, penicillin G benzathine, up to 2,400,000 units	0.00	1.72	1.72	0.00	1.72	1.72	XXX	■
J0585		E	Botulinum toxin type A, per unit	0.00	0.17	0.17	0.00	0.17	0.17	XXX	■
J0587		E	Botulinum toxin type b, per 100 units	0.00	0.36	0.36	0.00	0.36	0.36	XXX	■
J0600		E	Injection, edetate calcium disodium, up to 1000 mg	0.00	1.54	1.54	0.00	1.54	1.54	XXX	■
J0610		E	Injection, calcium gluconate, per 10 ml	0.00	0.04	0.04	0.00	0.04	0.04	XXX	■
J0620		E	Injection, calcium glycerophosphate and calcium lactate, per 10 ml	0.00	0.20	0.20	0.00	0.20	0.20	XXX	■
J0630		E	Injection, calcitonin-salmon, up to 400 units	0.00	1.28	1.28	0.00	1.28	1.28	XXX	■
J0635		E	Injection, calcitriol, 1 mcg ampule	0.00	0.51	0.51	0.00	0.51	0.51	XXX	■
J0640		E	Injection, leucovorin calcium, per 50 mg	0.00	0.82	0.82	0.00	0.82	0.82	XXX	■
J0670		E	Injection, mepivacaine HCl, per 10 ml	0.00	0.00	0.00	0.00	0.00	0.00	XXX	
J0690		E	Injection, cefazolin sodium, 500 mg	0.00	0.11	0.11	0.00	0.11	0.11	XXX	■
J0692		E	Injection, cefepime hydrochloride, 500 mg	0.00	0.31	0.31	0.00	0.31	0.31	XXX	■

■ RVU not developed by CMS. Gap-filled RVUs developed by CHEG.

Code	M	S	Description	Work Value	Non-Fac PE	Fac PE	Mal-practice	Non-Fac Total	Fac Total	Global	Gap
J0694		E	Injection, cefoxitin sodium, 1 g	0.00	0.44	0.44	0.00	0.44	0.44	XXX	■
J0696		E	Injection, ceftriaxone sodium, per 250 mg	0.00	0.59	0.59	0.00	0.59	0.59	XXX	■
J0697		E	Injection, sterile cefuroxime sodium, per 750 mg	0.00	0.40	0.40	0.00	0.40	0.40	XXX	■
J0698		E	Cefotaxime sodium, per g	0.00	0.50	0.50	0.00	0.50	0.50	XXX	■
J0702		E	Injection, betamethasone acetate and betamethasone sodium phosphate, per 3 mg	0.00	0.20	0.20	0.00	0.20	0.20	XXX	■
J0704		E	Injection, betamethasone sodium phosphate, per 4 mg	0.00	0.13	0.13	0.00	0.13	0.13	XXX	■
J0706		E	Injection, caffeine citrate, 5 mg	0.00	0.12	0.12	0.00	0.12	0.12	XXX	■
J0710		E	Injection, cephapirin sodium, up to 1 g	0.00	0.00	0.00	0.00	0.00	0.00	XXX	
J0713		E	Injection, ceftazidime, per 500 mg	0.00	0.33	0.33	0.00	0.33	0.33	XXX	■
J0715		E	Injection, ceftizoxime sodium, per 500 mg	0.00	0.29	0.29	0.00	0.29	0.29	XXX	■
J0720		E	Injection, chloramphenicol sodium succinate, up to 1 g	0.00	0.34	0.34	0.00	0.34	0.34	XXX	■
J0725		E	Injection, chorionic gonadotropin, per 1,000 USP units	0.00	0.13	0.13	0.00	0.13	0.13	XXX	■
J0735		E	Injection, clonidine hydrochloride, 1 mg	0.00	2.04	2.04	0.00	2.04	2.04	XXX	■
J0740		E	Injection, cidofovir, 375 mg	0.00	29.63	29.63	0.00	29.63	29.63	XXX	■
J0743		E	Injection, cilastatin sodium imipenem, per 250 mg	0.00	0.60	0.60	0.00	0.60	0.60	XXX	■
J0744		E	Injection, ciprofloxacin for intravenous infusion, 200 mg	0.00	0.57	0.57	0.00	0.57	0.57	XXX	■
J0745		E	Injection, codeine phosphate, per 30 mg	0.00	0.04	0.04	0.00	0.04	0.04	XXX	■
J0760		E	Injection, colchicine, per 1 mg	0.00	0.27	0.27	0.00	0.27	0.27	XXX	■
J0770		E	Injection, colistimethate sodium, up to 150 mg	0.00	1.58	1.58	0.00	1.58	1.58	XXX	■
J0780		E	Injection, prochlorperazine, up to 10 mg	0.00	0.31	0.31	0.00	0.31	0.31	XXX	■
J0800		E	Injection, corticotropin, up to 40 units	0.00	0.18	0.18	0.00	0.18	0.18	XXX	■
J0835		E	Injection, cosyntropin, per 0.25 mg	0.00	0.59	0.59	0.00	0.59	0.59	XXX	■
J0850		E	Injection, cytomegalovirus immune globulin intravenous (human), per vial	0.00	19.91	19.91	0.00	19.91	19.91	XXX	■
J0895		E	Injection, deferoxamine mesylate, 500 mg	0.00	0.52	0.52	0.00	0.52	0.52	XXX	■
J0900		E	Injection, testosterone enanthate and estradiol valerate, up to 1 cc	0.00	0.07	0.07	0.00	0.07	0.07	XXX	■
J0945		E	Injection, brompheniramine maleate, per 10 mg	0.00	0.04	0.04	0.00	0.04	0.04	XXX	■

■ RVU not developed by CMS. Gap-filled RVUs developed by CHEG.

Code	M	S	Description	Work Value	Non-Fac PE	Fac PE	Mal-practice	Non-Fac Total	Fac Total	Global	Gap
J0970		E	Injection, estradiol valerate, up to 40 mg	0.00	0.06	0.06	0.00	0.06	0.06	XXX	■
J1000		E	Injection, depo-estradiol cypionate, up to 5 mg	0.00	0.15	0.15	0.00	0.15	0.15	XXX	■
J1020		E	Injection, methylprednisolone acetate, 20 mg	0.00	0.09	0.09	0.00	0.09	0.09	XXX	■
J1030		E	Injection, methylprednisolone acetate, 40 mg	0.00	0.10	0.10	0.00	0.10	0.10	XXX	■
J1040		E	Injection, methylprednisolone acetate, 80 mg	0.00	0.17	0.17	0.00	0.17	0.17	XXX	■
J1050		E	Injection, medroxyprogesterone acetate, 100 mg	0.00	0.44	0.44	0.00	0.44	0.44	XXX	■
J1055		N	Injection, medroxyprogesterone acetate for contraceptive use, 150 mg	0.00	1.82	1.82	0.00	1.82	1.82	XXX	■
J1056		E	Injection, medroxyprogesterone acetate/ estradiol cypionate, 5 mg/25 mg	0.00	0.96	0.96	0.00	0.96	0.96	XXX	■
J1060		E	Injection, testosterone cypionate and estradiol cypionate, up to 1 ml	0.00	0.00	0.00	0.00	0.00	0.00	XXX	
J1070		E	Injection, testosterone cypionate, up to 100 mg	0.00	0.17	0.17	0.00	0.17	0.17	XXX	■
J1080		E	Injection, testosterone cypionate, 1 cc, 200 mg	0.00	0.46	0.46	0.00	0.46	0.46	XXX	■
J1095		E	Injection, dexamethasone acetate, per 8 mg	0.00	0.20	0.20	0.00	0.20	0.20	XXX	■
J1100		E	Injection, dexamethosone sodium phosphate, 1 mg	0.00	0.02	0.02	0.00	0.02	0.02	XXX	■
J1110		E	Injection, dihydroergotamine mesylate, per 1 mg	0.00	0.57	0.57	0.00	0.57	0.57	XXX	■
J1120		E	Injection, acetazolamide sodium, up to 500 mg	0.00	1.39	1.39	0.00	1.39	1.39	XXX	■
J1160		E	Injection, digoxin, up to 0.5 mg	0.00	0.09	0.09	0.00	0.09	0.09	XXX	■
J1165		E	Injection, phenytoin sodium, per 50 mg	0.00	0.03	0.03	0.00	0.03	0.03	XXX	■
J1170		E	Injection, hydromorphone, up to 4 mg	0.00	0.00	0.00	0.00	0.00	0.00	XXX	
J1180		E	Injection, dyphylline, up to 500 mg	0.00	0.31	0.31	0.00	0.31	0.31	XXX	■
J1190		E	Injection, dexrazoxane hydrochloride, per 250 mg	0.00	0.00	0.00	0.00	0.00	0.00	XXX	
J1200		E	Injection, diphenhydramine HCl, up to 50 mg	0.00	0.11	0.11	0.00	0.11	0.11	XXX	■
J1205		E	Injection, chlorothiazide sodium, per 500 mg	0.00	0.38	0.38	0.00	0.38	0.38	XXX	■
J1212		E	Injection, DMSO, dimethyl sulfoxide, 50%, 50 ml	0.00	1.62	1.62	0.00	1.62	1.62	XXX	■
J1230		E	Injection, methadone HCl, up to 10 mg	0.00	0.04	0.04	0.00	0.04	0.04	XXX	■
J1240		E	Injection, dimenhydrinate, up to 50 mg	0.00	0.03	0.03	0.00	0.03	0.03	XXX	■
J1245		E	Injection, dipyridamole, per 10 mg	0.00	0.83	0.83	0.00	0.83	0.83	XXX	■
J1250		E	Injection, dobutamine HCI, per 250 mg	0.00	0.14	0.14	0.00	0.14	0.14	XXX	■

■ RVU not developed by CMS. Gap-filled RVUs developed by CHEG.

Code	M	S	Description	Work Value	Non-Fac PE	Fac PE	Mal-practice	Non-Fac Total	Fac Total	Global	Gap
J1260		E	Injection, dolasetron mesylate, 10 mg	0.00	0.61	0.61	0.00	0.61	0.61	XXX	■
J1270		E	Injection, doxercalciferol, 1 mcg	0.00	0.43	0.43	0.00	0.43	0.43	XXX	■
J1320		E	Injection, amitriptyline HCl, up to 20 mg	0.00	0.08	0.08	0.00	0.08	0.08	XXX	■
J1325		E	Injection, epoprostenol, 0.5 mg	0.00	0.00	0.00	0.00	0.00	0.00	XXX	
J1327		E	Injection, eptifibatide, 5 mg	0.00	0.53	0.53	0.00	0.53	0.53	XXX	■
J1330		E	Injection, ergonovine maleate, up to 0.2 mg	0.00	0.21	0.21	0.00	0.21	0.21	XXX	■
J1364		E	Injection, erythromycin lactobionate, per 500 mg	0.00	0.28	0.28	0.00	0.28	0.28	XXX	■
J1380		E	Injection, estradiol valerate, up to 10 mg	0.00	0.19	0.19	0.00	0.19	0.19	XXX	■
J1390		E	Injection, estradiol valerate, up to 20 mg	0.00	0.27	0.27	0.00	0.27	0.27	XXX	■
J1410		E	Injection, estrogen conjugated, per 25 mg	0.00	2.14	2.14	0.00	2.14	2.14	XXX	■
J1435		E	Injection, estrone, per 1 mg	0.00	0.02	0.02	0.00	0.02	0.02	XXX	■
J1436		E	Injection, etidronate disodium, per 300 mg	0.00	2.47	2.47	0.00	2.47	2.47	XXX	■
J1438		E	Injection, etanercept, 25 mg (code may be used for Medicare when drug administered under the direct supervision of a physician, not for use when drug is self-administered)	0.00	5.47	5.47	0.00	5.47	5.47	XXX	■
J1440		E	Injection, filgrastim (G-CSF), 300 mcg	0.00	6.84	6.84	0.00	6.84	6.84	XXX	■
J1441		E	Injection, filgrastim (G-CSF), 480 mcg	0.00	11.07	11.07	0.00	11.07	11.07	XXX	■
J1450		E	Injection, fluconazole, 200 mg	0.00	3.36	3.36	0.00	3.36	3.36	XXX	■
J1452		E	Injection, fomivirsen sodium, intraocular, 1.65 mg	0.00	36.85	36.85	0.00	36.85	36.85	XXX	■
J1455		E	Injection, foscarnet sodium, per 1,000 mg	0.00	0.54	0.54	0.00	0.54	0.54	XXX	■
J1460		E	Injection, gamma globulin, intramuscular, 1 cc	0.00	0.00	0.00	0.00	0.00	0.00	XXX	
J1470		E	Injection, gamma globulin, intramuscular, 2 cc	0.00	0.00	0.00	0.00	0.00	0.00	XXX	
J1480		E	Injection, gamma globulin, intramuscular, 3 cc	0.00	0.00	0.00	0.00	0.00	0.00	XXX	
J1490		E	Injection, gamma globulin, intramuscular, 4 cc	0.00	0.00	0.00	0.00	0.00	0.00	XXX	
J1500		E	Injection, gamma globulin, intramuscular, 5 cc	0.00	0.00	0.00	0.00	0.00	0.00	XXX	
J1510		E	Injection, gamma globulin, intramuscular, 6 cc	0.00	0.00	0.00	0.00	0.00	0.00	XXX	
J1520		E	Injection, gamma globulin, intramuscular, 7 cc	0.00	0.00	0.00	0.00	0.00	0.00	XXX	
J1530		E	Injection, gamma globulin, intramuscular, 8 cc	0.00	0.00	0.00	0.00	0.00	0.00	XXX	
J1540		E	Injection, gamma globulin, intramuscular, 9 cc	0.00	0.00	0.00	0.00	0.00	0.00	XXX	
J1550		E	Injection, gamma globulin, intramuscular, 10 cc	0.00	0.00	0.00	0.00	0.00	0.00	XXX	

■ RVU not developed by CMS. Gap-filled RVUs developed by CHEG.

Code	M	S	Description	Work Value	Non-Fac PE	Fac PE	Mal-practice	Non-Fac Total	Fac Total	Global	Gap
J1560		E	Injection, gamma globulin, intramuscular, over 10 cc	0.00	0.00	0.00	0.00	0.00	0.00	XXX	
J1561		E	Injection, immune globulin, intravenous, 500 mg	0.00	1.17	1.17	0.00	1.17	1.17	XXX	■
J1563		E	Injection, immune globulin, intravenous, 1 g	0.00	3.09	3.09	0.00	3.09	3.09	XXX	■
J1565		E	Injection, respiratory syncytial virus immune globulin, intravenous, 50 mg	0.00	0.00	0.00	0.00	0.00	0.00	XXX	
J1570		E	Injection, ganciclovir sodium, 500 mg	0.00	1.34	1.34	0.00	1.34	1.34	XXX	■
J1580		E	Injection, Garamycin, gentamicin, up to 80 mg	0.00	0.21	0.21	0.00	0.21	0.21	XXX	■
J1590		E	Injection, gatifloxacin, 10 mg	0.00	0.35	0.35	0.00	0.35	0.35	XXX	■
J1600		E	Injection, gold sodium thiomalate, up to 50 mg	0.00	0.49	0.49	0.00	0.49	0.49	XXX	■
J1610		E	Injection, glucagon hydrochloride, per 1 mg	0.00	2.63	2.63	0.00	2.63	2.63	XXX	■
J1620		E	Injection, gonadorelin hydrochloride, per 100 mcg	0.00	7.46	7.46	0.00	7.46	7.46	XXX	■
J1626		E	Injection, granisetron hydrochloride, 100 mcg	0.00	0.72	0.72	0.00	0.72	0.72	XXX	■
J1630		E	Injection, haloperidol, up to 5 mg	0.00	0.30	0.30	0.00	0.30	0.30	XXX	■
J1631		E	Injection, haloperidol decanoate, per 50 mg	0.00	1.03	1.03	0.00	1.03	1.03	XXX	■
J1642		E	Injection, heparin sodium, (Heparin Lock Flush), per 10 units	0.00	0.02	0.02	0.00	0.02	0.02	XXX	■
J1644		E	Injection, heparin sodium, per 1,000 units	0.00	0.06	0.06	0.00	0.06	0.06	XXX	■
J1645		E	Injection, dalteparin sodium, per 2500 IU	0.00	0.57	0.57	0.00	0.57	0.57	XXX	■
J1650		E	Injection, enoxaparin sodium, 10 mg	0.00	0.66	0.66	0.00	0.66	0.66	XXX	■
J1655		E	Injection, tinzaparin sodium, 1000 IU	0.00	0.16	0.16	0.00	0.16	0.16	XXX	■
J1670		E	Injection, tetanus immune globulin, human, up to 250 units	0.00	3.93	3.93	0.00	3.93	3.93	XXX	■
J1700		E	Injection, hydrocortisone acetate, up to 25 mg	0.00	0.01	0.01	0.00	0.01	0.01	XXX	■
J1710		E	Injection, hydrocortisone sodium phosphate, up to 50 mg	0.00	0.20	0.20	0.00	0.20	0.20	XXX	■
J1720		E	Injection, hydrocortisone sodium succinate, up to 100 mg	0.00	0.13	0.13	0.00	0.13	0.13	XXX	■
J1730		E	Injection, diazoxide, up to 300 mg	0.00	4.54	4.54	0.00	4.54	4.54	XXX	■
J1742		E	Injection, ibutilide fumarate, 1 mg	0.00	8.56	8.56	0.00	8.56	8.56	XXX	■
J1745		E	Injection, infliximab, 10 mg	0.00	2.45	2.45	0.00	2.45	2.45	XXX	■
J1750		E	Injection, iron dextran, 50 mg	0.00	0.69	0.69	0.00	0.69	0.69	XXX	■
J1755		E	Injection, iron sucrose, 20 mg	0.00	0.53	0.53	0.00	0.53	0.53	XXX	■

■ RVU not developed by CMS. Gap-filled RVUs developed by CHEG.

Code	M	S	Description	Work Value	Non-Fac PE	Fac PE	Mal-practice	Non-Fac Total	Fac Total	Global	Gap
J1785		E	Injection, imiglucerase, per unit	0.00	0.15	0.15	0.00	0.15	0.15	XXX	■
J1790		E	Injection, droperidol, up to 5 mg	0.00	0.16	0.16	0.00	0.16	0.16	XXX	■
J1800		E	Injection, propranolol HCl, up to 1 mg	0.00	0.68	0.68	0.00	0.68	0.68	XXX	■
J1810		E	Injection, droperidol and fentanyl citrate, up to 2 ml ampule	0.00	0.00	0.00	0.00	0.00	0.00	XXX	
J1820		E	Injection, insulin, up to 100 units	0.00	0.17	0.17	0.00	0.17	0.17	XXX	■
J1825		E	Injection, interferon beta-1a, 33 mcg (code may be used for Medicare when drug administered under direct supervision of a physician, not for use when drug is self-administered)	0.00	8.74	8.74	0.00	8.74	8.74	XXX	■
J1830		E	Injection interferon beta-1b, 0.25 mg (code may be used for Medicare when drug administered under direct supervision of a physician, not for use when drug is self-administered)	0.00	0.00	0.00	0.00	0.00	0.00	XXX	
J1835		E	Injection, itraconazole, 50 mg	0.00	34.04	34.04	0.00	34.04	34.04	XXX	■
J1840		E	Injection, kanamycin sulfate, up to 500 mg	0.00	0.10	0.10	0.00	0.10	0.10	XXX	■
J1850		E	Injection, kanamycin sulfate, up to 75 mg	0.00	0.12	0.12	0.00	0.12	0.12	XXX	■
J1885		E	Injection, ketorolac tromethamine, per 15 mg	0.00	0.30	0.30	0.00	0.30	0.30	XXX	■
J1890		E	Injection, cephalothin sodium, up to 1 g	0.00	0.40	0.40	0.00	0.40	0.40	XXX	■
J1910		E	Injection, kutapressin, up to 2 ml	0.00	0.54	0.54	0.00	0.54	0.54	XXX	■
J1940		E	Injection, furosemide, up to 20 mg	0.00	0.05	0.05	0.00	0.05	0.05	XXX	■
J1950		E	Injection, leuprolide acetate (for depot suspension), per 3.75 mg	0.00	18.88	18.88	0.00	18.88	18.88	XXX	■
J1955		E	Injection, levocarnitine, per 1 g	0.00	1.37	1.37	0.00	1.37	1.37	XXX	■
J1956		E	Injection, levofloxacin, 250 mg	0.00	0.77	0.77	0.00	0.77	0.77	XXX	■
J1960		E	Injection, levorphanol tartrate, up to 2 mg	0.00	0.16	0.16	0.00	0.16	0.16	XXX	■
J1980		E	Injection, hyoscyamine sulfate, up to 0.25 mg	0.00	0.55	0.55	0.00	0.55	0.55	XXX	■
J1990		E	Injection, chlordiazepoxide HCl, up to 100 mg	0.00	1.00	1.00	0.00	1.00	1.00	XXX	■
J2000		E	Injection, lidocaine HCl, 50 cc	0.00	0.13	0.13	0.00	0.13	0.13	XXX	■
J2010		E	Injection, lincomycin HCl, up to 300 mg	0.00	0.04	0.04	0.00	0.04	0.04	XXX	■
J2020		E	Injection, linezolid, 200 mg	0.00	1.39	1.39	0.00	1.39	1.39	XXX	■
J2060		E	Injection, lorazepam, 2 mg	0.00	0.05	0.05	0.00	0.05	0.05	XXX	■
J2150		E	Injection, mannitol, 25% in 50 ml	0.00	0.18	0.18	0.00	0.18	0.18	XXX	■
J2175		E	Injection, meperidine HCl, per 100 mg	0.00	0.04	0.04	0.00	0.04	0.04	XXX	■

■ RVU not developed by CMS. Gap-filled RVUs developed by CHEG.

Code	M	S	Description	Work Value	Non-Fac PE	Fac PE	Mal-practice	Non-Fac Total	Fac Total	Global	Gap
J2180		E	Injection, meperidine and promethazine HCl, up to 50 mg	0.00	0.34	0.34	0.00	0.34	0.34	XXX	■
J2210		E	Injection, methylergonovine maleate, up to 0.2 mg	0.00	0.14	0.14	0.00	0.14	0.14	XXX	■
J2250		E	Injection, midazolam HCl, per 1 mg	0.00	0.09	0.09	0.00	0.09	0.09	XXX	■
J2260		E	Injection, milrinone lactate, per 5 ml	0.00	1.67	1.67	0.00	1.67	1.67	XXX	■
J2270		E	Injection, morphine sulfate, up to 10 mg	0.00	0.04	0.04	0.00	0.04	0.04	XXX	■
J2271		E	Injection, morphine sulfate, 100 mg	0.00	0.54	0.54	0.00	0.54	0.54	XXX	■
J2275		E	Injection, morphine sulfate (preservative-free sterile solution), per 10 mg	0.00	0.21	0.21	0.00	0.21	0.21	XXX	■
J2300		E	Injection, nalbuphine HCl, per 10 mg	0.00	0.15	0.15	0.00	0.15	0.15	XXX	■
J2310		E	Injection, naloxone HCl, per 1 mg	0.00	0.22	0.22	0.00	0.22	0.22	XXX	■
J2320		E	Injection, nandrolone decanoate, up to 50 mg	0.00	0.23	0.23	0.00	0.23	0.23	XXX	■
J2321		E	Injection, nandrolone decanoate, up to 100 mg	0.00	0.47	0.47	0.00	0.47	0.47	XXX	■
J2322		E	Injection, nandrolone decanoate, up to 200 mg	0.00	0.76	0.76	0.00	0.76	0.76	XXX	■
J2352		E	Injection, octreotide acetate, 1 mg	0.00	5.30	5.30	0.00	5.30	5.30	XXX	■
J2355		E	Injection, oprelvekin, 5 mg	0.00	9.08	9.08	0.00	9.08	9.08	XXX	■
J2360		E	Injection, orphenadrine citrate, up to 60 mg	0.00	0.07	0.07	0.00	0.07	0.07	XXX	■
J2370		E	Injection, phenylephrine HCl, up to 1 ml	0.00	0.11	0.11	0.00	0.11	0.11	XXX	■
J2400		E	Injection, chloroprocaine HCl, per 30 ml	0.00	0.64	0.64	0.00	0.64	0.64	XXX	■
J2405		E	Injection, ondansetron HCl, per 1 mg	0.00	0.23	0.23	0.00	0.23	0.23	XXX	■
J2410		E	Injection, oxymorphone HCl, up to 1 mg	0.00	0.11	0.11	0.00	0.11	0.11	XXX	■
J2430		E	Injection, pamidronate disodium, per 30 mg	0.00	9.82	9.82	0.00	9.82	9.82	XXX	■
J2440		E	Injection, papaverine HCl, up to 60 mg	0.00	0.11	0.11	0.00	0.11	0.11	XXX	■
J2460		E	Injection, oxytetracycline HCl, up to 50 mg	0.00	0.00	0.00	0.00	0.00	0.00	XXX	
J2500		E	Injection, paricalcitol, 5 mcg	0.00	1.01	1.01	0.00	1.01	1.01	XXX	■
J2510		E	Injection, penicillin G procaine, aqueous, up to 600,000 units	0.00	0.29	0.29	0.00	0.29	0.29	XXX	■
J2515		E	Injection, pentobarbital sodium, per 50 mg	0.00	0.03	0.03	0.00	0.03	0.03	XXX	■
J2540		E	Injection, penicillin G potassium, up to 600,000 units	0.00	0.00	0.00	0.00	0.00	0.00	XXX	
J2543		E	Injection, piperacillin sodium/tazobactam sodium, 1 gram/0.125 grams (1.125 grams)	0.00	0.00	0.00	0.00	0.00	0.00	XXX	

■ RVU not developed by CMS. Gap-filled RVUs developed by CHEG.

Code	M	S	Description	Work Value	Non-Fac PE	Fac PE	Mal-practice	Non-Fac Total	Fac Total	Global	Gap
J2545		E	Pentamidine isethionate, inhalation solution, per 300 mg, administered through a DME	0.00	4.29	4.29	0.00	4.29	4.29	XXX	■
J2550		E	Injection, promethazine HCl, up to 50 mg	0.00	0.08	0.08	0.00	0.08	0.08	XXX	■
J2560		E	Injection, phenobarbital sodium, up to 120 mg	0.00	0.30	0.30	0.00	0.30	0.30	XXX	■
J2590		E	Injection, oxytocin, up to 10 units	0.00	0.05	0.05	0.00	0.05	0.05	XXX	■
J2597		E	Injection, desmopressin acetate, per 1 mcg	0.00	0.26	0.26	0.00	0.26	0.26	XXX	■
J2650		E	Injection, prednisolone acetate, up to 1 ml	0.00	0.00	0.00	0.00	0.00	0.00	XXX	
J2670		E	Injection, tolazoline HCl, up to 25 mg	0.00	0.61	0.61	0.00	0.61	0.61	XXX	■
J2680		E	Injection, fluphenazine decanoate, up to 25 mg	0.00	0.53	0.53	0.00	0.53	0.53	XXX	■
J2690		E	Injection, procainamide HCl, up to 1 g	0.00	0.43	0.43	0.00	0.43	0.43	XXX	■
J2700		E	Injection, oxacillin sodium, up to 250 mg	0.00	0.20	0.20	0.00	0.20	0.20	XXX	■
J2710		E	Injection, neostigmine methylsulfate, up to 0.5 mg	0.00	0.03	0.03	0.00	0.03	0.03	XXX	■
J2720		E	Injection, protamine sulfate, per 10 mg	0.00	0.03	0.03	0.00	0.03	0.03	XXX	■
J2725		E	Injection, protirelin, per 250 mcg	0.00	1.89	1.89	0.00	1.89	1.89	XXX	■
J2730		E	Injection, pralidoxime chloride, up to 1 g	0.00	3.99	3.99	0.00	3.99	3.99	XXX	■
J2760		E	Injection, phentolamine mesylate, up to 5 mg	0.00	1.27	1.27	0.00	1.27	1.27	XXX	■
J2765		E	Injection, metoclopramide HCl, up to 10 mg	0.00	0.08	0.08	0.00	0.08	0.08	XXX	■
J2770		E	Injection, quinupristin/dalfopristin, 500 mg (150/350)	0.00	3.98	3.98	0.00	3.98	3.98	XXX	■
J2780		E	Injection, ranitidine hydrochloride, 25 mg	0.00	0.06	0.06	0.00	0.06	0.06	XXX	■
J2790		E	Injection, Rho (D) immune globulin, human, one dose package	0.00	4.33	4.33	0.00	4.33	4.33	XXX	■
J2792		E	Injection, rho D immune globulin, intravenous, human, solvent detergent, 100 IU	0.00	0.00	0.00	0.00	0.00	0.00	XXX	
J2795		E	Injection, ropivacaine hydrochloride, 1 mg	0.00	0.01	0.01	0.00	0.01	0.01	XXX	■
J2800		E	Injection, methocarbamol, up to 10 ml	0.00	0.45	0.45	0.00	0.45	0.45	XXX	■
J2810		E	Injection, theophylline, per 40 mg	0.00	0.00	0.00	0.00	0.00	0.00	XXX	
J2820		E	Injection, sargramostim (GM-CSF), 50 mcg	0.00	1.05	1.05	0.00	1.05	1.05	XXX	■
J2910		E	Injection, aurothioglucose, up to 50 mg	0.00	0.57	0.57	0.00	0.57	0.57	XXX	■
J2912		E	Injection, sodium chloride, 0.9%, per 2 ml	0.00	0.04	0.04	0.00	0.04	0.04	XXX	■
J2915		E	Injection, sodium ferric gluconate complex in sucrose injection, 62.5 mg	0.00	1.58	1.58	0.00	1.58	1.58	XXX	■

■ RVU not developed by CMS. Gap-filled RVUs developed by CHEG.

Code	M	S	Description	Work Value	Non-Fac PE	Fac PE	Mal-practice	Non-Fac Total	Fac Total	Global	Gap
J2920		E	Injection, methylprednisolone sodium succinate, up to 40 mg	0.00	0.08	0.08	0.00	0.08	0.08	XXX	■
J2930		E	Injection, methylprednisolone sodium succinate, up to 125 mg	0.00	0.13	0.13	0.00	0.13	0.13	XXX	■
J2940		E	Injection, somatrem, 1 mg	0.00	8.11	8.11	0.00	8.11	8.11	XXX	■
J2941		E	Injection, somatropin, 1 mg	0.00	1.59	1.59	0.00	1.59	1.59	XXX	■
J2950		E	Injection, promazine HCl, up to 25 mg	0.00	0.02	0.02	0.00	0.02	0.02	XXX	■
J2993		E	Injection, reteplase, 18.1 mg	0.00	0.00	0.00	0.00	0.00	0.00	XXX	
J2995		E	Injection, streptokinase, per 250,000 IU	0.00	4.69	4.69	0.00	4.69	4.69	XXX	■
J2997		E	Injection, alteplase recombinant, 1 mg	0.00	0.00	0.00	0.00	0.00	0.00	XXX	
J3000		E	Injection, streptomycin, up to 1 g	0.00	0.26	0.26	0.00	0.26	0.26	XXX	■
J3010		E	Injection, fentanyl citrate, 0.1 mg	0.00	0.08	0.08	0.00	0.08	0.08	XXX	■
J3030		E	Injection, sumatriptan succinate, 6 mg (code may not be used for Medicare when drug administered under direct supervision of a physician, not for use when drug is self-administered)	0.00	1.65	1.65	0.00	1.65	1.65	XXX	■
J3070		E	Injection, pentazocine HCl, up to 30 mg	0.00	0.15	0.15	0.00	0.15	0.15	XXX	■
J3100		E	Injection, tenecteplase, 50 mg	0.00	104.30	104.30	0.00	104.30	104.30	XXX	■
J3105		E	Injection, terbutaline sulfate, up to 1 mg	0.00	0.09	0.09	0.00	0.09	0.09	XXX	■
J3120		E	Injection, testosterone enanthate, up to 100 mg	0.00	0.14	0.14	0.00	0.14	0.14	XXX	■
J3130		E	Injection, testosterone enanthate, up to 200 mg	0.00	0.29	0.29	0.00	0.29	0.29	XXX	■
J3140		E	Injection, testosterone suspension, up to 50 mg	0.00	0.00	0.00	0.00	0.00	0.00	XXX	
J3150		E	Injection, testosterone propionate, up to 100 mg	0.00	0.04	0.04	0.00	0.04	0.04	XXX	■
J3230		E	Injection, chlorpromazine HCl, up to 50 mg	0.00	0.19	0.19	0.00	0.19	0.19	XXX	■
J3240		E	Injection, thyrotropin alpha, 0.9 mg	0.00	0.00	0.00	0.00	0.00	0.00	XXX	
J3245		E	Injection, tirofiban hydrochloride, 12.5 mg	0.00	15.54	15.54	0.00	15.54	15.54	XXX	■
J3250		E	Injection, trimethobenzamide HCl, up to 200 mg	0.00	0.07	0.07	0.00	0.07	0.07	XXX	■
J3260		E	Injection, tobramycin sulfate, up to 80 mg	0.00	0.27	0.27	0.00	0.27	0.27	XXX	■
J3265		E	Injection, torsemide, 10 mg/ml	0.00	0.17	0.17	0.00	0.17	0.17	XXX	■
J3280		E	Injection, thiethylperazine maleate, up to 10 mg	0.00	0.19	0.19	0.00	0.19	0.19	XXX	■
J3301		E	Injection, triamcinolone acetonide, per 10 mg	0.00	0.03	0.03	0.00	0.03	0.03	XXX	■

■ RVU not developed by CMS. Gap-filled RVUs developed by CHEG.

Code	M	S	Description	Work Value	Non-Fac PE	Fac PE	Mal-practice	Non-Fac Total	Fac Total	Global	Gap
J3302		E	Injection, triamcinolone diacetate, per 5 mg	0.00	0.02	0.02	0.00	0.02	0.02	XXX	■
J3303		E	Injection, triamcinolone hexacetonide, per 5 mg	0.00	0.11	0.11	0.00	0.11	0.11	XXX	■
J3305		E	Injection, trimetrexate glucoronate, per 25 mg	0.00	3.34	3.34	0.00	3.34	3.34	XXX	■
J3310		E	Injection, perphenazine, up to 5 mg	0.00	0.26	0.26	0.00	0.26	0.26	XXX	■
J3320		E	Injection, spectinomycin dihydrochloride, up to 2 g	0.00	1.04	1.04	0.00	1.04	1.04	XXX	■
J3350		E	Injection, urea, up to 40 g	0.00	3.23	3.23	0.00	3.23	3.23	XXX	■
J3360		E	Injection, diazepam, up to 5 mg	0.00	0.04	0.04	0.00	0.04	0.04	XXX	■
J3364		E	Injection, urokinase, 5,000 IU vial	0.00	2.21	2.21	0.00	2.21	2.21	XXX	■
J3365		E	Injection, IV, urokinase, 250,000 IU vial	0.00	18.52	18.52	0.00	18.52	18.52	XXX	■
J3370		R	Injection, vancomycin HCl, 500 mg	0.00	0.96	0.96	0.00	0.96	0.96	XXX	■
J3395		E	Injection, verteporfin, 15 mg	0.00	56.57	56.57	0.00	56.57	56.57	XXX	■
J3400		E	Injection, triflupromazine HCl, up to 20 mg	0.00	0.46	0.46	0.00	0.46	0.46	XXX	■
J3410		E	Injection, hydroxyzine HCl, up to 25 mg	0.00	0.03	0.03	0.00	0.03	0.03	XXX	■
J3420		E	Injection, vitamin B-12 cyanocobalamin, up to 1,000 mcg	0.00	0.01	0.01	0.00	0.01	0.01	XXX	■
J3430		E	Injection, phytonadione (vitamin K), per 1 mg	0.00	0.10	0.10	0.00	0.10	0.10	XXX	■
J3470		E	Injection, hyaluronidase, up to 150 units	0.00	0.80	0.80	0.00	0.80	0.80	XXX	■
J3475		E	Injection, magnesium sulphate, per 500 mg	0.00	0.06	0.06	0.00	0.06	0.06	XXX	■
J3480		E	Injection, potassium chloride, per 2 mEq	0.00	0.01	0.01	0.00	0.01	0.01	XXX	■
J3485		E	Injection, zidovudine, 10 mg	0.00	0.04	0.04	0.00	0.04	0.04	XXX	■
J3490		E	Unclassified drugs	0.00	0.00	0.00	0.00	0.00	0.00	XXX	
J3520		N	Edetate disodium, per 150 mg	0.00	0.02	0.02	0.00	0.02	0.02	XXX	■
J3530		E	Nasal vaccine inhalation	0.00	0.00	0.00	0.00	0.00	0.00	XXX	
J3535		N	Drug administered through a metered dose inhaler	0.00	0.00	0.00	0.00	0.00	0.00	XXX	
J3570		N	Laetrile, amygdalin, vitamin B-17	0.00	0.00	0.00	0.00	0.00	0.00	XXX	
J7030		E	Infusion, normal saline solution, 1,000 cc	0.00	0.40	0.40	0.00	0.40	0.40	XXX	■
J7040		E	Infusion, normal saline solution, sterile (500 ml = 1 unit)	0.00	0.44	0.44	0.00	0.44	0.44	XXX	■
J7042		E	5% dextrose/normal saline (500 ml = 1 unit)	0.00	0.00	0.00	0.00	0.00	0.00	XXX	
J7050		E	Infusion, normal saline solution, 250 cc	0.00	0.43	0.43	0.00	0.43	0.43	XXX	■

■ RVU not developed by CMS. Gap-filled RVUs developed by CHEG.

Code	M	S	Description	Work Value	Non-Fac PE	Fac PE	Mal-practice	Non-Fac Total	Fac Total	Global	Gap
J7051		E	Sterile saline or water, up to 5 cc	0.00	0.05	0.05	0.00	0.05	0.05	XXX	■
J7060		E	5% dextrose/water (500 ml = 1 unit)	0.00	0.39	0.39	0.00	0.39	0.39	XXX	■
J7070		E	Infusion, D-5-W, 1,000 cc	0.00	0.48	0.48	0.00	0.48	0.48	XXX	■
J7100		E	Infusion, dextran 40, 500 ml	0.00	5.39	5.39	0.00	5.39	5.39	XXX	■
J7110		E	Infusion, dextran 75, 500 ml	0.00	4.00	4.00	0.00	4.00	4.00	XXX	■
J7120		E	Ringer's lactate infusion, up to 1,000 cc	0.00	0.55	0.55	0.00	0.55	0.55	XXX	■
J7130		E	Hypertonic saline solution, 50 or 100 mEq, 20 cc vial	0.00	0.00	0.00	0.00	0.00	0.00	XXX	
J7190		X	Factor VIII (antihemophilic factor, human) per IU	0.00	0.03	0.03	0.00	0.03	0.03	XXX	■
J7191		X	Factor VIII (anti-hemophilic factor (porcine)), per IU	0.00	0.08	0.08	0.00	0.08	0.08	XXX	■
J7192		X	Factor VIII (antihemophilic factor, recombinant) per IU	0.00	0.05	0.05	0.00	0.05	0.05	XXX	■
J7193		E	Factor ix (antihemophilic factor, purified, non-recombinant) per IU	0.00	0.00	0.00	0.00	0.00	0.00	XXX	
J7194		X	Factor IX complex, per IU	0.00	0.02	0.02	0.00	0.02	0.02	XXX	■
J7195		E	Factor IX (antihemophilic factor, recombinant) per IU	0.00	0.00	0.00	0.00	0.00	0.00	XXX	
J7197		X	Antithrombin III (human), per IU	0.00	0.04	0.04	0.00	0.04	0.04	XXX	■
J7198		E	Anti-inhibitor, per IU	0.00	0.06	0.06	0.00	0.06	0.06	XXX	■
J7199		E	Hemophilia clotting factor, not otherwise classified	0.00	0.00	0.00	0.00	0.00	0.00	XXX	
J7300		N	Intrauterine copper contraceptive	0.00	0.00	0.00	0.00	0.00	0.00	XXX	
J7302		N	Levonorgestrel-releasing intrauterine contraceptive system, 52 mg	0.00	0.00	0.00	0.00	0.00	0.00	XXX	
J7308		E	Aminolevulinic acid HCL for topical administration, 20%, single unit dosage form (354 mg)	0.00	4.10	4.10	0.00	4.10	4.10	XXX	■
J7310		E	Ganciclovir, 4.5 mg, long-acting implant	0.00	184.26	184.26	0.00	184.26	184.26	XXX	■
J7316		E	Sodium hyaluronate, 5 mg for intra-articular injection	0.00	1.39	1.39	0.00	1.39	1.39	XXX	■
J7320		E	Hylan G-F 20, 16 mg, for intra-articular injection	0.00	0.00	0.00	0.00	0.00	0.00	XXX	
J7330		E	Autologous cultured chondrocytes, implant	0.00	0.00	0.00	0.00	0.00	0.00	XXX	
J7340		E	Dermal and epidermal, tissue of human origin, with or without bioengineered or processed elements, with metabolically active elements, per sq cm	0.00	0.00	0.00	0.00	0.00	0.00	XXX	

■ RVU not developed by CMS. Gap-filled RVUs developed by CHEG.

Code	M	S	Description	Work Value	Non-Fac PE	Fac PE	Mal-practice	Non-Fac Total	Fac Total	Global	Gap
J7500		X	Azathioprine, oral, 50 mg	0.00	0.05	0.05	0.00	0.05	0.05	XXX	■
J7501		X	Azathioprine, parenteral,100 mg	0.00	3.60	3.60	0.00	3.60	3.60	XXX	■
J7502		E	Cyclosporine, oral, 100 mg	0.00	0.26	0.26	0.00	0.26	0.26	XXX	■
J7504		X	Lymphocyte immune globulin, antithymocyte globulin, equine, parenteral, 250 mg	0.00	9.55	9.55	0.00	9.55	9.55	XXX	■
J7505		X	Muromonab-CD3, parenteral, 5 mg	0.00	30.13	30.13	0.00	30.13	30.13	XXX	■
J7506		X	Prednisone, oral, per 5 mg	0.00	0.00	0.00	0.00	0.00	0.00	XXX	
J7507		E	Tacrolimus, oral, per 1 mg	0.00	0.10	0.10	0.00	0.10	0.10	XXX	■
J7508		E	Tacrolimus, oral, per 5 mg	0.00	0.53	0.53	0.00	0.53	0.53	XXX	■
J7509		X	Methylprednisolone, oral, per 4 mg	0.00	0.02	0.02	0.00	0.02	0.02	XXX	■
J7510		X	Prednisolone, oral, per 5 mg	0.00	0.00	0.00	0.00	0.00	0.00	XXX	
J7511		E	Lymphocyte immune globulin, antithymocyte globulin, rabbit, parenteral, 25 mg	0.00	0.00	0.00	0.00	0.00	0.00	XXX	
J7513		E	Daclizumab, parenteral, 25 mg	0.00	15.41	15.41	0.00	15.41	15.41	XXX	■
J7515		E	Cyclosporine, oral, 25 mg	0.00	0.07	0.07	0.00	0.07	0.07	XXX	■
J7516		E	Cyclosporine, parenteral, 250 mg	0.00	0.97	0.97	0.00	0.97	0.97	XXX	■
J7517		E	Mycophenolate mofetil, oral, 250 mg	0.00	0.09	0.09	0.00	0.09	0.09	XXX	■
J7520		E	Sirolimus, oral, 1 mg	0.00	0.25	0.25	0.00	0.25	0.25	XXX	■
J7525		E	Tacrolimus, parenteral, 5 mg	0.00	4.47	4.47	0.00	4.47	4.47	XXX	■
J7599		X	Immunosuppressive drug, not otherwise classified	0.00	0.00	0.00	0.00	0.00	0.00	XXX	
J7608		E	Acetylcysteine, inhalation solution administered through DME, unit dose form, per gram	0.00	0.00	0.00	0.00	0.00	0.00	XXX	
J7618		E	Albuterol, all formulations including separated isomers, inhalation solution administered through DME, concentrated form, per 1 mg (Albuterol) or per 0.5 mg (Levalbuterol)	0.00	0.00	0.00	0.00	0.00	0.00	XXX	
J7619		E	Albuterol, all formulations including separated isomers, inhalation solution administered through DME, unit dose, per 1 mg (Albuterol) or per 0.5 mg (Levalbuterol)	0.00	0.00	0.00	0.00	0.00	0.00	XXX	
J7622		E	Bethamethasone, inhalation solution administered through DME, unit dose form, per milligram	0.00	0.00	0.00	0.00	0.00	0.00	XXX	
J7624		E	Bethamethasone, inhalation solution administered through DME, unit dose form, per milligram	0.00	0.00	0.00	0.00	0.00	0.00	XXX	

■ RVU not developed by CMS. Gap-filled RVUs developed by CHEG.

Code	M	S	Description	Work Value	Non-Fac PE	Fac PE	Mal-practice	Non-Fac Total	Fac Total	Global	Gap
J7626		E	Budesonide inhalation solution, administered through DME, unit dose form, 0.25 mg	0.00	0.16	0.16	0.00	0.16	0.16	XXX	■
J7628		E	Bitolterol mesylate, inhalation solution administered through DME, concentrated form, per milligram	0.00	0.00	0.00	0.00	0.00	0.00	XXX	
J7629		E	Bitolterol mesylate, inhalation solution administered through DME, unit dose form, per milligram	0.00	0.00	0.00	0.00	0.00	0.00	XXX	
J7631		E	Cromolyn sodium, inhalation solution administered through DME, unit dose form, per 10 milligrams	0.00	0.02	0.02	0.00	0.02	0.02	XXX	■
J7635		E	Atropine, inhalation solution administered through DME, concentrated form, per milligram	0.00	0.00	0.00	0.00	0.00	0.00	XXX	
J7636		E	Atropine, inhalation solution administered through DME, unit dose form, per milligram	0.00	0.00	0.00	0.00	0.00	0.00	XXX	
J7637		E	Dexamethasone, inhalation solution administered through DME, concentrated form, per milligram	0.00	0.00	0.00	0.00	0.00	0.00	XXX	
J7638		E	Dexamethasone, inhalation solution administered through DME, unit dose form, per milligram	0.00	0.00	0.00	0.00	0.00	0.00	XXX	
J7639		E	Dornase alpha, inhalation solution administered through DME, unit dose form, per milligram	0.00	1.54	1.54	0.00	1.54	1.54	XXX	■
J7641		E	Flunisolide, inhalation solution administered through DME, unit dose, per milligram	0.00	0.00	0.00	0.00	0.00	0.00	XXX	
J7642		E	Glycopyrrolate, inhalation solution administered through DME, concentrated form, per milligram	0.00	0.00	0.00	0.00	0.00	0.00	XXX	
J7643		E	Glycopyrrolate, inhalation solution administered through DME, unit dose form, per milligram	0.00	0.00	0.00	0.00	0.00	0.00	XXX	
J7644		E	Ipratropium bromide, inhalation solution administered through DME, unit dose form, per milligram	0.00	0.00	0.00	0.00	0.00	0.00	XXX	
J7648		E	Isoetharine HCl, inhalation solution administered through DME, concentrated form, per milligram	0.00	0.00	0.00	0.00	0.00	0.00	XXX	
J7649		E	Isoetharine HCl, inhalation solution administered through DME, unit dose form, per milligram	0.00	0.00	0.00	0.00	0.00	0.00	XXX	
J7658		E	Isoproterenol HCl, inhalation solution administered through DME, concentrated form, per milligram	0.00	0.00	0.00	0.00	0.00	0.00	XXX	

■ RVU not developed by CMS. Gap-filled RVUs developed by CHEG.

Code	M	S	Description	Work Value	Non-Fac PE	Fac PE	Mal-practice	Non-Fac Total	Fac Total	Global	Gap
J7659		E	Isoproterenol HCl, inhalation solution administered through DME, unit dose form, per milligram	0.00	0.00	0.00	0.00	0.00	0.00	XXX	
J7668		E	Metaproterenol sulfate, inhalation solution administered through DME, concentrated form, per 10 milligrams	0.00	0.00	0.00	0.00	0.00	0.00	XXX	
J7669		E	Metaproterenol sulfate, inhalation solution administered through DME, unit dose form, per 10 milligrams	0.00	0.00	0.00	0.00	0.00	0.00	XXX	
J7680		E	Terbutaline sulfate, inhalation solution administered through DME, concentrated form, per milligram	0.00	0.00	0.00	0.00	0.00	0.00	XXX	
J7681		E	Terbutaline sulfate, inhalation solution administered through DME, unit dose form, per milligram	0.00	0.00	0.00	0.00	0.00	0.00	XXX	
J7682		E	Tobramycin, unit dose form, 300 mg, inhalation solution, administered through DME	0.00	1.65	1.65	0.00	1.65	1.65	XXX	■
J7683		E	Triamcinolone, inhalation solution administered through DME, concentrated form, per milligram	0.00	0.00	0.00	0.00	0.00	0.00	XXX	
J7684		E	Triamcinolone, inhalation solution administered through DME, unit dose form, per milligram	0.00	0.00	0.00	0.00	0.00	0.00	XXX	
J7699		E	NOC drugs, inhalation solution administered through DME	0.00	0.00	0.00	0.00	0.00	0.00	XXX	
J7799		E	NOC drugs, other than inhalation drugs, administered through DME	0.00	0.00	0.00	0.00	0.00	0.00	XXX	
J8499		N	Prescription drug, oral, nonchemotherapeutic, not otherwise specified	0.00	0.00	0.00	0.00	0.00	0.00	XXX	
J8510		E	Bulsulfan; oral, 2 mg	0.00	0.07	0.07	0.00	0.07	0.07	XXX	■
J8520		E	Capecitabine, oral, 150 mg	0.00	0.09	0.09	0.00	0.09	0.09	XXX	■
J8521		E	Capecitabine, oral, 500 mg	0.00	0.31	0.31	0.00	0.31	0.31	XXX	■
J8530		E	Cyclophosphamide, oral, 25 mg	0.00	0.09	0.09	0.00	0.09	0.09	XXX	■
J8560		E	Etoposide, oral, 50 mg	0.00	1.97	1.97	0.00	1.97	1.97	XXX	■
J8600		E	Melphalan, oral 2 mg	0.00	0.08	0.08	0.00	0.08	0.08	XXX	■
J8610		E	Methotrexate, oral, 2.5 mg	0.00	0.12	0.12	0.00	0.12	0.12	XXX	■
J8700		E	Temozolmide, oral, 5 mg	0.00	0.23	0.23	0.00	0.23	0.23	XXX	■
J8999		E	Prescription drug, oral, chemotherapeutic, not otherwise specified	0.00	0.00	0.00	0.00	0.00	0.00	XXX	
J9000		E	Doxorubicin HCl, 10 mg	0.00	1.31	1.31	0.00	1.31	1.31	XXX	■

■ RVU not developed by CMS. Gap-filled RVUs developed by CHEG.

HCPCS

Code	M	S	Description	Work Value	Non-Fac PE	Fac PE	Mal-practice	Non-Fac Total	Fac Total	Global	Gap
J9001		E	Doxorubicin hydrochloride, all lipid formulations, 10 mg	0.00	13.92	13.92	0.00	13.92	13.92	XXX	■
J9015		E	Aldesleukin, per single use vial	0.00	24.88	24.88	0.00	24.88	24.88	XXX	■
J9017		E	Arsenic trioxide, 1 mg	0.00	9.66	9.66	0.00	9.66	9.66	XXX	■
J9020		E	Asparaginase, 10,000 units	0.00	2.32	2.32	0.00	2.32	2.32	XXX	■
J9031		E	BCG live (intravesical), per installation	0.00	6.20	6.20	0.00	6.20	6.20	XXX	■
J9040		E	Bleomycin sulfate, 15 units	0.00	11.27	11.27	0.00	11.27	11.27	XXX	■
J9045		E	Carboplatin, 50 mg	0.00	4.31	4.31	0.00	4.31	4.31	XXX	■
J9050		E	Carmustine, 100 mg	0.00	4.44	4.44	0.00	4.44	4.44	XXX	■
J9060		E	Cisplatin, powder or solution, per 10 mg	0.00	0.00	0.00	0.00	0.00	0.00	XXX	
J9062		E	Cisplatin, 50 mg	0.00	8.33	8.33	0.00	8.33	8.33	XXX	■
J9065		E	Injection, cladribine, per 1 mg	0.00	2.13	2.13	0.00	2.13	2.13	XXX	■
J9070		E	Cyclophosphamide, 100 mg	0.00	0.24	0.24	0.00	0.24	0.24	XXX	■
J9080		E	Cyclophosphamide, 200 mg	0.00	0.44	0.44	0.00	0.44	0.44	XXX	■
J9090		E	Cyclophosphamide, 500 mg	0.00	0.94	0.94	0.00	0.94	0.94	XXX	■
J9091		E	Cyclophosphamide, 1 g	0.00	1.85	1.85	0.00	1.85	1.85	XXX	■
J9092		E	Cyclophosphamide, 2 g	0.00	3.78	3.78	0.00	3.78	3.78	XXX	■
J9093		E	Cyclophosphamide, lyophilized, 100 mg	0.00	0.24	0.24	0.00	0.24	0.24	XXX	■
J9094		E	Cyclophosphamide, lyophilized, 200 mg	0.00	0.46	0.46	0.00	0.46	0.46	XXX	■
J9095		E	Cyclophosphamide, lyophilized, 500 mg	0.00	0.97	0.97	0.00	0.97	0.97	XXX	■
J9096		E	Cyclophosphamide, lyophilized, 1 g	0.00	1.94	1.94	0.00	1.94	1.94	XXX	■
J9097		E	Cyclophosphamide, lyophilized, 2 g	0.00	3.88	3.88	0.00	3.88	3.88	XXX	■
J9100		E	Cytarabine, 100 mg	0.00	0.23	0.23	0.00	0.23	0.23	XXX	■
J9110		E	Cytarabine, 500 mg	0.00	0.94	0.94	0.00	0.94	0.94	XXX	■
J9120		E	Dactinomycin, 0.5 mg	0.00	0.50	0.50	0.00	0.50	0.50	XXX	■
J9130		E	Dacarbazine, 100 mg	0.00	0.49	0.49	0.00	0.49	0.49	XXX	■
J9140		E	Dacarbazine, 200 mg	0.00	0.94	0.94	0.00	0.94	0.94	XXX	■
J9150		E	Daunorubicin HCl, 10 mg	0.00	3.10	3.10	0.00	3.10	3.10	XXX	■
J9151		E	Daunorubicin citrate, liposomal formulation, 10 mg	0.00	2.51	2.51	0.00	2.51	2.51	XXX	■
J9160		E	Denileukin diftitox, 300 mcg	0.00	38.34	38.34	0.00	38.34	38.34	XXX	■
J9165		E	Diethylstilbestrol diphosphate, 250 mg	0.00	0.56	0.56	0.00	0.56	0.56	XXX	■

■ RVU not developed by CMS. Gap-filled RVUs developed by CHEG.

Code	M	S	Description	Work Value	Non-Fac PE	Fac PE	Mal-practice	Non-Fac Total	Fac Total	Global	Gap
J9170		E	Docetaxel, 20 mg	0.00	11.55	11.55	0.00	11.55	11.55	XXX	■
J9180		E	Epirubicin hydrochloride, 50 mg	0.00	24.18	24.18	0.00	24.18	24.18	XXX	■
J9181		E	Etoposide, 10 mg	0.00	0.28	0.28	0.00	0.28	0.28	XXX	■
J9182		E	Etoposide, 100 mg	0.00	2.81	2.81	0.00	2.81	2.81	XXX	■
J9185		E	Fludarabine phosphate, 50 mg	0.00	10.04	10.04	0.00	10.04	10.04	XXX	■
J9190		E	Fluorouracil, 500 mg	0.00	0.08	0.08	0.00	0.08	0.08	XXX	■
J9200		E	Floxuridine, 500 mg	0.00	5.03	5.03	0.00	5.03	5.03	XXX	■
J9201		E	Gemcitabine HCl, 200 mg	0.00	3.96	3.96	0.00	3.96	3.96	XXX	■
J9202		E	Goserelin acetate implant, per 3.6 mg	0.00	17.32	17.32	0.00	17.32	17.32	XXX	■
J9206		E	Irinotecan, 20 mg	0.00	4.87	4.87	0.00	4.87	4.87	XXX	■
J9208		E	Ifosfamide, per 1 g	0.00	6.08	6.08	0.00	6.08	6.08	XXX	■
J9209		E	Mesna, 200 mg	0.00	1.57	1.57	0.00	1.57	1.57	XXX	■
J9211		E	Idarubicin HCl, 5 mg	0.00	13.90	13.90	0.00	13.90	13.90	XXX	■
J9212		E	Injection, interferon Alfacon-1, recombinant, 1 mcg	0.00	0.00	0.00	0.00	0.00	0.00	XXX	
J9213		E	Interferon alfa-2A, recombinant, 3 million units	0.00	1.33	1.33	0.00	1.33	1.33	XXX	■
J9214		E	Interferon alfa-2B, recombinant, 1 million units	0.00	0.43	0.43	0.00	0.43	0.43	XXX	■
J9215		E	Interferon alfa-N3, (human leukocyte derived), 250,000 IU	0.00	0.35	0.35	0.00	0.35	0.35	XXX	■
J9216		E	Interferon gamma-1B, 3 million units	0.00	12.19	12.19	0.00	12.19	12.19	XXX	■
J9217		E	Leuprolide acetate (for depot suspension), 7.5 mg	0.00	22.44	22.44	0.00	22.44	22.44	XXX	■
J9218		E	Leuprolide acetate, per 1 mg	0.00	0.00	0.00	0.00	0.00	0.00	XXX	
J9219		E	Leuprolide acetate implant, 65 mg	0.00	0.00	0.00	0.00	0.00	0.00	XXX	
J9230		E	Mechlorethamine HCl, (nitrogen mustard), 10 mg	0.00	0.44	0.44	0.00	0.44	0.44	XXX	■
J9245		E	Injection, melphalan HCl, 50 mg	0.00	14.80	14.80	0.00	14.80	14.80	XXX	■
J9250		E	Methotrexate sodium, 5 mg	0.00	0.02	0.02	0.00	0.02	0.02	XXX	■
J9260		E	Methotrexate sodium, 50 mg	0.00	0.22	0.22	0.00	0.22	0.22	XXX	■
J9265		E	Paclitaxel, 30 mg	0.00	6.73	6.73	0.00	6.73	6.73	XXX	■
J9266		E	Pegaspargase, per single dose vial	0.00	0.00	0.00	0.00	0.00	0.00	XXX	
J9268		E	Pentostatin, per 10 mg	0.00	64.17	64.17	0.00	64.17	64.17	XXX	■
J9270		E	Plicamycin, 2.5 mg	0.00	3.59	3.59	0.00	3.59	3.59	XXX	■

■ RVU not developed by CMS. Gap-filled RVUs developed by CHEG.

Code	M	S	Description	Work Value	Non-Fac PE	Fac PE	Mal-practice	Non-Fac Total	Fac Total	Global	Gap
J9280		E	Mitomycin, 5 mg	0.00	4.83	4.83	0.00	4.83	4.83	XXX	■
J9290		E	Mitomycin, 20 mg	0.00	16.35	16.35	0.00	16.35	16.35	XXX	■
J9291		E	Mitomycin, 40 mg	0.00	33.72	33.72	0.00	33.72	33.72	XXX	■
J9293		E	Injection, mitoxantrone HCl, per 5 mg	0.00	9.47	9.47	0.00	9.47	9.47	XXX	■
J9300		E	Gemtuzumab ozogamicin, 5 mg	0.00	78.46	78.46	0.00	78.46	78.46	XXX	■
J9310		E	Rituximab, 100 mg	0.00	17.12	17.12	0.00	17.12	17.12	XXX	■
J9320		E	Streptozocin, 1 g	0.00	4.56	4.56	0.00	4.56	4.56	XXX	■
J9340		E	Thiotepa, 15 mg	0.00	4.54	4.54	0.00	4.54	4.54	XXX	■
J9350		E	Topotecan, 4 mg	0.00	24.54	24.54	0.00	24.54	24.54	XXX	■
J9355		E	Trastuzumab, 10 mg	0.00	2.05	2.05	0.00	2.05	2.05	XXX	■
J9357		E	Valrubicin, intravesical, 200 mg	0.00	16.42	16.42	0.00	16.42	16.42	XXX	■
J9360		E	Vinblastine sulfate, 1 mg	0.00	0.16	0.16	0.00	0.16	0.16	XXX	■
J9370		E	Vincristine sulfate, 1 mg	0.00	1.35	1.35	0.00	1.35	1.35	XXX	■
J9375		E	Vincristine sulfate, 2 mg	0.00	2.04	2.04	0.00	2.04	2.04	XXX	■
J9380		E	Vincristine sulfate, 5 mg	0.00	6.00	6.00	0.00	6.00	6.00	XXX	■
J9390		E	Vinorelbine tartrate, per 10 mg	0.00	3.08	3.08	0.00	3.08	3.08	XXX	■
J9600		E	Porfimer sodium, 75 mg	0.00	101.00	101.00	0.00	101.00	101.00	XXX	■
J9999		E	Not otherwise classified, antineoplastic drug	0.00	0.00	0.00	0.00	0.00	0.00	XXX	
K0001	NU		Standard wheelchair	0.00	17.16	17.16	0.00	17.16	17.16	XXX	■
	RR			0.00	1.73	1.73	0.00	1.73	1.73	XXX	■
	UE			0.00	12.87	12.87	0.00	12.87	12.87	XXX	■
K0002	NU		Standard hemi (low seat) wheelchair	0.00	20.08	20.08	0.00	20.08	20.08	XXX	■
	RR			0.00	2.53	2.53	0.00	2.53	2.53	XXX	■
	UE			0.00	15.76	15.76	0.00	15.76	15.76	XXX	■
K0003	NU		Lightweight wheelchair	0.00	32.21	32.21	0.00	32.21	32.21	XXX	■
	RR			0.00	2.83	2.83	0.00	2.83	2.83	XXX	■
	UE			0.00	24.17	24.17	0.00	24.17	24.17	XXX	■
K0004	NU		High strength, lightweight wheelchair	0.00	40.05	40.05	0.00	40.05	40.05	XXX	■
	RR			0.00	3.37	3.37	0.00	3.37	3.37	XXX	■
	UE			0.00	30.04	30.04	0.00	30.04	30.04	XXX	■
K0005	NU		Ultralightweight wheelchair	0.00	49.62	49.62	0.00	49.62	49.62	XXX	■
	RR			0.00	4.65	4.65	0.00	4.65	4.65	XXX	■
	UE			0.00	37.22	37.22	0.00	37.22	37.22	XXX	■
K0006	NU		Heavy-duty wheelchair	0.00	35.70	35.70	0.00	35.70	35.70	XXX	■
	RR			0.00	3.92	3.92	0.00	3.92	3.92	XXX	■
	UE			0.00	26.91	26.91	0.00	26.91	26.91	XXX	■

■ RVU not developed by CMS. Gap-filled RVUs developed by CHEG.

Code	M S	Description	Work Value	Non-Fac PE	Fac PE	Mal-practice	Non-Fac Total	Fac Total	Global	Gap
K0007	NU	Extra heavy-duty wheelchair	0.00	45.59	45.59	0.00	45.59	45.59	XXX	■
	RR		0.00	4.56	4.56	0.00	4.56	4.56	XXX	■
	UE		0.00	44.64	44.64	0.00	44.64	44.64	XXX	■
K0009		Other manual wheelchair/base	0.00	0.00	0.00	0.00	0.00	0.00	XXX	
K0010	NU	Standard-weight frame motorized/power wheelchair	0.00	128.44	128.44	0.00	128.44	128.44	XXX	■
	RR		0.00	12.84	12.84	0.00	12.84	12.84	XXX	■
	UE		0.00	96.34	96.34	0.00	96.34	96.34	XXX	■
K0011	NU	Standard-weight frame motorized/power wheelchair with programmable control parameters for speed adjustment, tremor dampening, acceleration control and braking	0.00	211.13	211.13	0.00	211.13	211.13	XXX	■
	RR		0.00	15.59	15.59	0.00	15.59	15.59	XXX	■
K0012		Lightweight portable motorized/power wheelchair	0.00	90.86	90.86	0.00	90.86	90.86	XXX	■
K0014		Other motorized/power wheelchair base	0.00	0.00	0.00	0.00	0.00	0.00	XXX	
K0015	NU	Detachable, nonadjustable height armrest, each	0.00	5.07	5.07	0.00	5.07	5.07	XXX	■
	RR		0.00	1.07	1.07	0.00	1.07	1.07	XXX	■
	UE		0.00	3.78	3.78	0.00	3.78	3.78	XXX	■
K0016	NU	Detachable, adjustable height armrest, complete assembly, each	0.00	3.22	3.22	0.00	3.22	3.22	XXX	■
	RR		0.00	0.36	0.36	0.00	0.36	0.36	XXX	■
	UE		0.00	2.42	2.42	0.00	2.42	2.42	XXX	■
K0017	NU	Detachable, adjustable height armrest, base, each	0.00	1.37	1.37	0.00	1.37	1.37	XXX	■
	RR		0.00	0.15	0.15	0.00	0.15	0.15	XXX	■
	UE		0.00	1.04	1.04	0.00	1.04	1.04	XXX	■
K0018	NU	Detachable, adjustable height armrest, upper portion, each	0.00	1.82	1.82	0.00	1.82	1.82	XXX	■
	RR		0.00	0.18	0.18	0.00	0.18	0.18	XXX	■
	UE		0.00	1.16	1.16	0.00	1.16	1.16	XXX	■
K0019	NU	Arm pad, each	0.00	0.82	0.82	0.00	0.82	0.82	XXX	■
	RR		0.00	0.15	0.15	0.00	0.15	0.15	XXX	■
	UE		0.00	0.57	0.57	0.00	0.57	0.57	XXX	■
K0020	NU	Fixed, adjustable height armrest, pair	0.00	1.37	1.37	0.00	1.37	1.37	XXX	■
	RR		0.00	0.12	0.12	0.00	0.12	0.12	XXX	■
	UE		0.00	0.98	0.98	0.00	0.98	0.98	XXX	■
K0021	NU	Antitipping device, each	0.00	1.83	1.83	0.00	1.83	1.83	XXX	■
	RR		0.00	0.27	0.27	0.00	0.27	0.27	XXX	■
	UE		0.00	1.36	1.36	0.00	1.36	1.36	XXX	■
K0022	NU	Reinforced back upholstery	0.00	1.36	1.36	0.00	1.36	1.36	XXX	■
	RR		0.00	0.16	0.16	0.00	0.16	0.16	XXX	■
	UE		0.00	1.19	1.19	0.00	1.19	1.19	XXX	■
K0023	NU	Solid back insert, planar back, single density foam, attached with straps	0.00	4.00	4.00	0.00	4.00	4.00	XXX	■
	RR		0.00	0.27	0.27	0.00	0.27	0.27	XXX	■
	UE		0.00	2.15	2.15	0.00	2.15	2.15	XXX	■
K0024	NU	Solid back insert, planar back, single density foam, with adjustable hook-on hardware	0.00	4.71	4.71	0.00	4.71	4.71	XXX	■
	RR		0.00	0.47	0.47	0.00	0.47	0.47	XXX	■
	UE		0.00	3.53	3.53	0.00	3.53	3.53	XXX	■

■ RVU not developed by CMS. Gap-filled RVUs developed by CHEG.

Code	M	S	Description	Work Value	Non-Fac PE	Fac PE	Mal-practice	Non-Fac Total	Fac Total	Global	Gap
K0025	NU		Hook-on headrest extension	0.00	2.09	2.09	0.00	2.09	2.09	XXX	■
	RR			0.00	0.21	0.21	0.00	0.21	0.21	XXX	■
	UE			0.00	1.49	1.49	0.00	1.49	1.49	XXX	■
K0026	NU		Back upholstery for ultralightweight or high-strength lightweight wheelchair	0.00	2.12	2.12	0.00	2.12	2.12	XXX	■
	RR			0.00	0.21	0.21	0.00	0.21	0.21	XXX	■
	UE			0.00	1.39	1.39	0.00	1.39	1.39	XXX	■
K0027	NU		Back upholstery for wheelchair type other than ultralightweight or high-strength lightweight wheelchair	0.00	1.49	1.49	0.00	1.49	1.49	XXX	■
	RR			0.00	0.15	0.15	0.00	0.15	0.15	XXX	■
	UE			0.00	1.04	1.04	0.00	1.04	1.04	XXX	■
K0028	NU		Manual, fully reclining back	0.00	15.25	15.25	0.00	15.25	15.25	XXX	■
	RR			0.00	1.58	1.58	0.00	1.58	1.58	XXX	■
	UE			0.00	11.44	11.44	0.00	11.44	11.44	XXX	■
K0029	NU		Reinforced seat upholstery	0.00	1.39	1.39	0.00	1.39	1.39	XXX	■
	RR			0.00	0.12	0.12	0.00	0.12	0.12	XXX	■
	UE			0.00	1.05	1.05	0.00	1.05	1.05	XXX	■
K0030			Solid seat insert, planar seat, single density foam	0.00	4.05	4.05	0.00	4.05	4.05	XXX	■
K0031	NU		Safety belt/pelvic strap, each	0.00	1.22	1.22	0.00	1.22	1.22	XXX	■
	RR			0.00	0.12	0.12	0.00	0.12	0.12	XXX	■
	UE			0.00	1.04	1.04	0.00	1.04	1.04	XXX	■
K0032	NU		Seat upholstery for ultralightweight or high-strength lightweight wheelchair	0.00	1.22	1.22	0.00	1.22	1.22	XXX	■
	RR			0.00	0.12	0.12	0.00	0.12	0.12	XXX	■
	UE			0.00	0.92	0.92	0.00	0.92	0.92	XXX	■
K0033	NU		Seat upholstery for wheelchair type other than ultralightweight or high-strength lightweight wheelchair	0.00	1.22	1.22	0.00	1.22	1.22	XXX	■
	RR			0.00	0.12	0.12	0.00	0.12	0.12	XXX	■
	UE			0.00	0.92	0.92	0.00	0.92	0.92	XXX	■
K0034	NU		Heel loop, each	0.00	0.53	0.53	0.00	0.53	0.53	XXX	■
	RR			0.00	0.06	0.06	0.00	0.06	0.06	XXX	■
	UE			0.00	0.40	0.40	0.00	0.40	0.40	XXX	■
K0035	NU		Heel loop with ankle strap, each	0.00	0.71	0.71	0.00	0.71	0.71	XXX	■
	RR			0.00	0.06	0.06	0.00	0.06	0.06	XXX	■
	UE			0.00	0.56	0.56	0.00	0.56	0.56	XXX	■
K0036	NU		Toe loop, each	0.00	0.69	0.69	0.00	0.69	0.69	XXX	■
	RR			0.00	0.07	0.07	0.00	0.07	0.07	XXX	■
	UE			0.00	0.52	0.52	0.00	0.52	0.52	XXX	■
K0037	NU		High mount flip-up footrest, each	0.00	1.28	1.28	0.00	1.28	1.28	XXX	■
	RR			0.00	0.12	0.12	0.00	0.12	0.12	XXX	■
	UE			0.00	0.98	0.98	0.00	0.98	0.98	XXX	■
K0038	NU		Leg strap, each	0.00	0.66	0.66	0.00	0.66	0.66	XXX	■
	RR			0.00	0.06	0.06	0.00	0.06	0.06	XXX	■
	UE			0.00	0.48	0.48	0.00	0.48	0.48	XXX	■
K0039	NU		Leg strap, H style, each	0.00	1.46	1.46	0.00	1.46	1.46	XXX	■
	RR			0.00	0.15	0.15	0.00	0.15	0.15	XXX	■
	UE			0.00	1.07	1.07	0.00	1.07	1.07	XXX	■

■ RVU not developed by CMS. Gap-filled RVUs developed by CHEG.

Code	M	S	Description	Work Value	Non-Fac PE	Fac PE	Mal-practice	Non-Fac Total	Fac Total	Global	Gap
K0040	NU		Adjustable angle footplate, each	0.00	2.03	2.03	0.00	2.03	2.03	XXX	■
	RR			0.00	0.24	0.24	0.00	0.24	0.24	XXX	■
	UE			0.00	1.49	1.49	0.00	1.49	1.49	XXX	■
K0041	NU		Large size footplate, each	0.00	1.43	1.43	0.00	1.43	1.43	XXX	■
	RR			0.00	0.15	0.15	0.00	0.15	0.15	XXX	■
	UE			0.00	1.07	1.07	0.00	1.07	1.07	XXX	■
K0042	NU		Standard size footplate, each	0.00	0.98	0.98	0.00	0.98	0.98	XXX	■
	RR			0.00	0.09	0.09	0.00	0.09	0.09	XXX	■
	UE			0.00	0.75	0.75	0.00	0.75	0.75	XXX	■
K0043	NU		Footrest, lower extension tube, each	0.00	0.60	0.60	0.00	0.60	0.60	XXX	■
	RR			0.00	0.06	0.06	0.00	0.06	0.06	XXX	■
	UE			0.00	0.39	0.39	0.00	0.39	0.39	XXX	■
K0044	NU		Footrest, upper hanger bracket, each	0.00	0.45	0.45	0.00	0.45	0.45	XXX	■
	RR			0.00	0.06	0.06	0.00	0.06	0.06	XXX	■
	UE			0.00	0.33	0.33	0.00	0.33	0.33	XXX	■
K0045	NU		Footrest, complete assembly	0.00	1.58	1.58	0.00	1.58	1.58	XXX	■
	RR			0.00	0.15	0.15	0.00	0.15	0.15	XXX	■
	UE			0.00	1.19	1.19	0.00	1.19	1.19	XXX	■
K0046	NU		Elevating legrest, lower extension tube, each	0.00	0.60	0.60	0.00	0.60	0.60	XXX	■
	RR			0.00	0.06	0.06	0.00	0.06	0.06	XXX	■
	UE			0.00	0.39	0.39	0.00	0.39	0.39	XXX	■
K0047	NU		Elevating legrest, upper hanger bracket, each	0.00	2.15	2.15	0.00	2.15	2.15	XXX	■
	RR			0.00	0.21	0.21	0.00	0.21	0.21	XXX	■
	UE			0.00	1.64	1.64	0.00	1.64	1.64	XXX	■
K0048	NU		Elevating legrest, complete assembly	0.00	3.92	3.92	0.00	3.92	3.92	XXX	■
	RR			0.00	0.45	0.45	0.00	0.45	0.45	XXX	■
	UE			0.00	3.13	3.13	0.00	3.13	3.13	XXX	■
K0049	NU		Calf pad, each	0.00	0.89	0.89	0.00	0.89	0.89	XXX	■
	RR			0.00	0.09	0.09	0.00	0.09	0.09	XXX	■
	UE			0.00	0.69	0.69	0.00	0.69	0.69	XXX	■
K0050	NU		Ratchet assembly	0.00	0.92	0.92	0.00	0.92	0.92	XXX	■
	RR			0.00	0.09	0.09	0.00	0.09	0.09	XXX	■
	UE			0.00	0.75	0.75	0.00	0.75	0.75	XXX	■
K0051	NU		Cam release assembly, footrest or legrest, each	0.00	1.49	1.49	0.00	1.49	1.49	XXX	■
	RR			0.00	0.15	0.15	0.00	0.15	0.15	XXX	■
	UE			0.00	1.13	1.13	0.00	1.13	1.13	XXX	■
K0052	NU		Swingaway, detachable footrests, each	0.00	3.37	3.37	0.00	3.37	3.37	XXX	■
	RR			0.00	0.33	0.33	0.00	0.33	0.33	XXX	■
	UE			0.00	2.69	2.69	0.00	2.69	2.69	XXX	■
K0053	NU		Elevating footrests, articulating (telescoping), each	0.00	2.98	2.98	0.00	2.98	2.98	XXX	■
	RR			0.00	0.27	0.27	0.00	0.27	0.27	XXX	■
	UE			0.00	2.38	2.38	0.00	2.38	2.38	XXX	■
K0054	NU		Seat width of 10, 11, 12, 15, 17, or 20 inches for a high-strength, lightweight or ultralightweight wheelchair	0.00	2.80	2.80	0.00	2.80	2.80	XXX	■
	RR			0.00	0.27	0.27	0.00	0.27	0.27	XXX	■
	UE			0.00	2.12	2.12	0.00	2.12	2.12	XXX	■

■ RVU not developed by CMS. Gap-filled RVUs developed by CHEG.

Code	M	S	Description	Work Value	Non-Fac PE	Fac PE	Mal-practice	Non-Fac Total	Fac Total	Global	Gap
K0055	NU		Seat depth of 15, 17, or 18 inches for a high strength, lightweight or ultralightweight wheelchair	0.00	3.04	3.04	0.00	3.04	3.04	XXX	■
	RR			0.00	0.36	0.36	0.00	0.36	0.36	XXX	■
	UE			0.00	2.38	2.38	0.00	2.38	2.38	XXX	■
K0056	NU		Seat height less than 17 inches or equal to or greater than 21 inches for a high strength, lightweight, or ultralightweight wheelchair	0.00	3.04	3.04	0.00	3.04	3.04	XXX	■
	RR			0.00	0.36	0.36	0.00	0.36	0.36	XXX	■
	UE			0.00	2.38	2.38	0.00	2.38	2.38	XXX	■
K0057	NU		Seat width 19 or 20 inches for heavy duty or extra heavy-duty chair	0.00	3.73	3.73	0.00	3.73	3.73	XXX	■
	RR			0.00	0.45	0.45	0.00	0.45	0.45	XXX	■
	UE			0.00	2.68	2.68	0.00	2.68	2.68	XXX	■
K0058	NU		Seat depth 17 or 18 inches for a motorized/ power wheelchair	0.00	1.67	1.67	0.00	1.67	1.67	XXX	■
	RR			0.00	0.15	0.15	0.00	0.15	0.15	XXX	■
	UE			0.00	1.28	1.28	0.00	1.28	1.28	XXX	■
K0059	NU		Plastic coated handrim, each	0.00	0.92	0.92	0.00	0.92	0.92	XXX	■
	RR			0.00	0.09	0.09	0.00	0.09	0.09	XXX	■
	UE			0.00	0.69	0.69	0.00	0.69	0.69	XXX	■
K0060	NU		Steel handrim, each	0.00	0.80	0.80	0.00	0.80	0.80	XXX	■
	RR			0.00	0.09	0.09	0.00	0.09	0.09	XXX	■
	UE			0.00	0.63	0.63	0.00	0.63	0.63	XXX	■
K0061	NU		Aluminum handrim, each	0.00	1.10	1.10	0.00	1.10	1.10	XXX	■
	RR			0.00	0.12	0.12	0.00	0.12	0.12	XXX	■
	UE			0.00	0.86	0.86	0.00	0.86	0.86	XXX	■
K0062	NU		Handrim with 8 to 10 vertical or oblique projections, each	0.00	1.73	1.73	0.00	1.73	1.73	XXX	■
	RR			0.00	0.18	0.18	0.00	0.18	0.18	XXX	■
	UE			0.00	1.28	1.28	0.00	1.28	1.28	XXX	■
K0063	NU		Handrim with 12 to 16 vertical or oblique projections, each	0.00	2.24	2.24	0.00	2.24	2.24	XXX	■
	RR			0.00	0.21	0.21	0.00	0.21	0.21	XXX	■
	UE			0.00	1.73	1.73	0.00	1.73	1.73	XXX	■
K0064	NU		Zero pressure tube (flat free insert), any size, each	0.00	2.06	2.06	0.00	2.06	2.06	XXX	■
	RR			0.00	0.18	0.18	0.00	0.18	0.18	XXX	■
	UE			0.00	0.99	0.99	0.00	0.99	0.99	XXX	■
K0065	NU		Spoke protectors, each	0.00	1.25	1.25	0.00	1.25	1.25	XXX	■
	RR			0.00	0.12	0.12	0.00	0.12	0.12	XXX	■
	UE			0.00	0.95	0.95	0.00	0.95	0.95	XXX	■
K0066	NU		Solid tire, any size, each	0.00	0.89	0.89	0.00	0.89	0.89	XXX	■
	RR			0.00	0.10	0.10	0.00	0.10	0.10	XXX	■
	UE			0.00	0.69	0.69	0.00	0.69	0.69	XXX	■
K0067	NU		Pneumatic tire, any size, each	0.00	1.33	1.33	0.00	1.33	1.33	XXX	■
	RR			0.00	0.13	0.13	0.00	0.13	0.13	XXX	■
	UE			0.00	0.99	0.99	0.00	0.99	0.99	XXX	■
K0068	NU		Pneumatic tire tube, each	0.00	0.15	0.15	0.00	0.15	0.15	XXX	■
	UE			0.00	0.12	0.12	0.00	0.12	0.12	XXX	■
K0069	NU		Rear wheel assembly, complete, with solid tire, spokes or molded, each	0.00	2.86	2.86	0.00	2.86	2.86	XXX	■
	UE			0.00	2.15	2.15	0.00	2.15	2.15	XXX	■

■ RVU not developed by CMS. Gap-filled RVUs developed by CHEG.

Code	M	S	Description	Work Value	Non-Fac PE	Fac PE	Mal-practice	Non-Fac Total	Fac Total	Global	Gap
K0070	NU		Rear wheel assembly, complete with pneumatic tire, spokes or molded, each	0.00	5.07	5.07	0.00	5.07	5.07	XXX	■
	UE			0.00	3.90	3.90	0.00	3.90	3.90	XXX	■
K0071	NU		Front caster assembly, complete, with pneumatic tire, each	0.00	3.01	3.01	0.00	3.01	3.01	XXX	■
	UE			0.00	2.38	2.38	0.00	2.38	2.38	XXX	■
K0072	NU		Front caster assembly, complete, with semipneumatic tire, each	0.00	1.85	1.85	0.00	1.85	1.85	XXX	■
	UE			0.00	1.43	1.43	0.00	1.43	1.43	XXX	■
K0073	NU		Caster pin lock, each	0.00	1.01	1.01	0.00	1.01	1.01	XXX	■
	RR			0.00	0.09	0.09	0.00	0.09	0.09	XXX	■
	UE			0.00	0.77	0.77	0.00	0.77	0.77	XXX	■
K0074	NU		Pneumatic caster tire, any size, each	0.00	1.01	1.01	0.00	1.01	1.01	XXX	■
	RR			0.00	0.12	0.12	0.00	0.12	0.12	XXX	■
	UE			0.00	0.75	0.75	0.00	0.75	0.75	XXX	■
K0075	NU		Semipneumatic caster tire, any size, each	0.00	1.13	1.13	0.00	1.13	1.13	XXX	■
	RR			0.00	0.13	0.13	0.00	0.13	0.13	XXX	■
	UE			0.00	0.86	0.86	0.00	0.86	0.86	XXX	■
K0076	NU		Solid caster tire, any size, each	0.00	0.69	0.69	0.00	0.69	0.69	XXX	■
	RR			0.00	0.08	0.08	0.00	0.08	0.08	XXX	■
	UE			0.00	0.54	0.54	0.00	0.54	0.54	XXX	■
K0077	NU		Front caster assembly, complete, with solid tire, each	0.00	1.67	1.67	0.00	1.67	1.67	XXX	■
	RR			0.00	0.16	0.16	0.00	0.16	0.16	XXX	■
	UE			0.00	1.22	1.22	0.00	1.22	1.22	XXX	■
K0078	NU		Pneumatic caster tire tube, each	0.00	0.30	0.30	0.00	0.30	0.30	XXX	■
	RR			0.00	0.03	0.03	0.00	0.03	0.03	XXX	■
	UE			0.00	0.20	0.20	0.00	0.20	0.20	XXX	■
K0079	NU		Wheel lock extension, pair	0.00	1.67	1.67	0.00	1.67	1.67	XXX	■
	RR			0.00	0.19	0.19	0.00	0.19	0.19	XXX	■
	UE			0.00	0.56	0.56	0.00	0.56	0.56	XXX	■
K0080	NU		Antirollback device, pair	0.00	4.37	4.37	0.00	4.37	4.37	XXX	■
	RR			0.00	0.46	0.46	0.00	0.46	0.46	XXX	■
	UE			0.00	3.32	3.32	0.00	3.32	3.32	XXX	■
K0081	NU		Wheel lock assembly, complete, each	0.00	1.16	1.16	0.00	1.16	1.16	XXX	■
	UE			0.00	0.92	0.92	0.00	0.92	0.92	XXX	■
K0082			22 NF deep cycle lead acid battery, each	0.00	3.13	3.13	0.00	3.13	3.13	XXX	■
K0083			22 NF gel cell battery, each	0.00	3.90	3.90	0.00	3.90	3.90	XXX	■
K0084			Group 24 deep cycle lead acid battery, each	0.00	2.88	2.88	0.00	2.88	2.88	XXX	■
K0085			Group 24 gel cell battery, each	0.00	5.21	5.21	0.00	5.21	5.21	XXX	■
K0086			U-1 lead acid battery, each	0.00	3.13	3.13	0.00	3.13	3.13	XXX	■
K0087			U-1 gel cell battery, each	0.00	3.13	3.13	0.00	3.13	3.13	XXX	■
K0088			Battery charger, lead acid or gel cell	0.00	7.35	7.35	0.00	7.35	7.35	XXX	■
K0089	NU		Battery charger, dual mode	0.00	2.11	2.11	0.00	2.11	2.11	XXX	■
	UE			0.00	1.58	1.58	0.00	1.58	1.58	XXX	■

■ RVU not developed by CMS. Gap-filled RVUs developed by CHEG.

Code	M	S	Description	Work Value	Non-Fac PE	Fac PE	Mal-practice	Non-Fac Total	Fac Total	Global	Gap
K0090	NU		Rear wheel tire for power wheelchair, any size, each	0.00	2.06	2.06	0.00	2.06	2.06	XXX	■
	RR			0.00	0.21	0.21	0.00	0.21	0.21	XXX	■
	UE			0.00	1.52	1.52	0.00	1.52	1.52	XXX	■
K0091	NU		Rear wheel tire tube other than zero pressure for power wheelchair, any size, each	0.00	0.69	0.69	0.00	0.69	0.69	XXX	■
	RR			0.00	0.06	0.06	0.00	0.06	0.06	XXX	■
	UE			0.00	0.66	0.66	0.00	0.66	0.66	XXX	■
K0092	NU		Rear wheel assembly for power wheelchair, complete, each	0.00	6.71	6.71	0.00	6.71	6.71	XXX	■
	RR			0.00	0.66	0.66	0.00	0.66	0.66	XXX	■
	UE			0.00	5.04	5.04	0.00	5.04	5.04	XXX	■
K0093	NU		Rear wheel zero pressure tire tube (flat free insert) for power wheelchair, any size, each	0.00	4.20	4.20	0.00	4.20	4.20	XXX	■
	RR			0.00	0.42	0.42	0.00	0.42	0.42	XXX	■
	UE			0.00	3.07	3.07	0.00	3.07	3.07	XXX	■
K0094	NU		Wheel tire for power base, any size, each	0.00	1.34	1.34	0.00	1.34	1.34	XXX	■
	RR			0.00	0.12	0.12	0.00	0.12	0.12	XXX	■
	UE			0.00	0.98	0.98	0.00	0.98	0.98	XXX	■
K0095	NU		Wheel tire tube other than zero pressure for each base, any size, each	0.00	1.34	1.34	0.00	1.34	1.34	XXX	■
	RR			0.00	0.12	0.12	0.00	0.12	0.12	XXX	■
	UE			0.00	0.98	0.98	0.00	0.98	0.98	XXX	■
K0096	NU		Wheel assembly for power base, complete, each	0.00	7.57	7.57	0.00	7.57	7.57	XXX	■
	RR			0.00	0.75	0.75	0.00	0.75	0.75	XXX	■
	UE			0.00	5.66	5.66	0.00	5.66	5.66	XXX	■
K0097	NU		Wheel zero-pressure tire tube (flat free insert) for power base, any size, each	0.00	1.70	1.70	0.00	1.70	1.70	XXX	■
	RR			0.00	0.18	0.18	0.00	0.18	0.18	XXX	■
	UE			0.00	1.28	1.28	0.00	1.28	1.28	XXX	■
K0098	NU		Drive belt for power wheelchair	0.00	0.72	0.72	0.00	0.72	0.72	XXX	■
	RR			0.00	0.06	0.06	0.00	0.06	0.06	XXX	■
	UE			0.00	0.54	0.54	0.00	0.54	0.54	XXX	■
K0099	NU		Front caster for power wheelchair	0.00	2.18	2.18	0.00	2.18	2.18	XXX	■
	RR			0.00	0.21	0.21	0.00	0.21	0.21	XXX	■
	UE			0.00	1.64	1.64	0.00	1.64	1.64	XXX	■
K0100	NU		Wheelchair adapter for amputee, pair	0.00	2.68	2.68	0.00	2.68	2.68	XXX	■
	RR			0.00	0.33	0.33	0.00	0.33	0.33	XXX	■
	UE			0.00	2.09	2.09	0.00	2.09	2.09	XXX	■
K0101	NU		One-arm drive attachment, each	0.00	15.26	15.26	0.00	15.26	15.26	XXX	■
	RR			0.00	1.07	1.07	0.00	1.07	1.07	XXX	■
	UE			0.00	11.29	11.29	0.00	11.29	11.29	XXX	■
K0102	NU		Crutch and cane holder, each	0.00	1.16	1.16	0.00	1.16	1.16	XXX	■
	RR			0.00	0.12	0.12	0.00	0.12	0.12	XXX	■
	UE			0.00	0.86	0.86	0.00	0.86	0.86	XXX	■
K0103	NU		Transfer board, less than 25 inches	0.00	1.55	1.55	0.00	1.55	1.55	XXX	■
	RR			0.00	0.15	0.15	0.00	0.15	0.15	XXX	■
	UE			0.00	1.07	1.07	0.00	1.07	1.07	XXX	■
K0104	NU		Cylinder tank carrier, each	0.00	3.19	3.19	0.00	3.19	3.19	XXX	■
	RR			0.00	0.33	0.33	0.00	0.33	0.33	XXX	■
	UE			0.00	2.38	2.38	0.00	2.38	2.38	XXX	■

■ RVU not developed by CMS. Gap-filled RVUs developed by CHEG.

Code	M	S	Description	Work Value	Non-Fac PE	Fac PE	Mal-practice	Non-Fac Total	Fac Total	Global	Gap
K0105	NU		IV hanger, each	0.00	2.68	2.68	0.00	2.68	2.68	XXX	■
	RR			0.00	0.27	0.27	0.00	0.27	0.27	XXX	■
	UE			0.00	2.00	2.00	0.00	2.00	2.00	XXX	■
K0106	NU		Arm trough, each	0.00	2.89	2.89	0.00	2.89	2.89	XXX	■
	RR			0.00	0.30	0.30	0.00	0.30	0.30	XXX	■
	UE			0.00	2.15	2.15	0.00	2.15	2.15	XXX	■
K0107	NU		Wheelchair tray	0.00	2.80	2.80	0.00	2.80	2.80	XXX	■
	RR			0.00	0.27	0.27	0.00	0.27	0.27	XXX	■
	UE			0.00	2.09	2.09	0.00	2.09	2.09	XXX	■
K0108			Other accessories	0.00	0.00	0.00	0.00	0.00	0.00	XXX	
K0112			Trunk support device, vest type, with inner frame, prefabricated	0.00	7.36	7.36	0.00	7.36	7.36	XXX	■
K0113			Trunk support device, vest type, without inner frame, prefabricated	0.00	4.47	4.47	0.00	4.47	4.47	XXX	■
K0114	NU		Back support system for use with a wheelchair, with inner frame, prefabricated	0.00	22.86	22.86	0.00	22.86	22.86	XXX	■
	RR			0.00	2.32	2.32	0.00	2.32	2.32	XXX	■
	UE			0.00	17.14	17.14	0.00	17.14	17.14	XXX	■
K0115	NU		Seating system, back module, posterior-lateral control, with or without lateral supports, custom fabricated for attachment to wheelchair base	0.00	23.33	23.33	0.00	23.33	23.33	XXX	■
	RR			0.00	2.32	2.32	0.00	2.32	2.32	XXX	■
	UE			0.00	17.49	17.49	0.00	17.49	17.49	XXX	■
K0116	NU		Seating system, combined back and seat module, custom fabricated for attachment to wheelchair base	0.00	48.72	48.72	0.00	48.72	48.72	XXX	■
	RR			0.00	4.86	4.86	0.00	4.86	4.86	XXX	■
	UE			0.00	36.53	36.53	0.00	36.53	36.53	XXX	■
K0183			Nasal application device used with positive airway pressure device	0.00	2.22	2.22	0.00	2.22	2.22	XXX	■
K0184			Nasal single piece interface, replacement for nasal application device, pair or single piece interface	0.00	0.68	0.68	0.00	0.68	0.68	XXX	■
K0185			Headgear used with positive airway pressure device	0.00	1.10	1.10	0.00	1.10	1.10	XXX	■
K0186			Chin strap used with positive airway pressure device	0.00	0.51	0.51	0.00	0.51	0.51	XXX	■
K0187			Tubing used with positive airway pressure device	0.00	1.13	1.13	0.00	1.13	1.13	XXX	■
K0188			Filter, disposable, used with positive airway pressure device	0.00	0.15	0.15	0.00	0.15	0.15	XXX	■
K0189			Filter, nondisposable, used with positive airway pressure device	0.00	0.42	0.42	0.00	0.42	0.42	XXX	■
K0195			Elevating legrest, pair (for use with capped rental wheelchair base)	0.00	3.28	3.28	0.00	3.28	3.28	XXX	■
K0268			Humidifier, nonheated, used with positive airway pressure device	0.00	0.00	0.00	0.00	0.00	0.00	XXX	

■ RVU not developed by CMS. Gap-filled RVUs developed by CHEG.

Code	M	S	Description	Work Value	Non-Fac PE	Fac PE	Mal-practice	Non-Fac Total	Fac Total	Global	Gap
K0415			Prescription antiemetic drug, oral, per 1 mg, for use in conjunction with oral anti-cancer drug, not otherwise specified	0.00	0.00	0.00	0.00	0.00	0.00	XXX	
K0416			Prescription antiemetic drug, rectal, per 1 mg, for use in conjunction with oral anti-cancer drug, not otherwise specified	0.00	0.00	0.00	0.00	0.00	0.00	XXX	
K0452			Wheelchair bearings, any type	0.00	0.00	0.00	0.00	0.00	0.00	XXX	
K0455			Infusion pump used for uninterrupted administration of epoprostenol	0.00	0.00	0.00	0.00	0.00	0.00	XXX	
K0460			Power add-on, to convert manual wheelchair to motorized wheelchair, joystick control	0.00	0.00	0.00	0.00	0.00	0.00	XXX	
K0461			Power add-on, to convert manual wheelchair to power operated vehicle, tiller control	0.00	0.00	0.00	0.00	0.00	0.00	XXX	
K0462			Temporary replacement for patient owned equipment being repaired, any type	0.00	0.00	0.00	0.00	0.00	0.00	XXX	
K0531			Humidifier, heated, used with positive airway pressure device	0.00	0.00	0.00	0.00	0.00	0.00	XXX	
K0532			Respiratory assist device, bi-level pressure capability, without backup rate feature, used with noninvasive interface, e.g., nasal or facial mask (intermittent assist device with continuous positive airway pressure device)	0.00	0.00	0.00	0.00	0.00	0.00	XXX	
K0533			Respiratory assist device, bi-level pressure capability, with backup rate feature, used with noninvasive interface, e.g., nasal or facial mask (intermittent assist device with continuous positive airway pressure device)	0.00	0.00	0.00	0.00	0.00	0.00	XXX	
K0534			Respiratory assist device, bi-level pressure capacity, with backup rate feature, used with invasive interface, e.g., tracheostomy tube (intermittent assist device with continuous positive airway pressure device)	0.00	0.00	0.00	0.00	0.00	0.00	XXX	
K0538	**RR**		Negative pressure wound therapy electrical pump, stationary or portable	0.00	0.00	0.00	0.00	0.00	0.00	XXX	
K0539			Dressing set for negative pressure wound therapy electrical pump, stationary or portable, each	0.00	0.00	0.00	0.00	0.00	0.00	XXX	
K0540			Canister set for negative pressure wound therapy electrical pump, stationary or portable, each	0.00	0.00	0.00	0.00	0.00	0.00	XXX	
K0541			Speech generating device, digitized speech, using pre-recorded messages, less than or equal to eight minutes recording time	0.00	0.00	0.00	0.00	0.00	0.00	XXX	
K0542			Speech generating device, digitized speech, using pre-recorded messages, greater than 8 minutes recording time	0.00	0.00	0.00	0.00	0.00	0.00	XXX	

■ RVU not developed by CMS. Gap-filled RVUs developed by CHEG.

Code	M	S	Description	Work Value	Non-Fac PE	Fac PE	Mal-practice	Non-Fac Total	Fac Total	Global	Gap
K0543			Speech generating device, synthesized speech, requiring message formulation by spelling and access by physical contact with the device	0.00	0.00	0.00	0.00	0.00	0.00	XXX	
K0544			Speech generating device, synthesized speech, permitting multiple methods of message formulation and multiple methods of device access	0.00	0.00	0.00	0.00	0.00	0.00	XXX	
K0545			Speech generating software program, for personal computer or personal digital assistant	0.00	0.00	0.00	0.00	0.00	0.00	XXX	
K0546			Accessory for speech generating device, mounting system	0.00	0.00	0.00	0.00	0.00	0.00	XXX	
K0547			Accessory for speech generating device, not otherwise classified	0.00	0.00	0.00	0.00	0.00	0.00	XXX	
K0548		I	Nonemergency transportation: per mile — volunteer, with no vested or personal interest	0.00	0.06	0.06	0.00	0.06	0.06	XXX	
K0551			Residual limb support system, solid base with adjustable drop hooks, mounts to wheelchair frame, each	0.00	0.00	0.00	0.00	0.00	0.00	XXX	
L0100			Cranial orthosis (helmet), with or without soft interface, molded to patient model	0.00	14.91	14.91	0.00	14.91	14.91	XXX	■
L0110			Cranial orthosis (helmet), with or without soft-interface, non-molded	0.00	3.72	3.72	0.00	3.72	3.72	XXX	■
L0120			Cervical, flexible, nonadjustable (foam collar)	0.00	0.17	0.17	0.00	0.17	0.17	XXX	■
L0130			Cervical, flexible, thermoplastic collar, molded to patient	0.00	4.22	4.22	0.00	4.22	4.22	XXX	■
L0140			Cervical, semi-rigid, adjustable (plastic collar)	0.00	1.65	1.65	0.00	1.65	1.65	XXX	■
L0150			Cervical, semi-rigid, adjustable molded chin cup (plastic collar with mandibular/occipital piece)	0.00	0.71	0.71	0.00	0.71	0.71	XXX	■
L0160			Cervical, semi-rigid, wire frame occipital/ mandibular support	0.00	3.49	3.49	0.00	3.49	3.49	XXX	■
L0170			Cervical, collar, molded to patient model	0.00	16.70	16.70	0.00	16.70	16.70	XXX	■
L0172			Cervical, collar, semi-rigid thermoplastic foam, two piece	0.00	3.29	3.29	0.00	3.29	3.29	XXX	■
L0174			Cervical, collar, semi-rigid, thermoplastic foam, two piece with thoracic extension	0.00	7.12	7.12	0.00	7.12	7.12	XXX	■
L0180			Cervical, multiple post collar, occipital/ mandibular supports, adjustable	0.00	3.58	3.58	0.00	3.58	3.58	XXX	■
L0190			Cervical, multiple post collar, occipital/ mandibular supports, adjustable cervical bars (Somi, Guilford, Taylor types)	0.00	12.83	12.83	0.00	12.83	12.83	XXX	■

■ RVU not developed by CMS. Gap-filled RVUs developed by CHEG.

Code	M	S	Description	Work Value	Non-Fac PE	Fac PE	Mal-practice	Non-Fac Total	Fac Total	Global	Gap
L0200			Cervical, multiple post collar, occipital/ mandibular supports, adjustable cervical bars, and thoracic extension	0.00	13.37	13.37	0.00	13.37	13.37	XXX	■
L0210			Thoracic, rib belt	0.00	1.15	1.15	0.00	1.15	1.15	XXX	■
L0220			Thoracic, rib belt, custom fabricated	0.00	3.17	3.17	0.00	3.17	3.17	XXX	■
L0300			TLSO, flexible (dorso-lumbar surgical support)	0.00	4.50	4.50	0.00	4.50	4.50	XXX	■
L0310			TLSO, flexible (dorso-lumbar surgical support), custom fabricated	0.00	8.52	8.52	0.00	8.52	8.52	XXX	■
L0315			TLSO, flexible (dorso-lumbar surgical support), elastic type, with rigid posterior panel	0.00	6.81	6.81	0.00	6.81	6.81	XXX	■
L0317			TLSO, flexible (dorso-lumbar surgical support), hyperextension, elastic type, with rigid posterior panel	0.00	9.24	9.24	0.00	9.24	9.24	XXX	■
L0320			TLSO, anterior-posterior control (Taylor type), with apron front	0.00	3.19	3.19	0.00	3.19	3.19	XXX	■
L0321			TLSO, anterior-posterior control, with rigid or semi-rigid posterior panel, prefabricated (includes fitting and adjustment)	0.00	10.43	10.43	0.00	10.43	10.43	XXX	■
L0330			TLSO, anterior-posterior-lateral control (Knight-Taylor type), with apron front	0.00	11.87	11.87	0.00	11.87	11.87	XXX	■
L0331			TLSO, anterior-posterior-lateral control, with rigid or semi-rigid posterior panel, prefabricated (includes fitting and adjustment)	0.00	12.93	12.93	0.00	12.93	12.93	XXX	■
L0340			TLSO, anterior-posterior-lateral-rotary control (Arnold, Magnuson, Steindler types), with apron front	0.00	16.90	16.90	0.00	16.90	16.90	XXX	■
L0350			TLSO, anterior-posterior-lateral-rotary control, flexion compression jacket, custom fitted	0.00	24.79	24.79	0.00	24.79	24.79	XXX	■
L0360			TLSO, anterior-posterior-lateral-rotary control, flexion compression jacket molded to patient model	0.00	36.69	36.69	0.00	36.69	36.69	XXX	■
L0370			TLSO, anterior-posterior-lateral-rotary control, hyperextension (Jewett, Lennox, Baker, Cash types)	0.00	10.46	10.46	0.00	10.46	10.46	XXX	■
L0380			TLSO, anterior-posterior-lateral-rotary control, with extensions	0.00	16.11	16.11	0.00	16.11	16.11	XXX	■
L0390			TLSO, anterior-posterior-lateral control molded to patient model	0.00	36.87	36.87	0.00	36.87	36.87	XXX	■
L0391			TLSO, anterior-posterior-lateral-rotary control, with rigid or semi-rigid posterior panel, prefabricated (includes fitting and adjustment)	0.00	40.23	40.23	0.00	40.23	40.23	XXX	■
L0400			TLSO, anterior-posterior-lateral control molded to patient model, with interface material	0.00	40.15	40.15	0.00	40.15	40.15	XXX	■

■ RVU not developed by CMS. Gap-filled RVUs developed by CHEG.

Code	M	S	Description	Work Value	Non-Fac PE	Fac PE	Mal-practice	Non-Fac Total	Fac Total	Global	Gap
L0410			TLSO, anterior-posterior-lateral control, two-piece construction, molded to patient model	0.00	46.01	46.01	0.00	46.01	46.01	XXX	■
L0420			TLSO, anterior-posterior-lateral control, two-piece construction, molded to patient model, with interface material	0.00	48.81	48.81	0.00	48.81	48.81	XXX	■
L0430			TLSO, anterior-posterior-lateral control, with interface material, custom fitted	0.00	34.69	34.69	0.00	34.69	34.69	XXX	■
L0440			TLSO, anterior-posterior-lateral control, with overlapping front section, spring steel front, custom fitted	0.00	29.01	29.01	0.00	29.01	29.01	XXX	■
L0500			LSO, flexible (lumbo-sacral surgical support)	0.00	3.52	3.52	0.00	3.52	3.52	XXX	■
L0510			LSO, flexible (lumbo-sacral surgical support), custom fabricated	0.00	7.12	7.12	0.00	7.12	7.12	XXX	■
L0515			LSO, anterior-posterior control, with rigid or semi-rigid posterior panel, prefabricated	0.00	4.74	4.74	0.00	4.74	4.74	XXX	■
L0520			LSO, anterior-posterior-lateral control (Knight, Wilcox types), with apron front	0.00	3.13	3.13	0.00	3.13	3.13	XXX	■
L0530			LSO, anterior-posterior control (Macausland type), with apron front	0.00	10.73	10.73	0.00	10.73	10.73	XXX	■
L0540			LSO, lumbar flexion (Williams flexion type)	0.00	3.46	3.46	0.00	3.46	3.46	XXX	■
L0550			LSO, anterior-posterior-lateral control, molded to patient model	0.00	34.25	34.25	0.00	34.25	34.25	XXX	■
L0560			LSO, anterior-posterior-lateral control, molded to patient model, with interface material	0.00	37.41	37.41	0.00	37.41	37.41	XXX	■
L0561			LSO, anterior-posterior-lateral control, with rigid or semi-rigid posterior panel, prefabricated	0.00	40.02	40.02	0.00	40.02	40.02	XXX	■
L0565			LSO, anterior-posterior-lateral control, custom fitted	0.00	29.03	29.03	0.00	29.03	29.03	XXX	■
L0600			Sacroiliac, flexible (sacroiliac surgical support)	0.00	2.38	2.38	0.00	2.38	2.38	XXX	■
L0610			Sacroiliac, flexible (sacroiliac surgical support), custom fabricated	0.00	6.69	6.69	0.00	6.69	6.69	XXX	■
L0620			Sacroiliac, semi-rigid (Goldthwaite, Osgood types), with apron front	0.00	10.96	10.96	0.00	10.96	10.96	XXX	■
L0700			CTLSO, anterior-posterior-lateral control, molded to patient model (Minerva type)	0.00	52.34	52.34	0.00	52.34	52.34	XXX	■
L0710			CTLSO, anterior-posterior-lateral control, molded to patient model, with interface material (Minerva type)	0.00	54.07	54.07	0.00	54.07	54.07	XXX	■
L0810			Halo procedure, cervical halo incorporated into jacket vest	0.00	66.79	66.79	0.00	66.79	66.79	XXX	■

■ RVU not developed by CMS. Gap-filled RVUs developed by CHEG.

Code	M	S	Description	Work Value	Non-Fac PE	Fac PE	Mal-practice	Non-Fac Total	Fac Total	Global	Gap
L0820			Halo procedure, cervical halo incorporated into plaster body jacket	0.00	55.93	55.93	0.00	55.93	55.93	XXX	■
L0830			Halo procedure, cervical halo incorporated into Milwaukee type orthosis	0.00	81.19	81.19	0.00	81.19	81.19	XXX	■
L0860			Addition to halo procedure, magnetic resonance image compatible system	0.00	31.54	31.54	0.00	31.54	31.54	XXX	■
L0900			Torso support, ptosis support	0.00	4.14	4.14	0.00	4.14	4.14	XXX	■
L0910			Torso support, ptosis support, custom fabricated	0.00	9.00	9.00	0.00	9.00	9.00	XXX	■
L0920			Torso support, pendulous abdomen support	0.00	4.40	4.40	0.00	4.40	4.40	XXX	■
L0930			Torso support, pendulous abdomen support, custom fabricated	0.00	9.80	9.80	0.00	9.80	9.80	XXX	■
L0940			Torso support, postsurgical support	0.00	4.10	4.10	0.00	4.10	4.10	XXX	■
L0950			Torso support, postsurgical support, custom fabricated	0.00	8.91	8.91	0.00	8.91	8.91	XXX	■
L0960			Torso support, postsurgical support, pads for postsurgical support	0.00	1.79	1.79	0.00	1.79	1.79	XXX	■
L0970			TLSO, corset front	0.00	2.96	2.96	0.00	2.96	2.96	XXX	■
L0972			LSO, corset front	0.00	2.67	2.67	0.00	2.67	2.67	XXX	■
L0974			TLSO, full corset	0.00	4.63	4.63	0.00	4.63	4.63	XXX	■
L0976			LSO, full corset	0.00	4.14	4.14	0.00	4.14	4.14	XXX	■
L0978			Axillary crutch extension	0.00	4.98	4.98	0.00	4.98	4.98	XXX	■
L0980			Peroneal straps, pair	0.00	0.45	0.45	0.00	0.45	0.45	XXX	■
L0982			Stocking supporter grips, set of four (4)	0.00	0.42	0.42	0.00	0.42	0.42	XXX	■
L0984			Protective body sock, each	0.00	1.55	1.55	0.00	1.55	1.55	XXX	■
L0986			Addition to spinal orthosis, rigid or semi-rigid abdominal panel, prefabricated	0.00	0.00	0.00	0.00	0.00	0.00	XXX	
L0999			Addition to spinal orthosis, not otherwise specified	0.00	0.00	0.00	0.00	0.00	0.00	XXX	
L1000			CTLSO (Milwaukee), inclusive of furnishing initial orthosis, including model	0.00	52.57	52.57	0.00	52.57	52.57	XXX	■
L1005			Tension based scoliosis orthosis and accessory pads, includes fitting and adjustment	0.00	0.00	0.00	0.00	0.00	0.00	XXX	
L1010			Addition to CTLSO or scoliosis orthosis, axilla sling	0.00	1.74	1.74	0.00	1.74	1.74	XXX	■
L1020			Addition to CTLSO or scoliosis orthosis, kyphosis pad	0.00	2.24	2.24	0.00	2.24	2.24	XXX	■

■ RVU not developed by CMS. Gap-filled RVUs developed by CHEG.

Code	M	S	Description	Work Value	Non-Fac PE	Fac PE	Mal-prac-tice	Non-Fac Total	Fac Total	Global	Gap
L1025			Addition to CTLSO or scoliosis orthosis, kyphosis pad, floating	0.00	3.23	3.23	0.00	3.23	3.23	XXX	■
L1030			Addition to CTLSO or scoliosis orthosis, lumbar bolster pad	0.00	1.65	1.65	0.00	1.65	1.65	XXX	■
L1040			Addition to CTLSO or scoliosis orthosis, lumbar or lumbar rib pad	0.00	2.02	2.02	0.00	2.02	2.02	XXX	■
L1050			Addition to CTLSO or scoliosis orthosis, sternal pad	0.00	2.15	2.15	0.00	2.15	2.15	XXX	■
L1060			Addition to CTLSO or scoliosis orthosis, thoracic pad	0.00	2.47	2.47	0.00	2.47	2.47	XXX	■
L1070			Addition to CTLSO or scoliosis orthosis, trapezius sling	0.00	2.33	2.33	0.00	2.33	2.33	XXX	■
L1080			Addition to CTLSO or scoliosis orthosis, outrigger	0.00	1.43	1.43	0.00	1.43	1.43	XXX	■
L1085			Addition to CTLSO or scoliosis orthosis, outrigger, bilateral with vertical extensions	0.00	3.99	3.99	0.00	3.99	3.99	XXX	■
L1090			Addition to CTLSO or scoliosis orthosis, lumbar sling	0.00	2.38	2.38	0.00	2.38	2.38	XXX	■
L1100			Addition to CTLSO or scoliosis orthosis, ring flange, plastic or leather	0.00	4.12	4.12	0.00	4.12	4.12	XXX	■
L1110			Addition to CTLSO or scoliosis orthosis, ring flange, plastic or leather, molded to patient model	0.00	6.62	6.62	0.00	6.62	6.62	XXX	■
L1120			Addition to CTLSO, scoliosis orthosis, cover for upright, each	0.00	1.03	1.03	0.00	1.03	1.03	XXX	■
L1200			TLSO, inclusive of furnishing initial orthosis only	0.00	40.57	40.57	0.00	40.57	40.57	XXX	■
L1210			Addition to TLSO, (low profile), lateral thoracic extension	0.00	6.77	6.77	0.00	6.77	6.77	XXX	■
L1220			Addition to TLSO, (low profile), anterior thoracic extension	0.00	5.74	5.74	0.00	5.74	5.74	XXX	■
L1230			Addition to TLSO, (low profile), Milwaukee type superstructure	0.00	14.72	14.72	0.00	14.72	14.72	XXX	■
L1240			Addition to TLSO, (low profile), lumbar derotation pad	0.00	2.01	2.01	0.00	2.01	2.01	XXX	■
L1250			Addition to TLSO, (low profile), anterior ASIS pad	0.00	1.87	1.87	0.00	1.87	1.87	XXX	■
L1260			Addition to TLSO, (low profile), anterior thoracic derotation pad	0.00	1.96	1.96	0.00	1.96	1.96	XXX	■
L1270			Addition to TLSO, (low profile), abdominal pad	0.00	2.00	2.00	0.00	2.00	2.00	XXX	■
L1280			Addition to TLSO, (low profile), rib gusset (elastic), each	0.00	2.24	2.24	0.00	2.24	2.24	XXX	■

■ RVU not developed by CMS. Gap-filled RVUs developed by CHEG.

Code	M	S	Description	Work Value	Non-Fac PE	Fac PE	Mal-practice	Non-Fac Total	Fac Total	Global	Gap
L1290			Addition to TLSO, (low profile), lateral trochanteric pad	0.00	2.03	2.03	0.00	2.03	2.03	XXX	■
L1300			Other scoliosis procedure, body jacket molded to patient model .	0.00	43.25	43.25	0.00	43.25	43.25	XXX	■
L1310			Other scoliosis procedure, postoperative body jacket	0.00	44.51	44.51	0.00	44.51	44.51	XXX	■
L1499			Spinal orthosis, not otherwise specified	0.00	0.00	0.00	0.00	0.00	0.00	XXX	
L1500			THKAO, mobility frame (Newington, Parapodium types)	0.00	49.17	49.17	0.00	49.17	49.17	XXX	■
L1510			THKAO, standing frame, with or without tray and accessories	0.00	31.11	31.11	0.00	31.11	31.11	XXX	■
L1520			THKAO, swivel walker	0.00	59.07	59.07	0.00	59.07	59.07	XXX	■
L1600			HO, abduction control of hip joints, flexible, Frejka type with cover, prefabricated, includes fitting and adjustment	0.00	3.34	3.34	0.00	3.34	3.34	XXX	■
L1610			HO, abduction control of hip joints, flexible, (Frejka cover only), prefabricated, includes fitting and adjustment	0.00	1.14	1.14	0.00	1.14	1.14	XXX	■
L1620			HO, abduction control of hip joints, flexible, (Pavlik harness), prefabricated, includes fitting and adjustment	0.00	3.47	3.47	0.00	3.47	3.47	XXX	■
L1630			HO, abduction control of hip joints, semi-flexible (Von Rosen type), custom fabricated	0.00	4.39	4.39	0.00	4.39	4.39	XXX	■
L1640			HO, abduction control of hip joints, static, pelvic band or spreader bar, thigh cuffs, custom fabricated	0.00	11.95	11.95	0.00	11.95	11.95	XXX	■
L1650			HO, abduction control of hip joints, static, adjustable (Ilfled type), prefabricated, includes fitting and adjustment	0.00	5.99	5.99	0.00	5.99	5.99	XXX	■
L1660			HO, abduction control of hip joints, static, plastic, prefabricated, includes fitting and adjustment	0.00	4.44	4.44	0.00	4.44	4.44	XXX	■
L1680			HO, abduction control of hip joints, dynamic, pelvic control, adjustable hip motion control, thigh cuffs (Rancho hip action type), custom fabricated	0.00	31.55	31.55	0.00	31.55	31.55	XXX	■
L1685			HO, abduction control of hip joint, postoperative hip abduction type, custom fabricated	0.00	30.78	30.78	0.00	30.78	30.78	XXX	■
L1686			HO, abduction control of hip joint, postoperative hip abduction type, prefabricated, includes fitting and adjustments	0.00	23.62	23.62	0.00	23.62	23.62	XXX	■

■ RVU not developed by CMS. Gap-filled RVUs developed by CHEG.

Code	M	S	Description	Work Value	Non-Fac PE	Fac PE	Mal-practice	Non-Fac Total	Fac Total	Global	Gap
L1690			Combination, bilateral, lumbo-sacral, hip, femur orthosis providing adduction and internal rotation control, prefabricated, includes fitting and adjustment	0.00	0.00	0.00	0.00	0.00	0.00	XXX	
L1700			Legg Perthes orthosis, (Toronto type), custom fabricated	0.00	39.54	39.54	0.00	39.54	39.54	XXX	■
L1710			Legg Perthes orthosis, (Newington type), custom fabricated	0.00	46.29	46.29	0.00	46.29	46.29	XXX	■
L1720			Legg Perthes orthosis, trilateral, (Tachdijan type), custom fabricated	0.00	34.12	34.12	0.00	34.12	34.12	XXX	■
L1730			Legg Perthes orthosis, (Scottish Rite type), custom fabricated	0.00	29.30	29.30	0.00	29.30	29.30	XXX	■
L1750			Legg Perthes orthosis, Legg Perthes sling (Sam Brown type), prefabricated, includes fitting and adjustment	0.00	5.10	5.10	0.00	5.10	5.10	XXX	■
L1755			Legg Perthes orthosis, (Patten bottom type), custom fabricated	0.00	40.99	40.99	0.00	40.99	40.99	XXX	■
L1800			KO, elastic with stays, prefabricated, includes fitting and adjustment	0.00	1.22	1.22	0.00	1.22	1.22	XXX	■
L1810			KO, elastic with joints, prefabricated, includes fitting and adjustment	0.00	2.28	2.28	0.00	2.28	2.28	XXX	■
L1815			KO, elastic or other elastic type material with condylar pad(s), prefabricated, includes fitting and adjustment	0.00	2.13	2.13	0.00	2.13	2.13	XXX	■
L1820			KO, elastic with condylar pads and joints, prefabricated, includes fitting and adjustment	0.00	3.01	3.01	0.00	3.01	3.01	XXX	■
L1825			KO, elastic knee cap, prefabricated, includes fitting and adjustment	0.00	0.69	0.69	0.00	0.69	0.69	XXX	■
L1830			KO, immobilizer, canvas longitudinal, prefabricated, inlcudes fitting and adjustment	0.00	1.82	1.82	0.00	1.82	1.82	XXX	■
L1832			KO, adjustable knee joints, positional orthosis, rigid support, prefabricated, includes fitting and adjustment	0.00	14.30	14.30	0.00	14.30	14.30	XXX	■
L1834			KO, without knee joint, rigid, custom fabricated	0.00	18.30	18.30	0.00	18.30	18.30	XXX	■
L1840			KO, derotation, medial-lateral, anterior cruciate ligament, custom fabricated	0.00	21.28	21.28	0.00	21.28	21.28	XXX	■
L1843			KO, single upright, thigh and calf, with adjustable flexion and extension joint, medial-lateral and rotation control, prefabricated, includes fitting and adjustment	0.00	0.00	0.00	0.00	0.00	0.00	XXX	
L1844			KO, single upright, thigh and calf, with adjustable flexion and extension joint, medial-lateral and rotation control, custom fabricated	0.00	33.02	33.02	0.00	33.02	33.02	XXX	■

■ RVU not developed by CMS. Gap-filled RVUs developed by CHEG.

Code	M	S	Description	Work Value	Non-Fac PE	Fac PE	Mal-practice	Non-Fac Total	Fac Total	Global	Gap
L1845			KO, double upright, thigh and calf, with adjustable flexion and extension joint, medial-lateral and rotation control, prefabricated, includes fitting and adjustment	0.00	19.16	19.16	0.00	19.16	19.16	XXX	■
L1846			KO, double upright, thigh and calf, with adjustable flexion and extension joint, medial-lateral and rotation control, custom fabricated	0.00	25.85	25.85	0.00	25.85	25.85	XXX	■
L1847			KO, double upright with adjustable joint, with inflatable air support chamber(s), prefabricated, includes fitting and adjustment	0.00	0.00	0.00	0.00	0.00	0.00	XXX	
L1850			KO, Swedish type, prefabricated, includes fitting and adjustment	0.00	5.96	5.96	0.00	5.96	5.96	XXX	■
L1855			KO, molded plastic, thigh and calf sections, with double upright knee joints, custom fabricated	0.00	28.45	28.45	0.00	28.45	28.45	XXX	■
L1858			KO, molded plastic, polycentric knee joints, pneumatic knee pads (CTI), custom fabricated	0.00	27.42	27.42	0.00	27.42	27.42	XXX	■
L1860			KO, modification of supracondylar prosthetic socket, custom fabricated (SK)	0.00	27.78	27.78	0.00	27.78	27.78	XXX	■
L1870			KO, double upright, thigh and calf lacers, with knee joints, custom fabricated	0.00	27.10	27.10	0.00	27.10	27.10	XXX	■
L1880			KO, double upright, nonmolded thigh and calf cuffs/lacers with knee joints, custom fabricated	0.00	18.33	18.33	0.00	18.33	18.33	XXX	■
L1885			KO, single or double upright, thigh and calf, with funtional active resistance control, prefabricated, includes fitting and adjustment	0.00	21.61	21.61	0.00	21.61	21.61	XXX	■
L1900			AFO, spring wire, dorsiflexion assist calf band, custom fabricated	0.00	6.97	6.97	0.00	6.97	6.97	XXX	■
L1902			AFO, ankle gauntlet, prefabricated, includes fitting and adjustment	0.00	1.67	1.67	0.00	1.67	1.67	XXX	■
L1904			AFO, molded ankle gauntlet, custom fabricated	0.00	12.19	12.19	0.00	12.19	12.19	XXX	■
L1906			AFO, multiligamentus ankle support, prefabricated, includes fitting and adjustment	0.00	2.13	2.13	0.00	2.13	2.13	XXX	■
L1910			AFO, posterior, single bar, clasp attachment to shoe counter, prefabricated, includes fitting and adjustment	0.00	6.92	6.92	0.00	6.92	6.92	XXX	■
L1920			AFO, single upright with static or adjustable stop (Phelps or Perlstein type), custom fabricated	0.00	9.06	9.06	0.00	9.06	9.06	XXX	■
L1930			Ankle foot orthosis, plastic or other material, prefabricated, includes fitting and adjustment	0.00	6.12	6.12	0.00	6.12	6.12	XXX	■
L1940			Ankle foot orthosis, plastic or other material, custom-fabricated	0.00	12.81	12.81	0.00	12.81	12.81	XXX	■

■ RVU not developed by CMS. Gap-filled RVUs developed by CHEG.

Code	M	S	Description	Work Value	Non-Fac PE	Fac PE	Mal-practice	Non-Fac Total	Fac Total	Global	Gap
L1945			AFO, molded to patient model, plastic, rigid anterior tibial section (floor reaction), custom fabricated	0.00	23.96	23.96	0.00	23.96	23.96	XXX	■
L1950			AFO, spiral, (IRM type), plastic, custom fabricated	0.00	19.29	19.29	0.00	19.29	19.29	XXX	■
L1960			AFO, posterior solid ankle, plastic, custom fabricated	0.00	14.35	14.35	0.00	14.35	14.35	XXX	■
L1970			AFO, plastic, with ankle joint, custom fabricated	0.00	18.42	18.42	0.00	18.42	18.42	XXX	■
L1980			AFO, single upright free plantar dorsiflexion, solid stirrup, calf band/cuff (single bar "BK" orthosis), custom fabricated	0.00	9.51	9.51	0.00	9.51	9.51	XXX	■
L1990			AFO, double upright free plantar dorsiflexion, solid stirrup, calf band/cuff (double bar "BK" orthosis), custom fabricated	0.00	11.54	11.54	0.00	11.54	11.54	XXX	■
L2000			KAFO, single upright, free knee, free ankle, solid stirrup, thigh and calf bands/cuffs (single bar "AK" orthosis), custom fabricated	0.00	26.26	26.26	0.00	26.26	26.26	XXX	■
L2010			KAFO, single upright, free ankle, solid stirrup, thigh and calf bands/cuffs (single bar "AK" orthosis), without knee joint, custom fabricated	0.00	23.94	23.94	0.00	23.94	23.94	XXX	■
L2020			KAFO, double upright, free knee, free ankle, solid stirrup, thigh and calf bands/cuffs (double bar "AK" orthosis), custom fabricated	0.00	30.23	30.23	0.00	30.23	30.23	XXX	■
L2030			KAFO, double upright, free ankle, solid stirrup, thigh and calf bands/cuffs, (double bar "AK" orthosis), without knee joint, custom fabricated	0.00	26.22	26.22	0.00	26.22	26.22	XXX	■
L2035			KAFO, full plastic, static, (pediatric size), prefabricated, includes fitting and adjustment	0.00	1.64	1.64	0.00	1.64	1.64	XXX	■
L2036			KAFO, full plastic, double upright, free knee, custom fabricated	0.00	48.04	48.04	0.00	48.04	48.04	XXX	■
L2037			KAFO, full plastic, single upright, free knee, custom fabricated	0.00	43.12	43.12	0.00	43.12	43.12	XXX	■
L2038			KAFO, full plastic, without knee joint, multiaxis ankle, (Lively orthosis or equal), custom fabricated	0.00	37.01	37.01	0.00	37.01	37.01	XXX	■
L2039			KAFO, full plastic, single upright, poly-axial hinge, medial lateral rotation control, custom fabricated	0.00	0.00	0.00	0.00	0.00	0.00	XXX	
L2040			HKAFO, torsion control, bilateral rotation straps, pelvic band/belt, custom fabricated	0.00	4.60	4.60	0.00	4.60	4.60	XXX	■
L2050			HKAFO, torsion control, bilateral torsion cables, hip joint, pelvic band/belt, custom fabricated	0.00	12.34	12.34	0.00	12.34	12.34	XXX	■

■ RVU not developed by CMS. Gap-filled RVUs developed by CHEG.

Code	M	S	Description	Work Value	Non-Fac PE	Fac PE	Mal-practice	Non-Fac Total	Fac Total	Global	Gap
L2060			HKAFO, torsion control, bilateral torsion cables, ball bearing hip joint, pelvic band/ belt, custom fabricated	0.00	15.03	15.03	0.00	15.03	15.03	XXX	■
L2070			HKAFO, torsion control, unilateral rotation straps, pelvic band/belt, custom fabricated	0.00	3.49	3.49	0.00	3.49	3.49	XXX	■
L2080			HKAFO, torsion control, unilateral torsion cable, hip joint, pelvic band/belt, custom fabricated	0.00	9.31	9.31	0.00	9.31	9.31	XXX	■
L2090			HKAFO, torsion control, unilateral torsion cable, ball bearing hip joint, pelvic band/belt, custom fabricated	0.00	11.35	11.35	0.00	11.35	11.35	XXX	■
L2102			AFO, fracture orthosis, tibial fracture cast orthosis, plaster type casting material, custom fabricated	0.00	12.05	12.05	0.00	12.05	12.05	XXX	■
L2104			AFO, fracture orthosis, tibial fracture cast orthosis, synthetic type casting material, custom fabricated	0.00	12.78	12.78	0.00	12.78	12.78	XXX	■
L2106			AFO, fracture orthosis, tibial fracture cast orthosis, thermoplastic type casting material, custom fabricated	0.00	17.61	17.61	0.00	17.61	17.61	XXX	■
L2108			AFO, fracture orthosis, tibial fracture cast orthosis, custom fabricated	0.00	25.69	25.69	0.00	25.69	25.69	XXX	■
L2112			AFO, fracture orthosis, tibial fracture orthosis, soft, prefabricated, includes fitting and adjustment	0.00	12.08	12.08	0.00	12.08	12.08	XXX	■
L2114			AFO, fracture orthosis, tibial fracture orthosis, semi-rigid, prefabricated, includes fitting and adjustment	0.00	15.03	15.03	0.00	15.03	15.03	XXX	■
L2116			AFO, fracture orthosis, tibial fracture orthosis, rigid, prefabricated, includes fitting and adjustment	0.00	15.20	15.20	0.00	15.20	15.20	XXX	■
L2122			KAFO, fracture orthosis, femoral fracture cast orthosis, plaster type casting material, custom fabricated	0.00	21.23	21.23	0.00	21.23	21.23	XXX	■
L2124			KAFO, fracture orthosis, femoral fracture cast orthosis, synthetic type casting material, custom fabricated	0.00	25.37	25.37	0.00	25.37	25.37	XXX	■
L2126			KAFO, fracture orthosis, femoral fracture cast orthosis, thermoplastic type casting material, custom fabricated	0.00	28.40	28.40	0.00	28.40	28.40	XXX	■
L2128			KAFO, fracture orthosis, femoral fracture cast orthosis, custom fabricated	0.00	44.40	44.40	0.00	44.40	44.40	XXX	■
L2132			KAFO, fracture orthosis, femoral fracture cast orthosis, soft, prefabricated, includes fitting and adjustment	0.00	20.89	20.89	0.00	20.89	20.89	XXX	■

■ RVU not developed by CMS. Gap-filled RVUs developed by CHEG.

Code	M	S	Description	Work Value	Non-Fac PE	Fac PE	Mal-practice	Non-Fac Total	Fac Total	Global	Gap
L2134			KAFO, fracture orthosis, femoral fracture cast orthosis, semi-rigid, prefabricated, includes fitting and adjustment	0.00	25.04	25.04	0.00	25.04	25.04	XXX	■
L2136			KAFO, fracture orthosis, femoral fracture cast orthosis, rigid, prefabricated, includes fitting and adjustment	0.00	30.62	30.62	0.00	30.62	30.62	XXX	■
L2180			Addition to lower extremity fracture orthosis, plastic shoe insert with ankle joints	0.00	3.03	3.03	0.00	3.03	3.03	XXX	■
L2182			Addition to lower extremity fracture orthosis, drop lock knee joint	0.00	2.38	2.38	0.00	2.38	2.38	XXX	■
L2184			Addition to lower extremity fracture orthosis, limited motion knee joint	0.00	3.21	3.21	0.00	3.21	3.21	XXX	■
L2186			Addition to lower extremity fracture orthosis, adjustable motion knee joint, Lerman type	0.00	3.90	3.90	0.00	3.90	3.90	XXX	■
L2188			Addition to lower extremity fracture orthosis, quadrilateral brim	0.00	7.76	7.76	0.00	7.76	7.76	XXX	■
L2190			Addition to lower extremity fracture orthosis, waist belt	0.00	2.26	2.26	0.00	2.26	2.26	XXX	■
L2192			Addition to lower extremity fracture orthosis, hip joint, pelvic band, thigh flange, and pelvic belt	0.00	9.23	9.23	0.00	9.23	9.23	XXX	■
L2200			Addition to lower extremity, limited ankle motion, each joint	0.00	1.23	1.23	0.00	1.23	1.23	XXX	■
L2210			Addition to lower extremity, dorsiflexion assist (plantar flexion resist), each joint	0.00	1.74	1.74	0.00	1.74	1.74	XXX	■
L2220			Addition to lower extremity, dorsiflexion and plantar flexion assist/resist, each joint	0.00	2.12	2.12	0.00	2.12	2.12	XXX	■
L2230			Addition to lower extremity, split flat caliper stirrups and plate attachment	0.00	1.99	1.99	0.00	1.99	1.99	XXX	■
L2240			Addition to lower extremity, round caliper and plate attachment	0.00	2.17	2.17	0.00	2.17	2.17	XXX	■
L2250			Addition to lower extremity, foot plate, molded to patient model, stirrup attachment	0.00	9.20	9.20	0.00	9.20	9.20	XXX	■
L2260			Addition to lower extremity, reinforced solid stirrup (Scott-Craig type)	0.00	5.19	5.19	0.00	5.19	5.19	XXX	■
L2265			Addition to lower extremity, long tongue stirrup	0.00	3.04	3.04	0.00	3.04	3.04	XXX	■
L2270			Addition to lower extremity, varus/valgus correction ("T") strap, padded/lined or malleolus pad	0.00	1.49	1.49	0.00	1.49	1.49	XXX	■
L2275			Addition to lower extremity, varus/vulgus correction, plastic modification, padded/lined	0.00	3.25	3.25	0.00	3.25	3.25	XXX	■
L2280			Addition to lower extremity, molded inner boot	0.00	11.73	11.73	0.00	11.73	11.73	XXX	■

■ RVU not developed by CMS. Gap-filled RVUs developed by CHEG.

Code	M	S	Description	Work Value	Non-Fac PE	Fac PE	Mal-practice	Non-Fac Total	Fac Total	Global	Gap
L2300			Addition to lower extremity, abduction bar (bilateral hip involvement), jointed, adjustable	0.00	6.97	6.97	0.00	6.97	6.97	XXX	■
L2310			Addition to lower extremity, abduction bar, straight	0.00	3.19	3.19	0.00	3.19	3.19	XXX	■
L2320			Addition to lower extremity, nonmolded lacer	0.00	5.33	5.33	0.00	5.33	5.33	XXX	■
L2330			Addition to lower extremity, lacer molded to patient model	0.00	10.17	10.17	0.00	10.17	10.17	XXX	■
L2335			Addition to lower extremity, anterior swing band	0.00	5.89	5.89	0.00	5.89	5.89	XXX	■
L2340			Addition to lower extremity, pretibial shell, molded to patient model	0.00	11.57	11.57	0.00	11.57	11.57	XXX	■
L2350			Addition to lower extremity, prosthetic type, (BK) socket, molded to patient model, (used for "PTB," "AFO" orthoses)	0.00	23.07	23.07	0.00	23.07	23.07	XXX	■
L2360			Addition to lower extremity, extended steel shank	0.00	1.34	1.34	0.00	1.34	1.34	XXX	■
L2370			Addition to lower extremity, Patten bottom	0.00	6.65	6.65	0.00	6.65	6.65	XXX	■
L2375			Addition to lower extremity, torsion control, ankle joint and half solid stirrup	0.00	2.93	2.93	0.00	2.93	2.93	XXX	■
L2380			Addition to lower extremity, torsion control, straight knee joint, each joint	0.00	3.19	3.19	0.00	3.19	3.19	XXX	■
L2385			Addition to lower extremity, straight knee joint, heavy duty, each joint	0.00	3.47	3.47	0.00	3.47	3.47	XXX	■
L2390			Addition to lower extremity, offset knee joint, each joint	0.00	2.83	2.83	0.00	2.83	2.83	XXX	■
L2395			Addition to lower extremity, offset knee joint, heavy duty, each joint	0.00	4.05	4.05	0.00	4.05	4.05	XXX	■
L2397			Addition to lower extremity orthosis, suspension sleeve	0.00	2.91	2.91	0.00	2.91	2.91	XXX	■
L2405			Addition to knee joint, drop lock, each joint	0.00	1.32	1.32	0.00	1.32	1.32	XXX	■
L2415			Addition to knee lock with integrated release mechanism (bail, cable, or equal), any material, each joint	0.00	4.77	4.77	0.00	4.77	4.77	XXX	■
L2425			Addition to knee joint, disc or dial lock for adjustable knee flexion, each joint	0.00	4.72	4.72	0.00	4.72	4.72	XXX	■
L2430			Addition to knee joint, ratchet lock for active and progressive knee extension, each joint	0.00	0.00	0.00	0.00	0.00	0.00	XXX	
L2435			Addition to knee joint, polycentric joint, each joint	0.00	4.47	4.47	0.00	4.47	4.47	XXX	■
L2492			Addition to knee joint, lift loop for drop lock ring	0.00	2.64	2.64	0.00	2.64	2.64	XXX	■

■ RVU not developed by CMS. Gap-filled RVUs developed by CHEG.

Code	M	S	Description	Work Value	Non-Fac PE	Fac PE	Mal-practice	Non-Fac Total	Fac Total	Global	Gap
L2500			Addition to lower extremity, thigh/weight bearing, gluteal/ischial weight bearing, ring	0.00	5.99	5.99	0.00	5.99	5.99	XXX	■
L2510			Addition to lower extremity, thigh/weight bearing, quadri-lateral brim, molded to patient model	0.00	18.80	18.80	0.00	18.80	18.80	XXX	■
L2520			Addition to lower extremity, thigh/weight bearing, quadri-lateral brim, custom fitted	0.00	11.93	11.93	0.00	11.93	11.93	XXX	■
L2525			Addition to lower extremity, thigh/weight bearing, ischial containment/narrow M-L brim molded to patient model	0.00	31.56	31.56	0.00	31.56	31.56	XXX	■
L2526			Addition to lower extremity, thigh/weight bearing, ischial containment/narrow M-L brim, custom fitted	0.00	17.73	17.73	0.00	17.73	17.73	XXX	■
L2530			Addition to lower extremity, thigh/weight bearing, lacer, nonmolded	0.00	6.09	6.09	0.00	6.09	6.09	XXX	■
L2540			Addition to lower extremity, thigh/weight bearing, lacer, molded to patient model	0.00	10.94	10.94	0.00	10.94	10.94	XXX	■
L2550			Addition to lower extremity, thigh/weight bearing, high roll cuff	0.00	7.44	7.44	0.00	7.44	7.44	XXX	■
L2570			Addition to lower extremity, pelvic control, hip joint, Clevis type, two position joint, each	0.00	12.33	12.33	0.00	12.33	12.33	XXX	■
L2580			Addition to lower extremity, pelvic control, pelvic sling	0.00	12.02	12.02	0.00	12.02	12.02	XXX	■
L2600			Addition to lower extremity, pelvic control, hip joint, Clevis type, or thrust bearing, free, each	0.00	5.32	5.32	0.00	5.32	5.32	XXX	■
L2610			Addition to lower extremity, pelvic control, hip joint, Clevis or thrust bearing, lock, each	0.00	6.29	6.29	0.00	6.29	6.29	XXX	■
L2620			Addition to lower extremity, pelvic control, hip joint, heavy-duty, each	0.00	6.91	6.91	0.00	6.91	6.91	XXX	■
L2622			Addition to lower extremity, pelvic control, hip joint, adjustable flexion, each	0.00	7.94	7.94	0.00	7.94	7.94	XXX	■
L2624			Addition to lower extremity, pelvic control, hip joint, adjustable flexion, extension, abduction control, each	0.00	8.57	8.57	0.00	8.57	8.57	XXX	■
L2627			Addition to lower extremity, pelvic control, plastic, molded to patient model, reciprocating hip joint and cables	0.00	44.39	44.39	0.00	44.39	44.39	XXX	■
L2628			Addition to lower extremity, pelvic control, metal frame, reciprocating hip joint and cables	0.00	43.38	43.38	0.00	43.38	43.38	XXX	■
L2630			Addition to lower extremity, pelvic control, band and belt, unilateral	0.00	6.41	6.41	0.00	6.41	6.41	XXX	■
L2640			Addition to lower extremity, pelvic control, band and belt, bilateral	0.00	8.70	8.70	0.00	8.70	8.70	XXX	■

■ RVU not developed by CMS. Gap-filled RVUs developed by CHEG.

Code	M	S	Description	Work Value	Non-Fac PE	Fac PE	Mal-practice	Non-Fac Total	Fac Total	Global	Gap
L2650			Addition to lower extremity, pelvic and thoracic control, gluteal pad, each	0.00	3.11	3.11	0.00	3.11	3.11	XXX	■
L2660			Addition to lower extremity, thoracic control, thoracic band	0.00	4.83	4.83	0.00	4.83	4.83	XXX	■
L2670			Addition to lower extremity, thoracic control, paraspinal uprights	0.00	4.42	4.42	0.00	4.42	4.42	XXX	■
L2680			Addition to lower extremity, thoracic control, lateral support uprights	0.00	4.05	4.05	0.00	4.05	4.05	XXX	■
L2750			Addition to lower extremity orthosis, plating chrome or nickel, per bar	0.00	2.18	2.18	0.00	2.18	2.18	XXX	■
L2755			Addition to lower extremity orthosis, high strength, lightweight material, all hybrid lamination/prepreg composite, per segment	0.00	0.00	0.00	0.00	0.00	0.00	XXX	
L2760			Addition to lower extremity orthosis, extension, per extension, per bar (for lineal adjustment for growth)	0.00	1.57	1.57	0.00	1.57	1.57	XXX	■
L2768			Orthotic side bar disconnect device, per bar	0.00	0.00	0.00	0.00	0.00	0.00	XXX	
L2770			Addition to lower extremity orthosis, any material, per bar or joint	0.00	1.60	1.60	0.00	1.60	1.60	XXX	■
L2780			Addition to lower extremity orthosis, noncorrosive finish, per bar	0.00	1.76	1.76	0.00	1.76	1.76	XXX	■
L2785			Addition to lower extremity orthosis, drop lock retainer, each	0.00	0.82	0.82	0.00	0.82	0.82	XXX	■
L2795			Addition to lower extremity orthosis, knee control, full kneecap	0.00	2.21	2.21	0.00	2.21	2.21	XXX	■
L2800			Addition to lower extremity orthosis, knee control, kneecap, medial or lateral pull	0.00	2.77	2.77	0.00	2.77	2.77	XXX	■
L2810			Addition to lower extremity orthosis, knee control, condylar pad	0.00	2.03	2.03	0.00	2.03	2.03	XXX	■
L2820			Addition to lower extremity orthosis, soft interface for molded plastic, below knee section	0.00	2.38	2.38	0.00	2.38	2.38	XXX	■
L2830			Addition to lower extremity orthosis, soft interface for molded plastic, above knee section	0.00	2.43	2.43	0.00	2.43	2.43	XXX	■
L2840			Addition to lower extremity orthosis, tibial length sock, fracture or equal, each	0.00	1.13	1.13	0.00	1.13	1.13	XXX	■
L2850			Addition to lower extremity orthosis, femoral length sock, fracture or equal, each	0.00	1.60	1.60	0.00	1.60	1.60	XXX	■
L2860			Addition to lower extremity joint, knee or ankle, concentric adjustable torsion style mechanism, each	0.00	0.00	0.00	0.00	0.00	0.00	XXX	
L2999			Lower extremity orthoses, not otherwise specified	0.00	0.00	0.00	0.00	0.00	0.00	XXX	

■ RVU not developed by CMS. Gap-filled RVUs developed by CHEG.

Code	M	S	Description	Work Value	Non-Fac PE	Fac PE	Mal-practice	Non-Fac Total	Fac Total	Global	Gap
L3000			Foot insert, removable, molded to patient model, "UCB" type, Berkeley shell, each	0.00	5.87	5.87	0.00	5.87	5.87	XXX	■
L3001			Foot insert, removable, molded to patient model, Spenco, each	0.00	3.46	3.46	0.00	3.46	3.46	XXX	■
L3002			Foot insert, removable, molded to patient model, Plastazote or equal, each	0.00	2.86	2.86	0.00	2.86	2.86	XXX	■
L3003			Foot insert, removable, molded to patient model, silicone gel, each	0.00	3.52	3.52	0.00	3.52	3.52	XXX	■
L3010			Foot insert, removable, molded to patient model, longitudinal arch support, each	0.00	4.56	4.56	0.00	4.56	4.56	XXX	■
L3020			Foot insert, removable, molded to patient model, longitudinal/metatarsal support, each	0.00	5.78	5.78	0.00	5.78	5.78	XXX	■
L3030			Foot insert, removable, formed to patient foot, each	0.00	5.78	5.78	0.00	5.78	5.78	XXX	■
L3040			Foot, arch support, removable, premolded, longitudinal, each	0.00	1.03	1.03	0.00	1.03	1.03	XXX	■
L3050			Foot, arch support, removable, premolded, metatarsal, each	0.00	0.95	0.95	0.00	0.95	0.95	XXX	■
L3060			Foot, arch support, removable, premolded, longitudinal/metatarsal, each	0.00	1.85	1.85	0.00	1.85	1.85	XXX	■
L3070			Foot, arch support, nonremovable, attached to shoe, longitudinal, each	0.00	0.57	0.57	0.00	0.57	0.57	XXX	■
L3080			Foot, arch support, nonremovable, attached to shoe, metatarsal, each	0.00	0.23	0.23	0.00	0.23	0.23	XXX	■
L3090			Foot, arch support, nonremovable, attached to shoe, longitudinal/metatarsal, each	0.00	0.36	0.36	0.00	0.36	0.36	XXX	■
L3100			Hallus-Valgus night dynamic splint	0.00	0.60	0.60	0.00	0.60	0.60	XXX	■
L3140			Foot, abduction rotation bar, including shoes	0.00	1.73	1.73	0.00	1.73	1.73	XXX	■
L3150			Foot, abduction rotation bar, without shoes	0.00	1.45	1.45	0.00	1.45	1.45	XXX	■
L3160			Foot, adjustable shoe-styled positioning device	0.00	0.45	0.45	0.00	0.45	0.45	XXX	■
L3170			Foot, plastic heel stabilizer	0.00	0.76	0.76	0.00	0.76	0.76	XXX	■
L3201			Orthopedic shoe, oxford with supinator or pronator, infant	0.00	1.71	1.71	0.00	1.71	1.71	XXX	■
L3202			Orthopedic shoe, oxford with supinator or pronator, child	0.00	1.68	1.68	0.00	1.68	1.68	XXX	■
L3203			Orthopedic shoe, oxford with supinator or pronator, junior	0.00	1.64	1.64	0.00	1.64	1.64	XXX	■
L3204			Orthopedic shoe, hightop with supinator or pronator, infant	0.00	1.64	1.64	0.00	1.64	1.64	XXX	■

■ RVU not developed by CMS. Gap-filled RVUs developed by CHEG.

Code	M	S	Description	Work Value	Non-Fac PE	Fac PE	Mal-practice	Non-Fac Total	Fac Total	Global	Gap
L3206			Orthopedic shoe, hightop with supinator or pronator, child	0.00	1.71	1.71	0.00	1.71	1.71	XXX	■
L3207			Orthopedic shoe, hightop with supinator or pronator, junior	0.00	1.74	1.74	0.00	1.74	1.74	XXX	■
L3208			Surgical boot, each, infant	0.00	0.91	0.91	0.00	0.91	0.91	XXX	■
L3209			Surgical boot, each, child	0.00	1.29	1.29	0.00	1.29	1.29	XXX	■
L3211			Surgical boot, each, junior	0.00	1.37	1.37	0.00	1.37	1.37	XXX	■
L3212			Benesch boot, pair, infant	0.00	1.91	1.91	0.00	1.91	1.91	XXX	■
L3213			Benesch boot, pair, child	0.00	2.31	2.31	0.00	2.31	2.31	XXX	■
L3214			Benesch boot, pair, junior	0.00	2.46	2.46	0.00	2.46	2.46	XXX	■
L3215			Orthopedic footwear, woman's shoes, oxford	0.00	3.13	3.13	0.00	3.13	3.13	XXX	■
L3216			Orthopedic footwear, woman's shoes, depth inlay	0.00	3.78	3.78	0.00	3.78	3.78	XXX	■
L3217			Orthopedic footwear, woman's shoes, hightop, depth inlay	0.00	4.10	4.10	0.00	4.10	4.10	XXX	■
L3218			Orthopedic footwear, woman's surgical boot, each	0.00	0.75	0.75	0.00	0.75	0.75	XXX	■
L3219			Orthopedic footwear, man's shoes, oxford	0.00	3.52	3.52	0.00	3.52	3.52	XXX	■
L3221			Orthopedic footwear, man's shoes, depth inlay	0.00	4.22	4.22	0.00	4.22	4.22	XXX	■
L3222			Orthopedic footwear, man's shoes, hightop, depth inlay	0.00	4.66	4.66	0.00	4.66	4.66	XXX	■
L3223			Orthopedic footwear, man's surgical boot, each	0.00	1.04	1.04	0.00	1.04	1.04	XXX	■
L3224			Orthopedic footwear, woman's shoe, oxford, used as an integral part of a brace (orthosis)	0.00	0.00	0.00	0.00	0.00	0.00	XXX	
L3225			Orthopedic footwear, man's shoe, oxford, used as an integral part of a brace (orthosis)	0.00	0.00	0.00	0.00	0.00	0.00	XXX	
L3230			Orthopedic footwear, custom shoes, depth inlay	0.00	5.48	5.48	0.00	5.48	5.48	XXX	■
L3250			Orthopedic footwear, custom molded shoe, removable inner mold, prosthetic shoe, each	0.00	10.67	10.67	0.00	10.67	10.67	XXX	■
L3251			Foot, shoe molded to patient model, silicone shoe, each	0.00	1.47	1.47	0.00	1.47	1.47	XXX	■
L3252			Foot, shoe molded to patient model, Plastazote (or similar), custom fabricated, each	0.00	5.84	5.84	0.00	5.84	5.84	XXX	■
L3253			Foot, molded shoe Plastazote (or similar), custom fitted, each	0.00	1.46	1.46	0.00	1.46	1.46	XXX	■
L3254			Nonstandard size or width	0.00	0.00	0.00	0.00	0.00	0.00	XXX	
L3255			Nonstandard size or length	0.00	0.00	0.00	0.00	0.00	0.00	XXX	

■ RVU not developed by CMS. Gap-filled RVUs developed by CHEG.

Code	M	S	Description	Work Value	Non-Fac PE	Fac PE	Mal-practice	Non-Fac Total	Fac Total	Global	Gap
L3257			Orthopedic footwear, additional charge for split size	0.00	1.06	1.06	0.00	1.06	1.06	XXX	■
L3260			Ambulatory surgical boot, each	0.00	0.60	0.60	0.00	0.60	0.60	XXX	■
L3265			Plastazote sandal, each	0.00	0.65	0.65	0.00	0.65	0.65	XXX	■
L3300			Lift, elevation, heel, tapered to metatarsals, per inch	0.00	0.75	0.75	0.00	0.75	0.75	XXX	■
L3310			Lift, elevation, heel and sole, neoprene, per inch	0.00	1.49	1.49	0.00	1.49	1.49	XXX	■
L3320			Lift, elevation, heel and sole, cork, per inch	0.00	3.95	3.95	0.00	3.95	3.95	XXX	■
L3330			Lift, elevation, metal extension (skate)	0.00	6.39	6.39	0.00	6.39	6.39	XXX	■
L3332			Lift, elevation, inside shoe, tapered, up to one-half inch	0.00	0.45	0.45	0.00	0.45	0.45	XXX	■
L3334			Lift, elevation, heel, per inch	0.00	0.44	0.44	0.00	0.44	0.44	XXX	■
L3340			Heel wedge, SACH	0.00	1.07	1.07	0.00	1.07	1.07	XXX	■
L3350			Heel wedge	0.00	0.68	0.68	0.00	0.68	0.68	XXX	■
L3360			Sole wedge, outside sole	0.00	0.51	0.51	0.00	0.51	0.51	XXX	■
L3370			Sole wedge, between sole	0.00	0.61	0.61	0.00	0.61	0.61	XXX	■
L3380			Clubfoot wedge	0.00	1.05	1.05	0.00	1.05	1.05	XXX	■
L3390			Outflare wedge	0.00	1.46	1.46	0.00	1.46	1.46	XXX	■
L3400			Metatarsal bar wedge, rocker	0.00	1.40	1.40	0.00	1.40	1.40	XXX	■
L3410			Metatarsal bar wedge, between sole	0.00	2.37	2.37	0.00	2.37	2.37	XXX	■
L3420			Full sole and heel wedge, between sole	0.00	0.76	0.76	0.00	0.76	0.76	XXX	■
L3430			Heel, counter, plastic reinforced	0.00	1.91	1.91	0.00	1.91	1.91	XXX	■
L3440			Heel, counter, leather reinforced	0.00	1.28	1.28	0.00	1.28	1.28	XXX	■
L3450			Heel, SACH cushion type	0.00	1.04	1.04	0.00	1.04	1.04	XXX	■
L3455			Heel, new leather, standard	0.00	0.44	0.44	0.00	0.44	0.44	XXX	■
L3460			Heel, new rubber, standard	0.00	0.75	0.75	0.00	0.75	0.75	XXX	■
L3465			Heel, Thomas with wedge	0.00	0.54	0.54	0.00	0.54	0.54	XXX	■
L3470			Heel, Thomas extended to ball	0.00	1.31	1.31	0.00	1.31	1.31	XXX	■
L3480			Heel, pad and depression for spur	0.00	0.89	0.89	0.00	0.89	0.89	XXX	■
L3485			Heel, pad, removable for spur	0.00	0.60	0.60	0.00	0.60	0.60	XXX	■
L3500			Orthopedic shoe addition, insole, leather	0.00	0.66	0.66	0.00	0.66	0.66	XXX	■
L3510			Orthopedic shoe addition, insole, rubber	0.00	0.61	0.61	0.00	0.61	0.61	XXX	■

■ RVU not developed by CMS. Gap-filled RVUs developed by CHEG.

Code	M	S	Description	Work Value	Non-Fac PE	Fac PE	Mal-practice	Non-Fac Total	Fac Total	Global	Gap
L3520			Orthopedic shoe addition, insole, felt covered with leather	0.00	1.00	1.00	0.00	1.00	1.00	XXX	■
L3530			Orthopedic shoe addition, sole, half	0.00	0.30	0.30	0.00	0.30	0.30	XXX	■
L3540			Orthopedic shoe addition, sole, full	0.00	1.10	1.10	0.00	1.10	1.10	XXX	■
L3550			Orthopedic shoe addition, toe tap, standard	0.00	0.18	0.18	0.00	0.18	0.18	XXX	■
L3560			Orthopedic shoe addition, toe tap, horseshoe	0.00	0.24	0.24	0.00	0.24	0.24	XXX	■
L3570			Orthopedic shoe addition, special extension to instep (leather with eyelets)	0.00	0.98	0.98	0.00	0.98	0.98	XXX	■
L3580			Orthopedic shoe addition, convert instep to velcro closure	0.00	1.46	1.46	0.00	1.46	1.46	XXX	■
L3590			Orthopedic shoe addition, convert firm shoe counter to soft counter	0.00	1.13	1.13	0.00	1.13	1.13	XXX	■
L3595			Orthopedic shoe addition, March bar	0.00	0.33	0.33	0.00	0.33	0.33	XXX	■
L3600			Transfer of an orthosis from one shoe to another, caliper plate, existing	0.00	1.85	1.85	0.00	1.85	1.85	XXX	■
L3610			Transfer of an orthosis from one shoe to another, caliper plate, new	0.00	2.98	2.98	0.00	2.98	2.98	XXX	■
L3620			Transfer of an orthosis from one shoe to another, solid stirrup, existing	0.00	1.85	1.85	0.00	1.85	1.85	XXX	■
L3630			Transfer of an orthosis from one shoe to another, solid stirrup, new	0.00	2.26	2.26	0.00	2.26	2.26	XXX	■
L3640			Transfer of an orthosis from one shoe to another, Dennis Browne splint (Riveton), both shoes	0.00	0.75	0.75	0.00	0.75	0.75	XXX	■
L3649			Orthopedic shoe, modification, addition or transfer, not otherwise specified	0.00	0.00	0.00	0.00	0.00	0.00	XXX	
L3650			SO, figure of eight design abduction re- strainer, prefabricated, includes fitting and adjustment	0.00	1.50	1.50	0.00	1.50	1.50	XXX	■
L3660			SO, figure of eight design abduction restrainer, canvas and webbing, prefabricated, includes fitting and adjustment	0.00	2.59	2.59	0.00	2.59	2.59	XXX	■
L3670			SO, acromio/clavicular (canvas and webbing type), prefabricated, includes fitting and adjustment	0.00	2.86	2.86	0.00	2.86	2.86	XXX	■
L3675			SO, vest type abduction restrainer, canvas webbing type, or equal, prefabricated, includes fitting and adjustment	0.00	3.22	3.22	0.00	3.22	3.22	XXX	■
L3677			Shoulder orthosis, hard plastic, shoulder stabilizer, pre-fabricated, includes fitting and adjustment	0.00	4.32	4.32	0.00	4.32	4.32	XXX	■
L3700			EO, elastic with stays, prefabricated, includes fitting and adjustment	0.00	1.76	1.76	0.00	1.76	1.76	XXX	■

■ RVU not developed by CMS. Gap-filled RVUs developed by CHEG.

Code	M	S	Description	Work Value	Non-Fac PE	Fac PE	Mal-practice	Non-Fac Total	Fac Total	Global	Gap
L3710			EO, elastic with metal joints, prefabricated, includes fitting and adjustment	0.00	3.13	3.13	0.00	3.13	3.13	XXX	■
L3720			EO, double upright with forearm/arm cuffs, free motion, custom fabricated	0.00	16.57	16.57	0.00	16.57	16.57	XXX	■
L3730			EO, double upright with forearm/arm cuffs, extension/flexion assist, custom fabricated	0.00	22.84	22.84	0.00	22.84	22.84	XXX	■
L3740			EO, double upright with forearm/arm cuffs, adjustable position lock with active control, custom fabricated	0.00	27.09	27.09	0.00	27.09	27.09	XXX	■
L3760			Elbow orthosis, with adjustable position locking joint(s), prefabricated, includes fitting and adjustments, any type	0.00	0.00	0.00	0.00	0.00	0.00	XXX	
L3800			WHFO, short opponens, no attachments, custom fabricated	0.00	5.07	5.07	0.00	5.07	5.07	XXX	■
L3805			WHFO, long opponens, no attachment, custom fabricated	0.00	8.11	8.11	0.00	8.11	8.11	XXX	■
L3807			WHFO, without joint(s), prefabricated, includes fitting and adjustments, any type	0.00	0.00	0.00	0.00	0.00	0.00	XXX	
L3810			WHFO, addition to short and long opponens, thumb abduction ("C") bar	0.00	1.64	1.64	0.00	1.64	1.64	XXX	■
L3815			WHFO, addition to short and long opponens, second M.P. abduction assist	0.00	1.53	1.53	0.00	1.53	1.53	XXX	■
L3820			WHFO, addition to short and long opponens, I.P. extension assist, with M.P. extension stop	0.00	2.61	2.61	0.00	2.61	2.61	XXX	■
L3825			WHFO, addition to short and long opponens, M.P. extension stop	0.00	1.65	1.65	0.00	1.65	1.65	XXX	■
L3830			WHFO, addition to short and long opponens, M.P. extension assist	0.00	2.15	2.15	0.00	2.15	2.15	XXX	■
L3835			WHFO, addition to short and long opponens, M.P. spring extension assist	0.00	2.32	2.32	0.00	2.32	2.32	XXX	■
L3840			WHFO, addition to short and long opponens, spring swivel thumb	0.00	1.59	1.59	0.00	1.59	1.59	XXX	■
L3845			WHFO, addition to short and long opponens, thumb I.P. extension assist, with M.P. stop	0.00	2.06	2.06	0.00	2.06	2.06	XXX	■
L3850			WHO, addition to short and long opponens, action wrist, with dorsiflexion assist	0.00	2.94	2.94	0.00	2.94	2.94	XXX	■
L3855			WHFO, addition to short and long opponens, adjustable M.P. flexion control	0.00	2.97	2.97	0.00	2.97	2.97	XXX	■
L3860			WHFO, addition to short and long opponens, adjustable M.P. flexion control and I.P.	0.00	4.05	4.05	0.00	4.05	4.05	XXX	■
L3890			Addition to upper extremity joint, wrist or elbow, concentric adjustable torsion style mechanism, each	0.00	0.00	0.00	0.00	0.00	0.00	XXX	

■ RVU not developed by CMS. Gap-filled RVUs developed by CHEG.

Code	M	S	Description	Work Value	Non-Fac PE	Fac PE	Mal-prac-tice	Non-Fac Total	Fac Total	Global	Gap
L3900			WHFO, dynamic flexor hinge, reciprocal wrist extension/flexion, finger flexion/extension, wrist or finger driven, custom fabricated	0.00	32.79	32.79	0.00	32.79	32.79	XXX	■
L3901			WHFO, dynamic flexor hinge, reciprocal wrist extension/flexion, finger flexion/extension, cable driven, custom fabricated	0.00	40.71	40.71	0.00	40.71	40.71	XXX	■
L3902			WHFO, external powered, compressed gas, custom fabricated	0.00	61.72	61.72	0.00	61.72	61.72	XXX	■
L3904			WHFO, external powered, electric, custom fabricated	0.00	74.19	74.19	0.00	74.19	74.19	XXX	■
L3906			WHO, wrist gauntlet, molded to patient model, custom fabricated	0.00	10.01	10.01	0.00	10.01	10.01	XXX	■
L3907			WHFO, wrist gauntlet with thumb spica, molded to patient model, custom fabricated	0.00	12.87	12.87	0.00	12.87	12.87	XXX	■
L3908			WHO, wrist extension control cock-up, nonmolded, prefabricated, includes fitting and adjustment	0.00	1.19	1.19	0.00	1.19	1.19	XXX	■
L3910			WHFO, Swanson design, prefabricated, includes fitting and adjustment	0.00	5.92	5.92	0.00	5.92	5.92	XXX	■
L3912			HFO, flexion glove with elastic finger control, prefabricated, includes fitting and adjustment	0.00	2.28	2.28	0.00	2.28	2.28	XXX	■
L3914			WHO, wrist extension cock-up, prefabricated, includes fitting and adjustment	0.00	1.83	1.83	0.00	1.83	1.83	XXX	■
L3916			WHFO, wrist extension cock-up, with outrigger, prefabricated, includes fitting and adjustment	0.00	3.22	3.22	0.00	3.22	3.22	XXX	■
L3918			HFO, knuckle bender, prefabricated, includes fitting and adjustment	0.00	1.99	1.99	0.00	1.99	1.99	XXX	■
L3920			HFO, knuckle bender, with outrigger, prefabricated, includes fitting and adjustment	0.00	2.48	2.48	0.00	2.48	2.48	XXX	■
L3922			HFO, knuckle bender, two segment to flex joints, prefabricated, includes fitting and adjustment	0.00	2.26	2.26	0.00	2.26	2.26	XXX	■
L3923			Hand finger orthosis, without joint(s), prefabricated, includes fitting and adjustments, any type	0.00	0.00	0.00	0.00	0.00	0.00	XXX	
L3924			WHFO, Oppenheimer, prefabricated, includes fitting and adjustment	0.00	2.70	2.70	0.00	2.70	2.70	XXX	■
L3926			WHFO, Thomas suspension, prefabricated, includes fitting and adjustment	0.00	2.35	2.35	0.00	2.35	2.35	XXX	■
L3928			HFO, finger extension, with clock spring, prefabricated, includes fitting and adjustment	0.00	1.07	1.07	0.00	1.07	1.07	XXX	■
L3930			WHFO, finger extension, with wrist support, prefabricated, includes fitting and adjustment	0.00	1.56	1.56	0.00	1.56	1.56	XXX	■

■ RVU not developed by CMS. Gap-filled RVUs developed by CHEG.

Code	M	S	Description	Work Value	Non-Fac PE	Fac PE	Mal-practice	Non-Fac Total	Fac Total	Global	Gap
L3932			FO, safety pin, spring wire, prefabricated, includes fitting and adjustment	0.00	0.91	0.91	0.00	0.91	0.91	XXX	■
L3934			FO, safety pin, modified, prefabricated, includes fitting and adjustment	0.00	0.97	0.97	0.00	0.97	0.97	XXX	■
L3936			WHFO, Palmer, prefabricated, includes fitting and adjustment	0.00	2.26	2.26	0.00	2.26	2.26	XXX	■
L3938			WHFO, dorsal wrist, prefabricated, includes fitting and adjustment	0.00	2.36	2.36	0.00	2.36	2.36	XXX	■
L3940			WHFO, dorsal wrist, with outrigger attachment, prefabricated, includes fitting and adjustment	0.00	2.28	2.28	0.00	2.28	2.28	XXX	■
L3942			HFO, reverse knuckle bender, prefabricated, includes fitting and adjustment	0.00	1.88	1.88	0.00	1.88	1.88	XXX	■
L3944			HFO, reverse knuckle bender, with outrigger, prefabricated, includes fitting and adjustment	0.00	2.49	2.49	0.00	2.49	2.49	XXX	■
L3946			HFO, composite elastic, prefabricated, includes fitting and adjustment	0.00	1.84	1.84	0.00	1.84	1.84	XXX	■
L3948			FO, finger knuckle bender, prefabricated, includes fitting and adjustment	0.00	1.39	1.39	0.00	1.39	1.39	XXX	■
L3950			WHFO, combination Oppenheimer, with knuckle bender and two attachments, prefabricated, includes fitting and adjustment	0.00	3.80	3.80	0.00	3.80	3.80	XXX	■
L3952			WHFO, combination Oppenheimer, with reverse knuckle and two attachments, prefabricated, includes fitting and adjustment	0.00	4.22	4.22	0.00	4.22	4.22	XXX	■
L3954			HFO, spreading hand, prefabricated, includes fitting and adjustment	0.00	2.28	2.28	0.00	2.28	2.28	XXX	■
L3956			Addition of joint to upper extremity orthosis, any material; per joint	0.00	0.00	0.00	0.00	0.00	0.00	XXX	
L3960			SEWHO, abduction positioning, airplane design, prefabricated, includes fitting and adjustment	0.00	18.62	18.62	0.00	18.62	18.62	XXX	■
L3962			SEWHO, abduction positioning, Erb's palsey design, prefabricated, includes fitting and adjustment	0.00	18.18	18.18	0.00	18.18	18.18	XXX	■
L3963			SEWHO, molded shoulder, arm, forearm, and wrist, with articulating elbow joint, custom fabricated	0.00	42.26	42.26	0.00	42.26	42.26	XXX	■
L3964			SEO, mobile arm support attached to wheelchair, balanced, adjustable, prefabricated, includes fitting and adjustment	0.00	19.22	19.22	0.00	19.22	19.22	XXX	■
L3965			SEO, mobile arm support attached to wheelchair, balanced, adjustable Rancho type, prefabricated, includes fitting and adjustment	0.00	30.69	30.69	0.00	30.69	30.69	XXX	■

■ RVU not developed by CMS. Gap-filled RVUs developed by CHEG.

HCPCS

Code	M	S	Description	Work Value	Non-Fac PE	Fac PE	Mal-prac-tice	Non-Fac Total	Fac Total	Global	Gap
L3966			SEO, mobile arm support attached to wheelchair, balanced, reclining, prefabricated, includes fitting and adjustment	0.00	24.35	24.35	0.00	24.35	24.35	XXX	■
L3968			SEO, mobile arm support attached to wheelchair, balanced, friction arm support (friction dampening to proximal and distal joints), prefabricated, includes fitting and adjustment	0.00	26.98	26.98	0.00	26.98	26.98	XXX	■
L3969			SEO, mobile arm support, monosuspension arm and hand support, overhead elbow forearm hand sling support, yoke type arm suspension support, prefabricated, includes fitting and adjustment	0.00	19.70	19.70	0.00	19.70	19.70	XXX	■
L3970			SEO, addition to mobile arm support, elevating proximal arm	0.00	7.61	7.61	0.00	7.61	7.61	XXX	■
L3972			SEO, addition to mobile arm support, offset or lateral rocker arm with elastic balance control	0.00	7.09	7.09	0.00	7.09	7.09	XXX	■
L3974			SEO, addition to mobile arm support, supinator	0.00	4.38	4.38	0.00	4.38	4.38	XXX	■
L3980			Upper extremity fracture orthosis, humeral, prefabricated, includes fitting and adjustment	0.00	7.83	7.83	0.00	7.83	7.83	XXX	■
L3982			Upper extremity fracture orthosis, radius/ulnar, prefabricated, includes fitting and adjustment	0.00	9.46	9.46	0.00	9.46	9.46	XXX	■
L3984			Upper extremity fracture orthosis, wrist, prefabricated, includes fitting and adjustment	0.00	8.72	8.72	0.00	8.72	8.72	XXX	■
L3985			Upper extremity fracture orthosis, forearm, hand with wrist hinge, custom fabricated	0.00	14.81	14.81	0.00	14.81	14.81	XXX	■
L3986			Upper extremity fracture orthosis, combination of humeral, radius/ulnar, wrist (example: Colles' fracture), custom fabricated	0.00	14.20	14.20	0.00	14.20	14.20	XXX	■
L3995			Addition to upper extremity orthosis, sock, fracture or equal, each	0.00	0.83	0.83	0.00	0.83	0.83	XXX	■
L3999			Upper limb orthosis, not otherwise specified	0.00	0.00	0.00	0.00	0.00	0.00	XXX	
L4000			Replace girdle for spinal orthosis (CTLSO or SO)	0.00	30.40	30.40	0.00	30.40	30.40	XXX	■
L4010			Replace trilateral socket brim	0.00	17.37	17.37	0.00	17.37	17.37	XXX	■
L4020			Replace quadrilateral socket brim, molded to patient model	0.00	22.30	22.30	0.00	22.30	22.30	XXX	■
L4030			Replace quadrilateral socket brim, custom fitted	0.00	13.07	13.07	0.00	13.07	13.07	XXX	■
L4040			Replace molded thigh lacer	0.00	10.57	10.57	0.00	10.57	10.57	XXX	■
L4045			Replace nonmolded thigh lacer	0.00	8.49	8.49	0.00	8.49	8.49	XXX	■
L4050			Replace molded calf lacer	0.00	10.69	10.69	0.00	10.69	10.69	XXX	■
L4055			Replace nonmolded calf lacer	0.00	6.91	6.91	0.00	6.91	6.91	XXX	■

■ RVU not developed by CMS. Gap-filled RVUs developed by CHEG.

Code	M	S	Description	Work Value	Non-Fac PE	Fac PE	Mal-practice	Non-Fac Total	Fac Total	Global	Gap
L4060			Replace high roll cuff	0.00	8.22	8.22	0.00	8.22	8.22	XXX	■
L4070			Replace proximal and distal upright for KAFO	0.00	7.29	7.29	0.00	7.29	7.29	XXX	■
L4080			Replace metal bands KAFO, proximal thigh	0.00	2.62	2.62	0.00	2.62	2.62	XXX	■
L4090			Replace metal bands KAFO-AFO, calf or distal thigh	0.00	2.34	2.34	0.00	2.34	2.34	XXX	■
L4100			Replace leather cuff KAFO, proximal thigh	0.00	2.70	2.70	0.00	2.70	2.70	XXX	■
L4110			Replace leather cuff KAFO-AFO, calf or distal thigh	0.00	2.20	2.20	0.00	2.20	2.20	XXX	■
L4130			Replace pretibial shell	0.00	12.84	12.84	0.00	12.84	12.84	XXX	■
L4205			Repair of orthotic device, labor component, per 15 minutes	0.00	0.00	0.00	0.00	0.00	0.00	XXX	
L4210			Repair of orthotic device, repair or replace minor parts	0.00	0.00	0.00	0.00	0.00	0.00	XXX	
L4350			Pneumatic ankle control splint (e.g., aircast), prefabricated, includes fitting and adjustment	0.00	1.70	1.70	0.00	1.70	1.70	XXX	■
L4360			Pneumatic walking splint (e.g., aircast), prefabricated, includes fitting and adjustment	0.00	5.78	5.78	0.00	5.78	5.78	XXX	■
L4370			Pneumatic full leg splint (e.g., aircast), prefabricated, includes fitting and adjustment	0.00	4.89	4.89	0.00	4.89	4.89	XXX	■
L4380			Pneumatic knee splint (e.g., aircast), prefabricated, includes fitting and adjustment	0.00	2.00	2.00	0.00	2.00	2.00	XXX	■
L4392			Replacement soft interface material, static AFO	0.00	0.45	0.45	0.00	0.45	0.45	XXX	■
L4394			Replace soft interface material, foot drop splint	0.00	0.42	0.42	0.00	0.42	0.42	XXX	■
L4396			Static ankle foot orthosis, including soft interface material, adjustable for fit, for positioning, pressure reduction, may be used for minimal ambulation, prefabricated, includes fitting and adjustment	0.00	3.37	3.37	0.00	3.37	3.37	XXX	■
L4398			Foot drop splint, recumbent positioning device, prefabricated, includes fitting and adjustment	0.00	2.28	2.28	0.00	2.28	2.28	XXX	■
L5000			Partial foot, shoe insert with longitudinal arch, toe filler	0.00	13.94	13.94	0.00	13.94	13.94	XXX	■
L5010			Partial foot, molded socket, ankle height, with toe filler	0.00	33.58	33.58	0.00	33.58	33.58	XXX	■
L5020			Partial foot, molded socket, tibial tubercle height, with toe filler	0.00	54.65	54.65	0.00	54.65	54.65	XXX	■
L5050			Ankle, Symes, molded socket, SACH foot	0.00	63.30	63.30	0.00	63.30	63.30	XXX	■
L5060			Ankle, Symes, metal frame, molded leather socket, articulated ankle/foot	0.00	76.19	76.19	0.00	76.19	76.19	XXX	■
L5100			Below knee, molded socket, shin, SACH foot	0.00	64.11	64.11	0.00	64.11	64.11	XXX	■

■ RVU not developed by CMS. Gap-filled RVUs developed by CHEG.

Code	M	S	Description	Work Value	Non-Fac PE	Fac PE	Mal-practice	Non-Fac Total	Fac Total	Global	Gap
L5105			Below knee, plastic socket, joints and thigh lacer, SACH foot	0.00	95.83	95.83	0.00	95.83	95.83	XXX	■
L5150			Knee disarticulation (or through knee), molded socket, external knee joints, shin, SACH foot	0.00	96.86	96.86	0.00	96.86	96.86	XXX	■
L5160			Knee disarticulation (or through knee), molded socket, bent knee configuration, external knee joints, shin, SACH foot	0.00	105.37	105.37	0.00	105.37	105.37	XXX	■
L5200			Above knee, molded socket, single axis constant friction knee, shin, SACH foot	0.00	91.13	91.13	0.00	91.13	91.13	XXX	■
L5210			Above knee, short prosthesis, no knee joint ("stubbies"), with foot blocks, no ankle joints, each	0.00	66.94	66.94	0.00	66.94	66.94	XXX	■
L5220			Above knee, short prosthesis, no knee joint ("stubbies"), with articulated ankle/foot, dynamically aligned, each	0.00	76.09	76.09	0.00	76.09	76.09	XXX	■
L5230			Above knee, for proximal femoral focal deficiency, constant friction knee, shin, SACH foot	0.00	104.93	104.93	0.00	104.93	104.93	XXX	■
L5250			Hip disarticulation, Canadian type; molded socket, hip joint, single axis constant friction knee, shin, SACH foot	0.00	143.12	143.12	0.00	143.12	143.12	XXX	■
L5270			Hip disarticulation, tilt table type; molded socket, locking hip joint, single axis constant friction knee, shin, SACH foot	0.00	141.87	141.87	0.00	141.87	141.87	XXX	■
L5280			Hemipelvectomy, Canadian type; molded socket, hip joint, single axis constant friction knee, shin, SACH foot	0.00	140.45	140.45	0.00	140.45	140.45	XXX	■
L5301			Below knee, molded socket, shin, SACH foot, endoskeletal system	0.00	63.68	63.68	0.00	63.68	63.68	XXX	■
L5311			Knee disarticulation (or through knee), molded socket, external knee joints, shin, SACH foot, endoskeletal system	0.00	95.00	95.00	0.00	95.00	95.00	XXX	■
L5321			Above knee, molded socket, open end, SACH foot, endoskeletal system, single axis knee	0.00	95.12	95.12	0.00	95.12	95.12	XXX	■
L5331			Hip disarticulation, Canadian type, molded socket, endoskeletal system, hip joint, single axis knee, SACH foot	0.00	132.88	132.88	0.00	132.88	132.88	XXX	■
L5341			Hemipelvectomy, Canadian type, molded socket, endoskeletal system, hip joint, single axis knee, SACH foot	0.00	141.97	141.97	0.00	141.97	141.97	XXX	■
L5400			Immediate postsurgical or early fitting, application of initial rigid dressing, including fitting, alignment, suspension, and one cast change, below knee	0.00	33.20	33.20	0.00	33.20	33.20	XXX	■

■ RVU not developed by CMS. Gap-filled RVUs developed by CHEG.

Code	M	S	Description	Work Value	Non-Fac PE	Fac PE	Mal-practice	Non-Fac Total	Fac Total	Global	Gap
L5410			Immediate postsurgical or early fitting, application of initial rigid dressing, including fitting, alignment and suspension, below knee, each additional cast change and realignment	0.00	11.53	11.53	0.00	11.53	11.53	XXX	■
L5420			Immediate postsurgical or early fitting, application of initial rigid dressing, including fitting, alignment and suspension and one cast change "AK" or knee disarticulation	0.00	41.93	41.93	0.00	41.93	41.93	XXX	■
L5430			Immediate postsurgical or early fitting, application of initial rigid dressing, including fitting, alignment and suspension, "AK" or knee disarticulation, each additional cast change and realignment	0.00	13.86	13.86	0.00	13.86	13.86	XXX	■
L5450			Immediate postsurgical or early fitting, application of nonweight bearing rigid dressing, below knee	0.00	11.23	11.23	0.00	11.23	11.23	XXX	■
L5460			Immediate postsurgical or early fitting, application of nonweight bearing rigid dressing, above knee	0.00	15.04	15.04	0.00	15.04	15.04	XXX	■
L5500			Initial, below knee "PTB" type socket, non-alignable system, pylon, no cover, SACH foot, plaster socket, direct formed	0.00	35.43	35.43	0.00	35.43	35.43	XXX	■
L5505			Initial, above knee — knee disarticulation, ischial level socket, non-alignable system, pylon, no cover, SACH foot plaster socket, direct formed	0.00	47.98	47.98	0.00	47.98	47.98	XXX	■
L5510			Preparatory, below knee "PTB" type socket, non-alignable system, pylon, no cover, SACH foot, plaster socket, molded to model	0.00	41.06	41.06	0.00	41.06	41.06	XXX	■
L5520			Preparatory, below knee "PTB" type socket, non-alignable system, pylon, no cover, SACH foot, thermoplastic or equal, direct formed	0.00	39.67	39.67	0.00	39.67	39.67	XXX	■
L5530			Preparatory, below knee "PTB" type socket, non-alignable system, pylon, no cover, SACH foot, thermoplastic or equal, molded to model	0.00	47.64	47.64	0.00	47.64	47.64	XXX	■
L5535			Preparatory, below knee "PTB" type socket, non-alignable system, pylon, no cover, SACH foot, prefabricated, adjustable open end socket	0.00	46.79	46.79	0.00	46.79	46.79	XXX	■
L5540			Preparatory, below knee "PTB" type socket, non-alignable system, pylon, no cover, SACH foot, laminated socket, molded to model	0.00	49.93	49.93	0.00	49.93	49.93	XXX	■
L5560			Preparatory, above knee — knee disarticulation, ischial level socket, non-alignable system, pylon, no cover, SACH foot, plaster socket, molded to model	0.00	53.61	53.61	0.00	53.61	53.61	XXX	■
L5570			Preparatory, above knee — knee disarticulation, ischial level socket, non-alignable system, pylon, no cover, SACH foot, thermoplastic or equal, direct formed	0.00	55.74	55.74	0.00	55.74	55.74	XXX	■

■ RVU not developed by CMS. Gap-filled RVUs developed by CHEG.

Code	M	S	Description	Work Value	Non-Fac PE	Fac PE	Mal-prac-tice	Non-Fac Total	Fac Total	Global	Gap
L5580			Preparatory, above knee — knee disarticulation, ischial level socket, non-alignable system, pylon, no cover, SACH foot, thermoplastic or equal, molded to model	0.00	65.07	65.07	0.00	65.07	65.07	XXX	■
L5585			Preparatory, above knee — knee disarticulation, ischial level socket, non-alignable system, pylon, no cover, SACH foot, prefabricated adjustable open end socket	0.00	70.57	70.57	0.00	70.57	70.57	XXX	■
L5590			Preparatory, above knee — knee disarticulation, ischial level socket, non-alignable system, pylon, no cover, SACH foot, laminated socket, molded to model	0.00	66.31	66.31	0.00	66.31	66.31	XXX	■
L5595			Preparatory, hip disarticulation — hemipelvectomy, pylon, no cover, SACH foot, thermoplastic or equal, molded to patient model	0.00	111.07	111.07	0.00	111.07	111.07	XXX	■
L5600			Preparatory, hip disarticulation — hemipelvectomy, pylon, no cover, SACH foot, laminated socket, molded to patient model	0.00	122.66	122.66	0.00	122.66	122.66	XXX	■
L5610			Addition to lower extremity, endoskeletal system, above knee, hydracadence system	0.00	57.11	57.11	0.00	57.11	57.11	XXX	■
L5611			Addition to lower extremity, endoskeletal system, above knee — knee disarticulation, 4-bar linkage, with friction swing phase control	0.00	44.43	44.43	0.00	44.43	44.43	XXX	■
L5613			Addition to lower extremity, endoskeletal system, above knee — knee disarticulation, 4-bar linkage, with hydraulic swing phase control	0.00	67.62	67.62	0.00	67.62	67.62	XXX	■
L5614			Addition to lower extremity, endoskeletal system, above knee — knee disarticulation, 4-bar linkage, with pneumatic swing phase control	0.00	99.95	99.95	0.00	99.95	99.95	XXX	■
L5616			Addition to lower extremity, endoskeletal system, above knee, universal multiplex system, friction swing phase control	0.00	37.47	37.47	0.00	37.47	37.47	XXX	■
L5617			Addition to lower extremity, quick change self-aligning unit, above or below knee, each	0.00	14.36	14.36	0.00	14.36	14.36	XXX	■
L5618			Addition to lower extremity, test socket, Symes	0.00	7.75	7.75	0.00	7.75	7.75	XXX	■
L5620			Addition to lower extremity, test socket, below knee	0.00	7.66	7.66	0.00	7.66	7.66	XXX	■
L5622			Addition to lower extremity, test socket, knee disarticulation	0.00	10.00	10.00	0.00	10.00	10.00	XXX	■
L5624			Addition to lower extremity, test socket, above knee	0.00	10.04	10.04	0.00	10.04	10.04	XXX	■
L5626			Addition to lower extremity, test socket, hip disarticulation	0.00	13.15	13.15	0.00	13.15	13.15	XXX	■

Code	M	S	Description	Work Value	Non-Fac PE	Fac PE	Mal-prac-tice	Non-Fac Total	Fac Total	Global	Gap
L5628			Addition to lower extremity, test socket, hemipelvectomy	0.00	13.32	13.32	0.00	13.32	13.32	XXX	■
L5629			Addition to lower extremity, below knee, acrylic socket	0.00	8.76	8.76	0.00	8.76	8.76	XXX	■
L5630			Addition to lower extremity, Symes type, expandable wall socket	0.00	12.38	12.38	0.00	12.38	12.38	XXX	■
L5631			Addition to lower extremity, above knee or knee disarticulation, acrylic socket	0.00	12.13	12.13	0.00	12.13	12.13	XXX	■
L5632			Addition to lower extremity, Symes type, "PTB" brim design socket	0.00	6.14	6.14	0.00	6.14	6.14	XXX	■
L5634			Addition to lower extremity, Symes type, posterior opening (Canadian) socket	0.00	8.40	8.40	0.00	8.40	8.40	XXX	■
L5636			Addition to lower extremity, Symes type, medial opening socket	0.00	7.03	7.03	0.00	7.03	7.03	XXX	■
L5637			Addition to lower extremity, below knee, total contact	0.00	7.96	7.96	0.00	7.96	7.96	XXX	■
L5638			Addition to lower extremity, below knee, leather socket	0.00	13.41	13.41	0.00	13.41	13.41	XXX	■
L5639			Addition to lower extremity, below knee, wood socket	0.00	30.93	30.93	0.00	30.93	30.93	XXX	■
L5640			Addition to lower extremity, knee disarticulation, leather socket	0.00	17.64	17.64	0.00	17.64	17.64	XXX	■
L5642			Addition to lower extremity, above knee, leather socket	0.00	17.11	17.11	0.00	17.11	17.11	XXX	■
L5643			Addition to lower extremity, hip disarticulation, flexible inner socket, external frame	0.00	42.94	42.94	0.00	42.94	42.94	XXX	■
L5644			Addition to lower extremity, above knee, wood socket	0.00	16.30	16.30	0.00	16.30	16.30	XXX	■
L5645			Addition to lower extremity, below knee, flexible inner socket, external frame	0.00	22.02	22.02	0.00	22.02	22.02	XXX	■
L5646			Addition to lower extremity, below knee, air cushion socket	0.00	15.11	15.11	0.00	15.11	15.11	XXX	■
L5647			Addition to lower extremity, below knee, suction socket	0.00	21.93	21.93	0.00	21.93	21.93	XXX	■
L5648			Addition to lower extremity, above knee, air cushion socket	0.00	18.15	18.15	0.00	18.15	18.15	XXX	■
L5649			Addition to lower extremity, ischial containment/narrow M-L socket	0.00	52.51	52.51	0.00	52.51	52.51	XXX	■
L5650			Addition to lower extremity, total contact, above knee or knee disarticulation socket	0.00	13.47	13.47	0.00	13.47	13.47	XXX	■
L5651			Addition to lower extremity, above knee, flexible inner socket, external frame	0.00	33.14	33.14	0.00	33.14	33.14	XXX	■

■ RVU not developed by CMS. Gap-filled RVUs developed by CHEG.

Code	M	S	Description	Work Value	Non-Fac PE	Fac PE	Mal-practice	Non-Fac Total	Fac Total	Global	Gap
L5652			Addition to lower extremity, suction suspension, above knee or knee disarticulation socket	0.00	12.04	12.04	0.00	12.04	12.04	XXX	■
L5653			Addition to lower extremity, knee disarticulation, expandable wall socket	0.00	16.06	16.06	0.00	16.06	16.06	XXX	■
L5654			Addition to lower extremity, socket insert, Symes (Kemblo, Pelite, Aliplast, Plastazote or equal)	0.00	9.15	9.15	0.00	9.15	9.15	XXX	■
L5655			Addition to lower extremity, socket insert, below knee (Kemblo, Pelite, Aliplast, Plastazote or equal)	0.00	7.54	7.54	0.00	7.54	7.54	XXX	■
L5656			Addition to lower extremity, socket insert, knee disarticulation (Kemblo, Pelite, Aliplast, Plastazote or equal)	0.00	10.22	10.22	0.00	10.22	10.22	XXX	■
L5658			Addition to lower extremity, socket insert, above knee (Kemblo, Pelite, Aliplast, Plastazote or equal)	0.00	10.04	10.04	0.00	10.04	10.04	XXX	■
L5660			Addition to lower extremity, socket insert, Symes, silicone gel or equal	0.00	15.91	15.91	0.00	15.91	15.91	XXX	■
L5661			Addition to lower extremity, socket insert, multidurometer, Symes	0.00	16.78	16.78	0.00	16.78	16.78	XXX	■
L5662			Addition to lower extremity, socket insert, below knee, silicone gel or equal	0.00	14.57	14.57	0.00	14.57	14.57	XXX	■
L5663			Addition to lower extremity, socket insert, knee disarticulation, silicone gel or equal	0.00	19.01	19.01	0.00	19.01	19.01	XXX	■
L5664			Addition to lower extremity, socket insert, above knee, silicone gel or equal	0.00	18.33	18.33	0.00	18.33	18.33	XXX	■
L5665			Addition to lower extremity, socket insert, multidurometer, below knee	0.00	14.13	14.13	0.00	14.13	14.13	XXX	■
L5666			Addition to lower extremity, below knee, cuff suspension	0.00	1.94	1.94	0.00	1.94	1.94	XXX	■
L5668			Addition to lower extremity, below knee, molded distal cushion	0.00	2.77	2.77	0.00	2.77	2.77	XXX	■
L5670			Addition to lower extremity, below knee, molded supracondylar suspension ("PTS" or similar)	0.00	7.48	7.48	0.00	7.48	7.48	XXX	■
L5671			Addition to lower extremity, below knee/above knee suspension locking mechanism (shuttle, lanyard or equal), excludes socket insert	0.00	0.00	0.00	0.00	0.00	0.00	XXX	
L5672			Addition to lower extremity, below knee, removable medial brim suspension	0.00	8.22	8.22	0.00	8.22	8.22	XXX	■
L5674			Addition to lower extremity, below knee, suspension sleeve, any material, each	0.00	1.76	1.76	0.00	1.76	1.76	XXX	■

■ RVU not developed by CMS. Gap-filled RVUs developed by CHEG.

Code	M	S	Description	Work Value	Non-Fac PE	Fac PE	Mal-practice	Non-Fac Total	Fac Total	Global	Gap
L5675			Addition to lower extremity, below knee, suspension sleeve, heavy duty, any material, each	0.00	2.38	2.38	0.00	2.38	2.38	XXX	■
L5676			Addition to lower extremity, below knee, knee joints, single axis, pair	0.00	9.98	9.98	0.00	9.98	9.98	XXX	■
L5677			Addition to lower extremity, below knee, knee joints, polycentric, pair	0.00	13.59	13.59	0.00	13.59	13.59	XXX	■
L5678			Addition to lower extremity, below knee joint covers, pair	0.00	1.10	1.10	0.00	1.10	1.10	XXX	■
L5680			Addition to lower extremity, below knee, thigh lacer, nonmolded	0.00	8.40	8.40	0.00	8.40	8.40	XXX	■
L5682			Addition to lower extremity, below knee, thigh lacer, gluteal/ischial, molded	0.00	17.25	17.25	0.00	17.25	17.25	XXX	■
L5684			Addition to lower extremity, below knee, fork strap	0.00	1.34	1.34	0.00	1.34	1.34	XXX	■
L5686			Addition to lower extremity, below knee, back check (extension control)	0.00	1.40	1.40	0.00	1.40	1.40	XXX	■
L5688			Addition to lower extremity, below knee, waist belt, webbing	0.00	1.70	1.70	0.00	1.70	1.70	XXX	■
L5690			Addition to lower extremity, below knee, waist belt, padded and lined	0.00	2.71	2.71	0.00	2.71	2.71	XXX	■
L5692			Addition to lower extremity, above knee, pelvic control belt, light	0.00	3.67	3.67	0.00	3.67	3.67	XXX	■
L5694			Addition to lower extremity, above knee, pelvic control belt, padded and lined	0.00	5.01	5.01	0.00	5.01	5.01	XXX	■
L5695			Addition to lower extremity, above knee, pelvic control, sleeve suspension, neoprene or equal, each	0.00	4.50	4.50	0.00	4.50	4.50	XXX	■
L5696			Addition to lower extremity, above knee or knee disarticulation, pelvic joint	0.00	5.10	5.10	0.00	5.10	5.10	XXX	■
L5697			Addition to lower extremity, above knee or knee disarticulation, pelvic band	0.00	2.21	2.21	0.00	2.21	2.21	XXX	■
L5698			Addition to lower extremity, above knee or knee disarticulation, Silesian bandage	0.00	2.89	2.89	0.00	2.89	2.89	XXX	■
L5699			All lower extremity prostheses, shoulder harness	0.00	5.16	5.16	0.00	5.16	5.16	XXX	■
L5700			Replacement, socket, below knee, molded to patient model	0.00	70.15	70.15	0.00	70.15	70.15	XXX	■
L5701			Replacement, socket, above knee/knee disarticulation, including attachment plate, molded to patient model	0.00	93.78	93.78	0.00	93.78	93.78	XXX	■
L5702			Replacement, socket, hip disarticulation, including hip joint, molded to patient model	0.00	104.30	104.30	0.00	104.30	104.30	XXX	■

■ RVU not developed by CMS. Gap-filled RVUs developed by CHEG.

Code	M	S	Description	Work Value	Non-Fac PE	Fac PE	Mal-practice	Non-Fac Total	Fac Total	Global	Gap
L5704			Custom shaped protective cover, below knee	0.00	12.99	12.99	0.00	12.99	12.99	XXX	■
L5705			Custom shaped protective cover, above knee	0.00	24.32	24.32	0.00	24.32	24.32	XXX	■
L5706			Custom shaped protective cover, knee disarticulation	0.00	23.68	23.68	0.00	23.68	23.68	XXX	■
L5707			Custom shaped protective cover, hip disarticulation	0.00	27.03	27.03	0.00	27.03	27.03	XXX	■
L5710			Addition, exoskeletal knee-shin system, single axis, manual lock	0.00	8.68	8.68	0.00	8.68	8.68	XXX	■
L5711			Addition, exoskeletal knee-shin system, single axis, manual lock, ultra-light material	0.00	14.26	14.26	0.00	14.26	14.26	XXX	■
L5712			Addition, exoskeletal knee-shin system, single axis, friction swing and stance phase control (safety knee)	0.00	10.67	10.67	0.00	10.67	10.67	XXX	■
L5714			Addition, exoskeletal knee-shin system, single axis, variable friction swing phase control	0.00	10.70	10.70	0.00	10.70	10.70	XXX	■
L5716			Addition, exoskeletal knee-shin system, polycentric, mechanical stance phase lock	0.00	17.58	17.58	0.00	17.58	17.58	XXX	■
L5718			Addition, exoskeletal knee-shin system, polycentric, friction swing and stance phase control	0.00	21.99	21.99	0.00	21.99	21.99	XXX	■
L5722			Addition, exoskeletal knee-shin system, single axis, pneumatic swing, friction stance phase control	0.00	23.73	23.73	0.00	23.73	23.73	XXX	■
L5724			Addition, exoskeletal knee-shin system, single axis, fluid swing phase control	0.00	41.72	41.72	0.00	41.72	41.72	XXX	■
L5726			Addition, exoskeletal knee-shin system, single axis, external joints, fluid swing phase control	0.00	47.68	47.68	0.00	47.68	47.68	XXX	■
L5728			Addition, exoskeletal knee-shin system, single axis, fluid swing and stance phase control	0.00	65.62	65.62	0.00	65.62	65.62	XXX	■
L5780			Addition, exoskeletal knee-shin system, single axis, pneumatic/hydra pneumatic swing phase control	0.00	25.94	25.94	0.00	25.94	25.94	XXX	■
L5785			Addition, exoskeletal system, below knee, ultra-light material (titanium, carbon fiber or equal)	0.00	14.30	14.30	0.00	14.30	14.30	XXX	■
L5790			Addition, exoskeletal system, above knee, ultra-light material (titanium, carbon fiber or equal)	0.00	20.22	20.22	0.00	20.22	20.22	XXX	■
L5795			Addition, exoskeletal system, hip disarticulation, ultra-light material (titanium, carbon fiber or equal)	0.00	25.58	25.58	0.00	25.58	25.58	XXX	■
L5810			Addition, endoskeletal knee-shin system, single axis, manual lock	0.00	13.41	13.41	0.00	13.41	13.41	XXX	■

■ RVU not developed by CMS. Gap-filled RVUs developed by CHEG.

Code	M	S	Description	Work Value	Non-Fac PE	Fac PE	Mal-prac-tice	Non-Fac Total	Fac Total	Global	Gap
L5811			Addition, endoskeletal knee-shin system, single axis, manual lock, ultra-light material	0.00	17.98	17.98	0.00	17.98	17.98	XXX	■
L5812			Addition, endoskeletal knee-shin system, single axis, friction swing and stance phase control (safety knee)	0.00	13.95	13.95	0.00	13.95	13.95	XXX	■
L5814			Addition, endoskeletal knee-shin system, polycentric, hydraulic swing phase control, mechanical stance phase lock	0.00	0.00	0.00	0.00	0.00	0.00	XXX	
L5816			Addition, endoskeletal knee-shin system, polycentric, mechanical stance phase lock	0.00	16.18	16.18	0.00	16.18	16.18	XXX	■
L5818			Addition, endoskeletal knee-shin system, polycentric, friction swing and stance phase control	0.00	22.05	22.05	0.00	22.05	22.05	XXX	■
L5822			Addition, endoskeletal knee-shin system, single axis, pneumatic swing, friction stance phase control	0.00	36.27	36.27	0.00	36.27	36.27	XXX	■
L5824			Addition, endoskeletal knee-shin system, single axis, fluid swing phase control	0.00	37.25	37.25	0.00	37.25	37.25	XXX	■
L5826			Addition, endoskeletal knee-shin system, single axis, hydraulic swing phase control, with miniature high activity frame	0.00	0.00	0.00	0.00	0.00	0.00	XXX	
L5828			Addition, endoskeletal knee-shin system, single axis, fluid swing and stance phase control	0.00	77.78	77.78	0.00	77.78	77.78	XXX	■
L5830			Addition, endoskeletal knee-shin system, single axis, pneumatic/swing phase control	0.00	45.50	45.50	0.00	45.50	45.50	XXX	■
L5840			Addition, endoskeletal knee-shin system, 4-bar linkage or multiaxial, pneumatic swing phase control	0.00	53.42	53.42	0.00	53.42	53.42	XXX	■
L5845			Addition, endoskeletal knee-shin system, stance flexion feature, adjustable	0.00	80.46	80.46	0.00	80.46	80.46	XXX	■
L5846			Addition, endoskeletal knee-shin system, microprocessor control feature, swing phase only	0.00	116.22	116.22	0.00	116.22	116.22	XXX	■
L5847			Addition, endoskeletal knee-shin system, microprocessor control feature, stance phase	0.00	110.62	110.62	0.00	110.62	110.62	XXX	■
L5850			Addition, endoskeletal system, above knee or hip disarticulation, knee extension assist	0.00	2.71	2.71	0.00	2.71	2.71	XXX	■
L5855			Addition, endoskeletal system, hip disarticulation, mechanical hip extension assist	0.00	7.30	7.30	0.00	7.30	7.30	XXX	■
L5910			Addition, endoskeletal system, below knee, alignable system	0.00	8.58	8.58	0.00	8.58	8.58	XXX	■
L5920			Addition, endoskeletal system, above knee or hip disarticulation, alignable system	0.00	15.05	15.05	0.00	15.05	15.05	XXX	■

■ RVU not developed by CMS. Gap-filled RVUs developed by CHEG.

Code	M	S	Description	Work Value	Non-Fac PE	Fac PE	Mal-prac-tice	Non-Fac Total	Fac Total	Global	Gap
L5925			Addition, endoskeletal system, above knee, knee disarticulation or hip disarticulation, manual lock	0.00	7.78	7.78	0.00	7.78	7.78	XXX	■
L5930			Addition, endoskeletal system, high activity knee control frame	0.00	72.12	72.12	0.00	72.12	72.12	XXX	■
L5940			Addition, endoskeletal system, below knee, ultra-light material (titanium, carbon fiber or equal)	0.00	13.35	13.35	0.00	13.35	13.35	XXX	■
L5950			Addition, endoskeletal system, above knee, ultra-light material (titanium, carbon fiber or equal)	0.00	21.33	21.33	0.00	21.33	21.33	XXX	■
L5960			Addition, endoskeletal system, hip disarticulation, ultra-light material (titanium, carbon fiber or equal)	0.00	24.32	24.32	0.00	24.32	24.32	XXX	■
L5962			Addition, endoskeletal system, below knee, flexible protective outer surface covering system	0.00	13.60	13.60	0.00	13.60	13.60	XXX	■
L5964			Addition, endoskeletal system, above knee, flexible protective outer surface covering system	0.00	25.14	25.14	0.00	25.14	25.14	XXX	■
L5966			Addition, endoskeletal system, hip disarticulation, flexible protective outer surface covering system	0.00	32.39	32.39	0.00	32.39	32.39	XXX	■
L5968			Addition to lower limb prosthesis, multiaxial ankle with swing phase active dorsiflexion feature	0.00	0.00	0.00	0.00	0.00	0.00	XXX	
L5970			All lower extremity prostheses, foot, external keel, SACH foot	0.00	5.57	5.57	0.00	5.57	5.57	XXX	■
L5972			All lower extremity prostheses, flexible keel foot (Safe, Sten, Bock Dynamic or equal)	0.00	9.60	9.60	0.00	9.60	9.60	XXX	■
L5974			All lower extremity prostheses, foot, single axis ankle/foot	0.00	6.41	6.41	0.00	6.41	6.41	XXX	■
L5975			All lower extremity prosthesis, combination single axis ankle and flexible keel foot	0.00	0.00	0.00	0.00	0.00	0.00	XXX	
L5976			All lower extremity prostheses, energy storing foot (Seattle Carbon Copy II or equal)	0.00	15.44	15.44	0.00	15.44	15.44	XXX	■
L5978			All lower extremity prostheses, foot, multi-axial ankle/foot	0.00	8.14	8.14	0.00	8.14	8.14	XXX	■
L5979			All lower extremity prostheses, multi-axial ankle, dynamic response foot, one piece system	0.00	63.12	63.12	0.00	63.12	63.12	XXX	■
L5980			All lower extremity prostheses, flex-foot system	0.00	98.58	98.58	0.00	98.58	98.58	XXX	■
L5981			All lower extremity prostheses, flex-walk system or equal	0.00	76.53	76.53	0.00	76.53	76.53	XXX	■

■ RVU not developed by CMS. Gap-filled RVUs developed by CHEG.

Code	M	S	Description	Work Value	Non-Fac PE	Fac PE	Mal-practice	Non-Fac Total	Fac Total	Global	Gap
L5982			All exoskeletal lower extremity prostheses, axial rotation unit	0.00	15.94	15.94	0.00	15.94	15.94	XXX	■
L5984			All endoskeletal lower extremity prostheses, axial rotation unit	0.00	14.52	14.52	0.00	14.52	14.52	XXX	■
L5985			All endoskeletal lower extremity prostheses, dynamic prosthetic pylon	0.00	6.08	6.08	0.00	6.08	6.08	XXX	■
L5986			All lower extremity prostheses, multi-axial rotation unit ("MCP" or equal)	0.00	17.46	17.46	0.00	17.46	17.46	XXX	■
L5987			All lower extremity prosthesis, shank foot system with vertical loading pylon	0.00	0.00	0.00	0.00	0.00	0.00	XXX	
L5988			Addition to lower limb prosthesis, vertical shock reducing pylon feature	0.00	0.00	0.00	0.00	0.00	0.00	XXX	
L5989			Addition to lower extremity prosthesis, endoskeletal system, pylon with integrated electronic force sensors	0.00	0.00	0.00	0.00	0.00	0.00	XXX	
L5990			Addition to lower extremity prosthesis, user adjustable heel height	0.00	0.00	0.00	0.00	0.00	0.00	XXX	
L5999			Lower extremity prosthesis, not otherwise specified	0.00	0.00	0.00	0.00	0.00	0.00	XXX	
L6000			Partial hand, Robin-Aids, thumb remaining (or equal)	0.00	32.82	32.82	0.00	32.82	32.82	XXX	■
L6010			Partial hand, Robin-Aids, little and/or ring finger remaining (or equal)	0.00	34.28	34.28	0.00	34.28	34.28	XXX	■
L6020			Partial hand, Robin-Aids, no finger remaining (or equal)	0.00	35.05	35.05	0.00	35.05	35.05	XXX	■
L6050			Wrist disarticulation, molded socket, flexible elbow hinges, triceps pad	0.00	52.07	52.07	0.00	52.07	52.07	XXX	■
L6055			Wrist disarticulation, molded socket with expandable interface, flexible elbow hinges, triceps pad	0.00	66.10	66.10	0.00	66.10	66.10	XXX	■
L6100			Below elbow, molded socket, flexible elbow hinge, triceps pad	0.00	53.07	53.07	0.00	53.07	53.07	XXX	■
L6110			Below elbow, molded socket (Muenster or Northwestern suspension types)	0.00	56.38	56.38	0.00	56.38	56.38	XXX	■
L6120			Below elbow, molded double wall split socket, step-up hinges, half cuff	0.00	60.20	60.20	0.00	60.20	60.20	XXX	■
L6130			Below elbow, molded double wall split socket, stump activated locking hinge, half cuff	0.00	59.59	59.59	0.00	59.59	59.59	XXX	■
L6200			Elbow disarticulation, molded socket, outside locking hinge, forearm	0.00	65.32	65.32	0.00	65.32	65.32	XXX	■
L6205			Elbow disarticulation, molded socket with expandable interface, outside locking hinges, forearm	0.00	94.81	94.81	0.00	94.81	94.81	XXX	■

■ RVU not developed by CMS. Gap-filled RVUs developed by CHEG.

HCPCS

Code	M	S	Description	Work Value	Non-Fac PE	Fac PE	Mal-practice	Non-Fac Total	Fac Total	Global	Gap
L6250			Above elbow, molded double wall socket, internal locking elbow, forearm	0.00	70.03	70.03	0.00	70.03	70.03	XXX	■
L6300			Shoulder disarticulation, molded socket, shoulder bulkhead, humeral section, internal locking elbow, forearm	0.00	92.75	92.75	0.00	92.75	92.75	XXX	■
L6310			Shoulder disarticulation, passive restoration (complete prosthesis)	0.00	83.59	83.59	0.00	83.59	83.59	XXX	■
L6320			Shoulder disarticulation, passive restoration (shoulder cap only)	0.00	42.17	42.17	0.00	42.17	42.17	XXX	■
L6350			Interscapular thoracic, molded socket, shoulder bulkhead, humeral section, internal locking elbow, forearm	0.00	104.30	104.30	0.00	104.30	104.30	XXX	■
L6360			Interscapular thoracic, passive restoration (complete prosthesis)	0.00	75.81	75.81	0.00	75.81	75.81	XXX	■
L6370			Interscapular thoracic, passive restoration (shoulder cap only)	0.00	51.79	51.79	0.00	51.79	51.79	XXX	■
L6380			Immediate postsurgical or early fitting, application of initial rigid dressing, including fitting alignment and suspension of components, and one cast change, wrist disarticulation or below elbow	0.00	29.50	29.50	0.00	29.50	29.50	XXX	■
L6382			Immediate postsurgical or early fitting, application of initial rigid dressing including fitting alignment and suspension of components, and one cast change, elbow disarticulation or above elbow	0.00	39.78	39.78	0.00	39.78	39.78	XXX	■
L6384			Immediate postsurgical or early fitting, application of initial rigid dressing including fitting alignment and suspension of components, and one cast change, shoulder disarticulation or interscapular thoracic	0.00	54.15	54.15	0.00	54.15	54.15	XXX	■
L6386			Immediate postsurgical or early fitting, each additional cast change and realignment	0.00	9.51	9.51	0.00	9.51	9.51	XXX	■
L6388			Immediate postsurgical or early fitting, application of rigid dressing only	0.00	12.37	12.37	0.00	12.37	12.37	XXX	■
L6400			Below elbow, molded socket, endoskeletal system, including soft prosthetic tissue shaping	0.00	53.39	53.39	0.00	53.39	53.39	XXX	■
L6450			Elbow disarticulation, molded socket, endoskeletal system, including soft prosthetic tissue shaping	0.00	75.82	75.82	0.00	75.82	75.82	XXX	■
L6500			Above elbow, molded socket, endoskeletal system, including soft prosthetic tissue shaping	0.00	74.08	74.08	0.00	74.08	74.08	XXX	■
L6550			Shoulder disarticulation, molded socket, endoskeletal system, including soft prosthetic tissue shaping	0.00	88.10	88.10	0.00	88.10	88.10	XXX	■

■ RVU not developed by CMS. Gap-filled RVUs developed by CHEG.

Code	M	S	Description	Work Value	Non-Fac PE	Fac PE	Mal-practice	Non-Fac Total	Fac Total	Global	Gap
L6570			Interscapular thoracic, molded socket, endoskeletal system, including soft prosthetic tissue shaping	0.00	105.47	105.47	0.00	105.47	105.47	XXX	■
L6580			Preparatory, wrist disarticulation or below elbow, single wall plastic socket, friction wrist, flexible elbow hinges, figure of eight harness, humeral cuff, Bowden cable control, "USMC" or equal pylon, no cover, molded to patient model	0.00	44.25	44.25	0.00	44.25	44.25	XXX	■
L6582			Preparatory, wrist disarticulation or below elbow, single wall socket, friction wrist, flexible elbow hinges, figure of eight harness, humeral cuff, Bowden cable control, "USMC" or equal pylon, no cover, direct formed	0.00	37.92	37.92	0.00	37.92	37.92	XXX	■
L6584			Preparatory, elbow disarticulation or above elbow, single wall plastic socket, friction wrist, locking elbow, figure of eight harness, fair lead cable control, "USMC" or equal pylon, no cover, molded to patient model	0.00	56.89	56.89	0.00	56.89	56.89	XXX	■
L6586			Preparatory, elbow disarticulation or above elbow, single wall socket, friction wrist, locking elbow, figure of eight harness, fair lead cable control, "USMC" or equal pylon, no cover, direct formed	0.00	46.88	46.88	0.00	46.88	46.88	XXX	■
L6588			Preparatory, shoulder disarticulation or interscapular thoracic, single wall plastic socket, shoulder joint, locking elbow, friction wrist, chest strap, fair lead cable control, "USMC" or equal pylon, no cover, molded to patient model	0.00	78.90	78.90	0.00	78.90	78.90	XXX	■
L6590			Preparatory, shoulder disarticulation or interscapular thoracic, single wall socket, shoulder joint, locking elbow, friction wrist, chest strap, fair lead cable control, "USMC" or equal pylon, no cover, direct formed	0.00	62.86	62.86	0.00	62.86	62.86	XXX	■
L6600			Upper extremity additions, polycentric hinge, pair	0.00	4.92	4.92	0.00	4.92	4.92	XXX	■
L6605			Upper extremity additions, single pivot hinge, pair	0.00	3.94	3.94	0.00	3.94	3.94	XXX	■
L6610			Upper extremity additions, flexible metal hinge, pair	0.00	3.93	3.93	0.00	3.93	3.93	XXX	■
L6615			Upper extremity addition, disconnect locking wrist unit	0.00	5.62	5.62	0.00	5.62	5.62	XXX	■
L6616			Upper extremity addition, additional disconnect insert for locking wrist unit, each	0.00	1.64	1.64	0.00	1.64	1.64	XXX	■
L6620			Upper extremity addition, flexion-friction wrist unit	0.00	8.69	8.69	0.00	8.69	8.69	XXX	■
L6623			Upper extremity addition, spring assisted rotational wrist unit with latch release	0.00	17.67	17.67	0.00	17.67	17.67	XXX	■

■ RVU not developed by CMS. Gap-filled RVUs developed by CHEG.

Code	M	S	Description	Work Value	Non-Fac PE	Fac PE	Mal-prac-tice	Non-Fac Total	Fac Total	Global	Gap
L6625			Upper extremity addition, rotation wrist unit with cable lock	0.00	11.15	11.15	0.00	11.15	11.15	XXX	■
L6628			Upper extremity addition, quick disconnect hook adapter, Otto Bock or equal	0.00	11.13	11.13	0.00	11.13	11.13	XXX	■
L6629			Upper extremity addition, quick disconnect lamination collar with coupling piece, Otto Bock or equal	0.00	4.01	4.01	0.00	4.01	4.01	XXX	■
L6630			Upper extremity addition, stainless steel, any wrist	0.00	6.12	6.12	0.00	6.12	6.12	XXX	■
L6632			Upper extremity addition, latex suspension sleeve, each	0.00	1.64	1.64	0.00	1.64	1.64	XXX	■
L6635			Upper extremity addition, lift assist for elbow	0.00	4.86	4.86	0.00	4.86	4.86	XXX	■
L6637			Upper extremity addition, nudge control elbow lock	0.00	9.95	9.95	0.00	9.95	9.95	XXX	■
L6640			Upper extremity additions, shoulder abduction joint, pair	0.00	7.79	7.79	0.00	7.79	7.79	XXX	■
L6641			Upper extremity addition, excursion amplifier, pulley type	0.00	4.40	4.40	0.00	4.40	4.40	XXX	■
L6642			Upper extremity addition, excursion amplifier, lever type	0.00	5.82	5.82	0.00	5.82	5.82	XXX	■
L6645			Upper extremity addition, shoulder flexion-abduction joint, each	0.00	7.69	7.69	0.00	7.69	7.69	XXX	■
L6650			Upper extremity addition, shoulder universal joint, each	0.00	9.33	9.33	0.00	9.33	9.33	XXX	■
L6655			Upper extremity addition, standard control cable, extra	0.00	1.94	1.94	0.00	1.94	1.94	XXX	■
L6660			Upper extremity addition, heavy duty control cable	0.00	2.12	2.12	0.00	2.12	2.12	XXX	■
L6665			Upper extremity addition, Teflon, or equal, cable lining	0.00	1.16	1.16	0.00	1.16	1.16	XXX	■
L6670			Upper extremity addition, hook to hand, cable adapter	0.00	1.09	1.09	0.00	1.09	1.09	XXX	■
L6672			Upper extremity addition, harness, chest or shoulder, saddle type	0.00	4.77	4.77	0.00	4.77	4.77	XXX	■
L6675			Upper extremity addition, harness, figure of eight type, for single control	0.00	3.41	3.41	0.00	3.41	3.41	XXX	■
L6676			Upper extremity addition, harness, figure of eight type, for dual control	0.00	2.79	2.79	0.00	2.79	2.79	XXX	■
L6680			Upper extremity addition, test socket, wrist disarticulation or below elbow	0.00	6.38	6.38	0.00	6.38	6.38	XXX	■
L6682			Upper extremity addition, test socket, elbow disarticulation or above elbow	0.00	6.35	6.35	0.00	6.35	6.35	XXX	■

■ RVU not developed by CMS. Gap-filled RVUs developed by CHEG.

Code	M	S	Description	Work Value	Non-Fac PE	Fac PE	Mal-practice	Non-Fac Total	Fac Total	Global	Gap
L6684			Upper extremity addition, test socket, shoulder disarticulation or interscapular thoracic	0.00	8.87	8.87	0.00	8.87	8.87	XXX	■
L6686			Upper extremity addition, suction socket	0.00	16.75	16.75	0.00	16.75	16.75	XXX	■
L6687			Upper extremity addition, frame type socket, below elbow or wrist disarticulation	0.00	12.96	12.96	0.00	12.96	12.96	XXX	■
L6688			Upper extremity addition, frame type socket, above elbow or elbow disarticulation	0.00	14.60	14.60	0.00	14.60	14.60	XXX	■
L6689			Upper extremity addition, frame type socket, shoulder disarticulation	0.00	18.60	18.60	0.00	18.60	18.60	XXX	■
L6690			Upper extremity addition, frame type socket, interscapular-thoracic	0.00	18.95	18.95	0.00	18.95	18.95	XXX	■
L6691			Upper extremity addition, removable insert, each	0.00	9.54	9.54	0.00	9.54	9.54	XXX	■
L6692			Upper extremity addition, silicone gel insert or equal, each	0.00	15.44	15.44	0.00	15.44	15.44	XXX	■
L6693			Upper extremity addition, locking elbow, forearm counterbalance	0.00	0.00	0.00	0.00	0.00	0.00	XXX	
L6700			Terminal device, hook, Dorrance or equal, model #3	0.00	14.30	14.30	0.00	14.30	14.30	XXX	■
L6705			Terminal device, hook, Dorrance or equal, model #5	0.00	8.40	8.40	0.00	8.40	8.40	XXX	■
L6710			Terminal device, hook, Dorrance or equal, model #5X	0.00	9.51	9.51	0.00	9.51	9.51	XXX	■
L6715			Terminal device, hook, Dorrance or equal, model #5XA	0.00	9.45	9.45	0.00	9.45	9.45	XXX	■
L6720			Terminal device, hook, Dorrance or equal, model #6	0.00	23.54	23.54	0.00	23.54	23.54	XXX	■
L6725			Terminal device, hook, Dorrance or equal, model #7	0.00	11.38	11.38	0.00	11.38	11.38	XXX	■
L6730			Terminal device, hook, Dorrance or equal, model #7LO	0.00	18.16	18.16	0.00	18.16	18.16	XXX	■
L6735			Terminal device, hook, Dorrance or equal, model #8	0.00	8.22	8.22	0.00	8.22	8.22	XXX	■
L6740			Terminal device, hook, Dorrance or equal, model #8X	0.00	10.73	10.73	0.00	10.73	10.73	XXX	■
L6745			Terminal device, hook, Dorrance or equal, model #88X	0.00	9.80	9.80	0.00	9.80	9.80	XXX	■
L6750			Terminal device, hook, Dorrance or equal, model #10P	0.00	9.69	9.69	0.00	9.69	9.69	XXX	■
L6755			Terminal device, hook, Dorrance or equal, model #10X	0.00	9.66	9.66	0.00	9.66	9.66	XXX	■

■ RVU not developed by CMS. Gap-filled RVUs developed by CHEG.

Code	M	S	Description	Work Value	Non-Fac PE	Fac PE	Mal-prac-tice	Non-Fac Total	Fac Total	Global	Gap
L6765			Terminal device, hook, Dorrance or equal, model #12P	0.00	10.10	10.10	0.00	10.10	10.10	XXX	■
L6770			Terminal device, hook, Dorrance or equal, model #99X	0.00	9.74	9.74	0.00	9.74	9.74	XXX	■
L6775			Terminal device, hook, Dorrance or equal, model #555	0.00	11.53	11.53	0.00	11.53	11.53	XXX	■
L6780			Terminal device, hook, Dorrance or equal, model #SS555	0.00	12.34	12.34	0.00	12.34	12.34	XXX	■
L6790			Terminal device, hook, Accu hook or equal	0.00	12.46	12.46	0.00	12.46	12.46	XXX	■
L6795			Terminal device, hook, 2 load or equal	0.00	34.15	34.15	0.00	34.15	34.15	XXX	■
L6800			Terminal device, hook, APRL VC or equal	0.00	27.95	27.95	0.00	27.95	27.95	XXX	■
L6805			Terminal device, modifier wrist flexion unit	0.00	9.39	9.39	0.00	9.39	9.39	XXX	■
L6806			Terminal device, hook, TRS Grip, Grip III, VC, or equal	0.00	0.00	0.00	0.00	0.00	0.00	XXX	
L6807			Terminal device, hook, Grip I, Grip II, VC, or equal	0.00	0.00	0.00	0.00	0.00	0.00	XXX	
L6808			Terminal device, hook, TRS Adept, infant or child, VC, or equal	0.00	0.00	0.00	0.00	0.00	0.00	XXX	
L6809			Terminal device, hook, TRS Super Sport, passive	0.00	10.22	10.22	0.00	10.22	10.22	XXX	■
L6810			Terminal device, pincher tool, Otto Bock or equal	0.00	5.16	5.16	0.00	5.16	5.16	XXX	■
L6825			Terminal device, hand, Dorrance, VO	0.00	28.46	28.46	0.00	28.46	28.46	XXX	■
L6830			Terminal device, hand, APRL, VC	0.00	37.37	37.37	0.00	37.37	37.37	XXX	■
L6835			Terminal device, hand, Sierra, VO	0.00	32.54	32.54	0.00	32.54	32.54	XXX	■
L6840			Terminal device, hand, Becker Imperial	0.00	22.62	22.62	0.00	22.62	22.62	XXX	■
L6845			Terminal device, hand, Becker Lock Grip	0.00	20.98	20.98	0.00	20.98	20.98	XXX	■
L6850			Terminal device, hand, Becker Plylite	0.00	19.01	19.01	0.00	19.01	19.01	XXX	■
L6855			Terminal device, hand, Robin-Aids, VO	0.00	24.17	24.17	0.00	24.17	24.17	XXX	■
L6860			Terminal device, hand, Robin-Aids, VO soft	0.00	18.33	18.33	0.00	18.33	18.33	XXX	■
L6865			Terminal device, hand, passive hand	0.00	8.97	8.97	0.00	8.97	8.97	XXX	■
L6867			Terminal device, hand, Detroit Infant Hand (mechanical)	0.00	26.49	26.49	0.00	26.49	26.49	XXX	■
L6868			Terminal device, hand, passive infant hand, Steeper, Hosmer or equal	0.00	6.62	6.62	0.00	6.62	6.62	XXX	■
L6870			Terminal device, hand, child mitt	0.00	6.56	6.56	0.00	6.56	6.56	XXX	■

■ RVU not developed by CMS. Gap-filled RVUs developed by CHEG.

Code	M	S	Description	Work Value	Non-Fac PE	Fac PE	Mal-practice	Non-Fac Total	Fac Total	Global	Gap
L6872			Terminal device, hand, NYU child hand	0.00	25.99	25.99	0.00	25.99	25.99	XXX	■
L6873			Terminal device, hand, mechanical infant hand, Steeper or equal	0.00	12.90	12.90	0.00	12.90	12.90	XXX	■
L6875			Terminal device, hand, Bock, VC	0.00	21.43	21.43	0.00	21.43	21.43	XXX	■
L6880			Terminal device, hand, Bock, VO	0.00	13.92	13.92	0.00	13.92	13.92	XXX	■
L6881			Automatic grasp feature, addition to upper limb prosthetic terminal device	0.00	0.00	0.00	0.00	0.00	0.00	XXX	
L6882			Microprocessor control feature, addition to upper limb prosthetic terminal device	0.00	0.00	0.00	0.00	0.00	0.00	XXX	
L6890			Terminal device, glove for above hands, production glove	0.00	4.68	4.68	0.00	4.68	4.68	XXX	■
L6895			Terminal device, glove for above hands, custom glove	0.00	15.41	15.41	0.00	15.41	15.41	XXX	■
L6900			Hand restoration (casts, shading and measurements included), partial hand, with glove, thumb or one finger remaining	0.00	33.97	33.97	0.00	33.97	33.97	XXX	■
L6905			Hand restoration (casts, shading and measurements included), partial hand, with glove, multiple fingers remaining	0.00	40.50	40.50	0.00	40.50	40.50	XXX	■
L6910			Hand restoration (casts, shading and measurements included), partial hand, with glove, no fingers remaining	0.00	39.46	39.46	0.00	39.46	39.46	XXX	■
L6915			Hand restoration (shading and measurements included), replacement glove for above	0.00	17.25	17.25	0.00	17.25	17.25	XXX	■
L6920			Wrist disarticulation, external power, self-suspended inner socket, removable forearm shell, Otto Bock or equal switch, cables, two batteries and one charger, switch control of terminal device	0.00	0.00	0.00	0.00	0.00	0.00	XXX	
L6925			Wrist disarticulation, external power, self-suspended inner socket, removable forearm shell, Otto Bock or equal electrodes, cables, two batteries and one charger, myoelectronic control of terminal device	0.00	0.00	0.00	0.00	0.00	0.00	XXX	
L6930			Below elbow, external power, self-suspended inner socket, removable forearm shell, Otto Bock or equal switch, cables, two batteries and one charger, switch control of terminal device	0.00	0.00	0.00	0.00	0.00	0.00	XXX	
L6935			Below elbow, external power, self-suspended inner socket, removable forearm shell, Otto Bock or equal electrodes, cables, two batteries and one charger, myoelectronic control of terminal device	0.00	0.00	0.00	0.00	0.00	0.00	XXX	

■ RVU not developed by CMS. Gap-filled RVUs developed by CHEG.

Code	M	S	Description	Work Value	Non-Fac PE	Fac PE	Mal-practice	Non-Fac Total	Fac Total	Global	Gap
L6940			Elbow disarticulation, external power, molded inner socket, removable humeral shell, outside locking hinges, forearm, Otto Bock or equal switch, cables, two batteries and one charger, switch control of terminal device	0.00	0.00	0.00	0.00	0.00	0.00	XXX	
L6945			Elbow disarticulation, external power, molded inner socket, removable humeral shell, outside locking hinges, forearm, Otto Bock or equal electrodes, cables, two batteries and one charger, myoelectronic control of terminal device	0.00	0.00	0.00	0.00	0.00	0.00	XXX	
L6950			Above elbow, external power, molded inner socket, removable humeral shell, internal locking elbow, forearm, Otto Bock or equal switch, cables, two batteries and one charger, switch control of terminal device	0.00	0.00	0.00	0.00	0.00	0.00	XXX	
L6955			Above elbow, external power, molded inner socket, removable humeral shell, internal locking elbow, forearm, Otto Bock or equal electrodes, cables, two batteries and one charger, myoelectronic control of terminal device	0.00	0.00	0.00	0.00	0.00	0.00	XXX	
L6960			Shoulder disarticulation, external power, molded inner socket, removable shoulder shell, shoulder bulkhead, humeral section, mechanical elbow, forearm, Otto Bock or equal switch, cables, two batteries and one charger, switch control of terminal device	0.00	0.00	0.00	0.00	0.00	0.00	XXX	
L6965			Shoulder disarticulation, external power, molded inner socket, removable shoulder shell, shoulder bulkhead, humeral section, mechanical elbow, forearm, Otto Bock or equal electrodes, cables, two batteries and one charger, myoelectronic control of terminal device	0.00	0.00	0.00	0.00	0.00	0.00	XXX	
L6970			Interscapular-thoracic, external power, molded inner socket, removable shoulder shell, shoulder bulkhead, humeral section, mechanical elbow, forearm, Otto Bock or equal switch, cables, two batteries and one charger, switch control of terminal device	0.00	0.00	0.00	0.00	0.00	0.00	XXX	
L6975			Interscapular-thoracic, external power, molded inner socket, removable shoulder shell, shoulder bulkhead, humeral section, mechanical elbow, forearm, Otto Bock or equal electrodes, cables, two batteries and one charger, myoelectronic control of terminal device	0.00	0.00	0.00	0.00	0.00	0.00	XXX	
L7010			Electronic hand, Otto Bock, Steeper or equal, switch controlled	0.00	0.00	0.00	0.00	0.00	0.00	XXX	
L7015			Electronic hand, System Teknik, Variety Village or equal, switch controlled	0.00	0.00	0.00	0.00	0.00	0.00	XXX	

■ RVU not developed by CMS. Gap-filled RVUs developed by CHEG.

Code	M	S	Description	Work Value	Non-Fac PE	Fac PE	Mal-practice	Non-Fac Total	Fac Total	Global	Gap
L7020			Electronic greifer, Otto Bock or equal, switch controlled	0.00	0.00	0.00	0.00	0.00	0.00	XXX	
L7025			Electronic hand, Otto Bock or equal, myoelectronically controlled	0.00	0.00	0.00	0.00	0.00	0.00	XXX	
L7030			Electronic hand, System Teknik, Variety Village or equal, myoelectronically controlled	0.00	0.00	0.00	0.00	0.00	0.00	XXX	
L7035			Electronic greifer, Otto Bock or equal, myoelectronically controlled	0.00	0.00	0.00	0.00	0.00	0.00	XXX	
L7040			Prehensile actuator, Hosmer or equal, switch controlled	0.00	0.00	0.00	0.00	0.00	0.00	XXX	
L7045			Electronic hook, child, Michigan or equal, switch controlled	0.00	0.00	0.00	0.00	0.00	0.00	XXX	
L7170			Electronic elbow, Hosmer or equal, switch controlled	0.00	0.00	0.00	0.00	0.00	0.00	XXX	
L7180			Electronic elbow, Boston, Utah or equal, myoelectronically controlled	0.00	0.00	0.00	0.00	0.00	0.00	XXX	
L7185			Electronic elbow, adolescent, Variety Village or equal, switch controlled	0.00	0.00	0.00	0.00	0.00	0.00	XXX	
L7186			Electronic elbow, child, Variety Village or equal, switch controlled	0.00	0.00	0.00	0.00	0.00	0.00	XXX	
L7190			Electronic elbow, adolescent, Variety Village or equal, myoelectronically controlled	0.00	0.00	0.00	0.00	0.00	0.00	XXX	
L7191			Electronic elbow, child, Variety Village or equal, myoelectronically controlled	0.00	0.00	0.00	0.00	0.00	0.00	XXX	
L7260			Electronic wrist rotator, Otto Bock or equal	0.00	0.00	0.00	0.00	0.00	0.00	XXX	
L7261			Electronic wrist rotator, for Utah arm	0.00	0.00	0.00	0.00	0.00	0.00	XXX	
L7266			Servo control, Steeper or equal	0.00	0.00	0.00	0.00	0.00	0.00	XXX	
L7272			Analogue control, UNB or equal	0.00	0.00	0.00	0.00	0.00	0.00	XXX	
L7274			Proportional control, 6-12 volt, Liberty, Utah or equal	0.00	0.00	0.00	0.00	0.00	0.00	XXX	
L7360			Six volt battery, Otto Bock or equal, each	0.00	6.26	6.26	0.00	6.26	6.26	XXX	■
L7362			Battery charger, six volt, Otto Bock or equal	0.00	6.91	6.91	0.00	6.91	6.91	XXX	■
L7364			Twelve volt battery, Utah or equal, each	0.00	11.00	11.00	0.00	11.00	11.00	XXX	■
L7366			Battery charger, twelve volt, Utah or equal	0.00	14.81	14.81	0.00	14.81	14.81	XXX	■
L7499			Upper extremity prosthesis, not otherwise specified	0.00	0.00	0.00	0.00	0.00	0.00	XXX	
L7500			Repair of prosthetic device, hourly rate (excludes V5335 Repair of oral or laryngeal prosthesis or artificial larynx)	0.00	0.00	0.00	0.00	0.00	0.00	XXX	

■ RVU not developed by CMS. Gap-filled RVUs developed by CHEG.

Code	M	S	Description	Work Value	Non-Fac PE	Fac PE	Mal-practice	Non-Fac Total	Fac Total	Global	Gap
L7510			Repair of prosthetic device, repair or replace minor parts (excludes V5335 Repair of oral or laryngeal prosthesis or artificial larynx)	0.00	0.00	0.00	0.00	0.00	0.00	XXX	
L7520			Repair prosthetic device, labor component, per 15 minutes	0.00	0.00	0.00	0.00	0.00	0.00	XXX	
L7900			Vacuum erection system	0.00	8.79	8.79	0.00	8.79	8.79	XXX	■
L8000			Breast prosthesis, mastectomy bra	0.00	0.80	0.80	0.00	0.80	0.80	XXX	■
L8001			Breast prosthesis, mastectomy bra, with integrated breast prosthesis form, unilateral	0.00	1.34	1.34	0.00	1.34	1.34	XXX	■
L8002			Breast prosthesis, mastectomy bra, with integrated breast prosthesis form, bilateral	0.00	1.64	1.64	0.00	1.64	1.64	XXX	■
L8010			Breast prosthesis, mastectomy sleeve	0.00	1.34	1.34	0.00	1.34	1.34	XXX	■
L8015			External breast prosthesis garment, with mastectomy form, post-mastectomy	0.00	1.19	1.19	0.00	1.19	1.19	XXX	■
L8020			Breast prosthesis, mastectomy form	0.00	4.50	4.50	0.00	4.50	4.50	XXX	■
L8030			Breast prosthesis, silicone or equal	0.00	7.09	7.09	0.00	7.09	7.09	XXX	■
L8035			Custom breast prosthesis, post mastectomy, molded to patient model	0.00	0.00	0.00	0.00	0.00	0.00	XXX	
L8039			Breast prosthesis, not otherwise specified	0.00	0.00	0.00	0.00	0.00	0.00	XXX	
L8041			Midfacial prosthesis, provided by a non-physician	0.00	0.00	0.00	0.00	0.00	0.00	XXX	
L8042			Orbital prosthesis, provided by a non-physician	0.00	0.00	0.00	0.00	0.00	0.00	XXX	
L8043			Upper facial prosthesis, provided by a non-physician	0.00	0.00	0.00	0.00	0.00	0.00	XXX	
L8044			Hemi-facial prosthesis, provided by a non-physician	0.00	0.00	0.00	0.00	0.00	0.00	XXX	
L8045			Auricular prosthesis, provided by a non-physician	0.00	0.00	0.00	0.00	0.00	0.00	XXX	
L8046			Partial facial prosthesis, provided by a non-physician	0.00	0.00	0.00	0.00	0.00	0.00	XXX	
L8047			Nasal septal prosthesis, provided by a non-physician	0.00	0.00	0.00	0.00	0.00	0.00	XXX	
L8049			Repair or modification of maxillofacial prosthesis, labor component, 15 minute increments, provided by a non-physician	0.00	0.00	0.00	0.00	0.00	0.00	XXX	
L8100			Gradient compression stocking, below knee, 18-30 mmhg, each	0.00	0.57	0.57	0.00	0.57	0.57	XXX	■
L8110			Gradient compression stocking, below knee, 30-40 mmhg, each	0.00	0.58	0.58	0.00	0.58	0.58	XXX	■

■ RVU not developed by CMS. Gap-filled RVUs developed by CHEG.

Code	M	S	Description	Work Value	Non-Fac PE	Fac PE	Mal-practice	Non-Fac Total	Fac Total	Global	Gap
L8120			Gradient compression stocking, below knee, 40-50 mmhg, each	0.00	0.60	0.60	0.00	0.60	0.60	XXX	■
L8130			Gradient compression stocking, thigh length, 18-30 mmhg, each	0.00	0.89	0.89	0.00	0.89	0.89	XXX	■
L8140			Gradient compression stocking, thigh length, 30-40 mmhg, each	0.00	0.89	0.89	0.00	0.89	0.89	XXX	■
L8150			Gradient compression stocking, thigh length, 40-50 mmhg, each	0.00	0.77	0.77	0.00	0.77	0.77	XXX	■
L8160			Gradient compression stocking, full length/ chap style, 18-30 mmhg, each	0.00	1.00	1.00	0.00	1.00	1.00	XXX	■
L8170			Gradient compression stocking, full length/ chap style, 30-40 mmhg, each	0.00	1.00	1.00	0.00	1.00	1.00	XXX	■
L8180			Gradient compression stocking, full length/ chap style, 40-50 mmhg, each	0.00	1.00	1.00	0.00	1.00	1.00	XXX	■
L8190			Gradient compression stocking, waist length, 18-30 mmhg, each	0.00	4.02	4.02	0.00	4.02	4.02	XXX	■
L8195			Gradient compression stocking, waist length, 30-40 mmhg, each	0.00	0.00	0.00	0.00	0.00	0.00	XXX	
L8200			Gradient compression stocking, waist length, 40-50 mmhg, each	0.00	4.02	4.02	0.00	4.02	4.02	XXX	■
L8210			Gradient compression stocking, custom made	0.00	2.01	2.01	0.00	2.01	2.01	XXX	■
L8220			Gradient compression stocking, lymphedema	0.00	0.60	0.60	0.00	0.60	0.60	XXX	■
L8230			Gradient compression stocking, garter belt	0.00	0.63	0.63	0.00	0.63	0.63	XXX	■
L8239			Gradient compression stocking, not otherwise specified	0.00	0.00	0.00	0.00	0.00	0.00	XXX	
L8300			Truss, single with standard pad	0.00	2.30	2.30	0.00	2.30	2.30	XXX	■
L8310			Truss, double with standard pads	0.00	3.67	3.67	0.00	3.67	3.67	XXX	■
L8320			Truss, addition to standard pad, water pad	0.00	1.46	1.46	0.00	1.46	1.46	XXX	■
L8330			Truss, addition to standard pad, scrotal pad	0.00	1.37	1.37	0.00	1.37	1.37	XXX	■
L8400			Prosthetic sheath, below knee, each	0.00	0.45	0.45	0.00	0.45	0.45	XXX	■
L8410			Prosthetic sheath, above knee, each	0.00	0.57	0.57	0.00	0.57	0.57	XXX	■
L8415			Prosthetic sheath, upper limb, each	0.00	0.60	0.60	0.00	0.60	0.60	XXX	■
L8417			Prosthetic sheath/sock, including a gel cushion layer, below knee or above knee, each	0.00	0.00	0.00	0.00	0.00	0.00	XXX	
L8420			Prosthetic sock, multiple ply, below knee, each	0.00	0.54	0.54	0.00	0.54	0.54	XXX	■
L8430			Prosthetic sock, multiple ply, above knee, each	0.00	0.63	0.63	0.00	0.63	0.63	XXX	■
L8435			Prosthetic sock, multiple ply, upper limb, each	0.00	0.45	0.45	0.00	0.45	0.45	XXX	■

■ RVU not developed by CMS. Gap-filled RVUs developed by CHEG.

Code	M	S	Description	Work Value	Non-Fac PE	Fac PE	Mal-prac-tice	Non-Fac Total	Fac Total	Global	Gap
L8440			Prosthetic shrinker, below knee, each	0.00	1.16	1.16	0.00	1.16	1.16	XXX	■
L8460			Prosthetic shrinker, above knee, each	0.00	1.85	1.85	0.00	1.85	1.85	XXX	■
L8465			Prosthetic shrinker, upper limb, each	0.00	1.34	1.34	0.00	1.34	1.34	XXX	■
L8470			Prosthetic sock, single ply, fitting, below knee, each	0.00	0.18	0.18	0.00	0.18	0.18	XXX	■
L8480			Prosthetic sock, single ply, fitting, above knee, each	0.00	0.27	0.27	0.00	0.27	0.27	XXX	■
L8485			Prosthetic sock, single ply, fitting, upper limb, each	0.00	0.30	0.30	0.00	0.30	0.30	XXX	■
L8490			Addition to prosthetic sheath/sock, air seal suction retention system	0.00	3.67	3.67	0.00	3.67	3.67	XXX	■
L8499			Unlisted procedure for miscellaneous prosthetic services	0.00	0.00	0.00	0.00	0.00	0.00	XXX	
L8500			Artificial larynx, any type	0.00	0.00	0.00	0.00	0.00	0.00	XXX	
L8501			Tracheostomy speaking valve	0.00	3.34	3.34	0.00	3.34	3.34	XXX	■
L8505			Artificial larynx replacement battery/accessory, any type	0.00	0.00	0.00	0.00	0.00	0.00	XXX	
L8507			Tracheo-esophageal voice prosthesis, patient inserted, any type, each	0.00	0.00	0.00	0.00	0.00	0.00	XXX	
L8509			Tracheo-esophageal voice prosthesis, inserted by a licensed health care provider, any type	0.00	0.00	0.00	0.00	0.00	0.00	XXX	
L8510			Voice amplifier	0.00	0.00	0.00	0.00	0.00	0.00	XXX	
L8600			Implantable breast prosthesis, silicone or equal	0.00	28.87	28.87	0.00	28.87	28.87	XXX	■
L8603			Injectable bulking agent, collagen implant, urinary tract, 2.5 ml syringe, includes shipping and necessary supplies	0.00	0.00	0.00	0.00	0.00	0.00	XXX	
L8606			Injectable bulking agent, synthetic implant, urinary tract, 1 ml syringe, includes shipping and necessary supplies	0.00	0.00	0.00	0.00	0.00	0.00	XXX	
L8610			Ocular implant	0.00	0.00	0.00	0.00	0.00	0.00	XXX	
L8612			Aqueous shunt	0.00	0.00	0.00	0.00	0.00	0.00	XXX	
L8613			Ossicular implant	0.00	0.00	0.00	0.00	0.00	0.00	XXX	
L8614			Cochlear device/system	0.00	0.00	0.00	0.00	0.00	0.00	XXX	
L8619			Cochlear implant external speech processor, replacement	0.00	0.00	0.00	0.00	0.00	0.00	XXX	
L8630			Metacarpophalangeal joint implant	0.00	0.00	0.00	0.00	0.00	0.00	XXX	
L8641			Metatarsal joint implant	0.00	0.00	0.00	0.00	0.00	0.00	XXX	

■ RVU not developed by CMS. Gap-filled RVUs developed by CHEG.

Code	M	S	Description	Work Value	Non-Fac PE	Fac PE	Mal-prac-tice	Non-Fac Total	Fac Total	Global	Gap
L8642			Hallux implant	0.00	0.00	0.00	0.00	0.00	0.00	XXX	
L8658			Interphalangeal joint implant	0.00	0.00	0.00	0.00	0.00	0.00	XXX	
L8670			Vascular graft material, synthetic, implant	0.00	0.00	0.00	0.00	0.00	0.00	XXX	
L8699			Prosthetic implant, not otherwise specified	0.00	0.00	0.00	0.00	0.00	0.00	XXX	
L9900			Orthotic and prosthetic supply, accessory, and/or service component of another HCPCS L code	0.00	0.00	0.00	0.00	0.00	0.00	XXX	
M0064		A	Brief office visit for the sole purpose of monitoring or changing drug prescriptions used in the treatment of mental psychoneurotic and personality disorders	0.37	0.25	0.12	0.01	0.63	0.50	XXX	
M0075		N	Cellular therapy	0.00	0.00	0.00	0.00	0.00	0.00	XXX	
M0076		N	Prolotherapy	0.00	0.00	0.00	0.00	0.00	0.00	XXX	
M0100		N	Intragastric hypothermia using gastric freezing (MNP)	0.00	0.00	0.00	0.00	0.00	0.00	XXX	
M0300		N	IV chelation therapy (chemical endarterectomy)	0.00	0.00	0.00	0.00	0.00	0.00	XXX	
M0301		N	Fabric wrapping of abdominal aneurysm (MNP)	0.00	0.00	0.00	0.00	0.00	0.00	XXX	
P2028		X	Cephalin floculation, blood	0.00	0.00	0.00	0.00	0.00	0.00	XXX	
P2029		X	Congo red, blood	0.00	0.00	0.00	0.00	0.00	0.00	XXX	
P2031		N	Hair analysis (excluding arsenic)	0.00	0.00	0.00	0.00	0.00	0.00	XXX	
P2033		X	Thymol turbidity, blood	0.00	0.00	0.00	0.00	0.00	0.00	XXX	
P2038		X	Mucoprotein, blood (seromucoid) (medical necessity procedure)	0.00	0.40	0.40	0.00	0.40	0.40	XXX	■
P3000		X	Screening Papanicolaou smear, cervical or vaginal, up to three smears, by technician under physician supervision	0.00	0.51	0.51	0.00	0.51	0.51	XXX	■
P3001		A	Screening Papanicolaou smear, cervical or vaginal, up to three smears, requiring interpretation by physician	0.42	0.19	0.19	0.01	0.62	0.62	XXX	
P7001		I	Culture, bacterial, urine; quantitative, sensitivity study	0.00	0.98	0.98	0.00	0.98	0.98	XXX	■
P9010		E	Blood (whole), for transfusion, per unit	0.00	2.31	2.31	0.00	2.31	2.31	XXX	■
P9011		E	Blood (split unit), specify amount	0.00	3.30	3.30	0.00	3.30	3.30	XXX	■
P9012		E	Cryoprecipitate, each unit	0.00	0.00	0.00	0.00	0.00	0.00	XXX	
P9016		E	Red blood cells, leukocytes reduced, each unit	0.00	0.00	0.00	0.00	0.00	0.00	XXX	
P9017		E	Fresh frozen plasma (single donor), each unit	0.00	0.00	0.00	0.00	0.00	0.00	XXX	

■ RVU not developed by CMS. Gap-filled RVUs developed by CHEG.

Code	M	S	Description	Work Value	Non-Fac PE	Fac PE	Mal-practice	Non-Fac Total	Fac Total	Global	Gap
P9019		E	Platelets, each unit	0.00	0.00	0.00	0.00	0.00	0.00	XXX	
P9020		E	Platelet rich plasma, each unit	0.00	0.00	0.00	0.00	0.00	0.00	XXX	
P9021		E	Red blood cells, each unit	0.00	0.00	0.00	0.00	0.00	0.00	XXX	
P9022		E	Red blood cells, washed, each unit	0.00	0.00	0.00	0.00	0.00	0.00	XXX	
P9023		X	Plasma, pooled multiple donor, solvent/ detergent treated, frozen, each unit	0.00	0.00	0.00	0.00	0.00	0.00	XXX	
P9031		X	Platelets, leukocytes reduced, each unit	0.00	0.00	0.00	0.00	0.00	0.00	XXX	
P9032		X	Platelets, irradiated, each unit	0.00	0.00	0.00	0.00	0.00	0.00	XXX	
P9033		X	Platelets, leukocytes reduced, irradiated, each unit	0.00	0.00	0.00	0.00	0.00	0.00	XXX	
P9034		X	Platelets, pheresis, each unit	0.00	0.00	0.00	0.00	0.00	0.00	XXX	
P9035		X	Platelets, pheresis, leukocytes reduced, each unit	0.00	0.00	0.00	0.00	0.00	0.00	XXX	
P9036		X	Platelets, pheresis, irradiated, each unit	0.00	0.00	0.00	0.00	0.00	0.00	XXX	
P9037		X	Platelets, pheresis, leukocytes reduced, irradiated, each unit	0.00	0.00	0.00	0.00	0.00	0.00	XXX	
P9038		X	Red blood cells, irradiated, each unit	0.00	0.00	0.00	0.00	0.00	0.00	XXX	
P9039		X	Red blood cells, deglycerolized, each unit	0.00	0.00	0.00	0.00	0.00	0.00	XXX	
P9040		X	Red blood cells, leukocytes reduced, irradiated, each unit	0.00	0.00	0.00	0.00	0.00	0.00	XXX	
P9041		X	Infusion, albumin (human), 5%, 50 ml	0.00	1.26	1.26	0.00	1.26	1.26	XXX	■
P9043		X	Infusion, plasma protein fraction (human), 5%, 50 ml	0.00	0.94	0.94	0.00	0.94	0.94	XXX	■
P9044		X	Plasma, cryoprecipitate reduced, each unit	0.00	0.00	0.00	0.00	0.00	0.00	XXX	
P9045		X	Infusion, albumin (human), 5%, 250 ml	0.00	2.84	2.84	0.00	2.84	2.84	XXX	■
P9046		X	Infusion, albumin (human), 25%, 20 ml	0.00	1.20	1.20	0.00	1.20	1.20	XXX	■
P9047		X	Infusion, albumin (human), 25%, 50 ml	0.00	2.84	2.84	0.00	2.84	2.84	XXX	■
P9048		X	Infusion, plasma protein fraction (human), 5%, 250 ml	0.00	2.76	2.76	0.00	2.76	2.76	XXX	■
P9050		X	Granulocytes, pheresis, each unit	0.00	0.00	0.00	0.00	0.00	0.00	XXX	
P9603		X	Travel allowance one way in connection with medically necessary laboratory specimen collection drawn from homebound or nursing home bound patient; prorated miles actually travelled	0.00	0.00	0.00	0.00	0.00	0.00	XXX	

■ RVU not developed by CMS. Gap-filled RVUs developed by CHEG.

Code	M	S	Description	Work Value	Non-Fac PE	Fac PE	Mal-practice	Non-Fac Total	Fac Total	Global	Gap
P9604		X	Travel allowance one way in connection with medically necessary laboratory specimen collection drawn from homebound or nursing home bound patient; prorated trip charge	0.00	0.18	0.18	0.00	0.18	0.18	XXX	■
P9612		X	Catheterization for collection of specimen, single patient, all places of service	0.00	1.20	1.20	0.00	1.20	1.20	XXX	■
P9615		X	Catheterization for collection of specimen(s) (multiple patients)	0.00	0.00	0.00	0.00	0.00	0.00	XXX	
Q0035		A	Cardiokymography	0.17	0.44	0.44	0.03	0.64	0.64	XXX	
	26	A		0.17	0.07	0.07	0.01	0.25	0.25	XXX	
	TC	A		0.00	0.37	0.37	0.02	0.39	0.39	XXX	
Q0091		A	Screening Papanicolaou smear; obtaining, preparing and conveyance of cervical or vaginal smear to laboratory	0.37	0.68	0.15	0.01	1.06	0.53	XXX	
Q0092		A	Set-up portable x-ray equipment	0.00	0.30	0.30	0.01	0.31	0.31	XXX	
Q0111		X	Wet mounts, including preparations of vaginal, cervical or skin specimens	0.00	0.36	0.36	0.00	0.36	0.36	XXX	■
Q0112		X	All potassium hydroxide (KOH) preparations	0.00	0.42	0.42	0.00	0.42	0.42	XXX	■
Q0113		X	Pinworm examination	0.00	0.00	0.00	0.00	0.00	0.00	XXX	
Q0114		X	Fern test	0.00	0.00	0.00	0.00	0.00	0.00	XXX	
Q0115		X	Post-coital direct, qualitative examinations of vaginal or cervical mucous	0.00	0.00	0.00	0.00	0.00	0.00	XXX	
Q0136		E	Injection, epoetin alpha, (for non ESRD use), per 1,000 units	0.00	0.38	0.38	0.00	0.38	0.38	XXX	■
Q0163		X	Diphenhydramine hydrochloride, 50 mg, oral, FDA approved prescription anti-emetic, for use as a complete therapeutic substitute for an IV anti-emetic at time of chemotherapy treatment not to exceed a 48-hour dosage regimen	0.00	0.00	0.00	0.00	0.00	0.00	XXX	
Q0164		X	Prochlorperazine maleate, 5 mg, oral, FDA approved prescription anti-emetic, for use as a complete therapeutic substitute for an IV anti-emetic at the time of chemotherapy treatment, not to exceed a 48-hour dosage regimen	0.00	0.02	0.02	0.00	0.02	0.02	XXX	■
Q0165		X	Prochlorperazine maleate, 10 mg, oral, FDA approved prescription anti-emetic, for use as a complete therapeutic substitute for an IV anti-emetic at the time of chemotherapy treatment, not to exceed a 48-hour dosage regimen	0.00	0.03	0.03	0.00	0.03	0.03	XXX	■
Q0166		X	Granisetron hydrochloride, 1 mg, oral, FDA approved prescription anti-emetic, for use as a complete therapeutic substitute for an IV anti-emetic at the time of chemotherapy treatment, not to exceed a 24-hour dosage regimen	0.00	1.42	1.42	0.00	1.42	1.42	XXX	■

■ RVU not developed by CMS. Gap-filled RVUs developed by CHEG.

Code	M	S	Description	Work Value	Non-Fac PE	Fac PE	Mal-practice	Non-Fac Total	Fac Total	Global	Gap
Q0167		X	Dronabinol, 2.5 mg, oral, FDA approved prescription anti-emetic, for use as a complete therapeutic substitute for an IV anti-emetic at the time of chemotherapy treatment, not to exceed a 48-hour dosage regimen	0.00	0.11	0.11	0.00	0.11	0.11	XXX	■
Q0168		X	Dronabinol, 5 mg, oral, FDA approved prescription anti-emetic, for use as a complete therapeutic substitute for an IV anti-emetic at the time of chemotherapy treatment, not to exceed a 48-hour dosage regimen	0.00	0.24	0.24	0.00	0.24	0.24	XXX	■
Q0169		X	Promethazine hydrochloride, 12.5 mg, oral, FDA approved prescription anti-emetic, for use as a complete therapeutic substitute for an IV anti-emetic at the time of chemotherapy treatment, not to exceed a 48-hour dosage regimen	0.00	0.00	0.00	0.00	0.00	0.00	XXX	
Q0170		X	Promethazine hydrochloride, 25 mg, oral, FDA approved prescription anti-emetic, for use as a complete therapeutic substitute for an IV anti-emetic at the time of chemotherapy treatment, not to exceed a 48-hour dosage regimen	0.00	0.00	0.00	0.00	0.00	0.00	XXX	
Q0171		X	Chlorpromazine hydrochloride, 10 mg, oral, FDA approved prescription anti-emetic, for use as a complete therapeutic substitute for an IV anti-emetic at the time of chemotherapy treatment, not to exceed a 48-hour dosage regimen	0.00	0.01	0.01	0.00	0.01	0.01	XXX	■
Q0172		X	Chlorpromazine hydrochloride, 25 mg, oral, FDA approved prescription anti-emetic, for use as a complete therapeutic substitute for an IV anti-emetic at the time of chemotherapy treatment, not to exceed a 48-hour dosage regimen	0.00	0.01	0.01	0.00	0.01	0.01	XXX	■
Q0173		X	Trimethobenzamide hydrochloride, 250 mg, oral, FDA approved prescription anti-emetic, for use as a complete therapeutic substitute for an IV anti-emetic at the time of chemotherapy treatment, not to exceed a 48-hour dosage regimen	0.00	0.01	0.01	0.00	0.01	0.01	XXX	■
Q0174		X	Thiethylperazine maleate, 10 mg, oral, FDA approved prescription anti-emetic, for use as a complete therapeutic substitute for an IV anti-emetic at the time of chemotherapy treatment, not to exceed a 48-hour dosage regimen	0.00	0.02	0.02	0.00	0.02	0.02	XXX	■
Q0175		X	Perphenzaine, 4 mg, oral, FDA approved prescription anti-emetic, for use as a complete therapeutic substitute for an IV anti-emetic at the time of chemotherapy treatment, not to exceed a 48-hour dosage regimen	0.00	0.00	0.00	0.00	0.00	0.00	XXX	

■ RVU not developed by CMS. Gap-filled RVUs developed by CHEG.

Code	M	S	Description	Work Value	Non-Fac PE	Fac PE	Mal-practice	Non-Fac Total	Fac Total	Global	Gap
Q0176		X	Perphenzaine, 8mg, oral, FDA approved prescription anti-emetic, for use as a complete therapeutic substitute for an IV anti-emetic at the time of chemotherapy treatment, not to exceed a 48-hour dosage regimen	0.00	0.00	0.00	0.00	0.00	0.00	XXX	
Q0177		X	Hydroxyzine pamoate, 25 mg, oral, FDA approved prescription anti-emetic, for use as a complete therapeutic substitute for an IV anti-emetic at the time of chemotherapy treatment, not to exceed a 48-hour dosage regimen	0.00	0.00	0.00	0.00	0.00	0.00	XXX	
Q0178		X	Hydroxyzine pamoate, 50 mg, oral, FDA approved prescription anti-emetic, for use as a complete therapeutic substitute for an IV anti-emetic at the time of chemotherapy treatment, not to exceed a 48-hour dosage regimen	0.00	0.01	0.01	0.00	0.01	0.01	XXX	■
Q0179		X	Ondansetron hydrochloride 8 mg, oral, FDA approved prescription anti-emetic, for use as a complete therapeutic substitute for an IV anti-emetic at the time of chemotherapy treatment, not to exceed a 48-hour dosage regimen	0.00	0.00	0.00	0.00	0.00	0.00	XXX	
Q0180		X	Dolasetron mesylate, 100 mg, oral, FDA approved prescription anti-emetic, for use as a complete therapeutic substitute for an IV anti-emetic at the time of chemotherapy treatment, not to exceed a 24-hour dosage regimen	0.00	2.21	2.21	0.00	2.21	2.21	XXX	■
Q0181		X	Unspecified oral dosage form, FDA approved prescription anti-emetic, for use as a complete therapeutic substitute for an IV anti-emetic at the time of chemotherapy treatment, not to exceed a 48-hour dosage regimen	0.00	0.00	0.00	0.00	0.00	0.00	XXX	
Q0183		X	Dermal tissue, of human origin, with and without other bioengineered or processed elements, but without metabolically active elements, per square centimeter	0.00	0.00	0.00	0.00	0.00	0.00	XXX	
Q0184		X	Dermal tissue, of human origin, with or without other bioengineered or processed elements, with metabolically active elements, per square centimeter	0.00	0.00	0.00	0.00	0.00	0.00	XXX	
Q0187		E	Factor VIIa (coagulation factor, recombinant) per 1.2 mg	0.00	0.00	0.00	0.00	0.00	0.00	XXX	
Q1001		X	New technology intraocular lens category 1 as defined in Federal Register notice, Vol. 65, date May 3, 2000	0.00	0.00	0.00	0.00	0.00	0.00	XXX	
Q1002		X	New technology intraocular lens category 2 as defined in Federal Register notice, Vol. 65, dated May 3, 2000	0.00	0.00	0.00	0.00	0.00	0.00	XXX	
Q1003		X	New technology intraocular lens category 3 as defined in Federal Register notice	0.00	0.00	0.00	0.00	0.00	0.00	XXX	
Q1004		X	New technology intraocular lens category 4 as defined in Federal Register notice	0.00	0.00	0.00	0.00	0.00	0.00	XXX	

■ RVU not developed by CMS. Gap-filled RVUs developed by CHEG.

Code	M	S	Description	Work Value	Non-Fac PE	Fac PE	Mal-practice	Non-Fac Total	Fac Total	Global	Gap
Q1005		X	New technology intraocular lens category 5 as defined in Federal Register notice	0.00	0.00	0.00	0.00	0.00	0.00	XXX	
Q2001		N	Oral, cabergoline, 0.5 mg	0.00	0.94	0.94	0.00	0.94	0.94	XXX	■
Q2002		E	Injection, Elliott's B solution, per ml	0.00	0.45	0.45	0.00	0.45	0.45	XXX	■
Q2003		E	Injection, aprotinin, 10,000 kiu	0.00	0.07	0.07	0.00	0.07	0.07	XXX	■
Q2004		E	Irrigation solution for treatment of bladder calculi, for example renacidin, per 500 ml	0.00	0.78	0.78	0.00	0.78	0.78	XXX	■
Q2005		E	Injection, corticorelin ovine triflutate, per dose	0.00	11.67	11.67	0.00	11.67	11.67	XXX	■
Q2006		E	Injection, digoxin immune fab (ovine), per vial	0.00	17.50	17.50	0.00	17.50	17.50	XXX	■
Q2007		E	Injection, ethanolamine oleate, 100 mg	0.00	1.26	1.26	0.00	1.26	1.26	XXX	■
Q2008		E	Injection, fomepizole, 1.5 mg	0.00	0.00	0.00	0.00	0.00	0.00	XXX	
Q2009		E	Injection, fosphenytoin, 50 mg	0.00	0.00	0.00	0.00	0.00	0.00	XXX	
Q2010		E	Injection, glatiramer acetate, per dose	0.00	0.95	0.95	0.00	0.95	0.95	XXX	■
Q2011		E	Injection, hemin, per 1 mg	0.00	0.00	0.00	0.00	0.00	0.00	XXX	
Q2012		E	Injection, pegademase bovine, 25 IU	0.00	4.42	4.42	0.00	4.42	4.42	XXX	■
Q2013		E	Injection, pentastarch, 10% solution, per 100 ml	0.00	0.48	0.48	0.00	0.48	0.48	XXX	■
Q2014		E	Injection, sermorelin acetate, 0.5 mg	0.00	0.50	0.50	0.00	0.50	0.50	XXX	■
Q2017		E	Injection, teniposide, 50 mg	0.00	6.86	6.86	0.00	6.86	6.86	XXX	■
Q2018		E	Injection, urofollitropin, 75 IU	0.00	2.49	2.49	0.00	2.49	2.49	XXX	■
Q2019		E	Injection, basiliximab, 20 mg	0.00	41.55	41.55	0.00	41.55	41.55	XXX	■
Q2020		E	Injection, histrelin acetate, 10 mg	0.00	0.00	0.00	0.00	0.00	0.00	XXX	
Q2021		E	Injection, lepirudin, 50 mg	0.00	3.98	3.98	0.00	3.98	3.98	XXX	■
Q2022		E	von Willebrand factor complex, human, per IU	0.00	0.03	0.03	0.00	0.03	0.03	XXX	■
Q3001		E	Radioelements for brachytherapy, any type, each	0.00	0.00	0.00	0.00	0.00	0.00	XXX	
Q3002		E	Supply of radiopharmaceutical diagnostic imaging agent, gallium GA 67, per microcurie	0.00	0.00	0.00	0.00	0.00	0.00	XXX	
Q3003		E	Supply of radiopharmaceutical diagnostic imaging agent, technetium Tc 99m bicisate, per unit dose	0.00	0.00	0.00	0.00	0.00	0.00	XXX	
Q3004		E	Supply of radiopharmaceutical diagnostic imaging agent, xenon XE 133, per 10 microcurie	0.00	0.00	0.00	0.00	0.00	0.00	XXX	

■ RVU not developed by CMS. Gap-filled RVUs developed by CHEG.

Code	M	S	Description	Work Value	Non-Fac PE	Fac PE	Mal-practice	Non-Fac Total	Fac Total	Global	Gap
Q3005		E	Supply of radiopharmaceutical diagnostic imaging agent, technetium Tc 99m mertiatide, per microcurie	0.00	0.00	0.00	0.00	0.00	0.00	XXX	
Q3006		E	Supply of radiopharmaceutical diagnostic imaging agent, technetium Tc 99m glucepatate, per 5 microcurie	0.00	0.00	0.00	0.00	0.00	0.00	XXX	
Q3007		E	Supply of radiopharmaceutical diagnostic imaging agent, sodium phosphate P32, per microcurie	0.00	0.00	0.00	0.00	0.00	0.00	XXX	
Q3008		E	Supply of radiopharmaceutical diagnostic imaging agent, indium 111 — in pentetreotide, per 3 microcurie	0.00	0.00	0.00	0.00	0.00	0.00	XXX	
Q3009		E	Supply of radiopharmaceutical diagnostic imaging agent, technetium Tc 99m oxidronate, per microcurie	0.00	0.00	0.00	0.00	0.00	0.00	XXX	
Q3010		E	Supply of radiopharmaceutical diagnostic imaging agent, technetium Tc 99m — labeled red blood cells, per microcurie	0.00	0.00	0.00	0.00	0.00	0.00	XXX	
Q3011		E	Supply of radiopharmaceutical diagnostic imaging agent, chromic phosphate P32 suspension, per microcurie	0.00	0.00	0.00	0.00	0.00	0.00	XXX	
Q3012		E	Supply of oral radiopharmaceutical diagnostic imaging agent, cyanocobalamin cobalt Co57, per 0.5 microcurie	0.00	0.00	0.00	0.00	0.00	0.00	XXX	
Q3013		I	Injection, verteporfin, 15 mg	0.00	0.00	0.00	0.00	0.00	0.00	XXX	
Q3014		E	Telehealth originating site facility fee	0.00	0.00	0.00	0.00	0.00	0.00	XXX	
Q3017		E	Ambulance service, advanced life support (ALS) assessment, no other ALS services provided	0.00	0.00	0.00	0.00	0.00	0.00	XXX	
Q4001		X	Casting supplies, body cast adult, with or without head, plaster	0.00	4.99	4.99	0.00	4.99	4.99	XXX	■
Q4002		X	Cast supplies, body cast adult, with or without head, fiberglass	0.00	10.62	10.62	0.00	10.62	10.62	XXX	■
Q4003		X	Cast supplies, shoulder cast, adult (11 years +), plaster	0.00	2.70	2.70	0.00	2.70	2.70	XXX	■
Q4004		X	Cast supplies, shoulder cast, adult (11 years +), fiberglass	0.00	5.75	5.75	0.00	5.75	5.75	XXX	■
Q4005		X	Cast supplies, long arm cast, adult (11 years +), plaster	0.00	1.49	1.49	0.00	1.49	1.49	XXX	■
Q4006		X	Cast supplies, long arm cast, adult (11 years +), fiberglass	0.00	3.17	3.17	0.00	3.17	3.17	XXX	■
Q4007		X	Cast supplies, long arm cast, pediatric (0-10 years), plaster	0.00	0.74	0.74	0.00	0.74	0.74	XXX	■

■ RVU not developed by CMS. Gap-filled RVUs developed by CHEG.

Code	M	S	Description	Work Value	Non-Fac PE	Fac PE	Mal-practice	Non-Fac Total	Fac Total	Global	Gap
Q4008		X	Cast supplies, long arm cast, pediatric (0-10 years), fiberglass	0.00	1.58	1.58	0.00	1.58	1.58	XXX	■
Q4009		X	Cast supplies, short arm cast, adult (11 years +), plaster	0.00	1.14	1.14	0.00	1.14	1.14	XXX	■
Q4010		X	Cast supplies, short arm cast, adult (11 years +), fiberglass	0.00	2.45	2.45	0.00	2.45	2.45	XXX	■
Q4011		X	Cast supplies, short arm cast, pediatric (0-10 years), plaster	0.00	0.57	0.57	0.00	0.57	0.57	XXX	■
Q4012		X	Cast supplies, short arm cast, pediatric (0-10 years), fiberglass	0.00	1.23	1.23	0.00	1.23	1.23	XXX	■
Q4013		X	Cast supplies, gauntlet cast (includes lower forearm and hand), adult (11 years +), plaster	0.00	1.08	1.08	0.00	1.08	1.08	XXX	■
Q4014		X	Cast supplies, gauntlet cast (includes lower forearm and hand), adult (11 years +), fiberglass	0.00	2.31	2.31	0.00	2.31	2.31	XXX	■
Q4015		X	Cast supplies, gauntlet cast (includes lower forearm and hand), pediatric (0-10 years), plaster	0.00	0.54	0.54	0.00	0.54	0.54	XXX	■
Q4016		X	Cast supplies, gauntlet cast (includes lower forearm and hand), pediatric (0-10 years), fiberglass	0.00	1.15	1.15	0.00	1.15	1.15	XXX	■
Q4017		X	Cast supplies, long arm splint, adult (11 years +), plaster	0.00	0.94	0.94	0.00	0.94	0.94	XXX	■
Q4018		X	Cast supplies, long arm splint, adult (11 years +), fiberglass	0.00	2.01	2.01	0.00	2.01	2.01	XXX	■
Q4019		X	Cast supplies, long arm splint, pediatric (0-10 years), plaster	0.00	0.47	0.47	0.00	0.47	0.47	XXX	■
Q4020		X	Cast supplies, long arm splint, pediatric (0-10 years), fiberglass	0.00	1.01	1.01	0.00	1.01	1.01	XXX	■
Q4021		X	Cast supplies, short arm splint, adult (11 years +), plaster	0.00	0.94	0.94	0.00	0.94	0.94	XXX	■
Q4022		X	Cast supplies, short arm splint, adult (11 years +), fiberglass	0.00	2.01	2.01	0.00	2.01	2.01	XXX	■
Q4023		X	Cast supplies, short arm splint, pediatric (0-10 years), plaster	0.00	0.47	0.47	0.00	0.47	0.47	XXX	■
Q4024		X	Cast supplies, short arm splint, pediatric (0-10 years), fiberglass	0.00	1.01	1.01	0.00	1.01	1.01	XXX	■
Q4025		X	Cast supplies, hip spica (one or both legs), adult (11 years +), plaster	0.00	4.19	4.19	0.00	4.19	4.19	XXX	■
Q4026		X	Cast supplies, hip spica (one or both legs), adult (11 years +), fiberglass	0.00	8.92	8.92	0.00	8.92	8.92	XXX	■
Q4027		X	Cast supplies, hip spica (one or both legs), pediatric (0-10 years), plaster	0.00	2.10	2.10	0.00	2.10	2.10	XXX	■

■ RVU not developed by CMS. Gap-filled RVUs developed by CHEG.

Code	M	S	Description	Work Value	Non-Fac PE	Fac PE	Mal-practice	Non-Fac Total	Fac Total	Global	Gap
Q4028		X	Cast supplies, hip spica (one or both legs), pediatric (0-10 years), fiberglass	0.00	4.46	4.46	0.00	4.46	4.46	XXX	■
Q4029		X	Cast supplies, long leg cast, adult (11 years +), plaster	0.00	2.07	2.07	0.00	2.07	2.07	XXX	■
Q4030		X	Cast supplies, long leg cast, adult (11 years +), fiberglass	0.00	4.39	4.39	0.00	4.39	4.39	XXX	■
Q4031		X	Cast supplies, long leg cast, pediatric (0-10 years), plaster	0.00	1.03	1.03	0.00	1.03	1.03	XXX	■
Q4032		X	Cast supplies, long leg cast, pediatric (0-10 years), fiberglass	0.00	2.20	2.20	0.00	2.20	2.20	XXX	■
Q4033		X	Cast supplies, long leg cylinder cast, adult (11 years +), plaster	0.00	1.76	1.76	0.00	1.76	1.76	XXX	■
Q4034		X	Cast supplies, long leg cylinder cast, adult (11 years +), fiberglass	0.00	3.74	3.74	0.00	3.74	3.74	XXX	■
Q4035		X	Cast supplies, long leg cylinder cast, pediatric (0-10 years), plaster	0.00	0.88	0.88	0.00	0.88	0.88	XXX	■
Q4036		X	Cast supplies, long leg cylinder cast, pediatric (0-10 years), fiberglass	0.00	1.87	1.87	0.00	1.87	1.87	XXX	■
Q4037		X	Cast supplies, short leg cast, adult (11 years +), plaster	0.00	2.37	2.37	0.00	2.37	2.37	XXX	■
Q4038		X	Cast supplies, short leg cast, adult (11 years +), fiberglass	0.00	5.04	5.04	0.00	5.04	5.04	XXX	■
Q4039		X	Cast supplies, short leg cast, pediatric (0-10 years), plaster	0.00	1.18	1.18	0.00	1.18	1.18	XXX	■
Q4040		X	Cast supplies, short leg cast, pediatric (0-10 years), fiberglass	0.00	2.52	2.52	0.00	2.52	2.52	XXX	■
Q4041		X	Cast supplies, long leg splint, adult (11 years +), plaster	0.00	1.35	1.35	0.00	1.35	1.35	XXX	■
Q4042		X	Cast supplies, long leg splint, adult (11 years +), fiberglass	0.00	2.88	2.88	0.00	2.88	2.88	XXX	■
Q4043		X	Cast supplies, long leg splint, pediatric (0-10 years), plaster	0.00	0.68	0.68	0.00	0.68	0.68	XXX	■
Q4044		X	Cast supplies, long leg splint, pediatric (0-10 years), fiberglass	0.00	1.44	1.44	0.00	1.44	1.44	XXX	■
Q4045		X	Cast supplies, short leg splint, adult (11 years +), plaster	0.00	0.88	0.88	0.00	0.88	0.88	XXX	■
Q4046		X	Cast supplies, short leg splint, adult (11 years +), fiberglass	0.00	1.87	1.87	0.00	1.87	1.87	XXX	■
Q4047		X	Cast supplies, short leg splint, pediatric (0-10 years), plaster	0.00	0.44	0.44	0.00	0.44	0.44	XXX	■
Q4048		X	Cast supplies, short leg splint, pediatric (0-10 years), fiberglass	0.00	0.93	0.93	0.00	0.93	0.93	XXX	■

■ RVU not developed by CMS. Gap-filled RVUs developed by CHEG.

HCPCS

Code	M	S	Description	Work Value	Non-Fac PE	Fac PE	Mal-practice	Non-Fac Total	Fac Total	Global	Gap
Q4049		X	Finger splint, static	0.00	1.15	1.15	0.00	1.15	1.15	XXX	■
Q4050		X	Cast supplies, for unlisted types and materials of casts	0.00	0.00	0.00	0.00	0.00	0.00	XXX	
Q4051		X	Splint supplies, miscellaneous (includes thermoplastics, strapping, fasteners, padding and other supplies)	0.00	0.00	0.00	0.00	0.00	0.00	XXX	
Q9920		E	Injection of EPO, per 1000 units, at patient HCT of 20 or less	0.00	0.38	0.38	0.00	0.38	0.38	XXX	■
Q9921		E	Injection of EPO, per 1000 units, at patient HCT of 21	0.00	0.38	0.38	0.00	0.38	0.38	XXX	■
Q9922		E	Injection of EPO, per 1000 units, at patient HCT of 22	0.00	0.38	0.38	0.00	0.38	0.38	XXX	■
Q9923		E	Injection of EPO, per 1000 units, at patient HCT of 23	0.00	0.38	0.38	0.00	0.38	0.38	XXX	■
Q9924		E	Injection of EPO, per 1000 units, at patient HCT of 24	0.00	0.38	0.38	0.00	0.38	0.38	XXX	■
Q9925		E	Injection of EPO, per 1000 units, at patient HCT of 25	0.00	0.38	0.38	0.00	0.38	0.38	XXX	■
Q9926		E	Injection of EPO, per 1000 units, at patient HCT of 26	0.00	0.38	0.38	0.00	0.38	0.38	XXX	■
Q9927		E	Injection of EPO, per 1000 units, at patient HCT of 27	0.00	0.38	0.38	0.00	0.38	0.38	XXX	■
Q9928		E	Injection of EPO, per 1000 units, at patient HCT of 28	0.00	0.38	0.38	0.00	0.38	0.38	XXX	■
Q9929		E	Injection of EPO, per 1000 units, at patient HCT of 29	0.00	0.38	0.38	0.00	0.38	0.38	XXX	■
Q9930		E	Injection of EPO, per 1000 units, at patient HCT of 30	0.00	0.38	0.38	0.00	0.38	0.38	XXX	■
Q9931		E	Injection of EPO, per 1000 units, at patient HCT of 31	0.00	0.38	0.38	0.00	0.38	0.38	XXX	■
Q9932		E	Injection of EPO, per 1000 units, at patient HCT of 32	0.00	0.38	0.38	0.00	0.38	0.38	XXX	■
Q9933		E	Injection of EPO, per 1000 units, at patient HCT of 33	0.00	0.38	0.38	0.00	0.38	0.38	XXX	■
Q9934		E	Injection of EPO, per 1000 units, at patient HCT of 34	0.00	0.38	0.38	0.00	0.38	0.38	XXX	■
Q9935		E	Injection of EPO, per 1000 units, at patient HCT of 35	0.00	0.38	0.38	0.00	0.38	0.38	XXX	■
Q9936		E	Injection of EPO, per 1000 units, at patient HCT of 36	0.00	0.38	0.38	0.00	0.38	0.38	XXX	■
Q9937		E	Injection of EPO, per 1000 units, at patient HCT of 37	0.00	0.38	0.38	0.00	0.38	0.38	XXX	■

■ RVU not developed by CMS. Gap-filled RVUs developed by CHEG.

Code	M	S	Description	Work Value	Non-Fac PE	Fac PE	Mal-practice	Non-Fac Total	Fac Total	Global	Gap
Q9938		E	Injection of EPO, per 1000 units, at patient HCT of 38	0.00	0.38	0.38	0.00	0.38	0.38	XXX	■
Q9939		E	Injection of EPO, per 1000 units, at patient HCT of 39	0.00	0.38	0.38	0.00	0.38	0.38	XXX	■
Q9940		E	Injection of EPO, per 1000 units, at patient HCT of 40 or above	0.00	0.38	0.38	0.00	0.38	0.38	XXX	■
R0070		C	Transportation of portable x-ray equipment and personnel to home or nursing home, per trip to facility or location, one patient seen	0.00	1.85	1.85	0.00	1.85	1.85	XXX	■
R0075		C	Transportation of portable x-ray equipment and personnel to home or nursing home, per trip to facility or location, more than one patient seen, per patient	0.00	1.71	1.71	0.00	1.71	1.71	XXX	■
R0076		B	Transportation of portable EKG to facility or location, per patient	0.00	1.67	1.67	0.00	1.67	1.67	XXX	■
S0009		I	Injection, butorphanol tartrate, 1mg	0.00	0.20	0.20	0.00	0.20	0.20	XXX	■
S0012		I	Butorphanol tartrate, nasal spray, 25 mg	0.00	2.43	2.43	0.00	2.43	2.43	XXX	■
S0014		I	Tacrine hydrochloride, 10 mg	0.00	0.04	0.04	0.00	0.04	0.04	XXX	■
S0016		I	Injection, amikacin sulfate, 500 mg	0.00	3.85	3.85	0.00	3.85	3.85	XXX	■
S0017		I	Injection, aminocaproic acid, 5 grams	0.00	0.25	0.25	0.00	0.25	0.25	XXX	■
S0020		I	Injection, bupivicaine hydrochloride, 30 ml	0.00	0.00	0.00	0.00	0.00	0.00	XXX	
S0021		I	Injection, ceftoperazone sodium, 1 gram	0.00	0.00	0.00	0.00	0.00	0.00	XXX	
S0023		I	Injection, cimetidine hydrochloride, 300 mg	0.00	0.21	0.21	0.00	0.21	0.21	XXX	■
S0028		I	Injection, famotidine, 20 mg	0.00	0.14	0.14	0.00	0.14	0.14	XXX	■
S0030		I	Injection, metronidazole, 500 mg	0.00	0.76	0.76	0.00	0.76	0.76	XXX	■
S0032		I	Injection, nafcillin sodium, 2 grams	0.00	0.16	0.16	0.00	0.16	0.16	XXX	■
S0034		I	Injection, ofloxacin, 400 mg	0.00	0.00	0.00	0.00	0.00	0.00	XXX	
S0039		I	Injection, sulfamethoxazole and trimethoprim, 10 ml	0.00	0.31	0.31	0.00	0.31	0.31	XXX	■
S0040		I	Injection, ticarcillin disodium and clavulanate potassium, 3.1 grams	0.00	0.46	0.46	0.00	0.46	0.46	XXX	■
S0071		I	Injection, acyclovir sodium, 50 mg	0.00	0.07	0.07	0.00	0.07	0.07	XXX	■
S0072		I	Injection, amikacin sulfate, 100 mg	0.00	2.16	2.16	0.00	2.16	2.16	XXX	■
S0073		I	Injection, aztreonam, 500 mg	0.00	0.28	0.28	0.00	0.28	0.28	XXX	■
S0074		I	Injection, cefotetan disodium, 500 mg	0.00	0.01	0.01	0.00	0.01	0.01	XXX	■
S0077		I	Injection, clindamycin phosphate, 300 mg	0.00	0.41	0.41	0.00	0.41	0.41	XXX	■

■ RVU not developed by CMS. Gap-filled RVUs developed by CHEG.

Code	M	S	Description	Work Value	Non-Fac PE	Fac PE	Mal-prac-tice	Non-Fac Total	Fac Total	Global	Gap
S0078		I	Injection, fosphenytoin sodium, 750 mg	0.00	0.00	0.00	0.00	0.00	0.00	XXX	
S0079		I	Injection, octreotide acetate, 100 mCg (for doses over 1 mg use J2352 or C1207)	0.00	0.43	0.43	0.00	0.43	0.43	XXX	
S0080		I	Injection, pentamidine isethionate, 300 mg	0.00	2.98	2.98	0.00	2.98	2.98	XXX	■
S0081		I	Injection, piperacillin sodium, 500 mg	0.00	0.00	0.00	0.00	0.00	0.00	XXX	
S0085		I	Injection, gatifloxacin, 200 mg	0.00	0.54	0.54	0.00	0.54	0.54	XXX	■
S0087		I	Injection, alemtuzumab, 30 mg	0.00	0.00	0.00	0.00	0.00	0.00	XXX	
S0088		I	Imatinib, 100 mg	0.00	0.00	0.00	0.00	0.00	0.00	XXX	
S0090		I	Sildenafil citrate, 25 mg	0.00	0.28	0.28	0.00	0.28	0.28	XXX	■
S0091		I	Granisetron hydrochloride, 1 mg (for circumstances falling under the Medicare statute, use Q0166)	0.00	6.16	6.16	0.00	6.16	6.16	XXX	
S0092		I	Injection, hydromorphone hydrochloride, 250 mg (loading dose for infusion pump)	0.00	2.80	2.80	0.00	2.80	2.80	XXX	
S0093		I	Injection, morphine sulfate, 500 mg (loading dose for infusion pump)	0.00	1.45	1.45	0.00	1.45	1.45	XXX	
S0155		I	Sterile dilutant for epoprostenol, 50 ml	0.00	0.00	0.00	0.00	0.00	0.00	XXX	
S0156		I	Exemestane, 25 mg	0.00	0.21	0.21	0.00	0.21	0.21	XXX	■
S0157		I	Becaplermin gel 0.01%, 0.5 gm	0.00	0.00	0.00	0.00	0.00	0.00	XXX	
S0170		I	Anastrozole, oral, 1mg	0.00	0.20	0.20	0.00	0.20	0.20	XXX	
S0171		I	Injection, bumetanide, 0.5 mg	0.00	0.05	0.05	0.00	0.05	0.05	XXX	
S0172		I	Chlorambucil, oral, 2 mg	0.00	0.05	0.05	0.00	0.05	0.05	XXX	
S0173		I	Dexamethasone, oral, 4 mg	0.00	0.03	0.03	0.00	0.03	0.03	XXX	
S0174		I	Dolasetron mesylate, oral 50 mg (for circumstances falling under the Medicare statute, use Q0180)	0.00	2.03	2.03	0.00	2.03	2.03	XXX	
S0175		I	Flutamide, oral, 125 mg	0.00	0.08	0.08	0.00	0.08	0.08	XXX	
S0176		I	Hydroxyurea, oral, 500 mg	0.00	0.04	0.04	0.00	0.04	0.04	XXX	
S0177		I	Levamisole hydrochloride, oral, 50 mg	0.00	0.20	0.20	0.00	0.20	0.20	XXX	
S0178		I	Lomustine, oral, 10 mg	0.00	0.20	0.20	0.00	0.20	0.20	XXX	
S0179		I	Megestrol acetate, oral, 20 mg	0.00	0.02	0.02	0.00	0.02	0.02	XXX	
S0181		I	Ondansetron hydrochloride, oral, 4 mg (for circumstances falling under the Medicare statute, use Q0179)	0.00	0.53	0.53	0.00	0.53	0.53	XXX	
S0182		I	Procarbazine hydrochloride, oral, 50 mg	0.00	0.02	0.02	0.00	0.02	0.02	XXX	

■ RVU not developed by CMS. Gap-filled RVUs developed by CHEG.

Code	M	S	Description	Work Value	Non-Fac PE	Fac PE	Mal-practice	Non-Fac Total	Fac Total	Global	Gap
S0183		I	Prochlorperazine maleate, oral, 5 mg (for circumstances falling under the medicare statute, use Q0164-Q0165)	0.00	0.02	0.02	0.00	0.02	0.02	XXX	
S0187		I	Tamoxifen citrate, oral, 10 mg	0.00	0.07	0.07	0.00	0.07	0.07	XXX	
S0189		I	Testosterone pellet, 75 mg	0.00	0.47	0.47	0.00	0.47	0.47	XXX	
S0190			Mitepristone, oral, 200 mg	0.00	0.00	0.00	0.00	0.00	0.00	XXX	
S0191			Misoprostol, oral, 200 mcg	0.00	0.03	0.03	0.00	0.03	0.03	XXX	
S0199			Medically induced abortion by oral ingestion of medication including all	0.00	0.00	0.00	0.00	0.00	0.00	XXX	
S0206		I	Procedure performed in surgery suite in physician's office (list separately in addition to code for primary procedure to denote use of facility and equipment)	0.00	0.00	0.00	0.00	0.00	0.00	XXX	
S0208		I	Paramedic intercept, hospital-based ALS service (non-voluntary), non-transport	0.00	0.00	0.00	0.00	0.00	0.00	XXX	
S0209		I	Wheelchair van, mileage, per mile	0.00	0.00	0.00	0.00	0.00	0.00	XXX	
S0215		I	Non-emergency transportation; mileage	0.00	0.00	0.00	0.00	0.00	0.00	XXX	
S0220		I	Medical conference by a physician with interdisciplinary team of health professionals or representatives of community agencies to coordinate activities of patient care (patient is present); approximately 30 minutes	0.00	0.00	0.00	0.00	0.00	0.00	XXX	
S0221		I	Medical conference by a physician with interdisciplinary team of health professionals or representatives of community agencies to coordinate activities of patient care (patient is present); approximately 60 minutes	0.00	0.00	0.00	0.00	0.00	0.00	XXX	
S0250		I	Comprehensive geriatric assessment and treatment planning performed by assessment team	0.00	0.00	0.00	0.00	0.00	0.00	XXX	
S0255		I	Hospice referral visit (advising patient and family of care options) performed by nurse, social worker, or other designated staff	0.00	0.00	0.00	0.00	0.00	0.00	XXX	
S0260		I	History and physical (outpatient or office) related to surgical procedure (list separately in addition to code for appropriate evaluation and management service)	0.00	0.00	0.00	0.00	0.00	0.00	XXX	
S0302		I	Completed early periodic screening diagnosis and treatment (EPSDT) service (list in addition to code for appropriate evaluation and management service)	0.00	0.00	0.00	0.00	0.00	0.00	XXX	
S0310		I	Hospitalist services (list separately in addition to code for appropriate evaluation and management service)	0.00	0.00	0.00	0.00	0.00	0.00	XXX	

■ RVU not developed by CMS. Gap-filled RVUs developed by CHEG.

Code	M	S	Description	Work Value	Non-Fac PE	Fac PE	Mal-prac-tice	Non-Fac Total	Fac Total	Global	Gap
S0340		I	Lifestyle modification program for management of coronary artery disease, including all supportive services; first quarter/stage	0.00	0.00	0.00	0.00	0.00	0.00	XXX	
S0341		I	Lifestyle modification program for management of coronary artery disease, including all supportive services; second or third quarter/ stage	0.00	0.00	0.00	0.00	0.00	0.00	XXX	
S0342		I	Lifestyle modification program for management of coronary artery disease, including all supportive services; fourth quarter/stage	0.00	0.00	0.00	0.00	0.00	0.00	XXX	
S0395		I	Impression casting of a foot performed by a practitioner other than the manufacturer of the orthotic	0.00	0.00	0.00	0.00	0.00	0.00	XXX	
S0400		I	Global fee for extracorporeal shock wave lithotripsy treatment of kidney stone(s)	0.00	0.00	0.00	0.00	0.00	0.00	XXX	
S0500		I	Disposable contact lens, per lens	0.00	0.00	0.00	0.00	0.00	0.00	XXX	
S0504		I	Single vision prescription lens (safety, athletic, or sunglass), per lens	0.00	0.00	0.00	0.00	0.00	0.00	XXX	
S0506		I	Bifocal vision prescription lens (safety, athletic, or sunglass), per lens	0.00	0.00	0.00	0.00	0.00	0.00	XXX	
S0508		I	Trifocal vision prescription lens (safety, athletic, or sunglass), per lens	0.00	0.00	0.00	0.00	0.00	0.00	XXX	
S0510		I	Non-prescription lens (safety, athletic, or sunglass), per lens	0.00	0.00	0.00	0.00	0.00	0.00	XXX	
S0512		I	Daily wear specialty contact lens, per lens	0.00	0.00	0.00	0.00	0.00	0.00	XXX	
S0514		I	Color contact lens, per lens	0.00	0.00	0.00	0.00	0.00	0.00	XXX	
S0516		I	Safety eyeglass frames	0.00	0.00	0.00	0.00	0.00	0.00	XXX	
S0518		I	Sunglasses frames	0.00	0.00	0.00	0.00	0.00	0.00	XXX	
S0580		I	Polycarbonate lens (list this code in addition to the basic code for the lens)	0.00	0.00	0.00	0.00	0.00	0.00	XXX	
S0581		I	Nonstandard lens (list this code in addition to the basic code for the lens)	0.00	0.00	0.00	0.00	0.00	0.00	XXX	
S0590		I	Integral lens service, miscellaneous services reported separately	0.00	0.00	0.00	0.00	0.00	0.00	XXX	
S0592		I	Comprehensive contact lens evaluation	0.00	0.00	0.00	0.00	0.00	0.00	XXX	
S0601		I	Screening proctoscopy	0.00	0.00	0.00	0.00	0.00	0.00	XXX	
S0605		I	Digital rectal examination, annual	0.00	0.00	0.00	0.00	0.00	0.00	XXX	
S0610		I	Annual gynecological examination; new patient	0.00	0.00	0.00	0.00	0.00	0.00	XXX	
S0612		I	Annual gynecological examination; established patient	0.00	0.00	0.00	0.00	0.00	0.00	XXX	

■ RVU not developed by CMS. Gap-filled RVUs developed by CHEG.

Code	M	S	Description	Work Value	Non-Fac PE	Fac PE	Mal-practice	Non-Fac Total	Fac Total	Global	Gap
S0620		I	Routine ophthalmological examination including refraction; new patient	0.00	0.00	0.00	0.00	0.00	0.00	XXX	
S0621		I	Routine ophthalmological examination including refraction; established patient	0.00	0.00	0.00	0.00	0.00	0.00	XXX	
S0622		I	Physical exam for college, new or established patient (list separately in addition to appropriate evaluation and management code)	0.00	0.00	0.00	0.00	0.00	0.00	XXX	
S0630		I	Removal of sutures by a physician other than the physician who originally closed the wound	0.00	0.00	0.00	0.00	0.00	0.00	XXX	
S0800		I	Laser in situ keratomileusis (LASIK)	0.00	0.00	0.00	0.00	0.00	0.00	XXX	
S0810		I	Photorefractive keratectomy (PRK)	0.00	0.00	0.00	0.00	0.00	0.00	XXX	
S0812		I	Phototherapeutic keratectomy (PTK)	0.00	0.00	0.00	0.00	0.00	0.00	XXX	
S0820		I	Computerized corneal topography, unilateral	0.00	0.00	0.00	0.00	0.00	0.00	XXX	
S0830		I	Ultrasound pachymetry to determine corneal thickness, with interpretation and report, unilateral	0.00	0.00	0.00	0.00	0.00	0.00	XXX	
S1001		I	Deluxe item, patient aware (list in addition to code for basic item)	0.00	0.00	0.00	0.00	0.00	0.00	XXX	
S1002		I	Customized item (list in addition to code for basic item)	0.00	0.00	0.00	0.00	0.00	0.00	XXX	
S1015		I	IV tubing extension set	0.00	0.00	0.00	0.00	0.00	0.00	XXX	
S1016		I	Non-PVC (polyvinyl chloride) intravenous administration set, for use with drugs that are not stable in PVC e.g., paclitaxel	0.00	0.00	0.00	0.00	0.00	0.00	XXX	
S1025		I	Inhaled nitric oxide for the treatment of hypoxic respiratory failure in the neonate; per diem	0.00	0.00	0.00	0.00	0.00	0.00	XXX	
S1030		I	Continuous noninvasive glucose monitoring device, purchase (for physician interpretation of data, use CPT code)	0.00	0.00	0.00	0.00	0.00	0.00	XXX	
S1031		I	Continuous noninvasive glucose monitoring device, rental, including sensor, sensor replacement, and download to monitor (for physician interpretation of data, use cpt code)	0.00	0.00	0.00	0.00	0.00	0.00	XXX	
S2053		I	Transplantation of small intestine, and liver allografts	0.00	0.00	0.00	0.00	0.00	0.00	XXX	
S2054		I	Transplantation of multivisceral organs	0.00	0.00	0.00	0.00	0.00	0.00	XXX	
S2055		I	Harvesting of donor multivisceral organs, with preparation and maintenance of allografts; from cadaver donor	0.00	0.00	0.00	0.00	0.00	0.00	XXX	
S2060		I	Lobar lung transplantation	0.00	0.00	0.00	0.00	0.00	0.00	XXX	

■ RVU not developed by CMS. Gap-filled RVUs developed by CHEG.

HCPCS

Code	M	S	Description	Work Value	Non-Fac PE	Fac PE	Mal-prac-tice	Non-Fac Total	Fac Total	Global	Gap
S2061		I	Donor lobectomy (lung) for transplantation, living donor	0.00	0.00	0.00	0.00	0.00	0.00	XXX	
S2065		I	Simultaneous pancreas kidney transplantation	0.00	0.00	0.00	0.00	0.00	0.00	XXX	
S2080		I	Laser-assisted uvulopalatoplasty (LAUP)	0.00	0.00	0.00	0.00	0.00	0.00	XXX	
S2102		I	Islet cell tissue transplant from pancreas; allogeneic	0.00	0.00	0.00	0.00	0.00	0.00	XXX	
S2103		I	Adrenal tissue transplant to brain	0.00	0.00	0.00	0.00	0.00	0.00	XXX	
S2112		I	Arthroscopy, knee, surgical for harvesting of cartilage (chondrocyte cells)	0.00	0.00	0.00	0.00	0.00	0.00	XXX	
S2115		I	Osteotomy, periacetabular, with internal fixation	0.00	0.00	0.00	0.00	0.00	0.00	XXX	
S2120		I	Low density lipoprotein (LDL) apheresis using heparin-induced extracorporeal LDL precipitation	0.00	0.00	0.00	0.00	0.00	0.00	XXX	
S2140		I	Cord blood harvesting for transplantation, allogeneic	0.00	0.00	0.00	0.00	0.00	0.00	XXX	
S2142		I	Cord blood-derived stem-cell transplantation, allogeneic	0.00	0.00	0.00	0.00	0.00	0.00	XXX	
S2150		I	Bone marrow or blood-derived peripheral stem cell harvesting and transplantation, allogenic or autologous, including pheresis, high-dose chemotherapy, and 28 days of post-transplant care (including drugs; hospitalization; medical, surgical, diagnostic and emergency services)	0.00	0.00	0.00	0.00	0.00	0.00	XXX	
S2180		I	Donor leukocyte infusion (e.g., DLI, donor lymphocyte infusion, donor buffy coat cell transfusion, donor peripheral blood monocyte transfusion)	0.00	0.00	0.00	0.00	0.00	0.00	XXX	
S2202		I	Echosclerotherapy	0.00	0.00	0.00	0.00	0.00	0.00	XXX	
S2205		I	Minimally invasive direct coronary artery bypass surgery involving mini-thoracotomy or mini-sternotomy surgery, performed under direct vision; using arterial graft(s), single coronary arterial graft	0.00	0.00	0.00	0.00	0.00	0.00	XXX	
S2206		I	Minimally invasive direct coronary artery bypass surgery involving mini-thoracotomy or mini-sternotomy surgery, performed under direct vision; using arterial graft(s), two coronary arterial grafts	0.00	0.00	0.00	0.00	0.00	0.00	XXX	
S2207		I	Minimally invasive direct coronary artery bypass surgery involving mini-thoracotomy or mini-sternotomy surgery, performed under direct vision; using venous graft only, single coronary venous graft	0.00	0.00	0.00	0.00	0.00	0.00	XXX	

■ RVU not developed by CMS. Gap-filled RVUs developed by CHEG.

Code	M	S	Description	Work Value	Non-Fac PE	Fac PE	Mal-practice	Non-Fac Total	Fac Total	Global	Gap
S2208		I	Minimally invasive direct coronary artery bypass surgery involving mini-thoracotomy or mini-sternotomy surgery, performed under direct vision; using single arterial and venous graft(s), single venous graft	0.00	0.00	0.00	0.00	0.00	0.00	XXX	
S2209		I	Minimally invasive direct coronary artery bypass surgery involving mini-thoracotomy or mini-sternotomy surgery, performed under direct vision; using two arterial grafts and single venous graft	0.00	0.00	0.00	0.00	0.00	0.00	XXX	
S2250		I	Uterine artery embolization for uterine fibroids	0.00	0.00	0.00	0.00	0.00	0.00	XXX	
S2260		I	Induced abortion, 17 to 24 weeks, any surgical method	0.00	0.00	0.00	0.00	0.00	0.00	XXX	
S2300		I	Arthroscopy, shoulder, surgical; with thermally-induced capsulorrhaphy	0.00	0.00	0.00	0.00	0.00	0.00	XXX	
S2340		I	Chemodenervation of abductor muscle(s) of vocal cord	0.00	0.00	0.00	0.00	0.00	0.00	XXX	
S2341		I	Chemodenervation of adductor muscle(s) of vocal cord	0.00	0.00	0.00	0.00	0.00	0.00	XXX	
S2342		I	Nasal endoscopy for post-operative debridement following functional endoscopic sinus surgery, nasal and/or sinus cavity(s), unilateral or bilateral	0.00	0.00	0.00	0.00	0.00	0.00	XXX	
S2350		I	Diskectomy, anterior, with decompression of spinal cord and/or nerve root(s), including osteophytectomy; lumbar, single interspace	0.00	0.00	0.00	0.00	0.00	0.00	XXX	
S2351		I	Diskectomy, anterior, with decompression of spinal cord and/or nerve root(s), including osteophytectomy; lumbar, each additional interspace (list separately in addition to code for primary procedure)	0.00	0.00	0.00	0.00	0.00	0.00	XXX	
S2360		I	Percutaneous vertebroplasty, one vertebral body, unilateral or bilateral injection; cervical	0.00	0.00	0.00	0.00	0.00	0.00	XXX	
S2361		I	Each additional cervical vertebral body (list separately in addition to code for primary procedure)	0.00	0.00	0.00	0.00	0.00	0.00	XXX	
S2370		I	Intradiscal electrothermal therapy, single interspace	0.00	0.00	0.00	0.00	0.00	0.00	XXX	
S2371		I	Each additional interspace (list separately in addition to code for primary procedure)	0.00	0.00	0.00	0.00	0.00	0.00	XXX	
S2400		I	Repair, congenital hernia in the fetus, procedure performed in utero	0.00	0.00	0.00	0.00	0.00	0.00	XXX	
S2401		I	Repair, urinary tract obstruction in the fetus, procedure performed in utero	0.00	0.00	0.00	0.00	0.00	0.00	XXX	

■ RVU not developed by CMS. Gap-filled RVUs developed by CHEG.

Code	M	S	Description	Work Value	Non-Fac PE	Fac PE	Mal-practice	Non-Fac Total	Fac Total	Global	Gap
S2402		I	Repair, congenital cystic adenomatoid malformation in the fetus, procedure performed in utero	0.00	0.00	0.00	0.00	0.00	0.00	XXX	
S2403		I	Repair, extralobar pulmonary sequestration in the fetus, procedure performed in utero	0.00	0.00	0.00	0.00	0.00	0.00	XXX	
S2404		I	Repair, myelomeningocele in the fetus, procedure performed in utero	0.00	0.00	0.00	0.00	0.00	0.00	XXX	
S2409		I	Repair, congenital malformation of fetus, procedure performed in utero, not otherwise classified	0.00	0.00	0.00	0.00	0.00	0.00	XXX	
S2411		I	Fetoscopic laser therapy for treatment of twin-to-twin transfusion syndrome	0.00	0.00	0.00	0.00	0.00	0.00	XXX	
S3600		I	Stat laboratory request (situations other than S3601)	0.00	0.00	0.00	0.00	0.00	0.00	XXX	
S3601		I	Emergency stat laboratory charge for patient who is homebound or residing in a nursing facility	0.00	0.00	0.00	0.00	0.00	0.00	XXX	
S3620		I	Newborn metabolic screening panel, includes test kit, postage and the laboratory tests specified by the state for inclusion in this panel (e.g., galactose; hemoglobin, electrophoresis; hydroxyprogesterone, 17-d; phenylanine (PKU); and thyroxine, total)	0.00	0.00	0.00	0.00	0.00	0.00	XXX	
S3630		I	Eosinophil count, blood, direct	0.00	0.00	0.00	0.00	0.00	0.00	XXX	
S3645		I	HIV-1 antibody testing of oral mucosal transudate	0.00	0.00	0.00	0.00	0.00	0.00	XXX	
S3650		I	Saliva test, hormone level; during menopause	0.00	0.00	0.00	0.00	0.00	0.00	XXX	
S3652		I	Saliva test, hormone level; to assess preterm labor risk	0.00	0.00	0.00	0.00	0.00	0.00	XXX	
S3701		I	Immunoassay for nuclear matrix protein 22 (NMP-22), quantitative	0.00	0.00	0.00	0.00	0.00	0.00	XXX	
S3708		I	Gastrointestinal fat absorption study	0.00	0.00	0.00	0.00	0.00	0.00	XXX	
S3818		I	Complete gene sequence analysis; BRCA 1 gene	0.00	0.00	0.00	0.00	0.00	0.00	XXX	
S3819		I	Complete gene sequence analysis; BRCA2 gene	0.00	0.00	0.00	0.00	0.00	0.00	XXX	
S3830		I	Complete MLH1 and MLH2 gene sequence analysis for hereditary nonpolyposis colorectal cancer (HNPCC) genetic testing	0.00	0.00	0.00	0.00	0.00	0.00	XXX	
S3831		I	Single-mutation analysis (in individual with a known MLH1 and MLH2 mutation in the family) for hereditary nonpolyposis colorectal cancer (HNPCC) genetic testing	0.00	0.00	0.00	0.00	0.00	0.00	XXX	
S3835		I	Complete gene sequence analysis for cystic fibrosis genetic testing	0.00	0.00	0.00	0.00	0.00	0.00	XXX	

■ RVU not developed by CMS. Gap-filled RVUs developed by CHEG.

Code	M	S	Description	Work Value	Non-Fac PE	Fac PE	Mal-practice	Non-Fac Total	Fac Total	Global	Gap
S3837		I	Complete gene sequence analysis for hemochromatosis genetic testing	0.00	0.00	0.00	0.00	0.00	0.00	XXX	
S3900		I	Surface electromyography (EMG)	0.00	0.00	0.00	0.00	0.00	0.00	XXX	
S3902		I	Ballistocardiogram	0.00	0.00	0.00	0.00	0.00	0.00	XXX	
S3904		I	Masters two step	0.00	0.00	0.00	0.00	0.00	0.00	XXX	
S4011		I	In vitro fertilization; including but not limited to identification and incubation of mature oocytes, fertilization with sperm, incubation of embryo(s), and subsequent visualization for determination of development	0.00	0.00	0.00	0.00	0.00	0.00	XXX	
S4015		I	Complete in vitro fertilization cycle, case rate	0.00	0.00	0.00	0.00	0.00	0.00	XXX	
S4016		I	Frozen in vitro fertilization cycle, case rate	0.00	0.00	0.00	0.00	0.00	0.00	XXX	
S4018		I	Frozen embryo transfer procedure cancelled before transfer, case rate	0.00	0.00	0.00	0.00	0.00	0.00	XXX	
S4020		I	In vitro fertilization procedure cancelled before aspiration, case rate	0.00	0.00	0.00	0.00	0.00	0.00	XXX	
S4021		I	In vitro fertilization procedure cancelled after aspiration, case rate	0.00	0.00	0.00	0.00	0.00	0.00	XXX	
S4022		I	Assisted oocyte fertilization, case rate	0.00	0.00	0.00	0.00	0.00	0.00	XXX	
S4025		I	Donor services for in vitro fertilization (sperm or embryo), case rate	0.00	0.00	0.00	0.00	0.00	0.00	XXX	
S4026		I	Procurement of donor sperm from sperm bank	0.00	0.00	0.00	0.00	0.00	0.00	XXX	
S4027		I	Storage of previously frozen embryos	0.00	0.00	0.00	0.00	0.00	0.00	XXX	
S4028		I	Microsurgical epididymal sperm aspiration (mesa)	0.00	0.00	0.00	0.00	0.00	0.00	XXX	
S4030		I	Sperm procurement and cryopreservation services; initial visit	0.00	0.00	0.00	0.00	0.00	0.00	XXX	
S4031		I	Sperm procurement and cryopreservation services; subsequent visit	0.00	0.00	0.00	0.00	0.00	0.00	XXX	
S4980			Levonorgestrel — releasing intrauterine system, each	0.00	0.00	0.00	0.00	0.00	0.00	XXX	
S4981		I	Insertion of levonorgestrel-releasing intrauterine system	0.00	0.00	0.00	0.00	0.00	0.00	XXX	
S4989		I	Contraceptive intrauterine device (e.g., Progestacert IUD), including implants and supplies	0.00	0.00	0.00	0.00	0.00	0.00	XXX	
S4990		I	Nicotine patches, legend	0.00	0.00	0.00	0.00	0.00	0.00	XXX	
S4991		I	Nicotine patches, non-legend	0.00	0.00	0.00	0.00	0.00	0.00	XXX	
S5000		I	Prescription drug, generic	0.00	0.00	0.00	0.00	0.00	0.00	XXX	

■ RVU not developed by CMS. Gap-filled RVUs developed by CHEG.

Code	M	S	Description	Work Value	Non-Fac PE	Fac PE	Mal-practice	Non-Fac Total	Fac Total	Global	Gap
S5001		I	Prescription drug, brand name	0.00	0.00	0.00	0.00	0.00	0.00	XXX	
S5010		I	5% dextrose and 45% normal saline, 1000 ml	0.00	0.00	0.00	0.00	0.00	0.00	XXX	
S5011		I	5% dextrose in lactated ringer's, 1000 ml	0.00	0.00	0.00	0.00	0.00	0.00	XXX	
S5012		I	5% dextrose with potassium chloride, 1000 ml	0.00	0.00	0.00	0.00	0.00	0.00	XXX	
S5013		I	5% dextrose/45% normal saline with potassium chloride and magnesium sulfate, 1000 ml	0.00	0.00	0.00	0.00	0.00	0.00	XXX	
S5014		I	5% dextrose/0.45% normal saline with potassium chloride and magnesium sulfate, 1500 ml	0.00	0.00	0.00	0.00	0.00	0.00	XXX	
S5035		I	Home infusion therapy, routine service of infusion device (e.g., pump maintenance)	0.00	0.00	0.00	0.00	0.00	0.00	XXX	
S5036		I	Home infusion therapy, repair of infusion device (e.g., pump repair)	0.00	0.00	0.00	0.00	0.00	0.00	XXX	
S5497		I	Home infusion therapy, catheter care/ maintenance, not otherwise classified; includes administrative services, professional pharmacy services, care coordination, and all necessary supplies and equipment (drugs and nursing visits coded separately), per diem	0.00	0.00	0.00	0.00	0.00	0.00	XXX	
S5498		I	Home infusion therapy, catheter care/ maintenance, simple (single lumen), includes administrative services, professional pharmacy services, care coordination and all necessary supplies and equipment, (drugs and nursing visits coded separately), per diem	0.00	0.00	0.00	0.00	0.00	0.00	XXX	
S5501		I	Home infusion therapy, catheter care/ maintenance, complex (more than one lumen), includes administrative services, professional pharmacy services, care coordination, and all necessary supplies and equipment (drugs and nursing visits coded separately), per diem	0.00	0.00	0.00	0.00	0.00	0.00	XXX	
S5502		I	Home infusion therapy, catheter care/ maintenance, implanted access device, includes administrative services, professional pharmacy services, care coordination and all necessary supplies and equipment, (drugs and nursing visits coded separately), per diem (use this code for interim maintenance of vascular access not currently in use)	0.00	0.00	0.00	0.00	0.00	0.00	XXX	
S5517		I	Home infusion therapy, all supplies necessary for restoration of catheter patency or declotting	0.00	0.00	0.00	0.00	0.00	0.00	XXX	
S5518		I	Home infusion therapy, all supplies necessary for catheter repair	0.00	0.00	0.00	0.00	0.00	0.00	XXX	
S5520		I	Home infusion therapy, all supplies (including catheter) necessary for a peripherally inserted central venous catheter (PICC) line insertion	0.00	0.00	0.00	0.00	0.00	0.00	XXX	

■ RVU not developed by CMS. Gap-filled RVUs developed by CHEG.

Code	M	S	Description	Work Value	Non-Fac PE	Fac PE	Mal-practice	Non-Fac Total	Fac Total	Global	Gap
S5521		I	Home infusion therapy, all supplies (including catheter) necessary for a midline catheter insertion	0.00	0.00	0.00	0.00	0.00	0.00	XXX	
S5522		I	Home infusion therapy, insertion of peripherally inserted central venous catheter (PICC), nursing services only (no supplies or catheter included)	0.00	0.00	0.00	0.00	0.00	0.00	XXX	
S5523		I	Home infusion therapy, insertion of midline central venous catheter, nursing services only (no supplies or catheter included)	0.00	0.00	0.00	0.00	0.00	0.00	XXX	
S8030		I	Scleral application of tantalum ring(s) for localization of lesions for proton beam therapy	0.00	0.00	0.00	0.00	0.00	0.00	XXX	
S8035		I	Magnetic source imaging	0.00	0.00	0.00	0.00	0.00	0.00	XXX	
S8037		I	Magnetic resonance cholangiopancreatography (MRCP)	0.00	0.00	0.00	0.00	0.00	0.00	XXX	
S8040		I	Topographic brain mapping	0.00	0.00	0.00	0.00	0.00	0.00	XXX	
S8049		I	Intraoperative radiation therapy (single administration)	0.00	0.00	0.00	0.00	0.00	0.00	XXX	
S8055		I	Ultrasound guidance for multifetal pregnancy reduction(s), technical component (only to be used when the physician doing the reduction procedure does not perform the ultrasound, guidance is included in the CPT code for multifetal pregnancy reduction - 59866)	0.00	0.00	0.00	0.00	0.00	0.00	XXX	
S8080		I	Scintimammography (radioimmunoscintigraphy of the breast), unilateral, including supply of radiopharmaceutical	0.00	0.00	0.00	0.00	0.00	0.00	XXX	
S8085		I	Fluorine-18 fluorodeoxyglucose (F-18 FDG) imaging using dual-head coincidence detection system (non-dedicated PET scan)	0.00	0.00	0.00	0.00	0.00	0.00	XXX	
S8092		I	Electron beam computed tomography (also known as ultrafast CT, cine CT)	0.00	0.00	0.00	0.00	0.00	0.00	XXX	
S8095		I	Wig (for medically-induced or congenital hair loss)	0.00	0.00	0.00	0.00	0.00	0.00	XXX	
S8096		I	Portable peak flow meter	0.00	0.00	0.00	0.00	0.00	0.00	XXX	
S8097		I	Asthma kit (including but not limited to portable peak expiratory flow meter, instructional video, brochure, and/or spacer)	0.00	0.00	0.00	0.00	0.00	0.00	XXX	
S8100		I	Holding chamber or spacer for use with an inhaler or nebulizer; without mask	0.00	0.00	0.00	0.00	0.00	0.00	XXX	
S8101		I	Holding chamber or spacer for use with an inhaler or nebulizer; with mask	0.00	0.00	0.00	0.00	0.00	0.00	XXX	
S8105		I	Oximeter for measuring blood oxygen levels noninvasively	0.00	0.00	0.00	0.00	0.00	0.00	XXX	

■ RVU not developed by CMS. Gap-filled RVUs developed by CHEG.

Code	M	S	Description	Work Value	Non-Fac PE	Fac PE	Mal-prac-tice	Non-Fac Total	Fac Total	Global	Gap
S8110		I	Peak expiratory flow rate (physician services)	0.00	0.00	0.00	0.00	0.00	0.00	XXX	
S8180		I	Tracheostomy shower protector	0.00	0.00	0.00	0.00	0.00	0.00	XXX	
S8181		I	Tracheostomy tube holder	0.00	0.00	0.00	0.00	0.00	0.00	XXX	
S8182		I	Humidifier, heated, used with ventilator, non-servo-controlled	0.00	0.00	0.00	0.00	0.00	0.00	XXX	
S8183		I	Humidifier, heated, used with ventilator, dual servo-controlled with temperature monitoring	0.00	0.00	0.00	0.00	0.00	0.00	XXX	
S8185		I	Flutter device	0.00	0.00	0.00	0.00	0.00	0.00	XXX	
S8186		I	Swivel adaptor	0.00	0.00	0.00	0.00	0.00	0.00	XXX	
S8189		I	Tracheostomy supply, not otherwise classified	0.00	0.00	0.00	0.00	0.00	0.00	XXX	
S8190		I	Electronic spirometer (or microspirometer)	0.00	0.00	0.00	0.00	0.00	0.00	XXX	
S8200		I	Chest compression vest	0.00	0.00	0.00	0.00	0.00	0.00	XXX	
S8205		I	Chest compression system generator and hoses (for use with chest compression vest — S8200)	0.00	0.00	0.00	0.00	0.00	0.00	XXX	
S8210		I	Mucus trap	0.00	0.00	0.00	0.00	0.00	0.00	XXX	
S8260		I	Oral orthotic for treatment of sleep apnea, includes fitting, fabrication, and materials	0.00	0.00	0.00	0.00	0.00	0.00	XXX	
S8401		I	Child-size incontinence garment, diaper, each	0.00	0.00	0.00	0.00	0.00	0.00	XXX	
S8403		I	Adult-sized incontinence garment, disposable, pull-up brief, each	0.00	0.00	0.00	0.00	0.00	0.00	XXX	
S8404		I	Child-size incontinence garment, disposable, pull-up brief, each	0.00	0.00	0.00	0.00	0.00	0.00	XXX	
S8405		I	Disposable liner/shield for incontinence, each	0.00	0.00	0.00	0.00	0.00	0.00	XXX	
S8415		I	Supplies for home delivery of infant	0.00	0.00	0.00	0.00	0.00	0.00	XXX	
S8420		I	Gradient pressure aid (sleeve and glove combination), custom made	0.00	0.00	0.00	0.00	0.00	0.00	XXX	
S8421		I	Gradient pressure aid (sleeve and glove combination), ready made	0.00	0.00	0.00	0.00	0.00	0.00	XXX	
S8422		I	Gradient pressure aid (sleeve), custom made, medium weight	0.00	0.00	0.00	0.00	0.00	0.00	XXX	
S8423		I	Gradient pressure aid (sleeve), custom made, heavy weight	0.00	0.00	0.00	0.00	0.00	0.00	XXX	
S8424		I	Gradient pressure aid (sleeve), ready made	0.00	0.00	0.00	0.00	0.00	0.00	XXX	
S8425		I	Gradient pressure aid (glove), custom made, medium weight	0.00	0.00	0.00	0.00	0.00	0.00	XXX	
S8426		I	Gradient pressure aid (glove), custom made, heavy weight	0.00	0.00	0.00	0.00	0.00	0.00	XXX	

■ RVU not developed by CMS. Gap-filled RVUs developed by CHEG.

Code	M	S	Description	Work Value	Non-Fac PE	Fac PE	Mal-practice	Non-Fac Total	Fac Total	Global	Gap
S8427		I	Gradient pressure aid (glove), ready made	0.00	0.00	0.00	0.00	0.00	0.00	XXX	
S8428		I	Gradient pressure aid (gauntlet), ready made	0.00	0.00	0.00	0.00	0.00	0.00	XXX	
S8429		I	Gradient pressure exterior wrap	0.00	0.00	0.00	0.00	0.00	0.00	XXX	
S8430		I	Padding for compression bandage, roll	0.00	0.00	0.00	0.00	0.00	0.00	XXX	
S8431		I	Compression bandage, roll	0.00	0.00	0.00	0.00	0.00	0.00	XXX	
S8450		I	Splint, prefabricated, digit (specify digit by use of modifier)	0.00	0.00	0.00	0.00	0.00	0.00	XXX	
S8451		I	Splint, prefabricated, wrist or ankle	0.00	0.00	0.00	0.00	0.00	0.00	XXX	
S8452		I	Splint, prefabricated, elbow	0.00	0.00	0.00	0.00	0.00	0.00	XXX	
S8490		I	Insulin syringes (100 syringes, any size)	0.00	0.00	0.00	0.00	0.00	0.00	XXX	
S8950		I	Complex lymphedema therapy, each 15 minutes	0.00	0.00	0.00	0.00	0.00	0.00	XXX	
S8999		I	Resuscitation bag (for use by patient on artificial respiration during power failure or other catastropic event)	0.00	0.00	0.00	0.00	0.00	0.00	XXX	
S9001		I	Home uterine monitor with or without associated nursing services	0.00	0.00	0.00	0.00	0.00	0.00	XXX	
S9007		I	Ultrafiltration monitor	0.00	0.00	0.00	0.00	0.00	0.00	XXX	
S9015		I	Automated EEG monitoring	0.00	0.00	0.00	0.00	0.00	0.00	XXX	
S9022		I	Digital subtraction angiography (use in addition to CPT code for the procedure for further identification)	0.00	0.00	0.00	0.00	0.00	0.00	XXX	
S9024		I	Paranasal sinus ultrasound	0.00	0.00	0.00	0.00	0.00	0.00	XXX	
S9025		I	Omnicardiogram/cardiointegram	0.00	0.00	0.00	0.00	0.00	0.00	XXX	
S9055		I	Procuren or other growth factor preparation to promote wound healing	0.00	0.00	0.00	0.00	0.00	0.00	XXX	
S9056		I	Coma stimulation per diem	0.00	0.00	0.00	0.00	0.00	0.00	XXX	
S9061		I	Home administration of aerosolized drug therapy (e.g., pentamidine); administrative services, professional pharmacy services, care coordination, all necessary supplies and equipment (drugs and nursing visits coded separately), per diem	0.00	0.00	0.00	0.00	0.00	0.00	XXX	
S9075		I	Smoking cessation treatment	0.00	0.00	0.00	0.00	0.00	0.00	XXX	
S9083		I	Global fee urgent care centers	0.00	0.00	0.00	0.00	0.00	0.00	XXX	
S9088		I	Services provided in an urgent care center (list in addition to code for service)	0.00	0.00	0.00	0.00	0.00	0.00	XXX	
S9090		I	Vertebral axial decompression, per session	0.00	0.00	0.00	0.00	0.00	0.00	XXX	

■ RVU not developed by CMS. Gap-filled RVUs developed by CHEG.

Code	M	S	Description	Work Value	Non-Fac PE	Fac PE	Mal-practice	Non-Fac Total	Fac Total	Global	Gap
S9098		I	Home visit, phototherapy services (e.g., Bili-lite), including equipment rental, nursing services, blood draw, supplies, and other services, per diem	0.00	0.00	0.00	0.00	0.00	0.00	XXX	
S9109		I	Congestive heart failure telemonitoring, equipment rental, including telescale, computer system and software, telephone connections, and maintenance, per month	0.00	0.00	0.00	0.00	0.00	0.00	XXX	
S9117		I	Back school, per visit	0.00	0.00	0.00	0.00	0.00	0.00	XXX	
S9122		I	Home health aide or certified nurse assistant, providing care in the home; per hour	0.00	0.00	0.00	0.00	0.00	0.00	XXX	
S9123		I	Nursing care, in the home; by registered nurse, per hour	0.00	0.00	0.00	0.00	0.00	0.00	XXX	
S9124		I	Nursing care, in the home; by licensed practical nurse, per hour	0.00	0.00	0.00	0.00	0.00	0.00	XXX	
S9125		I	Respite care, in the home, per diem	0.00	0.00	0.00	0.00	0.00	0.00	XXX	
S9126		I	Hospice care, in the home, per diem	0.00	0.00	0.00	0.00	0.00	0.00	XXX	
S9127		I	Social work visit, in the home, per diem	0.00	0.00	0.00	0.00	0.00	0.00	XXX	
S9128		I	Speech therapy, in the home, per diem	0.00	0.00	0.00	0.00	0.00	0.00	XXX	
S9129		I	Occupational therapy, in the home, per diem	0.00	0.00	0.00	0.00	0.00	0.00	XXX	
S9131		I	Physical therapy; in the home, per diem	0.00	0.00	0.00	0.00	0.00	0.00	XXX	
S9140		I	Diabetic management program, follow-up visit to non-MD provider	0.00	0.00	0.00	0.00	0.00	0.00	XXX	
S9141		I	Diabetic management program, follow-up visit to MD provider	0.00	0.00	0.00	0.00	0.00	0.00	XXX	
S9208		I	Home management of preterm labor, including administrative services, professional pharmacy services, care coordination, and all necessary supplies or equipment (drugs and nursing visits coded separately), per diem (do not use this code with any home infusion per diem code)	0.00	0.00	0.00	0.00	0.00	0.00	XXX	
S9209		I	Home management of preterm premature rupture of membranes (pprom), including administrative services, professional pharmacy services, care coordination, and all necessary supplies or equipment (drugs and nursing visits coded separately), per diem (do not use this code with any home infusion per diem code)	0.00	0.00	0.00	0.00	0.00	0.00	XXX	
S9211		I	Home management of gestational hypertension, includes administrative services, professional pharmacy services, care coordination and all necessary supplies and equipment (drugs and nursing visits coded separately); per diem (do not use this code with any home infusion per diem code)	0.00	0.00	0.00	0.00	0.00	0.00	XXX	

■ RVU not developed by CMS. Gap-filled RVUs developed by CHEG.

Code	M	S	Description	Work Value	Non-Fac PE	Fac PE	Mal-practice	Non-Fac Total	Fac Total	Global	Gap
S9212		I	Home management of postpartum hypertension, includes administrative services, professional pharmacy services, care coordination, and all necessary supplies and equipment (drugs and nursing visits coded separately), per diem (do not use this code with any home infusion per diem code)	0.00	0.00	0.00	0.00	0.00	0.00	XXX	
S9213		I	Home management of preeclampsia, includes administrative services, professional pharmacy services, care coordination, and all necessary supplies and equipment (drugs and nursing services coded separately); per diem (do not use this code with any home infusion per diem code)	0.00	0.00	0.00	0.00	0.00	0.00	XXX	
S9214		I	Home management of gestational diabetes, includes administrative services, professional pharmacy services, care coordination, and all necessary supplies and equipment (drugs and nursing visits coded separately); per diem (do not use this code with any home infusion per diem code)	0.00	0.00	0.00	0.00	0.00	0.00	XXX	
S9216		I	Nursing services and all necessary equipment and supplies for gestational hypertension program (includes maternal assessment as needed, telephonic collection of blood pressure, urine protein, weight and fetal movement counting via a home data collection system, patient status reports, 24 hour/7 day a week nursing support, and all education to the patient and caregiver); per diem	0.00	0.00	0.00	0.00	0.00	0.00	XXX	
S9217		I	Nursing services and all necessary equipment and supplies for postpartum hypertension program (includes maternal assessment as needed, telephonic collection of blood pressure, urine protein, weight, compliance management support, patient status reports, 24 hour/7 day a week nursing support, and all education to the patient and caregiver); per diem	0.00	0.00	0.00	0.00	0.00	0.00	XXX	
S9218		I	Nursing services and all necessary equipment and supplies for preeclampsia program (includes maternal assessment as needed, telephonic collection of blood pressure, urine protein, weight and daily fetal movement counts via a home data collection system, compliance management support, patient status reports, 24 hour/7 day a week nursing support, and all education to the patient and caregiver); per diem	0.00	0.00	0.00	0.00	0.00	0.00	XXX	
S9325		I	Home infusion therapy, pain management infusion; administrative services, professional pharmacy services, care coordination, and all necessary supplies and equipment, (drugs and nursing visits coded separately), per diem (do not use this code with S9326, S9327 or S9328)	0.00	0.00	0.00	0.00	0.00	0.00	XXX	

HCPCS

Code	M	S	Description	Work Value	Non-Fac PE	Fac PE	Mal-practice	Non-Fac Total	Fac Total	Global	Gap
S9326		I	Home infusion therapy, continuous pain management infusion; administrative services, professional pharmacy services, care coordination and all necessary supplies and equipment (drugs and nursing visits coded separately), per diem	0.00	0.00	0.00	0.00	0.00	0.00	XXX	
S9327		I	Home infusion therapy, intermittent pain management infusion; administrative services, professional pharmacy services, care coordination, and all necessary supplies and equipment (drugs and nursing visits coded separately), per diem	0.00	0.00	0.00	0.00	0.00	0.00	XXX	
S9328		I	Home infusion therapy, implanted pump pain management infusion; administrative services, professional pharmacy services, care coordination, and all necessary supplies and equipment (drugs and nursing visits coded separately), per diem	0.00	0.00	0.00	0.00	0.00	0.00	XXX	
S9329		I	Home infusion therapy, chemotherapy infusion; administrative services, professional pharmacy services, care coordination, and all necessary supplies and equipment (drugs and nursing visits coded separately), per diem (do not use this code with S9330 or S9331)	0.00	0.00	0.00	0.00	0.00	0.00	XXX	
S9330		I	Home infusion therapy, continuous chemotherapy infusion; administrative services, professional pharmacy services, care coordination, and all necessary supplies and equipment (drugs and nursing visits coded separately), per diem	0.00	0.00	0.00	0.00	0.00	0.00	XXX	
S9331		I	Home infusion therapy, intermittent chemotherapy infusion; administrative services, professional pharmacy services, care coordination, and all necessary supplies and equipment (drugs and nursing visits coded separately), per diem	0.00	0.00	0.00	0.00	0.00	0.00	XXX	
S9336		I	Home infusion therapy, continuous anticoagulant infusion therapy (e.g., heparin), administrative services, professional pharmacy services, care coordination and all necessary supplies and equipment (drugs and nursing visits coded separately), per diem	0.00	0.00	0.00	0.00	0.00	0.00	XXX	
S9338		I	Home infusion therapy, immunotherapy therapy; administrative services, professional pharmacy services, care coordination, and all necessary supplies and equipment (drug and nursing visits coded separately), per diem	0.00	0.00	0.00	0.00	0.00	0.00	XXX	
S9339		I	Home therapy; peritoneal dialysis, administrative services, professional pharmacy services, care coordination and all necessary supplies and equipment (drugs and nursing visits coded separately), per diem	0.00	0.00	0.00	0.00	0.00	0.00	XXX	

■ RVU not developed by CMS. Gap-filled RVUs developed by CHEG.

Code	M	S	Description	Work Value	Non-Fac PE	Fac PE	Mal-practice	Non-Fac Total	Fac Total	Global	Gap
S9340		I	Home therapy; enteral nutrition; administrative services, professional pharmacy services, care coordination, and all necessary supplies and equipment (enteral formula and nursing visits coded separately), per diem	0.00	0.00	0.00	0.00	0.00	0.00	XXX	
S9341		I	Home therapy; enteral nutrition via gravity; administrative services, professional pharmacy services, care coordination, and all necessary supplies and equipment (enteral formula and nursing visits coded separately), per diem	0.00	0.00	0.00	0.00	0.00	0.00	XXX	
S9342		I	Home therapy; enteral nutrition via pump; administrative services, professional pharmacy services, care coordination, and all necessary supplies and equipment (enteral formula and nursing visits coded separately), per diem	0.00	0.00	0.00	0.00	0.00	0.00	XXX	
S9343		I	Home therapy; enteral nutrition via bolus; administrative services, professional pharmacy services, care coordination, and all necessary supplies and equipment (enteral formula and nursing visits coded separately), per diem	0.00	0.00	0.00	0.00	0.00	0.00	XXX	
S9345		I	Home infusion therapy, anti-hemophilic agent infusion therapy (e.g., factor VIII); administrative services, professional pharmacy services, care coordination, and all necessary supplies and equipment (drugs and nursing visits coded separately), per diem	0.00	0.00	0.00	0.00	0.00	0.00	XXX	
S9346		I	Home infusion therapy, alpha-1-proteinase inhibitor (e.g., Prolastin); administrative services, professional pharmacy services, care coordination, and all necessary supplies and equipment (drugs and nursing visits coded separately), per diem	0.00	0.00	0.00	0.00	0.00	0.00	XXX	
S9347		I	Home infusion therapy, uninterrupted, long-term, controlled rate intravenous infusion therapy (e.g., Epoprostenol); administrative services, professional pharmacy services, care coordination, all necessary supplies and equipment (drugs and nursing visits coded separately), per diem	0.00	0.00	0.00	0.00	0.00	0.00	XXX	
S9348		I	Home infusion therapy, sympathomimetic/ inotropic agent infusion therapy (e.g., Dobutamine); administrative services, professional pharmacy services, care coordination, all necessary supplies and equipment (drugs and nursing visits coded separately), per diem	0.00	0.00	0.00	0.00	0.00	0.00	XXX	
S9349		I	Home infusion therapy, tocolytic infusion therapy; administrative services, professional pharmacy services, care coordination, and all necessary supplies and equipment (drugs and nursing visits coded separately), per diem	0.00	0.00	0.00	0.00	0.00	0.00	XXX	

■ RVU not developed by CMS. Gap-filled RVUs developed by CHEG.

HCPCS

Code	M	S	Description	Work Value	Non-Fac PE	Fac PE	Mal-practice	Non-Fac Total	Fac Total	Global	Gap
S9351		I	Home infusion therapy, continuous anti-emetic infusion therapy; administrative services, professional pharmacy services, care coordination, all necessary supplies and equipment (drugs and nursing visits coded separately), per diem	0.00	0.00	0.00	0.00	0.00	0.00	XXX	
S9353		I	Home infusion therapy, continuous insulin infusion therapy; administrative services, professional pharmacy services, care coordination, and all necessary supplies and equipment (drugs and nursing visits coded separately), per diem	0.00	0.00	0.00	0.00	0.00	0.00	XXX	
S9355		I	Home infusion therapy, chelation therapy; administrative services, professional pharmacy services, care coordination, and all necessary supplies and equipment (drugs and nursing visits coded separately), per diem	0.00	0.00	0.00	0.00	0.00	0.00	XXX	
S9357		I	Home infusion therapy, enzyme replacement intravenous therapy; (e.g., Imiglucerase); administrative services, professional pharmacy services, care coordination, and all necessary supplies and equipment (drugs and nursing visits coded separately), per diem	0.00	0.00	0.00	0.00	0.00	0.00	XXX	
S9359		I	Home infusion therapy, anti-tumor necrosis factor intravenous therapy; (e.g., Infliximab); administrative services, professional pharmacy services, care coordination, and all necessary supplies and equipment (drugs and nursing visits coded separately), per diem	0.00	0.00	0.00	0.00	0.00	0.00	XXX	
S9361		I	Home infusion therapy, diuretic intravenous therapy; administrative services, professional pharmacy services, care coordination, and all necessary supplies and equipment (drugs and nursing visits coded separately), per diem	0.00	0.00	0.00	0.00	0.00	0.00	XXX	
S9363		I	Home infusion therapy, anti-spasmotic intravenous therapy; administrative services, professional pharmacy services, care coordination, and all necessary supplies and equipment (drugs and nursing visits coded separately), per diem	0.00	0.00	0.00	0.00	0.00	0.00	XXX	
S9364		I	Home infusion therapy, total parenteral nutrition (TPN); administrative services, professional pharmacy services, care coordination, and all necessary supplies and equipment (includes standard TPN formula - lipids, specialty amino acid formulas, drugs, and nursing visits coded separately), per diem (do not use with home infusion codes S9365-S9368 using daily volume scales)	0.00	0.00	0.00	0.00	0.00	0.00	XXX	

■ RVU not developed by CMS. Gap-filled RVUs developed by CHEG.

Code	M	S	Description	Work Value	Non-Fac PE	Fac PE	Mal-practice	Non-Fac Total	Fac Total	Global	Gap
S9365		I	Home infusion therapy, total parenteral nutrition (TPN); one liter per day, administrative services, professional pharmacy services, care coordination, and all necessary supplies and equipment (includes standard TPN formula; lipids, specialty amino acid formulas, drugs, and nursing visits coded separately), per diem	0.00	0.00	0.00	0.00	0.00	0.00	XXX	
S9366		I	Home infusion therapy, total parenteral nutrition (TPN); more than one liter but no more than two liters per day, administrative services, professional pharmacy services, care coordination, and all necessary supplies and equipment (includes standard TPN formula; lipids, specialty amino acid formulas, drugs, and nursing visits coded separately), per diem	0.00	0.00	0.00	0.00	0.00	0.00	XXX	
S9367		I	Home infusion therapy, total parenteral nutrition (TPN); more than two liters but no more than three liters per day, administrative services, professional pharmacy services, care coordination, and all necessary supplies and equipment (includes standard TPN formula; lipids, specialty amino acids, drugs, and nursing visits coded separately), per diem	0.00	0.00	0.00	0.00	0.00	0.00	XXX	
S9368		I	Home infusion therapy, total parenteral nutrition (TPN); more than three liters per day, administrative services, professional pharmacy services, care coordination, and all necessary supplies and equipment (includes standard TPN formula; lipids, specialty amino acid formulas, drugs, and nursing visits coded separately), per diem	0.00	0.00	0.00	0.00	0.00	0.00	XXX	
S9370		I	Home therapy, intermittent anti-emetic injection therapy; administrative services, professional pharmacy services, care coordination, and all necessary supplies and equipment (drugs and nursing visits coded separately), per diem	0.00	0.00	0.00	0.00	0.00	0.00	XXX	
S9372		I	Home therapy; intermittent anticoagulant injection therapy (e.g., Heparin); administrative services, professional pharmacy services, care coordination, and all necessary supplies and equipment (drugs and nursing visits coded separately), per diem (do not use this code for flushing of infusion devices with heparin to maintain patency)	0.00	0.00	0.00	0.00	0.00	0.00	XXX	
S9373		I	Home infusion therapy, hydration therapy; administrative services, professional pharmacy services, care coordination, and all necessary supplies and equipment (drugs and nursing visits coded separately), per diem (do not use with hydration therapy codes S9374-S9377 using daily volume scales)	0.00	0.00	0.00	0.00	0.00	0.00	XXX	

■ RVU not developed by CMS. Gap-filled RVUs developed by CHEG.

Code	M	S	Description	Work Value	Non-Fac PE	Fac PE	Mal-practice	Non-Fac Total	Fac Total	Global	Gap
S9374		I	Home infusion therapy, hydration therapy; one liter per day, administrative services, professional pharmacy services, care coordination, and all necessary supplies and equipment (drugs and nursing visits coded separately), per diem	0.00	0.00	0.00	0.00	0.00	0.00	XXX	
S9375		I	Home infusion therapy, hydration therapy; more than one liter but no more than two liters per day, administrative services, professional pharmacy services, care coordination, and all necessary supplies and equipment (drugs and nursing visits coded separately), per diem	0.00	0.00	0.00	0.00	0.00	0.00	XXX	
S9376		I	Home infusion therapy, hydration therapy; more than two liters but no more than three liters per day, administrative services, professional pharmacy services, care coordination, and all necessary supplies and equipment (drugs and nursing visits coded separately), per diem	0.00	0.00	0.00	0.00	0.00	0.00	XXX	
S9377		I	Home infusion therapy, hydration therapy; more than three liters per day, administrative services, professional pharmacy services, care coordination, and all necessary supplies (drugs and nursing visits coded separately), per diem	0.00	0.00	0.00	0.00	0.00	0.00	XXX	
S9379		I	Home infusion therapy, infusion therapy, not otherwise classified; administrative services, professional pharmacy services, care coordination, and all necessary supplies and equipment (drugs and nursing visits coded separately), per diem	0.00	0.00	0.00	0.00	0.00	0.00	XXX	
S9381		I	Delivery or service to high risk areas requiring escort or extra protection, per visit	0.00	0.00	0.00	0.00	0.00	0.00	XXX	
S9435		I	Medical foods for inborn errors of metabolism	0.00	0.00	0.00	0.00	0.00	0.00	XXX	
S9441		I	Asthma education, non-physician provider, per session	0.00	0.00	0.00	0.00	0.00	0.00	XXX	
S9442		I	Birthing classes, non-physician provider, per session	0.00	0.00	0.00	0.00	0.00	0.00	XXX	
S9443		I	Lactation classes, non-physician provider, per session	0.00	0.00	0.00	0.00	0.00	0.00	XXX	
S9445		I	Patient education, not otherwise classified, non-physician provider, individual, per session	0.00	0.00	0.00	0.00	0.00	0.00	XXX	
S9446		I	Patient education, not otherwise classified, non-physician provider, group, per session	0.00	0.00	0.00	0.00	0.00	0.00	XXX	
S9455		I	Diabetic management program, group session	0.00	0.00	0.00	0.00	0.00	0.00	XXX	
S9460		I	Diabetic management program, nurse visit	0.00	0.00	0.00	0.00	0.00	0.00	XXX	
S9465		I	Diabetic management program, dietitian visit	0.00	0.00	0.00	0.00	0.00	0.00	XXX	

■ RVU not developed by CMS. Gap-filled RVUs developed by CHEG.

Code	M	S	Description	Work Value	Non-Fac PE	Fac PE	Mal-prac-tice	Non-Fac Total	Fac Total	Global	Gap
S9470		I	Nutritional counseling, dietitian visit	0.00	0.00	0.00	0.00	0.00	0.00	XXX	
S9472		I	Cardiac rehabilitation program, non-physician provider, per diem	0.00	0.00	0.00	0.00	0.00	0.00	XXX	
S9473		I	Pulmonary rehabilitation program, non-physician provider, per diem	0.00	0.00	0.00	0.00	0.00	0.00	XXX	
S9474		I	Enterostomal therapy by a registered nurse certified in enterostomal therapy, per diem	0.00	0.00	0.00	0.00	0.00	0.00	XXX	
S9475		I	Ambulatory setting substance abuse treatment or detoxification services, per diem	0.00	0.00	0.00	0.00	0.00	0.00	XXX	
S9480		I	Intensive outpatient psychiatric services, per diem	0.00	0.00	0.00	0.00	0.00	0.00	XXX	
S9485		I	Crisis intervention mental health services, per diem	0.00	0.00	0.00	0.00	0.00	0.00	XXX	
S9494		I	Home infusion therapy, antibiotic, antiviral, or antifungal therapy; administrative services, professional pharmacy services, care coordination, and all necessary supplies and equipment (drug and nursing visits coded separately), per diem (do not use with home infusion codes for hourly dosing schedules S9497-S9504)	0.00	0.00	0.00	0.00	0.00	0.00	XXX	
S9497		I	Home infusion therapy, antibiotic, antiviral, or antifungal therapy; once every three hours; administrative services, professional pharmacy services, care coordination, and all necessary supplies and equipment (drugs and nursing visits coded separately), per diem	0.00	0.00	0.00	0.00	0.00	0.00	XXX	
S9500		I	Home infusion therapy, antibiotic, antiviral, or antifungal therapy; once every 24 hours; administrative services, professional pharmacy services, care coordination, and all necessary supplies and equipment (drugs and nursing visits coded separately), per diem	0.00	0.00	0.00	0.00	0.00	0.00	XXX	
S9501		I	Home infusion therapy, antibiotic, antiviral, or antifungal therapy; once every 12 hours; administrative services, professional pharmacy services, care coordination, and all necessary supplies and equipment (drugs and nursing visits coded separately), per diem	0.00	0.00	0.00	0.00	0.00	0.00	XXX	
S9502		I	Home infusion therapy, antibiotic, antiviral, or antifungal therapy; once every eight hours, administrative services, professional pharmacy services, care coordination, and all necessary supplies and equipment (drugs and nursing visits coded separately), per diem	0.00	0.00	0.00	0.00	0.00	0.00	XXX	

■ RVU not developed by CMS. Gap-filled RVUs developed by CHEG.

Code	M	S	Description	Work Value	Non-Fac PE	Fac PE	Mal-prac-tice	Non-Fac Total	Fac Total	Global	Gap
S9503		I	Home infusion therapy, antibiotic, antiviral, or antifungal; once every six hours; administrative services, professional pharmacy services, care coordination, and all necessary supplies and equipment (drugs and nursing visits coded separately), per diem	0.00	0.00	0.00	0.00	0.00	0.00	XXX	
S9504		I	Home infusion therapy, antibiotic, antiviral, or antifungal; once every four hours; administrative services, professional pharmacy services, care coordination, and all necessary supplies and equipment (drugs and nursing visits coded separately), per diem	0.00	0.00	0.00	0.00	0.00	0.00	XXX	
S9524		I	Nursing services related to home iv therapy, per diem	0.00	0.00	0.00	0.00	0.00	0.00	XXX	
S9529		I	Routine venipuncture for collection of specimen(s), single home bound, nursing home, or skilled nursing facility patient	0.00	0.00	0.00	0.00	0.00	0.00	XXX	
S9537		I	Home therapy; hematopoietic hormone injection therapy (e.g., Crythropoietin, G-CSF, GM-CSF); administrative services, professional pharmacy services, care coordination, and all necessary supplies and equipment (drugs and nursing visits coded separately), per diem	0.00	0.00	0.00	0.00	0.00	0.00	XXX	
S9538		I	Home transfusion of blood product(s); administrative services, professional pharmacy services, care coordination and all necessary supplies and equipment (blood products, drugs, and nursing visits coded separately), per diem	0.00	0.00	0.00	0.00	0.00	0.00	XXX	
S9542		I	Home injectable therapy; not otherwise classified, including administrative services, professional pharmacy services, coordination of care, and all necessary supplies and equipment (drugs and nursing visits coded separately), per diem	0.00	0.00	0.00	0.00	0.00	0.00	XXX	
S9543		I	Administration of medication, intramuscularly, epidurally or subcutaneously, in the home setting, including all nursing care, equipment, and supplies; per diem	0.00	0.00	0.00	0.00	0.00	0.00	XXX	
S9558		I	Home injectable therapy; growth hormone, including administrative services, professional pharmacy services, coordination of care, and all necessary supplies and equipment (drugs and nursing visits coded separately), per diem	0.00	0.00	0.00	0.00	0.00	0.00	XXX	
S9559		I	Home injectable therapy; interferon, including administrative services, professional pharmacy services, coordination of care, and all necessary supplies and equipment (drugs and nursing visits coded separately), per diem	0.00	0.00	0.00	0.00	0.00	0.00	XXX	

■ RVU not developed by CMS. Gap-filled RVUs developed by CHEG.

Code	M	S	Description	Work Value	Non-Fac PE	Fac PE	Mal-practice	Non-Fac Total	Fac Total	Global	Gap
S9560		I	Home injectable therapy; hormonal therapy (e.g.; leuprolide, goserelin), including administrative services, professional pharmacy services, care coordination, and all necessary supplies and equipment (drugs and nursing visits coded separately), per diem	0.00	0.00	0.00	0.00	0.00	0.00	XXX	
S9800		I	Home therapy; provision of infusion, specialty drug administration, and/or associated nursing services and procedures, by highly technical R.N., per hour (do not use this code with S9524)	0.00	0.00	0.00	0.00	0.00	0.00	XXX	
S9810		I	Home therapy; professional pharmacy services for provision of infusion, specialty drug administration, and/or disease state management, not otherwise classified, per hour (do not use this code with any per diem code)	0.00	0.00	0.00	0.00	0.00	0.00	XXX	
S9981		I	Medical records copying fee, administrative	0.00	0.00	0.00	0.00	0.00	0.00	XXX	
S9982		I	Medical records copying fee, per page	0.00	0.00	0.00	0.00	0.00	0.00	XXX	
S9986		I	Not medically necessary service (patient is aware that service not medically necessary)	0.00	0.00	0.00	0.00	0.00	0.00	XXX	
S9989		I	Services provided outside of the united states of america (list in addition to code(s) for services(s))	0.00	0.00	0.00	0.00	0.00	0.00	XXX	
S9990		I	Services provided as part of a phase II clinical trial	0.00	0.00	0.00	0.00	0.00	0.00	XXX	
S9991		I	Services provided as part of a phase III clinical trial	0.00	0.00	0.00	0.00	0.00	0.00	XXX	
S9992		I	Transportation costs to and from trial location and local transportation costs (e.g., fares for taxicab or bus) for clinical trial participant and one caregiver/companion	0.00	0.00	0.00	0.00	0.00	0.00	XXX	
S9994		I	Lodging costs (e.g., hotel charges) for clinical trial participant and one caregiver/companion	0.00	0.00	0.00	0.00	0.00	0.00	XXX	
S9996		I	Meals for clinical trial participant and one caregiver/companion	0.00	0.00	0.00	0.00	0.00	0.00	XXX	
S9999		I	Sales tax	0.00	0.00	0.00	0.00	0.00	0.00	XXX	
T1000		I	Private duty/independent nursing service(s) - licensed, up to 15 minutes	0.00	0.00	0.00	0.00	0.00	0.00	XXX	
T1001		I	Nursing assessment/evaluation	0.00	0.00	0.00	0.00	0.00	0.00	XXX	
T1002		I	RN services, up to 15 minutes	0.00	0.00	0.00	0.00	0.00	0.00	XXX	
T1003		I	LPN/LVN services, up to 15 minutes	0.00	0.00	0.00	0.00	0.00	0.00	XXX	
T1004		I	Services of a qualified nursing aide, up to 15 minutes	0.00	0.00	0.00	0.00	0.00	0.00	XXX	
T1005		I	Respite care services, up to 15 minutes	0.00	0.00	0.00	0.00	0.00	0.00	XXX	

■ RVU not developed by CMS. Gap-filled RVUs developed by CHEG.

Code	M	S	Description	Work Value	Non-Fac PE	Fac PE	Mal-practice	Non-Fac Total	Fac Total	Global	Gap
T1006		I	Alcohol and/or substance abuse services, family/couple counseling	0.00	0.00	0.00	0.00	0.00	0.00	XXX	
T1007		I	Alcohol and/or substance abuse services, treatment plan development and/or modification	0.00	0.00	0.00	0.00	0.00	0.00	XXX	
T1008		I	Day treatment for individual alcohol and/or substance abuse services	0.00	0.00	0.00	0.00	0.00	0.00	XXX	
T1009		I	Child sitting services for children of the individual receiving alcohol and/or substance abuse services	0.00	0.00	0.00	0.00	0.00	0.00	XXX	
T1010		I	Meals for individuals receiving alcohol and/or substance abuse services (when meals not included in the program)	0.00	0.00	0.00	0.00	0.00	0.00	XXX	
T1011		I	Alcohol and/or substance abuse services, not otherwise classified	0.00	0.00	0.00	0.00	0.00	0.00	XXX	
T1012		I	Alcohol and/or substance abuse services, skills development	0.00	0.00	0.00	0.00	0.00	0.00	XXX	
T1013		I	Sign language or oral interpreter services	0.00	0.00	0.00	0.00	0.00	0.00	XXX	
T1014		I	Telehealth transmission, per minute, professional services bill separately	0.00	0.00	0.00	0.00	0.00	0.00	XXX	
T1015		I	Clinic visit/encounter, all-inclusive	0.00	0.00	0.00	0.00	0.00	0.00	XXX	
V2020		X	Frames, purchases	0.00	1.77	1.77	0.00	1.77	1.77	XXX	■
V2025		N	Deluxe frame	0.00	0.00	0.00	0.00	0.00	0.00	XXX	
V2100		X	Sphere, single vision, plano to plus or minus 4.00, per lens	0.00	1.71	1.71	0.00	1.71	1.71	XXX	■
V2101		X	Sphere, single vision, plus or minus 4.12 to plus or minus 7.00d, per lens	0.00	1.17	1.17	0.00	1.17	1.17	XXX	■
V2102		X	Sphere, single vision, plus or minus 7.12 to plus or minus 20.00d, per lens	0.00	1.70	1.70	0.00	1.70	1.70	XXX	■
V2103		X	Spherocylinder, single vision, plano to plus or minus 4.00d sphere, 0.12 to 2.00d cylinder, per lens	0.00	1.14	1.14	0.00	1.14	1.14	XXX	■
V2104		X	Spherocylinder, single vision, plano to plus or minus 4.00d sphere, 2.12 to 4.00d cylinder, per lens	0.00	1.45	1.45	0.00	1.45	1.45	XXX	■
V2105		X	Spherocylinder, single vision, plano to plus or minus 4.00d sphere, 4.25 to 6.00d cylinder, per lens	0.00	1.16	1.16	0.00	1.16	1.16	XXX	■
V2106		X	Spherocylinder, single vision, plano to plus or minus 4.00d sphere, over 6.00d cylinder, per lens	0.00	1.13	1.13	0.00	1.13	1.13	XXX	■

■ RVU not developed by CMS. Gap-filled RVUs developed by CHEG.

Code	M	S	Description	Work Value	Non-Fac PE	Fac PE	Mal-practice	Non-Fac Total	Fac Total	Global	Gap
V2107		X	Spherocylinder, single vision, plus or minus 4.25 to plus or minus 7.00 sphere, 0.12 to 2.00d cylinder, per lens	0.00	1.22	1.22	0.00	1.22	1.22	XXX	■
V2108		X	Spherocylinder, single vision, plus or minus 4.25d to plus or minus 7.00d sphere, 2.12 to 4.00d cylinder, per lens	0.00	1.25	1.25	0.00	1.25	1.25	XXX	■
V2109		X	Spherocylinder, single vision, plus or minus 4.25 to plus or minus 7.00d sphere, 4.25 to 6.00d cylinder, per lens	0.00	1.40	1.40	0.00	1.40	1.40	XXX	■
V2110		X	Spherocylinder, single vision, plus or minus 4.25 to 7.00d sphere, over 6.00d cylinder, per lens	0.00	1.37	1.37	0.00	1.37	1.37	XXX	■
V2111		X	Spherocylinder, single vision, plus or minus 7.25 to plus or minus 12.00d sphere, 0.25 to 2.25d cylinder, per lens	0.00	1.43	1.43	0.00	1.43	1.43	XXX	■
V2112		X	Spherocylinder, single vision, plus or minus 7.25 to plus or minus 12.00d sphere, 2.25d to 4.00d cylinder, per lens	0.00	1.59	1.59	0.00	1.59	1.59	XXX	■
V2113		X	Spherocylinder, single vision, plus or minus 7.25 to plus or minus 12.00d sphere, 4.25 to 6.00d cylinder, per lens	0.00	1.77	1.77	0.00	1.77	1.77	XXX	■
V2114		X	Spherocylinder, single vision sphere over plus or minus 12.00d, per lens	0.00	1.92	1.92	0.00	1.92	1.92	XXX	■
V2115		X	Lenticular (myodisc), per lens, single vision	0.00	2.32	2.32	0.00	2.32	2.32	XXX	■
V2116		X	Lenticular lens, nonaspheric, per lens, single vision	0.00	1.86	1.86	0.00	1.86	1.86	XXX	■
V2117		X	Lenticular, aspheric, per lens, single vision	0.00	2.64	2.64	0.00	2.64	2.64	XXX	■
V2118		X	Aniseikonic lens, single vision	0.00	2.07	2.07	0.00	2.07	2.07	XXX	■
V2199		X	Not otherwise classified, single vision lens	0.00	0.00	0.00	0.00	0.00	0.00	XXX	
V2200		X	Sphere, bifocal, plano to plus or minus 4.00d, per lens	0.00	2.33	2.33	0.00	2.33	2.33	XXX	■
V2201		X	Sphere, bifocal, plus or minus 4.12 to plus or minus 7.00d, per lens	0.00	1.59	1.59	0.00	1.59	1.59	XXX	■
V2202		X	Sphere, bifocal, plus or minus 7.12 to plus or minus 20.00d, per lens	0.00	1.86	1.86	0.00	1.86	1.86	XXX	■
V2203		X	Spherocylinder, bifocal, plano to plus or minus 4.00d sphere, 0.12 to 2.00d cylinder, per lens	0.00	1.46	1.46	0.00	1.46	1.46	XXX	■
V2204		X	Spherocylinder, bifocal, plano to plus or minus 4.00d sphere, 2.12 to 4.00d cylinder, per lens	0.00	1.46	1.46	0.00	1.46	1.46	XXX	■
V2205		X	Spherocylinder, bifocal, plano to plus or minus 4.00d sphere, 4.25 to 6.00d cylinder, per lens	0.00	1.77	1.77	0.00	1.77	1.77	XXX	■
V2206		X	Spherocylinder, bifocal, plano to plus or minus 4.00d sphere, over 6.00d cylinder, per lens	0.00	1.77	1.77	0.00	1.77	1.77	XXX	■

■ RVU not developed by CMS. Gap-filled RVUs developed by CHEG.

Code	M	S	Description	Work Value	Non-Fac PE	Fac PE	Mal-practice	Non-Fac Total	Fac Total	Global	Gap
V2207		X	Spherocylinder, bifocal, plus or minus 4.25 to plus or minus 7.00d sphere, 0.12 to 2.00d cylinder, per lens	0.00	1.77	1.77	0.00	1.77	1.77	XXX	■
V2208		X	Spherocylinder, bifocal, plus or minus 4.25 to plus or minus 7.00d sphere, 2.12 to 4.00d cylinder, per lens	0.00	1.71	1.71	0.00	1.71	1.71	XXX	■
V2209		X	Spherocylinder, bifocal, plus or minus 4.25 to plus or minus 7.00d sphere, 4.25 to 6.00d cylinder, per lens	0.00	1.83	1.83	0.00	1.83	1.83	XXX	■
V2210		X	Spherocylinder, bifocal, plus or minus 4.25 to plus or minus 7.00d sphere, over 6.00d cylinder, per lens	0.00	2.01	2.01	0.00	2.01	2.01	XXX	■
V2211		X	Spherocylinder, bifocal, plus or minus 7.25 to plus or minus 12.00d sphere, 0.25 to 2.25d cylinder, per lens	0.00	2.07	2.07	0.00	2.07	2.07	XXX	■
V2212		X	Spherocylinder, bifocal, plus or minus 7.25 to plus or minus 12.00d sphere, 2.25 to 4.00d cylinder, per lens	0.00	2.41	2.41	0.00	2.41	2.41	XXX	■
V2213		X	Spherocylinder, bifocal, plus or minus 7.25 to plus or minus 12.00d sphere, 4.25 to 6.00d cylinder, per lens	0.00	1.89	1.89	0.00	1.89	1.89	XXX	■
V2214		X	Spherocylinder, bifocal, sphere over plus or minus 12.00d, per lens	0.00	2.78	2.78	0.00	2.78	2.78	XXX	■
V2215		X	Lenticular (myodisc), per lens, bifocal	0.00	2.41	2.41	0.00	2.41	2.41	XXX	■
V2216		X	Lenticular, nonaspheric, per lens, bifocal	0.00	2.59	2.59	0.00	2.59	2.59	XXX	■
V2217		X	Lenticular, aspheric lens, bifocal	0.00	2.47	2.47	0.00	2.47	2.47	XXX	■
V2218		X	Aniseikonic, per lens, bifocal	0.00	2.43	2.43	0.00	2.43	2.43	XXX	■
V2219		X	Bifocal seg width over 28mm	0.00	1.25	1.25	0.00	1.25	1.25	XXX	■
V2220		X	Bifocal add over 3.25d	0.00	1.01	1.01	0.00	1.01	1.01	XXX	■
V2299		X	Specialty bifocal (by report)	0.00	0.00	0.00	0.00	0.00	0.00	XXX	
V2300		X	Sphere, trifocal, plano to plus or minus 4.00d, per lens	0.00	3.14	3.14	0.00	3.14	3.14	XXX	■
V2301		X	Sphere, trifocal, plus or minus 4.12 to plus or minus 7.00d per lens	0.00	2.44	2.44	0.00	2.44	2.44	XXX	■
V2302		X	Sphere, trifocal, plus or minus 7.12 to plus or minus 20.00, per lens	0.00	2.62	2.62	0.00	2.62	2.62	XXX	■
V2303		X	Spherocylinder, trifocal, plano to plus or minus 4.00d sphere, 0.12 to 2.00d cylinder, per lens	0.00	1.94	1.94	0.00	1.94	1.94	XXX	■
V2304		X	Spherocylinder, trifocal, plano to plus or minus 4.00d sphere, 2.25 to 4.00d cylinder, per lens	0.00	1.89	1.89	0.00	1.89	1.89	XXX	■
V2305		X	Spherocylinder, trifocal, plano to plus or minus 4.00d sphere, 4.25 to 6.00 cylinder, per lens	0.00	2.20	2.20	0.00	2.20	2.20	XXX	■

■ RVU not developed by CMS. Gap-filled RVUs developed by CHEG.

Code	M	S	Description	Work Value	Non-Fac PE	Fac PE	Mal-practice	Non-Fac Total	Fac Total	Global	Gap
V2306		X	Spherocylinder, trifocal, plano to plus or minus 4.00d sphere, over 6.00d cylinder, per lens	0.00	2.26	2.26	0.00	2.26	2.26	XXX	■
V2307		X	Spherocylinder, trifocal, plus or minus 4.25 to plus or minus 7.00d sphere, 0.12 to 2.00d cylinder, per lens	0.00	2.17	2.17	0.00	2.17	2.17	XXX	■
V2308		X	Spherocylinder, trifocal, plus or minus 4.25 to plus or minus 7.00d sphere, 2.12 to 4.00d cylinder, per lens	0.00	1.95	1.95	0.00	1.95	1.95	XXX	■
V2309		X	Spherocylinder, trifocal, plus or minus 4.25 to plus or minus 7.00d sphere, 4.25 to 6.00d cylinder, per lens	0.00	2.12	2.12	0.00	2.12	2.12	XXX	■
V2310		X	Spherocylinder, trifocal, plus or minus 4.25 to plus or minus 7.00d sphere, over 6.00d cylinder, per lens	0.00	2.51	2.51	0.00	2.51	2.51	XXX	■
V2311		X	Spherocylinder, trifocal, plus or minus 7.25 to plus or minus 12.00d sphere, 0.25 to 2.25d cylinder, per lens	0.00	2.50	2.50	0.00	2.50	2.50	XXX	■
V2312		X	Spherocylinder, trifocal, plus or minus 7.25 to plus or minus 12.00d sphere, 2.25 to 4.00d cylinder, per lens	0.00	2.48	2.48	0.00	2.48	2.48	XXX	■
V2313		X	Spherocylinder, trifocal, plus or minus 7.25 to plus or minus 12.00d sphere, 4.25 to 6.00d cylinder, per lens	0.00	2.95	2.95	0.00	2.95	2.95	XXX	■
V2314		X	Spherocylinder, trifocal, sphere over plus or minus 12.00d, per lens	0.00	3.02	3.02	0.00	3.02	3.02	XXX	■
V2315		X	Lenticular (myodisc), per lens, trifocal	0.00	3.60	3.60	0.00	3.60	3.60	XXX	■
V2316		X	Lenticular nonaspheric, per lens, trifocal	0.00	3.17	3.17	0.00	3.17	3.17	XXX	■
V2317		X	Lenticular, aspheric lens, trifocal	0.00	3.39	3.39	0.00	3.39	3.39	XXX	■
V2318		X	Aniseikonic lens, trifocal	0.00	4.15	4.15	0.00	4.15	4.15	XXX	■
V2319		X	Trifocal seg width over 28 mm	0.00	1.40	1.40	0.00	1.40	1.40	XXX	■
V2320		X	Trifocal add over 3.25d	0.00	1.46	1.46	0.00	1.46	1.46	XXX	■
V2399		X	Specialty trifocal (by report)	0.00	0.00	0.00	0.00	0.00	0.00	XXX	
V2410		X	Variable asphericity lens, single vision, full field, glass or plastic, per lens	0.00	2.53	2.53	0.00	2.53	2.53	XXX	■
V2430		X	Variable asphericity lens, bifocal, full field, glass or plastic, per lens	0.00	3.29	3.29	0.00	3.29	3.29	XXX	■
V2499		X	Variable sphericity lens, other type	0.00	0.00	0.00	0.00	0.00	0.00	XXX	
V2500		X	Contact lens, PMMA, spherical, per lens	0.00	2.93	2.93	0.00	2.93	2.93	XXX	■
V2501		X	Contact lens, PMMA, toric or prism ballast, per lens	0.00	3.93	3.93	0.00	3.93	3.93	XXX	■
V2502		X	Contact lens, PMMA, bifocal, per lens	0.00	3.23	3.23	0.00	3.23	3.23	XXX	■

■ RVU not developed by CMS. Gap-filled RVUs developed by CHEG.

Code	M	S	Description	Work Value	Non-Fac PE	Fac PE	Mal-practice	Non-Fac Total	Fac Total	Global	Gap
V2503		X	Contact lens, PMMA, color vision deficiency, per lens	0.00	3.97	3.97	0.00	3.97	3.97	XXX	■
V2510		X	Contact lens, gas permeable, spherical, per lens	0.00	3.23	3.23	0.00	3.23	3.23	XXX	■
V2511		X	Contact lens, gas permeable, toric, prism ballast, per lens	0.00	4.70	4.70	0.00	4.70	4.70	XXX	■
V2512		X	Contact lens, gas permeable, bifocal, per lens	0.00	5.31	5.31	0.00	5.31	5.31	XXX	■
V2513		X	Contact lens, gas permeable, extended wear, per lens	0.00	4.64	4.64	0.00	4.64	4.64	XXX	■
V2520		P	Contact lens, hydrophilic, spherical, per lens	0.00	2.84	2.84	0.00	2.84	2.84	XXX	■
V2521		X	Contact lens, hydrophilic, toric, or prism ballast, per lens	0.00	5.12	5.12	0.00	5.12	5.12	XXX	■
V2522		X	Contact lens, hydrophilic, bifocal, per lens	0.00	5.00	5.00	0.00	5.00	5.00	XXX	■
V2523		X	Contact lens, hydrophilic, extended wear, per lens	0.00	3.93	3.93	0.00	3.93	3.93	XXX	■
V2530		X	Contact lens, scleral, gas impermeable, per lens (for contact lens modification, see CPT Level I code 92325)	0.00	5.49	5.49	0.00	5.49	5.49	XXX	■
V2531		X	Contact lens, scleral, gas permeable, per lens (for contact lens modification, see CPT Level I code 92325)	0.00	6.91	6.91	0.00	6.91	6.91	XXX	■
V2599		X	Contact lens, other type	0.00	0.00	0.00	0.00	0.00	0.00	XXX	
V2600		X	Hand held low vision aids and other nonspectacle mounted aids	0.00	0.00	0.00	0.00	0.00	0.00	XXX	
V2610		X	Single lens spectacle mounted low vision aids	0.00	0.00	0.00	0.00	0.00	0.00	XXX	
V2615		X	Telescopic and other compound lens system, including distance vision telescopic, near vision telescopes and compound microscopic lens system	0.00	0.00	0.00	0.00	0.00	0.00	XXX	
V2623		X	Prosthetic eye, plastic, custom	0.00	25.35	25.35	0.00	25.35	25.35	XXX	■
V2624		X	Polishing/resurfacing of ocular prosthesis	0.00	1.27	1.27	0.00	1.27	1.27	XXX	■
V2625		X	Enlargement of ocular prosthesis	0.00	10.46	10.46	0.00	10.46	10.46	XXX	■
V2626		X	Reduction of ocular prosthesis	0.00	5.64	5.64	0.00	5.64	5.64	XXX	■
V2627		X	Scleral cover shell	0.00	35.01	35.01	0.00	35.01	35.01	XXX	■
V2628		X	Fabrication and fitting of ocular conformer	0.00	8.60	8.60	0.00	8.60	8.60	XXX	■
V2629		X	Prosthetic eye, other type	0.00	0.00	0.00	0.00	0.00	0.00	XXX	
V2630		X	Anterior chamber intraocular lens	0.00	0.00	0.00	0.00	0.00	0.00	XXX	
V2631		X	Iris supported intraocular lens	0.00	0.00	0.00	0.00	0.00	0.00	XXX	

■ RVU not developed by CMS. Gap-filled RVUs developed by CHEG.

Code	M	S	Description	Work Value	Non-Fac PE	Fac PE	Mal-practice	Non-Fac Total	Fac Total	Global	Gap
V2632		X	Posterior chamber intraocular lens	0.00	0.00	0.00	0.00	0.00	0.00	XXX	
V2700		X	Balance lens, per lens	0.00	1.31	1.31	0.00	1.31	1.31	XXX	■
V2710		X	Slab off prism, glass or plastic, per lens	0.00	1.77	1.77	0.00	1.77	1.77	XXX	■
V2715		X	Prism, per lens	0.00	0.35	0.35	0.00	0.35	0.35	XXX	■
V2718		X	Press-on lens, Fresnell prism, per lens	0.00	0.79	0.79	0.00	0.79	0.79	XXX	■
V2730		X	Special base curve, glass or plastic, per lens	0.00	0.61	0.61	0.00	0.61	0.61	XXX	■
V2740		X	Tint, plastic, rose 1 or 2, per lens	0.00	0.38	0.38	0.00	0.38	0.38	XXX	■
V2741		X	Tint, plastic, other than rose 1 or 2, per lens	0.00	0.30	0.30	0.00	0.30	0.30	XXX	■
V2742		X	Tint, glass, rose 1 or 2, per lens	0.00	0.29	0.29	0.00	0.29	0.29	XXX	■
V2743		X	Tint, glass, other than rose 1 or 2, per lens	0.00	0.44	0.44	0.00	0.44	0.44	XXX	■
V2744		X	Tint, photochromatic, per lens	0.00	0.46	0.46	0.00	0.46	0.46	XXX	■
V2750		X	Antireflective coating, per lens	0.00	0.55	0.55	0.00	0.55	0.55	XXX	■
V2755		X	U-V lens, per lens	0.00	0.46	0.46	0.00	0.46	0.46	XXX	■
V2760		X	Scratch resistant coating, per lens	0.00	0.52	0.52	0.00	0.52	0.52	XXX	■
V2770		X	Occluder lens, per lens	0.00	0.58	0.58	0.00	0.58	0.58	XXX	■
V2780		X	Oversize lens, per lens	0.00	0.40	0.40	0.00	0.40	0.40	XXX	■
V2781		X	Progressive lens, per lens	0.00	0.00	0.00	0.00	0.00	0.00	XXX	
V2785		X	Processing, preserving and transporting corneal tissue	0.00	0.00	0.00	0.00	0.00	0.00	XXX	
V2790		X	Amniotic membrane for surgical reconstruction, per procedure	0.00	0.00	0.00	0.00	0.00	0.00	XXX	
V2799		X	Vision service, miscellaneous	0.00	0.00	0.00	0.00	0.00	0.00	XXX	
V5008		N	Hearing screening	0.00	1.37	1.37	0.00	1.37	1.37	XXX	■
V5010		N	Assessment for hearing aid	0.00	1.80	1.80	0.00	1.80	1.80	XXX	■
V5011		N	Fitting/orientation/checking of hearing aid	0.00	2.81	2.81	0.00	2.81	2.81	XXX	■
V5014		N	Repair/modification of a hearing aid	0.00	3.39	3.39	0.00	3.39	3.39	XXX	■
V5020		N	Conformity evaluation	0.00	1.58	1.58	0.00	1.58	1.58	XXX	■
V5030		N	Hearing aid, monaural, body worn, air conduction	0.00	24.92	24.92	0.00	24.92	24.92	XXX	■
V5040		N	Hearing aid, monaural, body worn, bone conduction	0.00	18.94	18.94	0.00	18.94	18.94	XXX	■
V5050		N	Hearing aid, monaural, in the ear	0.00	21.90	21.90	0.00	21.90	21.90	XXX	■
V5060		N	Hearing aid, monaural, behind the ear	0.00	18.30	18.30	0.00	18.30	18.30	XXX	■

■ RVU not developed by CMS. Gap-filled RVUs developed by CHEG.

Code	M	S	Description	Work Value	Non-Fac PE	Fac PE	Mal-prac-tice	Non-Fac Total	Fac Total	Global	Gap
V5070		N	Glasses, air conduction	0.00	10.17	10.17	0.00	10.17	10.17	XXX	■
V5080		N	Glasses, bone conduction	0.00	25.56	25.56	0.00	25.56	25.56	XXX	■
V5090		N	Dispensing fee, unspecified hearing aid	0.00	9.09	9.09	0.00	9.09	9.09	XXX	■
V5100		N	Hearing aid, bilateral, body worn	0.00	41.00	41.00	0.00	41.00	41.00	XXX	■
V5110		N	Dispensing fee, bilateral	0.00	9.24	9.24	0.00	9.24	9.24	XXX	■
V5120		N	Binaural, body	0.00	35.84	35.84	0.00	35.84	35.84	XXX	■
V5130		N	Binaural, in the ear	0.00	38.13	38.13	0.00	38.13	38.13	XXX	■
V5140		N	Binaural, behind the ear	0.00	39.65	39.65	0.00	39.65	39.65	XXX	■
V5150		N	Binaural, glasses	0.00	42.33	42.33	0.00	42.33	42.33	XXX	■
V5160		N	Dispensing fee, binaural	0.00	11.06	11.06	0.00	11.06	11.06	XXX	■
V5170		N	Hearing aid, CROS, in the ear	0.00	29.45	29.45	0.00	29.45	29.45	XXX	■
V5180		N	Hearing aid, CROS, behind the ear	0.00	24.92	24.92	0.00	24.92	24.92	XXX	■
V5190		N	Hearing aid, CROS, glasses	0.00	29.13	29.13	0.00	29.13	29.13	XXX	■
V5200		N	Dispensing fee, CROS	0.00	9.17	9.17	0.00	9.17	9.17	XXX	■
V5210		N	Hearing aid, BICROS, in the ear	0.00	31.99	31.99	0.00	31.99	31.99	XXX	■
V5220		N	Hearing aid, BICROS, behind the ear	0.00	30.74	30.74	0.00	30.74	30.74	XXX	■
V5230		N	Hearing aid, BICROS, glasses	0.00	31.78	31.78	0.00	31.78	31.78	XXX	■
V5240		N	Dispensing fee, BICROS	0.00	9.49	9.49	0.00	9.49	9.49	XXX	■
V5241		N	Dispensing fee, monaural hearing aid, any type	0.00	0.00	0.00	0.00	0.00	0.00	XXX	
V5242		N	Hearing aid, analog, monaural, CIC (completely in the ear canal)	0.00	0.00	0.00	0.00	0.00	0.00	XXX	
V5243		N	Hearing aid, analog, monaural, ITC (in the canal)	0.00	0.00	0.00	0.00	0.00	0.00	XXX	
V5244		N	Hearing aid, digitally programmable analog, monaural, CIC	0.00	0.00	0.00	0.00	0.00	0.00	XXX	
V5245		N	Hearing aid, digitally programmable, analog, monaural, ITC	0.00	0.00	0.00	0.00	0.00	0.00	XXX	
V5246		N	Hearing aid, digitally programmable analog, monaural, ITE (in the ear)	0.00	0.00	0.00	0.00	0.00	0.00	XXX	
V5247		N	Hearing aid, digitally programmable analog, monaural, BTE (behind the ear)	0.00	0.00	0.00	0.00	0.00	0.00	XXX	
V5248		N	Hearing aid, analog, binaural, CIC	0.00	0.00	0.00	0.00	0.00	0.00	XXX	
V5249		N	Hearing aid, analog, binaural, ITC	0.00	0.00	0.00	0.00	0.00	0.00	XXX	

■ RVU not developed by CMS. Gap-filled RVUs developed by CHEG.

Code	M	S	Description	Work Value	Non-Fac PE	Fac PE	Mal-practice	Non-Fac Total	Fac Total	Global	Gap
V5250		N	Hearing aid, digitally programmable analog, binaural, CIC	0.00	0.00	0.00	0.00	0.00	0.00	XXX	
V5251		N	Hearing aid, digitally programmable analog, binaural, ITC	0.00	0.00	0.00	0.00	0.00	0.00	XXX	
V5252		N	Hearing aid, digitally programmable, binaural, ITE	0.00	0.00	0.00	0.00	0.00	0.00	XXX	
V5253		N	Hearing aid, digitally programmable, binaural, BTE	0.00	0.00	0.00	0.00	0.00	0.00	XXX	
V5254		N	Hearing aid, digital, monaural, CIC	0.00	0.00	0.00	0.00	0.00	0.00	XXX	
V5255		N	Hearing aid, digital, monaural, ITC	0.00	0.00	0.00	0.00	0.00	0.00	XXX	
V5256		N	Hearing aid, digital, monaural, ITE	0.00	0.00	0.00	0.00	0.00	0.00	XXX	
V5257		N	Hearing aid, digital, monaural, BTE	0.00	0.00	0.00	0.00	0.00	0.00	XXX	
V5258		N	Hearing aid, digital, binaural, CIC	0.00	0.00	0.00	0.00	0.00	0.00	XXX	
V5259		N	Hearing aid, digital, binaural, ITC	0.00	0.00	0.00	0.00	0.00	0.00	XXX	
V5260		N	Hearing aid, digital, binaural, ITE	0.00	0.00	0.00	0.00	0.00	0.00	XXX	
V5261		N	Hearing aid, digital, binaural, BTE	0.00	0.00	0.00	0.00	0.00	0.00	XXX	
V5262		N	Hearing aid, disposable, any type, monaural	0.00	0.00	0.00	0.00	0.00	0.00	XXX	
V5263		N	Hearing aid, disposable, any type, binaural	0.00	0.00	0.00	0.00	0.00	0.00	XXX	
V5264		N	Ear mold/insert, not disposable, any type	0.00	0.00	0.00	0.00	0.00	0.00	XXX	
V5265		N	Ear mold/insert, disposable, any type	0.00	0.00	0.00	0.00	0.00	0.00	XXX	
V5266		N	Battery for use in hearing device	0.00	0.00	0.00	0.00	0.00	0.00	XXX	
V5267		N	Hearing aid supplies/accessories	0.00	0.00	0.00	0.00	0.00	0.00	XXX	
V5268		N	Assistive listening device, telephone amplifier, any type	0.00	0.00	0.00	0.00	0.00	0.00	XXX	
V5269		N	Assistive listening device, alerting, any type	0.00	0.00	0.00	0.00	0.00	0.00	XXX	
V5270		N	Assistive listening device, television amplifier, any type	0.00	0.00	0.00	0.00	0.00	0.00	XXX	
V5271		N	Assistive listening device, television caption decoder	0.00	0.00	0.00	0.00	0.00	0.00	XXX	
V5272		N	Assistive listening device, TDD	0.00	0.00	0.00	0.00	0.00	0.00	XXX	
V5273		N	Assistive listening device, for use with cochlear implant	0.00	0.00	0.00	0.00	0.00	0.00	XXX	
V5274		N	Assistive learning device, not otherwise specified	0.00	0.00	0.00	0.00	0.00	0.00	XXX	
V5275		N	Ear impression, each	0.00	0.00	0.00	0.00	0.00	0.00	XXX	

■ RVU not developed by CMS. Gap-filled RVUs developed by CHEG.

Code	M	S	Description	Work Value	Non-Fac PE	Fac PE	Mal-prac-tice	Non-Fac Total	Fac Total	Global	Gap
V5299		R	Hearing service, miscellaneous	0.00	0.00	0.00	0.00	0.00	0.00	XXX	
V5336		N	Repair/modification of augmentative communicative system or device (excludes adaptive hearing aid)	0.00	0.00	0.00	0.00	0.00	0.00	XXX	
V5362		R	Speech screening	0.00	0.00	0.00	0.00	0.00	0.00	XXX	
V5363		R	Language screening	0.00	0.00	0.00	0.00	0.00	0.00	XXX	
V5364		R	Dysphagia screening	0.00	0.00	0.00	0.00	0.00	0.00	XXX	

■ RVU not developed by CMS. Gap-filled RVUs developed by CHEG.